£120·00
2e1996.

190

FEMALE UROLOGY

SHLOMO RAZ, M.D.

Professor of Surgery/Urology
University of California at Los Angeles School of Medicine
Los Angeles, California

FEMALE UROLOGY

SECOND EDITION

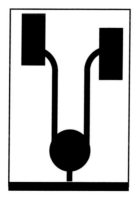

W.B. SAUNDERS COMPANY
A Division of Harcourt Brace & Company

Philadelphia   London   Toronto   Montreal   Sydney   Tokyo

W.B. SAUNDERS COMPANY
A Division of
Harcourt Brace & Company

The Curtis Center
Independence Square West
Philadelphia, Pennsylvania 19106

Library of Congress Cataloging-in-Publication Data

Female urology / [edited by] Shlomo Raz.—2nd ed.

p.   cm.

Includes bibliographical references and index.

ISBN 0–7216–6723–6

1. Urogynecology.   I. Raz, Shlomo.
    [DNLM: 1. Genital Diseases, Female.   2. Urologic
    Diseases.   WJ 190 F329 1996]   RG484.F46 1996
    616.6′0082—dc20

DNLM/DLC   95–17714

Female Urology   ISBN 0–7216–6723–6

Printed in the United States of America.

Last digit is the print number: 9   8   7   6   5   4   3   2   1

To my wife
Sylvia
and my children
Alan, Yael, Daniela, and Karyn
for your support, understanding, and forgiveness
for time not spent with you.

Contributors

Rodney A. Appell, M.D.
Head, Section of Voiding Dysfunction and Female Urology, Cleveland Clinic Foundation, Cleveland, Ohio
Collagen Injections

Joseph W. Babiarz, M.D.
Director, Urodynamics and Incontinence Center, Wausau Hospital, Wausau, Wisconsin
Pelvic Floor Relaxation

Zoran L. Barbaric, M.D.
Professor of Radiology, University of California at Los Angeles School of Medicine; Attending Radiologist, UCLA Medical Center, Los Angeles, California
Female Uroradiology; Endoscopic and Percutaneous Management of Ureteral Injuries, Fistulas, Obstruction, and Strictures

David M. Barrett, M.D.
Professor of Urology, Mayo Graduate School of Medicine; Chair, Department of Urology, Mayo Clinic, Rochester, Minnesota
Use of Silicon Particles for the Treatment of Urinary Incontinence; Artificial Sphincter: Abdominal Approach

Jerry G. Blaivas, M.D., F.A.C.S.
Clinical Professor of Urology, Cornell University Medical School; Attending Surgeon, New York Hospital, New York, New York
Evaluation of Urinary Tract Dysfunction; Periurethral Injections of Autologous Fat for the Treatment of Incontinence; Reconstruction of the Damaged Urethra

Alain P. Bourcier, M.D.
Director of Training Program and Instructor, Institut Français de Réadaptation Uro-Génitale; Director, Urodynamic Laboratory, and Consultant Biomedical, Mutuelle Générale P.T.T., Paris, France
Pelvic Floor Rehabilitation

Eugene J. Carter, M.D.
Fellow, Plastic and Reconstructive Surgery, Harbor/UCLA Medical Center, Torrance, California
Vaginal Reconstruction

Mauro Cervigni, M.D.
Uro-gynecology Unit, S. Carlo Di Nancy-Hospital, Rome, Italy
Hormonal Influences in the Lower Urinary Tract

Ashok Chopra, M.D.
Fellow in Female and Reconstructive Urology, University of California at Los Angeles School of Medicine, Los Angeles, California
Laparoscopic Bladder Neck Suspension; Stamey Needle Suspension for Female Stress Incontinence; Pathogenesis of Cystoceles: Anterior Colporrhaphy; Raz Techniques for Anterior Vaginal Wall Repair; Technique of Rectangular Fascial Sling; Anterior Vaginal Wall Sling; Uterine Prolapse; Enterocele and Vault Prolapse; Vesicovaginal Fistula; Surgical Closure of the Bladder Neck; Benign Cystic Lesions of the Vagina and Vulva

L. L. Christensen, M.D.
Research Fellow, Aarhus University, Aarhus, Denmark; Fellow, Institute of Experimental and Clinical Research, Skejby, Denmark
Urethral Pressures in the Study of Female Incontinence

C. E. Constantinou, Ph.D.
Associate Professor, Department of Urology, Stanford University School of Medicine, Stanford, California
Urethral Pressures in the Study of Female Incontinence

William C. de Groat, Ph.D.
Professor, Departments of Pharmacology and Neuroscience, University of Pittsburgh School of Medicine, Pittsburgh, Pennsylvania
Neuroanatomy and Neurophysiology: Innervation of the Lower Urinary Tract

Ananias C. Diokno, M.D.

Associate Professor, University of Michigan Medical School, Ann Arbor, Michigan; Chief, Department of Urology, William Beaumont Hospital, Royal Oak, Michigan

Epidemiology of Female Incontinence

Richard M. Ehrlich, M.D.

Clinical Professor of Surgery/Urology, University of California at Los Angeles School of Medicine; Attending Urologist, UCLA Medical Center, Los Angeles, California

Management of Vesicoureteral Reflux in Adults and Children

Ahmad Elbadawi, M.D.

Professor of Pathology and Urology, State University of New York Health Science Center at Syracuse College of Medicine, Syracuse, New York

Structural Basis of Voiding Dysfunction

Denise M. Elser, M.D.

Director of Urogynecology, Assistant Residency Director, Christ Hospital, Oak Lawn, Illinois

Bladder Training in the Management of Urinary Incontinence in Community-Dwelling Women

J. Andrew Fantl, M.D.

Professor and Vice Chairman, Department of Obstetrics, Gynecology and Reproductive Medicine; Director, Division of Gynecology and General Obstetrics, State University of New York at Stony Brook, Stony Brook, New York

Bladder Training in the Management of Urinary Incontinence in Community-Dwelling Women

Gerhard J. Fuchs, M.D.

Director, Stone Treatment Center and Section of Endourology and Laparoscopic Urology, Division of Urology, University of California at Los Angeles School of Medicine, Los Angeles, California

Endoscopic and Percutaneous Management of Ureteral Injuries, Fistulas, Obstruction, and Strictures

Ruben F. Gittes, M.D.

Clinical Professor of Surgery/Urology, University of California at San Diego School of Medicine, San Diego, California; Chairman, Department of Surgery, Scripps Clinic and Research Foundation, La Jolla, California

No-Incision Urethropexy

Jacob Golomb, M.D.

Lecturer, Sackler School of Medicine, Tel Aviv University, Tel Aviv, Israel; Attending Urologist and Head of Section of Female Urology and Urodynamic Laboratory, Department of Urology, Chaim Sheba Medical Center, Tel Hashomer, Israel

Uroflowmetry

E. Ann Gormley, M.D.

Assistant Professor, Surgery [Urology], Section of Urology, Department of Surgery, Dartmouth-Hitchcock Medical Center; Attending, Mary Hitchcock Hospital, Lebanon, New Hampshire

Clinical Assessment of Urethral Sphincter and Conduit Function by Measurement of Abdominal and Detrusor Pressures Required to Induce Leakage; Abdominal Fascial Slings

David S. Grapey, M.D.

Active Staff, Moses Cone Memorial Hospital, and Wesley Long Community Hospital, Greensboro, North Carolina

Urinary Tract Infections

H. Roger Hadley, M.D.

Professor, Division of Urology, Department of Surgery, Loma Linda University School of Medicine; Chief, Division of Urology, Department of Surgery, Loma Linda University Medical Center, Loma Linda, California

Artificial Sphincter: Transvaginal Approach

David R. Henly, M.D.

Private Practice, Northland Urology Associates, Duluth, Minnesota

Use of Silicon Particles for the Treatment of Urinary Incontinence

Dianne M. Heritz, M.D., F.R.C.S.C.

Lecturer, University of Toronto, Division of Urology; Attending Surgeon, Women's College Hospital, Toronto, Ontario, Canada

Evaluation of Urinary Tract Dysfunction; Periurethral Injections of Autologous Fat for the Treatment of Incontinence; Reconstruction of the Damaged Urethra

Katherine F. Jeter, Ed.D., E.T., C.E.T.N.

Clinical Assistant Professor, Mary Black School of Nursing, University of South Carolina at Spartanburg; Staff Affiliate, Spartanburg Regional Medical Center, Spartanburg, South Carolina; Adjunct Professor of Nursing, Medical University of South Carolina, Charleston, South Carolina

The Social Impact of Urinary Incontinence

Lindsey A. Kerr, M.D.

Assistant Professor, George Washington University School of Medicine and Health Sciences; Director, Continence and Urodynamic Program, George Washington University Medical Center, Washington, District of Columbia

Use of Artificial Material for Sling Surgery in the Treatment of Female Stress Urinary Incontinence

Carl G. Klutke, M.D.

Assistant Professor, Department of Surgery, Division of Urology, Washington University School of Medicine, St. Louis, Missouri

Endoscopic Evaluation of the Female Lower Urinary Tract

Gary E. Leach, M.D.

Associate Clinical Professor, University of California at Los Angeles; Chief of Urology, Kaiser Permanente Medical Center, Los Angeles, California

Use of Fascia Lata for Pubovaginal Sling

Malcolm A. Lesavoy, M.D.

Professor of Plastic and Reconstructive Surgery, University of California at Los Angeles School of Medicine, Los Angeles, California; Chief of Plastic and Reconstructive Surgery, Harbor/UCLA Medical Center, Torrance, California

Vaginal Reconstruction

Robert M. Levin, Ph.D.

Resident Professor of Pharmacology in Urology, University of Pennsylvania School of Medicine; Pharmacologist, Veterans Affairs Medical Center, Philadelphia, Pennsylvania

Pharmacologic Basis of Bladder and Urethral Function and Dysfunction

Robert L. Long, M.D.

Assistant Professor of Surgery, Division of Urology, University of Louisville School of Medicine; Attending Urologist, University of Louisville Medical Center, Alliant Medical Pavilion, Jewish Hospital, Louisville, Kentucky; Attending Urologist, Fort Walton Beach Medical Center, Fort Walton Beach, Florida

Artificial Sphincter: Abdominal Approach

Penelope A. Longhurst, Ph.D.

Research Associate Professor, Department of Pharmacology, University of Pennsylvania School of Medicine; Research Associate Professor, Division of

Urology, Hospital of the University of Pennsylvania, Philadelphia, Pennsylvania

Pharmacologic Basis of Bladder and Urethral Function and Dysfunction

Stephen D. Mark, M.B., F.R.A.C.S.

Fellow, Reconstructive Urology and Urodynamics, Duke University Medical Center, Durham, North Carolina

Detrusor Hyperactivity; Continent Urinary Diversion

Edward J. McGuire, M.D.

Professor of Surgery (Urology) and Director, Division of Urology, University of Texas Medical School at Houston; Clinical Professor, The University of Texas M.D. Anderson Cancer Center, Houston, Texas

Clinical Assessment of Urethral Sphincter and Conduit Function by Measurement of Abdominal and Detrusor Pressures Required to Induce Leakage; Abdominal Fascial Slings

Victor W. Nitti, M.D.

Assistant Professor, Department of Urology, and Director, Neurourology and Female Urology, New York University School of Medicine; Attending Urologist, Tisch Hospital, New York University Medical Center, New York, New York

Urinary Retention

Pat D. O'Donnell, M.D.

Professor, Division of Urology, University of Cincinnati College of Medicine; Attending Urologist, University of Cincinnati Medical Center; Chief of Urology, Cincinnati Veterans Hospital, Cincinnati, Ohio

Biofeedback Therapy

Joseph G. Ouslander, M.D.

Associate Professor of Medicine, Multicampus Program in Geriatric Medicine and Gerontology, University of California at Los Angeles School of Medicine, Los Angeles, California; Vice President, Medical Affairs, Jewish Home for the Aging, Reseda, California

Lower Urinary Tract Disorders in the Elderly Female

C. Lowell Parsons, M.D.

Professor of Surgery/Urology, University of California at San Diego School of Medicine; Staff Physician, Veterans Affairs Medical Center, San Diego, California

Interstitial Cystitis

J. Kellogg Parsons

Student, University of Pennsylvania School of Medicine, Philadelphia, Pennsylvania

Interstitial Cystitis

Anup Patel, M.S., F.R.C.S.(Urol.)

Clinical Fellow in Endourology and Laparoscopic Urology, Division of Urology, University of California at Los Angeles School of Medicine, Los Angeles, California

Endoscopic and Percutaneous Management of Ureteral Injuries, Fistulas, Obstruction, and Strictures

Christopher K. Payne, M.D.

Assistant Professor of Urology, Stanford University School of Medicine; Director, Center for Neurourology, Stanford University Medical Center, Stanford, California

Ureteral Injuries in the Female: Fistulas and Obstruction

David F. Penson, M.D.

Resident, Division of Urology, University of California at Los Angeles School of Medicine, Los Angeles, California

Why Anti-incontinence Surgery Succeeds or Fails

Shlomo Raz, M.D.

Professor of Surgery/Urology, University of California at Los Angeles School of Medicine, Los Angeles, California

Anatomy and Pathophysiology of Pelvic Support; Urinary Retention; Laparoscopic Bladder Neck Suspension; Stamey Needle Suspension for Female Stress Incontinence; Pathogenesis of Cystoceles: Anterior Colporrhaphy; Raz Techniques for Anterior Vaginal Wall Repair; Technique of Rectangular Fascial Sling; Anterior Vaginal Wall Sling; Why Anti-incontinence Surgery Succeeds or Fails; Pelvic Floor Relaxation; Uterine Prolapse; Enterocele and Vault Prolapse; Female Urethral Diverticulum; Vesicovaginal Fistula; Surgical Closure of the Bladder Neck; Complications of Vaginal Surgery; Benign Cystic Lesions of the Vagina and Vulva

Dieter H. Sauerwein, M.D.

Werner Wicker Hospital, Bad Widungen, Germany

Use of Nerve Deafferentation and Stimulation in the Paraplegic Female Patient

Anthony J. Schaeffer, M.D.

Professor of Urology and Chairman, Department of Urology, Northwestern University Medical School, Division of Urology, Chicago, Illinois

Urinary Tract Infections

Richard A. Schmidt, M.D.

Professor of Urology, University of Colorado Health Sciences Center, Denver, Colorado

Clinical Value of Neurostimulation: A Urologic Viewpoint

Larry T. Sirls, M.D.

Assistant Clinical Professor, Case Western Reserve University School of Medicine, Cleveland, Ohio; Co-Director, Urodynamics Laboratory, Department of Urology, Henry Ford Hospital, Detroit, Michigan

Use of Fascia Lata for Pubovaginal Sling

David R. Staskin, M.D.

Assistant Professor of Surgery/Urology, Harvard Medical School and Beth Israel Hospital, Boston, Massachusetts

Use of Artificial Material for Sling Surgery in the Treatment of Female Stress Urinary Incontinence

Lynn Stothers, M.D., M.H.Sc., F.R.C.S.C.

Fellow of Reconstructive Urology, Neurourology and Urodynamics, Division of Urology, University of California at Los Angeles School of Medicine, Los Angeles, California

Laparoscopic Bladder Neck Suspension; Stamey Needle Suspension for Female Stress Incontinence; Pathogenesis of Cystoceles: Anterior Colporrhaphy; Raz Techniques for Anterior Vaginal Wall Repair; Technique of Rectangular Fascial Sling; Anterior Vaginal Wall Sling; Uterine Prolapse; Enterocele and Vault Prolapse; Vesicovaginal Fistula; Surgical Closure of the Bladder Neck; Benign Cystic Lesions of the Vagina and Vulva

Maryrose P. Sullivan, Ph.D.

Lecturer, Health Sciences and Technology, Massachusetts Institute of Technology, Cambridge, Massachusetts; Instructor, Division of Urology, Harvard Medical School, Boston, Massachusetts; Associate Director of Urology Research, West Roxbury Veterans Affairs Medical Center, West Roxbury, Massachusetts

Micturition Profilometry

Emil A. Tanagho, M.D.

Professor and Chairman, Department of Urology, University of California at San Francisco School of Medicine, San Francisco, California

Developmental Anatomy and Urogenital Abnormalities; Colpocystourethropexy

Samir S. Taneja, M.D.

Resident in Surgery/Urology, University of California at Los Angeles School of Medicine, Los Angeles, California

Management of Vesicoureteral Reflux in Adults and Children

Remigio Vela-Navarrete, M.D.

Professor of Urology and Chief, Department of Urology, Fundacion Jimenez Diaz, Universidad Autonoma, Madrid, Spain

Caruncle and Prolapse of the Urethral Mucosa

Gregory R. Wahle, M.D.

Assistant Professor of Urology, Indiana University School of Medicine; Staff Urologist, Indiana University Medical Center, Indianapolis, Indiana

Anatomy and Pathophysiology of Pelvic Support; Female Urethral Diverticulum; Complications of Vaginal Surgery

Yu Wang, M.D.

Attending Physician, Department of Urology, Southern California Kaiser Permanente Medical Group, Fontana, California

Artificial Sphincter: Transvaginal Approach

George D. Webster, M.B., F.R.C.S.

Professor of Surgery, Division of Urology, Duke University School of Medicine; Attending Urologist, Duke University Medical Center, Durham, North Carolina

Detrusor Hyperactivity; Continent Urinary Diversion

Alan J. Wein, M.D.

Professor and Chair, University of Pennsylvania School of Medicine; Chief of Urology, Hospital of the University of Pennsylvania, Philadelphia, Pennsylvania

Principles of Pharmacologic Therapy: Practical Drug Treatment of Voiding Dysfunction in the Female

Philip E. Werthman, M.D.

Chief Resident, Division of Urology, Department of Surgery, University of California at Los Angeles School of Medicine, Los Angeles, California

Endoscopic and Percutaneous Management of Ureteral Injuries, Fistulas, Obstruction, and Strictures

Subbarao V. Yalla, M.D.

Associate Professor of Surgery in Urology, Harvard Medical School, Boston, Massachusetts; Chief of Urology, Brockton/West Roxbury Veterans Affairs Medical Center, Boston, Massachusetts

Micturition Profilometry

George P. H. Young, M.D.

Assistant Professor of Surgery (Urology), Cornell University Medical College; Assistant Attending Surgeon (Urology) and Director of Female Urology, Neurourology, Urodynamics, and Reconstructive Urology Unit, The New York Hospital, New York, New York

Anatomy and Pathophysiology of Pelvic Support; Female Urethral Diverticulum; Complications of Vaginal Surgery

Philippe E. Zimmern, M.D., F.A.C.S.

Associate Clinical Professor of Urology, University of California at Los Angeles School of Medicine; Staff Urologist and Co-Director of Urodynamic Laboratory, Kaiser Sunset Medical Center, Los Angeles, California

Bladder Dysfunction After Radiation and Radical Pelvic Surgery

Foreword

When I began my training in surgery and urology in 1966 (and when I finished in 1972), the subject matter of female urology included urinary tract infection, the urethral syndrome, and a few retropubic or abdominal procedures to treat stress urinary incontinence and various fistulas. Even though we urologists regarded the treatment of all urinary incontinence as our divine right, the subjects of female pelvic anatomy, support, and prolapse were accorded little attention in our texts and literature. The female bladder was considered analogous to that of the male, and the area of the female bladder neck and urethra was generally described as a condensation of that of the male, minus the prostate. The "urethral syndrome" described virtually every combination of symptoms that emanated from the area between the umbilicus and the knees that was unassociated with cancer, culture-documented infection, and urinary incontinence. The uterus, fallopian tubes, and ovaries were "female organs" either that were a nuisance during surgery or that the gynecologists had already removed, and the vagina was a structure to surgically avoid, except during a few oncologic procedures.

For the current generation of graduating urologists, female urology has quite a different meaning. The concept properly includes the specialized anatomy, physiology, and pharmacology of the lower urinary tract in the female and all associated diseases and dysfunctions, and it includes the nononcologic and nonendocrinologic aspects of the female genital tract that are related to lower urinary tract function, its restoration, and its repair.

No one has been more instrumental in this fundamental shift of urologic thinking than the author/editor of this book, Shlomo Raz. As an individual whose first contributions to urologic science included prostatic receptor pharmacology (and the suggestion that alpha receptors might be useful to treat BPH-induced voiding dysfunction) and study of the effects of estrogen and progesterone on urinary tract smooth muscle, Dr. Raz was no stranger to innovation and to the scientific method. As a skilled scientist and surgeon who was frustrated with the state of urologic expertise in the realm of female lower urinary tract dysfunction and urinary incontinence, he has worked over the past 20 years to advance the knowledge of the pathophysiology, evaluation, and medical and surgical management of these problems, and to redefine the role of the urologist in addressing these areas. The first edition of his "bible," enunciating these principles, was planned in 1980 and published in 1983. Since that time, Dr. Raz has continued to expand the limits of female urology. There has been a continuing questioning of established "principles" and a steady progression of scholarly achievements in this area. Continuing to draw on his own expertise and experience, that of other independent pioneers in this field (Drs. Blaivas, McGuire, Tanagho, and others), and that of many of his former students (fellows), Dr. Raz has put together this second edition. Simply put, some broad strokes have been narrowed, the scope of female urology has been more precisely defined, and an all-inclusive text of principles, practice, and application has emerged. His philosophy of what this subject matter includes is now the rule, rather than the exception.

ALAN J. WEIN

Preface

Perhaps no aspect of urologic practice has flourished in the past decade as has female genitourinary dysfunction and reconstruction. A great number of changes have taken place since the publication of our first edition of *Female Urology* in 1983. This new edition represents our effort to update these developments for urologists, gynecologists, and those health care providers focusing on the female genitourinary tract.

The book is divided into nine parts for easy orientation. Part I highlights fundamental aspects of the female genitourinary tract, including the embryology, neuroanatomy, pharmacology, and physiology of the bladder and urethra. The anatomy and the pathophysiology of continence mechanisms, as well as the epidemiology and social impact of urinary incontinence, are discussed.

Part II is dedicated to diagnostic techniques. We recognize that not every woman requires sophisticated evaluation for a proper diagnosis. Careful documentation of the medical history, physical examination, and simple clinical tests should be the first line of investigation. Endoscopy of the urethra and the bladder has advanced greatly owing to the advent of newer optics and the use of urethroscopy. Videourodynamic evaluation has equipped us with an improved understanding of the function of the lower urinary tract in its filling, storage, and voiding phases. There has also been an emergence of newer diagnostic techniques such as abdominal leak pressures and micturition pressures. Finally, this section presents a review of the techniques and developments in uroradiology as they apply to the female bladder and urethra.

Part III deals with urinary tract infections and a group of diverse conditions pertaining to voiding dysfunction. Leaders in the field discuss our current understanding of the diagnosis and treatment of interstitial cystitis and urinary tract infections. Chapters on urinary retention and obstruction, bladder instability, and geriatric voiding dysfunction discuss the best treatments for these difficult problems.

Part IV relates to nonsurgical treatment of lower urinary tract dysfunction. In planning therapy, an array of nonsurgical treatments is available, including behavior modification, biofeedback, pelvic floor rehabilitation, and pharmacologic treatment. We have included a group of chapters dedicated to the role of noninvasive treatments on voiding dysfunction. There is no doubt that they are effective in selected cases and should be used prior to surgery.

Part V deals with the surgical treatment of anatomic incontinence and anterior vaginal wall prolapse. The treatment of stress incontinence should be tailored to the clinical findings and the social impact of stress incontinence on the individual patient. Mild incontinence to one patient may have no social significance, while the same degree of incontinence to another may be devastating. Our choice of surgery is based mainly on the degree of prolapse of the anterior vaginal wall and not on the type of incontinence (anatomic or resulting from intrinsic dysfunction). As noted in this section, we have abandoned the use of simple bladder neck suspension procedures for stress incontinence patients with minimal or mild urethral hypermobility, in favor of the vaginal wall sling, regardless of the type of incontinence.

Part VI deals with the treatment of intrinsic sphincter dysfunction, including the use of the different slings, injectables, and the artificial sphincter. Although in most cases we can properly diagnose intrinsic sphincter dysfunction, the diagnosis frequently is difficult to formulate because of the lack of correlation between the patient's symptoms and the findings on the urodynamic evaluation. Good clinical judgment should prevail in the selection of the most appropriate therapy.

Part VII covers pelvic prolapse. Prolapse of the

pelvic organs is a common occurrence and results from multiple deliveries, hysterectomy, and hormonal deprivation. Prolapse may affect the anterior wall, the posterior vaginal wall, or the vaginal dome. We must recognize that, in most cases, anatomic stress incontinence is a manifestation of pelvic prolapse and is thus untreatable as an isolated condition. When planning surgery for stress incontinence, we must consider the degree of anterior vaginal prolapse and the repair of any other concomitant pelvic prolapse, including rectocele, enterocele, or uterine prolapse. Repair of pelvic floor relaxation has a great impact on the long-term success of stress incontinence surgery and on the prevention of postoperative enterocele or rectocele.

Part VIII deals with a group of conditions that, in most cases, require reconstructive procedures. The incidence of urethral diverticula has decreased in recent years with the advent of newer and more powerful antibiotics. Improved surgical techniques for hysterectomy have diminished the incidence of vesicovaginal fistula. Nevertheless, controversies concerning fistula management, such as timing of surgery (early or late), abdominal versus vaginal approach, and the need for excision of the fistulous tract and the use of adjuvant techniques such as Martius flaps or peritoneal flaps, still flourish. Controversies on the treatment of ureteric injury, repair of the destroyed urethra, and construction of a neovagina are also discussed.

Part IX covers emerging technologies in the treatment of the hyperactive bladder and voiding dysfunction. Both are based on the use of implantable devices to modulate sacral roots function.

Readers of this book will likely encounter old and new information, weaknesses and strengths, shortcomings, and subjectivity. As with any multiauthored book, the material is destined, at some points, to overlap and dissent. At the same time, it is clearly beneficial to present more than one opinion, so that both areas of agreement and those of contention are evident. Our intent in this new edition is to present a forum of different opinions and to provide an updated resource concerning current practice in the field.

SHLOMO RAZ

Contents

PART IV
Nonsurgical Treatment of Lower Urinary Tract Dysfunction, 245

PART V
Surgery for Anatomic Incontinence, 317

PART VI
Treatment of Intrinsic Sphincter Dysfunction, 367

PART I

Basic Concepts

CHAPTER 1

Developmental Anatomy and Urogenital Abnormalities

Emil A. Tanagho, M.D.

Knowledge of the sequence of events in the development of the lower urinary tract is important to understanding some of the common urogenital anomalies encountered in clinical practice. The lower urinary tract in its earlier phases of development is closely related to the gastrointestinal tract as well as to the genital system. Progressive development and differentiation separates these three systems from one another. However, not infrequently, this differentiation is interrupted at one phase or another of the embryologic sequence, thus creating a variety of congenital anomalies.

During the fourth week of intrauterine life, the blind end of the hindgut caudal to the point of origin of the allantois expands to initiate the formation of what is known as the *cloaca.* As it develops, the cloaca is separated from the outside by an ectodermal depression under the root of the tail, called the *proctodeum,* and by a thin plate of tissue closing the hindgut and known as the *cloacal membrane.* Soon after the expansion of the hindgut to form the cloaca, the subdivision of the latter is initiated by development of a crescentic fold—the *urorectal fold*—that eventually separates the urinary system from the gastrointestinal tract (Fig. 1–1). The urorectal fold develops cephalad to the cloaca, where the allantois meets the hindgut, and progressively grows caudally and medially until the two folds meet each other and continue to bulge into the lumen of the cloaca from either side; finally, the folds meet and fuse with the cloacal membrane, thus dividing the cloaca into a ventral *urogenital sinus* and a dorsal *rectum* by the seventh week of intrauterine life.

As the urorectal septum grows, subdividing the cloaca into two compartments, other changes take place, essentially in the infraumbilical segment of the abdominal wall, and at the same time there is regression of the tail end. As a result of the combination of these two events, the cloacal membrane undergoes a reverse rotation, so that the ectodermal surface is no longer directed to the developing anterior abdominal wall but gradually moves caudally and posteriorly; usually this is its position by the time the dividing urorectal septum meets the cloacal membrane. The division of the cloaca is completed before the rupture of the cloacal membrane. There are now two separate openings, a ventral opening that represents a primitive urogenital sinus, and a dorsal opening—that of the hindgut. Until this point, the urogenital sinus was directly continuous with the allantois and had a tubular configuration, moving caudally into the cloacal membrane. During the process of its separation from the cloaca, the ventral division of the cloaca—the urogenital sinus—receives the mesonephric duct as well as the müllerian duct. Earlier, the müllerian ducts had fused toward the caudal end, and they meet with the urogenital sinus as one unit. Their point of meeting with the urogenital sinus is known as the müllerian tubercle, which is one of the most fixed points in the development of the entire lower urinary tract and a landmark of the urogenital sinus.

The mesonephric ducts grow forward and medially, bending rather sharply to meet the urogenital sinus separately. Right at the bend of the mesonephric duct the ureteral bud will develop (Fig. 1–2). The segment of the mesonephric duct between the ureteral bud and the urogenital sinus is known as the common nephric duct, which is progressively absorbed into the urogenital sinus, thus transporting an island of mesodermal tissue into the midst of the endodermal structure of the urogenital sinus. With complete absorption of the common nephric duct, the mesonephric duct assumes a separate opening into the urogenital sinus from the ureteral bud, with the latter moving upward and laterally and the mesonephric duct moving downward and medially. The absorbed tissue between the mesonephric duct and ureteral

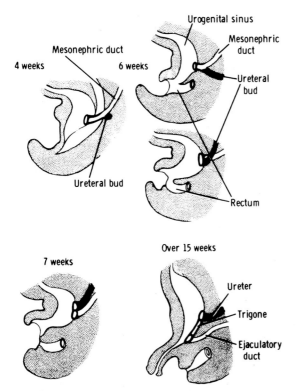

Figure 1-1 Development of the lower urinary tract. At 4 weeks the cloaca is dividing by a septum into an anterior urogenital sinus and posterior rectum. The mesonephric duct is already joining the anterior portion of the cloaca, and the ureteral bud has started to develop at the bend of the mesonephric duct as it turns forward and medially to join the urogenital sinus. At 6 weeks the urorectal septum is progressively separating the urogenital sinus anteriorly from the rectum posteriorly. By the seventh week the separation is complete, and the ureter and the mesonephric duct each acquire a separate opening in the urogenital sinus. After the twelfth week the ureter starts its upward and lateral descent as the mesonephric duct moves downward and medially. Tissue absorbed in between is forming the trigone.

bud expands to form the trigonal structure, which extends between the two ureteral orifices all the way down to the termination of the mesonephric duct; this becomes an ejaculatory duct in the male and a Gartner's duct in the female. It is worth noting that the trigonal body is the only mesodermal inclusion into the endodermal vesicourethral unit. As indicated before, the müllerian ducts fuse together and meet the urogenital sinus in the midline as one ductal system at the müllerian tubercle. The urogenital sinus itself is divided into two main segments, and the dividing line is the point of meeting of the combined müllerian ducts with the urogenital sinus (Müller's tubercle). In the female, the segment of the urogenital sinus caudal to Müller's tubercle expands and opens up to become the vaginal vestibule, whereas in the male it becomes the phallic portion of the male urethra. The segment of the urogenital sinus cranial to Müller's tubercle forms the bladder and part of the urethra in the male; in the female it forms the bladder and the entire urethra (Fig. 1–3).

The tubular configuration of the urogenital sinus

remains until approximately the third month of intrauterine life (Fig. 1–4). At that time the ventral part of the urogenital sinus starts to expand to form a saccular structure, the apex of which is tapered and directly continuous with the allantois. This is the future urinary bladder. The pelvic part of the urogenital sinus remains narrow and tubular and forms the entire urethra in the female and the supramontanal part of the prostatic urethra in the male. The segment distal to the meeting of the müllerian duct becomes the distal inframontanal segment of the prostatic urethra and the membranous urethra in the male; in the female it expands and is absorbed into the genital system, forming the distal one-fourth of the vagina.

After the expansion of the ventral segment of the urogenital sinus, the splanchnic mesoderm begins to accumulate around this saccular formation (including its tubular pelvic part) and progressively differentiates into interlacing bands of smooth muscle fibers. By the fifth week, the characteristic layers of the urinary bladder and urethra are recognizable.

Genital Development

The mesoderm originally accumulating around the cloacal membrane toward its caudal attachment to the umbilical cord proliferates while the cloacal membrane undergoes its change in orientation as a result of the development of the infraumbilical abdominal wall. Accumulation of this mesoderm results in the formation of two surface elevations known as the *genital tubercles*. Later, these two tubercles meet and fuse in the midline and differentiate into either phallus or clitoris, according to the sexual differentiation of the embryo.

In the male, the genital tubercle becomes elongated to form the primitive phallus. The corpora cavernosa are seen at the seventh week as paired mesenchymal columns within the shaft of the penis. Underneath the phallus is the opening of the primitive urogenital sinus that extends to the urethral folds toward the tip of the penis. It is the progressive fusion of these two urethral folds, starting proximally and moving caudally toward the tip of the penis, that completes the formation of the penile urethra. The corpus spongiosum results from the differentiation of the two chymal masses around these two fusing urethral folds (Fig. 1–5).

In the female, the genital tubercles dip caudally and develop much less than in the male; the future clitoris has all the essential elements of the penile structure but on a smaller scale. The mesenchymal columns differentiate into the corpora cavernosa, and a coronary sulcus identifies the glans clitoris. The most caudal part of the urogenital sinus, the opening of the genital tubercle, later widens and shortens to form the vaginal vestibule. On either side, the urethral folds that do not fuse remain separate and form the labia minora (see Fig. 1–5). The two genital

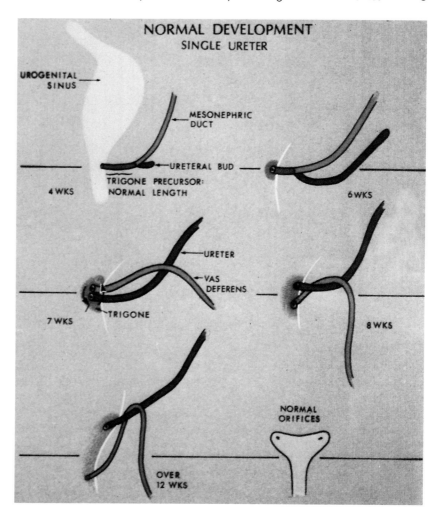

Figure 1-2 The lower end of the mesonephric duct as it joins the anterior division of the cloaca. Note that the common nephric duct is progressively absorbed into the urogenital sinus. By the seventh week the ureter and the mesonephric duct have separate openings, and the rotation takes place: the ureter moves upward and laterally, while the mesonephric duct moves downward and medially, expanding the absorbed tissue to form the trigonal structure.

swellings (which in the male form the scrotum after fusing in the midline) likewise remain separate, developing into the labia majora after they unite in the midline posteriorly, just in front of the anus, to form the posterior commissure.

GONADAL DEVELOPMENT

It has been established that each embryo is at first morphologically bisexual, with all the necessary elements for development of either sex. Differentiation of one set of sex primordia and gradual involution of the other is determined by the sex type of the gonad.

The primitive gonad is undifferentiated in its structure; it has the potential to become either a male or a female gonad by the development of specific histologic elements having different roles in gonadal genesis. Normal differentiation involves a gradual predominance of one component over the other. The primitive sex glands make their appearance by the fifth and sixth weeks within a localized region of thickening known as the urogenital ridge. At 6 weeks the gonad consists of a superficial germinal epithelium and an internal blastema. The blastemal mass

is derived mainly from the proliferative ingrowth from the superficial epithelium that comes loose from its basement membrane. During the seventh week the gonad begins to differentiate into either a testis or an ovary. If it is destined to develop into a testis, it will increase in size and shorten into a more compact organ while achieving a more caudal location. The attachment to the mesonephros becomes the gonadal mesentery, known as the mesorchium. The mass of the germinal epithelium grows into the underlying mesenchyme and forms cordlike masses. These are radially arranged and converge to the mesorchium, where a dense portion of the blastemal mass is also emerging as the primordium of the rete testis. A network of strands soon forms, which is continuous with the testis cords. The testis cords also split into three or four daughter cords; the latter eventually differentiate into the seminiferous tubules, which produce the spermatozoa. The rete testis unites with the mesonephric component that will form the male genital duct system.

If the gonad is going to develop into an ovary, it acquires a mesentery, known as the mesovarium, and settles in a more caudal position. The internal blastema differentiates in the ninth week into a pri-

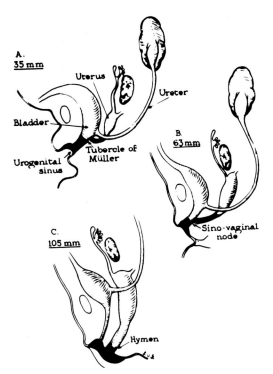

Figure 1-3 Differentiation of the urogenital sinus in the female. The müllerian ducts have fused in the midline and joined the urogenital sinus at the tubercle of Müller. The segment of the urogenital sinus distal to this müllerian tubercle will open and expand to become the vaginal vestibule; thus the combined müllerian ducts become separated from the urogenital sinus and will differentiate later to form most of the vagina and the uterus as well as the fallopian tubes. *A,* 35 mm. *B,* 63 mm. *C,* 105 mm.

mary cortex beneath the germinal epithelium and a loose primary medulla. A compact cellular mass bulges from the medulla into the mesovarium and establishes a primitive rete ovary. At 3 to 4 months the internal mass differentiates into the young ova. A new definitive cortex is formed from the germinal epithelium as well as from the blastema in the form of distinct cellular cords (Pflüger's tubes), and a permanent medulla is formed. The cortex differentiates into ovarian follicles containing ova.

As they develop, the undifferentiated gonads start high up in the abdominal cavity and eventually descend downward. By the third month the testis is located retroperitoneally in the true pelvis. The fibromuscular bands—the gubernaculum—are responsible for the further downward caudal migration of the testis through the abdominal wall to its final destination at the bottom of the scrotum. The testis, however, remains at the abdominal end of the inguinal canal until the seventh month, when it passes through the canal to the outside of the abdomen, dragging with it the processus vaginalis; it normally reaches the scrotal sac by the end of the eighth month. The ovary does not descend so far down; it undergoes an earlier internal descent, becomes attached through the gubernaculum to the tissues of the genital fold, and then attaches itself to the developing uterovaginal canal at its junction with the uterine tube. This part of the gubernaculum be-

tween the ovary and the uterus becomes the ovarian ligament. The part between the uterus and the labia majora becomes the round ligament of the uterus; this prevents extra-abdominal descent. When the ovary enters the true pelvis and remains there, it eventually lies posterior to the uterine tubes on the superior surface of the urogenital mesentery, which has descended with the ovary and now forms the broad ligament. The small processus vaginalis forms and passes toward the labial swelling, but it is usually obliterated at full term.

GENITAL DUCT SYSTEM

In embryonic life there are two sets of embryonic duct systems, each of which relates in its own way to the final genital duct system. These are (1) the *nephric duct system,* also known as the wolffian duct system, and (2) the *müllerian duct system,* a primarily genital structure. The nephric duct system is a combined urinary and genital duct system, but the müllerian duct system is genital from the start. These ducts grow caudally, eventually joining the urogenital sinus. The müllerian ducts meet the urogenital sinus in the midline, where they join as a single tube. Each mesonephric duct, on the other hand, remains separate and joins individually with the ventral division of the cloaca (the urogenital si-

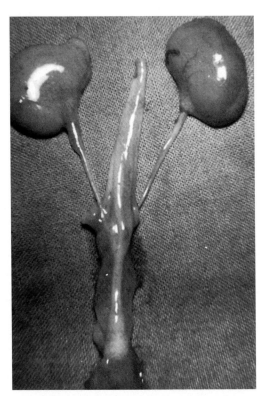

Figure 1-4 Midterm fetal genitourinary system in the female. Note that the tubular structure of the bladder is directly continuous with the urethra, with very minimal constriction at the level of the internal meatus. The ureters are still short, and the kidneys are differentiated. The tubular bladder is still continuous with the allantois via the umbilicus.

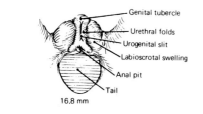

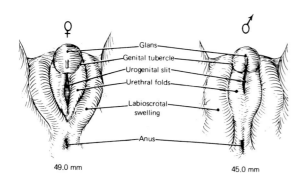

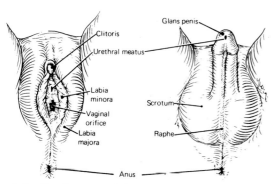

Figure 1-5 Development of the external genitalia in both male and female. Note that the genital tubercles that develop on the undersurface of the cloacal membrane will progressively enlarge and fuse—in the male to form the body of the penis and in the female to form the clitoris. The fusion of the urethral folds will complete the urethral formation in the male, whereas the folds will remain as the labia in the female. The post-tubercle segment of the urogenital sinus will open to become the vaginal vestibule of the female, whereas in the male it will form part of the urethra, which is completed by the urethral fold fusion.

nus) (Fig. 1–6). This happens at the 4-mm stage; by the 15-mm stage, or seventh week, the mesonephric duct has a separate opening into the urogenital sinus after the ureteral bud has attained its own independent opening. The müllerian duct reaches the urogenital sinus rather late, at about the 30-mm embryonic stage, at the ninth week.

Depending on the development of the embryo, the gonadal differentiation determines the development of the duct system. If the gonad becomes a testis, the wolffian duct system starts to differentiate into the male duct system, forming the epididymis and vas deferens, the seminal vesicle, and the ejaculatory duct; at the same time the müllerian duct system proceeds toward its junction with the urogenital si-

nus; however, it progressively degenerates, and a rudimentary structure remains. On the other hand, if the gonad develops into an ovary, the mesonephric duct system is the one that undergoes degenerative changes, whereas the müllerian duct system continues to grow and meet with the urogenital sinus, as mentioned before. However, its fused portion forms the upper part of the vagina and the uterus, and the two separate ducts remain as the fallopian tubes.

Initially, the müllerian duct develops lateral to the mesonephric duct and arises from the vagination of the coelomic epithelium into the parenchyma lateral to the cranial extremity of the mesonephric duct. This opening with the coelomic cavity remains as the fimbriated end of the uterine tube and later develops the characteristic fimbria. The ends grow caudally as a solid tip, cross in front of the mesonephric duct, continue to grow downward and medially, and finally meet and fuse in the midline. This fusion is partial at first, so that there is a temporary septum between the two tubes; progressively they become one canal. The disappearing septum was the potential lumen of the uterine vaginal canal. The solid end of the fused tubes is what meets the urogenital sinus in what is known as Müller's tubercle (or the sinovaginal node) (Fig. 1–7); this tubercle receives a limited contribution from the urogenital sinus, which later differentiates into the most distal fourth or fifth of the vaginal canal. The urogenital sinus itself, distal to Müller's tubercle, becomes shallow, and widens and opens up to form the floor of the vulval cleft. This results in separate urethral and vaginal openings, with the vaginal canal being brought out to its final position near the surface. The vaginal segment increases appreciably and becomes the vaginal vestibule, associated in its various elements with the expansion of the distal inframontanal segment of the urogenital sinus. This segment unfolds, and the genital swellings differentiate into labia minora and labia majora; the hymen is actually the remnant of the müllerian tubercle, differentiating the vaginal vestibule from the vaginal canal proper. It is estimated that the lower fifth of the vaginal canal is derived from the genital sinus with the sinovaginal node, while the remainder of the vagina and the uterus are formed from the fused distal third of the müllerian ducts. The fallopian tubes (or oviducts) are formed from the cephalad two-thirds of the müllerian duct system.

In the male, the müllerian duct system completely degenerates; all that is left of it is the blind pouch seen at the müllerian tubercle, situated at the prostatic utricle; on either side are the openings of the mesonephric ducts—now the ejaculatory ducts.

Congenital Abnormalities of the Genitourinary Tract

Failure of division of the cloaca, whether partial or complete, is rather rare; when it happens it is known as *persistent cloaca*. The rectum and the bladder

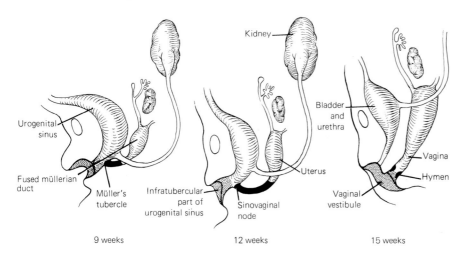

Figure 1-6   Expansion of the post-tubercle segment of the urogenital sinus to form the vaginal vestibule, with the sinovaginal node achieving a separate opening constituting the entrance to the vaginal canal, formed from the fused segment of the two müllerian ducts. The remaining part of the fused segment will form the uterus, while the unfused part will become the fallopian tubes. (From Tanagho EA: Embryology of the genitourinary system. *In* Tanagho EA, McAninch JW [eds]: General Urology, 14th ed. Norwalk, CT, Appleton & Lange, 1995.)

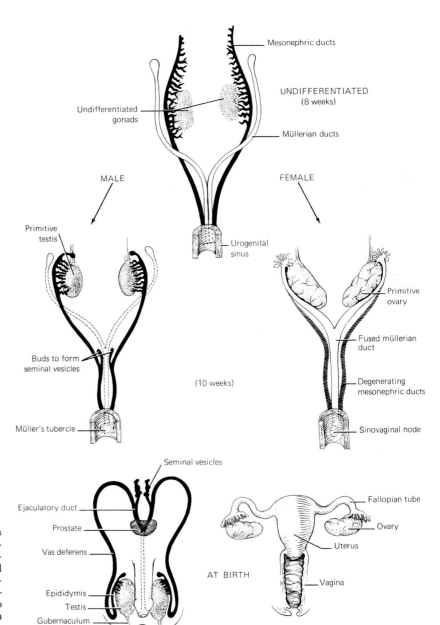

Figure 1-7   Undifferentiated sexual structures early in embryonic life (eighth week) as the embryo grows and differentiates into either a female or a male; the representative segments and their future course (depending on sexual differentiation) are seen. (From Tanagho EA: Embryology of the genitourinary system. *In* Tanagho EA, McAninch JW [eds]: General Urology, 14th ed. Norwalk, CT, Appleton & Lange, 1995.)

open into one receptacle. Minor forms of this abnormality result in rectovesical fistula or rectovestibular fistula. These are commonly associated with imperforate anus or anal atresia.

Development of the genital primordia in an area more caudal than normal can result in the formation of the corpora cavernosa just caudal to the urogenital sinus outlet, with the urethral groove lying on its dorsal rather than on its ventral surface. The extreme degree of such an abnormal development results in bladder exstrophy; in a minor degree it produces epispadias. This can happen in both males and females. In the female it usually is associated with lack of complete fusion of the genital tubercles, bifid clitoris, and failure of fusion of the labia minora ventrally. In the male the same phenomenon is associated with lack of complete fusion of the urethral folds, and the urogenital sinus opens in the dorsum of the penis, a condition known as incomplete epispadias.

Abnormalities in the lower end of the mesonephric duct and the developing ureteral bud, whether in number or in location, can result in several anomalies, mainly duplicated system or ectopic ureteral endings, sometimes all the way out to the vaginal vestibule or even into the vaginal canal itself.

Lack of development of the gonads is termed *gonadal agenesis;* poor development is known as *hypogenesis.* Other abnormalities of the gonadal duct system can result from arrest in the development of the infratubercular segment of the urogenital sinus, which, if it persists, results in the urethra and vagina sharing a common duct. Lack of absorption of the septum between the fusing müllerian ducts can produce a bicornuate uterus, either partial or complete; if it is complete, a double vaginal canal might ensue.

BIBLIOGRAPHY

Amar AD, Hutch JA: Anomalies of the ureter. *In* Alken CE, Dix VW, Goodwin WE, et al (eds): Encyclopedia of Urology, vol 7: Malformations. New York, Springer-Verlag, 1968, p 98.

Brosman SA: Mixed gonadal dysgenesis. J Urol 121:344, 1979.

Burns RK: Hormones and the differentiation of sex. *In* Avery GS (ed): Survey of Biological Progress, vol. 1. New York, Academic Press, 1949.

Callan NA, Blakemore K, Park J, et al: Fetal genitourinary tract anomalies: Evaluation, operative correction, and follow-up. Obstet Gynecol 75:67, 1990.

Chwalle R: The process of formation of cystic dilatations of the vesical end of the ureter and of diverticula at the ureteral ostium. Urol Cutan Rev 31:499, 1927.

Gambino J, Caldwell B, Dietrich R, et al: Congenital disorders of sexual differentiation: MR findings. AJR 158:363, 1992.

Gruenwald P: The relation of the growing müllerian duct to the wolffian duct and its importance for the genesis of malformations. Anat Rec 81:1, 1949.

Lenaghan D: Bifid ureters in children: An anatomical, physiological and clinical study. J Urol 87:808, 1962.

Lewis BV, Brant HA: Obstetric and gynecologic complications associated with müllerian duct abnormalities. Obstet Gynecol 28:315, 1966.

Magee MC, Lucey DT, Fried FA: A new embryologic classification for urogynecologic malformations: The syndrome of mesonephric duct induced müllerian deformities. J Urol 121:265, 1979.

Marshall FF: Embryology of the lower genitourinary tract. Urol Clin North Am 5:3, 1978.

Meyer R: Normal and abnormal development of the ureter in the human embryo: A mechanistic consideration. Anat Rec 96:355, 1946.

Mostwin JL: Current concepts of female pelvic anatomy and physiology. Urol Clin North Am 18:175, 1991.

Sugrue D: Male urogenital hypoplasia. Am J Surg 115:390, 1968.

Tanagho EA: Embryologic basis for lower ureteral anomalies: A hypothesis. Urology 7:451, 1976.

Tanagho EA: Embryology of the genitourinary system. *In* Smith DR (ed): General Urology, 9th ed. Los Altos, CA, Lange Medical Publications, 1978, p 14.

Walsh PC: The differential diagnosis of ambiguous genitalia in the newborn. Urol Clin North Am 5:213, 1978.

Woods MS, Sheppard RG, Hardman DA, Woods HJ: Congenital genitourinary anomalies. Is there a predilection for multiple primary malignant neoplasms? Cancer 69:546, 1992.

Structural Basis of Voiding Dysfunction

Ahmad Elbadawi, M.D.

Functional behavior of the urinary bladder has been investigated for over a century. Yet, several aspects of the mechanism of voiding and the way it is altered in vesical dysfunction remain unresolved. This can largely be attributed to the complexity of structural organization of the bladder and its outlet and the matching complexity of their function.[1–7]

The storage (filling) and expulsion (voiding) phases of micturition involve essentially opposite functions of the bladder and urethra.[8] The bladder acts as a reservoir for urine during filling and as a pump for expelling its stored urine during voiding. The urethra during bladder filling is closed, sealed, and noncompliant, acting as a sphincter to maintain continence, but it opens, dilates, and becomes compliant during voiding, acting as a conduit for the urinary stream. Efficient urine storage requires a compliant and stable detrusor together with a continent bladder outlet.[5, 9] Compliance of the detrusor allows distention of the bladder to capacity, and its stability ensures absence of untimely contractions that could involuntarily force some urine past the closed outlet, resulting in incontinence. Complete emptying of the full bladder depends on[9] (1) optimal contractility of the detrusor so that it can mount a strong, speedy, sustained, and unitary voiding contraction; (2) coordinated opening of the bladder outlet; and (3) maintenance of the opened outlet as a free conduit for an uninterrupted and strong urinary stream.

It is obvious that the anatomy and structure of the bladder and urethra must be optimally suited to the complex dynamic events in the micturition cycle.[6] Important elements in this regard are the inherent physical and biomechanical properties of the tissue components of both vesical and urethral walls and their bearing on organ distensibility and contractility.[8, 10–12] Two crucial elements, however, are (1) the topographic and microstructural organization of the musculature of the bladder wall and urethra, and (2) the elaborate system of vesicourethral innervation,

with complex central cephalospinal control and intricate peripheral pathways.[1–6, 13, 14]

Various disciplines have contributed through experimental and clinical investigation to our current knowledge of bladder function and dysfunction. Gross anatomy was the natural start during the previous century, and it prevailed for many decades. It resulted in some fundamental concepts that have been expanded and refined in the current century as the result of improved methods of dissection, neuroanatomic tracing techniques, and microscopic staining procedures. Following the initial era of anatomic investigation, the principal approach to studies on voiding has been the characterization of physiologic and muscular responses of the lower urinary tract, mainly the bladder. It is undeniable that definition and measurement of these responses are important for understanding the overall nature of neuromuscular function of the bladder and urethra. Nonetheless, such an approach cannot define the factors that determine function of the effector organ (i.e., smooth muscle of detrusor and urethral wall) in regard to the exact mechanism and balance of their contractility, distensibility, and stability during the filling and expulsion phases of micturition. Attempts to define these factors based purely on physiopharmacologic studies are largely inferential and have generated some misconceptions. One such misconception is the idea that the sympathetic autonomic nervous system has little or no role in either vesical or urethral function.[15, 16] This dogma prevailed through the mid 1960s until it was invalidated by microscopic proof of sympathetic innervation of the vesicourethral muscularis, and was subsequently confirmed by innumerable physiopharmacologic observations.[1, 4, 5, 7]

Landmarks in our knowledge of muscular anatomy of the lower urinary tract include[3, 6, 17, 18] (1) continuation of the muscularis of the terminal ureters as the vesical "trigone," and beyond, into the dorsal wall of the urethra; (2) the nonlayered, interwoven organization of muscle bundles of the detrusor[13]; (3) identification of a vesical sheath around the terminal ureters,[19] which was eventually refined as the concept of dual ureteral sheath[20, 21]; and (4) the concept of the rhabdosphincter as an integral striated muscle component of urethral muscularis.[1, 3, 6, 22] Milestones in our knowledge of the innervation and neural control of the bladder and urethra include[1–5] (1) definition in the spinal cord of a sacral parasympathetic and a lumbar sympathetic nucleus for subcephalic bladder control as well as a sacral cord nucleus supplying peripheral somatomotor innervation of the volitional urinary sphincter[23–26]; (2) multilevel localization of centers of bladder control in the brain, their interconnections, and their spinal neurotract projections[27–30]; (3) description of the topographic organization of peripheral sympathetic and parasympathetic outflows, respectively, through the hypogastric and pelvic nerve/plexus pathways and their differences in different species[23, 31, 32]; (4) recognition of dual sympathetic and parasympathetic innervation of the bladder and urethra, and introduction of the functional concept of bladder body versus bladder base[33, 34]; (5) localization of the origin of intrinsic vesicourethral innervation in peripheral ganglia close to and within the organs, including the concept of sympathetic and parasympathetic effector short neurons[35, 36]; (6) concepts of infraspinal interaction of sympathetic and parasympathetic pathways within peripheral ganglia (via collaterals and interneurons)[34–39] as well as the vesicourethral muscularis (via axoaxonal synapses at the effector cell level)[40–42]; (7) recognition of auxiliary autonomic innervation of the rhabdosphincter in animals and humans[22, 43–45]; and (8) recognition of neuropeptides as a class of putative neurotransmitters or modulatory cotransmitters in peripheral vesicourethral innervation.[5–7, 46, 47]

It is axiomatic that full knowledge of the structure of an organ is key to the understanding of how it functions. An obvious corollary of this axiom is that alteration of the structure of an organ is reflected in alteration of its function. Both the axiom and its corollary should be fundamental premises in studies of the bladder in particular, in view of its unique function and intimate anatomic relationship to two other organs of different but closely integrated function—the ureter supplying it with urine and the urethra serving as the conduit for its expulsion. Tacit awareness of these premises stimulated research at the biochemical and molecular levels during the past few decades. This research has yielded important information on the biomechanics, energetics, and neuroreceptor attributes of the bladder and urethra. Not unexpectedly, however, such information has not fully clarified the basis of normal or abnormal smooth muscle function of either organ.

Microscopic study of the vesicourethral muscularis has yet to attain its full potential for determining the true basis of normal and abnormal voiding. Routine tissue histology and histochemistry have provided only limited information about tissue topography and general organization of this system. The notoriously tedious nature of electron microscopy has in part been responsible for its lagging use in investigation of bladder function and dysfunction until recently. Another major stumbling block has been the lack of clear guidelines and precisely defined criteria for such ultrastructural approach.

In this chapter, current knowledge of the microstructure of the vesicourethral muscularis and its functional correlates will be reviewed. In addition, observations on microstructural defects in various forms of voiding dysfunction will be presented, and their bearing on the pathophysiology and management of such disorders will be discussed. The information presented is derived largely from overlapping studies on bladder ultrastructure in normal experimental animals, experimental voiding dysfunction, and various clinical disorders of micturition.

Normal Ultrastructure of Vesicourethral Muscularis

Until the previous decade, the urinary bladder had received little attention by students of tissue ultrastructure, unlike organs such as the intestine. The rather simplistic ideas about bladder function and its neural control that prevailed until the mid 1960s probably thwarted interest in serious electron microscopic investigation. Or, perhaps, no one suspected that bladder structure and function were sufficiently complex to justify such investigation.

The few reports on vesical ultrastructure available before the 1980s presented general, vague, or imprecise information and therefore were largely noncontributory. A notable exception, however, was a study on the distribution of intrinsic afferent (sensory) nerves in the cat bladder, including the relative contributions of sympathetic and parasympathetic pathways.[48, 49] The observations reported in this study confirmed and supplemented earlier accounts of the cholinergic and adrenergic suburothelial nerves demonstrated histochemically in the cat bladder.[33] The existence of nerve terminals within the urothelium is ultrastructurally indisputable in animals and humans.[1] A proposal for distinguishing suburothelial sensory nerves by electron microscopic counting of axonal synaptic vesicles[50] remains unconfirmed.

Recent studies on the detrusor and "internal sphincter"[51–53] have provided detailed information about their intrinsic innervation and have shown that their muscle cells have the ultrastructural features of smooth muscle in general.[54–56] Definitions of the various terms and structural parameters have been provided in other reports.[51, 56–58]

MUSCLE CELLS

Ultrastructurally, each of the grossly recognizable bundles of vesicourethral muscularis in various animals and humans is composed of incompletely separated and imperfectly outlined compact groups (fascicles) of muscle cells.[51, 56, 58] The muscle cell profile (Fig. 2–1) has a smooth contour and a polygonal to cylindrical configuration, depending on the plane of sectioning relative to its long axis. Nuclei of typical

appearance are centrally located and rarely have nucleoli. Mitoses are ordinarily absent in muscle cells of the adult bladder.[59]

The perimeter of each cell profile is delineated by a continuous cell membrane (sarcolemma) that displays alternating thick electron-dense and thin-

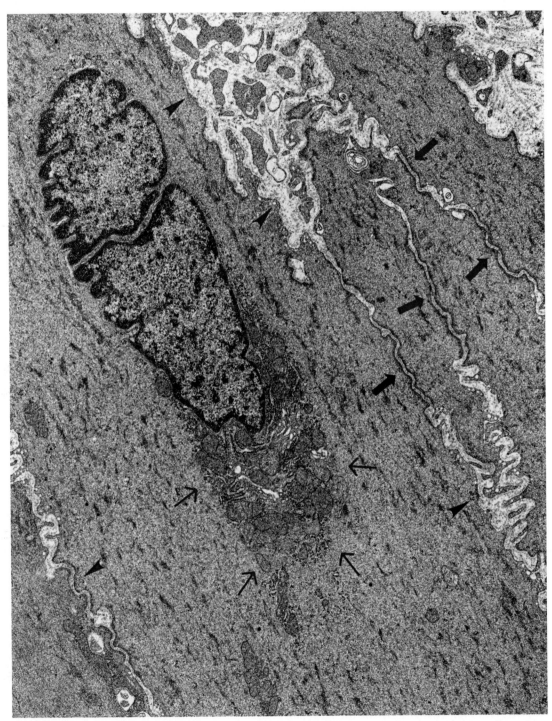

Figure 2-1   Muscle cells of normal detrusor. Sarcolemma (cell membrane) has alternating thick dense bands and interposed thin zones with caveolae, with outlying basal laminae *(arrowheads)*. Cells are adjoined by intermediate junctions *(thick arrows)* and separated by narrow spaces. Nucleus is capped on one side by endoplasmic reticulum and mitochondria *(thin arrows)*. Sarcoplasm is packed with myofilaments, with evenly distributed cigar-shaped dense bodies and scattered mitochondria. (Neg #P-34289) Final magnification ×13,890. (From Elbadawi A: Functional pathology of urinary bladder muscularis: The new frontier in diagnostic uropathology. Semin Diagn Pathol 10[4]:319, 1993.)

ner, less dense zones, with an outlying basal lamina of even thickness and moderate electron density. The thick sarcolemmal zones (dense bands) are composed of sarcolemma plus subjacent highly dense material in sarcoplasm. The interposed thinner zones consist only of sarcolemma, with strings of caveolae that appear as rows of flask-shaped surface vesicles of uniform size.

The sarcoplasm is packed with evenly distributed myofilaments of uniform orientation and alignment, with evenly dispersed dense bodies of uniform cigar-shaped appearance in cylindrical cell profiles of longitudinally sectioned cells. The myofilaments are slanted at approximately a 10-degree angle with the long cell axis and are anchored to dense bands of sarcolemma. Organelles of typical structure, mainly mitochondria and endoplasmic reticulum, are aggregated in a conical zone capping each nuclear pole (in cylindrical profiles); some mitochondria, cisternae of reticulum, and clusters of ribosomes are also scattered in sarcoplasm, particularly beneath sarcolemmal caveolae.

Inter-relationship of Muscle Cells

Individual cells within muscle fascicles are separated by spaces of uniform width (generally <200 nm). The intercellular space contains small amounts of amorphous material similar to basal lamina and a few isolated collagen fibrils that are mainly attached to sarcolemmal dense bands of related muscle cells. Contiguous muscle cells have intermediate-type junctions (attachment plaques, zonulae adherentes) of typical appearance, length, and 30- to 60-nm separation gaps. Some also have zones (with approximately 15-nm gaps) of simple apposition of sarcolemma.[57, 60] Contrary to one report,[61] it is generally accepted that gap junctions (nexus) are absent or only sparsely encountered in the normal vesicourethral muscularis of animals and humans.[51, 53, 60, 62]

INTRINSIC NERVES

Ultrastructural studies have confirmed dual innervation of the normal bladder and urethra by cholinergic and adrenergic axons and provided morphologic details of the relationships between these axons and muscle cells.[1–5] Nerve elements within the vesicourethral muscularis course in its interstitium as Schwann cell–ensheathed axon bundles. Varicosities of some axons become exposed along their course in these bundles to face smooth muscle cells. The main vehicle of muscular innervation, however, is provided by individual preterminal axons that "break away" from the bundles to establish contact with the muscle cells. Many muscle cells have either cholinergic or adrenergic neuroeffector junctions, some have both (diautonomic junctions), and some have neither.[2, 4, 51] Clefts of neuroeffector junctions (i.e., spaces between axon and muscle cell) are generally 15 to 80 nm wide.

It seems certain that no part of the vesicourethral muscularis has a 1:1 nerve-muscle ratio,[1, 5, 59] as inferred in the original histochemical study on vesical innervation.[33] The basis for upholding that impression in one study on the human bladder[53] is questionable.[4, 6, 59] Synaptic contacts between cholinergic and adrenergic or probable copeptidergic axons (axoaxonal synapses) have been discovered as a unique feature of intrinsic neuroplexuses of vesicourethral muscularis in animals[40, 41] and humans (Elbadawi A—unpublished data).

INTERSTITIUM

Collagen and elastic fibers are the main components of interstitium in vesicourethral muscularis. Partitions of interstitium surround and separate muscle bundles.[56, 58] These partitions extend into each bundle as microsepta that incompletely delineate its component fascicles. Vascular and neural elements supplying the muscularis are contained in interstitium between and within the muscle bundles.

Microstructural Basis of Vesicourethral Muscular Function

Conceptually, the vesicourethral muscularis comprises three integrated microstructural compartments: one for generating, another for modulating, and a third for coordinating its functional responses.[9, 63]

The *generator compartment* consists of smooth muscle cells, which enable the vesicourethral muscularis to respond appropriately to various stimuli, particularly to generate the neurally triggered unitary detrusor contraction of voiding. Several microstructural elements play specific roles in the excitation-contraction coupling mechanism of smooth muscle.[9, 52, 54–56] Proper composition, organization, and intracellular disposition of myofilaments bearing the contractile proteins actin and myosin ensure generation of an optimal contractile force. A sufficient complement of intact mitochondria provides the enzymes necessary for generating the necessary ATP-dependent energy. Mitochondria and an intact endoplasmic reticulum provide and store intracellular Ca^{2+}, which is necessary for muscle cell contraction. An intact sarcolemma provides anchorage for myofilaments at its dense bands, to transmit the contractile force to the cell surface. The function of sarcolemmal caveolae has not yet been established. The close spatial association between caveolae and cisternae of subsarcolemmal endoplasmic reticulum, a site of Ca^{2+} binding and storage,[54, 64] suggests that they are involved in the mechanism of muscle contraction. There is evidence that caveolae are sites of active ion (Na^+, K^+, Ca^{2+}) transport, Na^+-Ca^{2+} exchange, or passive Ca^{2+} binding, all of which are involved in the excitation-contraction coupling mechanism.[65]

The *modulator compartment* comprises intrinsic neuroplexuses and their neuroeffector junctions. Neural influence through the latter involves induction, facilitation, inhibition, or disinhibition of chemical neurotransmission to muscle cells under central cephalospinal and peripheral autonomic ganglionic control.[1, 5, 9] Intact structure of intrinsic axons is necessary for conduction of neural impulses throughout their course within the detrusor. Structural integrity of neuroeffector junctions, including the predominant small (clear or dense-core) vesicle content of their axonal components, is necessary for chemical neurotransmission to the target muscle cells. Axoaxonal synapses modulate prejunctional, reciprocal cholinergic ⇄ adrenergic inhibition of effector neural influence in the normal mammalian vesical muscularis, including that of humans.[9, 40, 41] From the structural standpoint, the efficacy and net effect of neural influence on this muscularis depend mainly on (1) the distribution and relative density of the various functional types of structurally intact axons (i.e., cholinergic versus adrenergic), and (2) the width and content of junctional clefts of preserved neuroeffector junctions. Alteration of the inherent structure or spatial relationship of axons within the bladder may hinder one normal neurally triggered neural response or another, or may generate incongruous, uncoordinated, or spurious muscle cell responses.[9]

The *coordinator compartment* is in part muscular and in part interstitial. It is responsible for maintaining spatial topographic organization of muscle cells relative to each other within muscle fascicles and bundles of the detrusor and urethral muscularis. Moreover, it provides the basis for tridimensional distensibility of the bladder, which allows it to be filled to capacity with minimal rise in luminal pressure (i.e., compliance).[11, 66] Compliance is determined by the relative proportions of muscular and interstitial elements as well as the delicate balance of the rigid and elastic components of interstitium—i.e., collagen and elastin, respectively.[10, 66–68]

The main role of the coordinator compartment, however, is to synergize and unify muscle cell responses in the entire detrusor or urethral wall. The most important functional expression of this role is the neurally triggered, coordinated, unitary detrusor contraction that initiates voiding.[1, 4, 9] As indicated earlier, only a fraction of muscle cells of the detrusor are innervated and directly excitable by neural stimuli, despite its overall dense innervation.[1, 4, 6] Voiding contraction of the detrusor, which is in essence a synergized, summated, and sustained contraction of its component fascicles and bundles, thus requires transmittal of contraction from the innervated to all noninnervated muscle cells (i.e., muscle cell coupling).

It is known that cell coupling in smooth muscle is either electrical or mechanical.[54, 55, 69] Electrical coupling *propagates the electrical signal* (action potential) heralding contraction of a muscle cell through gap junctions (and to some extent through simple sarcolemmal appositions) of muscle cells; these junctions (or appositions) provide low-resistance pathways that directly "connect," and allow exchange of ions between sarcoplasms of the adjoined muscle cells. A smooth muscle system endowed with an electrical coupling mechanism thus behaves functionally as a virtual syncytium through which contraction of the component cells can be elicited in near synchrony. The relatively slower mechanical coupling, on the other hand, *transmits the force* generated in a contracting muscle cell through intermediate junctions with adjacent cells. Contrary to one review,[61] cell coupling in normal vesicourethral muscularis is achieved by mechanical cell coupling because its muscle cells have intermediate junctions but no or sparse gap junctions.[51, 53, 60] Active force generated by the contractile apparatus of a muscle cell is discharged to the entire cell surface through insertions of myofilaments into sarcolemmal dense bands, resulting in cell shortening. The consequently developed tension is transmitted through intermediate junctions to adjoined cells, resulting in their deformation and subsequent contraction. Collagen fibrils juxtaposed to the cell surface in the intercellular space contribute to mechanical transmittal of force from the contracting cell to adjacent cells. Summation of minuscule tensions transmitted from cell to cell and from muscle cells to microsepta of interstitium culminates in contraction of entire muscle bundles, and ultimately in contraction of the entire organ in unison—by subsequent force transmittal through partitions of interstitium between the bundles.[60]

It is thus obvious that normal contractility of vesicourethral muscularis, in regard to complete emptying of the bladder, depends on three factors in addition to the inherent topographic organization and structural integrity of its cells. These are the ability of a contracting muscle cell to shorten (thus generating a contraction force), mechanical cell coupling to transmit that force, and a vehicle to summate the transmitted force through the muscularis. All three factors have recognizable ultrastructural correlates. Effective cell shortening requires a normal cylindrical configuration of the muscle cell and a normal complement of myofilaments optimally aligned at a narrow angle with sarcolemma. Mechanical cell coupling is largely determined by the geometric spatial disposition of detrusor muscle cells as well as their structural inter-relationship in regard to their compact arrangement within fascicles, intermediate cell junctions, and narrow interspaces containing few collagen fibrils. Collagen fibers in microsepta and partitions of interstitium, respectively between muscle fascicles and bundles, play a key role in eliciting the summated, unitary voiding contraction.

Ultrastructure of Rhabdosphincter

The feline rhabdosphincter is composed of a mixture of fast- and slow-twitch myofibers, which have the same distinguishable ultrastructure as ordinary somatic mammalian striated muscle.[44] Contrary to one report,[70] the human rhabdosphincter appears to be composed of both types of myofibers (Mathews, Light, Wheeler et al, data to be published).

The concept of triple (i.e., somatomotor plus dual parasympathetic-sympathetic autonomic) innervation of the feline rhabdosphincter based on histochemical study[22] was validated by electron microscopy in the cat,[44, 71] and its adrenergic autonomic component was also confirmed in the human.[45] Two forms of nerve-myofiber relationship are present in the feline rhabdosphincter with intact innervation. One has the classic sole plate differentiation of the myofiber facing a cholinergic neuroterminal, which is characteristic of somatomotor neuromuscular junctions at large. In the other, a cholinergic or adrenergic axon terminal is closely apposed to the surface of a myofiber and has a functionally plausible, narrow neuromuscular cleft but no sole plate differentiation. These surface contacts are considered autonomic because (1) their morphology is identical to those of autonomic neuroeffector junctions in the vesicourethral muscularis and other mammalian smooth muscle systems; (2) they persist, despite disappearance of axons innervating sole plates, following bilateral sacral ventral rhizotomy—the known source of somatomotor innervation through the pudendal nerves (see later discussion).[71–73]

Functional Pathology of Detrusor

Changes in the three microstructural compartments of the detrusor have been described in various forms of voiding dysfunction. Those described in histologic preparations are largely nonspecific and have been of limited usefulness in regard to correlation with the functional abnormalities.[56, 58] On the other hand, the constellations of changes identified ultrastructurally in different dysfunctions tend to predominate in one compartment or another and are distinctive for each dysfunction.[56, 58] For this reason, to define the microstructural correlates of a voiding dysfunction fully and accurately, one needs to study the smooth muscle, interstitium, and intrinsic neural compartments of the detrusor with equal attention and scrutiny.[9, 56]

NEUROPATHIC VOIDING DYSFUNCTION

Practically all information on the microstructural basis of this dysfunction available so far has been derived from experimental studies in the cat. These studies have dispelled some traditionally held dogmas and have laid the foundation for a new concept in pathophysiology of the lower motor neuropathic bladder.[74–79] According to this concept, abnormal behavior of such a bladder does not merely reflect its release from cephalospinal neural control but is largely the result of dynamic, profound changes in

intrinsic nerves and to some extent muscle cells—the two structural elements that jointly determine that behavior. These neuropathic structural changes can be defined fully and accurately only by electron microscopy,[79] and readily distinguish a decentralization from a "denervation" functional type of lower motor neuropathic bladder. The same studies also validate the concept of triple innervation of the feline rhabdosphincter.[71–73, 80]

The Decentralized Bladder

For decades, belief that postganglionic nerves within the bladder are unchanged following decentralization by parasympathetic preganglionic neurectomy (sacral roots, pelvic nerve trunks) remained universal and absolute. The underlying logic was that such neurectomy leaves untouched and structurally intact the ganglion cells that provide the intrinsic vesical nerves. Studies on models of the decentralized bladder, however, revealed dynamic structural changes in intrinsic postganglionic nerves of the detrusor—namely, initial degeneration with eventual regeneration.

Occurring beyond and across preganglionic synapses, short-term degeneration of axons duplicates the well-known phenomenon of primary transsynaptic nerve degeneration in the brain,[81] and represents the first example of this phenomenon in the peripheral autonomic nervous system.[74] The axonal degeneration results in loss of cholinergic neuroeffector junctions, and is associated with transjunctional degeneration of detrusor muscle cells—a previously unknown phenomenon.[76] The term transjunctional underscores the fact that the muscle cell degeneration occurs at a site two levels of anatomic discontinuity peripheral to the sacral spinal cord nucleus (i.e., the preganglionic synapse in the peripheral ganglia and the neuroeffector junction at the terminal effector tissue level). The initially degenerating axons eventually regenerate. This regeneration expresses yet another previously unrecognized phenomenon because it is not a simple restitution of the original complement of cholinergic axons but is also associated with[75] (1) sprouting of adrenergic (postganglionic sympathetic) axons with adrenergic hyperinnervation (also documented histochemically[71, 82]), and (2) emergence of peptide-replete axons and axon terminals. Neuroeffector junctions become reestablished by the latter axonal population in addition to the regenerating cholinergic and sprouting adrenergic axons; muscle cell regeneration occurs concomitantly.[76] Ultrastructural profiles of regenerating muscle cells have expanded rough endoplasmic reticulum replete with clustered ribosomes, prominent subsarcolemmal reticulum, numerous intact paranuclear and subsarcolemmal mitochondria, and frequent nucleoli. It appears that an intact preganglionic sympathetic pathway is necessary for the long-term axonal changes to take place after decentralization because they do not occur when decentralization is combined with hypogastric neurectomy.[78] This fact, together with available pharmacologic evidence,[83] suggests that adrenergic hyperinnervation of the detrusor is an important factor in development of hypertonicity in the lower motor neuropathic bladder.[78]

The "Denervated" Bladder

Changes in intrinsic axons and muscle cells of the detrusor also occur after postganglionic neurectomy,[77] that is, severing of the pelvic plexus (parasympathetic plus sympathetic extrinsic nerves) very close to the bladder. Such neurectomy mimics the clinical situation of severe neural deficit following major extirpative pelvic surgery.[84] The resultant short-term degenerative changes in axons and muscle cells are similar to those seen in the decentralized bladder but are more profound in both scope and degree. Long-term changes, however, are different, including little cholinergic axonal regeneration, sparse adrenergic innervation, and no appreciable population of peptide-rich axons. Similar sparsity of adrenergic nerves has been reported in bladder biopsy specimens from patients who had had abdominoperineal resection of the rectum.[85]

The "Denervated" Rhabdosphincter

Decentralization of the bladder by bilateral sacral ventral rhizotomy deprives the rhabdosphincter of its somatomotor innervation. The somatomotor-denervated rhabdosphincter loses its population of classic neuromuscular junctions, and the ultrastructure of its sole plates becomes markedly simplified, but the autonomic axon contacts with the myofibers lacking sole plates persist.[71] Eventually, the autonomic junctions become both prominent and widespread, and, in addition, many of the residual simplified sole plates become newly innervated by a cholinergic axon, an adrenergic axon, or both.[72] These changes indicate permanent degeneration of somatomotor nerves and persistence plus long-term "propagation" of autonomic innervation in denervated territories of the rhabdosphincter. Along with the axonal changes, the myofibers display a combination of degeneration and regeneration.[80]

The somatomotor-denervated rhabdosphincter thus appears to be under exclusive autonomic neural control. The nature of this control has not as yet been investigated. Nor have responses to autonomic neural stimuli been demonstrated either physiologically or pharmacologically in the normal rhabdosphincter, although they are unequivocal in the cat and their adrenergic component has been proved in the human. The autonomic component may have a subtle, very specific, or precisely timed function in normal micturition that is difficult to duplicate in an investigative setting. Or it may be functionally operative or discernible only in abnormal voiding. Currently available physiopharmacologic methods of study may or may not be sufficiently sensitive to segregate autonomic responses of the rhabdosphincter from those of the intimately associated urethral smooth muscularis, in either the normal or the neuropathic rhabdosphincter.

The Upper Motor Neuropathic Bladder

As described in the brain, the phenomenon of transsynaptic degeneration may be primary, secondary, tertiary, and so on, depending on the number of synaptic relays between the injured neuron and the neuron providing degenerating terminals in the same pathway.[81] Transsynaptic degeneration in the decentralized bladder is primary because, as far as is known, only one relay station (in a peripheral vesicourethral ganglion) is interposed between the interrupted preganglionic neuron (ventral root) and the corresponding postganglionic neuron providing the degenerating terminals within the bladder. It is conceivable that comparable degeneration may follow interruption of central neuraxial pathways as an expression of secondary or tertiary transsynaptic degeneration (across one or two central plus the peripheral relay stations). Observations in one study on a spinal cord transection model suggest that such degeneration may occur,[86] but it needs to be confirmed by detailed investigation in experimental models and clinical settings. If such confirmation is obtained, a new important concept would emerge—namely, that functional derangement in the bladder deprived of cephalic control is in part due to structural changes in vesicourethral muscularis despite preserved anatomic integrity of the sacral cord as well as infraspinal neural pathways.

POORLY CONTRACTILE DETRUSOR

Impaired contractility may be the only manifestation of a non-neuropathic detrusor dysfunction (e.g., in the elderly[87, 88]) or it may occur as an additional abnormality in an obstructed or unstable detrusor.[89, 90] The ultrastructural hallmark of a poorly contractile detrusor is the *degeneration pattern* (Fig. 2–2), characterized by widespread degeneration of muscle cells and intrinsic nerves.[52, 58] Degeneration of muscle cells can be recognized ultrastructurally by a spectrum of features that reflect its severity. Mild degeneration results in such subtle features as malalignment of myofilaments with patchy stacking, crisscross or swerving patterns, and uneven crowding or clumping of sarcoplasmic dense bodies. Features of moderate degeneration include disorganization or disruption of myofilaments, disruption of sarcoplasmic dense bodies and mitochondria, distention of cisternae of endoplasmic reticulum with loss of ribosomes, appearance in sarcoplasm of highly electron-dense patches or laminate bodies, and occasionally large deposits of glycogen particles. Severe degeneration is manifested by sequestration, extrusion (bleb-

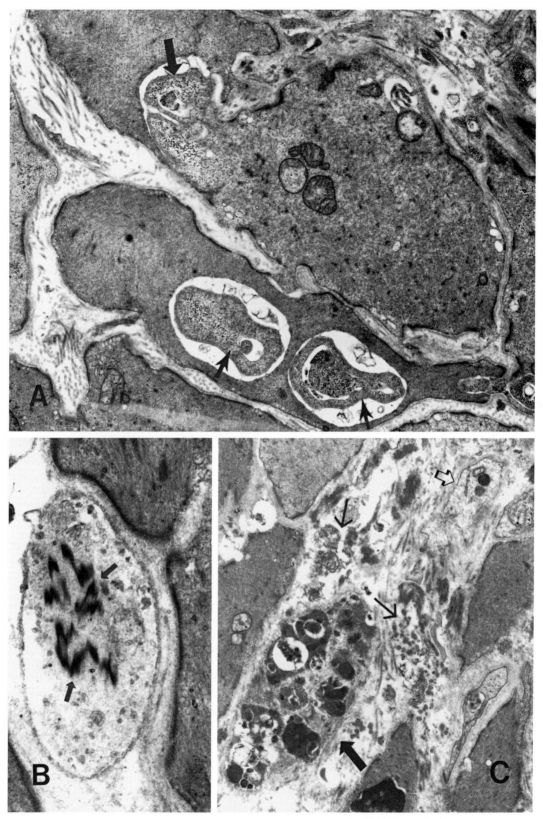

Figure 2-2 Degeneration in poor detrusor contractility. *A*, Degenerating muscle cells, one with sequestered sarcoplasm *(arrows)*, another with sarcoplasmic bleb intruding on adjacent cell *(thick arrow)*. (Neg #J-23425) Final magnification ×16,500. *B*, Degenerating muscle cell, showing sarcoplasm of rarefied appearance with disrupted myofilaments and clustered, thickened, and confluent dense bodies *(arrows)*. (Neg #J-10542) Final magnification × 27,300. *C*, Severe degeneration of muscle cell *(thick arrow)*. Sarcoplasm is completely disrupted and replaced by irregular, large, highly electron-dense patches and multivesiculated bodies; abundant cell debris *(arrows)* is evident in adjacent interstitium. Note profile of degenerating axon *(open arrow)* with depleted vesicles, disrupted mitochondria, and highly electron-dense patch. (Neg #J-26811) Final magnification ×14,000. (From Elbadawi A: Pathology and pathophysiology of detrusor in incontinence. Urol Clin North Am 22:3, 1995.)

bing), vacuolation, or floccular appearance of sarcoplasm, loss or electron-dense homogenization of myofilaments, distortion of the nucleus with irregular clumping of chromatin, and thickening or breaching of sarcolemma with replication of the basal lamina. Severely degenerating cells ultimately become shrivelled or disintegrated.

Degeneration in intrinsic nerves can be recognized only ultrastructurally by a constellation of features that include[52, 58] depletion of synaptic vesicles, axoplasmic dense bodies, breaching of axolemma, and disruption of mitochondria in axon terminals and varicosities of neuroeffector junctions. Severe degeneration of axons results in their retraction from related muscle cells and ultimately in fragmentation or lysis. Axons ensheathed by Schwann cells may undergo vacuolar or floccular change, with disruption of their axoplasmic content of neurofilaments and neurotubules. Loss of ensheathed axons results in the distinctive appearance of collapsed Schwann cells with redundant and replicated basal laminae.

The features of the degeneration pattern can easily explain impaired contractility of the detrusor.[9, 52, 58] Degeneration of the intrinsic nerves would impede transmission of neural impulses along axons as well as neuroeffector transmission to muscle cells at their terminals. Degeneration of muscle cells would disrupt their contractile elements, energetic machinery, and Ca^{2+} stores, rendering them unable to generate an efficient contraction, or any contraction, whether in response to a propagated neural impulse or secondary to mechanical "pull" by a contracting adjacent muscle cell with preserved structure.

DETRUSOR OVERACTIVITY (INSTABILITY)

Several factors have been implicated in the pathogenesis of detrusor instability. Some of these factors are functional, whereas others revolve around a structural change in the unstable detrusor. A change in density of one functional type of intrinsic nerves or another has been reported in histochemical preparations,[91, 92] but the methods used to determine nerve density in these studies are questionable.[8, 59, 89, 93] Recent electron microscopic studies have revealed that the principal structural change in the unstable detrusor, whether obstructed or not, is in the inter-relationship of its muscle cells.[58, 60, 63, 89]

Reduction of vasoactive intestinal polypeptide (VIP)-reactive nerves in the detrusor with idiopathic instability (i.e., no outlet obstruction or neural deficit) has been described in one histochemical study.[91] Loss of such nerves was thus suggested as the cause of instability on the premise that it would deprive the detrusor of an inhibitory role of the neuropeptide as a neurotransmitter or neuromodulator.[94, 95] Histochemical observations on "VIPergic" nerves are not sufficient to determine their structural status; only electron microscopy can determine such status, particularly the content and type of axonal synaptic vesicles.[1, 9] No correlation between detrusor function

and immunohistochemical reactivity of VIP was found in a recent study of human bladder biopsies.[96] Loss of inhibitory VIP-reactive nerves as the cause of involuntary detrusor contractions is difficult to reconcile with the clinical observation that they are susceptible to neurally mediated inhibition.[97]

In a more recent study, "increased appreciation of bladder filling" due to "relative abundance" of "presumptive sensory nerves" in suburothelium was suggested as an explanation for idiopathic instability.[92] Aside from the questionable counting method used, no adjustment for thickness of suburothelium in the specimens studied was mentioned; such thickness varies in different subjects and can easily be altered even by minor pathologic changes in the bladder wall such as mild cystitis, vascular congestion, or edema.[8] Moreover, there is no basis for the postulated association between the number of nerves and the degree of sensory excitability or perception.[8]

Muscle cells of the overactive (unstable) aging detrusor, whether obstructed or not, have some distinctive ultrastructural features, collectively designated the *dysjunction pattern*.[58, 60, 89] This pattern is characterized by moderately widened spaces between individual muscle cells, scarce intermediate muscle cell junctions, and abundant distinctive protrusion junctions and ultraclose cell abutments (Figs. 2–3 and 2–4) that are not found in the normal detrusor. The only difference between the obstructed and unobstructed overactive detrusor is a superimposed myohypertrophy pattern (see later discussion) in the former (see Fig. 2–4). The dysjunction pattern is not associated with any particular change in intrinsic nerves of the overactive detrusor, whether obstructed or not, except degenerative changes when the detrusor is also poorly contractile.

The protrusion junctions and ultraclose abutments of the dysjunction pattern resemble gap junctions in having a very narrow separation cleft ($\leq$10 nm) and no sarcolemmal thickening at the contact zone of the adjoined muscle cells. These features suggest that both types of junction serve as a vehicle for electrical muscle cell coupling in the overactive detrusor in lieu of the normal mechanism of mechanical cell coupling that is curtailed by reduction of intermediate cell junctions.[58, 60] This introduces a new concept of pathogenesis of detrusor overactivity (instability), whether it is associated with outlet obstruction or not. According to this concept, involuntary detrusor contractions in either setting are elicited by a bipartite myogenic mechanism, consisting of irritable loci and a final common pathway. The irritable locus represents muscle cells with heightened inherent spontaneous activity with or without increased responsiveness to a "trigger for contraction," such as stretch or excitatory neural stimuli. The final common pathway is served by muscle cells "linked" by protrusion junctions and abutments to acquire the functional properties of a "syncytium" in and around the irritable loci. Limited, small contractions originating independently in one or more loci, whether spontaneous or triggered, are propagated electrically through that

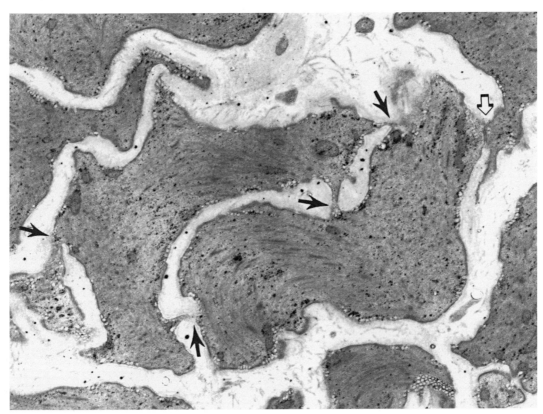

Figure 2-3 Dysjunction pattern in detrusor overactivity. Muscle cells are separated by mildly widened spaces with depleted normal intermediate junctions, adjoined by protrusion junctions *(arrows)* with indiscernible gaps between cells and overall appearance of pseudosyncytium at the junctions. Profile of the residual intermediate junction *(open arrow)* is distinctly different from that of protrusion junction. (Neg #J-11762) Final magnification ×13,500. (From Elbadawi A: Pathology and pathophysiology of detrusor in incontinence. Urol Clin North Am 22:3, 1995.)

syncytium to outlying muscle cells, recruiting them to contract in near-synchrony. If the electrical propagation involves a sufficiently large muscle territory, the result would be significant, urodynamically measurable contractions that, by definition, are involuntary. Electrical cell coupling remains partially suppressible by neurally mediated inhibition, insofar as its completion, progression, or even initiation is concerned,[60] and it does not hinder the development of neurally triggered, unitary, effective voiding contractions. Preliminary studies so far indicate the presence of the dysjunction pattern in "idiopathic" instability in young adults as well as in the overactive neuropathic (i.e., hyperreflexic) detrusor.

OBSTRUCTED DETRUSOR

Until the last decade, structure of the obstructed detrusor was investigated almost exclusively by routine histologic methods. The only convincing changes reported were in the interstitium,[98–106] which, not surprisingly, failed to explain why or how the obstructed bladder become dysfunctional. Changes in intrinsic nerves of the obstructed detrusor were described in a few histochemical studies, but no meaningful correlation was made with its abnormal functional behavior.[107–111] The validity and significance of these neural changes remain debatable.[8, 59, 89, 93]

Ultrastructural studies revealed characteristic changes in the experimentally or clinically obstructed detrusor,[89, 112–116] including the rare entity of outlet obstruction in women.[89] Collectively designated the *myohypertrophy pattern,* these changes predominate in muscle cells and interstitium and can explain practically all functional abnormalities in the obstructed detrusor.[89] Additional changes in the obstructed human detrusor have been correlated with specific superimposed, urodynamically defined derangements of its function.[52, 60, 89] Contrary to some reports,[104, 105] there is no correlation between the scope and degree of ultrastructural changes in the detrusor and the degree of bladder trabeculation as observed cystoscopically.[58, 89]

Myohypertrophy Pattern

The myohypertrophy pattern has three features (Fig. 2–5): muscle cell hypertrophy, markedly widened spaces between individual muscle cells, and "collagenosis."[58, 63, 89] Characteristically, the extent of cell separation and collagenosis is nonuniform, so that muscle fascicles with different degrees of loosened structure exist side by side in the same section or even microscopic field.

Muscle cell hypertrophy (i.e., increased cell size)

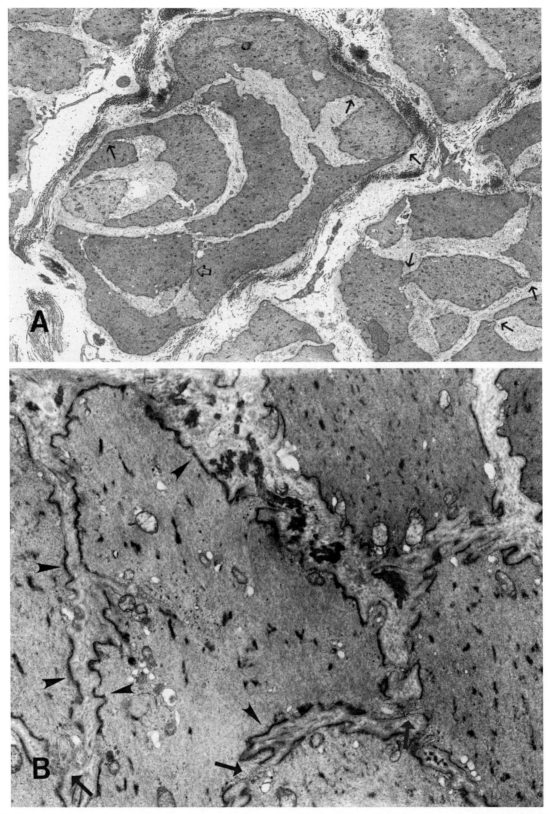

Figure 2-4 Myohypertrophy plus dysjunction pattern of overactive (unstable) obstructed detrusor. *A,* Overview showing widely variable size and shape of muscle cell profiles, markedly widened intercellular spaces containing abundant collagen, depleted intermediate cell junctions, and numerous protrusion junctions *(arrows);* open arrow marks residual intermediate junction. (Neg #J-28754) Final magnification ×4,090. (Modified from Elbadawi A: Functional pathology of urinary bladder muscularis: The new frontier in diagnostic uropathology. Semin Diagn Pathol 10[4]:348, 1993.) *B,* Muscle cell profiles adjoined as pseudosyncytium by ultraclose abutments *(arrows);* sarcolemmas (cell membranes) are dominated by dense bands *(arrowheads)* with depleted caveolae in interposed thinner zones. (Neg #J-22725) Final magnification ×11,800. (From Elbadawi A: Pathology and pathophysiology of detrusor in incontinence. Urol Clin North Am 22:3, 1995.)

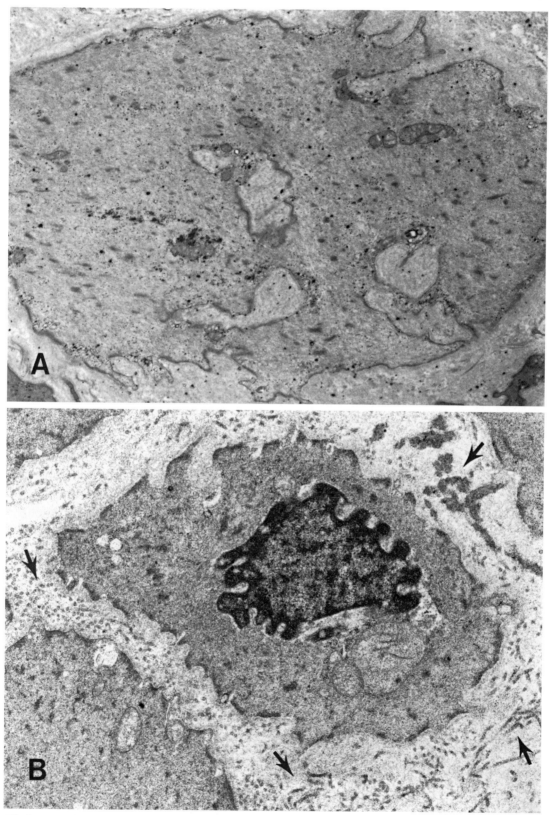

Figure 2-5 Myohypertrophy pattern of obstructed detrusor. *A,* Bizarre twisted profile of hypertrophic muscle cell. (Neg #J-11768) Final magnification ×13,000. *B,* Markedly widened spaces between individual muscle cells containing abundant collagen fibrils and some elastic fibers *(arrows).* (Neg #P-40013) Final magnification ×18,600.

is the traditional hallmark of obstruction in hollow viscera.[117, 118] Because of its nonlayered meshwork organization,[3, 6, 13] the detrusor does not lend itself to traditional methods for estimating muscle cell size in the intestine, such as diameter or length of muscle cell profiles, number of muscle cell nuclei per area, volume density of muscle cells, and so on.[59, 93, 114] This fact casts doubt on the validity of data indicating the presence of hypertrophy of obstructed detrusor in several studies.[99, 103, 105, 119–121]

A hypertrophied muscle cell cannot be recognized qualitatively on light microscopy but has a distinctive, easily discernible ultrastructural profile[58, 63, 89, 113, 116] characterized by branching of the tapering ends of the cell, deformed or bizarre cell configuration with irregular infoldings or contortions (see Fig. 2–5A), and occasional "reflexive" intermediate junctions[122] between contortions or branches of the same cell. Branches of hypertrophic muscle cells appear to interlock as a braid in tridimensional perspective.

"Collagenosis" designates the presence of abundant collagen fibrils *and fibers* in markedly widened spaces between *individual* muscle cells (see Figs. 2–4A and 2–5B).[58, 89] These features cannot be recognized by light microscopy. Abundant collagen fibers also expand microsepta and partitions of interstitium, respectively, between muscle fascicles and bundles. This corresponds to the "fibrosis" mentioned as the main structural change in earlier studies on the obstructed detrusor. Intercellular collagen is generally associated with deposits of basal lamina–like material and a variable number of elastic fibers. Separation of muscle cells results in shearing of their junctions, which, consequently, become fewer and unevenly distributed. Muscle cell separation results in loosening of the normally compact arrangement of muscle cells in fascicles and bundles of the detrusor. When such separation is excessive, the fascicular arrangement is lost, and the cells lie individually, wide apart, amid a dominant background of collagen.

Structural/Functional Correlations

Traditionally, it has been thought that the obstructed detrusor undergoes "compensatory" muscular hypertrophy and thus becomes stronger to overcome the obstruction.[123] This dogma is fallacious. It is now recognized that the obstructed detrusor is not stronger, if not actually weaker, and has a slower velocity (speed) of contraction than the norm—even in the presence of adequate bladder emptying and absence of retained urine.[63, 124–127] Theoretically, a hypertrophic smooth muscle cell can generate a stronger contraction than a normal cell. This, however, does not necessarily mean a stronger contraction of the detrusor as a whole. Several ultrastructural features of the myohypertrophy pattern limit the ability of hypertrophic muscle cells to shorten (that is, contract). Loss of intermediate cell junctions between widely separated muscle cells greatly restricts the main vehicle for mechanical cell coupling,

so that the force of contraction of muscle cells would not be transmitted effectively to outlying cells. Such hindrance of force transmittal is accentuated by excessive collagen in the widened intercellular spaces as well as the expanded interstitium. The net effect of these impediments would be inability of the obstructed detrusor to mount the speedy, strong, coordinated, or sustained contraction necessary for complete emptying of the full bladder.

Superimposed Structural Changes

Muscle cell degeneration has been described as a constant feature of experimental acute, transient overdistention of the rabbit detrusor,[113, 114] the human detrusor after repeated episodes of acute retention with bladder overdistention,[128] and the chronically obstructed human detrusor of both genders when its contractility is overtly impaired with considerable residual urine.[89] Degeneration of intrinsic nerves has also been observed ultrastructurally in the rabbit model as well as the chronically obstructed, poorly contractile human detrusor. Widespread degenerative changes, superimposed on myohypertrophy and collagenosis, further weaken an obstructed detrusor.[89] Reduction in density of intrinsic nerves has been reported in some light microscopic histochemical studies on the obstructed human detrusor[107, 109, 111] as well as in a pig model intended to reproduce long-term bladder outlet obstruction.[108] Based primarily on such "reduction" and on in vitro detrusor responses in the pig model, it was proposed that "cholinergic denervation" with subsequent supersensitivity was the cause of obstruction-associated instability.[129] It should be pointed out, however, that the methods used to assess nerve density in the histochemical studies were questionable.[8, 59, 93] Furthermore, the conclusion in most of these studies that the observed changes were the result of nerve loss (or "denervation") was not substantiated by direct evidence of structural nerve damage or degeneration in any. More reservations about the denervation concept of instability have been raised in a recent ultrastructural study of the obstructed human detrusor,[89] which attributed instability in such detrusor to presence of the same protrusion junctions and abutments (see Fig. 2–5) that are the cardinal feature of the overactive unobstructed bladder (see earlier discussion).

A variable number of elastic fibers accompany deposits of collagen in intercellular spaces (see Figs. 2–4A and 2–5B) and interstitium of the obstructed detrusor.[89, 112] Massive deposits of elastic fibers (designated *hyperelastosis*) have been observed in the excessively distended detrusor of patients with chronic urinary retention secondary to bladder outlet obstruction (Fig. 2–6).[58, 89] Such detrusors also have excessive collagenosis, marked expansion of interstitium, and severe muscle cell degeneration, with scattered residual hypertrophic muscle cells. These changes markedly obscure or eliminate orderly or-

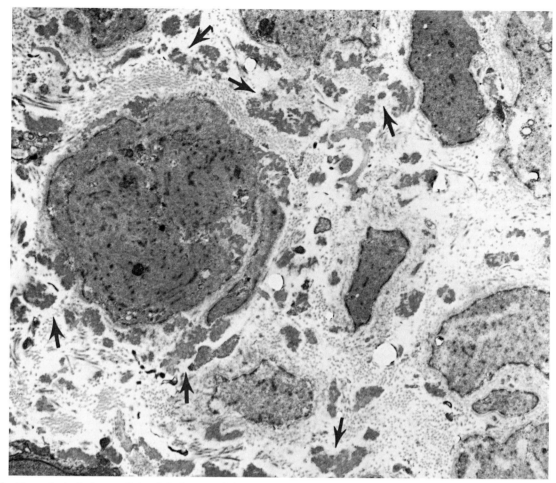

Figure 2-6 Hyperelastosis in overdistended obstructed detrusor. Muscle cell profiles are far apart (up to 6 μm) in interstitium with abundant collagen and elastic fibers *(arrows)*. (Neg #J11922) Final magnification ×10,550. (Modified from Elbadawi A: Functional pathology of urinary bladder muscularis: The new frontier in diagnostic uropathology. Semin Diagn Pathol 10[4]:349, 1993.)

ganization of detrusor muscular elements as fascicles.[58, 89]

Regeneration of muscle cells and intrinsic axons in the detrusor accompanies degeneration of the corresponding elements following obstruction in the experimental rabbit model of acute transient overdistention and is the most prominent change following relief of that obstruction.[113, 114] No regenerative changes were observed in the chronically obstructed human detrusor of either gender, even when degeneration of its muscle cells and axons was evident and widespread in association with overt impaired contractility.[58, 63, 89] Muscle cell regeneration, therefore, is not a part of the process leading to myohypertrophy in the obstructed detrusor and probably is not a manifestation of hyperplasia in the rabbit model. In this model, both muscle cell regeneration and hypertrophy are probably manifestations of structural adaptation, eventually leading to recovery, that follows the initial damage induced by acute distention of the bladder.[130] Similarly, regeneration of axonal elements in the same model probably represents their eventual structural recovery, as observed earlier in the experimentally decentralized bladder.[75]

THE AGING DETRUSOR

Knowledge of microstructure of the aging detrusor is crucial for our understanding of the pathology and pathophysiology of voiding dysfunctions and incontinence in the elderly. It has been shown biochemically that collagen content of the detrusor increases with advancing age in women,[131] resulting in reduction of its contractility.[11, 68, 126] In one report it was stated that neither the amount of smooth muscle nor the size of its individual cells is altered by age, but the "density" of cholinergic innervation is markedly reduced by age.[132] The validity of these observations has been questioned in a recent ultrastructural study of truly aging detrusors.[52, 56, 58] This study defined the microstructural norm of the aging detrusor, which was obtained from asymptomatic subjects who had no urodynamic evidence of obstruction, detrusor hyperactivity, impaired detrusor contractility, or altered bladder compliance.[52, 53] In such a detrusor, muscle cells and axons remain virtually intact except for a few subtle ultrastructural changes. These include moderate widening of spaces between individual muscle cells, modest intercellular deposits of basal lamina, considerable depletion of sarcolemmal caveolae with marked elongation of sarcolemmal dense bands, and normal (often elongated) intermediate cell junctions. These changes may be manifestations of a process of dedifferentiation of detrusor muscle cells associated with aging.[52]

Conclusion

The foregoing review reinforces the premise that morphologic evaluation of detrusor microstructure can be truly objective and functionally meaningful only if it includes an analysis of its muscular, interstitial, and neural (MIN) microstructural compartments. Practically all structural parameters that have direct impact on detrusor function can be defined only by electron microscopy. Studies done so far indicate that the data necessary for correlation of detrusor structure and function can be obtained readily and reproducibly from an endoscopic biopsy, which appears to be truly representative of the whole detrusor insofar as the fine structure of its smooth muscle elements is concerned. The parameters sought are basic and have been defined clearly so that they can be studied and evaluated by any pathologist with a knowledge of diagnostic electron microscopy and smooth muscle ultrastructure.[58]

It is now clear that different forms of human detrusor dysfunction are associated, in common, with one or more changes in one or more of the three MIN compartments but at the same time differ in one or more. This fact emphasizes the great potential of study of detrusor microstructure as the means of better understanding the pathophysiology of various voiding dysfunctions and of developing a valuable tool in the clinical diagnosis and management of such disorders. To gain the full benefit of such study, its goal should be to determine in each dysfunction not only the presence but, more important, also the spectrum, degree, and extent of distribution of the changes seen in each microstructural compartment. Only through pursuit of this approach can the natural history and the outcome of treatment of various voiding dysfunctions be explained, understood, and perhaps predicted with reasonable accuracy. To this end, the material needed for microstructural study should ideally be obtained at the time of patient presentation, during follow-up of patients managed conservatively, and at various intervals following surgical intervention or other specific therapy aimed at manipulation of bladder behavior. From such information one can begin to (1) understand the basis for differences in clinical presentation between patients with the same disorder as well as between different disorders; (2) recognize patterns of the natural course and evolution of different presentations of the same disorder as well as different disorders; (3) define structural markers of reversibility versus permanence of each disorder; (4) identify the structural correlates of successful versus ineffective treatment in patients with the same disorder and patient groups with different disorders. As information on the various dysfunctional disorders is gathered and correlated, one can begin to identify trends in the natural evolution and prognosis of each dysfunction and to methodically set appropriate indications, contraindications, and predictive indices for its available treatment modalities. Eventually, the stage will be set for the use of detrusor structural morphology as a routine if not a key modality in the clinical management of vesical dysfunction in general.

REFERENCES

1. Elbadawi A: Neuromorphologic basis of vesicourethral function. I. Histochemistry, ultrastructure and function of intrinsic nerves of the bladder and urethra. Neurourol Urodyn 1:3–50, 1982.
2. Elbadawi A: Autonomic innervation of the vesical outlet and its role in micturition. *In* Hinman F Jr (ed): Benign Prostatic Hypertrophy. New York, Springer-Verlag, 1983, pp 330–348.
3. Elbadawi A: Neuromorphology. Comparative neuromorphology in animals. *In* Torrens M, Morrison JFB (eds): The Physiology of the Lower Urinary Tract. London, Springer-Verlag, 1987, pp 23–52.
4. Elbadawi A: Le support anatomique de la physiologie des voies urinaires. *In* Buzelin JM, Richard F, Susset JG (eds): Physiologie et Pathologie de la Dynamique des Voies Urinaires (Haut et Bas Appareil). Paris, FIIS, 1987, pp 43–66.
5. Elbadawi A: Neuromuscular mechanisms of micturition. *In* Yalla SV, McGuire EJ, Elbadawi A, Blaivas JG (eds): Neurourology and Urodynamics. Principles and Practice. New York, Macmillan, 1988, pp 3–36.
6. Elbadawi A: Anatomy of the neuromuscular apparatus of micturition. *In* Krane RJ, Siroky MB (eds): Clinical Neurology, 2nd ed. Boston, Little, Brown, 1991, pp 5–24.
7. Van Arsdalen K, Wein AJ: Physiology of micturition and continence. *In* Krane RJ, Siroky MB (eds): Clinical Neurourology, 2nd ed. Boston, Little, Brown, 1991, pp 25–82.
8. Elbadawi A: Neurophysiology of storage and voiding function. Curr Opin Urol 3:255–261, 1993.
9. Elbadawi A: Structural basis of detrusor contractility. The 'MIN' approach to its understanding and study. Neurourol Urodyn 10:77–86, 1989.
10. Coolsaet BLRA: Bladder compliance and detrusor activity during the collection phase. Neurourol Urodyn 4:263–273, 1985.
11. Susset JG, Regnier CH: Viscoelastic properties of the bladder and urethra. *In* Yalla SV, McGuire EJ, Elbadawi A, Blaivas JG (eds): Neurourology and Urodynamics. Principles and Practice. New York, Macmillan, 1988, pp 106–121.
12. Lose LG: Simultaneous recording of pressure and cross-sectional area in the female urethra: A study of urethral closure function in healthy and stress incontinent women. Neurourol Urodyn 11:55–89, 1992.
13. Hunter deWT: A new concept of the urinary bladder musculature. J Urol 71:695–704, 1954.
14. Uhlenhuth E, Hunter deWT, Loechel WF: Problems in the Anatomy of the Pelvis. Philadelphia, Lippincott, 1953, pp 1–157.
15. Langworthy OR, Kolb LC, Lewis LG: Physiology of Micturition. Baltimore, Williams & Wilkins, 1940.
16. Tanagho EA, Meyers FH: The "internal sphincter." Is it under sympathetic control? Invest Urol 7:79–89, 1969.
17. Gil Vernet S: Morphology and Function of Vesico-Prostato-Urethral Musculature. Treviso, Libreria Editrice Canova, 1968, pp 11–328.
18. Hutch JA: Anatomy and Physiology of the Bladder, Trigone and Urethra. New York, Appleton-Century-Crofts, 1972, pp 71–122.
19. Waldeyer W: Über die sogennante Ureterscheide. Verhandl Anat Gesellsch 6:259–260, 1892.

20. Elbadawi A: Anatomy and function of the ureteral sheath. J Urol 107:224–229, 1972.
21. Elbadawi A, Amaku EO, Frank IN: Trilaminar musculature of the submucosal ureter. Anatomy and functional implications. Urology 2:409–417, 1973.
22. Elbadawi A, Schenk EA: A new theory of the innervation of bladder musculature. Part IV. Innervation of the vesicourethral junction and external urethral sphincter. J Urol 111:613–615, 1974.
23. Morrison JFB: Neural connections between the lower urinary tract and the spinal cord. In Torrens M, Morrison JFB (eds): The Physiology of the Lower Urinary Tract. London, Springer-Verlag, 1987, pp 53–88.
24. Onufrowicz B: On the arrangement and function of the cell groups in the sacral region of the spinal cord. Arch Neurol Psychopathol 3:387–411, 1900.
24. Shrøder HD: Anatomical and pathoanatomical studies on the spinal efferent systems innervating pelvic structures. J Auton Nerv Syst 14:23–48, 1985.
26. Ueyama T, Mizuno N, Nomura S, et al: Central distribution of afferent and efferent components of the pudendal nerve in the cat. J Comp Neurol 222:38–46, 1984.
27. Kuru M: Nervous control of micturition. Physiol Rev 45:425–494, 1965.
28. Bors E, Comarr AE: Neurological Urology. New York, Karger, 1971, pp 61–128.
29. Morrison JFB: Reflex control of the lower urinary tract. In Torrens M, Morrison JFB (eds): The Physiology of the Lower Urinary Tract. London, Springer-Verlag, 1987, pp 193–235.
30. Morrison JFB: Bladder control: Role of higher levels of the central nervous system. In Torrens M, Morrison JFB (eds): The Physiology of the Lower Urinary Tract. London, Springer-Verlag, 1987, pp 237–274.
31. Kuntz A: The Autonomic Nervous System. Philadelphia, Lea & Febiger, 1945, pp 284–303.
32. Mitchell GAG: Anatomy of the Autonomic Nervous System. Edinburgh, E & S Livingstone, 1853, pp 297–310.
33. Elbadawi A, Schenk EA: Dual innervation of the mammalian urinary bladder. A histochemical study of the distribution of cholinergic and adrenergic nerves. Am J Anat 119:405–428, 1966.
34. Elbadawi A, Schenk EA: A new theory of the innervation of urinary bladder musculature. I. Morphology of the intrinsic vesical innervation apparatus. J Urol 99:585–587, 1968.
35. Elbadawi A, Schenk EA: Intra- and extraganglionic peripheral cholinergic neurons in urogenital organs of the cat. Z Zellforsch 103:26–33, 1970.
36. Elbadawi A, Schenk EA: A new theory of the innervation of urinary bladder musculature. II. The innervation apparatus of the ureterovesical junction. J Urol 105:368–371, 1971.
37. Elbadawi A, Schenk EA: A new theory of the innervation of urinary bladder musculature. III. Postganglionic synapses in ureterovesico-urethral autonomic pathways. J Urol 105:372–374, 1971.
38. deGroat WC, Saum WR: Sympathetic inhibition of the urinary bladder and of pelvic ganglionic transmission in the cat. J Physiol 220:297–314, 1972.
39. Elbadawi A, Schenk EA: Parasympathetic and sympathetic postganglionic synapses in ureterovesical autonomic pathways. Z Zellforsch 146:147–156, 1973.
40. Elbadawi A: Ultrastructure of vesicourethral innervation. II. Postganglionic axoaxonal synapses in intrinsic innervation of the vesicourethral lissosphincter: A new structural and functional concept in micturition. J Urol 131:781–790, 1984.
41. Elbadawi A. Ultrastructure of vesicourethral innervation. III. Axoaxonal synapses between postganglionic cholinergic axons and probably SIF-cell derived processes in the feline lissosphincter. J Urol 133:524–528, 1985.
42. Mattiasson A, Andersson K-E, Elbadawi A, et al: Interaction between adrenergic and cholinergic nerve terminals in the urinary bladder of rabbit, cat and man. J Urol 137:1017–1019, 1987.
43. Watanabe H, Yamamoto T: Autonomic innervation of the muscles in the wall of the bladder and proximal urethra of male rats. J Anat 128:873–886, 1979.
44. Elbadawi A, Atta MA: Ultrastructure of vesicourethral innervation. IV. Evidence for somatomotor plus autonomic innervation of the male feline rhabdosphincter. Neurourol Urodyn 4:23–26, 1985.
45. Kumagai A, Koyanagi T, Takahasi Y: The innervation of the external urethral sphincter. An ultrastructural study in male human subjects. Eur Res 15:39–43, 1987.
46. Morrison JFB: The functions of efferent nerves to the lower urinary tract. In Torrens M, Morrison JFB (eds): The Physiology of the Lower Urinary Tract. London, Springer-Verlag, 1987, pp 133–159.
47. deGroat WC, Kawatani M, Hisamitsu T, et al: Neural control of micturition: The role of neuropeptides. J Auton Nerv Syst Suppl:369–387, 1986.
48. Uemura E, Fletcher TF, Dirks VA, et al: Distribution of sacral afferent axons in cat urinary bladder. Am J Anat 136:305–314, 1973.
49. Uemura E, Fletcher TF, Bradley WE: Distribution of lumbar and sacral afferent axons in submucosa of cat urinary bladder. Anat Rec 183:579–588, 1975.
50. Dixon JS, Gilpin CJ: Presumptive sensory axons of the human urinary bladder: A fine structural study. J Anat 151:199–207, 1987.
51. Elbadawi A: Ultrastructure of vesicourethral innervation. I. Neuroeffector and cell junctions in the male internal sphincter. J Urol 128:180–188, 1982.
52. Elbadawi A, Yalla SV, Resnick NM: Structural basis of geriatric voiding dysfunction. II. Aging detrusor: Normal vs impaired contractility. J Urol 150:1657–1667, 1993.
53. Daniel EE, Cowan W, Daniel VP: Structural bases for neural and myogenic control of human detrusor muscle. Can J Physiol Pharmacol 61:1247–1272, 1983.
54. Gabella G: Structure of smooth muscles. In Bülbring E, Brading AF, Jones AW, Tomita T (eds): Smooth muscle: An assessment of current knowledge. Austin, University of Texas Press, 1981, pp 1–46.
55. Gabella G: General aspects of the fine structure of smooth muscles. In Motta PM (ed): Ultrastructure of Smooth Muscle. Boston, Kluwer Academic Publishers, 1990, pp 1–22.
56. Elbadawi A, Yalla SV, Resnick NM: Structural basis of geriatric voiding dysfunction. I. Methods of a prospective ultra-structural/urodynamic study, and an overview of the findings. J Urol 150:1650–1656, 1993.
57. Henderson RM: Cell-to-cell contacts. In Daniel EE, Paton DM (eds): Methods in Pharmacology, vol 3. New York, Plenum Press, 1975, pp 47–77.
58. Elbadawi A: Functional pathology of urinary bladder muscularis: The new frontier in diagnostic uropathology. Semin Diagn Pathol 10:314–354, 1993.
59. Elbadawi A, Meyer S: Morphometry of the obstructed detrusor: I. Review of the issues. Neurourol Urodyn 8:163–171, 1989.
60. Elbadawi A, Yalla SV, Resnick NM: Structural basis of geriatric voiding dysfunction. III. Detrusor overactivity. J Urol 150:1668–1680, 1993.
61. Brading AF: Physiology of bladder smooth muscle. In Torrens M, Morrison JFB (eds): The Physiology of the Lower Urinary Tract. London, Springer-Verlag, 1987, pp 161–191.
62. Dixon JS, Gosling JA: Ultrastructure of smooth muscle cells in the urinary system. In Motta PM (ed): Ultrastructure of Smooth Muscle. Boston, Kluwer Academic Publishers, 1990, pp 153–169.
63. Elbadawi A: Pathology and pathophysiology of the obstructed detrusor. In Jardin A (ed): Prostate and α-Blockers. Chester, Adis International, 1990, pp 1–25.
64. Inoué T: The three-dimensional ultrastructure of intracellular organization of smooth muscle cells by scanning electron microscopy. In Motta PM (ed): Ultrastructure of Smooth Muscle. Boston, Kluwer Academic Publishers, 1990, pp 63–77.
65. Grover AK: Calcium-handling studies using isolated smooth muscle membranes. In Grover AK, Daniel EE (eds): Calcium and Contractility: Smooth Muscle. Clifton, Humana Press, 1985, pp 245–269.
66. Kondo A, Susset JG, Lefaivre J: Viscoelastic properties of bladder. I. Mechanical model and its mathematical analysis. Invest Urol 10:154–163, 1972.

67. Regnier CH, Kolsky H, Richardson PD, et al: The elastic behavior of the urinary bladder for large deformations. J Biomech 16:915–922, 1983.

68. Susset JG, Regnier CH: Physiologie vésico-sphinctérienne. La phase de remplissage: Properties visco-elastiques de la vessie et de l'urèthre. *In* Buzelin JM, Richard F, Susset JG (eds): Physiologie et Pathologie de la Dynamique des Voies Urinaires (Haut et Bas Appareil). Paris, FIIS, 1987, pp 66–83.

69. Tomita T: Electrical properties of mammalian smooth muscle. *In* Bülbring E, Brading AF, Jones AW, Tomita T (eds): Smooth Muscle. Baltimore: Williams & Wilkins, 1970, pp 197–243.

70. Gosling JA, Dixon JS, Critchley HOD, Thompson S-A: A comparative study of the human external sphincter and periurethral levator ani muscles. Br J Urol 53:35–41, 1981.

71. Elbadawi A, Atta MA: Intrinsic neuromuscular defects in the neurogenic bladder. IV. Loss of somatomotor and preservation of autonomic innervation of the male feline rhabdosphincter following bilateral sacral ventral rhizotomy. Neurourol Urodyn 4:219–229, 1985.

72. Elbadawi A, Atta MA: Intrinsic neuromuscular defects in the neurogenic bladder. V. Autonomic re-innervation of the male feline rhabdosphincter following somatic denervation by bilateral sacral ventral rhizotomy. Neurourol Urodyn 5:65–85, 1986.

73. Atta MA, Elbadawi A: Intrinsic neuromuscular defects in the neurogenic bladder. VII. Neurohistochemistry of the somatically denervated male feline rhabdosphincter. Neurourol Urodyn 6:47–56, 1987.

74. Elbadawi A, Atta MA, Franck JI: Intrinsic neuromuscular defects in the neurogenic bladder. I. Short-term ultrastructural changes in muscular innervation of the decentralized feline bladder base following unilateral sacral ventral rhizotomy. Neurourol Urodyn 3:93–113, 1984.

75. Atta MA, Franck JI, Elbadawi A: Intrinsic neuromuscular defects in the neurogenic bladder. II. Long-term innervation of the unilaterally decentralized feline bladder base by regenerated cholinergic, increased adrenergic, and emergent probable "peptidergic" nerves. Neurourol Urodyn 3:185–200, 1984.

76. Elbadawi A, Atta MA: Intrinsic neuromuscular defects in the neurogenic bladder. III. Transjunctional, short- and long-term ultrastructural changes in muscle cells of the decentralized bladder base following unilateral sacral ventral rhizotomy. Neurourol Urodyn 3:245–270, 1984.

77. Elbadawi A, Atta MA, Hanno AG-E: Intrinsic neuromuscular defects in the neurogenic bladder. VIII. Effects of unilateral pelvic and pelvic plexus neurectomy on ultrastructure of the feline bladder base. Neurourol Urodyn 7:77–92, 1988.

78. Hanno AG-E, Atta MA, Elbadawi A: Intrinsic neuromuscular defects in the neurogenic bladder. IX. Effects of combined parasympathetic decentralization and hypogastric neurectomy on neuromuscular ultrastructure of the feline bladder base. Neurourol Urodyn 7:93–111, 1988.

79. Elbadawi A, Atta MA: Intrinsic neuromuscular defects in the neurogenic bladder. X. Value and limitations of neurohistochemistry. Neurourol Urodyn 8:263–276, 1989.

80. Elbadawi A, Atta MA: Intrinsic neuromuscular defects in the neurogenic bladder. VI. Myofiber ultrastructure in the somatically denervated male feline rhabdosphincter. Neurourol Urodyn 5:453–473, 1986.

81. Cowan WM: Antegrade and retrograde transneuronal degeneration in the central and peripheral nervous system. *In* Nauta WJH, Ebbesson SOE (eds): Contemporary Research Methods in Neuroanatomy. New York, Springer-Verlag, 1978, pp 217–251.

82. Sundin T, Dahlström A: The sympathetic innervation of the urinary bladder and urethra in the normal state and after parasympathetic denervation at the spinal root level. An experimental study in cats. Scand J Urol Nephrol 7:131–149, 1973.

83. Kawatani M, deGroat WC: The effect of partial denervation on the efferent pathways to the urinary bladder. Proceedings of the 6th Annual Symposium of the Urodynamics Society, 1984, p 35.

84. McGuire EJ, Yalla SV, Elbadawi A: Abnormalities of vesico-urethral dysfunction following radical pelvic extirpative surgery. *In* Yalla SV, McGuire EJ, Elbadawi A, Blaivas JG (eds): Neurourology and Urodynamics. Principles and Practice. New York, Macmillan, 1988, pp 331–337.

85. Neal DE, Bogue PR, Williams RE: Histological appearances of the nerves of the bladder in patients with denervation of the bladder after excision of the rectum. Br J Urol 54:658–666, 1982.

86. Elbadawi A, Miller LF, Liu JS, et al: Structural detrusor damage in a spinal dog neurostimulation model. Neurourol Urodyn 9:199–200, 1990.

87. Resnick NM: Voiding dysfunction in the elderly. *In* Yalla SV, McGuire EJ, Elbadawi A, Blaivas JG (eds): Neurourology and Urodynamics, Principles and Practice. New York, Macmillan, 1988, pp 303–330.

88. Resnick NM, Yalla SV, Laurino E: The pathophysiology of urinary incontinence among institutionalized elderly persons. N Engl J Med 320:1–7, 1989.

89. Elbadawi A, Yalla SV, Resnick NM: Structural basis of geriatric voiding dysfunction. IV. Bladder outlet obstruction. J Urol 150:1681–1695, 1993.

90. Resnick NM, Yalla, SV: Detrusor hyperactivity with impaired contractile function. An unrecognized but common cause of incontinence in elderly patients. JAMA 257:3076–3081, 1987.

91. Gu J, Restorick JM, Blank MA, et al: Vasoactive intestinal polypeptide in the normal and unstable bladder. Br J Urol 55:645–647, 1983.

92. Moore KH, Gilpin SA, Dixon JS, et al: Increase in presumptive sensory nerves of the urinary bladder in idiopathic detrusor instability. Br J Urol 70:370–372, 1992.

93. Meyer S, Elbadawi A: Morphometry of the obstructed detrusor. II. Principles of a comprehensive protocol. Neurourol Urodyn 8:173–191, 1989.

94. Kinder RB, Mundy AR: Pathophysiology of idiopathic detrusor instability and detrusor hyper-reflexia. An *in vitro* study of human detrusor muscle. Br J Urol 60:509–515, 1987.

95. Mundy AR: Detrusor instability. Br J Urol 62:393–397, 1988.

96. Van Poppel H, Stessens R, Baert L, et al: Vasoactive intestinal peptide innervation of human urinary bladder in normal and pathologic conditions. Urol Int 43:205–210, 1988.

97. McGuire EJ: Evaluation of urinary incontinence. *In* Yalla SV, McGuire EJ, Elbadawi A, Blaivas JG (eds): Neurourology and Urodynamics. Principles and Practice. New York, Macmillan, 1988, pp 211–220.

98. Magasi P, Csontai A, Ruszinkó B: Beiträge zur Blasenwanddegeneration. Z Urol Nephrol 62:209–216, 1969.

99. Brent L, Stephens FD: The response of smooth muscle cells in the rabbit urinary bladder to outflow obstruction. Invest Urol 12:494–502, 1975.

100. Ghoniem GM, Regnier CH, Biancani P, et al: The effect of vesical outlet obstruction on detrusor contractility and passive properties in rabbits. J Urol 135:1284–1289, 1986.

101. Clermont A: Etude Ultrastructurale du Muscle Vésical chez l'Homme. Thèse, Docteur de Médecin, Nice, France, 1978, pp 1–88.

102. Cortivo R, Pagano F, Passerini G, et al: Elastin and collagen in the normal and obstructed bladder. Br J Urol 53:134–137, 1981.

103. Gilpin SA, Gosling JA, Barnard RJ: Morphological and morphometric studies of the human obstructed, trabeculated urinary bladder. Br J Urol 57:525–529, 1985.

104. Gosling JA, Dixon JS: Structure of the trabeculated detrusor smooth muscle in cases of prostatic hypertrophy. Urol Int 35:351–354, 1980.

105. Gosling JA, Dixon JS: Detrusor morphology in relation to bladder outflow obstruction and instability. *In* Hinman F Jr (ed): Benign prostatic hypertrophy. New York, Springer-Verlag, 1983, pp 666–671.

106. Mayo ME, Lloyd-Davies RW, Shuttleworth KED, Tighe JR: The damaged human detrusor: Functional and electron microscopic changes in disease. Br J Urol 45:116–125, 1973.

107. Gosling JA, Gilpin SA, Dixon JS, Gilpin CJ: Decrease in autonomic innervation of the human detrusor muscle in outflow obstruction. J Urol 136:501–505, 1986.

108. Dixon JS, Gilpin CJ, Gilpin SA, et al: Sequential morphological changes in the pig detrusor in response to chronic partial urethral obstruction. Br J Urol 64:385–390, 1989.
109. Cumming JA, Chisholm GD: Changes in detrusor innervation with relief of outflow tract obstruction. Br J Urol 69:7–11, 1992.
110. Chapple CR, Milner P, Moss HE, Burnstock G: Loss of sensory neuropeptides in the obstructed human bladder. Br J Urol 70:373–381, 1992.
111. Williams JH, Turner WH, Sainsbury GM, Brading AF: Experimental model of bladder outflow tract obstruction in the guinea-pig. Br J Urol 71:543–554, 1993.
112. Mayo ME, Hinman F: Structure and function of the rabbit bladder altered by chronic obstruction or cystitis. Invest Urol 14:6–9, 1976.
113. Elbadawi A, Meyer S, Malkowicz SB, et al: Effects of short-term partial outlet obstruction on the rabbit detrusor: An ultrastructural study. Neurourol Urodyn 8:89–116, 1989.
114. Meyer S, Atta MA, Wein AJ, et al: Morphometric analysis of muscle cell changes in the short-term partially obstructed rabbit detrusor. Neurourol Urodyn 8:117–131, 1989.
115. Meyer S, Levin RM, Ruggieri MR, et al: Quantitative analysis of intercellular changes in the short-term partially obstructed rabbit detrusor. Neurourol Urodyn 8:133–140, 1989.
116. Meyer S, Hassouna M, Mokhless I, et al: Ultrastructural changes in the obstructed pig detrusor: A preliminary report. Neurourol Urodyn 8:141–150, 1989.
117. Gabella G: Hypertrophy of intestinal smooth muscle. Cell Tis Res 163:199–214, 1975.
118. Gabella G: Hypertrophic smooth muscle. I. Size and shape of cells, occurrence of mitoses. Cell Tis Res 201:63–78, 1979.
119. Jaske G, Hoffstäder F: Changes in the bladder wall muscle associated with benign prostatic enlargement. Urol Res 5:149–152, 1977.
120. Hoekstra JW, Griffiths DJ, Tauecchio EA, Shroeder T-KF: Effects of long-term catheter implantation on the contractile and histological properties of the canine bladder. J Urol 133:709–712, 1985.
121. Uvelius B, Persson L, Mattiasson A: Smooth muscle cell hypertrophy and hyperplasia in the rat detrusor after short-term infravesical outflow obstruction. J Urol 131:173–176, 1984.
122. Gabella G: Hypertrophic smooth muscle. III. Increase in number and size of gap junctions. Cell Tis Res 201:263–276, 1979.
123. Leriche A: Mécanisme des symptômes fonctionnels de l'hypertrophie bénigne de la prostate. Physiopathologie et symptômes. In Prostate et Alpha-bloquants. Amsterdam, Excerpta Medica, 1989, pp 76–98.
124. Coolsaet B, Elbadawi A: Urodynamics in the management of benign prostatic hypertrophy. World J Urol 6:215–224, 1989.
125. McGuire EJ: Detrusor responses to obstruction. In Rodgers C, Coffey DS, Cuhna G, et al (eds): Benign Prostatic Hypertrophy, II. Bethesda, NIH Publication No 87-2881, 1987, pp 211–220.
126. Susset JG: Effects of aging and prostatic obstruction on detrusor morphology and function. In Hinman F Jr (ed): Benign Prostatic Hypertrophy. New York, Springer-Verlag, 1983, pp 653–665.
127. Susset JG: Effet de l'hypertrophie prostatique bénigne sur la contractilité vésicale. In Prostate et Alpha-bloquants. Amsterdam, Excerpta Medica, 1989, pp 49–72.
128. Lloyd-Davies RW, Hinman F Jr: Structural and functional changes leading to impaired bacterial elimination after overdistension of the rabbit bladder. Invest Urol 9:136–142, 1971.
129. Speakman MJ, Brading AF, Gilpin CJ, et al: Bladder outflow obstruction—a cause of denervation supersensitivity. J Urol 138:1461–1466, 1987.
130. Elbadawi A, Meyer S, Regnier CH: The role of ischemia in structural changes in the rabbit detrusor following partial bladder outlet obstruction. A working hypothesis and a biomechanical/structural model proposal. Neurourol Urodyn 8:151–162, 1989.
131. Susset JG, Servot-Viguier D, Lamy F, et al: Collagen in 155 human bladders. Invest Urol 16:204–206, 1978.
132. Gilpin SA, Gilpin CJ, Dixon JS, et al: The effect of age on the autonomic innervation of the urinary bladder. Br J Urol 58:378–381, 1986.

CHAPTER 3

Neuroanatomy and Neurophysiology: Innervation of the Lower Urinary Tract

William C. de Groat, Ph.D.

The storage and periodic elimination of urine depend on the coordinated activity of two functional units in the lower urinary tract: (1) a reservoir (the urinary bladder) and (2) an outlet consisting of the bladder neck, the urethra, and the urethral sphincter. Coordination between these organs is mediated by a complex neural control system located in the brain, spinal cord, and peripheral ganglia. Thus, urine storage and release are highly dependent on central nervous system pathways. This distinguishes the lower urinary tract from many other visceral structures (e.g., the gastrointestinal tract and cardiovascular system) that maintain a certain level of function even after extrinsic neural input has been eliminated.

The lower urinary tract is also unusual in its pattern of activity and organization of neural control mechanisms. For example, the urinary bladder has only two modes of operation: storage and elimination. Thus, many of the neural circuits have switchlike or phasic patterns of activity, unlike the tonic patterns characteristic of the autonomic pathways to cardiovascular organs. In addition, micturition is under voluntary control and depends on learned behavior that develops during maturation of the nervous system, whereas many other visceral functions are regulated involuntarily. Micturition also requires the integration of autonomic and somatic efferent mechanisms to coordinate the activity of visceral organs (the bladder and urethra) with that of urethral striated muscles.

Due to the complexity of the neural mechanisms regulating the lower urinary tract, micturition is sensitive to a wide variety of injuries, diseases, and chemicals that affect the nervous system. Thus, neurologic mechanisms are an important consideration in the diagnosis and treatment of voiding disorders. This chapter reviews (1) the innervation of the urinary bladder and urethra, (2) the organization of the reflex pathways controlling urine storage and elimination, (3) the neurotransmitters involved in micturition reflex pathways, and (4) neurogenic dysfunctions of the lower urinary tract.

Innervation

The innervation of the lower urinary tract is derived from three sets of peripheral nerves: sacral parasympathetic (pelvic nerves), thoracolumbar sympathetic (hypogastric nerves and sympathetic chain), and sacral somatic nerves (primarily the pudendal nerves) (Fig. 3–1).[1–6]

SACRAL PARASYMPATHETIC PATHWAYS

The sacral parasympathetic nerves, which in humans originate from the S2 to S4 segments of the spinal cord, provide the major excitatory input to the bladder. Cholinergic preganglionic neurons located in the intermediolateral region of the sacral spinal cord send axons to ganglionic cells in the pelvic plexus and the bladder wall (see Fig. 3–1). Transmission in bladder ganglia is mediated by a nicotinic cholinergic mechanism. In some species (cats and rabbits) ganglionic synapses act like gating circuits, exhibiting marked facilitation during repetitive preganglionic activity and modulation by various transmitter systems, including muscarinic, adrenergic, purinergic, and enkephalinergic systems (Table 3–1).[7, 8] Thus, the ganglia appear to have an important role in regulating neural input to the bladder. Whether bladder ganglia in humans have similar properties is not known. Ganglion cells in turn excite the bladder smooth muscle. Histochemical studies have shown that a large proportion of ganglion cells contain acetylcholinesterase (AChE) and therefore are presum-

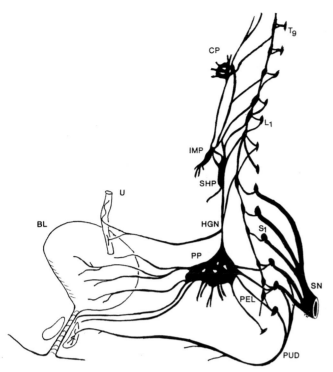

Figure 3-1 Diagram showing the innervation of the female lower urinary tract. BL, urinary bladder; CP, celiac plexus; HGN, hypogastric nerve; IMP, inferior mesenteric plexus; L_1, first lumbar root; PEL, pelvic nerves; PP, pelvic plexus; PUD, pudendal nerve; S_1, first sacral root; SN, sciatic nerve; SHP, superior hypogastric plexus; T_9, ninth thoracic root; U, ureter. (Modified from de Groat WC, Booth AM: Autonomic systems to bladder and sex organs. *In* Dyck PJ, Thomas PK, Griffin JW, et al [eds]: Peripheral Neuropathy, 3rd ed. Philadelphia, WB Saunders, 1993, p 198.)

tagonizes the contraction elicited by stimulation of the pelvic nerves. Thus, other substances that stimulate bladder smooth muscle, such as adenosine triphosphate (ATP) (see Table 3–1) have been considered possible cotransmitters in the parasympathetic excitatory pathway.[6] In animals, ATP is released by electrical stimulation of vesical nerves, and ATP antagonists depress bladder contractions elicited by nerve stimulation. Exogenous ATP also has an excitatory effect on human bladder smooth muscle; however, the ATP-mediated component of excitatory transmission is not prominent, suggesting that this type of transmission is less important in humans.[9]

SACRAL SOMATIC PATHWAYS

Somatic efferent pathways to the external urethral sphincter are carried in the pudendal nerve from anterior horn cells in the third and fourth sacral segments. Branches of the pudendal nerve and other sacral somatic nerves also carry efferent impulses to muscles of the pelvic floor.

THORACOLUMBAR SYMPATHETIC PATHWAYS

Sympathetic preganglionic pathways that arise from the T11 to L2 spinal segments pass to the sympathetic chain ganglia and then to prevertebral ganglia in the superior hypogastric and pelvic plexus and also to short adrenergic neurons in the bladder and urethra. Sympathetic postganglionic nerves that release norepinephrine provide an excitatory input to smooth muscle of the urethra and bladder base, an inhibitory input to smooth muscle in the body of the bladder, and inhibitory and facilitory input to vesical parasympathetic ganglia.[1, 7, 10] The adrenergic receptors mediating these responses are listed in Table 3–1.

ably cholinergic. AChE-positive nerves are abundant in all parts of the bladder but are less extensive in the urethra. Exogenous acetylcholine produces a contraction of bladder smooth muscle, which is blocked by atropine and is therefore considered to be mediated by muscarinic receptors (see Table 3–1). However, in many species atropine only partially an-

TABLE 3–1
Receptors for Putative Transmitters in the Lower Urinary Tract

Tissue	Cholinergic	Adrenergic	Other
Bladder body	+ (M_2) + (M_3)	− (β_2)	+ Adenosine triphosphate (P_2) − Vasoactive intestinal peptide + Substance P
Cholinergic nerve terminals	− (M_2) + (M_1)	+ (α_1)	− Neuropeptide Y
Bladder base	+ (M_2)	+ (α_1)	− Vasoactive intestinal peptide
Ganglia	+ (N) + (M_1)	+ (α_1) − (α_2) + (β)	− Enkephalinergic (δ) − Purinergic (P_1) + Substance P
Urethra	+ (M)	+ (α_1) + (α_2) − (β_2)	+ Purinergic (P_2) − Vasoactive intestinal peptide − Nitric oxide
Adrenergic nerve terminals	− (M_2)	− (α_2)	− Neuropeptide Y
Sphincter striated muscle	+ (N)		

Letters in parentheses indicate receptor type, e.g., M (muscarinic) and N (nicotinic). Plus and minus signs indicate excitatory and inhibitory effects.

NEURAL MODULATION

Postganglionic nerve terminals are sites of "cross-talk" between sympathetic and parasympathetic nerves and also possible sites of gating mechanisms. For example, in the rat lower urinary tract, activation of M-2 (muscarinic) cholinergic receptors on nerve terminals suppresses acetylcholine and norepinephrine release, whereas activation of M-1 cholinergic receptors or alpha-1-adrenergic receptors enhances acetylcholine release.[11–13]

Other putative transmitters, including neuropeptide Y (NPY), vasoactive intestinal polypeptide (VIP), and nitric oxide, have also been identified in efferent pathways to the lower urinary tract of animals and humans (see Table 3–1).[6, 7, 14, 15] NPY is present in adrenergic and cholinergic neurons[15] and when administered exogenously acts prejunctionally to suppress the release of norepinephrine and acetylcholine from postganglionic nerve terminals.[16] Nitric oxide and VIP have smooth muscle relaxant effects. Nitric oxide has been implicated in neurally mediated relaxation of the proximal urethra,[14] whereas VIP that is released with acetylcholine may function as an inhibitory transmitter in the bladder. Thus, efferent control of the bladder and urethra is potentially complex and involves multiple transmitters and multiple synaptic gating mechanisms in ganglia as well as at postganglionic nerve terminals.

LUMBOSACRAL AFFERENT PATHWAYS

Afferent activity arising in the bladder is transmitted to the central nervous system by both sets of autonomic nerves.[1, 17] The afferent nerves most important for initiating micturition are those passing in the pelvic nerve to the sacral spinal cord. These afferents consist of small myelinated (A-delta) and unmyelinated (C) fibers that convey impulses from tension receptors and nociceptors in the bladder wall.[2, 18–20] Electrophysiologic studies in the cat have shown that A-delta bladder afferents respond in a graded manner to passive distention as well as active contraction of the bladder.[20, 21] The intravesical pressure threshold for activation of these afferents ranges from 5 to 15 mmHg, which is consistent with pressures at which humans report the first sensation of bladder filling during cystometry. A-delta afferents in the cat show a linear increase in firing with increasing intravesical pressures that extend into the noxious range, suggesting that nociceptive stimuli in the bladder may be encoded in part by high rates of firing in polymodal afferents, which also transmit non-noxious information.

High-threshold C-fiber afferents have also been detected in the cat bladder. Under normal conditions the large majority of these afferents do not respond to bladder distention and therefore have been termed silent C fibers, but many can be activated by chemical irritation of the bladder mucosa[18–20] or cold temperatures.[22] Following chemical irritation, C-fiber afferents exhibit spontaneous firing with the bladder empty and increased firing during bladder distention.[17–20] Activation of C-fiber afferents by chemical irritation facilitates the micturition reflex and decreases bladder capacity.[1, 23, 24] Administration of capsaicin, a neurotoxin that desensitizes C-fiber afferents, blocks this facilitation but does not block micturition reflexes in normal animals, indicating that C-fiber afferent pathways are not essential for normal voiding.[1, 25]

Mechanoreceptor afferents from the bladder and urethra have also been identified in sympathetic nerves passing to the lumbar spinal cord. These afferent pathways consist of myelinated as well as unmyelinated axons that respond to similar stimulus modalities as afferents in the pelvic nerve.[2, 21] The function of sympathetic nerve afferents in the control of micturition is uncertain; however, based on clinical observations it is clear that in humans they carry nociceptive information from the lower urinary tract.

Afferent pathways from the urethra, which induce the sensations of temperature, pain, and passage of urine, travel in the pudendal nerve to the lumbosacral spinal cord. Afferents from the female sex organs, including the clitoris, vagina, and part of the innervation of the uterine cervix, also travel in the pudendal nerve.[26] These afferents, as well as pudendal nerve afferents from the striated sphincter muscles, are known to have a modulating influence on micturition.

Immunohistochemical studies have shown that a large percentage of bladder afferent neurons contain peptides: calcitonin gene–related peptide (CGRP), VIP, substance P, enkephalins, and cholecystokinin (CCK).[6, 17, 27, 28] In the spinal cord, peptidergic afferent terminals have a distribution that is very similar to that of bladder afferents. In the bladder, these peptides are also common in nerves in the submucosal and subepithelial layers and around blood vessels. The neurotoxin capsaicin, when applied locally to the bladder in experimental animals, releases peptides from peripheral afferent terminals and produces inflammatory responses, including plasma extravasation and vasodilatation.[25] Afferent peptides can also modulate the release of acetylcholine from postganglionic nerves. These findings suggest that the neuropeptides may be important neurotransmitters in afferent pathways in the lower urinary tract.

Anatomy of Spinal Pathways

EFFERENT NEURONS

Preganglionic neurons in the lumbosacral parasympathetic nucleus have been identified in the intermediolateral region of the spinal cord in various species.[1] In the cat the sacral parasympathetic nucleus is divided into two groups of cells; a dorsal band and a lateral band. Neurons innervating the urinary bladder are located in the lateral band.[1] These neu-

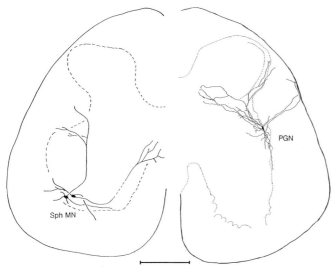

Figure 3–2 Comparison of the dendritic distributions of external urethral sphincter motoneurons (Sph MN) *(left)* and a sacral parasympathetic preganglionic neuron (PGN) *(right)* in the cat. The sacral preganglionic neuron, which was filled intracellularly with neurobiotin, has dendrites that extend into the lateral funiculus, the lateral lamina I, the dorsal commissure, and the sacral autonomic nucleus. Dendrites were reconstructed from serial sections extending 500 μm rostral and caudal to the cell body. Two sphincter motoneurons *(left)* were labeled by retrograde axonal transport following injections of cholera toxin–horseradish peroxidase (HRP) into the external urethral sphincter. Although the dendritic distributions are incomplete, they show prominent dendritic projections of one cell to lamina X around the central canal and projections of another cell to the intermediolateral region. Right and left sides are at slightly different rostrocaudal levels. Calibration represents 500 μm.

rons send dendrites to discrete regions of the spinal cord including (1) the lateral and dorsal lateral funiculus, (2) lamina I on the lateral edge of the dorsal horn, (3) the dorsal gray commissure, and (4) the gray matter and lateral funiculus ventral to the autonomic nucleus (Fig. 3–2).[29] It has been suggested that the dendrites in the lateral funiculus receive inputs from descending pathways from the brain, whereas the other dendrites receive segmental inputs from interneurons or primary afferents. Lumbar sympathetic preganglionic neurons and motor neurons innervating the external urethral sphincter have similar dendritic distributions.

AFFERENT PROJECTIONS

Afferent pathways from the lower urinary tract project to discrete regions of the dorsal horn that contain the soma or dendrites of efferent neurons innervating the lower urinary tract. Pelvic nerve afferent pathways from the urinary bladder of the cat[1, 17] and the rat[30] project into Lissauer's tract at the apex of the dorsal horn and then pass rostrocaudally, giving off collaterals that extend laterally and medially through the superficial layer of the dorsal horn (lamina I) into the deeper layers (laminae V to VII and X) at the base of the dorsal horn (Figs. 3–3 and 3–4). The lateral pathway, which is the most prominent projection, terminates in the region of the sacral parasympathetic nucleus and also sends some axons to the dorsal commissure (see Figs. 3–3 and 3–4).

Pudendal nerve afferent pathways from the external urethral sphincter of the cat have central terminations that overlap in part with those of bladder afferents in lateral laminae I, V to VII, and X.[31, 32] Afferents from the female sexual organs also terminate in these areas. For example, uterine cervix afferents in the cat project primarily to lateral lamina I,[26, 33] whereas clitoral afferents terminate primarily in lamina X and the dorsal commissure.[34] These afferents differ markedly from cutaneous pudendal nerve afferents, which terminate in the middle layers of the dorsal horn (laminae II to IV; see Fig. 3–3B). The overlap of the central projections of bladder afferents and the afferents in the pudendal nerve to the sex organs, urethra, and skin is of interest because

Figure 3–3 The central projection in the sacral spinal cord of visceral afferents in the pelvic nerve *(A)* and somatic afferents in the pudendal nerve *(B)* of the monkey. Afferents were labeled by the transganglionic transport of HRP. Bar = 400 μm. MP, medial pathway; LP, lateral pathway. (From Roppolo JR, Nadelhaft I, de Groat WC: The organization of pudendal motoneurons and primary afferent projections in the spinal cord of the rhesus monkey revealed by horseradish peroxidase. J Comp Neurol 234:475, 1985. Reprinted by permission of John Wiley & Sons, Inc.)

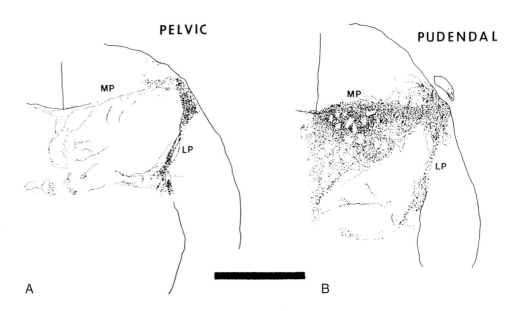

PELVIC

PUDENDAL

A

B

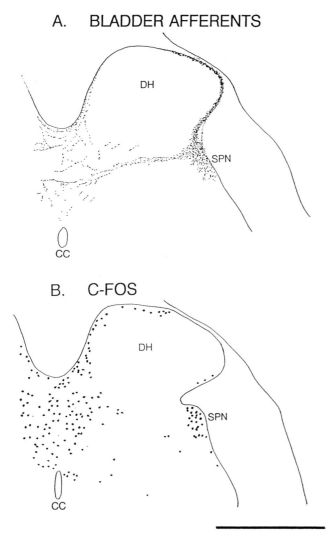

A.   BLADDER AFFERENTS

DH

SPN

CC

B.   C-FOS

DH

SPN

CC

Figure 3–4 Comparison of the distribution of bladder afferent projections to the L₆ spinal cord of the rat *(A)* with the distribution of *c-fos* positive cells in the L₆ spinal segment following chemical irritation of the lower urinary tract of the rat *(B)*. Afferents were labeled by wheat germ agglutinin–horseradish peroxidase injected into the urinary bladder. *C-fos* immunoreactivity is present in the nuclei of cells. DH, dorsal horn; SPN, sacral parasympathetic nucleus; CC, central canal. Calibration represents 500 μm.

activation of the latter afferents can markedly influence bladder function.[1]

SPINAL INTERNEURONS

The spinal neurons involved in processing[1, 35, 36] afferent input from the lower urinary tract and the sex organs have been identified by physiologic and anatomic tracing techniques. Interneurons that fire in response to bladder distention or mechanical stimulation of the vagina or uterine cervix have been detected in lateral intermediate gray matter near the sacral parasympathetic nucleus and in the region of the dorsal commissure (lamina X).[35] Commonly, stimulation of sex organ afferents inhibits neurons activated by bladder distention, which is consistent

with the inhibitory effect of these afferents on bladder reflexes.[36]

Spinal interneurons have also been identified by the expression of the immediate early gene *c-fos* (see Fig. 3–4B)[24, 37–39] and by transneuronal transport of pseudorabies virus from the bladder.[40–42] The protein product of the *c-fos* gene can be detected immunocytochemically in the nuclei of neurons within 30 to 60 minutes after synaptic activation. In the rat, noxious or non-noxious stimulation of the bladder and urethra as well as electrical stimulation of the pelvic or pudendal nerves increased the levels of *c-fos* protein, primarily in the dorsal commissure and in the area of the sacral parasympathetic nucleus, the major sites of termination of afferents from the lower urinary tract (see Fig. 3–4A).[24, 37–39] Neurons in these same regions were labeled by the pseudorabies virus, which passes transsynaptically in a sequential manner from postganglionic to preganglionic efferent neurons and then to segmental interneurons and eventually to neurons in the brain (Fig. 3–5) (see later discussion). Interneurons in the dorsal commissure region also project to the sphincter motor nucleus.[1, 43] These results indicate that interneurons in restricted regions of the intermediate gray matter and dorsal commissure play a major role in coordinating the different aspects of lower urinary tract function.

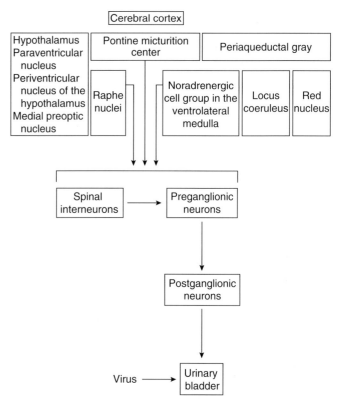

Figure 3–5 Structures in the brain and spinal cord of the adult and neonatal rat labeled after injection of pseudorabies virus into the urinary bladder. Virus is transported transneuronally in a retrograde direction. Based on studies of Nadelhaft et al,[41] Roppolo et al,[40] and de Groat et al.[42]

MICTURITION REFLEX

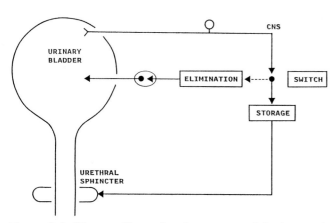

Figure 3-6 Diagram illustrating the anatomy of the lower urinary tract and the switchlike function of the micturition reflex pathway. During urine storage a low level of afferent activity activates efferent input to the urethral sphincter. A high level of afferent activity induced by bladder distention activates the switching circuit in the central nervous system (CNS), producing firing in the efferent pathways to the bladder, inhibition of the efferent outflow to the sphincter, and urine elimination.

Reflex Mechanisms Controlling the Lower Urinary Tract

The central pathways controlling lower urinary tract function are organized as simple on-off switching circuits (Fig. 3–6) that maintain a reciprocal relationship between the urinary bladder and the urethral outlet. The principal reflex components of these switching circuits are listed in Table 3–2 and are illustrated in Figure 3–7. Intravesical pressure measurements during bladder filling in both humans and animals reveal that bladder pressure is maintained at a low and relatively constant level when bladder volume is below the threshold for inducing voiding (see Fig. 3–7A). Accommodation of the bladder to increasing volumes of urine is primarily a passive phenomenon that depends on the intrinsic properties of the vesical smooth muscle and the quiescence of the parasympathetic efferent pathway.[1–5, 44–45] In addition, in some species urine storage is also facilitated by sympathetic reflexes that mediate inhibition of bladder activity and closure of the urethral outlet (see Table 3–2 and Fig. 3–8). During bladder filling the activity of the sphincter electromyogram (EMG) also increases (see Fig. 3–7B), reflecting an increase in efferent firing in the pudendal nerve and an increase in outlet resistance that contributes to the maintenance of urinary continence.

The storage phase of the urinary bladder can be switched to the voiding phase either involuntarily (by reflex) or voluntarily (see Fig. 3–7B). The former is readily demonstrated in the human infant (see Fig. 3–7A) and in the anesthetized animal when the volume of urine exceeds the micturition threshold. At this point, increased afferent firing from tension receptors in the bladder reverses the pattern of efferent outflow, producing firing in the sacral parasympathetic pathways and inhibition of sympathetic and somatic pathways. The expulsion phase consists of an initial relaxation of the urethral sphincter (see Fig. 3–7A) followed in a few seconds by a contraction of the bladder, an increase in bladder pressure, and flow of urine. Secondary reflexes elicited by the flow of urine through the urethra facilitate bladder emptying.[2, 4]

These reflexes require the integrated action of neuronal populations at various levels of the neuraxis (Figs. 3–8 and 3–9). Certain reflexes, for example, those mediating the excitatory input to the sphincters and the sympathetic inhibitory input to the bladder, are organized at the spinal level (see Fig. 3–8), whereas the parasympathetic transmission to the de-

TABLE 3–2
Reflexes to the Lower Urinary Tract

Afferent Pathway	Efferent Pathway	Central Pathway
Urine storage, low-level vesical afferent activity (pelvic nerve)	1. External sphincter contraction (somatic nerves) 2. Internal sphincter contraction (sympathetic nerves) 3. Detrusor inhibition (sympathetic nerves) 4. Ganglionic inhibition (sympathetic nerves) 5. Sacral parasympathetic outflow inactive	Spinal reflexes
Micturition, high-level vesical activity (pelvic nerve)	1. Inhibition of external sphincter activity 2. Inhibition of sympathetic outflow 3. Activation of parasympathetic outflow	Spinobulbospinal reflexes

From de Groat WC, Booth AM: Autonomic systems to the urinary bladder and sexual organs. *In* Dyck PJ, Thomas PK, Griffin JW, et al (eds): Peripheral Neuropathy, 3rd ed, vol 1. Philadelphia, W. B. Saunders, 1993, p 202.

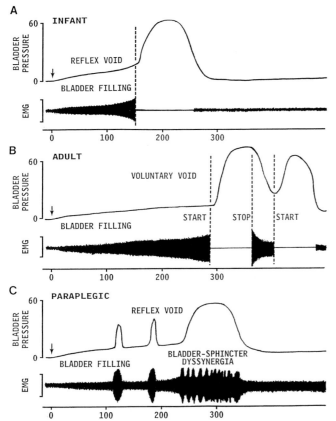

Figure 3-7 Combined cystometrograms and sphincter electromyograms (EMG) comparing reflex voiding responses in an infant *(A)* and a paraplegic patient *(C)* with a voluntary voiding response in an adult *(B)*. The abscissa in all records represents bladder volume in milliliters, and the ordinates represent bladder pressure in centimeters of water and electrical activity of the EMG recording. On the left side of each trace the arrows indicate the start of a slow infusion of fluid into the bladder (bladder filling). Vertical dashed lines indicate the start of sphincter relaxation, which precedes by a few seconds the bladder contraction in *A* and *B*. In *B* note that a voluntary cessation of voiding (stop) is associated with an initial increase in sphincter EMG followed by a reciprocal relaxation of the bladder. Resumption of voiding is again associated with sphincter relaxation and a delayed increase in bladder pressure. On the other hand, in the paraplegic patient *(C)* the reciprocal relationship between bladder and sphincter is abolished. During bladder filling, transient uninhibited bladder contractions occur in association with sphincter activity. Further filling leads to more prolonged and simultaneous contractions of the bladder and sphincter (bladder-sphincter dyssynergia). Loss of the reciprocal relationship between bladder and sphincter in paraplegic patients interferes with bladder emptying. (From de Groat WC, Steers WD: Autonomic regulation of the urinary bladder and sex organs. *In* Loewy AD, Spyer KM [eds]: Central Regulation of Autonomic Functions. Oxford, Oxford University Press, 1990, p 310.)

trusor has a more complicated central organization involving spinal and spinobulbospinal pathways (see Fig. 3–9).

STORAGE REFLEXES

SYMPATHETIC PATHWAYS   Studies in animals indicate that sympathetic input to the lower urinary tract is tonically active during bladder filling.[1] Surgical or

pharmacologic blockade of the sympathetic pathways can reduce urethral resistance, bladder capacity, and bladder wall compliance and increase the frequency and amplitude of bladder contractions.[1]

Sympathetic firing is initiated at least in part by a sacrolumbar intersegmental spinal reflex pathway triggered by vesical afferent activity in the pelvic nerves[1, 46] (see Fig. 3–8). This vesicosympathetic reflex represents a negative feedback mechanism whereby an increase in bladder pressure triggers an increase in inhibitory input to the bladder, thus allowing the bladder to accommodate larger volumes of urine. The reflex pathway is inhibited during mic-

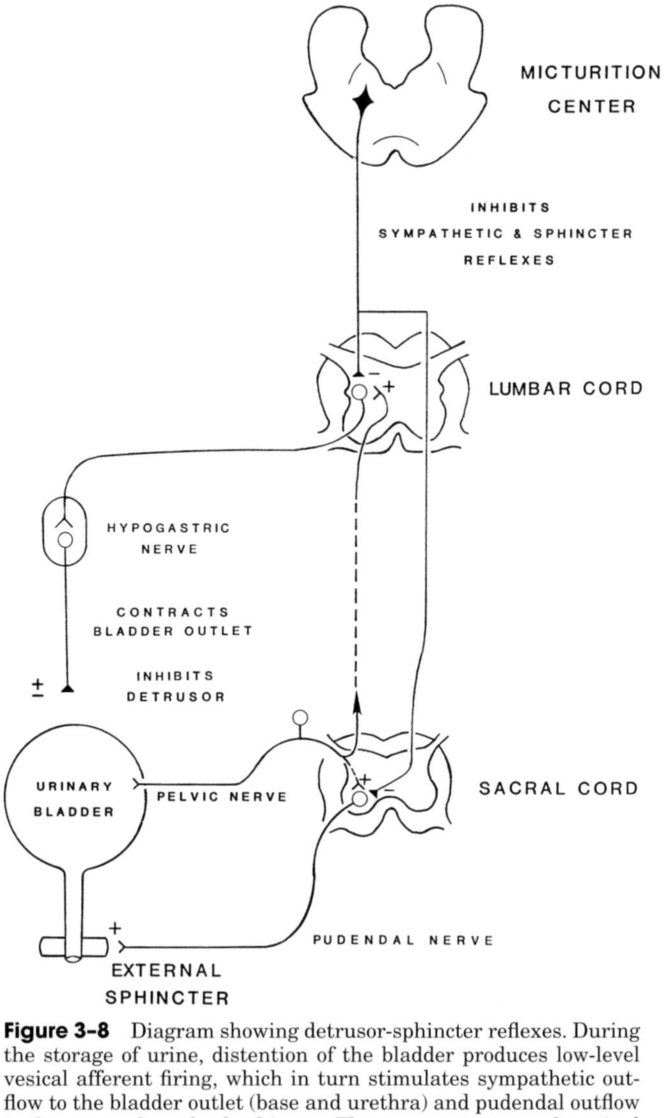

Figure 3-8 Diagram showing detrusor-sphincter reflexes. During the storage of urine, distention of the bladder produces low-level vesical afferent firing, which in turn stimulates sympathetic outflow to the bladder outlet (base and urethra) and pudendal outflow to the external urethral sphincter. These responses occur by spinal reflex pathways and represent "guarding reflexes," which promote continence. Sympathetic firing also inhibits detrusor muscle and transmission in bladder ganglia. At initiation of micturition, intense vesical afferent activity activates the brain stem micturition center, which inhibits the spinal guarding reflexes. (From de Groat WC, Booth AM: Autonomic systems to bladder and sex organs. *In* Dyck PJ, Thomas PK, Griffin JW, et al [eds]: Peripheral Neuropathy, 3rd ed. Philadelphia, WB Saunders, 1993, p 198.)

MICTURITION REFLEX PATHWAYS

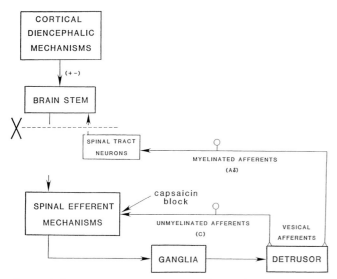

Figure 3-9 Diagram of the central reflex pathways regulating micturition in the cat. In an animal with an intact neuraxis, micturition is initiated by a supraspinal reflex pathway passing through a center in the brain stem. The pathway is triggered by myelinated afferents (Aδ) connected to tension receptors in the bladder wall. In animals with spinal injury connections between the brain stem and the sacral spinal cord are interrupted (X), and micturition is initially blocked. However, in animals with chronic spinal injury a spinal reflex mechanism emerges that is triggered by unmyelinated (C-fiber) vesical afferents. The C-fiber reflex pathway is usually weak or undetectable in animals with an intact nervous system. Capsaicin (20 to 30 mg/kg, subcutaneous) blocks the C-fiber reflex in cats with chronic spinal injury but does not block micturition reflexes in intact cats. (From de Groat WC, Kawatani M, Hisamitsu T, et al: Mechanisms underlying the recovery of urinary bladder function following spinal cord injury. J Auton Nerv Syst 30 (Suppl), S71, 1990.)

turition, and the inhibition in turn is abolished by transection of the spinal cord at the thoracic level, indicating that it originates at a supraspinal site, possibly the pontine micturition center (see Fig. 3–8).[46]

SOMATIC EFFERENT PATHWAYS TO THE URETHRAL SPHINCTER Reflex control of the striated urethral sphincter is similar to control of sympathetic pathways to the lower urinary tract (see Fig. 3–8). During bladder filling pudendal motor neurons are activated by vesical afferent input, whereas during micturition motor neurons are reciprocally inhibited. Inhibition depends in part on supraspinal mechanisms because in animals with chronic spinal lesions and paraplegic patients it is weak or absent. In paraplegics the uninhibited spinal vesicosphincter excitatory reflex pathway commonly initiates a striated sphincter contraction in concert with a contraction of the bladder (bladder-sphincter dyssynergia) (see Fig. 3–7C). This reflex interferes with bladder emptying.[2, 5]

Supraspinal control of sphincter motor neurons has been studied with electrophysiological techniques in animals. Electrical stimulation of the lateral funiculus of the spinal cord or stimulation of various areas of the brain evokes excitatory post-synaptic potentials and firing in sphincter motor neurons and an increase in the sphincter EMG in the cat.[47, 48] Stimulation of the lateral pontine reticular formation, an area that has been designated the "urine storage center," elicits an increase in sphincter EMG and also inhibits bladder activity.[1, 2, 49–53] Stimulation of dorsal medial pontine sites (the pontine micturition center) excites the bladder and inhibits sphincter EMG at latencies of 40 to 50 msec.[49, 51, 53] These findings indicate that the spinal reflex pathways that mediate urine storage are strongly modulated by descending input from the brain.

VOIDING REFLEXES

SPINOBULBOSPINAL MICTURITION REFLEX PATHWAY Micturition is mediated by activation of the sacral parasympathetic efferent pathway to the bladder and reciprocal inhibition of the somatic pathway to the urethral sphincter (see Table 3–1 and Fig. 3–7B). Studies in animals using brain lesioning techniques have revealed that neurons in the brain stem at the level of the inferior colliculus play an essential role in the control of the parasympathetic component of micturition (see Figs. 3–9 and 3–10). Removal of areas of the brain above the inferior colliculus by intercollicular

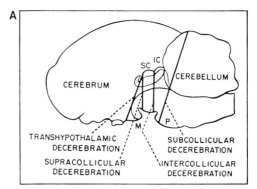

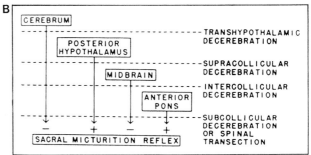

Figure 3-10 A, Sagittal section of the cat brain showing various levels of brain transections made in the study of the supraspinal control of micturition. SC, IC, superior and inferior colliculi, respectively; M, midbrain; P, pons. B, Diagram indicating the net facilitory and inhibitory actions of various levels of the brain identified by the transection procedures shown in A. (From Tang PC: Levels of the brain stem and diencephalon controlling the micturition reflex. J Neurophysiol 18:583, 1955; and Tang PC, Ruch TC: Localization of brain stem and diencephalic areas controlling the micturition reflex. J Comp Neurol 106:213, 1956. Reprinted by permission of John Wiley & Sons, Inc.)

decerebration usually facilitates micturition by eliminating inhibitory inputs from more rostral areas of
the brain.[54, 55] However, transection at any point below the colliculi abolishes micturition. Bilateral lesions in the rostral pons abolish micturition, whereas
electrical stimulation at these sites triggers bladder
contractions and micturition.[1, 2, 4, 49, 53, 56] These observations led to the concept of a spinobulbospinal micturition reflex pathway that passes through a center
in the rostral brain stem (the pontine micturition
center [PMC]) (see Fig. 3–9). This pathway functions
as an on-off switch (see Fig. 3–6) that is activated by
a critical level of afferent activity arising from tension receptors in the bladder.[4] This switch in turn is
modulated by inhibitory and excitatory influences
from areas of the brain rostral to the pons (e.g., the
diencephalon and cerebral cortex) and from other
areas of the brain stem (see Figs. 3–9, 3–10, and 3–
11).

PONTINE MICTURITION CENTER

Physiologic and pharmacologic experiments have
provided substantial support for the concept that
neuronal circuitry in the PMC functions as a switch
in the micturition reflex pathway. The switch seems
to regulate bladder capacity and coordinate the activity of the bladder and external urethral sphincter.[1,
49, 51] Electrical or chemical stimulation in the PMC of
the rat, cat, or dog induces (1) suppression of urethral
sphincter EMG activity, (2) firing of sacral preganglionic neurons, (3) bladder contractions, and (4) release
of urine.[1, 2, 4, 49, 51, 53] Microinjections of putative inhibitory transmitters into the PMC of the cat can increase the volume threshold for inducing micturition
and in high doses completely block reflex voiding,
indicating that synapses in this region are important
for regulating the set-point for reflex voiding and
also are an essential link in the reflex pathway (Fig.
3–12).[23] The pontine micturition center receives inputs from neurons located in lateral laminae I, V,
and VII of the sacral spinal cord.[1] Neurons in these
areas of the spinal cord receive dense projections
from bladder afferent pathways[17, 30] (see Figs. 3–3,
3–4, and 3–11) and respond to distention or contraction of the bladder.[35, 39] It is assumed that these neurons represent the spinal ascending limb of the micturition reflex pathway.

Descending projections from the PMC to the spinal
cord have also been identified in the cat and rat[1, 49]
(see Fig. 3–11). In the cat, neurons in the dorsolateral
pons send direct projections to the sacral parasympathetic nucleus and to lamina I on the lateral edge of
the sacral dorsal horn, an area that contains dendritic projections from the sacral preganglionic neurons and afferent inputs from the bladder.[17, 29, 30]
Thus, the sites of termination of descending projections from the PMC are optimally located to regulate reflex mechanisms at the spinal level. A second
area located somewhat more laterally in the pons,
where electrical stimulation activates the urethral

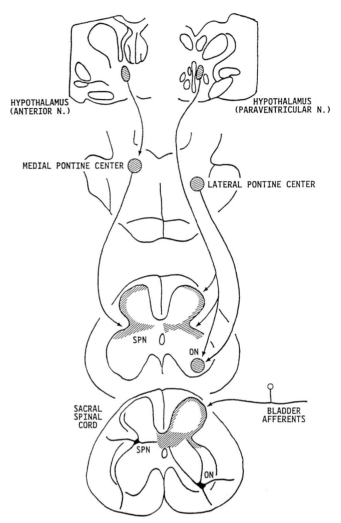

Figure 3-11   Neural connections between the brain and the sacral spinal cord that may be involved in the regulation of the
lower urinary tract in the cat. Lower section of spinal cord shows
the location and morphology of a preganglionic neuron in the
sacral parasympathetic nucleus (SPN), a sphincter motoneuron in
Onuf's nucleus (ON), and the sites of central termination of afferent projections from the urinary bladder. Upper section of spinal
cord shows the sites of termination of descending pathways arising
in the pontine micturition center (medial), the pontine sphincter
or urine storage center (lateral), and the paraventricular nuclei of
the hypothalamus. Section through the pons shows projection for
anterior hypothalamic nuclei to the pontine micturition center.
Based on studies of Holstege G, et al.[49] (From de Groat WC:
Neural control of urinary bladder and sexual organs. *In* Bannister
R, Mathias CJ [eds]: Autonomic Failure, 3rd ed. Oxford, Oxford
University Press, 1992, p 129.)

sphincter, sends projections to the sphincter motor
nucleus in the sacral spinal cord[49] (see Fig. 3–11).

SPINAL MICTURITION REFLEX PATHWAY

Reflex mechanisms in the spinal cord can also mediate bladder contractions and voiding.[1, 35, 56, 57] In most
species these mechanisms are weak or absent in
adults with an intact nervous system; however, they
are prominent in neonates or in mature animals fol-

PONTINE MICTURITION CENTER

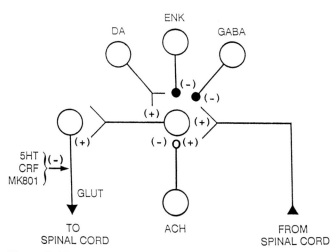

Figure 3-12 Diagram showing the variety of neurotransmitters that may regulate transmission in the pontine micturition center and in the descending limb of the micturition reflex pathway. DA, dopamine; ENK, enkephalins; GABA, γ-aminobutyric acid; GLUT, glutamic acid; ACH, acetylcholine; 5-HT, 5-hydroxytryptamine; CRF, corticotropin-releasing factor; MK-801, a noncompetitive NMDA glutamate receptor antagonist; (+), excitatory; (−), inhibitory synapse (indicated by filled circles). ACH has both excitatory and inhibitory effects in the pontine micturition center (synapse indicated by open circle). Descending limb of the reflex can be depressed by 5-HT agonists, CRF, and MK-801. (From de Groat WC, Booth AM, Yoshimura N: Neurophysiology of micturition and its modification in animal models of human disease. *In* Maggi CA [ed]: The Autonomic Nervous System, vol 3. Nervous Control of the Urogenital System. London, Harwood Academic Publishers, 1993. © 1993 by Harwood Academic Publishers.)

lowing spinal cord injury above the lumbosacral level. In the cat the spinal micturition reflex is mediated by C-fiber afferents (see Fig. 3–9), whereas the spinobulbospinal reflex in normal animals is triggered by A-delta afferent input from tension receptors in the urinary bladder. Somatic afferent pathways, particularly afferents with receptors in the perineum, can also induce voiding reflexes.[35] Thus, spinal pathways mediate involuntary or automatic micturition, whereas the spinobulbospinal pathways are involved in voluntary micturition.

Modulation of the Micturition Reflex Pathway by Other Centers in the Brain

Experiments in animals as well as clinical studies in humans indicate that various sites in the brain in addition to those directly involved in the micturition reflex pathway influence lower urinary tract function. Detailed reviews[1, 2, 4, 5] of the clinical and animal literature concerning the regulation of micturition by the brain have been published.

Recent axonal tracing studies in rats using trans-synaptic transport of pseudorabies virus have revealed the presence of direct connections from neurons in multiple brain areas to the reflex circuitry that regulates bladder function.[40–42] As illustrated in Figure 3–5, following injection of the virus into the bladder wall, preganglionic neurons and interneurons in the spinal cord are labeled at short transport times; then, at longer transport times, neurons in various areas of the brain including the PMC, paraventricular and medial preoptic nuclei of the hypothalamus, cerebral cortex, red nucleus, and periaqueductal gray and raphe nuclei in the brain stem are labeled by the virus. The possible functions of these neurons in the regulation of lower urinary tract function have been revealed primarily by lesion and electrophysiologic studies in animals.

CEREBRAL CORTEX AND DIENCEPHALON

Studies in humans indicate that voluntary control of micturition depends on connections between (1) the frontal cortex and the septal or preoptic region of the hypothalamus, and (2) connections between the paracentral lobule and the brain stem and spinal cord.[58] Lesions to these areas of cortex resulting from tumors, aneurysms, or cerebrovascular disease appear to increase bladder activity indirectly by removing cortical inhibitory control over the anterior hypothalamic area, which normally provides an excitatory input to micturition centers in the brain stem.[2]

Lesion studies in cats have also revealed an inhibitory role for the cerebral cortex. For example, removal of the motor cortex on one side reduced bladder capacity, and removal of the contralateral cortex further decreased capacity.[59] Subsequent decerebration did not elicit any additional change in bladder function. This study suggests that the predominent facilitory effect of decerebration in animals with an intact neuraxis[4, 54, 55] results in large part from the removal of tonic inhibitory impulses originating at the cortical level (see Fig. 3–10). Cortical influences may be mediated by a number of projections to subcortical sites including the hypothalamus, pons, extrapyramidal pathways to the brain stem, and the corticospinal system. The literature on the hypothalamic influences on lower urinary tract function is extensive (see references 2 and 4). Electrical stimulation of the anterior or lateral hypothalamus of animals activates the sacral parasympathetic excitatory pathway to the bladder and induces bladder contractions and voiding. In the cat the effects of hypothalamic stimulation are probably mediated by actions in the brain stem as well as direct projections to the spinal cord.

Axonal tracing studies in cats have shown that hypothalamic areas have diverse projections to areas of the brain stem that have an important role in the control of bladder function. For example, the anterior hypothalamic area projects directly through the medial forebrain bundle to the pontine micturition center (see Fig. 3–11).[60, 61] The lateral hypothalamic area projects to the parabrachial nucleus,[61] which reportedly has facilitory effects on micturition.[2] The anterior, medial, and paraventricular areas of the hypothalamus project to the central gray matter and medullary raphe nuclei. Electrical stimulation of the latter areas and adjacent reticular formation (e.g., the nucleus reticularis gigantocellularis) has been shown to exert prominent modulatory effects on bladder and urethral sphincter activity.[2, 62] Medial and posterior hypothalamic areas including the paraventricular nucleus have direct projections to the sacral parasympathetic nucleus, the sphincter motor nucleus (Onuf's nucleus), and certain sites in the spinal cord where bladder afferents terminate (laminae I and X).[60] Thus, hypothalamic control may be mediated by direct inputs to pontine and sacral micturition centers or by indirect mechanisms through other brain stem regions.

The influence of the hypothalamus on bladder function may in turn be modulated by afferent input from the bladder. Tracing studies in rats have identified a spinohypothalamic pathway arising from neurons in the region of the sacral parasympathetic nucleus.[63, 64] C-fos studies have shown that a large percentage of these neurons (60%) receive afferent input from the lower urinary tract.[64] This spinohypothalamic pathway may provide one route by which changes in bladder pressure modulate the firing of hypothalamic neurons.[65] This pathway also provides the anatomic substrate for putative spinohypothalamospinal and spinohypothalamopontine loops that could provide important modulatory control over micturition.

MIDBRAIN

Lesion studies[54, 55] indicate that the predominant effect of midbrain circuitry on bladder function is inhibition. However, electrical stimulation in the midbrain can produce excitatory as well as inhibitory effects.[1, 4, 53, 66] One area of the midbrain that has attracted attention as a possible facilitory micturition center is the periaqueductal gray (PAG). Electrical stimulation in the dorsolateral portion of the PAG and in the adjacent segmental reticular formation produced bladder contractions in the cat[51] and reduced the volume threshold for inducing micturition in the rat.[53] Because the PAG receives afferent input from the bladder[66] via spinal tract neurons in the intermediolateral region of the lumbosacral cord[1] and also receives prominent inputs from the hypothalamus, it may play a pivotal role in processing information before it is received by the PMC. Neurons in the ventrolateral PAG project to the PMC, raising the possibility that PAG neurons may be an important link in the micturition reflex pathway.

MEDULLA

Medullary centers have been implicated in both inhibitory and facilitory modulation of the micturition

reflex pathway. The two most prominent modulatory mechanisms are mediated by descending bulbospinal projections from the nucleus gigantocellularis reticularis (NGR) and the caudal raphe nuclei.[4, 67, 68] Electrical stimulation in the NGR (1) inhibits bladder motility, (2) reduces reflex firing in the pelvic nerve efferent pathways,[2] and (3) elicits both excitatory postsynaptic potentials and inhibitory postsynaptic potentials in sphincter motoneurons.[47]

Electrical or chemical stimulation of the nucleus raphe magnus (NRM), which is the origin of descending serotonergic projections to the spinal cord, inhibits reflex bladder contractions and reflex firing in the sacral efferent pathways to the bladder of the cat.[67, 68] Stimulation of the NRM also inhibits the firing of spinal dorsal horn neurons activated by afferents in the pelvic nerve.[69] Thus, descending raphe spinal pathways may modulate bladder sensory mechanisms in the spinal cord, and this in turn may account for the inhibitory effect of raphe stimulation on bladder reflexes. In the rat and cat, raphe neurons are activated by bladder distention.[69, 70] This raises the possibility that afferent input from the bladder may trigger a reflex loop, resulting in activation of a raphe-spinal inhibitory pathway that could suppress the micturition reflex pathway at the spinal level.

Neurotransmitters in Micturition Reflex Pathways

Because the sacral parasympathetic reflex pathway to the bladder is essentially a positive feedback circuit, it requires tonic inhibitory modulation to store urine properly and to prevent voiding at low bladder volumes. Damage to central inhibitory mechanisms following disease or injury to the nervous system leads to failure of urine storage and bladder hyperactivity and incontinence. Animal studies indicate that multiple transmitters may be involved in regulating transmission in the PMC (see Fig. 3–12) and in the spinal cord (see references 1 and 3 for detailed summaries).

INHIBITORY TRANSMITTERS

Several types of inhibitory transmitters including (1) opioid peptides (enkephalins), (2) inhibitory amino acids (gamma-aminobutyric acid [GABA], glycine), (3) 5-hydroxytryptamine (serotonin), (4) acetylcholine, (5) dopamine, and (6) nonopioid peptides (corticotropin-releasing factor [CRF], motilin, and NPY) can inhibit the micturition reflex when they are applied to the central nervous system. Experimental evidence in anesthetized animals indicates that GABA and enkephalins exert tonic inhibitory control in the PMC and regulate bladder capacity. The inhibitory effects are mediated by GABA-A and mu opioid receptors, respectively.[1, 51] Administration of GABA-

A or opioid receptor antagonists into the PMC reduced the micturition volume threshold, indicating that the set-point for reflex voiding is regulated by inhibitory mechanisms in the brain.

GABA and enkephalins also have inhibitory actions in the spinal cord. Baclofen, a GABA-B agonist that mimicks the inhibitory effect of GABA, has been used clinically via intrathecal administration in patients with hyperactive bladders to suppress bladder activity and promote urine storage.[71]

Intrathecal administration of CRF, which is a peptide contained in PMC neurons and in descending pathways from the PMC to the lumbosacral parasympathetic nucleus in the rat, inhibits the micturition reflex in the rat, raising the possibility that CRF may be an inhibitory cotransmitter in the descending limb of the micturition reflex pathway.

5-Hydroxytryptamine (5-HT), which is present in a dense collection of terminals in the lumbosacral spinal autonomic nuclei and in the sphincter motor nucleus,[72, 73] probably has a complex role in the regulation of lower urinary tract function. The 5-HT-containing terminals are part of an extensive bulbospinal projection system that arises in the medullary raphe nuclei. Pharmacologic studies in animals indicate that this system may promote urine storage by exciting sympathetic and sphincter efferent pathways and by inhibiting parasympathetic excitatory outflow to the bladder.[1]

Interest in the role of dopamine in the control of bladder function arises from the clinical observation that patients with idiopathic Parkinson's disease often have bladder hyperactivity. Parkinson's disease is a disorder of basal ganglia function caused by degeneration of dopamine-containing neurons. An animal model for Parkinson's disease has been developed in monkeys by administration of a neurotoxin (MPTP) that destroys dopamine-containing neurons. Animals treated with MPTP show motor symptoms typical of Parkinson's disease and also have hyperactive bladders. Pharmacologic studies[74] in MPTP-treated monkeys have revealed that bladder hyperactivity was due to the loss of dopaminergic inhibition mediated by D_1 dopaminergic receptors. On the other hand, D_2 dopaminergic receptors can mediate a facilitation of micturition.

EXCITATORY NEUROTRANSMITTERS

Excitatory neurotransmission in the central pathways to the lower urinary tract may depend on several types of transmitters including (1) glutamic acid, (2) neuropeptides (substance P, VIP), (3) norepinephrine, and (4) acetylcholine.

Glutamic acid[75] and norepinephrine[76] have been implicated as transmitters in bulbospinal excitatory pathways arising in the region of the PMC. The excitatory effects of these agents are mediated by N-methyl-D-aspartic acid (NMDA) glutamatergic receptors and alpha-1-adrenergic receptors, respectively. Glutamic acid has also been identified as a mediator

of a spinal micturition reflex pathway triggered by perineal afferents in neonatal rats.[77] Another type of glutamate receptor (AMPA) is involved in this reflex.

Neuropeptides, such as substance P and VIP, which are contained in a considerable percentage of bladder afferents,[25, 27, 28] can modulate the micturition reflex when they are injected intrathecally. Intrathecal administration of substance P antagonists in rats suppresses reflex bladder activity induced by distention or chemical irritation of the bladder, indicating that the peptide may be involved as an excitatory transmitter in several types of bladder reflexes in this species.[78, 79] In the cat, VIP has been implicated as a C-fiber afferent transmitter that mediates automatic micturition in chronic paraplegic animals.[1, 80]

Alterations in Bladder Reflex Pathways Following Neural Injury or Disease

SPINAL CORD INJURY

Electrophysiologic studies in animals have shown that the micturition reflex pathways in neurally intact animals and those with chronic spinal injuries are markedly different. The most prominent change occurs in the afferent limb of the micturition reflex, which in cats with chronic spinal injuries consists of unmyelinated (C-fiber) axons.[1, 35, 80] However, in cats with an intact spinal cord, myelinated (A-delta) afferents activate the micturition reflex (see Fig. 3–9).[1, 56, 57] This change in the afferent limb was demonstrated by electrophysiologic recording and also by administering capsaicin,[1, 81] a neurotoxin known to disrupt the function of C-fiber afferents.[20] In normal cats, capsaicin did not block reflex contractions of the bladder or the A-delta-fiber evoked bladder reflex. However, in cats with chronic spinal injury capsaicin completely blocked both the rhythmic bladder contractions induced by bladder distention and the C-fiber-evoked reflex firing recorded on bladder postganglionic nerves.[1, 81]

The emergence of the C-fiber-evoked reflex in animals with chronic spinal injuries is consistent with the emergence of other types of reflexes in paraplegic humans. For example, introduction of cold water into the bladder of paraplegic patients induces reflex voiding.[82] However, cold stimulation has no effect in normal patients. Studies in cats indicate that cold temperatures activate C-fiber afferents.[22] Thus, the positive cold response in paraplegic humans may also reflect emergence of C-fiber-evoked bladder reflexes.

OTHER NEUROLOGIC CONDITIONS

The cold water test is also positive in other situations including (1) infants,[83] (2) patients with multiple sclerosis and Parkinson's disease, and (3) elderly patients with hyperactive bladders.[84] The presence of the cold reflex in neonates, its disappearance with maturation of the nervous system, and its reemergence under conditions in which higher brain functions are disrupted suggests that it may reflect a primitive involuntary voiding reflex organized at the spinal level. Direct evidence of the contribution of C-fiber bladder afferents to bladder hyperactivity and involuntary voiding has been obtained in clinical studies in which capsaicin, the C-fiber afferent neurotoxin,[3] was administered intravesically to multiple sclerosis patients with hyperreflexic bladders.[85] In these patients capsaicin increased bladder capacity and reduced the frequency of incontinence. Intravesical administration of capsaicin has also been reported to increase bladder capacity and reduce irritative symptoms in patients with hypersensitive bladders.[86] These observations suggest that capsaicin-sensitive, C-fiber bladder afferents may be involved in several pathologic conditions associated with bladder hyperactivity.

The emergence of C-fiber bladder reflexes is probably mediated by several mechanisms including changes in central synaptic connections and alterations in the properties of the peripheral afferent receptors that lead to sensitization of the "silent" C fibers and the unmasking of responses to mechanical stimuli.[93, 94] As noted earlier, C-fiber bladder afferents in the cat normally do not respond to bladder distention[19] but do respond to this stimulus following spinal injury.[80] In rats it has been shown that bladder afferent neurons undergo both morphologic (neuronal hypertrophy)[87, 93, 94] and physiologic changes following spinal cord injury.[88] It has been speculated that this neuroplasticity is mediated by the actions of neurotrophic factors released within the spinal cord or the urinary bladder. Neurotrophic factors have also been implicated in the neuroplasticity of the bladder innervation that accompanies other types of disorders, including partial urethral obstruction,[89, 90] streptozotocin-induced diabetes,[91] and peripheral nerve damage.[92] More detailed discussions of neuroplasticity in bladder reflex pathways can be found in several recent reviews.[1, 58, 91, 92]

Summary

The lower urinary tract has two main functions: storage and periodic elimination of urine. These functions are regulated by a complex neural control system located in the brain and spinal cord. This control system performs like a simple switching circuit to maintain a reciprocal relationship between the reservoir (bladder) and the outlet components (urethra and urethral sphincter) of the urinary tract. The switching circuit is modulated by several neurotransmitter systems and is therefore sensitive to a variety of drugs and neurologic diseases. A more complete understanding of the neurohumoral mechanisms involved in bladder and urethral control will no doubt facilitate the development of new diagnostic methods and therapies for lower urinary tract dysfunction.

Acknowledgments

Research supported by NIH grants DK 37241, DK 42369, and DK 49430.

REFERENCES

1. De Groat WC, Booth AM, Yoshimura N: Neurophysiology of micturition and its modification in animal models of human disease. *In* Maggi CA (ed): The Autonomic Nervous System, vol 3. Nervous Control of the Urogenital System. London, Harwood Academic Publishers, 1993, pp 227–290.
2. Torrens M, Morrison JFB: The Physiology of the Lower Urinary Tract. Berlin, Springer-Verlag, 1987.
3. De Groat WC, Steers WD: Autonomic regulation of the urinary bladder and sex organs. *In* Loewy AD, Spyer KM (eds): Central Regulation of Autonomic Functions. Oxford, Oxford University Press, 1990, pp 310–333.
4. Kuru M: Nervous control of micturition. Physiol Rev 45:425, 1965.
5. Van Arsdalen K, Wein AJ: Physiology of micturition and continence. *In* Krane RJ, Siroky M (eds): Clinical Neuro-Urology, 2nd ed. New York, Little Brown, 1991, pp 25–82.
6. Lincoln J, Burnstock G: Autonomic innervation of the urinary bladder and urethra. *In* Maggi CA (ed): The Autonomic Nervous System, vol. 3. Nervous Control of the Urogenital System. London, Harwood Academic Publishers, 1993, pp 33–68.
7. De Groat WC, Booth AM: Synaptic transmission in pelvic ganglia. *In* Maggi CA (ed): The Autonomic Nervous System, vol. 3. Nervous Control of the Urogenital System. London, Harwood Academic Publishers, 1993, pp 291–347.
8. Keast JR, Kawatani M, de Groat WC: Sympathetic modulation of cholinergic transmission in cat vesical ganglia is mediated by alpha-1 and alpha-2 adrenoceptors. Am J Physiol 258:R44, 1990.
9. Levin RM, Longhurst PA: Pharmacological basis of bladder and urethral function and dysfunction. *In* Raz S (ed): Female Urology: Female Genitourinary Dysfunction and Reconstruction, 2nd ed. Philadelphia, W.B. Saunders, 1995.
10. De Groat WC, Theobald RJ: Reflex activation of sympathetic pathways to vesical smooth muscle and parasympathetic ganglia by electrical stimulation of vesical afferents. J Physiol (Lond) 259:223, 1976.
11. Somogyi GT, de Groat WC: Modulation of the release of ³H-norepinephrine from the base and body of the rat urinary bladder by endogenous adrenergic and cholinergic mechanisms. J Pharmacol Exp Ther 255:204, 1990.
12. Somogyi GT, de Groat WC: Evidence for inhibitory nicotinic and facilitatory muscarinic receptors in cholinergic nerve terminals of the rat urinary bladder. J Auton Nerv Syst 37:89, 1992.
13. Somogyi GT, Tanowitz M, de Groat WC: Evidence for facilitatory α_1 adrenoceptors on nerve terminals of the rat urinary bladder. Soc Neurosci Abstr 18:252, 1992.
14. Andersson K-E, Garcia-Pascual A, Persson K, et al: Electrically-induced, nerve-mediated relaxation of rabbit urethra involves nitric oxide. J Urol 147:253, 1992.
15. Keast JR, de Groat WC: Immunohistochemical characterization of pelvic neurons which project to the bladder, colon, or penis in rats. J Comp Neurol 288:387, 1989.
16. Zoubek JA, Somogyi GT, de Groat WC: A comparison of inhibitory effects of neuropeptide Y on rat urinary bladder, urethra and vas deferens. Am J Physiol 265:R537–43, 1993.
17. De Groat WC: Spinal cord projections and neuropeptides in visceral afferent neurons. Prog Brain Res 67:165, 1986.
18. Jänig W, Koltzenburg M: Pain arising from the urogenital tract. *In* Maggi CA (ed): The Autonomic Nervous System, vol.

3. Nervous Control of the Urogenital System. London, Harwood Academic Publishers, 1993, pp 525–578.

19. Häbler HJ, Jänig W, Koltzenburg M: Activation of unmyelinated afferent fibres by mechanical stimuli and inflammation of the urinary bladder in the cat. J Physiol (Lond) 425:545, 1990.

20. Jänig W, Koltzenburg M: On the function of spinal primary afferent fibres supplying colon and urinary bladder. J Auton Nerv Syst 30 Suppl:S89, 1990.

21. Jänig W, Morrison JFB: Functional properties of spinal visceral afferents supplying abdominal and pelvic organs, with special emphasis on visceral nociception. Prog Brain Res 67:87, 1986.

22. Fall M, Lindström S, Mazieres L: A bladder-to-bladder cooling reflex in the cat. J Physiol (Lond) 427:281, 1990.

23. McMahon SB, Abel C: A model for the study of visceral pain states: Chronic inflammation of the chronic decerebrate rat urinary bladder by irritant chemicals. Pain 28:109, 1987.

24. Birder LA, de Groat WC: Increased c-fos expression in spinal neurons after chemical irritation of the lower urinary tract of the rat. J Neurosci 12:4878, 1992.

25. Maggi CA: The dual, sensory and efferent function of the capsaicin-sensitive primary sensory nerves in the bladder and urethra. In Maggi CA (ed): The Autonomic Nervous System, vol. 3. Nervous Control of the Urogenital System. London, Harwood Academic Publishers, 1993, pp 383–422.

26. Kawatani M, Takeshige C, de Groat WC: Central distribution of afferent pathways from the uterus of the cat. J Comp Neurol 288:81, 1989.

27. Keast JR, de Groat WC: Segmental distribution and peptide content of primary afferent neurons innervating the urogenital organs and colon of male rats. J Comp Neurol 319:615, 1992.

28. De Groat WC: Neuropeptides in pelvic afferent pathways. Experientia Suppl 56:334, 1989.

29. Morgan CW, de Groat WC, Felkins LA, et al: Intracellular injection of neurobiotin or horseradish peroxidase reveals separate types of preganglionic neurons in the sacral parasympathetic nucleus of the cat. J Comp Neurol 331:161, 1993.

30. Steers WD, Ciambotti J, Etzel B, et al: Alterations in afferent pathways from the urinary bladder of the rat in response to partial urethral obstruction. J Comp Neurol 310:401, 1991.

31. Thor KB, Morgan C, Nadelhaft I, et al: Organization of afferent and efferent pathways in the pudendal nerve of the female cat. J Comp Neurol 288:263, 1989.

32. Roppolo JR, Nadelhaft I, de Groat WC: The organization of pudendal motoneurons and primary afferent projections in the spinal cord of the rhesus monkey revealed by horseradish peroxidase. J Comp Neurol 234:475, 1985.

33. Kawatani M, de Groat WC: A large proportion of afferent neurons innervating the uterine cervix of the cat contain VIP and other neuropeptides. Cell Tissue Res 266:191, 1991.

34. Kawatani M, de Groat WC: Segmental distribution and central projections of clitoral afferent pathways of the cat. Soc Neurosci Abstr 16:882, 1990.

35. De Groat WC, Nadelhaft I, Milne RJ, et al: Organization of the sacral parasympathetic reflex pathways to the urinary bladder and large intestine. J Auton Nerv Syst 3:135, 1981.

36. De Groat WC: Excitation and inhibition of sacral parasympathetic neurons by visceral and cutaneous stimuli in the cat. Brain Res 33:499, 1971.

37. Birder LA, de Groat WC: Induction of c-fos gene expression in spinal neurons in the rat by nociceptive and non-nociceptive stimulation of the lower urinary tract. Am J Physiol 265:R643, 1993.

38. Birder LA, Roppolo JR, Iadarola MJ, et al: Electrical stimulation of visceral afferent pathways in the pelvic nerve increases c-fos in the rat lumbosacral spinal cord. Neurosci Lett 129:193, 1991.

39. Birder LA, de Groat WC: The effect of glutamate antagonists on c-fos expression induced in spinal neurons by irritation of the lower urinary tract. Brain Res 580:115, 1992.

40. Roppolo JR, Card P, Sugaya K, et al: Identification of the central nervous system pathways controlling bladder function in the neonatal rat using transneuronal tracing with pseudorabies virus. Soc Neurosci Abstr 18:126, 1992.

41. Nadelhaft I, Vera PL, Card JP, et al: Central nervous system neurons labelled following the injection of pseudorabies virus into the rat urinary bladder. Neurosci Lett 143:271, 1992.

42. De Groat WC, Roppolo JR, Yoshimura N, et al: Neural control of the urinary bladder and colon. In Taché Y, Wingate D, Burks T (eds): Proceedings of the Second International Symposium on Brain-Gut Interactions. Boca Raton, FL, CRC Press, 1993, pp 167–190.

43. Konishi A, Itoh K, Sugimoto T, et al: Leucine-enkephalin-like immunoreactive afferent fibers to pudendal motoneurons in the cat. Neurosci Lett 61:109, 1985.

44. De Groat WC, Booth AM: Autonomic systems to bladder and sex organs. In Dyck PJ, Thomas PK, Griffin JW, et al (eds): Peripheral Neuropathy, 3rd ed. Philadelphia, W.B. Saunders, 1993, pp 198–207.

45. De Groat WC: Neural control of urinary bladder and sexual organs. In Bannister R, Mathias CJ (eds): Autonomic Failure, 3rd ed. Oxford, Oxford University Press, 1992, pp 129–159.

46. De Groat WC, Lalley PM: Reflex firing in the lumbar sympathetic outflow to activation of vesical afferent fibres. J Physiol (Lond) 226:289, 1972.

47. Mackel R: Segmental and descending control of the external urethral and anal sphincters in the cat. J Physiol (Lond) 294:105, 1979.

48. Shefchyk SJ: The effects of lumbosacral deafferentation on pontine micturition centre-evoked voiding in the decerebrate cat. Neurosci Lett 99:175, 1989.

49. Holstege G, Griffiths D, De Wall H, et al: Anatomical and physiological observations on supraspinal control of bladder and urethral sphincter muscles in the cat. J Comp Neurol 250:449, 1986.

50. Kruse MN, Mallory BS, Noto H, et al: Properties of the descending limb of the spinobulbospinal micturition reflex pathway in the cat. Brain Res 556:6, 1991.

51. Mallory BS, Roppolo JR, de Groat WC: Pharmacological modulation of the pontine micturition center. Brain Res 546:310, 1991.

52. Holstege G, Tan J: Supraspinal control of motoneurons innervating the striated muscles of the pelvic floor including urethral and anal sphincters in the cat. Brain 110:1323, 1987.

53. Kruse MN, Noto H, Roppolo JR, et al: Pontine control of the urinary bladder and external urethral sphincter in the rat. Brain Res 532:182, 1990.

54. Tang PC, Ruch TC: Localization of brain stem and diencephalic areas controlling the micturition reflex. J Comp Neurol 106:213, 1956.

55. Tang PC: Levels of the brain stem and diencephalon controlling the micturition reflex. J Neurophysiol 18:583, 1955.

56. De Groat WC: Nervous control of the urinary bladder of the cat. Brain Res 87:201, 1975.

57. De Groat WC, Ryall RW: Reflexes to sacral parasympathetic neurons concerned with micturition in the cat. J Physiol (Lond) 200:87, 1969.

58. Nathan PW: The central nervous connections of the bladder. In Williams DI, Chisholm GD (eds): Scientific Foundations of Urology, vol. II. Chicago, Year Book, 1976, pp 51–58.

59. Langworthy OR, Kolb LC: The encephalic control of tone in the musculature of the urinary bladder. Brain 56:371, 1933.

60. Holstege G: Some anatomical observations on the projections from the hypothalamus to brainstem and spinal cord: An HRP and autoradiographic tracing study in the cat. J Comp Neurol 260:98, 1987.

61. Moga MM, Herbert H, Hurley KM, et al: Organization of cortical, basal forebrain, and hypothalamic afferents to the parabrachial nucleus in the rat. J Comp Neurol 295:624, 1990.

62. McMahon SB, Spillane K: Brain stem influences on the parasympathetic supply to the urinary bladder of the cat. Brain Res 234:237, 1982.

63. Burstein R, Wang JL, Elde RP, et al: Neurons in the sacral parasympathetic nucleus that project to the hypothalamus do not also project through the pelvic nerve—a double labeling study combining Fluoro-gold and cholera toxin B in the rat. Brain Res 506:159, 1990.

64. Birder LA, Roppolo JR, Iadarola MJ, et al: C-fos as a marker for subsets of visceral second order neurons in the rat lumbosacral spinal cord. Soc Neurosci Abstr 16:703, 1990.

65. Stuart DG, Porter RW, Adey WR, et al: Hypothalamic unit activity. I. Visceral and somatic influences. Electroencephalogr Clin Neurophysiol 16:237, 1964.

66. Noto H, Roppolo JR, Steers WD, et al: Excitatory and inhibitory influences on bladder activity elicited by electrical stimulation in the pontine micturition center in rat. Brain Res 492:99, 1989.

67. Morrison JFB, Spillane K: Neuropharmacological studies on descending inhibitory controls over the micturition reflex. J Auton Nerv Syst Suppl 393, 1986.

68. Chen SY, Wang SD, Cheng CL, et al: Glutamate activation of neurons in cardiovascular reactive areas of the cat brain stem affects urinary bladder motility. Am J Physiol 265:F520, 1993.

69. Lumb BM: Brainstem control of visceral afferent pathways in the spinal cord. Prog Brain Res 67:279, 1986.

70. Oh UT, Hobbs SF, Garrison D, et al: Responses of raphe-spinal neurons (RSN) to urinary bladder distension (UBD) and sympathetic nerve stimulation. Soc Neurosci Abstr 12:375, 1986.

71. Nanninga JB, Frost F, Penn R: Effect of intrathecal baclofen on bladder and sphincter function. J Urol 142:101, 1989.

72. Dahlström A, Fuxe K: The distribution of monoamine terminals in the central nervous system. II. Experimentally induced changes in the interneuronal amine levels of the bulbospinal neuron systems. Acta Physiol Scand 64 Suppl 274:1, 1965.

73. Tashiro T, Satoda T, Matsushima R, et al: Convergence of serotonin-, enkephalin- and substance P-like immunoreactive afferent fibers on single pudendal motoneurons in Onuf's nucleus of the cat: A light microscope study combining the triple immunocytochemical staining technique with the retrograde HRP-tracing method. Brain Res 481:392, 1989.

74. Yoshimura N, Mizuta E, Kuno S, et al: The dopamine D_1 receptor agonist SKF 38393 suppresses detrusor hyperreflexia in the monkey with parkinsonism induced by 1-methyl-4-phenyl-1,2,3,6-tetrahydropyridine (MPTP). Neuropharmacology 32:315, 1993.

75. Yoshiyama M, Roppolo JR, de Groat WC: Effects of MK-801 on the micturition reflex in the rat: Possible sites of action. J Pharmacol Exp Ther 265:844, 1993.

76. Yoshimura N, Sasa M, Yoshida O, et al: α_1-Adrenergic receptor-mediated excitation from the locus coeruleus of the sacral parasympathetic preganglionic neuron. Life Sci 47:789, 1990.

77. Sugaya K, de Groat WC: Effects of MK-801 and CNQX, glutamate receptor antagonists on bladder activity in neonatal rats. Brain Res 640:1–10, 1994.

78. Lecci A, Giuliani S, Maggi CA: Effect of the NK-1 receptor antagonist GR 82,334 on reflexly-induced bladder contractions. Life Sci 51:277, 1992.

79. Kawatani M, Matsumoto G, Birder LA, et al: Intrathecal administration of NK1 receptor antagonist, CP96345, inhibits the micturition reflex in the rat. Regulatory Peptides 46:392, 1993.

80. De Groat WC, Kawatani M, Hisamitsu T, et al: Mechanisms underlying the recovery of urinary bladder function following spinal cord injury. J Auton Nerv Syst 30 Suppl: S71, 1990.

81. McMahon SB, Morrison JFB: Spinal neurones with long projections activated from the abdominal viscera of the cat. J Physiol (Lond) 322:1, 1982.

82. Bors E, Comarr AE: Neurological Urology, Physiology of Micturition, Its Neurological Disorders and Sequelae. Baltimore, University Park Press, 1971.

83. Geirsson G, Glad G, Fall M, et al: The bladder cooling test in neurologically normal infants and children. ICCS Proc 2:12, 1993.

84. Fall M, Geirsson G, Lindström S: The overactive bladder: Insight into neurophysiology by analysis of cystometric abnormalities. Neurourol Urodynamics 10:337, 1991.

85. Fowler CJ, Jewkes D, McDonald WI, et al: Intravesical capsaicin for neurogenic bladder dysfunction. Lancet 339:1239, 1992.

86. Maggi CA, Barbanti G, Santicioli P, et al: Cystometric evidence that capsaicin-sensitive nerves modulate the afferent branch of micturition reflex in humans. J Urol 142:150, 1991.

87. Kruse MN, Erdman SL, Tanowitz M, et al: Differential effects of spinal cord injury on the morphology of bladder afferent and efferent neurons. Soc Neurosci Abstr 18:127, 1992.

88. Yoshimura N, de Groat WC: Plasticity of sodium and potassium channels in rat afferent neurons following spinal cord injury or partial urethral obstruction. Soc Neurosci Abstr 19:1762, 1993.

89. Steers WD, Ciambotti J, Erdman S, et al: Morphological plasticity in efferent pathways to the urinary bladder of the rat following urethral obstruction. J Neurosci 10:1943, 1990.

90. Steers WD, Kolbeck S, Creedon D, et al: Nerve growth factor in the urinary bladder of the adult regulates neuronal form and function. J Clin Invest 88:1709, 1991.

91. Steers WD, Mackway AM, Ciambotti J, et al: Alterations in neural pathways to the urinary bladder of the rat in response to streptozotocin-induced diabetes. J Auton Nerv Syst 47:83, 1993.

92. DelGaudio W, Booth AM, Stewart R, et al: Hypertrophy of bladder pelvic ganglion cells following chronic parasympathetic decentralization. Soc Neurosci Abstr 17:1002, 1991.

93. Kruse MN, de Groat WC: Changes in lower urinary tract function following spinal cord injury. J Restor Neurol Neurosci 5:79, 1993.

94. De Groat WC, Kruse MN: Central processing and morphological plasticity in lumbosacral afferent pathways from the lower urinary tract. In Mayer EA, Raybould HE (eds): Basic and Clinical Aspects of Chronic Abdominal Pain, vol 9. Pain Research and Clinical Management. Amsterdam, Elsevier Science Publishers, 1993, pp 219–235.

CHAPTER 4

Pharmacologic Basis of Bladder and Urethral Function and Dysfunction

Robert M. Levin, Ph.D.
Penelope A. Longhurst, Ph.D.

The function of the urinary bladder is to collect and store urine at low intravesical pressures and then, under voluntary control, to expel the urine by means of a sustained contraction.[1-3] Efficient bladder emptying requires coordinated contraction by the smooth muscle elements of the bladder body and relaxation of the bladder neck and urethra.[3, 4] To a large extent, urinary bladder function depends on the underlying structure of the organ as a whole, relying on the interrelationships among smooth muscle, connective tissue, and epithelial elements. Frequently, bladder dysfunction in women is related to differences in the anatomy and structure of the female lower urinary tract compared to that of the male. Specifically, the female urethra is considerably shorter than that of the male, the external sphincter is smaller and does not completely encircle the urethra, and women do not have a prostate to add to urethral resistance.[1, 2] These factors make women much more subject to incontinence than men but less likely to develop partial outlet obstruction. The details of these anatomic differences are covered in detail elsewhere in this book.

An alteration in the ratio of connective tissue to smooth muscle can significantly alter compliance and functional capacity and can impair the bladder's ability to empty efficiently and fully.[5] Thus, a change in structural compartmentalization can affect bladder function independent of autonomic receptor density and distribution and the contractile capabilities of the smooth muscle elements.[2, 3, 5] Thus, any discussion of the relationship between smooth muscle function, receptor distribution and density, and the functional ability of the bladder to empty must take into account the status of the bladder as a whole, not just the contractile response of isolated sections of bladder smooth muscle to specific forms of stimulation.

Intracellularly, detrusor contraction, like that of all smooth muscle, is dependent on the interaction between the smooth muscle contractile proteins actin and myosin as a result of phosphorylation of myosin light chains by myosin light chain kinase.[6, 7] In turn, phosphorylation of myosin filaments depends on the translocation of calcium from the extracellular space and the release of bound intracellular calcium.[8, 9] The rate and magnitude of pressure generation depends on the active interaction of actin and myosin with calcium, mediated by myosin light chain kinase and the net breakdown of cytosolic adenosine 5′-triphosphate (ATP). In addition, bladder emptying requires maintenance of pressure during the tonic phase of bladder contraction.[2, 5, 10-12] A defect in the ability to sustain a contraction can seriously reduce the bladder's ability to empty while not affecting its ability to generate pressure.[5, 13, 14]

Most of the basic information available on the pharmacology and physiology of bladder function has been derived from studies using male animals. Males have been used because of the changes in sex hormones that occur during estrus in females and the hormonal changes that occur during pregnancy and lactation. It has been recognized for a long time that alterations in sex hormones can have profound effects on smooth muscle function, autonomic receptor distribution and density, muscle metabolism and biochemistry, and protein synthesis, and thus may lead to variable responses in otherwise well-controlled animal experiments.[15-25] The basic method of controlling for these hormone-induced alterations has consisted primarily of excluding females from scientific studies, both at the experimental level using animals and at the clinical level using humans.

The specific aim of this review is twofold: first, the presentation of information on the basic physiology and pharmacology of the mammalian lower urinary tract, and second, a review of the current literature on the modulations of these basic functions in the female. Thus, the emphasis of this article is on how female hormones modify the basic response of the lower urinary tract to neurohumoral and pharmacologic stimulation.

Pharmacologic treatment of bladder contractile dysfunction is largely based on our knowledge of the autonomic innervation of the bladder and related structures. The drugs used are, in general, those developed for use in other organ systems.[2, 4] Their efficacy in the lower urinary tract is frequently considered a side effect of their use in the treatment of other disorders. Possible targets for pharmacologic intervention include nerve terminals and the release of specific neurotransmitters, specific receptor subtypes in the bladder and urethra, and specific ion channels in the bladder and urethra.

Bladder function depends on a number of factors, including (1) the status of neuronal innervation, (2) the structure of the organ as a whole, and (3) the contractile response of the smooth muscle elements. These three factors are intimately associated with each other, and an alteration in one factor can induce substantial adaptive changes in the other two. Thus, hormonally mediated changes in neuronal distribution, receptor density and distribution, smooth muscle size and number (hypertrophy and hyperplasia), connective tissue density and distribution, and urothelial cell proliferation and permeability can significantly affect bladder function and may be directly involved in the generation of specific disorders primarily observed in women (i.e., stress or urge incontinence and interstitial cystitis).

Autonomic Innervation

Smooth muscle contraction is dependent on the autonomic nervous system. The terms sympathetic and parasympathetic refer to anatomic divisions of the autonomic nervous system.[4, 26] The sympathetic division consists of fibers originating in the thoracic and lumbar regions of the spinal cord, and the parasympathetic division consists of fibers originating in the cranial and sacral spinal nerves.

For many years the only autonomic neurotransmitters recognized were acetylcholine and norepinephrine. However, it became obvious that other transmitters might also be present in components of the autonomic nervous system. Burnstock has repeatedly emphasized the possibility of cotransmitter release and the concept of modulatory transmitter mechanisms, including prejunctional inhibition or enhancement of transmitter release, postjunctional modulation of transmitter action, and secondary involvement of locally synthesized hormones and prostaglandins.[27–29] Cotransmitters may be released along with a classic neurotransmitter in response to nervous activation and may interact at the level of

the receptor or second messenger before evoking functional responses. The cotransmitter may have a direct action on postjunctional cells or may facilitate the action of the classic neurotransmitter or act as an inhibitor of its release. Cotransmitters and classic transmitters may be stored in the same vesicle, thereby being released in a parallel fashion at all impulse frequencies, or they can be stored in separate vesicle types, in which case differential release at different impulse frequencies may be possible. This concept may explain why pharmacologic blockade of classic receptors sometimes only partially abolishes the effects of neural stimulation. These somewhat complicated concepts and possibilities are nicely summarized by Lundberg and Hokfelt.[30]

The postganglionic nerve-evoked contractile response of the urinary bladder of nearly all vertebrate species, including humans, is only partially blocked by antimuscarinic agents such as atropine and scopolamine[29, 31–33] and is relatively unaffected by alpha- and beta-adrenergic[34, 35] or nicotinic antagonists.[35] The most likely explanation for this response is that in addition to acetylcholine released from cholinergic nerves, another neurotransmitter is released by nonadrenergic, noncholinergic nerves and contributes to the contraction. The presence of these neurons was alluded to in the early literature by Langley[36, 37] and has been suggested to exist throughout the gastrointestinal tract[38, 39] as well as other organs including the lung, trachea, esophagus, cardiovascular system, and seminal vesicles.[40–42] In the human female bladder these nerves have been estimated to be responsible for up to 50% of the contractile response.[34] Evidence accumulated during the past few decades suggests that the neurotransmitter used by these neurons is most likely a purine nucleotide or analog, and these nerves have therefore been termed "purinergic" by Burnstock (for review, see reference 40).

Studies that have desensitized the P_2-purinergic receptors or have used the photoaffinity analog of ATP, arylazidoaminopropionyl adenosine 5′-triphosphate (ANAPP$_3$), have provided strong evidence that supports the purinergic innervation of the urinary bladder. These studies have demonstrated that the atropine-resistant portion of the response to both field stimulation in vitro and pelvic nerve stimulation in vivo is at least partially mediated by ATP.[43–46] Although there is good evidence that purinergic innervation participates in the neuronally induced contractile response of the bladder of the rat, rabbit, guinea pig, and cat, the role of purinergic innervation in the normal function of the pig and human bladder is questionable.[47]

Although a wide variety of neurohumoral agents such as vasoactive intestinal polypeptide (VIP), substance P, prostaglandins, 5-hydroxytryptamine, histamine, endogenous opioids, galanin, and neuropeptide Y (NPY) have potent direct actions on bladder and urethral smooth muscle,[48, 49] their roles in bladder function are unclear. Some of these agents may be released as cotransmitters, some may be produced within the bladder and act as local hormones, and some may have no in vivo function. Furthermore, their importance in micturition is questionable because the major portion of the contractile response to parasympathetic stimulation (in humans) can be blocked by muscarinic inhibition, and most responses to sympathetic (hypogastric) stimulation can be blocked by alpha- or beta-adrenergic inhibition.[2, 4]

Autonomic Receptors: Distribution and Response

Stimulation of autonomic nerves initiates responses in target tissues that result from release of specific neurohumoral transmitters and their subsequent binding to postjunctional receptors. In the lower urinary tract, the major receptor types are cholinergic muscarinic receptors (responding to transmitter release from parasympathetic nerves), alpha- and beta-adrenergic receptors (responding to transmitter release from sympathetic nerves), and, in various animal species, purinergic receptors (responding to transmitter release from purinergic nerves).[2, 4]

Pharmacologically, the bladder can be divided into two sections—the bladder body and the bladder base.[50–52] Both the responses to autonomic agonists and the distribution of autonomic receptors follow this division. Table 4–1 presents a comparison of the density of cholinergic and adrenergic receptors with the contractile response of the rabbit bladder body and base.[50, 51] Muscarinic receptors and the contractile response to cholinergic stimulation are greatest in the bladder body and lowest in the bladder base. Similarly, beta-adrenergic receptors and relaxant responses of bladder smooth muscle to beta-receptor stimulation are greatest in the bladder body and lowest in the bladder base, whereas alpha-adrenergic receptors and contractile responses to alpha-receptor stimulation are greatest in the bladder base and

weakest in the bladder body. In addition, cholinergic innervation is dense in both the bladder body and the bladder base, whereas adrenergic innervation is dense in the bladder base and sparse in the bladder body.[50–53]

Based on this distribution of autonomic receptors and contractile responses, muscarinic agonists theoretically should be effective in improving bladder contraction and emptying; alpha-adrenergic agonists should be effective in increasing urethral tone and reducing incontinence; and beta-adrenergic agonists should be effective in increasing bladder capacity. Conversely, muscarinic antagonists should be effective in reducing bladder hyperactivity; alpha-adrenergic antagonists should be effective in reducing urethral pressure and improving conditions such as benign prostatic hyperplasia (BPH); and beta-adrenergic antagonists would not be expected to have much therapeutic value. Although there are data showing that these pharmacologic agents have the expected actions in in vitro experiments on isolated tissues, their clinical effectiveness is limited by their lack of selectivity.[2]

In an attempt to determine whether bladder and urethral tissues have specific receptor subtypes that can be used to develop more selective agents, several investigators have investigated the autonomic receptor subtype distribution in the bladder and urethra. The initial methods used to identify receptor subtypes were based on the pharmacologic potency of a series of agents that specifically bind to the receptor. Classically, there exist at least two alpha-adrenergic (alpha-1 and alpha-2), two beta-adrenergic (beta-1 and beta-2), and two muscarinic receptor (M_1 and M_2) subtypes.[54–58] Alpha-1 receptors were originally described as "postsynaptic receptors," and alpha-2 receptors were originally designated as "presynaptic receptors."[54, 55] However, recent studies have demonstrated that this anatomic description is incorrect, and it is no longer used. Molecular cloning has indicated that adrenergic and cholinergic receptors can be further subdivided into more subtypes. However,

TABLE 4–1
Autonomic Receptor Distribution and Contractile Response in the Rabbit Bladder Body and Bladder Base

	Receptor Density (fmole/mg protein)	Contractile Response (g tension)
Bladder body		
Cholinergic muscarinic	22 ± 3	6.3 ± 1.0
Beta-adrenergic	91 ± 10	−1.0 ± 0.2[a]
Alpha-adrenergic	21 ± 4	0.4 ± 0.2
Bladder base		
Cholinergic muscarinic	8 ± 1[b]	1.5 ± 0.5[b]
Beta-adrenergic	47 ± 6[b]	−0.4 ± 0.1[a, b]
Alpha-adrenergic	88 ± 9[b]	3.0 ± 0.4[b]

Receptor densities of bladders from adult male New Zealand White rabbits were determined in filtered whole homogenate using ^{3}H-DHE and prazosin for measurement of alpha-adrenergic receptors, ^{3}H-DHA and propranolol for beta-adrenergic receptors, and ^{3}H-QNB and atropine for muscarinic cholinergic receptors.[50, 51] The bladders were separated at the ureteral orifices into bladder body and bladder base. Each point represents the mean ± SEM of six to eight individual observations.
[a]Decrease in tension from a baseline of 1.2 g
[b]Significantly different from the corresponding value for the bladder body ($p < .05$)

in general, the classic pharmacologically derived definitions are used in this review.

Receptor-binding studies of alpha-adrenergic receptors often use the specific alpha-1 antagonist prazosin and the alpha-2 antagonist yohimbine to distinguish between the two receptor subtypes. One study by Levin and colleagues demonstrated that male rabbit and human bladders contain 80% alpha-1 receptors and 20% alpha-2 receptors.[59] This distribution is similar to that reported by Ueda and associates in the rabbit bladder.[60] Tsujimoto and associates[61] and Honda and coworkers[62] showed that the contractile response of the rabbit bladder base to a variety of alpha agonists is mediated primarily by alpha-1 receptors. Using similar methodology, Kunisawa and colleagues[63] came to the same conclusion using isolated strips of human urinary bladder base.

Beta receptors can be differentiated into beta-1 and beta-2 subtypes using specific antagonists such as ICI-118, ICI-89, ICI-118,551, metoprolol, practolol, or zinterol.[59, 64] Studies in our laboratory demonstrated that the bladder body in both the rabbit and the human contains primarily beta-2 receptors.[59] The density of beta-1 receptors was below the level of detection. In similar studies using other agents, Anderson and Marks demonstrated that the rabbit bladder detrusor contained primarily beta-2 receptors with a very small beta-1 component.[64] Similarly, Morita and colleagues demonstrated that the relaxant responses of isolated strips of rabbit bladder to a variety of beta agonists were mediated by beta-2 receptors.[65]

Currently, three types of muscarinic receptors have been identified pharmacologically: M-1, M-2, and M-3.[66] In general, M-1 receptors predominate at ganglia and secretory glands, M-2 receptors are found in the myocardium and smooth muscle, and M-3 receptors are found in smooth muscle and secretory glands. Two further receptor subtypes, M-4 and M-5, may be present in some cells.[66] Classically, M-1 and M-2 muscarinic receptors were separated into two groups using the selective antagonist pirenzepine (PZP).[58] Pirenzepine has a high affinity for the M-1 type muscarinic receptor, which blocks gastric secretion and other M-1–mediated responses, but a low affinity for the M-2 receptor, which regulates heart rate and smooth muscle contraction. Using both direct ^{3}H-PZP binding studies and indirect inhibition of binding of the nonspecific muscarinic antagonist ^{3}H-QNB by unlabeled PZP, studies by several investigators demonstrated that neither the human nor the rabbit urinary bladder contains high-affinity PZP sites; rather, muscarinic responses are mediated through the low-affinity M_2 receptor.[59, 67] More recently, however, it has been shown that the urinary bladder also contains M-3 muscarinic receptors, which were previously defined as M-2β.[68]

The techniques of molecular cloning have been used to detect additional subtypes of adrenergic and cholinergic receptors. At least five subtypes of the muscarinic cholinergic receptor have been identified. Like the pharmacologic classification, the cloned subtypes have a distinct anatomic localization and agonist-antagonist specificities and, when stimulated, may produce their effects through different mechanisms. The cloned muscarinic receptors are identified as m-1, m-2, m-3, m-4, and m-5. More clones may be identified in the future.[66, 69] The locations and specificity of the m-1, m-2, and m-3 receptors appear to correspond well with those of the M-1, M-2, and M-3 receptors.[70] Functional and binding studies, similarly, indicate that both alpha-1- and alpha-2-adrenergic receptors can be further subdivided into at least two additional subtypes (alpha-1$_A$ and alpha-1$_B$, alpha-2$_A$ and alpha-2$_B$), and molecular cloning has produced six different alpha receptors. Genes for the beta-1 and beta-2 receptors have been cloned.[71] More recently, a human gene that encodes a beta-3 receptor has been isolated.[72] The identification of these different receptor subtypes in urologic tissues and the production of drugs with the ability to distinguish between the different subtypes opens a new door to the therapy of disorders of the lower urinary tract.

Bladder Contraction and Calcium and Potassium Ion Channels

Contraction of the urinary bladder after agonist stimulation results from an increase in intracellular calcium, which then interacts with the contractile proteins. The major source of this activator calcium is extracellular calcium, which enters the smooth muscle cells through receptor-operated channels or voltage-operated calcium channels opened as a result of membrane depolarization. Additional calcium is supplied by release from intracellular stores. Calcium entry through the voltage-gated L-type calcium channels is prevented by the group of drugs called the calcium antagonists. There are three different classes of calcium antagonists, each having a wide variety of selectivity for smooth muscle and different pharmacologic properties, factors that are of important clinical significance.[73] Calcium entry can also be reduced, indirectly, by the potassium channel openers, a group of drugs that hyperpolarize the cell membrane.[74]

Calcium channel antagonists reduce in vitro spontaneous activity and the contractile response of bladder strips to field stimulation and a variety of agonists.[75-79] In general, the response of the bladder to field stimulation (or neuronal stimulation) is biphasic, consisting of a rapid increase in tension (phasic contraction) followed by a prolonged period of increased tension that is maintained for the duration of the stimulation (tonic contraction). Bladder emptying occurs almost entirely during tonic bladder contraction.[10] Calcium channel antagonists preferentially inhibit the tonic phase of the contractile response to field stimulation, as demonstrated in Figures 4–1 and 4–2.[79] This property of calcium channel blocking agents may limit their therapeutic usefulness in bladder dysfunction. Calcium antagonists altered the

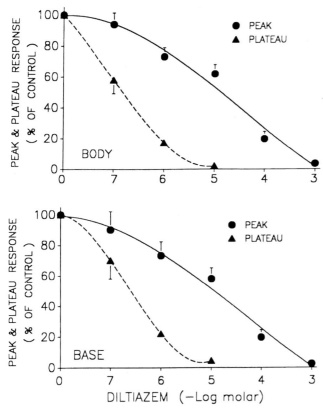

Figure 4-1 Effects of diltiazem on the peak (phasic) and plateau (tonic) responses of rabbit bladder body and base strips to field stimulation. Each point represents the mean ± SEM of six to eight individual observations. (Reprinted from Zhao Y, Wein AJ, Levin RM: Role of calcium in mediating the biphasic contraction of the rabbit urinary bladder. Gen Pharmacol 24:727–731, 1993, Copyright 1993, with kind permission from Elsevier Science Ltd, The Boulevard, Langford Lane, Kidlington OX5 IGB, UK.)

in vivo micturition reflex in rats by increasing the volume threshold and decreasing the amplitude of the micturition contraction.[80] At higher doses, the bladder was unable to empty, and micturition was incomplete. Clinically, it was hoped that calcium antagonists would be useful in the treatment of uninhibited detrusor contractions or incontinence resulting from bladder hyperactivity. Although nifedipine was reported to be useful in the treatment of urge incontinence, in which it caused subjective improvement and inhibited detrusor contractions and increased bladder capacity during urodynamic investigations,[81] other studies have found that side effects and a limited efficacy restrict use of the calcium antagonists in the treatment of bladder hyperactivity.[82]

The response of the urinary bladder to potassium channel openers is similar to the response to calcium channel antagonists.[83] In normal rats in vivo, pinacidil and cromakalim reduce micturition pressure. However, these agents had no effects on bladder capacity, residual urine, or compliance. In rats with bladder hypertrophy secondary to obstruction, potassium channel openers decreased spontaneous activity and caused a tendency toward residual urine

development.[84] In vivo potassium channel openers decrease the amplitude and frequency of experimentally induced hyperreflexia,[85] and in vitro they reduce spontaneous activity and the contractile responses of bladder strips to muscarinic agonists, methoxamine, potassium, and field stimulation.[85, 86] However, potassium channel openers have been disappointing clinically in the treatment of detrusor instability secondary to BPH, in which their use produced no subjective or objective improvement in symptoms.[87]

Urethral Function and Nitric Oxide

Bladder emptying is associated with inhibition of alpha-adrenergic tone, resulting in a decrease in outlet resistance.[1–3] In addition, urethral smooth muscle relaxation may occur in response to activation of beta-adrenergic receptors or stimulation of inhibitory nonadrenergic noncholinergic (NANC) nerves. Electrical stimulation of urethral preparations that were previously stimulated to a high tone results in relaxation (Fig. 4–3).[88] The relaxant response is sensitive to tetrodotoxin, suggesting that the transmitter re-

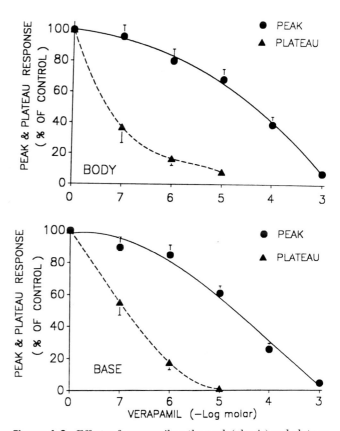

Figure 4-2 Effects of verapamil on the peak (phasic) and plateau (tonic) responses of rabbit bladder base and body strips to field stimulation. Each point represents the mean ± SEM of six to eight individual observations. (Reprinted from Zhao Y, Wein AJ, Levin RM: Role of calcium in mediating the biphasic contraction of the rabbit urinary bladder. Gen Pharmacol 24:727–731, 1993, Copyright 1993, with kind permission from Elsevier Science Ltd, The Boulevard, Langford Lane, Kidlington OX5 IGB, UK.)

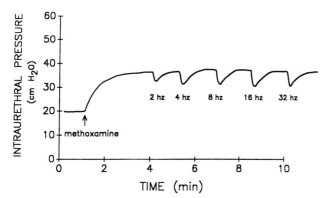

Figure 4-3 Representative trace showing the effects of field stimulation on the isolated cat whole urethra preparation in the presence of methoxamine prestimulation. (From Levin RM, Hayes L, Eika B, et al: Comparative autonomic responses of the cat and rabbit bladder and urethra. J Urol 148:216, 1992.)

sponsible is released from nerves. Recently, several studies have suggested that nitric oxide is the transmitter substance responsible for urethral relaxation. The relaxant response of the urethra to field stimulation is mimicked by nitric oxide[89] and prevented by N^G-monomethyl-L-arginine (L-NMMA), N^G-nitro-L-arginine (L-NOARG), and methylene blue, substances that prevent the formation of nitric oxide from L-arginine (L-NMMA and L-NOARG) or prevent activation of guanylate cyclase (methylene blue).[89–91] Recently, intra-arterial administration of N^G-nitro-L-arginine methyl ester (L-NAME) and L-NOARG has been shown to increase intravesical spontaneous activity and decrease bladder capacity and micturition volume in conscious rats.[91] These effects were prevented by coadministration of L-arginine. Electrically induced contractions of bladder detrusor were unaffected by L-NAME or L-arginine,[91] suggesting that although nitric oxide may play a role in micturition, it most likely acts by exerting an inhibitory influence on the bladder outlet.

Alteration of Autonomic Function in the Urinary Bladder Caused by Sex Hormones

The major problems associated with studies of the effects of sex hormones on urinary bladder function are the variety of different hormone treatments used and the frequent lack of appropriate controls. Most studies have examined the responses of bladders from female animals to estradiol treatment. Generally, the studies compared bladders from ovariectomized or intact controls with those of similar animals treated with estradiol. However, in many studies both intact and ovariectomized controls were not included. Furthermore, the hormone dosages ranged from subphysiologic to suprapharmacologic, and the duration of treatment, depending on the aim of the study, ranged from hours to several months. These

differences make cross-study interpretation of the data very difficult. If sex hormones are important for the function of any organ, castration should alter function, and replacement of the hormones should prevent the altered function. However, in the few studies in which intact controls were included, ovariectomy often had no effect on bladder function, indicating that sex hormones have little or no role in normal bladder function. Furthermore, subsequent estradiol treatment often did produce changes in bladder function, suggesting that the effects seen were not simply the result of hormone replacement or that the dose used was inappropriate. Rarely do the studies report a parameter (serum estradiol levels, uterine weight, and so on) that could indicate whether the dose of estradiol used was adequate to replace ovarian hormones. Additionally, in many studies estradiol treatment was given to intact animals, resulting in supraphysiologic dosage.

Almost all experimental studies have concentrated on the effects of estradiol on bladder function. However, progesterone is also produced by the ovaries and is generally considered a physiologic antagonist to estradiol. Progesterone levels as well as estradiol levels increase during pregnancy. Progesterone receptors, as well as estrogen receptors, are present in the bladder and urethra, but their role in the maintenance of continence is largely unknown.

HORMONES AND BLADDER MASS

In general, studies have shown that estradiol treatment increases bladder and urethral mass (Table 4–2). These findings are in close agreement with clinical studies showing increases in urethral mucosal thickness in postmenopausal women after estrogen therapy. Although it is likely that the increases in urethral weight are primarily the result of stimulation of estrogen receptors, which are present in much greater density than in the bladder, Longhurst and colleagues suggested that estradiol treatment causes a diuresis that contributes to increased bladder mass.[98] However, because no other studies have monitored urine output after treatment of animals with estrogens, this hypothesis remains speculative. Furthermore, increases in bladder mass may make interpretation of contractile data difficult if bladder strips from treated animals have a greater mass than those of controls or if the ratio of smooth muscle to connective tissue or epithelium changes.

HORMONES AND CONTRACTILE RESPONSES OF THE URETHRA

Four studies have examined contractile responses of the rabbit urethra to alpha-adrenergic stimulation after hormone treatment (Table 4–3). Hodgson and coworkers found a decreased sensitivity of bladder strips to phenylephrine 14 days after ovariectomy compared to bladders from rabbits in natural es-

TABLE 4–2
Effects of Estrogens on Bladder Weight

Ref	Treatment[a]	Species	Response
15	1	Rabbit	↑ urethra weight after OVX + E vs. OVX, NC bladder weight after OVX + E vs. OVX
92	2	Rabbit	NC urethra or bladder weight after OVX + E or OVX + EP vs. OVX
93	3	Rabbit	NC bladder weight after OVX + E vs. OVX
17	4	Rabbit	↑ bladder weight after OVX + E vs. FMC, NC after OVX vs. FMC
94	5	Rabbit	NC bladder weight after MMT or CAS or CAS + T vs. MMT
95	6	Rabbit	↑ bladder weight after OVX + E vs. OVX
96	7	Rat	↑ bladder weight MIC vs. FIC, ↑ bladder weight MMC vs. FMC
97	8	Rat	↓ bladder weight after OVX vs. FOC, NC after OVX + E or FOE vs. FOC
98	9	Rat	↑ bladder weight after OVX + E vs. FMC, NC after OVX vs. FMC
99	10	Rat	↑ bladder weight MMC vs. FMC

Abbreviations: NC, no change
[a]Treatment:
1. Mature ovariectomized females × 2 weeks (OVX); mature ovariectomized females + polyestradiol phosphate (4 mg, 4 days before use) (OVX + E)
2. Mature ovariectomized females × 3 weeks (OVX); mature ovariectomized females + polyestradiol phosphate (1.6 mg/kg, 5 days before use) (OVX + E); mature ovariectomized females + polyestradiol phosphate (4 mg, 5 days before use) + progesterone (0.7 mg/kg, 2 days before use) (OVX + EP)
3. Mature ovariectomized females × 3 weeks (OVX); mature ovariectomized females + 17β-estradiol (20 μg/kg, 2 or 24 hours before use) (OVX + E)
4. Mature intact female controls (FMC); ovariectomized females (OVX); OVX + estradiol (250-mg pellet, 21 days before use) (OVX + E)
5. Mature intact male controls (MMC); mature intact males + testosterone (MMT); castrated males (CAS); CAS + testosterone propionate (10 mg/day × 14 days) (CAS + T)
6. Mature ovariectomized females (OVX); mature ovariectomized females × 2 weeks, then + estradiol polyphosphate (1 mg/week for 1–8 weeks) (OVX + E)
7. Immature intact female controls (FIC); mature intact female controls (FMC); immature intact male controls (MIC); mature intact male controls (MMC)
8. Old intact female controls (FOC); old intact females + 17β-estradiol valerate (2 μg/week × 18 months) (FOE); mature ovariectomized females × 18 months (OVX); OVX + 17β-estradiol valerate (2 μg/week × 18 months) (OVX + E)
9. Mature intact female controls (FMC); mature ovariectomized females × 4 months (OVX); OVX + estradiol cypionate (100 mg/kg/month × 4 months) (OVX + E)
10. Mature intact female controls (FMC); mature intact male controls (MMC)

TABLE 4–3
Effects of Estrogens on Urethral Contractility

Ref	Treatment[a]	Response
100	1	↓ sensitivity to phenylephrine after OVX vs. FMC NC in sensitivity to phenylephrine after P or OVX + E vs. FMC
101	2	NC in sensitivity to norepinephrine after OVX vs. FMC ↑ sensitivity to norepinephrine after FME vs. FMC
102	3	Reduction of spontaneous activity after OVX + E vs. OVX NC in sensitivity or amplitude of response to phenylephrine after OVX vs. OVX + E NC in amplitude of response to acetylcholine after OVX vs. OVX + E
102	4	Reduction of spontaneous activity after OVX + E vs. OVX Enhanced response to phenylephrine after OVX + E vs. OVX ↑ sensitivity to phenylephrine after OVX + E vs. OVX
102	5	↑ sensitivity to phenylephrine after OVX + E vs. OVX
102	6	NC in contractile responses to hypogastric nerve stimulation, norepinephrine, phenylephrine, or isoproterenol of MMC vs. FMC
103	7	↑ amplitude of response to phenylephrine in MMC vs. FMC ↓ amplitude of response to clonidine in MMC vs. FMC

Abbreviations: NC, no change
[a]Treatment:
1. Mature intact female rabbits in natural estrus (FMC); mature ovariectomized females × 14 days (OVX); OVX + estradiol (1 μg/kg/day × 14 days) (OVX + E); pregnant (28 days' gestation) (P)
2. Mature intact female rabbit controls (FMC); mature ovariectomized females (OVX); mature intact females + polyestradiol phosphate (3 mg, 4–5 days before use) (FME)
3. Mature ovariectomized female rabbits × 8 days (OVX); OVX + stilbestrol (4 × 400 μg on alternate days) (OVX + E)
4. Female ovariectomized Tamar wallabies (OVX); OVX + estradiol (100 μg/day) (OVX + E)
5. Mature ovariectomized female dogs (OVX); OVX + stilbestrol (1 mg/day × 7 days) (OVX + E)
6. Mature intact male (MMC) and female (FMC) control rabbits
7. Mature intact male (MMC) and female (FMC) control rabbits

trus.[100] Estradiol treatment prevented the changes in sensitivity. There were no differences in contractile force. These are logical results: ovariectomy decreased sensitivity to phenylephrine, and this was prevented by hormone replacement. Larsson and co-workers, using a perfused urethra preparation, in which responses of circular and longitudinal muscles could be monitored simultaneously, found that poly-estradiol treatment of mature intact female rabbits increased their sensitivity to norepinephrine compared to age-matched controls.[101] Ovariectomy was previously shown to have no effects on sensitivity to norepinephrine. These findings are less easily explained. Because ovariectomy had no effects on contractility, the effects of estrogen treatment in this study are probably the result of supraphysiologic levels. To complete the confusion, Callahan and Creed found no change in sensitivity or maximal contraction of urethral strips from ovariectomized rabbits treated with stilbestrol to phenylephrine compared to ovariectomized controls and no change in response to acetylcholine.[102] However, without intact controls,

in this study it is impossible to tell whether ovariectomy alone altered the responses. In the same paper, Callahan and Creed reported that there were no differences between mature intact male and female rabbits in the responsiveness of the urethra to hypogastric nerve stimulation, norepinephrine, phenylephrine, or isoproterenol.[102] They also examined the influence of estrogen treatment on urethral preparations from female guinea pigs, wallabies, and dogs. As in rabbits, there were no differences in maximal responsiveness to phenylephrine of urethral strips from any of these species. However, there were significant increases in the sensitivity of strips from estrogen-treated wallabies and dogs compared to ovariectomized controls. Therefore, estrogen treatment seems to cause a tendency toward increased urethral sensitivity to alpha-adrenergic agonists. A more recent study examined the contractile responses of the proximal urethra from male and female rabbits to different alpha-adrenergic agonists.[103] The magnitude of the increase in urethral pressure in response to alpha-1 agonists was twofold

TABLE 4–4
Effects of Estrogens on Bladder Body Contractility

Ref	Treatment[a]	Response
16, 104	1	↑ contractile responses to epinephrine, methoxamine, bethanechol, ATP after FIE vs. FIC NC in responses to isoproterenol or KCl
95	2	↓ in sensitivity to field stimulation after OVX + E vs. OVX, NC in contractile response ↓ in contractile response to KCl after OVX + E vs. OVX NC in contractile response or sensitivity to carbachol after OVX + E vs. OVX
94	3	NC in contractile response or sensitivity to carbachol after CAS or CAS + T or MMT vs. MMC
105	4	NC in contractile responses to field stimulation, ATP, acetylcholine, or histamine after CAS vs. MMC
106	5	↓ contractile response and sensitivity to PGE$_1$ and PGE$_2$ after OVX vs. FMC ↑ contractile response and sensitivity to PGE$_1$ and PGE$_2$ after OVX + E vs. OVX
107	6	NC in in vivo contractile responses to hypogastric or pelvic nerve stimulation after OVX + E or OVX + P or OVX + EP vs. OVX
98	7	↓ contractile response to field stimulation, ATP, carbachol, KCl after OVX vs. FMC NC in contractile response to field stimulation, ATP, KCl; ↑ response to carbachol after OVX + E vs. FMC
108	8	NC in contractile response to field stimulation, ATP, KCl, carbachol after CAS vs. MMC ↓ contractile response to field stimulation, ATP after OVX vs. FMC NC in contractile response to carbachol, KCl after OVX vs. FMC
97	9	NC in contractile response to field stimulation after OVX or OVX + E or FOE vs. FOC
109	10	↓ contractile response to field stimulation, acetylcholine, carbachol after FME vs. FMC NC in contractile response to KCl or serotonin after FME vs. FMC

Abbreviations: NC, no change; KCl, potassium chloride
[a]Treatment:
1. Immature intact female control rabbits (FIC); immature females + estradiol (150 µg/kg twice daily × 4 days) (FIE)
2. Mature ovariectomized female rabbits (OVX); mature ovariectomized females × 2 weeks, then + estradiol polyphosphate (1 mg/week × 1–8 weeks) (OVX + E)
3. Mature intact male control rabbits (MMC); mature intact males + testosterone (MMT); castrated males (CAS); CAS + testosterone propionate (10 mg/day × 14 days) (CAS + T)
4. Mature intact male control hamsters (MMC); mature castrated males × 12 weeks (CAS)
5. Mature intact female control rats in natural estrus (FMC); mature ovariectomized females × 20 days (OVX); OVX + 17β-estradiol (50 µg/180–130 g animal) 24 hours before use (OVX + E)
6. Mature ovariectomized female rats (OVX); OVX × 21 days then + 17β-estradiol (50 µg/day × 4 days) (OVX + E); OVX + progesterone (2 mg/day × 4 days) (OVX + P); OVX + estradiol + progesterone (OVX + EP)
7. Mature intact female control rats (FMC); mature ovariectomized females × 4 months (OVX); OVX + estradiol cypionate (100 mg/kg/month × 4 months) (OVX + E)
8. Mature intact female control rats (FMC); mature ovariectomized females × 2 months (OVX); mature intact male rat controls (MMC); mature castrated males × 2 months (CAS)
9. Old intact female control rats (FOC); old intact females + 17β-estradiol valerate (2 µg/week × 19 months) (FOE); old ovariectomized females × 18 months (OVX); OVX + 17β-estradiol valerate (2 µg/week × 18 months) (OVX + E)
10. Mature intact female control rats (FMC); mature female rats in diestrus + estradiol benzoate (150 µg/kg twice daily × 8 days) (FME)

greater in males than in females, whereas the response to alpha-2 agonists was greater in females than in males. Alpha-1 agonists caused a rapid contraction, whereas the response to alpha-2 agonists was more gradual. The authors suggest that the slow, prolonged response to alpha-2 stimulation is important for the maintenance of continence in females.

HORMONES AND CONTRACTILE RESPONSES OF THE BLADDER

Studies examining the effects of hormone treatment on bladder contractile function have also produced conflicting results (Table 4–4). Short-term (4-day) high-dose treatment of immature female rabbits with estradiol caused increased contractile responses of bladder body strips to epinephrine, ATP, methoxamine, and bethanechol compared to immature intact controls.[16, 104] However, Batra and Andersson found no change in sensitivity or maximal contractile response to field stimulation or carbachol of bladder strips from female rabbits treated with estradiol polyphosphate for up to 8 weeks compared to ovariectomized controls.[95] Two studies examined the influence of castration of male animals on bladder contractility. Anderson and Navarro could find no differences in sensitivity or maximal responses of rabbit detrusor strips to carbachol or of bladder base to phenylephrine after castration or castration plus testosterone replacement.[94] Similarly, Belis and Longhurst found that castration had no influence on the contractile responsiveness of hamster bladder body to field stimulation, ATP, acetylcholine, or histamine.[105]

A few studies have also been done in rats. Borda and coworkers found a decreased maximal response and sensitivity of bladder body strips from 20-day ovariectomized female rats to prostaglandins E_2 and E_1 compared to those from rats in natural estrus.[106] No differences were found in responses to prostaglandin $F_{2\alpha}$. Sato and associates ovariectomized rats for 21 days before treating them with 17β-estradiol with and without progesterone for 4 days. Using an in vivo catheterized bladder preparation, they could find no effects of the treatments on the intravesical response to hypogastric or pelvic nerve stimulation.[107] Recent studies by Longhurst and colleagues found a decreased contractile responsiveness of bladder strips from ovariectomized rats to field stimulation and ATP after 2 months, and to field stimulation, carbachol, ATP, and potassium chloride after 4 months, suggesting that responses to ATP were more sensitive to the loss of sex hormones than were those to muscarinic agonists. The ovariectomy-induced changes were prevented by estradiol treatment.[98] No changes in bladder contractility were seen in males 2 months after orchiectomy.[108]

The only really long-term study reported in the literature found no difference in the contractile response of bladder body strips to field stimulation 18 months after ovariectomy or 10 months after ovariectomy followed by 8 months of estradiol treatment.[97] However, bladder strips from ovariectomized rats showed a greater atropine-sensitive portion (about 45%) of the response to field stimulation compared to intact controls (25%). This finding contrasts with the data of Elliott and coworkers, who examined the contractility of bladder strips from intact rats with and without in vivo estradiol treatment.[109] They found a decreased response to field stimulation, carbachol, and acetylcholine after estradiol treatment, and the atropine-sensitive portion of the response to field stimulation was reduced from approximately 20% in controls to zero in the estradiol-treated group. Whether these differences can be attributed to animal age or whether the duration of ovariectomy and treatment schedule are more important is not clear.

Two studies compared bladder micturition and strip contractility in age-matched male and female rats. Both Chun and associates, using 1- and 3-month-old rats,[96] and Longhurst and colleagues, using 6- and 24-month-old rats,[99] found that mature males consumed and excreted larger volumes of fluid than age-matched females and had larger bladders (Tables 4–5 and 4–6). No differences were found in

TABLE 4–5
General and Micturition Characteristics of 1- and 3-Month Sprague-Dawley Rats

	Immature (1 mo)		Mature (3 mo)	
	Male	Female	Male	Female
Body weight (g)	179 ± 10	170 ± 9	452 ± 11[a]	238 ± 6
Bladder weight (mg)	104 ± 5	102 ± 6	167 ± 11[a]	141 ± 8
Volume consumed per 24 hours (ml)	29.7 ± 2.7	32.7 ± 1.2	53.4 ± 4.5[a]	31.2 ± 2.3
Volume excreted per 24 hours (ml)	4.2 ± 0.7	6.3 ± 1.1	16.0 ± 1.7[a]	7.4 ± 1.4
Number of micturitions per 24 hours	11.9 ± 1.6	14.2 ± 2.7	18.8 ± 1.0	13.0 ± 2.1
Mean micturition volume (ml)	0.38 ± 0.03	0.46 ± 0.03	0.85 ± 0.08[a]	0.57 ± 0.04
In vitro bladder capacity (ml)	1.02 ± 0.16	1.12 ± 0.13	1.53 ± 0.11	1.48 ± 0.10

Each point represents the mean ± SEM of seven to 10 individual observations.
[a] $p < .05$ (vs. females at same age)
Modified from Chun AL, Wein AJ, Harkaway R, Levin RM: Comparison of urinary bladder function in sexually mature and immature male and female rats. J Urol 143:1267, 1990.

TABLE 4–6
General and Micturition Characteristics of 6- and 24-Month Fischer 344 Rats

	6 Month		24 Month	
	Male	Female	Male	Female
Body weight (g)	363 ± 3[a]	201 ± 5	402 ± 9[a]	272 ± 7
Bladder weight (mg)	95.7 ± 5.1[a]	71.6 ± 3.5	120.1 ± 5.5[a]	86.6 ± 1.2
(mg/kg body weight)	(255.4 ± 15.6[a])	(350.2 ± 20.6)	(214.7 ± 13.3)	(318.0 ± 3.8)
Volume consumed per 24 hours (ml)	23.7 ± 1.1[a]	18.1 ± 1.2	19.6 ± 1.3	16.5 ± 1.8
(ml/kg body weight)	(65.4 ± 3.1[a])	(90.4 ± 7.0)	(48.9 ± 3.6)	(60.7 ± 6.5)
Volume excreted per 24 hours (ml)	9.1 ± 0.6	6.6 ± 0.5	10.2 ± 1.0[a]	6.9 ± 1.8
(ml/kg body weight)	(25.0 ± 1.7)	(32.8 ± 2.7)	(25.2 ± 2.2)	(25.1 ± 4.2)
Number of micturitions per 24 hours				
During light cycle	3.4 ± 0.4[b]	3.7 ± 0.5†	3.7 ± 0.7	3.6 ± 0.6[b]
During dark cycle	8.3 ± 0.8	8.4 ± 0.9	4.7 ± 0.5[a]	8.3 ± 0.8
Mean micturition volume (ml)				
During light cycle	0.92 ± 0.11	0.63 ± 0.04	1.32 ± 0.11[a]	0.73 ± 0.12[a]
During dark cycle	0.67 ± 0.07	0.44 ± 0.03	1.29 ± 0.15[a]	0.58 ± 0.06
Maximal micturition volume (ml)				
During light cycle	1.24 ± 0.09	0.87 ± 0.04	1.88 ± 0.21[a]	1.00 ± 0.14
During dark cycle	1.11 ± 0.15	0.92 ± 0.06	1.81 ± 0.16[a]	1.00 ± 0.13

Each point represents the mean ± SEM of seven or eight individual observations
Light cycle 07:00 to 19:00, dark cycle 19:00 to 07:00
[a] $p < .05$ (vs. females at same age)
[b] $p < .05$ (vs. dark cycle)
Modified from Longhurst PA, Kauer J, Leggett RE, Levin RM: The influence of ovariectomy and estradiol replacement on urinary bladder function in rats. J Urol 148:915, 1992.

immature males and females.[96] However, although 3-month males excreted twice as much urine and had a significantly increased micturition volume compared to age-matched females, there were no differences in in vitro bladder capacity.[96] Both studies found increased contractile responsiveness of strips from age-matched males compared to females. However, Longhurst and colleagues attributed those differences to the larger mass of the bladder strips from the males.

PREGNANCY AND THE BLADDER

Perhaps the best example of the ways in which hormonal alterations can affect bladder function, physi-

ology, and pharmacology is the changes that accompany pregnancy. There is no doubt that pregnancy increases micturition frequency. Even in rabbits, micturition frequency increases during pregnancy (Fig. 4–4). In studies comparing age-matched virgin and pregnant rabbits there were no differences in maximal response of isolated bladder strips to field stimulation (Fig. 4–5).[110] However, the relative contributions of the cholinergic and purinergic components were altered substantially (Fig. 4–6). The maximal response of the bladder body to cholinergic stimula-

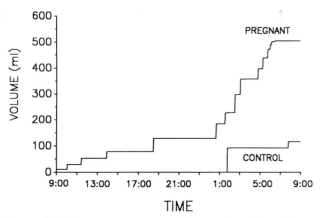

Figure 4–4 Representative trace showing the effects of pregnancy (day 21 of gestation) on micturition in age-matched rabbits. Light cycle 07:00 to 19:00.

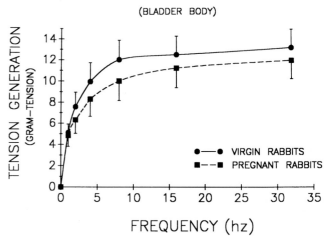

Figure 4–5 Effects of pregnancy on the contractile response to field stimulation. Each point represents the mean ± SEM of four to six individual observations. (From Tong Y-C, Wein AJ, Levin RM: Effects of pregnancy on adrenergic function in the rabbit urinary bladder. Neurourol Urodyn 11:525, 1992. Reprinted by permission of John Wiley & Sons, Inc.)

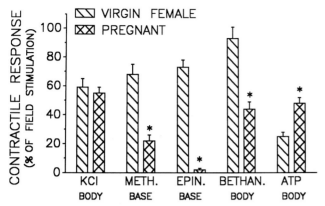

Figure 4–6 Effects of pregnancy on the contractile response to potassium chloride, methoxamine, epinephrine, bethanechol, and ATP. Each bar represents the mean ± SEM of four to six individual observations. *Significantly different from virgin female at $p < .05$.

tion was decreased by approximately 50%, and the maximal response to purinergic stimulation was increased by approximately 50% (see Fig. 4–6). Furthermore, the ability of isolated whole bladders from pregnant rabbits to empty in response to field stimulation, a function of cholinergic stimulation,[10] was decreased significantly (Fig. 4–7). The decreased response of the bladders from pregnant rabbits to cholinergic stimulation was associated with a significant decrease in muscarinic cholinergic receptor density.[111] The second major observation from these studies was that pregnancy resulted in a significant decrease in the response of isolated strips of bladder base (see Fig. 4–6) and urethra to alpha-adrenergic stimulation.[111–113] A decrease in the muscarinic responsiveness of the bladder body would be consistent with an increase in urine retention, whereas a decrease in the alpha-adrenergic response of the bladder base would be consistent with an increase in stress incontinence, both of which are associated clinically with pregnancy.

In other studies, the changes in hormone levels associated with pregnancy in rabbits (twenty-eighth day of gestation) were shown to increase the contractile response of bladder body strips to phenylephrine compared to natural estrus, causing an increase in sensitivity.[100] One study could find no influence of

pregnancy on in vivo bladder responses to hypogastric or pelvic nerve stimulation in rats.[107]

HORMONES AND AUTONOMIC RECEPTORS

Many studies have examined the changes that occur in autonomic receptors in the lower urinary tract after ovariectomy or estrogen treatment. Again, like the data on contractility, the results are conflicting, although all studies agree unanimously that there are no changes in the affinity of autonomic ligands for the different receptor types. In the rabbit urethra, polyestradiol treatment of mature female rabbits causes an increase in the density of alpha receptors,[101] but estradiol treatment of immature females has no effect on the density of alpha, beta, or muscarinic receptors of the rabbit base.[16, 104] Similarly, Shapiro could find no influence of ovariectomy or estradiol treatment on muscarinic receptor density of the female rabbit urethra/base compared to mature intact controls (Table 4–7).[17]

Three separate studies of autonomic receptors in the rabbit bladder show conflicting results (see Table 4–7). Levin and colleagues found that estradiol treatment of immature female rabbits caused an increase in bladder body alpha and muscarinic receptor densities but no change in beta receptor density.[16, 104] However, Shapiro found no change in bladder muscarinic receptor density after ovariectomy and a decrease after ovariectomy plus estradiol treatment.[17] Two weeks after ovariectomy of rabbits Batra and Andersson treated them with estradiol polyphosphate.[95] One week after ovariectomy decreases in muscarinic receptor density became evident and were not reversed by estradiol treatment.

Summary

The contractile responses of urinary bladder body, base, and urethra strips of sexually immature male and female animals to pharmacologic stimulation are qualitatively similar. In association with the hormonal changes that accompany sexual maturity, autonomic receptor density and distribution and con-

Figure 4–7 Effects of pregnancy on the ability of field stimulation and bethanechol to empty the isolated in vitro rabbit whole bladder.[111] Bladders were filled with 20 ml of saline before the response to 32-Hz field stimulation or 500-μM bethanechol was measured. Each bar represents the mean ± SEM of five to seven individual observations. *Significantly different from virgin female at $p < .05$. (From Levin RM, Zderic SA, Ewalt DH, et al: Effects of pregnancy on muscarinic receptor density and function in the rabbit urinary bladder. Pharmacology 43:69, 1991, with permission from S. Karger AG, Basel.)

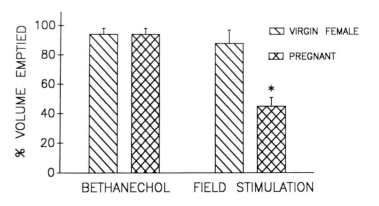

TABLE 4–7
**Influence of Hormones on Autonomic Receptor Density in
the Rabbit Bladder**

Ref	Treatment[a]	Tissue	α	β	Muscarinic
101	1	Urethra	↑ α_2 after FME vs. FMC	ND	ND
17	2	Urethra	ND	ND	NC after OVX or OVX + E vs. FMC
113	3	Urethra	↓ α_1 after CAS or CAS + E vs. MMC ↑ α_2 after CAS or CAS + E vs. MMC	NC after CAS or CAS + E vs. MMC	↓ after CAS or CAS + E vs. MMC
16, 104	4	Bladder	↑ α after FIE vs. FIC	NC after FIE vs. FIC	↑ after FIE vs. FIC
17	2	Bladder	ND	ND	NC after OVX or OVX + E vs. FMC
94	5	Bladder	↓ after CAS vs. MMC NC after MMT or CAS + T vs. MMC	NC after CAS or CAS + T or MMT vs. MMC	NC after CAS vs. MMC ↑ after CAS + T or MMT vs. MMC
95	6	Bladder	ND	ND	↓ after OVX + E vs. OVX

Abbreviations: ND, not determined; NC, no change

[a]Treatment:
1. Mature intact female controls (FMC); mature intact females + polyestradiol phosphate (3 mg, 4–5 days before use) (FME)
2. Mature intact female controls (FMC); ovariectomized females (OVX); OVX + estradiol (250-mg pellet, 21 days before use) (OVX + E)
3. Mature intact male controls (MMC); castrated males (CAS); CAS + estradiol (5 mg/kg Premarin, 3 × week for 6–8 weeks) (CAS + E)
4. Immature intact female controls (FIC); immature females + estradiol (150 µg/kg twice daily × 4 days) (FIE)
5. Mature intact male controls (MMC); mature intact males + testosterone (MMT); castrated males (CAS); CAS + testosterone propionate (10 mg/day × 14 days) (CAS + T)
6. Mature ovariectomized female controls (OVX); mature ovariectomized females × 2 weeks, then + estradiol polyphosphate (1 mg/week × 1–8 weeks) (OVX + E)

tractile responsiveness of the urinary bladder and urethra of the female are altered. These autonomic functions are again modulated during pregnancy in association with the alterations in circulating hormones. The physician should keep these points in mind when prescribing a therapeutic drug that acts by either activating or blocking specific autonomic receptors of the bladder body, base, or urethra.

REFERENCES

1. Mundy AR: Structure and function of the lower urinary tract. *In* Mundy AR (ed): Scientific Basis of Urology. New York, Churchill Livingstone, 1987, pp 48–73.
2. Wein AJ, Levin RM, Barrett DM: Voiding function: Relevant anatomy, physiology, and pharmacology. *In* Gillenwater JY, Grayhack JT, Howards SS, Duckett JD (eds): Adult and Pediatric Urology, 2nd ed. Chicago, Year Book, 1991, pp 933–999.
3. Sterling AM, Ritter RC, Zinner NR: The physical basis of obstructive uropathy. *In* Hinman F Jr (ed): Benign Prostatic Hypertrophy. New York, Springer-Verlag, 1983, pp 433–442.
4. Wein AJ, Raezer DM: Physiology of micturition. *In* Krane RJ, Siroky MB (eds): Clinical Neurourology. Boston, Little, Brown, 1979, pp 1–33.
5. Levin RM, Longhurst PA, Monson FC, et al: Effect of bladder outlet obstruction on the morphology, physiology, and pharmacology of the bladder. Prostate Suppl 3:9, 1990.
6. Hathaway DR, Konicki MV, Coolical SA: Phosphorylation of myosin light chain kinase from vascular smooth muscle by cAMP- and cGMP-dependent protein kinases. J Mol Cell Cardiol 17:841, 1985.
7. Kamm KE, Leachman SA, Michnoff CH, et al: Myosin light chain kinases and kinetics of myosin phosphorylation in smooth muscle cells. *In* Siegman MJ, Somlyo AP, Stephens NL (eds): Regulation and Contraction of Smooth Muscle. New York, Alan R. Liss, 1987, pp 183–194.
8. Stull JT, Kamm KE, Taylor DA: Calcium control of smooth muscle contraction. Am J Med Sci 31:241, 1988.
9. Ebashi S, Mikawa T, Kuwayama H, et al: Calcium regulation in smooth muscle. *In* Siegman MJ, Somlyo AP, Stephens NL (eds): Regulation and Contraction of Smooth Muscle. New York, Alan R. Liss, 1987, pp 109–118.
10. Levin RM, Ruggieri MR, Wein AJ: Functional effects of the purinergic innervation of the rabbit urinary bladder. J Pharmacol Exp Ther 236:452, 1986.
11. Levin RM, Wein AJ: Response of the in-vitro whole bladder (rabbit) preparation to autonomic agonists. J Urol 128:1087, 1982.
12. Levin RM, Hypolite J, Ruggieri MR, et al: Effects of muscarinic stimulation on intracellular calcium in the rabbit bladder: Comparison with metabolic response. Pharmacology 39:69, 1989.
13. Kato K, Wein AJ, Kitada S, et al: The functional effect of mild outlet obstruction on the rabbit urinary bladder. J Urol 140:880, 1988.
14. Kato K, Wein AJ, Longhurst PA, et al: The functional effects of long-term outlet obstruction on the rabbit urinary bladder. J Urol 143:600, 1990.
15. Batra SW, Iosif CS: Female urethra: A target for estrogen action. J Urol 129:418, 1983.
16. Levin RM, Shofer FS, Wein AJ: Estrogen-induced alterations in the autonomic responses of the rabbit urinary bladder. J Pharmacol Exp Ther 215:614, 1980.
17. Shapiro E: Effect of estrogens on the weight and muscarinic cholinergic receptor density of the rabbit bladder and urethra. J Urol 135:1084, 1986.
18. Huszar G, Roberts JM: Biochemistry and pharmacology of the myometrium and labor: Regulation at the cellular and molecular levels. Am J Obstet Gynecol 142:225, 1982.
19. Varol FG, Hadjiconstantinou M, Zuspan FP, Neff NH: Gestational alterations in phospholipase C coupled muscarinic response. Life Sci 45:1739, 1989.
20. Andriole VT: Urinary tract in pregnancy. Urol Clin North Am 2:285, 1975.
21. Waltzer WC: The urinary tract in pregnancy. J Urol 125:271, 1981.
22. Stanton SL, Kerr-Wilson R, Harris VG: The incidence of

urological symptoms in normal pregnancy. Br J Obstet Gynaecol 87:897, 1980.

23. Roberts JM, Insel PA, Goldfien RD, Goldfien A: Alpha receptors but not beta receptors increase in rabbit uterus with oestrogen. Nature 270:624, 1977.

24. Raz S, Zeigler M, Caine M: The effect of progesterone on the adrenergic receptors of the urethra. Br J Urol 45:131, 1973.

25. Qayyum MA, Fatani JA, Abbas MO: Degeneration of adrenergic nerves in the urinary bladder during pregnancy. Acta Anat 136:303, 1989.

26. Guyton AC: Textbook of Medical Physiology, 7th ed. Philadelphia, WB Saunders, 1986, pp 120–135, 136–149, 686–696.

27. Burnstock G: Evolution of the autonomic innervation of visceral and cardiovascular systems in vertebrates. Pharmacol Rev 21:247, 1969.

28. Burnstock G: Purinergic nerves. Pharmacol Rev 24:509, 1972.

29. Burnstock G, Dumsday B, Smythe A: Atropine resistant excitation of the urinary bladder: The possibility of transmission via nerves releasing a purine nucleotide. Br J Pharmacol 44:451, 1972.

30. Lundberg JM, Hokfelt T: Coexistence of peptides and classical neurotransmitters. Trends Neurosci 6:325, 1983.

31. Sjögren C, Andersson K-E, Husted S, et al: Atropine resistance of transmurally stimulated isolated human bladder muscle. J Urol 128:1368, 1982.

32. Luheshi GN, Zar MA: Presence of non-cholinergic motor transmission in human isolated bladder. J Pharm Pharmacol 42:223, 1990.

33. Krell RD, McCoy JL, Ridley PT: Pharmacological characterization of the excitatory innervation to the guinea-pig urinary bladder in vitro: Evidence for both cholinergic and non-adrenergic-non-cholinergic neurotransmission. Br J Pharmacol 74:15, 1981.

34. Cowan WD, Daniel EE: Human female bladder and its non-cholinergic contractile function. Can J Physiol Pharmacol 61:1236, 1983.

35. Downie JW, Dean DM: The contribution of cholinergic postganglionic neurotransmission to contractions of rabbit detrusor. J Pharmacol Exp Ther 203:417, 1977.

36. Langley JN, Anderson HK: The innervation of the pelvic and adjoining viscera. IV. The internal generative organs. J Physiol 19:122, 1885.

37. Langley JN: On inhibitory fibers in the vagus for the end of the oesophagus and the stomach. J Physiol 23:407, 1898.

38. Burnstock G, Campbell G, Rand MJ: The inhibitory innervation of the taenia of the guinea-pig caecum. J Physiol 182:504, 1966.

39. Campbell G, Burnstock G: Comparative physiology of gastrointestinal motility. In American Physiological Society: Handbook of Physiology. Section 6, Alimentary Canal; IV, Motility. Washington, American Physiological Society, 1968, pp 2213–2266.

40. Burnstock G: Past and current evidence for the purinergic nerve hypothesis. In Baer HP, Drummond GI (eds): Physiological and Regulatory Functions of Adenine Nucleotides. New York, Raven Press, 1979, pp 3–32.

41. Campbell G: Autonomic nervous supply to effector tissues. In Bulbring E, Brading A, Tomita T (eds): Smooth Muscle. London, Edward Arnold, 1970, pp 451–495.

42. Furness JB, Costa M: The nervous release and the actions of substances which affect intestinal muscle through neither adrenoceptors nor cholinoceptors. Recent developments in vertebrate smooth muscle physiology. Philos Trans R Soc 265:123, 1973.

43. Longhurst PA, Belis JA, O'Donnell JP, et al: A study of the atropine-resistant component of the neurogenic response of the rabbit urinary bladder. Eur J Pharmacol 99:295, 1984.

44. Theobald RJ: The effect of arylazido aminopropionyl ATP on atropine resistant contractions of the cat urinary bladder. Life Sci 32:2479, 1983.

45. Brading AF, Williams JH: Contractile responses of smooth muscle strips from rat and guinea-pig urinary bladder to transmural stimulation: Effects of atropine and α,β-methylene ATP. Br J Pharmacol 99:493, 1990.

46. Westfall D, Fedan JS, Colby J, et al: Evidence for a contribution by purines to the neurogenic response of the guinea-pig bladder. Eur J Pharmacol 87:415, 1983.

47. Brading A: Physiology of bladder smooth muscle. In Torrens M, Morrison JFB (eds): The Physiology of the Lower Urinary Tract. New York, Springer-Verlag, 1987, pp 161–192.

48. Klarskov P, Gerstenberg TC, Ramirez D, Hald T: Non-cholinergic, non-adrenergic nerve mediated relaxation of trigone, bladder neck and urethral smooth muscle in vitro. J Urol 129:848, 1983.

49. Klarskov P, Horby-Petersen J: Influence of serotonin on lower urinary tract smooth muscle in vitro. Br J Urol 58:507, 1986.

50. Levin RM, Shofer F, Wein AJ: Cholinergic, adrenergic, and purinergic response of sequential strips of rabbit urinary bladder. J Pharmacol Exp Ther 212:536, 1980.

51. Levin RM, Wein AJ: Distribution and function of adrenergic receptors in the urinary bladder of the rabbit. Mol Pharmacol 16:441, 1979.

52. Downie JW, Dean DM, Carro-Ciampi G, Awad SA: A difference in sensitivity to alpha-adrenergic agonists exhibited by detrusor and bladder neck of the rabbit. Can J Physiol Pharmacol 53:525, 1975.

53. Dean DM, Downie JW: Contribution of adrenergic and purinergic neurotransmission to contraction in rabbit detrusor. J Pharmacol Exp Ther 207:431, 1978.

54. Hoffman BB, Lefkowitz RJ: Agonist interactions with alpha-adrenergic receptors. J Cardiovasc Pharmacol 4:S14, 1982.

55. Lavin TN, Hoffman BB, Lefkowitz RJ: Determination of subtype selectivity of alpha-adrenergic antagonists. Mol Pharmacol 20:28, 1981.

56. Neve KA, McGonigle P, Molinoff PB: Quantitative analysis of the selectivity of radioligands for subtypes of beta adrenergic receptors. J Pharmacol Exp Ther 238:46, 1986.

57. Liang BT, Molinoff PB: Beta-adrenergic receptor subtypes in the atria: Evidence for close coupling of beta-1 and beta-2 adrenergic receptors to adenylate cyclase. J Pharmacol Exp Ther 238:886, 1986.

58. Gil DW, Wolfe BB: Pirenzepine distinguishes between muscarinic receptor mediated phosphoinositide breakdown and inhibition of adenylate cyclase. J Pharmacol Exp Ther 232:608, 1985.

59. Levin RM, Ruggieri MR, Wein AJ: Identification of receptor subtypes in the rabbit and human urinary bladder. J Urol 139:844, 1988.

60. Ueda S, Satake N, Shibata S: Alpha-1 and alpha-2 adrenoceptors in the smooth muscle of isolated rabbit urinary bladder and urethra. Eur J Pharmacol 103:249, 1984.

61. Tsujimoto G, Timmins PV, Hoffman BB: Alpha-adrenergic receptors in the rabbit bladder base smooth muscle: Alpha-1 adrenergic receptors mediate contractile responses. J Pharmacol Exp Ther 236:384, 1986.

62. Honda K, Osawa AM, Takenaka T: Alpha-1 adrenoceptor subtype mediating contraction of smooth muscle in the lower urinary tract and prostate of rabbits. Naunyn Schmiedebergs Arch Pharmacol 330:16, 1985.

63. Kunisawa Y, Kawabe K, Niijima T, et al: A pharmacological study of alpha adrenergic receptor subtypes in smooth muscle of human urinary bladder base and prostatic urethra. J Urol 134:396, 1985.

64. Anderson GF, Marks BH: Beta adrenoreceptors in the rabbit bladder detrusor muscle. J Pharmacol Exp Ther 228:283, 1984.

65. Morita T, Kondo S, Tsuchida S, Weiss RM: Characterization of functional beta adrenoceptor subtypes in rabbit urinary bladder smooth muscle. Tohoku J Exp Med 149:389, 1986.

66. Hulme EC, Birdsall MJM, Buckley NJ: Muscarinic receptor subtypes. Annu Rev Pharmacol Toxicol 30:633, 1990.

67. Nilvebrant L, Sparf B: Dicyclomine, benzhexol and oxybutynin distinguish between subclasses of muscarinic binding sites. Eur J Pharmacol 123:133, 1986.

68. Noronha-Blob L, Kachur JF: Enantiomers of oxybutynin: In vitro pharmacological characterization at M_1, M_2 and M_3 muscarinic receptors and in vivo effects on urinary bladder contraction, mydriasis and salivary secretion in guinea pigs. J Pharmacol Exp Ther 256:562, 1990.

69. Levine RR, Birdsall NJM (eds): Subtypes of muscarinic receptors. Proceedings of the 4th International Symposium on Subtypes of Muscarinic Receptors. Trends Pharmacol Sci Suppl 1–119, 1989.

70. Bonner TI: The molecular basis of muscarinic receptor diversity. Trends Neurosci 12:148, 1989.

71. Frielle T, Kobilka B, Lefkowitz RJ, Caron MG: Human beta$_1$- and beta$_2$-adrenergic receptors: Structurally and functionally related receptors derived from distinct genes. Trends Neurosci 11:321, 1988.

72. Emorine LJ, Marullo S, Briend-Sutren M-M, et al: Molecular characterization of the human beta$_3$-adrenergic receptor. Science 245:1118, 1989.

73. Triggle DJ: Calcium channel drugs: Antagonists and activators. ISI Atlas of Science. Pharmacology 1:319, 1987.

74. Cook NS: The pharmacology of potassium channels and their therapeutic potential. Trends Pharmacol Sci 9:21, 1988.

75. Batra S, Sjögren C, Andersson K-E, Fovaeus M: Source of calcium for contractions induced by depolarization and muscarinic receptor stimulation in rabbit urinary bladder. Acta Physiol Scand 130:545, 1987.

76. Mostwin JL: Receptor operated intracellular calcium stores in the smooth muscles of the guinea pig bladder. J Urol 133:905, 1985.

77. Bhat MB, Mishra SK, Raviprakash V: Differential susceptibility of cholinergic and noncholinergic neurogenic response to calcium channel blockers and low Ca^{++} medium in rat urinary bladder. Br J Pharmacol 86:837, 1989.

78. Yousif FB, Bolger GT, Ruzycky A, Triggle DJ: Ca^{2+} channel antagonist actions in bladder smooth muscle: Comparative pharmacologic and [^{3}H]nifedipine binding studies. Can J Physiol Pharmacol 63:453, 1985.

79. Zhao Y, Wein AJ, Levin RM: Role of calcium in mediating the biphasic contraction of the rabbit urinary bladder. Gen Pharmacol 24:727, 1993.

80. Maggi CA, Manzini S, Parlani M, et al: The effects of nifedipine on spontaneous, drug-induced and reflexly activated contractions of the rat urinary bladder: Evidence for the participation of an intracellular calcium store to micturition contraction. Gen Pharmacol 19:73, 1988.

81. Rud T, Andersson K-E, Ulmsten U: Effects of nifedipine in women with unstable bladders. Urol Int 34:421, 1979.

82. Andersson K-E, Forman A: Effects of calcium channel blockers on urinary tract smooth muscle. Acta Pharmacol Toxicol 58 (Suppl 2):193, 1986.

83. Andersson K-E, Andersson P-O, Fovaeus M, et al: Effects of pinacidil on bladder muscle. Drugs 36(Suppl 7):41, 1988.

84. Malmgren A, Andersson K-E, Sjögren C, Andersson PO: Effects of pinacidil and cromakalim (BRL 34915) on bladder function in rats with detrusor instability. J Urol 142:1134, 1989.

85. Levin RM, Hayes L, Zhao Y, Wein AJ: The effect of pinacidil on spontaneous and evoked contractile activity. Pharmacology 45:1, 1992.

86. Fujii K, Foster CD, Brading AF, Parekh AB: Potassium channel blockers and the effects of cromakalim on the smooth muscle of the guinea-pig bladder. Br J Pharmacol 99:779, 1990.

87. Andersson K-E, Mattiasson A: Lack of effect of pinacidil on detrusor instability in men with bladder outlet obstruction (abstract). J Urol 143:369A, 1990.

88. Levin RM, Hayes L, Eika B, et al: Comparative autonomic responses of the cat and rabbit bladder and urethra. J Urol 148:216, 1992.

89. Andersson K-E, Pascual AG, Persson K, et al: Electrically induced, nerve-mediated relaxation of rabbit urethra involves nitric oxide. J Urol 147:253, 1992.

90. Dokita S, Morgan WR, Wheeler MA, et al: N^G-nitro-L-arginine inhibits non-adrenergic, non-cholinergic relaxation in rabbit urethral smooth muscle. Life Sci 48:2429, 1991.

91. Persson K, Igawa Y, Mattiasson A, Andersson K-E: Effects of inhibition of the L-arginine/nitric oxide pathway in the rat lower urinary tract in vivo and in vitro. Br J Pharmacol 107:178, 1992.

92. Batra S, Bjellin L, Iosif S, et al: Effect of oestrogen and progesterone on the blood flow in the lower urinary tract of the rabbit. Acta Physiol Scand 123:191, 1985.

93. Batra S, Bjellin L, Sjögren C, et al: Increases in blood flow of the female rabbit urethra following low dose estrogens. J Urol 136:1360, 1986.

94. Anderson GF, Navarro SP: The response of autonomic receptors to castration and testosterone in the urinary bladder of the rabbit. J Urol 140:885, 1988.

95. Batra S, Andersson K-E: Oestrogen-induced changes in muscarinic receptor density and contractile responses in the female rabbit urinary bladder. Acta Physiol Scand 137:135, 1989.

96. Chun AL, Wein AJ, Harkaway R, Levin RM: Comparison of urinary bladder function in sexually mature and immature male and female rats. J Urol 143:1267, 1990.

97. Eika B, Salling LN, Christensen LL, et al: Long-term observation of the detrusor smooth muscle in rats. Its relationship to ovariectomy and estrogen treatment. Urol Res 18:439, 1990.

98. Longhurst PA, Kauer J, Leggett RE, Levin RM: The influence of ovariectomy and estradiol replacement on urinary bladder function in rats. J Urol 148:915, 1992.

99. Longhurst PA, Eika B, Leggett RE, Levin RM: Comparison of urinary bladder function in 6 and 24 month male and female rats. J Urol 148:1615, 1992.

100. Hodgson BJ, Dumas S, Bolling DR, Heesch CM: Effect of estrogen on sensitivity of rabbit bladder and urethra to phenylephrine. Invest Urol 16:67, 1978.

101. Larsson B, Andersson K-E, Batra S, et al: Effects of estradiol on norepinephrine-induced contraction, *alpha* adrenoceptor number and norepinephrine content in the female rabbit urethra. J Pharmacol Exp Ther 229:557, 1984.

102. Callahan SM, Creed KE: The effects of oestrogens on spontaneous activity and responses to phenylephrine of the mammalian urethra. J Physiol 358:35, 1985.

103. Yamaguchi T, Kitada S, Osada Y: Role of adrenoceptors in the proximal urethral function of female and male rabbits using an in vivo model of isovolumetric pressure generation. Neurourol Urodyn 12:49, 1993.

104. Levin RM, Jakobowitz D, Wein AJ: Autonomic innervation of rabbit urinary bladder following estrogen treatment. Urology 17:449, 1981.

105. Belis JA, Longhurst PA: Hormonal influence on the neurogenic response of the hamster vas deferens. J Urol 133:729, 1985.

106. Borda E, Chaud M, Gutnisky R, et al: Relationships between prostaglandins and estrogens on the motility of isolated rings from the rat urinary bladder. J Urol 129:1250, 1983.

107. Sato S, Hayashi RH, Garfield RE: Mechanical responses of the rat uterus, cervix, and bladder to stimulation of hypogastric and pelvic nerves in vivo. Biol Reprod 40:209, 1989.

108. Eika B, Levin RM, Longhurst PA: Modulation of urinary bladder function by sex hormones in streptozotocin-diabetic rats. J Urol 152:537, 1994.

109. Elliott RA, Castleden CM, Miodrag A: The effect of in vivo oestrogen pretreatment on the contractile response of rat isolated detrusor muscle. Br J Pharmacol 107:766, 1992.

110. Tong Y-C, Wein AJ, Levin RM: Effects of pregnancy on adrenergic function in the rabbit urinary bladder. Neurourol Urodyn 11:525, 1992.

111. Levin RM, Zderic SA, Ewalt DH, et al: Effects of pregnancy on muscarinic receptor density and function in the rabbit urinary bladder. Pharmacology 43:69, 1991.

112. Zderic SA, Plzak JE, Duckett JW, et al: Effect of pregnancy on rabbit urinary bladder physiology. 1. Effects of extracellular calcium. Pharmacology 41:124, 1990.

113. Morita T, Tsuchiya N, Tsujii T, Kondo S: Changes of autonomic receptors following castration and estrogen administration in the male rabbit urethral smooth muscle. Tohoku J Exp Med 166:403, 1992.

CHAPTER 5

Anatomy and Pathophysiology of Pelvic Support

Gregory R. Wahle, M.D.
George P. H. Young, M.D.
Shlomo Raz, M.D.

Women who experience significant changes in support of the pelvic floor often present with primary complaints related to urinary function. Although the mechanisms of urinary continence remain incompletely understood, several basic factors are known to act in concert to maintain normal urinary control in women. These include adequate bladder wall compliance to allow filling and low-pressure storage of urine in the bladder, and outlet resistance that is sufficient to prevent unintended leakage of urine. Causes of urinary incontinence related to the bladder, including processes that result in uninhibited detrusor activity or loss of normal compliance, are discussed in detail in other chapters of this book. Urinary incontinence related to the bladder outlet is more prevalent by far in women than in men,[1] in whom it is most commonly related to surgical damage or neurogenic alterations. Clinically significant incontinence in women most commonly is outlet-related and results from compromised anatomic support of the bladder neck and proximal urethra, which leads to stress urinary leakage.[2-4] In addition, the forces involved in the pathophysiology of stress urinary incontinence in women generally are not limited in their effects to the bladder outlet alone but result in other associated manifestations of deficiencies of pelvic support, including cystocele, uterine prolapse, enterocele, and rectocele.[5]

Clinicians involved in the care of women should possess a clear conceptual understanding of the anatomy and pathophysiology of pelvic support to evaluate and treat disorders of pelvic floor relaxation effectively. This chapter provides a basic review of the anatomy and musculofascial support of major pelvic structures and discusses their importance in clinically significant disorders of pelvic prolapse.

Anatomy of Pelvic Support

BLADDER

The bladder is a hollow muscular pelvic organ, for the purposes of study usually divided into three anatomic layers—the inner mucosa, the middle smooth muscle detrusor, and the outer adventitia consisting of fat and connective tissue. The mucosa consists of transitional cell epithelium and is continuous with the epithelium of the proximal urethra and both ureters. The muscular middle layer of the bladder is composed of a smooth muscle mesh, occasionally described as having three layers—the outlet, or bladder neck, the inner and outer longitudinal layer, and the middle circular layer[6] (Fig. 5–1). The function and innervation of the bladder are better understood if the structure of the bladder is thought of in terms of two divisions, the *body* and the *trigone*. The body of the bladder is primarily involved in compliant distention during gradual ureteral filling from the ureters, resulting in low-pressure filling and storage of urine and the generation of efficient detrusor muscle contraction during voiding. The trigone is a triangular region extending from the floor to apex of the bladder formed by both ureteral orifices and the bladder outlet. It has an embryologic origin different from that of the body of the bladder and has two muscular layers, superficial and deep, separate from the detrusor. The deep layer is a continuation of the fibromuscular outer layer, sometimes called *Waldeyer's sheath*, of the distal ureters, and the superficial layer is an extension of the inner ureteral musculature. The muscular layers of the trigone also continue distally into the posterior aspect of the proximal ure-

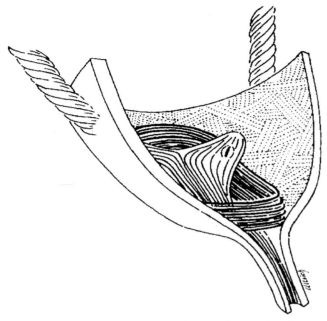

Figure 5-1 Schematic coronal section of the bladder showing circular orientation of detrusor muscle fibers at the bladder neck, and continuation of the apical trigonal musculature into the posterior urethra. (From Blaivas JG: Urodynamic testing. *In* Raz S [ed]: Female Urology. Philadelphia, WB Saunders, 1983, p 81.)

thra.[7] The bladder is richly innervated by the autonomic nervous system (Fig. 5–2). Cholinergic receptors from postganglionic parasympathetic fibers and beta-adrenergic receptors from postganglionic sympathetic fibers predominate in the body of the bladder, and alpha-adrenergic receptors from the

sympathetic system predominate in the trigone and proximal urethra.[8]

URETHRA

In the female, the urethra consists of a 4-cm tube of inner epithelium (transitional cell at the bladder neck and squamous cell at the meatus) and outer muscularis, including both smooth muscle in continuity with the trigonal musculature and striated muscle oriented circularly, particularly in the middle third.[9] The infolded epithelium is enclosed by a rich vascular sponge, which in turn is surrounded by a coat of smooth muscle and fibroelastic tissue (Fig. 5–3). The submucosa, consisting of loosely woven connective tissue scattered throughout with smooth muscle bundles and an elaborate vascular plexus,

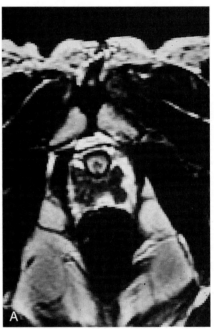

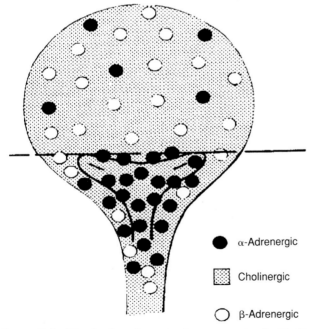

Figure 5-2 Distribution of autonomic receptors in the bladder and proximal urethra. (From Blaivas JG: Urodynamic testing. *In* Raz S [ed]: Female Urology. Philadelphia, WB Saunders, 1983, p 81.)

- ● α-Adrenergic
- ▦ Cholinergic
- ○ β-Adrenergic

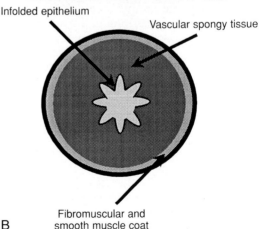

Infolded epithelium

Vascular spongy tissue

Fibromuscular and smooth muscle coat

Figure 5-3 Female urethra. *A*, MRI scan of the female pelvis, showing cross-sectional urethral anatomy. *B*, Schematic cross section of the urethra, showing epithelium, spongy tissue, and fibromuscular and smooth muscle coat.

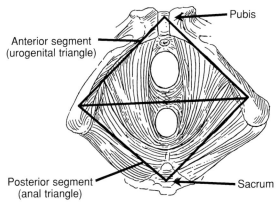

Figure 5-4 Pelvic floor. A transverse line between the ischial spines divides the pelvic floor into an anterior segment (urogenital triangle) and a posterior segment (anal triangle).

provides a compressive "washer effect" vital to the mechanism of continence.[10] Functionally, the integrity of the surrounding smooth muscle coat maintains this mechanism by directing submucosal expansile pressures inward toward the mucosa. Healthy, normal smooth muscle and the vascular spongy tissue of the urethra together provide a major contribution to the closure mechanism of the urethra and are therefore of great importance in normal passive urinary continence. Striated muscle fibers extrinsic to the urethra at the level of the urogenital diaphragm provide reflex and voluntary sphincteric activity and contribute primarily to active continence.

SPHINCTERIC STRUCTURES

Bladder outlet resistance is a complex mechanism that receives contributions from the bladder neck and proximal urethral smooth musculature, the anatomic support of the bladder base and urethra, and the striated muscle of the midurethral area in the female. A proximal or internal sphincter is often described, formed by circular fibers of smooth muscle at the bladder neck and, in the male, at the proximal prostatic urethra. It is sometimes also referred to as the smooth muscle sphincter.[9] The distal or external sphincter is composed of smooth muscle fibers, elastic tissue, intrinsic striated slow-twitch muscle fibers that provide baseline tonic activity, and extrinsic striated fast-twitch fibers that are responsible for reflex and voluntary sphincteric activity.[11] This is sometimes referred to as the striated sphincter and is under partial voluntary control separate from anal sphincter function.

SKELETAL SUPPORT

The bony pelvis provides the framework from which the pelvic structures ultimately draw support. The pelvic floor may be viewed from above as a diamond, with the symphysis pubis and sacrum at the anterior

and posterior apices and the ischial spines as the lateral anchors of ligamentous support (Fig. 5–4). A line drawn between the ischial spines is used to divide the pelvic floor into posterior and anterior segments. The sacrospinous ligaments fan out from the posterior aspect of the ischial spines to connect with the anterolateral surface of the sacrum and coccyx and provide a broad area for support of the posterior pelvic segment[12] (Fig. 5–5). Between the ischial spine and the lower portion of the symphysis pubis, the tendinous arch, a linear condensation of pelvic fascia (arising predominantly from the obturator internus muscle), provides the musculofascial origin for a large portion of the anterior pelvic diaphragm[13] (Fig. 5–6).

More superficial musculofascial support at the level of the perineum takes origin from the ischiopubic rami, the ischial tuberosities, the sacrotuberous ligaments (which run between the posterior aspect of the sacroiliac area and the inner surface of the tuberosities), and the coccyx. In addition, the perineal body, a tendinous structure located in the midline between the anus and the vaginal introitus, provides a point of central insertion for muscles and fascia of the perineum.[13]

PELVIC DIAPHRAGM

Directly beneath the pelvic viscera and their investing endopelvic fascia lies a layer of striated muscle and fascia, the pelvic diaphragm, which provides primary support for the contents of the abdominopelvic cavity.

The coccygeus muscles (see Fig. 5–6) run between the ischial spines and the lateral aspect of the sacrum and coccyx (and therefore both originate and insert on immobile structures) overlying the sacro-

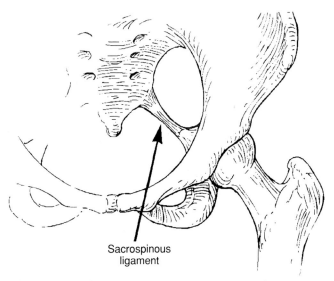

Figure 5-5 Sacrospinous ligament. This structure provides origin for musculofascial support of the posterior pelvic segment. (From Raz S: Vaginal prolapse. *In* Raz S [ed]: Atlas of Transvaginal Surgery. Philadelphia, WB Saunders, 1992, p 134.)

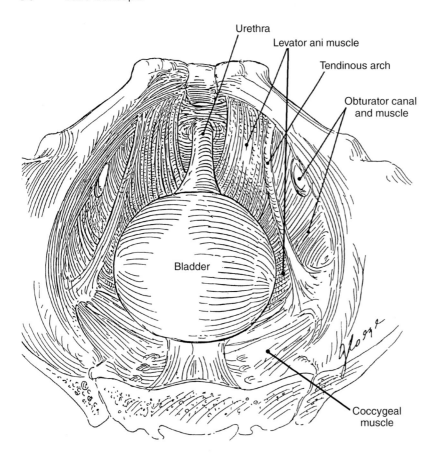

Figure 5-6 Pelvic floor, including tendinous arch (arcus tendineus) of the obturator fascia, and coccygeus and levator ani musculature. (From Raz S, Little NA, and Juma S: Female urology. *In* Walsh PC, Retik AB, Stamey TA, and Vaughan ED Jr. [eds]: Campbell's Urology, 6th ed. Philadelphia, WB Saunders, 1992, p 2783.)

spinous ligaments. They help support the posterior pelvic segment.[12]

The most important structure contributing to support of the pelvic viscera is the levator ani muscle group (see Fig. 5–6) and its fascia, which, together with the coccygeus muscles, compose the pelvic diaphragm. The levator ani muscle group is often divided into three component parts—the pubococcygeus, iliococcygeus, and ischiococcygeus—according to their origin from the pelvic sidewall.[14] The levator ani is perhaps best understood if it is considered as an integrated broad sheet of muscle extending from the inner surface of the pubis just lateral to the symphysis anteriorly to the pelvic surface of the ischial spines posteriorly. Between these points it takes origin from the tendinous arch of the obturator fascia. The levator fibers extend posteromedially from their point of origin and eventually join with corresponding fibers from the contralateral side between the rectum and coccyx in a midline raphe, and to the lateral aspect of the tip of the coccyx as well. The most medial and inferior fibers of the levator ani (which are part of its pubococcygeal portion and are sometimes referred to as the puborectalis) travel posteriorly alongside the urethra, vagina, and rectum to fuse anteriorly and laterally to the rectum, providing perineal support.

The urethra, vagina, and rectum pass through mid-line apertures in the levator ani, collectively called the levator hiatus (Fig. 5–7). Fascial attachments from the adjacent portions of the levators pro-

vide support to these pelvic structures as they exit the pelvis. Normally, the levator muscles hold the pelvic viscera like a hammock, providing a nearly horizontal floor of pelvic support[5] (Fig. 5–8). The bladder, proximal vagina, and intrapelvic rectum rest on the levator floor and are coapted against it during periods of increased intra-abdominal pressure, thus providing stability and contributing to urinary and fecal continence.

The fascia associated with the levator muscle group

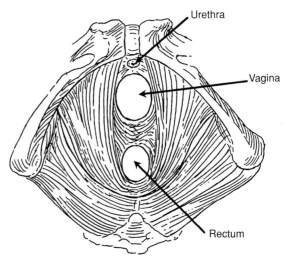

Figure 5-7 Pelvic floor, showing hiatuses in levator ani for urethra, vagina, and rectum.

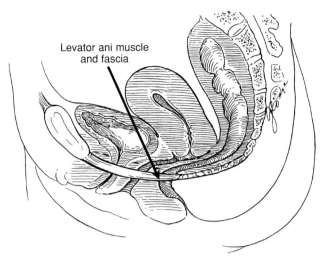

Figure 5-8 Sagittal section of pelvis, showing horizontal support of pelvic viscera by levator ani muscle and fascia. (Adapted from Raz S, Little NA, and Juma S: Female urology. *In* Walsh PC, Retik AB, Stamey TA, and Vaughan ED Jr. [eds]: Campbell's Urology, 6th ed. Philadelphia, WB Saunders, 1992, p 2782.)

Levator ani muscle and fascia

plays a crucial role in maintaining pelvic support. The fascia of the pelvic floor is often described as having different layers, and the abdominal portion is usually referred to as the *endopelvic fascia*. To avoid confusion, the authors prefer to avoid distinguishing between the endopelvic and other layers of fascia of the levator musculature and refer to them collectively as the *levator fascia*. Although the levator fascia (like the musculature) works in an integrated fashion to provide pelvic support, certain areas of the levator-endopelvic fascia have been separately described because of their importance in supporting individual pelvic structures and their role in the surgical correction of pelvic support defects. Four of these condensations—the pubourethral ligaments, the urethropelvic ligaments, the pubocervical fascia, and the cardinal-sacrouterine ligament complex—are discussed in detail in the following section.

ANTERIOR VAGINAL SUPPORT

Pubourethral Ligaments

The *pubourethral ligaments* are a condensation of the levator fascia that connect the inner surface of the inferior pubis to the midportion of the urethra[15] (Fig. 5–9). They support and stabilize the urethra and associated part of the anterior vaginal wall and divide the urethra into two halves—the proximal, which is intra-abdominal and is responsible for passive or involuntary continence—and the distal, which is outside the abdomen. Because the striated muscle fibers of the external urethral sphincter are located just distal to these ligaments, this midurethral area is responsible for active or voluntary continence. The distal urethra functions mainly as a conduit, and damage to or resection of the distalmost third of the

urethra usually results in no significant change in continence. In addition to the previously mentioned pubourethral ligaments, fascial support of the urethra in its midportion is provided laterally on each side by segments of the levator fascia just below their attachments to the pubis (see Fig. 5–9). These areas of levator fascia are continuous with the adjacent, more proximal urethropelvic ligaments (to be described subsequently). The pubourethral ligaments and the lateral levator fascial support of the midurethra may be referred to collectively as the *midurethral complex*.

Urethropelvic Ligaments

The most important source of anatomic support of the bladder neck and proximal urethra is a two-layered condensation of levator fascia that the authors call the *urethropelvic* ligaments.[16] One layer, the *periurethral fascia*, is encountered just beneath the epithelium during vaginal surgery as a glistening white layer that covers the vaginal side of the urethra. It is continuous with the pubocervical fascia (to be discussed later) proximally under the vaginal side of the bladder (Fig. 5–10). The second layer of the urethropelvic ligament consists of the levator fascia covering the abdominal side of the urethra. The fascia fuses laterally with the periurethral fascia and attaches as a unit to the tendinous arch of the obturator fascia along the pelvic sidewall on each side (Fig. 5–11). These lateral fusions (one on each side) of the periurethral and levator fasciae in the region of the bladder neck and proximal urethra provide critical elastic musculofascial support to the bladder outlet. These structures are therefore essential in maintaining passive continence in women, particularly during periods of increased intra-abdominal pressure. In addition, voluntary or reflex contractions of the levator or obturator musculature increase the tensile forces of these ligamentous areas, improving outlet resistance and continence. The urethropelvic ligaments are considered by the authors to be of great importance in the surgical therapy of anatomic stress incontinence.

Pubocervical Fascia

Just deep to the anterior vaginal wall in the region of the bladder base lies the *pubocervical fascia*, a layer of fascia formed from the fusion of the fasciae of the bladder wall and anterior vagina. It is continuous with the periurethral fascia distally and fuses proximally with the uterine cervix and cardinal ligament complex (to be discussed later) (see Fig. 5–10). The pubocervical fascia fuses laterally with the levator-endopelvic fascia covering the abdominal side of the bladder in a manner similar to that in the ligamentous support of the bladder neck and proximal urethra. These lateral fusions, which are analogous to the urethropelvic ligaments and are occasionally re-

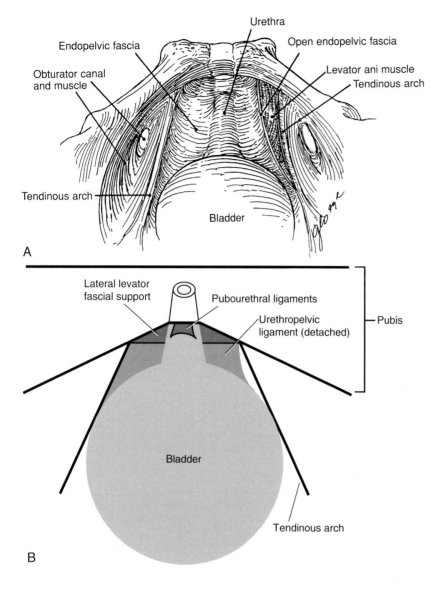

Urethra

Endopelvic fascia

Open endopelvic fascia

Obturator canal and muscle

Levator ani muscle

Tendinous arch

Tendinous arch

Bladder

A

Lateral levator fascial support

Pubourethral ligaments

Urethropelvic ligament (detached)

Pubis

Bladder

Tendinous arch

B

Figure 5-9 *A*, View of pelvis from above. (From Raz S, Little NA, and Juma S: Female urology. *In* Walsh PC, Retik AB, Stamey TA, and Vaughan ED Jr. [eds]: Campbell's Urology, 6th ed. Philadelphia, WB Saunders, 1992, p 2783.) *B*, Corresponding schematic diagram showing musculofascial support of the bladder neck and proximal urethra, including the mid-urethral complex (pubourethral ligaments and lateral levator attachments of the midportion of the urethra) and the urethropelvic ligaments. The urethropelvic ligament is detached from the tendinous arch (arcus tendineus) on the right side.

ferred to as the *vesicopelvic ligaments*[17] (Fig. 5–12), attach laterally on each side to the pelvic wall at the tendinous arch to support the base of the bladder and the anterior vaginal wall. Attenuation of support of the bladder at the attachment of the pubocervical fascia to the pelvic wall results in a *lateral* (or para-vaginal) *cystocele defect*, which is discussed later in this chapter in the section on anterior vaginal support defects.

The anteriormost aspect of the cardinal-sacrouterine ligament complex (described later) fuses with the medial portion of the pubocervical fascia, which is continuous distally with the periurethral fascia. Thus, when viewed from a vaginal perspective with the epithelium removed, these structures together form a rectangle of anterior vaginal fascial support beneath the base of the bladder[5] (see Fig. 5–22A). Herniation of the bladder through a midline defect in this fascial rectangle results in a *central cystocele defect*, which is discussed later in this chapter in the section on anterior vaginal support defects.

UTERUS AND VAGINAL VAULT SUPPORT

Cardinal-Sacrouterine Ligament Complex

The *cardinal ligaments*, also called Mackenrodt's ligaments, are thick, triangular condensations of pelvic fascia that originate from the pelvic fascia in the region of the greater sciatic foramina. They insert into the lateral aspects of a ring of fascia encircling the uterine cervix and isthmus and into the adjacent vaginal wall as well, providing major uterine and apical vaginal support. The cardinal ligaments fuse posteriorly with the *sacrouterine ligaments* (also called *uterosacral ligaments*), which originate off the second, third, and fourth sacral vertebrae and insert into the posterolateral aspect of the pericervical fascial ring and lateral vaginal fornices.[12] When viewed as a unit, the posterior aspect of the pubocervical fascia together with the cardinal-sacrouterine complex fan out superolaterally on each side like butterfly wings to provide two integrated sheets of fascial

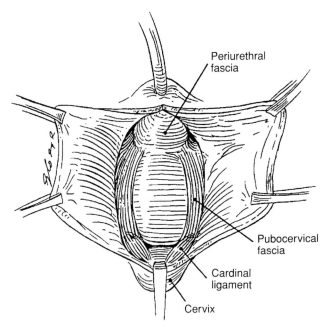

Figure 5-10 View of the rectangle of the anterior vaginal fascial support, which is found beneath the vaginal wall (shown retracted). The periurethral fascia, which forms the vaginal layer of the urethropelvic ligaments, is continuous with the pubocervical fascia proximally. (From Raz S, Little NA, and Juma S: Female urology. *In* Walsh PC, Retik AB, Stamey TA, and Vaughan ED Jr [eds]: Campbell's Urology, 6th ed. Philadelphia, WB Saunders, 1992, p 2785.)

support from the vaginal dome, uterine isthmus, and cervix to the pelvis[18] (Fig. 5–13).

Further uterine support is provided by the *broad ligaments*, which are more superiorly located, covered by anterior and posterior folds of peritoneum, and attach the lateral walls of the uterine body to the pelvic sidewall. They contain the fallopian tubes, the round and ovarian ligaments, and the uterine and ovarian vessels.

POSTERIOR VAGINA AND PERINEAL SUPPORT

Rectovaginal Septum

The cul-de-sac of the peritoneal cavity between the apex of the vagina and the anterior wall of the rectum continues as a fascial extension referred to as the rectovaginal septum. The two fascial layers of the rectovaginal septum, the *posterior vaginal fascia* and the *prerectal fascia*, fuse distally at their insertion into the perineal body (Fig. 5–14). Proximally, the layers blend with the cardinal-sacrouterine complex to provide support to the posterior apex of the vagina. Laterally, the layers fuse and continue posterolaterally as the *pararectal fascia* (also called the *rectal pillars*) on each side, eventually encircling the rectum by joining behind it (Fig. 5–15). When viewed through a posterior vaginal incision, the pararectal fascia lateral to the rectum separates the *prerectal space* from the *pararectal space*[17] (Fig. 5–16).

Support of the proximal vagina and intrapelvic rectum is provided by the medial fibers (pubococcygeus portion) of the levator ani musculature, which insert into the midline raphe between the vagina and rectum and posterior to the rectum (the *anococcygeal ligament*). As discussed previously, the proximal vagina and intrapelvic rectum lie on a nearly horizontal levator floor in conditions of normal pelvic support.

Perineum

A second level of pelvic support exists at the perineum (Fig. 5–17). A tendinous structure located in the midline between the anus and the vestibule of the vagina, the *perineal body*, provides a central point

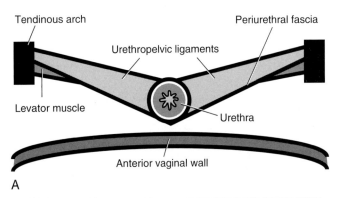

A

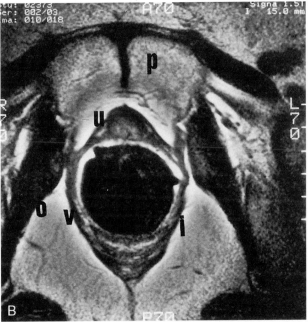

B

Figure 5-11 Urethropelvic ligaments. *A*, Schematic coronal section at the level of the proximal urethra, showing the two layers of the urethropelvic ligaments that enclose the urethra and fuse laterally to attach to the tendinous arch of the obturator fascia. *B*, MRI scan of the urethropelvic ligaments, which stretch from the urethra to the tendinous arch of the obturator on each side. The vaginal lumen is round and is distended by an intravaginal coil. p, Pubic bone; u, urethra; v, vaginal wall (distended by coil); o, obturator muscle; l, levator musculature. (From Raz S: Anatomy of pelvic support and stress incontinence. *In* Raz S [ed]: Atlas of Transvaginal Surgery. Philadelphia, WB Saunders, 1992, p 9.)

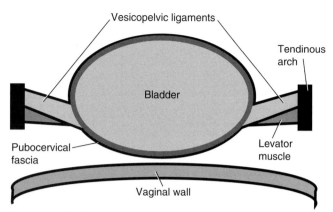

Figure 5-12 Vesicopelvic ligaments. Analogous to the urethropelvic ligaments, these two-layered fusions of levator fascia attach laterally to the tendinous arch to provide lateral support to the bladder base.

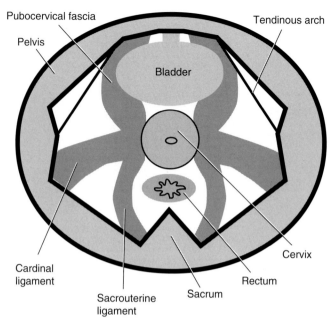

Figure 5-13 Schematic diagram of uterine support. Although depicted here as isolated structures, the pubocervical fascia, cardinal ligaments, and sacrouterine (also called uterosacral) ligaments are condensed regions of two integrated wings of fascial support that fan out on each side to attach to the pelvis and provide support to the uterus and adjacent vaginal wall.

of musculofascial insertion. A line drawn between the ischial tuberosities divides the perineum into anterior urogenital and posterior anal triangles (see Fig. 5-4).

The *urogenital triangle* in the female is divided in half longitudinally by the clitoris, urethra, and vaginal vestibule. Beneath the subcutaneous fascia, a superficial layer of muscle and membranous tissue is encountered. The *ischiocavernosus muscles* cover the two clitoral crura as they attach to the ischia of the pubis. The *bulbocavernosus muscles* run on each side of the vestibule beneath the labia between the clitoris anteriorly and the perineal body posteriorly. There are also two paired *superficial transverse perineal muscles* that run on each side of the perineal body to the ischial tuberosities laterally.

In the center of the *anal triangle* of the perineum is the anal canal. The muscle fibers of the superficial

anal sphincter enclose the anus as they run between the anococcygeal ligament and the perineal body. The deep anal sphincter fibers completely encircle the anal canal and fuse superiorly with inferomedial fibers of the levator ani (pubococcygeus-puborectalis).

A deeper musculofascial layer, the *urogenital diaphragm*, is located just inferior to the lowest portion of the levators. Striated muscle fibers encircle the

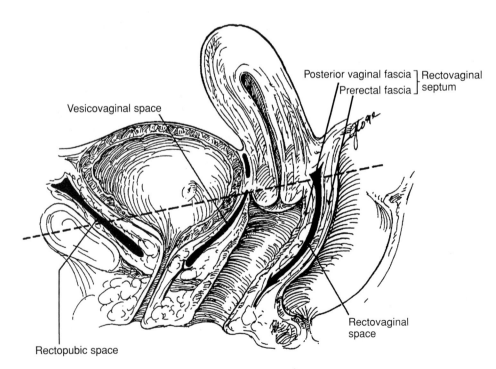

Figure 5-14 Sagittal section of the pelvis, showing the two layers of the rectovaginal septum (posterior vaginal fascia and prerectal fascia) and the rectovaginal space between them. These two layers fuse distally to insert into the perineal body. (From Raz S: Anatomy of pelvic support and stress incontinence. *In* Raz S [ed]: Atlas of Transvaginal Surgery. Philadelphia, WB Saunders, 1992, p 3.)

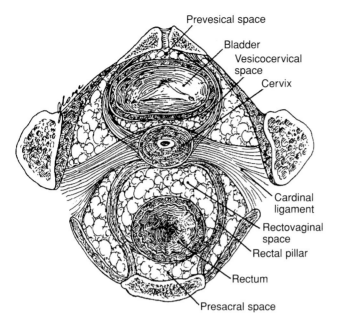

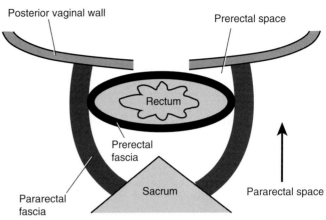

Figure 5-15 Cross section of the lower pelvis, showing the posterolateral extensions of the rectovaginal septa, the rectal pillars (pararectal fascia), which encircle the rectum. (From Raz S, Little NA, and Juma S: Female urology. *In* Walsh PC, Retik AB, Stamey TA, and Vaughan ED Jr [eds]: Campbell's Urology, 6th ed. Philadelphia, WB Saunders, 1992, p 2785.)

Figure 5-16 Schematic diagram of the separation of the prerectal and pararectal spaces by the pararectal fascia (rectal pillars). This relationship may be used to gain access to the pararectal space through a posterior vaginal incision during sacrospinalis fixation procedures.

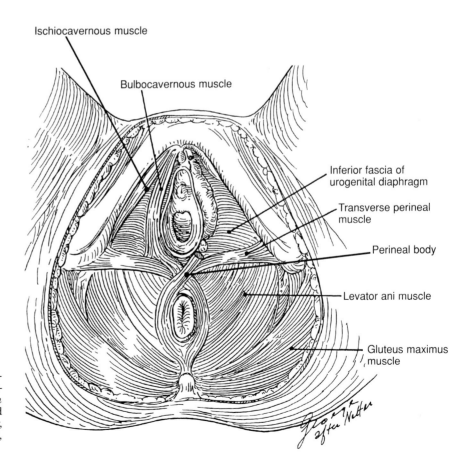

Figure 5-17 Superficial perineal musculature and perineal body. (From Raz S, Little NA, and Juma S: Female urology. *In* Walsh PC, Retik AB, Stamey TA, and Vaughan ED Jr [eds]: Campbell's Urology, 6th ed. Philadelphia, WB Saunders, 1992, p 2783.)

vagina and urethra at this level, providing voluntary urinary sphincteric function. Posteriorly, two paired *deep transverse perineal muscles* run between the perineal body and the ischial tuberosities, superior to their more superficial counterparts.[13]

Pathophysiology of Deficient Pelvic Support

Alterations in the normal support of pelvic structures may occur as a result of several processes. Congenital defects of pelvic support are uncommon and usually present in childhood. Traumatic or surgical injury may also cause various degrees of pelvic prolapse, as can heavy physical labor. Nulliparous women may experience genitourinary symptoms related to pelvic floor relaxation due to postmenopausal tissue atrophy.[19] Some authors have stressed the importance of denervation of the pelvic floor musculature in the genesis of pelvic relaxation.[20]

The most common source of significant pelvic support deficiency appears to be related to trauma from childbirth or hysterectomy. The fact that stress urinary incontinence and other manifestations of pelvic support compromise occur more often during or shortly after menopause rather than at the time of obstetric or gynecologic trauma further implicates trophic changes from hormonal alterations in the loss of pelvic support.[5]

Stress urinary incontinence is often the first symptom experienced during a gradual loss of pelvic support in women and frequently leads them to seek medical attention. It occurs when intravesical pressure exceeds that of outlet resistance during periods of increased intra-abdominal pressure, such as during coughing, sneezing, or straining. Before the pathophysiology of pelvic support defects is discussed in detail, the forces responsible for maintaining outlet resistance in women will be reviewed.

MECHANISMS OF OUTLET RESISTANCE IN WOMEN

Normal outlet resistance in women is achieved by several factors working in concert that provide continence both at rest and during stress. These factors can be organized into four categories.

Anatomic and Functional Urethral Length

Anatomic urethral length is defined as the distance between the internal meatus and external urethral meatus. Congenital anomalies and traumatic injuries resulting in loss of a portion of urethra may result in incontinence. Functional urethral length refers to the total length of the urethra measured during urethral pressure profilometry in which urethral pressure exceeds bladder pressure[21] and therefore correlates better with the physiology of outlet continence. Certain observations argue against the clinical usefulness of the concept of urethral lengths. Twenty percent of asymptomatic nulliparous women have open bladder necks at rest during transvaginal ultrasonography,[22] and up to 50% of normal continent women demonstrate funneling of the bladder neck and proximal urethra on straining cystograms.[23] Y-V plasty or incision of the bladder neck does not produce incontinence in women with otherwise healthy and well-supported outlets. As previously discussed in the section on anatomy, resection of the distal third of the female urethra does not typically influence continence. In addition, surgical elongation of a poorly coapted urethra does not restore continence. Despite these observations, certain critical lengths of healthy, functional urethra are required to provide the coaptation necessary to achieve passive continence and continence during abdominal stress. Although bladder neck suspension procedures do not change anatomic urethral length, their success in improving continence may be considered to result from an increase in or, more accurately, a restoration of functional urethral length.

Closing Forces of the Urethra

As discussed previously, the healthy infolded urethral mucosa and spongy vascular tissue of the normal female urethra (both under trophic hormonal influence), surrounded by a thin musculofascial envelope, create an effective coaptive seal, like the washer of a faucet.[10] The tensile forces of the urethropelvic ligaments (which enclose the urethra) and, indirectly, the levator musculature also result in compression of the proximal and midurethra. In addition, the resting tone of the striated musculature in the mid-urethral area provides further closing pressure to the urethra.

Pelvic Floor Muscular Activity During Stress

A sudden change in abdominal pressures produces reflex contraction of the muscles of both the levator group and the urogenital diaphragm in neurologically intact women, resulting in an increase in midurethral pressures. Voluntary or reflex contraction of the levator and obturator muscles also increases tension on the urethropelvic ligaments, thereby elevating and compressing the proximal urethra[5] (Fig. 5–18).

Position and Anatomic Support of the Outlet

A true valvular effect is created by the high retropubic fixation of the bladder neck and urethra in relation to the more dependent position of the bladder base. Limited posterior rotation of the bladder base against a well-supported urethra during stress in-

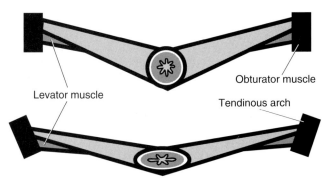

Figure 5-18 Schematic diagram of the urethra and its supporting fascia at rest *(above)* and during voluntary or reflex contraction of the obturator and levator musculature *(below)*. The subsequent increase in tension on the urethropelvic ligaments and the midurethral levator support results in elevation and compression of the bladder neck and urethra.

creases this valvular effect of the bladder neck.[5] In addition, direct through-transmission of intra-abdominal forces to the area of the proximal urethra in a woman with well-supported pelvic structures increases its resistance during periods of abdominal stress as well.[24]

In a normal healthy woman, this complex set of interrelated compensatory mechanisms exists to maintain sufficient outlet resistance to prevent urine leakage, even with the abdominal stress incurred during coughing, sneezing, walking, and straining. Proccesses that result in deterioration of these mechanisms can result in variable degrees of incontinence. Urethral function may be compromised by atrophy of urethral spongy tissue secondary to menopausal hormonal changes, compromised neuromuscular function, or damage from surgery, trauma, or radiation therapy. A weakened levator musculature is not as efficient at increasing midurethral pressures during stress. Although loss of intrinsic urethral resistance or pelvic floor muscular activity can adversely influence continence, the most common process resulting in impairment of the mechanisms of outlet resistance in women is loss of anatomic support of the bladder neck and urethra. Pelvic floor relaxation and weakening of the urethropelvic ligaments and midurethral complex produces significant posterior and downward rotation of the urethra and bladder neck. This laxity transfers the bladder neck and urethra to a dependent position in the pelvis, eliminating the previously described valvular function. Sudden increases in intra-abdominal pressure facilitate funneling and opening of a poorly supported outlet. In addition, intra-abdominal forces are not transmitted efficiently to the poorly supported proximal urethra owing to its extra-abdominal location and the loss of the backboard effect of the strong normal support of the urethropelvic ligaments.

The forces responsible for pelvic relaxation rarely affect only isolated anatomic zones, and stress urinary incontinence resulting from hypermobility of the bladder neck and urethra is therefore often accompanied by associated defects of pelvic support. It is nevertheless useful to organize defects in support according to their effects on various pelvic structures to allow logically planned evaluation and treatment.

ANTERIOR VAGINAL WALL

Bladder Neck and Urethral Prolapse

As discussed previously, normal support of the bladder outlet in women is provided by the levator fascia in the region of the bladder neck and urethra, referred to by the authors as the urethropelvic ligaments and the midurethral complex. Bladder neck hypermobility resulting in stress urinary incontinence is most commonly related to attenuation of the urethropelvic ligaments or their attachment to the pelvic sidewall at the tendinous arch of the obturator fascia. In general, little attention has been given to the support of the midportion of the urethra in the genesis of stress urinary incontinence. Videourodynamic evaluation reveals that in most patients with stress incontinence resulting from loss of pelvic support there is separation of the midportion of the urethra from its normal attachment to the underside of the symphysis pubis as well as hypermobility of the bladder neck and proximal urethra (Fig. 5–19). Although based on preliminary clinical work, the authors believe that further improvements in treatment may be achieved by incorporating concepts of midurethral support and use of the midurethral complex in designing and modifying surgical approaches for use in outlet-related incontinence.

Surgical procedures designed to restore an intrinsically normal but poorly supported outlet to a well-supported intrapelvic position can be expected to have an 80 to 90% rate of success in eliminating stress incontinence in women.[25–27] Although the importance of restoring anatomic position and support of the bladder neck and urethra in the treatment of stress incontinence is undeniable, one must keep in mind that the majority of women with bladder neck

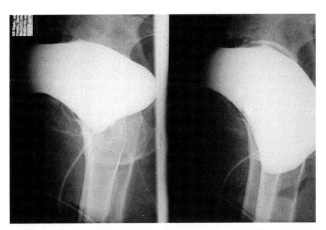

Figure 5-19 Lateral upright cystograms at rest *(left)* and during straining *(right)* showing hypermobility of the bladder neck and proximal urethra as well as separation of the midurethra from the underside of the pubis.

hypermobility do not experience significant incontinence. Intrinsic urethral function is critical to continence as well and may make up for loss of support of the bladder neck and proximal urethra. In fact, it is reasonable to argue that all women with outlet hypermobility and stress incontinence have a component of intrinsic urethral dysfunction. Conversely, anatomic support is not sufficient to achieve continence, and inadequate urethral resistance not uncommonly leads to nearly complete incontinence despite perfect support of the bladder neck and urethra.

Intrinsic Urethral Dysfunction

Although an understanding of the anatomic support of the bladder neck and urethra is essential in considering female urinary continence, knowledge of the anatomy and intrinsic function of the urethra is also required. The plasticity of the highly efficient mucosal seal mechanism discussed in the section on anatomy normally allows perfect continence even when a grooved sound is inserted into the urethra. The intrinsic urethral tissues are affected by trophic hormonal influences, and lack of estrogen at menopause may lead to thinning and flattening of the urethral epithelium and atrophy of the vascular sponge with substitution by fibrous tissue. Multiple surgical procedures, pelvic trauma, radiation therapy, and neurogenic disease may also impair the ability of the urethra to achieve or maintain a perfect seal. Outlet-related incontinence is frequently divided into anatomic incontinence (thought to be more common and present in up to 90% of cases of stress leakage at presentation), which is due to inadequate support of the bladder neck and urethra, and intrinsic sphincteric dysfunction, which is due to inadequacy of the urethra's contribution to resistance.[28] As previously discussed, when the continence mechanisms of intrinsic urethral function are compromised, stress incontinence may result despite adequate pelvic support. Simple bladder neck and proximal urethral suspension in such cases is insufficient to achieve continence, and treatment must be aimed at providing urethral coaptation and compression (by means of such procedures as sling procedures, injection of bulking agents into the envelope of the urethra, or implantation of hydraulic sphincter devices) as well as restoring anatomic support.

Cystocele

Hypermobility of the bladder neck and urethra is only one manifestation of anterior vaginal wall prolapse. Most women with stress urinary incontinence due to bladder neck hypermobility have an associated cystocele that must also be addressed at the time of evaluation and treatment.

Many classification systems have been used to grade cystocele defects.[29, 30] The authors prefer to describe four degrees of anterior vaginal wall pro-

lapse. In grade I and grade II cystourethrocele, there is a mild to moderate degree of hypermobility of the anterior vaginal wall during straining. In grade III the anterior vaginal wall reaches through the introitus on straining, and in grade IV the bladder base protrudes through the introitus.

As previously discussed, two different types of anterior vaginal wall support defects in the region of the base of the bladder can be identified (1) lateral defects, due to loss or attenuation of the lateral (or paravaginal) attachment of the pubocervical fascia–vesicopelvic ligament at the tendinous arch of the obturator, and (2) central defects, resulting from separation of the pubocervical fascia and cardinal ligaments in the midline, allowing herniation of the bladder base into the vagina (Fig. 5–20). These two types of support compromise may occur in conjunction, as seen in women with grade IV cystoceles who generally have combined lateral and central support defects, both of which must be corrected at the time of surgical repair (Fig. 5–21).

As discussed in the previous section on anatomy, the cardinal-sacrouterine complex combined with the periurethral and pubocervical fascia form a rectangle of support of the anterior vaginal wall (Fig. 5–22A), with fibers of the pubocervical fascia on each side fusing with the anteriormost aspect of the cardinal ligaments. In women with good uterine support from strong cardinal ligaments, the base of this rectangle is short and centrally located. In cases of uterine prolapse or laxity of the cardinal-sacrouterine complex following hysterectomy, the rectangle's base elongates and the pubocervical fascia widens, facilitating the formation of a central cystocele defect (Fig. 5–22).

UTERUS AND VAGINAL VAULT

The most important supporting structures of the vaginal vault and uterus are the sacrouterine and cardinal ligaments. In addition to contributing to anterior vaginal wall defects as mentioned previously, relaxation of the cardinal ligaments facilitates the formation of uterine or vaginal vault prolapse and enterocele.

Uterine or Vaginal Vault Prolapse

Uterine prolapse results from weakening of the supporting ligaments, particularly the cardinal-sacrouterine complex, owing to the same etiologic factors previously discussed in the pathophysiology of pelvic relaxation. Uterine prolapse is generally graded in the same way as for cystocele defects, grade I being minimal mobility, grade II descent with strain to the level of the midvagina, grade III descent with strain to the vaginal introitus, and grade IV (procidentia) prolapse through the introitus. After hysterectomy, deficient cardinal-sacrouterine fascial support may result in prolapse of the vaginal dome and region of

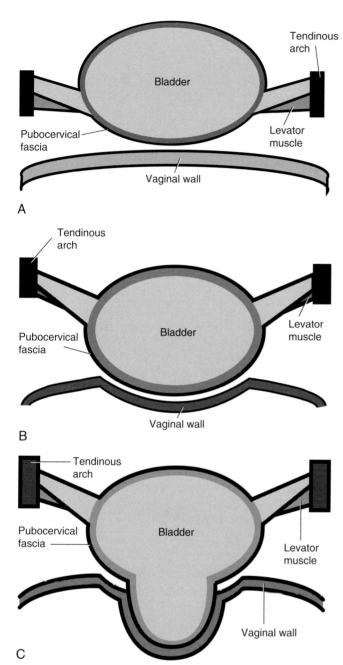

Figure 5-20 Schematic diagram of anterior vaginal support defects. *A*, Normal anterior vaginal support. *B*, Compromise of support of the bladder at the attachment of the pubocervical fascia to the pelvis, resulting in a lateral cystocele defect. *C*, Herniation of the base of the bladder through separated, attenuated pubocervical fascia and adjacent cardinal-sacrouterine ligament support, resulting in a central cystocele defect.

the closed cuff. Uterine prolapse infrequently occurs in isolation and may be managed by either suspension procedures or hysterectomy in conjunction with treatment of the accompanying pelvic support defects. Vaginal vault prolapse generally requires surgical fixation of the vaginal apex to the sacrum or sacrospinous ligament, or suspension in conjunction with repair of associated anterior vaginal wall support defects, if present.[17]

Enterocele

An enterocele is defined as a true hernia of peritoneum and its contents (usually small bowel), and generally occurs in the upper posterior portion of the vagina in association with the cul-de-sac of Douglas. Although an enterocele may occur through the pouch of Douglas in women with no history of vaginal surgery, most enteroceles are acquired and occur as "pulsion" defects at the vaginal dome created by separation of the cardinal-sacrouterine complex after hysterectomy[31] (Fig. 5–23). "Traction" enteroceles may be associated with uterine prolapse and generally occur posterior to the uterus and extending into the rectouterine space[32] (Fig. 5–24). Repair may be performed using an abdominal or vaginal approach.

POSTERIOR VAGINAL WALL AND PERINEUM

The complex fascial and muscular arrangement providing support to the posterior vagina, rectum, perineum, and anal sphincter was described earlier in the section on anatomy. Although the fascial support includes the prerectal and pararectal fasciae, it is helpful to consider two levels of musculofascial support—the pelvic floor or levator sling (particularly its puboccygeal portion), and the perineum, including the bulbocavernous, superficial, and deep transverse perineal muscles, the external anal sphincter, and the central tendon of the perineum.[33, 34]

Rectocele

In a normal woman the pelvic floor provides a strong, nearly horizontal platform of support for the pelvic

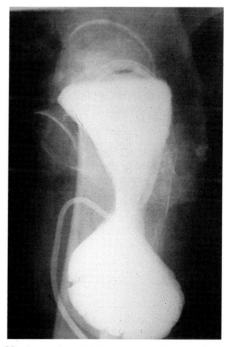

Figure 5-21 Lateral upright cystogram, showing grade IV cystocele with both lateral and central defects.

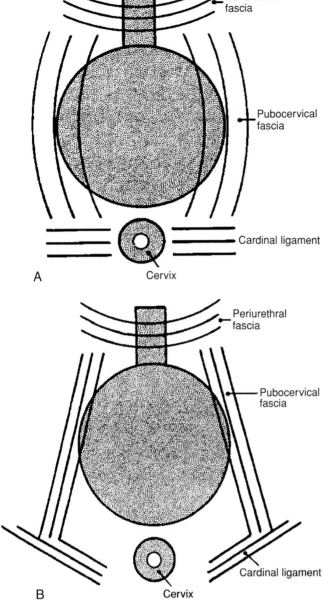

Figure 5–22 Schematic diagram of the pathophysiology of central cystocele defects. *A,* Normal rectangle of anterior vaginal fascial support. *B,* Attenuation or separation of the cardinal-sacrouterine ligament complex results in widening of the base of the rectangle of fascial support under the bladder, facilitating the formation of a central cystocele defect. (From Raz S, Little NA, and Juma S: Female urology. *In* Walsh PC, Retik AB, Stamey TA, and Vaughan ED Jr [eds]: Campbell's Urology, 6th ed. Philadelphia, WB Saunders, 1992, p 2785.)

structures, the levator hiatus is narrow, and the levator fibers provide separation between the posterior aspect of the distal vagina and the rectum. As a result, in the erect position two vaginal angles can be described. In its midportion the vagina forms a posterior angle of approximately 110 degrees with the axis of the distal vagina at the point where the vagina crosses the pelvic floor. The proximal half of the vagina lies on the horizontal plane of the levator plate. The second angle defines the relationship be-

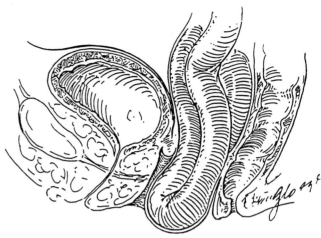

Figure 5–23 Schematic diagram of upright sagittal section of pelvis, showing pulsion enterocele defect through the cul-de-sac in a patient following hysterectomy.

tween the distal half of the vagina and the vertical line and is approximately 45 degrees, again reflecting the degree of support of the pelvic floor and perineum (Fig. 5–25). In women with significant pelvic floor prolapse, the levator plate relaxes and becomes convex instead of horizontal, the levator hiatus enlarges, and the normal midvaginal angulation disappears (Fig. 5–26). The vagina is now rotated downward and posteriorly and is no longer in a well-supported horizontal position. Intravaginal herniation of the rectum through an attenuated rectovaginal septum may also ensue, creating a rectocele[5] (Fig. 5–27).

Perineal Laxity

In women with damage to the second level of muscular support at the perineum, the vaginal introitus

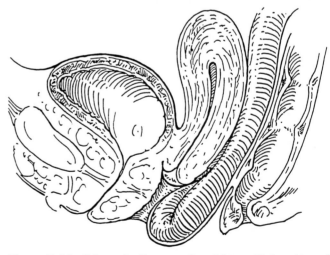

Figure 5–24 Schematic diagram of upright sagittal section of pelvis, showing traction enterocele defect through the rectouterine space, which may occur in conjunction with uterine prolapse. (From Raz S, Little NA, and Juma S: Female urology. *In* Walsh PC, Retik AB, Stamey TA, and Vaughan ED Jr [eds]: Campbell's Urology, 6th ed. Philadelphia, WB Saunders, 1992, p 2810.)

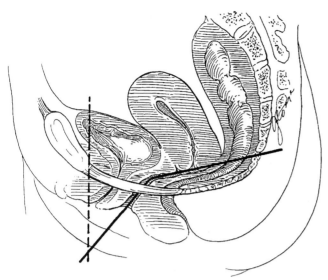

Figure 5-25 Schematic diagram of upright sagittal section of pelvis, showing normal vaginal support. The proximal vagina rests horizontally on the levator plate, forming an angle of approximately 110 degrees with the axis of the distal vagina. The distal vagina forms an angle of approximately 45 degrees with the vertical axis. (Modified from Raz S, Little NR, and Juma S: Female urology. *In* Walsh PC, Retik AB, Stamey TA, and Vaughan ED Jr [eds]: Campbell's Urology, 6th ed. Philadelphia, WB Saunders, 1992, p 2782.)

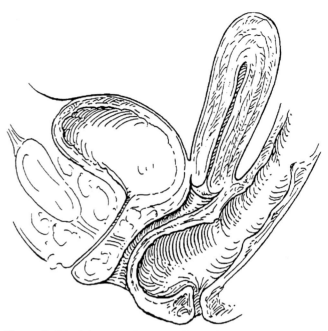

Figure 5-27 Schematic diagram of upright sagittal section of pelvis, showing herniation of the rectum through an attenuated rectovaginal septum (rectocele).

widens, and the distance between the urethra and posterior fourchette increases. Different degrees of perineal tears may be seen, ranging from minimal separation of the perineum to severe defects in which

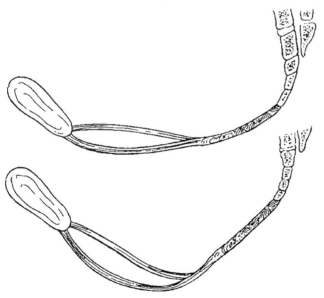

Figure 5-26 Upright sagittal diagram of levator hiatus and pelvic floor. Normally *(top)*, the floor is horizontal and the posterior portion of the hiatus supports the angulation between the distal and proximal vagina (see Fig. 5–25). In patients with deficient support *(bottom)*, the pelvic floor is weakened and convex, and the hiatus is attenuated and widened, resulting in loss of the midvaginal angulation. (From Raz S, Little NA, and Juma S: Female urology. *In* Walsh PC, Retik AB, Stamey TA, and Vaughan ED Jr [eds]: Campbell's Urology, 6th ed. Philadelphia, WB Saunders, 1992, p 2787.)

the normal perineal architecture has been destroyed and the posterior aspect of the vaginal introitus reaches the anterior anal wall.

As is the case with central and lateral anterior vaginal wall defects, combined defects of posterior vaginal support at both the level of the pelvic floor and the perineum often occur, particularly in cases of severe prolapse. Three defects are generally present; weakness of the prerectal and pararectal fasciae of the rectovaginal septum, widening of the levator hiatus and loss of separation of the midvagina and rectum (Fig. 5–28), and laxity of the perineal musculature and fascia. Corrective surgery of the posterior vaginal wall should include correction of the rectocele by reinforcing the attenuated prerectal and pararectal fasciae, repair of the defect of the levator muscles by reapproximating the levator hiatus and restoring the horizontal supporting plate of the proximal portion of the vagina, and repair of the fascia and musculature of the perineum, thereby providing normal introital size and improved vaginal support.[5]

Although stress urinary incontinence is frequently the incentive leading to a woman's initial visit to a physician, pelvic surgeons in general and urologists in particular have failed to recognize that stress urinary incontinence is only one manifestation of pelvic relaxation and have been remiss in addressing it without paying concomitant attention to the pelvic defects that often accompany it. By arming themselves with a fundamental grasp of the anatomy and pathophysiology of pelvic support, concerned clinicians will be able to treat effectively their female patients who present with complaints related to deficiencies in pelvic support and apply appropriately the current methods of evaluation and treatment discussed in other chapters of this book.

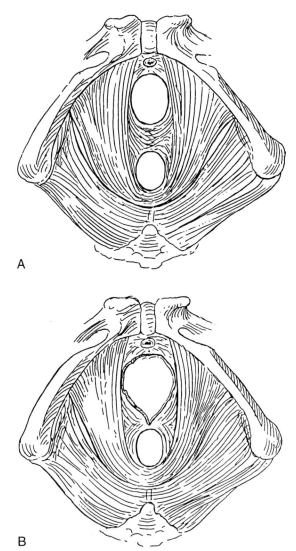

A

B

Figure 5-28 Pelvic floor defect. *A*, Normal levator floor and vaginal hiatus. There is good support in the region of the midvaginal angulation, and wide separation between the posterior vagina and anterior rectum. *B*, Attenuation and separation of the levator fibers that cross and join prerectally results in widening of the posterior aspect of the hiatus of the vagina. The midvaginal angulation and separation between the vagina and rectum are lost. (From Raz S, Little NA, and Juma S: Female urology. *In* Walsh PC, Retik AB, Stamey TA, and Vaughan ED Jr [eds]: Campbell's Urology, 6th ed. Philadelphia, WB Saunders, 1992, p 2807.)

REFERENCES

1. Diokno AC, Brock BM, Brown MB, Herzog AR: Prevalence of urinary incontinence and other urological symptoms in the non-institutionalized elderly. J Urol 136:1022, 1986.
2. Marshall VF, Marchetti AA, Krantz KE: The correction of stress incontinence by simple vesicourethral suspension. Surg Gynecol Obstet 88:509, 1949.
3. Hodgkinson CP: Stress urinary incontinence. Am J Obstet Gynecol 108:1141, 1970.
4. McGuire EJ, Lyton B, Pepe V, Kohorn EI: Stress urinary incontinence. Obstet Gynecol 47:255, 1976.
5. Raz S, Little NA, Juma S: Female urology. *In* Walsh PC, Retik AB, Stamey TA, Vaughan ED Jr (eds): Campbell's Urology, 6th ed. Philadelphia, WB Saunders Co, 1992, pp 2782–2829.
6. Hutch JA: A new theory of the anatomy of the internal sphincter and the physiology of micturition. Invest Urol 3:36, 1965.
7. Tanagho EA, Pugh RCB: The anatomy and function of the ureterovesical junction. Br J Urol 35:151, 1963.
8. Gosling JA: The structure of the bladder and urethra in relation to function. Urol Clin North Am 6(1):31, 1979.
9. Redman JF: Anatomy of the genitourinary system. *In* Gillenwater JY, Grayback JT, Howards S, Duckett JW (eds): Adult and Pediatric Urology, 2nd ed. St. Louis, Mosby–Year Book, 1991, pp 3–62.
10. Staskin DR, Zimmern PE, Hadley HR, Raz S: The pathophysiology of stress incontinence. Urol Clin North Am 12:271, 1985.
11. Elbadawi A: Neuromuscular mechanisms of micturition. *In* Yalla SV, McGuire EJ, Elbadawi A, Blaivas JG (eds): Neurology and Urodynamics. New York, Macmillan, 1988, pp 3–35.
12. DeLancey JOL, Richardson AC: Anatomy of genital support. *In* Hurt WG (ed): Urogynecologic Surgery. Gaithersburg, IL, Rockville, MD, Aspen Publishers, 1992, pp 19–33.
13. Tanagho EA: Anatomy of the lower urinary tract. *In* Walsh PC, Retik AB, Stamey TA, Vaughan ED (eds): Campbell's Urology, 6th ed. Philadelphia, WB Saunders, 1992, pp 40–69.
14. Redman JF: Surgical anatomy of the female genitourinary system. *In* Buchsbaum HJ, Schmidt JD: Gynecologic and Obstetric Urology, 3rd ed. Philadelphia, WB Saunders, 1993, pp 25–60.
15. Zacharin RF: The anatomic supports of the female urethra. Obstet Gynecol 21:754, 1968.
16. Klutke C, Golomb J, Barbaric Z, Raz S: The anatomy of stress incontinence: Magnetic resonance imaging of the female bladder neck and urethra. J Urol 143:563, 1989.
17. Raz S: The anatomy of pelvic support and stress incontinence. *In* Raz S (ed): Atlas of Transvaginal Surgery. Philadelphia, WB Saunders, 1992, pp 1–22.
18. Baden WF, Walker T: The anatomy of uterovaginal support. *In* Vaginal Defects. JB Lippincott, 1992, pp 25–50.
19. Stanton SL: Vaginal prolapse. *In* Raz S (ed): Female Urology. Philadelphia, WB Saunders, 1983, pp 229–240.
20. Snooks SJ, Swash M, Henry MM, Setchell ME: Injury to innervation of the pelvic floor sphincter musculature in childbirth. Lancet 2:546, 1984.
21. Bruskewitz R: Urethral pressure profile in female lower urinary tract dysfunction. *In* Raz S (ed): Female Urology. Philadelphia, WB Saunders, 1983, pp 113–122.
22. Chapple CR, Helm CW, Blease S, et al: Asymptomatic bladder neck incompetence in nulliparous females. Br J Urol 64:357, 1989.
23. Versi E, Cardozo LD, Studd JWW, et al: Internal urinary sphincter in maintenance of female continence. Br Med J 292:166, 1986.
24. Enhörning G: Simultaneous recording of intravesical and intraurethral pressure. Acta Chir Scand 276:3, 1961.
25. Green DF, McGuire EJ, Lyton B: A comparison of endoscopic suspension of the vesical neck versus anterior urethropexy for the treatment of stress urinary incontinence. J Urol 136:1205, 1986.
26. Spencer JR, O'Connor VJ, Schaeffer AJ: A comparison of endoscopic suspension of the vesical neck with suprapubic vesicourethropexy for treatment of stress urinary incontinence. J Urol 137:411, 1987.
27. Siegel AL, Raz S: Surgical treatment of stress urinary incontinence. Neurourol Urodyn 7:569, 1988.
28. Raz S, Siegel AL, Short JL, Snyder JA: Vaginal wall sling. J Urol 141:43, 1989.
29. Hughes EC: American College of Obstetricians and Gynecologists Book on Obstetric-Gynecologic Terminology. Philadelphia, FA Davis, 1972.
30. Beecham CT: Classification of vaginal relaxation. Am J Obstet Gynecol 136:957, 1980.
31. Zacharin RF: Pulsion enterocele: Review of the functional anatomy of the pelvic floor. Obstet Gynecol 55:135, 1980.
32. McCall ML: Posterior culdoplasty: Surgical correction of enterocele during vaginal hysterectomy: A preliminary report. Obstet Gynecol 10:595, 1957.
33. Huisman AB: Aspects of the anatomy of the female urethra with special relation to urinary continence. Contrib Gynecol Obstet 10:1, 1983.
34. Joseph J: Female genital structure and function. The bones, joints, and ligaments of the female pelvis. *In* Phillip E, Barnes J, Newton M (eds): Scientific Foundations of Obstetrics and Gynecology, 3rd ed. Chicago, Year Book, 1986, pp 86–94.

CHAPTER 6

Epidemiology of Female Incontinence

Ananias C. Diokno, M.D.

In the study of any condition it is imperative that the distribution and nature of the condition as well as the risk factors affecting it are understood. This is especially true of urinary incontinence, a condition that is multifactorial in origin. Although there is still a major gap in our knowledge of the various issues involved in the epidemiology of urinary incontinence, recent acquisition of information has made it possible to understand the extent to which this condition affects our patients.

Prevalence Rates

The *prevalence* of urinary incontinence is the probability of *being* incontinent within a defined population group within a specific period of time. The *incidence* of urinary incontinence is the probability of *becoming* incontinent during a defined period of time. Incidence may be reported as a 1-year or 5-year incidence or other period of time.

Knowledge of prevalence rates is helpful in projecting the need for health and medical services, whereas information on incidence is more helpful in studying the onset and course of the condition or disease. Early reports on the prevalence and incidence of urinary incontinence came from European studies, most of which involved elderly people living in the community.

Any studies on the epidemiology of urinary incontinence or, for that matter, any condition or disease, are significantly dependent on the definition of the condition as well as the method used to obtain the information. So when one reads the rates obtained from one study and compares them to another study, one must be cautious in interpreting the differences between studies.

The most comprehensive study to date on the prev-

alence of urinary incontinence in the general population was the one reported by Thomas and colleagues in 1980.[1] This study was carried out in two London boroughs through a postal survey of 22,430 people aged 5 years and over. The response rate in this postal survey was 89%. The survey team defined regular incontinence as two or more episodes of urinary incontinence occurring in the past month, whereas occasional incontinence was defined as less than two incontinence episodes per month. The results showed that the prevalence of incontinence in all age groups in women (5 to over 85 years old) was 8.5%. The breakdown of the prevalence rates according to the various age groups is presented in Table 6–1.

When incontinence was correlated with previous pregnancy as well as with number of pregnancies, nulliparous women were found to have a lower preva-

TABLE 6–1
Prevalence of Urinary Incontinence in Women Living in London

Age (Years)	Regular Incontinence (%)	Occasional Incontinence (%)
5–14	5.1	11.2
15–24	4.0	11.9
25–34	5.5	20.0
35–44	10.2	20.7
45–54	11.8	21.9
55–64	11.9	18.6
65–74	8.8	14.6
75–84	16.0	13.6
≥85	16.2	16.2
Total	16.6	8.5

From Thomas TM, Plymat KR, Blannin J, et al: Prevalence of urinary incontinence. BMJ 281:1243, 1980. Published by BMJ Publishing Group.

lence than those who had had one or more babies. The number of pregnancies did not make any difference among the incontinent respondents except those in the 45- to 54-year age group, in which those who had had four or more babies were most likely to report regular incontinence. Incontinence was also reported to be moderate or severe in approximately 20% of the respondents, of whom less than a third were receiving health or social services for the condition.

Elving and associates reported that 26% of women 30 to 59 years old had experienced urinary incontinence at some time in adult life.[2] They also reported that 14% perceived urinary incontinence as a social or hygienic problem.

Urinary incontinence is much more prevalent among institutionalized patients than among those living in the community. European hospital surveys of older people have revealed that as many as 48% of institutionalized elderly may be incontinent.[3] A survey sponsored by the United States Department of Health, Education and Welfare in 1975 on long-term facilities reported that 55% of patients surveyed had some problems with urinary control, and an additional 5% were using a catheter or other collecting device.[4] Similarly, the National Nursing Home Survey sponsored by the National Center for Health statistics in 1979 confirmed a prevalence of urinary incontinence of 50% among the more than 1.5 million nursing facility residents in the United States.[5] Willington estimated that 30% of unselected elderly admissions are incontinent of urine.[6]

Urinary incontinence in elderly people living in the community is much more prevalent than in any other age group. Several European studies have reported that the prevalence of incontinence in the elderly varies from 1.6 to 49%.[7-9] In the United States the most comprehensive epidemiologic study on urinary incontinence in the elderly living in the community was the survey called Medical Epidemiologic and Social Aspects of Aging (MESA) conducted in Washtenaw County, Michigan, headed by Diokno and colleagues, and sponsored by the National Institute on Aging.[10] This was a cross-sectional and longitudinal study on elderly respondents 60 years and older. A multistage stratified area probability sample of Washtenaw County identified 13,912 households that were screened by interviewers to identify those households containing one or more persons 60 years of age or older. At the baseline interview, 66% of potential respondents agreed to be interviewed, for a total of 1955 respondents. At the two subsequent resurveys, the reinterview response rates were 69% and 72% of the original respondents who were still alive.

The prevalence of urinary incontinence among all women 60 years and older interviewed for the study was 37.6%. The total number of women interviewed was 1145. When the prevalence rate was analyzed according to the various age groups, no significant difference was found between the prevalence rates of the various age groups from 60 years to over 85 years old.

Details of the clinical type of urinary incontinence were also obtained during the interview. Stress-type incontinence was defined as urine loss experienced at a time of physical exertion such as coughing or laughing. Urge incontinence was defined as involuntary loss of urine preceded by sudden urge to void. When the urine loss was associated with both stress and urge, it was considered mixed type. When urine loss was associated with neither stress nor urge, the incontinence was labeled other. The MESA study reported stress incontinence in 26.7%, urge in 9.1%, mixed in 55.3%, and other in 8.9% of female respondents.

The prevalence of associated bladder symptoms was also reported by the MESA study. Specifically, difficult bladder emptying symptoms included hesitancy, poor stream, interrupted stream, straining to void, and use of a catheter to drain the bladder. The overall prevalence of difficult bladder emptying symptoms, commonly known as symptoms of prostatism, among female respondents 60 years and older was 10.9% compared with 22.1% among men of a similar age group. The prevalence of irritative bladder symptoms including a history of urinary infection was reported to be 17.4% among women respondents compared to 11.8% among men. The difficult bladder emptying symptoms observed among elderly women were believed to be due most likely to an underactive bladder (weak detrusor muscle), whereas in men they are most likely related to an outlet obstruction.

The MESA study established the distribution of frequency of voiding in the elderly. Approximately 88% of all women respondents who were asymptomatic (no self-reported incontinence or irritative or obstructive symptoms) void no more than eight times per day (12% void nine times or more per day), whereas 70% of incontinent women void no more than eight times per day (30% void nine times or more per day). In terms of nocturia, 93% of asymptomatic women and 83% of incontinent women void no more than two times at night. The frequency of nocturia increased among women with bladder symptoms. Nocturia of three times or more was reported by 25% of women with irritative bladder symptoms and 24% of women with difficult bladder emptying symptoms. The increased frequency reported among symptomatic respondents compared to asymptomatic respondents was statistically significant.

The severity of urinary incontinence was analyzed according to the quantity of urine loss per day and the frequency of urine loss in 365 days. Almost two-thirds of women (64%) reported losing at least $1\frac{1}{2}$ teaspoons of urine a day when losing urine. About 15.8% reported losing at least $\frac{1}{4}$ cup or more of urine per day when having an incontinent episode. About 16.1% of women claimed they lost urine an average of 300 to 365 days a year, and one-third (33.4%) claimed they lost urine at least once a week.

Incidence and Remission Rates

The MESA study established the incidence rates of urinary incontinence in the elderly in the United States.[11] The incidence of women who were continent at the initial baseline interview and became incontinent a year later was 22.4%. The incidence at the third interview (third year) of respondents who were still continent during the second interview was 20.2%.

Of the incontinent respondents at the initial (baseline) interview, 11.2% became continent during the second interview. Similarly, 13.3% of the incontinent respondents at the second interview became continent at the third interview. These conversions represent the remission rates for incontinent women within a year.

When a continent person becomes incontinent in the subsequent year the most likely pattern is a mild form of incontinence. About half the cases of mild incontinence at the beginning of the survey remained mild; a few became severe. Interestingly, women with severe incontinence usually remained severely incontinent after 1 year of follow-up. Half of the cases of moderate incontinence remained moderate, and the rest became either mild or severe.

In terms of the type of incontinence, women who originally had the stress type of urinary incontinence either remained the same or developed the mixed type. Women with the mixed type usually stayed the same. Most continent women who became incontinent developed the stress type or a mixed stress-urge type of incontinence.

Correlates of Urinary Incontinence

It is well known that urinary incontinence is a condition with a multifactorial origin. The MESA study investigated and reported the many suspected correlates[12] of urinary incontinence. The factors investigated extended beyond the medical correlates into the social and psychological aspects. Among women, measures of depression, negative affect balance, and life satisfaction reflect to a statistically significant degree the effect of urinary incontinence.[13] Continent older women reported the highest levels of psychological well-being (i.e., the least depression and negative affect balance) and the most life satisfaction. Psychological well-being declines monotonically with increasing severity of urinary incontinence—that is, the more severely incontinent women experience higher depression and negative affect balance and lower life satisfaction than the less severely incontinent women or continent women. The overall effects are statistically significant, and the pairwise comparisons indicate that, generally, women with the more severe levels of urinary incontinence are significantly different from those who are continent. Changes in the measures of happiness and positive affect balance

are not as clear and do not reach statistical significance. Herzog and colleagues suggested that these relationships are partly explained by the fact that incontinent respondents are less healthy than are continent respondents.[13]

Miller presented data from the New Haven EPESE study showing that respondents who reported difficulty holding their urine "all of the time" or "most of the time" scored highest on a scale of depressive symptoms, followed by respondents who had difficulty "sometimes" or "hardly ever."[14] Continent respondents scored the lowest of the three groups. This pattern persisted when functional disabilities and chronic disabilities were controlled.

Because urinary incontinence in itself is not a life-threatening condition, many incontinent individuals have found ways of managing their own condition. The MESA respondents preferred using absorbent pads (55%) and locating a toilet on reaching a destination (42%).[15] Fewer respondents manipulated their voiding patterns (28%) or diet and fluid intake (16%), performed pelvic muscle exercises (12%), or took medication (6%). Among the MESA respondents, 41.8% of those with severe incontinence had talked with a doctor in the past year, whereas only 25.7% of those with moderate incontinence and 18.9% of those with mild incontinence had done so. In regard to the type of incontinence, 29.9% of those with the mixed type of incontinence had talked with their doctors in the past year, whereas only 20% of those with either urge or stress incontinence had talked with their doctors.

Study of the medical correlates of urinary incontinence confirmed that incontinence in elderly individuals is associated with many debilitating medical conditions.[12] Surveys showed that physical mobility problems, specific neurologic symptoms, lower urinary tract problems, bowel problems, respiratory problems, and a history of genital surgery are more prevalent among those who are incontinent than among those who are not. Other factors associated with female geriatric incontinence include a history of parent or sibling incontinence, incontinence either during pregnancy or postpartum, hearing problems, use of female hormones, and vaginal infections. Mobility problems among the elderly were identified by the use of a wheelchair or walking aids, the presence of any health problems that restrict the patient from going visiting, the presence of diagnosed arthritis or rheumatism, and whether the respondent fell during the last year. The results showed that the proportion of respondents who reported mobility limitations was significantly greater among those who were incontinent than among those who were not. Among incontinent women, those with urge symptoms reported more difficulty with mobility than those with other symptoms. For example, among women with urge incontinence, 28.2% had mobility problems, in contrast to only 6.8% of those with stress incontinence.

Questions on neurologic conditions asked of the respondents included queries about any disease of the nerves or muscles or numbness in any part of body in the past year. Incontinence in women was associated significantly more often with these neurologic factors than incontinence. With regard to respiratory symptoms, incontinent women reported that they cough or sneeze more often than continent women. Women with mixed-type incontinence were more likely to report sneezing than those with other types of incontinence.

Bowel problems, including lost control of stools in the past year, as well as problems with constipation were also significantly more prevalent among the incontinent respondents than among their continent counterparts. Vaginal infections were reported much more frequently by incontinent women.

As expected, more incontinent than continent respondents reported urinary tract problems. The largest differences were found among those who reported urinary tract infections, the presence of blood, cloudiness, or foul smell in the urine, slow and weak stream of urine, and the presence of pain, burning, or stinging during urination.

To identify causal relationships between urinary incontinence and its correlates, it is important to follow these respondents over a period of time. Because we have followed our respondents for several years, our preliminary data suggest a clear relationship among the onset of poor health, mobility problems, and urinary symptoms. These factors appear to be significant risk factors for the development of urinary incontinence in the elderly.

The MESA study confirmed the widespread use of diuretics among the elderly population.[16] Approximately one in four men and one in three women 60 years and older use diuretics. Wells and coworkers reported that diuretics were used in 29% of incontinent elderly women seen in a continence clinic.[17] Ouslander, in his study of nursing home patients, observed no significant difference in the use of diuretics between continent and incontinent patients. Shimp and colleagues reported the influence of diuretics on bladder symptoms in a study of 200 incontinent women recruited from a continence program clinic.[19] It was observed that incontinent women taking diuretics have a positive correlation with nocturia and a trend toward significant urge incontinence ($p = .056$) compared with incontinent women not taking diuretics.

The MESA study showed that there was no significant difference in the prevalence of incontinence in users and nonusers of diuretics. However, it was found that diuretic users who had uninhibited bladder contractions on cystometry had a significantly higher prevalence of urinary incontinence (85%) compared with nonusers with similar bladder abnormalities (25%). Among respondents who did not have uninhibited bladder contractions on cystometry, the use or nonuse of diuretics resulted in no difference between the two groups ($p = .085$). Although these comparisons were made in men because there were not enough women with uninhibited bladder contractions to compare, there is no reason not to expect similar relationships in women.

The correlation between diuretics and the presence of uninhibited bladder contractions has significant implications. When one is confronted with an elderly patient who has recently experienced the onset of urinary incontinence, especially of the urge type, one should specifically ask about the concomitant use of diuretics. If diuretic use correlates with the onset of incontinence, one may discontinue the diuretic and change to a nondiuretic therapy if this is medically feasible. If the diuretic cannot be discontinued, the use of bladder relaxants should be considered as long as the patient has adequate detrusor contractility and can empty the bladder adequately. As part of the overall management of incontinence in patients with mobility and dexterity problems, easier access to the toilet should be considered; otherwise, provisions for toilet supplements, such as commodes or urinals, should be encouraged.

Urodynamic Tests on Survey Respondents

Most urodynamic tests currently in use for the evaluation of female urinary incontinence have not been applied to a community-based sample to determine their specificity. Use of a community-based sample rather than studies conducted among groups of inpatients and/or outpatients allows calculation of prevalence estimates in a community.[20-22] To accomplish this goal, the MESA study invited 1108 women who were interviewed in the household to a free clinic evaluation; 258 self-reported continent and 198 incontinent women 60 years or older accepted and were examined. The clinic evaluation included a 40-minute interview (history), a physical examination including a pelvic examination, a noninstrumented provocative stress test, and urinalysis. Based on this information, a clinician determined each subject's continence status and the type of incontinence—stress, urge, mixed, or other. At the conclusion of the clinic visit, all subjects were invited to participate in a thorough urodynamic test. A total of 67 clinic-diagnosed continent and 100 incontinent respondents accepted. The urodynamic test consisted of an initial noninstrumented uroflowmetric test, catheterized measurement of the postvoid residual volume, filling and voiding cystometry with abdominal pressure monitoring, passive and dynamic urethral pressure measurements, and lateral resting and stress urethrocystograms.

The uroflowmetric measures of peak flow rate (PFR) and average flow rate (AFR) were analyzed according to the volume voided at increments of 100 ml. When volume was controlled, the mean PFR and AFR were not significantly different between the continent and incontinent subjects. There was also no significant difference in the flow rates of the four clinical types of incontinence. Continuity of the urinary stream was not associated with continence status or with the clinical type of incontinence. This

TABLE 6-2
**Estimated Prevalences (Percent) of
Female Subjects Classified by
Amount of Residual Urine and by
Clinical Diagnosis**

Clinical Diagnosis	Residual Urine (ml)[a]				Total No.
	0-50	51-100	101-150	151+	
Continent	78.1 ± 5.8	9.7 ± 3.2	2.4 ± 1.7	9.7 ± 3.7	69
Incontinent	86.5 ± 5.4	8.4 ± 2.9	1.6 ± 1.5	3.5 ± 2.0	92
Overall	81.6 ± 4.5	9.2 ± 2.2	2.1 ± 1.2	7.1 ± 2.3	161

[a]Estimated proportions and their standard errors are presented.

lack of correlation between flow rate and continence status was similar to the observation of Fantl and his group.[23] Because of the lack of discriminatory power of the uroflow test, uroflow measurements should not be used as a routine test in the diagnosis of an incontinent elderly woman except when concomitant obstructive symptoms are also being evaluated.

The volume of postvoid residual urine did not correlate with either continence status or clinical type of incontinence. Estimates of the proportion of subjects within the various ranges of postvoid residual urine measurements are presented in Table 6-2. The prevalence of a postvoid residual urine specimen greater than 50 ml among women 60 years and older is 16.3%. There was no statistically significant difference between continent and incontinent women with regard to prevalence of a residual urine volume of more than 50 ml. These findings are significant because it has always been assumed that at residual volumes of more than 150 ml urinary incontinence of the overflow type would be more prevalent. Because there were as many continent as incontinent respondents at any level of residual urine elevation it appears that an elevated volume of residual urine alone does not cause urinary incontinence. It is possible that incontinence may develop in someone with a high residual urine volume only when there is total detrusor failure, superimposed detrusor overactivity, or sphincteric dysfunction.

There are a few more data in the literature on the prevalence of uninhibited detrusor contractions in the elderly. However, most of the published data were obtained from limited and selected groups such as clinic patients or referrals to a specialist rather than from community-dwelling subjects. Brocklehurst and Dillane reported a 53% prevalence of uninhibited detrusor contractions among their incontinent subjects.[24] Castleden and associates reported a 61% prevalence, and Hilton and Stanton reported a 39% rate.[25, 26] These prevalence rates of uninhibited bladder contractions are significantly higher than those reported by the MESA study.[20] The MESA prevalence rate of uninhibited detrusor contractions among incontinent respondents of 12% may be explained by the fact that the subjects of the MESA study were community dwellers who were relatively healthy

compared with the hospital patients and stroke victims in the Brocklehurst series and the highly selected referred incontinent patients in the other two series. The prevalence in the MESA continent group of 4.9% is closer to the figure reported by Jones and Schoenberg,[27] who found an 11.1% prevalence among 38 hospitalized women without any urologic symptoms but far lower than the 30% prevalence rate of "large" uninhibited contractions among continent subjects reported by Brocklehurst and Dillane.[24] However, 40% of their subjects had central nervous system disease (predominantly cerebrovascular accidents). See Table 6-3 for the MESA prevalence rate of uninhibited bladder contractions.

There was no significant difference in the prevalence of uninhibited bladder contractions among women with no voiding symptoms and women with either irritative voiding or bladder emptying symptoms. Of the 166 women tested, the prevalence rates of uninhibited bladder contractions were 7% for asymptomatic respondents, 8% for those with irritative bladder symptoms, and 7% for those with bladder emptying symptoms. These findings suggest that uninhibited detrusor contractions are uncommon among healthy noninstitutionalized elderly women. The high prevalence among hospitalized or institutionalized patients with multiple health problems suggests that uninhibited detrusor contractions are more likely related to these medical conditions than to aging per se.

The use of urethral pressure profilometry (UPP) in the evaluation of female urinary incontinence is extremely controversial. The two tests used are the passive or static UPP and the dynamic UPP. The MESA study showed that static and dynamic UPP performed in the supine position did not distinguish (no significant difference) between continent and incontinent subjects.[21] However, static and dynamic UPP performed in the standing position did show a significant difference between continent and incontinent subjects, although there was so much overlap in the values recorded that it is impossible to adopt a specific range of values that can be used to identify patients with urethral insufficiency in elderly women.

Supine length of the urethra, both functional and anatomic, and the standing anatomic length did not distinguish between subjects with continence and incontinence or between those with stress and nonstress incontinence.[21] Although the functional ure-

TABLE 6-3
**Estimated Prevalences of Female
Subjects Classified by Uninhibited
Bladder and Clinical Diagnosis**

	Continent	Incontinent	Overall
Percentage with uninhibited bladder[a]	4.9 ± 2.9	12.2 ± 3.7	7.9 ± 2.3
Total no.	65	99	164

[a]Mean ± standard error.

thral lengths in the standing position of continent and incontinent subjects were significantly different, the amount of overlap between groups prevents the use of any specific length as a reliable guide to diagnosis of urethral insufficiency in elderly women.

Lateral stress urethrocystography showed that location of the bladder neck above or below the urogenital diaphragm (UGD) and the urethral axis did not correlate with continence status.[21, 22] This lack of correlation between the location of the bladder neck and continence status raises some doubt about the theory that the descent of the bladder neck below the urogenital diaphragm is a major factor in the development of stress urinary incontinence.

The posterior urethrovesical angle (PUV) was strongly associated with continence status. This finding supports the view that the PUV is significantly wider in incontinent women, probably due to loss of support or weakness of the posterior floor of the urethrovesical junction, a condition that supports the observations made by Jeffcoate and Roberts.[28] However, although there was a significant difference between the average PUV values in continent and incontinent respondents, it did not distinguish between stress and nonstress urinary incontinence. In addition, there was significant overlap in PUV values between continent and incontinent subjects, so that this test cannot be used alone in the diagnosis of urinary incontinence. This test may be more useful in assessing the type of repair to be done than in diagnosis.

The provocative stress test was an extremely specific test, producing only one false-positive result among 68 women when compared with self-reported continence status. Of greater importance is the fact that it was 100% specific for subjects who have nonstress incontinence symptoms. However, the sensitivity of the stress test is low, and it has an expected false-negative rate in the population of 28.5%. Sensitivity is further reduced if the severity of stress urine loss is minimal; the stress test was positive in only 13.9% of such subjects. This is a significant observation in that when the result of the stress test is positive, it suggests a moderate or severe type of stress incontinence.

Final analysis of the results of urodynamic tests in elderly noninstitutionalized women suggests that the symptom of stress urine loss, either alone or in combination with other symptoms, makes it likely that the patient will have urethral insufficiency or urethral sphincteric dysfunction. On the other hand, urge incontinence is a much more nonspecific symptom, with only 13.1% manifesting uninhibited bladder contractions on cystometry. Unless one opts for a therapeutic trial of an anticholinergic-antispasmodic agent, cystometry is the only direct test available to identify involuntary detrusor contractions.

The rest of the battery of urodynamic tests, including the uroflow study, static and dynamic urethral pressure profile, and lateral urethrocystography, should be used mainly as confirmatory studies when the diagnosis is suspected but not well established.

These tests may also help, when the diagnosis is already established, to determine the therapeutic approach to be used and to assess or predict the outcome of therapy.

REFERENCES

1. Thomas TM, Plymat KR, Blannin J, et al: Prevalence of urinary incontinence. BMJ 281:1243, 1980.
2. Elving LB, Foldspang A, Lam GW, et al: Descriptive epidemiology of urinary incontinence in 3,100 women age 30–59. Scand J Urol Nephrol 125 (Suppl): 37, 1989.
3. Wells T, Brink C: Urinary incontinence: Assessment and management. In Burnside M (ed): Nursing and the Aged. New York, McGraw-Hill, 1981, pp 519–548.
4. U.S. Department of Health, Education and Welfare: Long-Term Care Facility Improvement Study. Washington, DC, U.S. Government Printing Office, 1975.
5. Van Nostrand JF, et al (ed): The National Nursing Home Survey: Summary for the United States. DHEW Publication No. 79-1794. Vital and Health Statistics Series 13, No. 43. Washington DC, National Center for Health Statistics, Health Resources Administration, 1977.
6. Willington FL: Significance of incompetence of personal sanitary habits. Nurs Times 71:340, 1975.
7. Brocklehurst JC, Griffiths L, Fry J: The prevalence and symptomatology of urinary infection in an aged population. Gerontol Clin 10:242, 1968.
8. Akhtar AJ, Broe GA, Crombie A, et al: Disability and dependence in the elderly at home. Age Aging 2:102, 1973.
9. Yarnell JWG, Voyle GJ: The prevalence and severity of urinary incontinence in women. J Epidemiol Community Health 35:71, 1981.
10. Diokno AC, Brock BM, Brown MB, et al: Prevalence of urinary incontinence and other urological symptoms in the noninstitutionalized elderly. J Urol 136:1022, 1986.
11. Herzog AR, Diokno AC, Brown MB, et al: Two-year incidence, remission, and change patterns of urinary incontinence in noninstitutionalized older adults. J Geront Med Sci 45:67, 1990.
12. Diokno AC, Brock BM, Brown MB, et al: Medical correlates of urinary incontinence in the elderly. Urology 36:129, 1990.
13. Herzog AR, Fultz NG, Brock BM, et al: Urinary incontinence and psychological distress among older adults. Psychology Aging 3:115, 1988.
14. Miller RL: Urinary incontinence in the community elderly: Functional status, cognitive function and depressive symptoms: Findings from the Yale Health and Aging Study. Paper presented at the 113th Annual Meeting of the American Public Health Association, Washington, DC, 1985.
15. Herzog AR, Fultz NH, Normolle DP, et al: Methods used to manage urinary incontinence by older adults in the community. J Am Geriatr Soc 37: 339, 1989.
16. Diokno AC, Brown MB, Herzog AR: Relationship between use of diuretics and continence status in the elderly. Urology 38(1):39–42, 1991.
17. Wells TJ, Brink CA, Diokno AC: Urinary incontinence in the elderly women: Clinical findings. J Am Geriatr Soc 35:933, 1987.
18. Ouslander JG: Diagnostic evaluation of geriatric urinary incontinence. Geriatr Med 2(4):715, 1986.
19. Shimp LA, Wells TJ, Brink CA, et al: Relationship between drug use and urinary incontinence in elderly women. Drug Intel Clin Pharmacol 22:786, 1988.
20. Diokno AC, Brown MB, Brock BM, et al: Clinical and cystometric characteristics of continent and incontinent noninstitutionalized elderly. J Urol 140:567, 1988.
21. Diokno AC, Normolle DP, Brown MB, et al: Urodynamic tests for female geriatric urinary incontinence. Urology 36:431, 1990.
22. Diokno AC: Diagnostic categories of incontinence and the role of urodynamic testing. J Am Geriatr Soc 38:300, 1990.

23. Fantl JA, Smith PJ, Scheider V, et al: Fluid weight uroflowmetry in women. Am J Obstet Gynecol 145:1017, 1983.
24. Brocklehurst JC, Dillane JB: Studies of the female bladder in old age. Cystometrograms in non-incontinent women. Gerontol Clin 8:285, 1966.
25. Castleden CM, Duffin HM, Asher MJ: Clinical and urodynamic studies in 100 elderly incontinent patients. BMJ 282:1103, 1981.
26. Hilton P, Stanton SL: Algorithmic method for assessing urinary incontinence in elderly women. BMJ 282:940, 1981.
27. Jones KW, Schoenberg HW: Comparison of the incidence of bladder hyperreflexia in patients with benign prostatic hyperplasia and age-matched female controls. J Urol 133:425, 1985.
28. Jeffcoate TNA, Roberts H: Stress incontinence of urine. J Obstet Gynecol Br Emp 59:685, 1952.

CHAPTER 7

The Social Impact of Urinary Incontinence

Katherine F. Jeter, Ed.D., E.T., C.E.T.N.

The deleterious psychological, social, and economic sequelae of urinary incontinence have been widely considered and frequently reported in recent years.[1-15] However, it is difficult to draw conclusions from the literature because of disparate research methods, population samples, and definitions of incontinence. This chapter has several purposes. It begins with a brief review of prevalence and psychosocial impact studies. Findings from two extensive surveys of people with incontinence will be described, and, finally, suggestions for improving current clinical practices in the management of incontinent women will be discussed.

Prevalence and Psychosocial Impact Studies

Incontinence of some degree affects many women in all age groups. In various studies in this country and abroad the prevalence of incontinence in women has been estimated to be between 9 and 74%.[3, 8, 15-19] Currently, the Clinical Practice Guideline on Urinary Incontinence in Adults, published by the Agency for Health Care Policy and Research (AHCPR) of the U.S. Public Health Service, estimates that 10 million Americans are affected by incontinence.[15] The majority are women. The Guideline panel acknowledges that this estimate may be low. The number of incontinent people in the United States could be twice that if one considers the actual number of women who are incontinent but have never told anyone, the number of those who still leak after incontinence operations or begin leaking again several years after surgery, and the limitations of previous prevalence studies.

Despite the fact that urinary incontinence is esti-

mated to affect up to 74% of the female population, there are relatively few studies that measure the social impact of urinary incontinence on the daily lives of women.[20] These studies, like prevalence studies, use varying definitions of incontinence and varying scales and tools to measure impact. It seems obvious that attitudes toward voiding dysfunction vary widely among individuals and in different age groups, but research to verify this has been limited.[21] Wyman and colleagues summarized the results of 19 studies in 1990.[20] In these and other studies, avoidance of specific activities was a recurrent finding.[6, 10, 18, 22, 23] Decreased outings from home, less participation in social activities, and avoidance of sexual intimacy were frequently reported. Despite a decade that has seen an enormous increase in the amount of attention given to the prevalence, incidence, and impact of incontinence by the scientific community, governmental agencies, and the media, women with this condition in 1995 may not be receiving the treatment that they need or desire.[24, 25]

The Problem of Defining Incontinence

The concept of incontinence still eludes definition. Currently, there are three commonly used definitions, and numerous others are used occasionally. The International Continence Society (ICS) defines incontinence as ". . . involuntary loss of urine which is a social or hygienic problem and which is objectively demonstrable."[26] The Clinical Practice Guideline on Urinary Incontinence in Adults eschewed the ICS definition in favor of ". . . the involuntary loss of urine which is sufficient to be a problem."[15] In publications targeted to lay people, the definition may be different from these. A common explanation of incontinence is "the unexpected loss of urine in any amount, on a regular basis, in an inconvenient place. . . ."[1, 27] Because previous studies have not shown a correlation between the amount or frequency of urine loss and emotional distress, still other definitions might be considered, such as, "Incontinence is the inability to go to the bathroom when you want to and where you want to." Recognizing that loss of bladder control may not be a problem to patients with dementia, but that it is a leading cause of admission to nursing homes when families find it too taxing to care for an incontinent relative, another accurate definition might be, "Urinary incontinence refers to the uncontrolled passage of urine."

Social Influences That Affect Attitudes and Bladder Habits in Different Age Groups

The cause of incontinence in women remains unclear, but in most cases it is multifactorial.[19, 28] In the past efforts have been made to discover a psychogenic component.[2, 4, 29–36] Although several studies have shown that neuroticism and psychological factors may coexist with incontinence, there probably is not a cause-and-effect relationship.[2, 4, 29, 35] However, a reduction in sensory urgency and urine leakage has been shown to reduce psychological symptoms and improve the quality of life.[2, 37–38] Practically speaking, elimination of the "fear of accidents" and the comfort and confidence of being able to toilet predictably every 2 to 3 hours rather than unpredictably every 30 minutes to $1\frac{1}{2}$ hours certainly enhance psychological well-being and facilitate the opportunity to participate in social activities. Although it is doubtful that urinary incontinence in women has psychogenic origins, there are nevertheless psychological and social influences that exert a powerful impact on attitudes toward toileting and toward loss of bladder control.

CHILDHOOD AND ADOLESCENCE

Bowel and bladder control are highly prized in early childhood because they connote maturity, intelligence, and discipline. Children with nocturnal enuresis usually will not sleep at friends' homes or go away to camp because of the fear of ostracism or taunting. During adolescence, girls report an unwillingness to use the toilets at school because there are no doors on the stalls to give them privacy during urination. Schools explain that they must be able to maintain surveillance for drug use and cigarette smoking in the bathrooms. There is often inadequate time for girls to use the toilet between classes. Students report being reprimanded when their use of the bathroom between classes causes them to be late for the next class. School officials say they cannot allow pupils unrestricted access to bathrooms between and during classes because this would be disruptive, and most students would abuse the privilege. It is not uncommon for middle school and high school girls to void only before and after school. Such common practices do not tend to engender healthy attitudes toward elimination or reasonable bladder habits in adulthood.

ADULTHOOD

In adult women there are environmental and occupational impediments to good bladder habits. Although several states have introduced "potty parity" laws to increase the number of women's toilets in public places, it is not unusual to see long lines in ladies' restrooms at cultural and sporting events, airports, and meeting sites where the audience is predominantly female. Some women report restricting the amount and types of fluids they consume in anticipation of particular activities. Some employers restrict access to toilets. Assembly line workers, stenographers, and teachers may be required to urinate by the job's schedule rather than by their bladder capacity. Even without published policy guidelines governing toilet use, nurses, waitresses, and secretaries may find it difficult to urinate at reasonable intervals. Symptoms of sensory urgency, frequency, and incontinence may preclude a woman from taking or keeping certain jobs. A recent tongue-in-cheek article in a popular women's magazine describes the inadequacy of women's restrooms in office and government buildings and asserts that "the American economy is not going to appreciate the importance of a decent restroom to the average female worker until the American economy is run by women."[39] In fact, until recently in the U.S. Capitol, female senators have had to wait in line with tourists downstairs from the Senate chamber for want of access to a closer toilet because those outside the Senate chamber used to be for men only.

LATER LIFE

In the ever-increasing elderly population there are myriad social influences on bladder habits and serious repercussions for women who become incontinent or whose continence is marginal. Many public facilities and churches do not have accessible bathrooms. A woman with precarious bladder control or irritable voiding symptoms will soon determine "safe environments" in which she can get to the bathroom quickly. Consciously or subconsciously, she will eliminate places and programs where toileting would be difficult. Buses and vans that transport senior citizens to social functions and medical appointments usually do not have toilets. Older women report being unable to take advantage of transportation services because of this. Incontinence is not just a leading cause of admission to nursing homes; it may affect the living arrangements of tens of thousands of other older women. In the burgeoning retirement community industry, in which there are usually three levels of care—independent living, personal care, and skilled care—loss of bladder or bowel control usually results in a resident being moved from an independent living arrangement to a unit that provides more personal services. This loss of independence with enforced and increased professional assistance is a demeaning and expensive consequence of urinary incontinence.

How Women Have Reported the Experience of Incontinence in the Decade from 1983–1993

In 1983, a year after Help for Incontinent People (HIP),* a national nonprofit advocacy organization, was founded, the popular advice columnist "Dear Abby" discussed incontinence and advised her readers to write HIP for more information. Nearly 50,000 people wrote for help. They complained of embarrassment, loneliness, isolation, and frustration with the medical profession. In 1986 HIP developed a six-page, 34-item questionnaire, which was mailed to 33,500 people. Completed surveys were returned by 10,427 individuals.[10] The majority were reasonably healthy women 60 years of age or older who were living at home. The average length of time they had been incontinent was 9 years. Many of their management or coping strategies were self-devised. Modifying drinking habits and toileting practices were the two methods most commonly used to control urine loss. Feminine hygiene products and paper towels were the products most often used. Incontinence was described as a major problem with important social implications by 17.3% of them. This is consistent with the findings of a number of investigators.[38, 40, 41] However, the fact that *most* women say that they are not severely burdened by incontinence does not mean that *all* patients should not be carefully assessed to determine the impact of incontinence on their health and quality of life.[19, 28, 42, 43] Several worrisome findings appeared in the 1986 HIP survey. Nearly 40% of respondents believed that they were incontinent because they were old; another 20% said that they did not know why they were incontinent. These misconceptions may account for some women's failure to report incontinence to a physician or to articulate their symptoms during an office visit. The medical profession received poor marks from this sample population. Half of the respondents described doctors or

nurses as not helpful or too busy; 37.5% did not think that the health care provider was informative or knowledgeable. Nearly one-fourth (24.4%) thought that the doctor was embarrassed or unsympathetic. Only 9.7% said they were helped very much by their doctor, and 56.5% reported that their treatment was "no help at all." Findings from this survey cannot be generalized because the population represented a unique group. The majority of those surveyed were readers of an advice column and recipients of a quarterly newsletter about incontinence. However, the survey gave valuable insight into the lived experience of women with incontinence.

In 1992 a similar survey was sent to 115,000 people.[25] Half of them were members of HIP, and half had made one request for information from the organization but had not had sustained contact. Analyses of 3986 (4%) completed surveys were tabulated. Again the survey population was predominantly healthy older women living in the community. Some attitudes and behaviors had changed noticeably since the 1986 survey. More than 86% of the women had seen a physician about their incontinence. This is a marked increase from previous studies, which reported that only 25 to 50% of women had consulted a physician.[10, 14, 18, 24] As in the earlier HIP survey, incontinence was perceived quite differently within the group. Women whose incontinence was characterized by urgency and frequency were most likely to consider it a major problem. Dissatisfaction with the medical profession was high but not as high as in the earlier survey. More people became worse (6%) with treatment than were improved by it (3.2%). Women who elected to have surgery had both the highest levels of success and the highest levels of treatment failure. This finding is consistent with that of Diokno and associates in a study of 51 women in which it was reported that only 39% of those who had undergone surgery to correct urine loss had achieved absolute continence during a median follow-up period of 12 years.[44] Diokno and his colleagues also found that urologic symptoms were reported more frequently by respondents who had had surgery than by nonoperated respondents, suggesting that symptoms may have been induced by the operation. HIP's 1992 survey supported this finding, although it was impossible to determine whether the bothersome symptoms of frequency and urgency were caused by the operation or simply became more noticeable after symptoms of stress incontinence had been alleviated. Respondents to HIP's 1992 survey were asked to rate their bladder control problems on a scale of 1 to 5, with 5 being the greatest and 1 being the least of their concerns. Embarrassment was ranked highest, and odor was ranked second. Isolation from friends and family was the least worrisome to the respondents (Table 7–1). These data refute earlier reports that isolation from friends and family is common among incontinent people and may reflect an attitudinal change resulting from a decade of public education and perhaps improved management options.[11, 15] In their daily lives, 55% of respondents termed their

---

*Help for Incontinent People is a not-for-profit organization dedicated to improving the quality of life of people with incontinence. HIP is a leading source of education, advocacy, and support to the public and the health professions about the causes, prevention, diagnosis, treatments, and management alternatives for incontinence. For additional information, write HIP, P.O. Box 8306, Spartanburg, South Carolina 29305.

TABLE 7–1
Rating of Bladder Control Problems

Types of Worry	Numerical Rating	Mean Score All Respondents
Embarrassment	5 = Greatest worry	3.4
Odor	4	3.0
Cost	3	2.6
Isolation—friends	2	2.3
Isolation—family	1 = Least worry	2.0

loss of bladder control "always bothersome but manageable." Only 13.5% described it as a major problem, and 26% described it as an occasional nuisance. More than twice as many respondents in 1992 had been taught to do Kegel exercises than had been taught in the earlier population. Ideally, this change indicates a shift toward behavioral interventions for women with mild to moderate stress and urge incontinence.

The Difficulty of Measuring the Social Impact of Incontinence

Evaluating the social impact of incontinence requires scrutiny of both the social milieu and the cultural and historical attitudes of patients and health care providers. Early definitions of incontinence refer to it as an inability to suppress sexual appetite.[5] By 1976, English dictionaries added urine and fecal loss to the earlier definition, but incontinence was still defined primarily in terms of sexual promiscuity and bad temper. Thus, the term incontinence bespeaks lack of restraint and control and is a value-laden term. Furthermore, the time, place, and method of urination are culturally proscribed. The age of expected continence and toilet training and the point at which incontinence is no longer tolerated vary between cultures, within cultures, and between generations. In the 1950s and 1960s in the United States, early toilet training was the mode. Children in most states, even as late as the 1970s, were not allowed to attend public schools until they had achieved continence. Social attitudes and laws have changed remarkably in the past three to four decades. In the 1990s young parents are less likely to attempt toilet training as early as their parents did. They are less likely to be punitive toward preschoolers who have not achieved bladder control. Incontinent children, by virtue of legislation ensuring that all children have equal access to education in the least restrictive environment, now are ensured entry into public schools. The popular press, however, continues to refer to the subject of incontinence as "a closet issue" and the "last taboo," reinforcing the social stigma that continues to be associated with lack of bladder control.

Relating the Social Implications of Urinary Incontinence to Clinical Practice

To interpret the social implications of incontinence in women and apply them to current clinical practices to improve care for women with this pervasive condition, the *lived* experience of urine leakage must be separated from the *fact* of urine loss.[45] The fact and the lived experience may be quite dissimilar within groups, and it certainly varies between age groups.[18, 45] Urine leakage during intercourse in a 25-year-old newly married female cannot be equated with urine leakage in a 19-year-old paraplegic in her work setting, an 84-year-old woman who wants to travel with a church group, and a severely cognitively impaired 78-year-old nursing home resident. However, despite individual differences, varying urinary symptoms, and changing social mores, incontinent women currently share several unique burdens:

1. They do not report the onset of incontinence promptly and may "put up with it" for 6 to 9 years before seeking medical treatment.[7, 10, 18, 38, 42]
2. Women are accustomed to using feminine hygiene products and choose them in many instances instead of products specifically designed for urine absorption.[10, 18]
3. When they do seek treatment, women are likely to have their incontinence symptoms dismissed and to be dissatisfied with the results of their treatment. When their symptoms cannot be verified objectively by pad tests or urodynamic methods, they may be referred for psychological counseling or labeled neurotic.[36]
4. Despite mounting evidence that behavioral interventions promise improvement and even cure in many women with voiding dysfunction and urinary incontinence, American women are seldom offered this therapy.[25, 28, 38, 46, 47, 48]

DIAGNOSIS

The reasons why women tolerate incontinence for many years before seeking medical care remain unclear. Bayliss and Norton and associates found embarrassment to be the major factor causing delay.[38, 42] Both of these study populations were English, and the majority (79%) of general practitioners in England are men. Because embarrassment is acutely felt among incontinent American women and 81.9% of physicians in the United States are men, this factor may explain the similar delay in seeking treatment among American women. Norton and associates found that elderly women waited twice as long to seek treatment as younger women because they feared that surgery would be required. Other studies indicate that many women think that urine leakage is normal and not a condition that warrants medical treatment.[38] Others believe it to be, or are told that it is, an expected part of getting old. It is possible that some women do not deem their incontinence troublesome enough to spend the money or time needed for medical care. This latter attitude merits future research. These various attitudes have important implications for health providers.

A sensitive approach to the subject of urine leakage is required while taking a woman's history and performing the physical examination. It is helpful to send history forms and voiding diaries to the patient prior to the initial office visit. These imply that incontinence is common and may put patients at ease with the subject. It may also help them describe their urinary history better when they are given adequate time to think about it and spared the embarrassment of having to describe it in a face-to-face encounter with a health professional of the opposite sex. A prescreening intake or incontinence history might best be taken by another woman. Patients may be more comfortable with an office or clinic nurse, a physical therapist, or even a medical social worker whom they perceive to be an ally who would be less critical or scornful of this embarrassing condition.

Continuing public information and patient education are essential to cause women to recognize incontinence as a treatable symptom and to seek solutions for it aggressively. Consumers need to be taught how to access a health provider with a special interest in the diagnosis and treatment of incontinence and to request a second opinion if their primary physician does not take the complaint seriously or dismisses it as part of being female or as an expected complaint of aging.

TREATMENT

Once urinary incontinence has been identified as a symptom, the cause and the impact of the symptom on the patient's quality of life merit equal attention. Symptoms that are not secondary to anatomic displacement, concomitant medical conditions, or pharmacologic therapy required by another illness can be minimized or eliminated completely by modifying toileting behavior, daily activities, diet, and lifestyle.[48] The patient's active participation is required. Women are most likely to become involved and be compliant and to achieve success with treatment if their bladder symptoms interfere with social, intimate, or occupational activities *and* when a therapeutic relationship is developed between the caregiver and the patient.[20, 37, 41] Psychotherapy has been shown to improve bladder symptoms even in the absence of cystometric changes.[35] Might the sympathetic and proactive attitude of a physician or nurse be equally therapeutic? Various types of behavioral interventions have been shown to be effective in reducing incontinence in women.[25, 28, 38, 46, 49] Although cost comparison data are not yet available, it seems obvious that two to six sessions with a patient conducted by a nurse or licensed allied health professional to teach toileting procedures, describe dietary

influences on bladder habits, teach pelvic muscle exercises, monitor progress, and reinforce desired outcomes would be less expensive than medication or surgery.[35, 48, 49, 50] Other obvious advantages are that many of these interventions might have an additive effect with pharmacologic therapy or surgery. Rosenzweig and colleagues attempted to evaluate psychological status before and after surgery for stress incontinence.[36] They concluded that women who continued to experience urinary symptoms and psychological distress after surgery that had been deemed to be curative by urodynamic measures should be considered for psychological evaluation. Perhaps these women could have benefited from a therapeutic relationship with a health care provider who could help them improve their bladder habits with behavioral therapy. Experiences in programs that offer *only* behavioral therapy suggest that patients are not as frustrated when behavioral therapy yields only partial success as they are when expensive medications or surgical procedures do not result in complete resolution of symptoms.[37, 38, 49]

A caveat to urologists and gynecologists is that they must be enthusiastic proponents of behavioral interventions as first-line therapy. This offers assurance to their patients that the initiation of behavioral treatment rather than drugs or surgery does not imply that their symptoms are unimportant or "not bad enough for medicine or surgery."

Because symptoms of frequency and urgency are so troubling to patients, bladder training to increase the intervals between toileting coupled with dietary modification to minimize irritative voiding symptoms should improve patients' psychological well-being.[25, 28, 35, 37, 48] Several factors have been identified as impediments to the success of behavioral interventions: duration of incontinence, poor compliance, and obesity.[2, 28] Addressing each of these issues with patients and assisting them with printed materials, record-keeping forms, and personnel to monitor and reward success as well as encouraging a weight control program may improve treatment outcomes. Reaching women in health clubs, beauty salons, and health education forums who are just beginning to have problems with incontinence may be the key to improving the success of behavioral therapies. Bavendam and colleagues, in a study of women who used weighted vaginal cones, found that those women who referred themselves for cone use had the most successful outcome.[51] In a recent survey of women who completed a 4-hour educational program about the causes, treatments, and management alternatives for or pertaining to urinary incontinence, 24 of 40 women who completed the course were interviewed. One participant (5.8%) was cured; 47% rated their improvement as 20 to 90% better; two (11.6%) elected to have surgery, and one patient (5.8%) rated her incontinence as worse after the class. Five women (29%) had no change in their symptoms but also had made no change in their daily activities or bladder habits.[49] All women expressed satisfaction with the program and said they would recommend it to a friend. The cost to the hospital to conduct the classes, including simple refreshments, was $34.00 per person. Such classes warrant investigation, refinement, and pilot programs to investigate their efficacy.

DEFINING AND PREPARING HEALTH PROFESSIONALS

Family physicians and internists should be encouraged to include a sensitive and thorough continence evaluation in their routine patient assessments.[8, 19, 43] Nurse practitioners, nurse specialists, and some physical therapists practice in settings where an incontinence evaluation would be appropriate. With some advanced training, these health professionals should be able to evaluate patients' voiding dysfunction and recognize those for whom behavioral intervention would be appropriate and those for whom referral to a specialist would be preferable. Women admitted to the hospital for other conditions should have a thorough continence evaluation.

All health workers, school administrators, employers, and lawmakers should be educated to view bladder health and bladder control as a woman's right. Every effort should be made to construct enough toilet facilities, to provide adequate time for toileting, and to offer sufficient privacy and respect to encourage females to understand the importance of developing good bladder habits.

Implications for Future Research

Regardless of the difficulties inherent in defining the social impact of urinary incontinence on the lives of women of all ages, it is obvious that loss of bladder control results in restricted activities and other physical and social limitations. However, fewer than 20% of women describe incontinence as a major problem. There is no explanation for why women tolerate incontinence for an average of 7 to 9 years before seeking treatment. Are they resigned to their "female lot"?[52] Have they felt rebuffed by a health professional? Are they unaware that treatments are available that may improve or cure their symptoms? Do they fear that the cure would be worse than the disease? Why are tens of thousands of women calling nonprofit advocacy organizations and government agency numbers for help? Why are so many women dissatisfied with their medical treatment and the care they receive? What accounts for the difference between a study conducted by medical researchers, which showed that consumers believe that physicians could help them with their incontinence even after surgery has failed, and studies conducted by nonmedical groups, in which women perceived physicians as "not helpful"?[10, 25, 44, 52]

Prospective studies to identify strategies that maintain continence and prevent incontinence are urgently needed. Efforts must be continued to destigmatize incontinence and to develop more reasonable attitudes toward bladder function and dysfunction in different age groups. Now that behavioral interventions have proved effective, future research should be directed toward comparing the relative effects of different treatments and identifying factors associated with treatment failure.[5] Rather than continuing to select study subjects by age or symptoms, it is time to change the focus to determine how the lived experience of incontinence varies during the life span and how treatment choices—surgical, pharmacologic, and behavioral—affect the quality of life. It is not difficult to teach allied health professionals to recognize urinary symptoms that warrant referral to a urologist or urogynecologist for management, but it may be a significant challenge to teach surgeons to recognize patients for whom behavioral intervention would be most therapeutic and to refer these women to an individual qualified to provide this care.

Rather than separating subjective complaints of incontinence from objective demonstration of bladder leakage in a laboratory, self-reporting of bladder dysfunction and its effect on daily activities must be considered reliable data and treatment outcomes should be measured according to patient expectation and patient satisfaction. In most studies the social impact of incontinence varies widely and does not correlate with the amount of leakage or the duration of symptoms. Thus, in the majority of cases, the first-line intervention for women with urinary incontinence should be education to prepare them to choose the therapy that they believe will offer the most benefit in the context of their social setting. Surgery, in the absence of physical abnormalities that threaten renal function or cause debilitating symptoms, should be presented as an elective procedure.

REFERENCES

1. Gartley CB: Managing Incontinence. Ottawa, IL, Jameson Books, 1985, p 11.
2. Oldenburg B, Millard RJ: Predictors of longterm outcome following a bladder retraining program. J Psychosom Res 30(6):691–698, 1986.
3. Mohide EA: The prevalence and scope of urinary incontinence. Clin Geriatr Med 2(4):639–654, 1986.
4. Morrison M, Morrison LM, McAlister A, Glen ES: Visual analog scores and urinary incontinence. Br Med J 295:854, 1987.
5. Smith PS, Smith LJ: Continence and Incontinence. London, Croom Helm, 1987, p 27.
6. Breakwell SL, Walker SN: Differences in physical health, social interaction, and personal adjustment between continent and incontinent homebound aged women. J Community Health Nurs 5(1):19–31, 1988.
7. U.S. National Institutes of Health: Urinary Incontinence in Adults: Consensus conference. JAMA 261:2685–2690, 1989.
8. Jolleys JV: Reported prevalence of urinary incontinence in a general practice. BMJ 296:1300–1302, 1988.
9. Teasdale TA, Taffet GE, Luchi RJ, et al: Urinary incontinence in a community-residing elderly population. J Am Geriatr Soc 36(7):600–606, 1988.
10. Jeter KF, Wagner DB: Incontinence in the American home: A survey of 36,500 people. J Am Geriatr Soc 38(3):379–383, 1990.

11. Mitteness LS: Knowledge and beliefs about urinary incontinence in adulthood and old age. J Am Geriatr Soc 38(3):374–378, 1990.
12. Wyman JF, Fantl JA: Bladder training in ambulatory care management of urinary incontinence. Urol Nurs 11(3):11–17, 1991.
13. Sommer P, Bauer T, Nielsen KK, et al: Voiding patterns and prevalence of incontinence in women. Br J Urol 66:12–15, 1990.
14. Thiede HA: Prevalence of pelvic floor dysfunction in women. Conference on Pelvic Floor Dysfunction—An Initiative for Curriculum Enhancement in Residency Education. Chicago, The American Board of Obstetrics and Gynecology, 1992.
15. Urinary Incontinence Guideline Panel: Urinary Incontinence in Adults—Clinical Practice Guideline. AHCPR Publ 92-0038. Rockville, MD, U.S. Public Health Service, Agency for Health Care Policy and Research, 1992.
16. Versi E: Incontinence in the climacteric. Clin Obstet Gynecol 33(2):392–398, 1990.
17. Herzog AR, Fultz NH: Prevalence and incidence of urinary incontinence in community-dwelling populations. J Am Geriatr Soc 38(3):273–281, 1990.
18. Burgio KL, Matthews KA, Engel BT: Prevalence, incidence and correlates of urinary incontinence in healthy, middle-aged women. J Urol 146:1255–1259, 1991.
19. O'Connell HE, MacGregor RJ, Russell JM: Female urinary incontinence management in healthy, middle-aged women. Med J Aust 157(8):537–544, 1992.
20. Wyman JF, Harkins SW, Fantl JA: Psychosocial impact of urinary incontinence in the community-dwelling population. J Am Geriatr Soc 38(3):282–288, 1990.
21. Hunskaar S, Vinsnes A: The quality of life in women with urinary incontinence as measured by the sickness impact profile. J Am Geriatr Soc 39:378–382, 1991.
22. Norton PA: Prevalence and social impact of urinary incontinence in women. Clin Obstet Gynecol 33(2):295–297, 1990.
23. Lam GW, Foldspang A, Elving LB, Mommsen S: Social contacts, social abstention, and problem recognition correlated with adult female urinary incontinence. Danish Med Bull 39(6):565–570, 1992.
24. Norton PA: Non-surgical management. Conference on Pelvic Floor Dysfunction: An Initiative for Curriculum Enhancement in Residency Education. Chicago, The American Board of Obstetrics and Gynecology, 1992, pp 35–37.
25. Jeter KF, Verdell LL: Consumer focus '93: A survey of community-dwelling incontinent people. Union, SC, Help for Incontinent People, 1993.
26. Abrams P, Blaivas JG, Stanton SL, Andersen JT: The standardization of terminology of lower urinary tract dysfunction. Scand J Urol Nephrol Suppl 114:5–19, 1988.
27. Chalker R, Whitmore KE. Overcoming Bladder Disorders. New York, Harper-Collins, 1990, p 62.
28. Woodruff J, Thomas S: Behavioral medicine and the treatment of urinary symptoms. American Uro-Gynecologic Society Q Rep 11(1):1–5, 1993.
29. Norton KR, Bhat AV, Stanton SL: Psychiatric aspects of urinary incontinence in women attending an outpatient urodynamic clinic. BMJ 301(6746):271–272, 1990.
30. Hafner RJ, Stanton SL, Guy J: A psychiatric study of women with urgency and urge incontinence. Br J Urol 49:211–214, 1977.
31. Frewen WK: An objective assessment of the unstable bladder of psychosomatic origin. Br J Urol 50:246–249, 1978.
32. Stone CB, Judd GE: Psychogenic aspects of urinary incontinence in women. Clin Obstet Gynecol 21(3):807–815, 1978.
33. Crisp A, Sutherst J: Psychological factors in women with urinary incontinence. Proceedings of the International Continence Society and Urodynamic Society 1:174–176, 1983.
34. Morrison LM, Eadie AS, McAlister A, et al: Personality testing in 226 patients with urinary incontinence. Br J Urol 58:387–389, 1986.
35. Macaulay AJ, Stern RS, Holmes DM, Stanton SL: Micturition and the mind: Psychological factors in the etiology and treatment of urinary symptoms in women. BMJ 294:540–543, 1987.
36. Rosenzweig BA, Hirschke D, Thomas S, et al: Stress incontinence in women, psychological status before and after treatment. J Reprod Med 36(12):835–838, 1991.
37. Fantl JA, Wyman JF, McClish DK, et al: Efficacy of bladder training in older women with urinary incontinence. JAMA 265(5):609–613, 1991.
38. Bayliss V: Female incontinence: "The Basingstroke project." J R Soc Health 6:207–208, 1988.
39. Collins G: Potty politics: The gender gap. Working Woman, March 1993, p 93.
40. Lagro-Janssen ALM, Debruyne FMJ, Van Weel C: Psychologic aspects of female urinary incontinence in general practice. Br J Urol 70:499–502, 1992.
41. Wyman JF, Harkins SW, Choi SC, et al: Psycho-social impact of urinary incontinence in women. Obstet Gynecol 70(3):378–381, 1987.
42. Norton PA, MacDonald LD, Sedgwick PM, Stanton SL: The stress and delay associated with urinary incontinence, frequency, and urgency in women. BMJ 297:1187–1189, 1988.
43. Ouslander JG: Urinary incontinence: Out of the closet. JAMA 261(18):2695–2696, 1989.
44. Diokno AC, Brown MB, Brock BM, et al: Prevalence and outcome of surgery for female incontinence. Urology 33(4):285–290, 1989.
45. Klemm LW, Creason NS: Self-care practices of women with urinary incontinence—a preliminary study. Health Care Women Int 12:199–209, 1991.
46. Jeter K: Pelvic muscle exercises with and without biofeedback for the treatment of urinary incontinence. Probl Urol 5(1):72–83, 1991.
47. Newman DK, Smith DA: Pelvic muscle re-education as a nursing treatment for incontinence. Urol Nurs 12(1):9–15, 1992.
48. Bavendam TG: Geriatric female incontinence. Probl Urol 5(1):42–71, 1991.
49. Jeter KF, Tintle TE: Behavioral therapy in a group setting to promote continence in women: A test of efficacy and economy. Research Poster, American Urological Association Allied 25th Annual Meeting, San Antonio, Texas, May 16–20, 1993.
50. Forneret E, Leach GE: Cost-effective treatment of female stress urinary incontinence: Modified Pereyra bladder neck suspension. Urology 25:365–367, 1985.
51. Bavendam TG, Kallhoff JM, Gibbs CJ: Feminine vaginal cones for the treatment of stress urinary incontinence. Poster American Uro-Gynecologic Society 13th Annual Meeting, Boston, Massachusetts, August 27–30, 1992.
52. Glew J: A woman's lot? Nursing Times, April 9, 1986, pp 69–71.

PART II

Evaluation

CHAPTER 8

Evaluation of Urinary Tract Dysfunction

Dianne M. Heritz, M.D., F.R.C.S.C.
Jerry G. Blaivas, M.D., F.A.C.S.

Diagnostic evaluation of voiding dysfunction in women commences with a focused but detailed history and physical examination. Subjective information is derived from the patient's history as obtained from interviews or questionnaires. Semiobjective data are obtained from self-reported diaries and pad tests. Objective data are obtained by physical examination, laboratory tests, radiologic studies, ultrasound, urodynamic studies, and cystoscopy. Collection of subjective, semiobjective, and objective data should continue during and after treatment to assess outcomes.

The spectrum of voiding dysfunction ranges from mild stress urinary incontinence to severe neurologic disease resulting in upper urinary tract deterioration. Because the patient's symptoms are not necessarily proportional to the degree of bladder or renal involvement, a systematic approach should be used to include all aspects of voiding dysfunction.

Incontinence

Urinary incontinence is defined as an involuntary loss of urine that is objectively demonstrable and is a social or hygienic problem to the patient or caregiver. Urinary incontinence denotes a symptom, a sign, and a condition. The symptom indicates the patient's (or caregiver's) statement of involuntary urine loss. The sign is the objective demonstration of urine loss. The condition is the pathophysiologic condition underlying incontinence as demonstrated by clinical or urodynamic techniques.

ETIOLOGY OF URINARY INCONTINENCE

Urinary incontinence can be further divided into urethral and extraurethral incontinence. Urethral in-continence is caused by either bladder abnormalities or sphincter abnormalities. Both cognitive abnormalities and physical immobility, although not the proximate causes of incontinence, can be considered cofactors. Extraurethral causes of incontinence include ectopic ureter opening into the vagina and urinary fistula.

The conditions causing urinary incontinence may be presumed or definite. Definite conditions are documented by urodynamic techniques. Presumed conditions are documented clinically. For example, a neurologically normal woman who complains of urge incontinence despite a normal cystometrogram has presumed detrusor instability provided that sphincter abnormalities and overflow incontinence have been excluded. If the cystometrogram documents involuntary detrusor contractions, the diagnosis is definite detrusor instability. When reporting results, it should be clearly stated whether the conditions causing urinary incontinence are definite or presumed. The technique by which the condition is documented should always be specified.

Bladder Abnormalities Causing Urinary Incontinence

DETRUSOR OVERACTIVITY Detrusor overactivity is a generic term for involuntary detrusor contractions and should be used when the cause of the involuntary detrusor contractions is unclear.

DETRUSOR INSTABILITY This term denotes involuntary detrusor contractions not due to neurologic disorders.

DETRUSOR HYPERREFLEXIA This term denotes involuntary detrusor contractions that are due to neurologic conditions.

LOW BLADDER COMPLIANCE Low bladder compliance

TABLE 8–1
Detrusor Overactivity (Involuntary Detrusor Contractions)

Detrusor Instability
1. Idiopathic
2. Bladder outlet obstruction
3. Infection
4. Bladder stones
5. Bladder cancer

Detrusor Hyperreflexia
1. Supraspinal neurologic lesions (stroke, Parkinson's disease, hydrocephalus, brain tumor, multiple sclerosis)
2. Suprasacral neurologic lesions (spinal cord injury, multiple sclerosis, spina bifida, transverse myelitis)

Low Bladder Compliance
1. Neurogenic (myelodysplasia, pelvic surgery)
2. Non-neurogenic (indwelling catheter, radiation, interstitial cystitis, tuberculosis)

denotes an abnormal (decreased) volume-pressure relationship during bladder filling. In simple terms, low bladder compliance is recognizable by a steep rise in detrusor pressure during bladder filling.

The causes of detrusor overactivity are listed in Table 8–1.

Sphincter Abnormalities Causing Urinary Incontinence

From a physiologic standpoint, sphincter abnormalities that cause urinary incontinence are of two generic types—urethral hypermobility and intrinsic sphincter deficiency. In urethral hypermobility, the basic abnormality is a weakness of the pelvic floor. When abdominal pressure is increased, rotational descent of the vesical neck and proximal urethra occurs. If the urethra opens concomitantly, stress urinary incontinence ensues. Urethral hypermobility is often present in women who are not incontinent. Thus, the mere presence of urethral hypermobility is not sufficient to make a diagnosis of a sphincter abnormality unless incontinence is also demonstrated.

Intrinsic sphincteric deficiency (ISD) denotes an intrinsic malfunction of the urethral sphincter itself. Clinically, ISD is most commonly seen in three circumstances: (1) after surgery on the urethra, vagina, or bladder neck, (2) as a consequence of a neurologic lesion that involves the nerves to the vesical neck and proximal urethra, and (3) in the elderly.[1, 2]

Overflow Incontinence

Overflow incontinence is the leakage of urine due to incomplete bladder emptying caused by either impaired detrusor contractility or bladder outlet obstruction. The pathophysiology of overflow incontinence has not been studied very well. Conceptually, the actual leakage must be caused by either an overactive detrusor or a relative sphincter deficiency.

SYMPTOMS, SIGNS, AND CONDITIONS OF INCONTINENCE

The symptoms of incontinence are elicited by the patient's history, voiding diaries, and pad test. Furthermore, symptoms can (and should) be reproduced during urodynamic studies. The signs are assessed by examination and urodynamic studies. The conditions are the underlying pathophysiologic conditions (Table 8–2).

TABLE 8–2
Conditions and Causes of Incontinence

Symptom	Condition	Medical-Surgical Causes
Urge incontinence	Detrusor overactivity	Idiopathic
		Neurogenic
		Outlet obstruction
		Urinary tract infection
		Bladder or prostate cancer
Stress incontinence	1. Sphincter hypermobility	Pelvic floor relaxation
	2. Intrinsic sphincter deficiency	Urethral, bladder, or pelvic surgery
	3. Stress hyperreflexia	Neurogenic
		Detrusor overactivity
Unconscious incontinence	1. Detrusor overactivity	Same as above
	2. Sphincter abnormality	Same as above
	3. Extraurethral incontinence	Fistula
		Ectopic ureter
Continuous leakage	1. Sphincter abnormality	Same as above
	2. Impaired detrusor contractility	
	3. Extraurethral incontinence	Same as above
Nocturnal enuresis	1. Sphincter abnormality	Same as above
	2. Detrusor overactivity	Same as above
Postvoid dribble	Postsphincteric collection of urine	Idiopathic
		Urethral diverticulum
Extraurethral incontinence	1. Vesicovaginal, ureterovaginal, or urethrovaginal fistula	Trauma, surgical, obstetric, or other cause
	2. Ectopic ureter	Congenital

Urge Incontinence

SYMPTOM   The symptom of urge incontinence is the complaint of involuntary loss of urine associated with a sudden, strong desire to void (urgency).

SIGN   The sign is the observation of involuntary urine loss from the urethra synchronous with an uncontrollable urge to void.

CONDITION   The condition underlying urge incontinence is detrusor overactivity.

Stress Incontinence

SYMPTOM   The symptom is the complaint of involuntary loss of urine during coughing, sneezing, or physical exertion such as sport activities, sudden changes of position, and so on.

SIGN   The sign is the observation of loss of urine from the urethra synchronous with coughing, sneezing, or physical exertion.

CONDITION   The condition of stress incontinence is a sphincter abnormality.

Unconscious Incontinence

SYMPTOM   The symptom of unconscious incontinence is involuntary loss of urine unaccompanied by either urge or stress. The patient may become aware of the incontinent episode by feeling wetness or by other associated symptoms such as the onset of autonomic dysreflexia in patients with spinal cord injury.

SIGN   The sign is the observation of loss of urine without patient awareness of urge or stress.

CONDITION   The underlying condition may be detrusor overactivity, sphincter abnormality, or the conditions leading to overflow or extraurethral incontinence.

Continuous Leakage

SYMPTOM   Continuous leakage is the complaint of a continuous involuntary loss of urine.

SIGN   The sign is observation of a continuous urinary loss.

CONDITION   The condition may be a sphincter abnormality or extraurethral leakage.

Nocturnal Enuresis

SYMPTOM   The symptom of nocturnal enuresis is the complaint of urinary loss occurring only during sleep.

SIGN   The sign is observation of urinary loss during sleep.

CONDITION   The underlying condition is a sphincter abnormality, detrusor overactivity, or extraurethral leakage.

Postvoid Dribble

SYMPTOM   Postvoid dribble is the complaint of a dribbling loss of urine that occurs after voiding.

SIGN   The sign is observation of a dribbling loss of urine after voiding.

CONDITION   The condition underlying postvoid dribble has not been adequately defined but is thought to be retained urine in the urethra distal to the sphincter in men. In women urine may be retained in the vagina or in a urethral diverticulum.

Extraurethral Incontinence

Extraurethral incontinence is not a symptom; it is a sign and a condition.

SIGN   The sign is the observation of urine loss from a site other than the urethral meatus.

CONDITION   Continuous leakage of urine may be due to a congenital ectopic ureter or an acquired injury resulting in a ureterovaginal, vesicovaginal, or urethrovaginal fistula.

A precise diagnosis of urinary incontinence is best attained when it is actually witnessed by the examiner. In most instances, it makes little difference whether the urine loss is visualized during physical examination with a full bladder (the Marshall or Bonney test) or on cystoscopy, cystometry, or radiography. Regardless of the method of observation, when urinary loss from the urethral meatus is visualized, the observations and measurements made by the astute clinician usually serve to pinpoint the underlying abnormality and direct appropriate treatment.

Voiding Dysfunction and Frequency-Urgency Syndromes

Voiding dysfunction and frequency-urgency syndromes are imprecise terms that, in our opinion, represent a broad spectrum of underlying causes that have as a common denominator a high incidence of other vague symptoms such as abdominal or pelvic pressure, dyspareunia, and gastrointestinal complaints. In addition, each of these diagnoses is associated with a plethora of myths shared by physician and patient and burdened by an excess of presumed psychological overlay. Although we do not presume to understand the underlying cause of these conditions, we have developed a straightforward approach to diagnosis and treatment of urinary frequency and urgency.

Voiding dysfunction denotes an abnormality of micturition wherein there is a lack of coordination between the detrusor and the sphincter that mimicks detrusor–external sphincter dyssynergia. However, detrusor–external sphincter dyssynergia is seen only in patients with neurologic lesions of the spinal cord such as spinal cord injury or multiple sclerosis.

The hallmark of voiding dysfunction is a markedly interrupted or undulating flow of urine; the patient is essentially starting and stopping when she voids. We believe that this is a learned behavior, usually due to an underlying organic condition such as urinary tract infection or urethral obstruction; sometimes it is the result of improper methods of toilet training or trauma. Voiding dysfunction may coexist with frequency-urgency syndromes.

Women with refractory symptoms of urinary frequency, urgency, and pelvic pain pose a considerable diagnostic and therapeutic challenge. After more serious conditions such as bladder cancer have been excluded, these patients are often branded with the diagnosis of exclusion—interstitial cystitis. We prefer to use the term painful bladder syndrome or sensory urgency rather than many of the other near-synonyms for interstitial cystitis because the former terms are simply descriptive. Interstitial cystitis is associated with connotations of pathoanatomic changes, "incurability," and "chronicity"—allusions that are not necessarily warranted in many of the patients who are burdened by such a diagnosis. The typical patient is a young to middle-aged woman with normal results on urinalysis and urine culture and an unremarkable physical examination. Slow-fill cystometry or cystourethroscopy reveals only increasing pain during bladder filling that is relieved by emptying. Under anesthesia the classic findings of glomerulations, "Hunner's ulcer," and bleeding may or may not be present.

Pelvic Prolapse

Prolapse refers to a protrusion of the bladder (cystocele), urethra (urethrocele), rectum (rectocele), intestine (enterocele), or uterus (uterine prolapse) past the ordinary anatomic confines of the affected organ. At present, there is no universally accepted classification system to describe the extent of pelvic prolapse. We use the following system, which is based on the lowest extent of protrusion with a maximum Valsalva maneuver in the position (lithotomy, sitting, standing) that causes the greatest descent: Grade 1, mobility within the vagina; grade 2, extension to the introitus; grade 3, extension beyond the introitus; and grade 4, extension well beyond the introitus. Enteroceles may be classified as congenital or acquired, and acquired enteroceles are further classified as pulsion or traction. Congenital enteroceles are due to an "incomplete closure of the rectovaginal septum." Acquired enteroceles occur after bladder suspension procedures that cause widening of the pouch or cul-de-sac of Douglas. Traction enteroceles are associated with uterine prolapse, and pulsion enteroceles occur after hysterectomy and are associated with weakness of the vaginal vault. Another term for a pulsion enterocele is a true enterocele because it is filled with bowel, whereas a traction enterocele may contain only the cul-de-sac.[3]

Women with pelvic prolapse may be asymptomatic or may complain of concomitant voiding, bowel, or other pelvic symptoms. The severity of symptoms may not correlate at all with the degree of prolapse. A large prolapse can cause extrinsic ureteral obstruction with resultant hydronephrosis and recurrent urinary tract infection due to incomplete bladder emptying.

Evaluation of Urinary Tract Dysfunction

SUBJECTIVE DATA

History

The history begins with a detailed account of the precise nature of the patient's symptoms. Each symptom should be characterized and quantified as accurately as possible. When more than one symptom is present, the patient's assessment of the relative severity of each should be noted. The patient should be asked how often she urinates during the day and night, how long she can comfortably go between urinations, and how long micturition can be postponed once the urge is present. The reason for the frequency of urination should be determined. Is it because of a severe urge, or is it merely for convenience or an attempt to prevent incontinence? The severity of incontinence should be graded. Does stress incontinence occur during coughing, sneezing, or rising from a sitting to a standing position, or only during heavy physical exercise? If incontinence is associated with stress, is urine lost only for an instant during the stress, or does uncontrollable voiding occur? The latter suggests stress hyperreflexia. Is the incontinence positional? Does it ever occur in the lying or sitting position? Is there a sense of urgency first? Does urge incontinence occur? Is the patient aware of the act of incontinence, or does she just find herself wet (unconscious incontinence)? Is there continuous involuntary loss of urine? Does the patient lose only a few drops, or is her outer clothing saturated? Does she have postvoid dribbling or enuresis? Are protective pads worn? If so, do they become saturated? How often are they changed? Is there difficulty in initiating the stream, requiring pushing or straining to start? Is the stream weak or interrupted? Is there postvoid dribbling? Has the patient ever had urinary retention?

The symptoms of prolapse do not necessarily correlate with the degree of prolapse. The patient may notice or feel the protrusion, which may cause a feeling like "sitting on a ball." There may be a sensation of pressure in the vagina, rectum, or groin. The woman may feel a perineal wetness or bleeding from a vaginal ulceration, or she may have a sensation of "pelvic insecurity."[4] There may be a sacral backache that resolves when the patient is lying down.

Women with cystocele may present with a spectrum of symptoms ranging from urinary retention to overt stress incontinence. Between the two ends of this spectrum lie the symptoms of urgency, frequency, straining to void, and a dribbling stream. Some women with cystocele may be less symptomatic during the night because the cystocele is reduced in the supine position. Other lesions may enhance voiding by applying pressure on the anterior wall of the vagina. Symptoms of obstructive voiding may be replaced by stress incontinence when a pessary is inserted.

Symptoms due to rectocele include the sensation of incomplete evacuation of stool from the rectum or the need to apply digital pressure on the posterior vaginal wall to evacuate. Constipation per se does not usually result from a rectocele, although the patient may misinterpret her symptoms as constipation. Of course, blood in the stool or changes in the caliber of the stools should prompt colon and rectal examination to rule out neoplasm.

Past Medical History

The patient should be specifically queried about neurologic conditions that are known to affect bladder and sphincteric function, such as multiple sclerosis, spinal cord injury, lumbar disc disease, myelodysplasia, diabetes, stroke, or Parkinson's disease. If she does not have a previously diagnosed neurologic disease it is important to ask about double vision, muscular weakness, paralysis or poor coordination, tremor, numbness, and tingling. A history of vaginal surgery or previous surgical repair of incontinence should suggest the possibility of sphincteric injury. Abdominoperineal resection of the rectum or radical hysterectomy may be associated with neurologic injury to the bladder and sphincter. Radiation therapy may cause a small-capacity, low-compliance bladder or radiation cystitis.

Medications are a rare cause of urinary incontinence. Sympatholytic agents such as clonidine and prazosin may cause stress incontinence. Sympathomimetic and tricyclic antidepressants such as ephedrine or imipramine may cause bladder outlet obstruction, urinary retention, and overflow incontinence. Parasympathomimetics such as bethanechol may cause involuntary detrusor contractions.

Bladder Questionnaire

A questionnaire can expedite the retrieval of all of this information. We use two questionnaires, one directed toward bladder symptoms and the other toward past medical history, medications, and allergies. These questionnaires are sent to the patient before the first office visit. The patient has an opportunity to consider the questions and acquire the information, such as the names of medications and dates of previous surgeries, prior to the office visit.

SEMIOBJECTIVE DATA

Voiding Diary

To document the nature and severity of urinary incontinence, a voiding diary is indispensable. The reproducibility of a diary has been previously confirmed.[5] The particular information recorded in the diary depends on the patient's symptoms, but all diaries should include at least the time and amount of each micturition. From such a diary, the following information can be acquired or calculated: (1) the total 24-hour urinary output, (2) the number of voids, (3) the longest intervoiding interval, (4) the largest single void, and (5) the diurnal distribution. In addition, depending on the patient's complaint, notations about the character, time, and severity of incontinence, the need to push or strain to void, and associated pain or urgency can be compiled. The International Continence Society (ICS) has advised that the inclusion of a frequency-volume chart is an essential component of the patient's clinical assessment. The definition of functional bladder capacity by the ICS is the largest voided volume recorded in the patient's voiding diary.[6]

Can the voiding diary actually provide more data than a patient's history? Focusing on nocturia, we performed a retrospective review of randomly selected charts of 50 male and female patients presenting with a history of voiding dysfunction, including nocturia. These 50 patients had completed a bladder questionnaire, and a history was taken before the patient completed a 24-hour voiding diary. The diary recording of the number of times voided during sleep was compared with the number of times reported on the patient questionnaire. There was poor correlation between nocturia according to the patient's history and the number of voids during sleep ($r = 0.29$), and these results were statistically significant ($p = .038$). This study obviously has implications for the accuracy of the patient's report of symptoms alone, without objective or semiobjective validation.

Pad Tests

A number of pad tests have been described,[6, 7] but none have achieved widespread approval,[8, 9] and none have met scientific standards for good test-retest reliability. Nevertheless, we believe that the pad test is exceedingly useful but must be kept in perspective with the patient's symptoms. The most direct way of doing this is simply to ask the patient whether the pad test is representative of the usual symptoms; if not, it should be repeated.

OBJECTIVE DATA

Physical Examination

The physical examination begins by observing the patient's gait and demeanor as she first enters the office. A slight limp or lack of coordination, an abnormal speech pattern, facial asymmetry, or other abnormalities may be subtle signs of a neurologic condition.

The abdomen and flanks should be examined for masses, hernias, and a distended bladder. A pelvic examination is performed with the bladder comfortably full in the lithotomy position and generally should be repeated with the patient standing or sitting. The patient is asked to cough or strain to reproduce the symptoms of incontinence. The degree of hypermobility may be assessed both by examination with a full bladder and by the Q-tip test. The Q-tip test is performed by inserting a well-lubricated, sterile cotton-tipped applicator gently into the urethra while the patient is in the lithotomy position. During a Valsalva maneuver or while the patient is coughing, the arc of the end of the Q-tip may be estimated or measured from the resting position with a goniometer or approximated by the examiner in terms of degrees from the 0 axis (the position of the applicator at rest). Some examiners use a shortened red rubber catheter to obtain a residual volume and then check for mobility during stress. Mobility of the end of the instrument from the resting position to more than 15 degrees with straining indicates hypermobility of the bladder and urethra.

The anterior vaginal wall can be clearly seen by applying gentle pressure on the posterior vaginal wall with the posterior blade of a split vaginal speculum. The blade, if metal, should be warmed with water and inserted into the vagina toward the posterior wall. While the patient strains, the mobility of the bladder, urethra, and cervix is assessed for prolapse. The cervix is normally mobile; however, descent to the introitus is abnormal. Women with cystocele require careful examination in both the lithotomy and the sitting or standing positions. The design of our urodynamic chair allows the perineum to be visualized and examined while the patient is sitting. In many instances, incontinence is produced only in one or the other position, and prolapse is usually much worse in the sitting or standing position than in the lithotomy position. Moreover, in some patients incontinence can be reproduced only when the cystocele is reduced.

After examination of the anterior vaginal wall, the speculum blade is then rotated. The posterior vaginal wall and vault are examined for the presence of enterocele and rectocele. As the speculum is slowly withdrawn, a transverse groove separating an enterocele from a rectocele below may be visible. A finger inserted into the rectum can "tent up" a rectocele but not an enterocele.

The sacral dermatomes are evaluated by assessing anal sphincter tone and control, perianal sensation, and the bulbocavernosus reflex. With a finger placed in the rectum, the patient is asked to squeeze as if she were in the middle of urinating and were trying to stop. A lax or weakened anal sphincter or an inability to contract and relax it voluntarily is a sign of neurologic damage. The bulbocavernosus reflex is checked by suddenly squeezing the clitoris and feeling (or seeing) the anal sphincter and perineal muscles contract. Alternatively, the reflex may be initiated by suddenly pulling the balloon of a Foley catheter against the vesical neck. The absence of this reflex in men is almost always associated with a neurologic lesion, but the reflex is not detectable in up to 30% of otherwise normal women.[10]

If incontinence is not demonstrated in the lithotomy or sitting position, the patient is asked to cough or strain while standing to reproduce incontinence. Similarly, the distinction between an enterocele and a rectocele may best be assessed while the patient is standing. She should be positioned standing in front of the examiner with one foot elevated on a short standing stool. An enterocele is palpable between the forefinger (in the rectum) and the thumb (in the vagina). If bowel is not palpable between the index finger and the thumb, the posterior protrusion is probably a high rectocele. The perineal body and vaginal rectal septum are examined by palpating the septum through the vagina and rectum.

If a patient has been fitted with a pessary, it should be removed. In some patients even massive prolapse may not be appreciated immediately after the pessary is removed. It may be necessary to reexamine the patient after she has been standing for 30 minutes or more to allow an accurate assessment of the degree of prolapse. The vagina should be examined for any erosions or pudendal nerve injury from an ill-fitting pessary. Pudendal nerve injury is associated with paravaginal anesthesia, incontinence, worsening prolapse, and decreased anal sphincter tone.

Diagnosis of a urinary fistula depends on a high index of suspicion and should be suspected if there is new onset of incontinence after pelvic surgery or childbirth or after pelvic irradiation for gynecologic malignancy. In most instances, vesicovaginal and urethrovaginal fistulas are apparent on examination with a full bladder or at the time of cystoscopy, but ectopic ureter or a ureterovaginal or vesicouterine fistula is usually not apparent on examination.

If a vesicovaginal fistula is suspected but not seen at the time of cystoscopy, the bladder should be filled with fluid to which a dye such as indigo carmine or methylene blue has been added. The vagina should then be inspected for signs of urinary leakage with the urethra occluded by a Foley balloon catheter or the surgeon's examining finger to prevent urethral leakage.

To confirm the presence of an ectopic ureter or a ureterovaginal or vesicouterine fistula, intravenous pyelography, retrograde pyelography, cystography, or hysterosalpingography may be necessary. In doubtful cases, pyridium may be given orally and the patient instructed to wear a tampon and pads. If the pyridium stains the tampon but not the pad, a vaginal fistula or ectopic ureter should be excluded.

Routine Urologic Assessment

Routine laboratory tests include urinalysis, urine culture, and renal function tests. Positive urine cultures should be treated with culture-specific antibiotics, but patients with persistent bacteriuria or recurrent infections may require invasive testing while taking antibiotics. Hematuria should be evaluated by urinary cytology, intravenous pyelography, or cystourethroscopy.

Urodynamic Studies

The main purpose of urodynamic investigation is to determine the precise cause of the patient's voiding dysfunction. Obviously, to achieve this goal, her symptoms should be reproduced during the examination.

Urodynamic techniques vary from "eyeball" urodynamics to sophisticated multichannel synchronous video pressure-flow electromyographic studies. We believe that synchronous multichannel video urodynamic studies offer the most comprehensive artifact-free means of arriving at a precise diagnosis and perform them routinely when urodynamic tests are indicated. When multichannel studies are not performed routinely, they should be considered in the following circumstances:

1. Simpler diagnostic tests have been inconclusive
2. The patient complains of incontinence, but incontinence cannot be demonstrated clinically
3. The patient has previously undergone corrective surgery for incontinence
4. The patient has previously undergone radical pelvic surgery, such as abdominoperineal resection of the rectum or radical hysterectomy
5. The patient has a known or suspected neurologic disorder that might interfere with bladder or sphincter function (myelodysplasia, spinal cord injury, multiple sclerosis, herniated disc, cerebrovascular accident, Parkinson's disease, or the Shy-Drager syndrome).

Eyeball Urodynamics

Eyeball urodynamic tests are performed with the patient in the lithotomy position immediately after a uroflow study. A Foley catheter is inserted and the postvoid residual urine measured. A regional neurologic examination, including assessment of perineal sensation, anal tone and control, and bulbocavernosus reflex, is performed. A 60-ml catheter tip syringe is connected to the Foley catheter, and its barrel is removed. Water or saline is then poured in through the open end of the syringe and allowed to drip into the bladder by gravity. As the water level in the syringe falls, its meniscus represents the intravesical pressure, which can be estimated in centimeters of water above the symphysis pubis. When the water level in the syringe falls to the level of the catheter tip, the syringe is refilled.

During bladder filling the patient is told to neither void nor try to inhibit micturition; rather, she should simply report her sensations to the examiner. When she perceives the urge to void she is asked if that is the usual feeling experienced when she needs to urinate. Changes in intravesical pressure are apparent as a slowing of the rate of fall or a rise in the level of the fluid meniscus. A change in pressure may be caused by a detrusor contraction, an increase in abdominal pressure, or low bladder wall compliance. As soon as a change in pressure is noted, the examiner should attempt to determine the cause. Visual inspection usually indicates abdominal straining, but in doubtful cases the abdomen should be palpated. In most instances the cause of the rise in intravesical pressure is obvious, but when doubt exists, formal cystometry with rectal pressure monitoring is necessary.

Any sudden rise in pressure accompanied by either an urge to void or incontinence indicates an involuntary detrusor contraction. In some instances, the cause of the patient's incontinence is easily discernible because she voids uncontrollably around the catheter during an involuntary detrusor contraction. If involuntary detrusor contractions do not occur, the bladder is filled until a normal urge to void is experienced. The bladder is left full and the catheter removed. The presence or absence of gravitational urinary loss is then noted. The patient is asked to cough and bear down with gradually increasing force to determine the ease with which incontinence is produced. In women, the introitus is observed for signs of cystourethrocele, rectocele, enterocele, and uterine prolapse, as outlined earlier under physical examination.

Incontinence that occurs during stress is not always due to a sphincter abnormality. In some patients, stress initiates a reflex detrusor contraction. This condition has been termed stress hyperreflexia. Thus, it is important to determine whether leakage is accompanied by descent of the bladder base and urethra. It should be further noted whether the leakage stops as soon as the stress ceases or whether the patient actually continues to void uncontrollably. In the former case, the patient has the condition of stress incontinence; in the latter, it is stress hyperreflexia. If the patient has leakage that is clearly accompanied by descent of the bladder base and proximal urethra (a cystourethrocele) and the leakage stops as soon as the cough or strain is over, she has type I or II stress incontinence. If the leakage occurs without descent or with minimal provocation, she may have sphincteric incontinence (type III stress incontinence).

If the patient complains of urinary incontinence that has not been demonstrated, the examination should be repeated in the standing position. It is best performed by having the patient stand with one foot on a small stool. The examiner sits beside her and performs a vaginal examination while she coughs and strains. If the examiner is still unable to demonstrate incontinence, the patient is given a prescription for a urinary dye such as pyridium and asked to wear incontinence pads and tampons that she changes every 2 hours for a single representative day. She is instructed to bring the stained pads and tampons with her to the next office visit. The amount and location of the stains may help to determine the site and degree of urinary loss. It is axiomatic that, under ordinary circumstances, no patient should undergo invasive or irreversible treatment until the cause of incontinence has been clearly demonstrated.

Voiding Dysfunction

Women with voiding dysfunction are evaluated as outlined previously. However, urodynamic studies are generally not performed until the patient has undergone a course of behavior modification, sometimes with biofeedback. The purpose of the behavioral modification is to teach the patient to relax during micturition. In many cases, after completing behavioral therapy, the patient is no longer symptomatic. If symptoms persist, urodynamic studies are done. In some patients urodynamic studies are used as a biofeedback tool.

Frequency-Urgency and Painful Bladder Syndromes

The diagnostic approach to these patients commences with a history, physical examination, urinalysis and representative voiding diaries as outlined previously. We believe that cystoscopy should be performed with local anesthesia to assess the relationship of bladder filling to symptoms and to exclude neoplasm, stones, urethral diverticulum, and foreign bodies. We decry the practice of routinely performing cystoscopy under anesthesia and reserve bladder biopsy only for patients in whom there is a suspicion of bladder cancer. Urodynamic studies are performed to determine whether the symptoms are due to bladder filling, detrusor instability, or low bladder compliance. Voiding cystourethrography is performed to exclude urethral diverticulum. Ideally, the two studies can be combined in videourodynamic studies.

REFERENCES

1. Barbalias GA, Blaivas JG: Neurologic implications of the pathologically open bladder neck. J Urol 129:780, 1983.
2. Blaivas JG, Olssen CA: Stress incontinence: Classification and surgical approach. J Urol 139:727, 1988.
3. Zacharin RF: The clinical features of enterocoele. *In* Zacharin RF (ed): Pelvic Floor Anatomy and the Surgery of Pulsion Enterocoele. Vienna, Springer-Verlag, 1985, pp 77–101.
4. Wall LL, Norton PA, DeLancey JOL: Prolapse and the lower urinary tract. *In* Wall LL, Norton PA, DeLancey JOL (eds): Practical Urogynecology. Baltimore, Williams & Wilkins, 1993, pp 293–315.
5. Larsson G, Victor A: Micturition patterns in a female population studied with a frequency/volume chart. Scand J Urol Nephrol Suppl 114:53, 1988.
6. Abrams P, Blaivas JG, Stanton SL, Andersen JT: The standardization of terminology of lower urinary tract function. Scand J Urol Nephrol Suppl 114:5, 1988.
7. Hahn I, Fall M: Objective quantification of stress urinary incontinence: A short, reproducible, provocative pad-test. Neurourol Urodyn 10:475, 1991.
8. Lose G, Gammelgaard J, Jorgensen TJ: The one-hour pad-weighing test: Reproducibility and the correlation between the test result, start volume in the bladder and the diuresis. Neurourol Urodyn 5:17, 1986.
9. Christensen SJ, Colstrup H, Hertz JB, et al: Inter and intradepartmental variations of the perineal pad-weighing test. Neurourol Urodyn 5:23, 1986.
10. Blaivas JG: The bulbocavernosus reflex in urology: A prospective study of 299 patients. J Urol 126:197, 1981.

CHAPTER 9

Uroflowmetry

Jacob Golomb, M.D.

Uroflowmetry measures the volume of urine expelled per unit of time, usually expressed as milliliters per second. Urinary flow pattern is determined by both bladder pressure and bladder outlet resistance. Bladder voiding pressure is generated either by active detrusor contraction or by abdominal straining and the Credé maneuver. Resistance to flow is encountered at the bladder neck and urethra and is determined by urethral cross-sectional area and length. The normal female urethra is shorter and wider than the normal male urethra and offers less resistance to flow.

Free (noninvasive) uroflowmetry is a simple and inexpensive way of integrating the activity of the bladder and the outlet during the emptying phase of micturition. As such, it constitutes an extremely useful screening study, especially when combined with residual urine volume measurement, and it aids in the investigation of incontinence, obstruction, or detrusor dysfunction in men and women. Although normal results generally rule out any significant disorder in the process of bladder emptying, a flow pattern considerably in excess of normal usually indicates decreased outlet resistance, and low flow rates are secondary to either increased outlet resistance, decreased detrusor contractility, or both. In selected cases, flow rate recordings can be combined with measurements of substracted detrusor pressure during voiding to differentiate between detrusor-related and outlet-related decreased flow rates.

In this chapter we will discuss the hydrodynamic principles of urination essential to understanding urinary flow measurements, the various methods available for measuring urinary flow, and the application and interpretation of uroflowmetry in various clinical situations in female urology.

Basic Principles and Hydrodynamics of Urination

Micturition is a mechanical process that is under neuromuscular control. It is accomplished by a sustained active contraction of the detrusor muscle working against the hydrodynamic resistance of the bladder outlet and urethra. To appreciate the clinical significance of urinary flow evaluation, one must understand the principles of fluid dynamics involved in the process.

Conceptually, Ohm's law may be applied to urinary flow. This law states that flow is directly proportional to pressure and inversely proportional to resistance, namely,

$$\text{Flow} = \frac{\text{Pressure}}{\text{Resistance}}$$

The expulsive action of the bladder is represented by intravesical pressure (P_{ves}), which has two components, an extrinsic component (P_{abd}), which represents the contribution from the surrounding intra-abdominal structures and is grouped under the term abdominal pressure, and an intrinsic component (P_{det}), which represents forces in the detrusor itself and is called the detrusor pressure. The mathematical relation is

$$P_{ves} = P_{abd} + P_{det}$$

In urodynamic practice, P_{ves} is measured directly, P_{abd} is estimated indirectly by measuring the pressure in the rectum, and P_{det} is estimated by subtracting P_{abd} from P_{ves}.

Resistance is determined by the length and cross-sectional area (πr^2) of the urethra. Because cross-sectional area is related to the square of the radius, small decreases in caliber may have a profound effect after a critical diminished level is reached by any process that narrows the urethral lumen. It is important to remember that because flow equals cross-sectional area (cm^2) times velocity (cm/second), it follows that when cross-sectional area decreases, the particle velocity must increase to maintain the same flow. Thus, a considerable amount of energy is required to produce the pressure necessary to compensate for subtle reductions in urinary flow rate.

One modification is necessary in applying Ohm's law to the urethra because it has been demonstrated that flow in the urethra is turbulent rather than laminar.[1] In the case of turbulent flow, resistance is proportional to pressure/(flow)^2. Uroflow measurements can be used to quantitate urethral resistance if intravesical pressure is known.

In addition, it should be noted that flow rate is directly related to the intravesical urine volume as well as to the contraction velocity of the detrusor muscle. Thus, during micturition, the flow rate is affected by the decreasing intravesical volume regardless of changes in outflow resistance. Similarly, a higher initial bladder volume produces a higher flow rate if outflow resistance is unchanged. For this reason, if one wishes to use the flow rate as an index of outflow obstruction, one must account for the effect of intravesical volume.

Flow rate nomograms, relating average and maximum flow rate to intravesical volume, were developed by Siroky and associates[2] and were found to be highly accurate in separating individuals with obstructed urine flow from normal individuals (Fig. 9–1). Use of these flow nomograms permits one to incorporate the peak flow rate and the intravesical volume into a single measurement, expressed as a standard deviation (SD) above or below the mean. The nomogram allows comparison of flow rates when intravesical volume differs, and, more important, it neutralizes the effect of intravesical volume on flow rate, leaving outflow resistance as the major determinant.

It should be clear from this discussion that a poor urinary stream in a patient who voids only small amounts of urine may well be attributed to the small voided volume itself rather than to any obstruction. With a larger voided volume the urinary stream may become entirely normal.

Equipment and Measuring Techniques

Numerous methods and devices for measuring urinary flow have been developed. The simplest, direct observation of the casting distance of the stream, has been described in the urologic literature,[3] but its merit is questionable because as in the case of a stricture of the fossa navicularis, the patient who urinates farthest is not necessarily the most normal.

Requirements for devices that measure urinary flow rate vary with the goal of the investigation. Depending on the type of transducer used, the following measuring methods are used most commonly:[4]

1. *Weight transducers* measure the mass and hence the volume of urine voided. By differentiation with respect to time, they can produce a measure of urine flow rate.

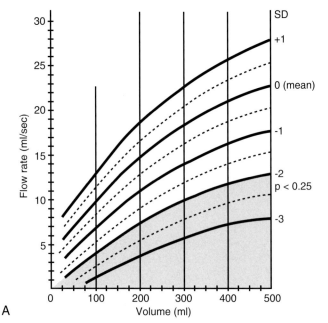

A

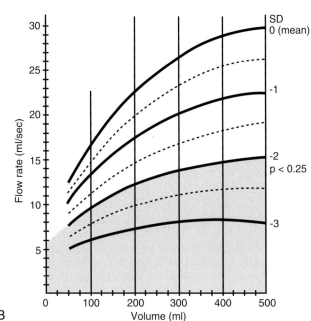

B

Figure 9–1 Flow rate nomograms, relating average *(A)* and maximum *(B)* flow rates to intravesical volume. (From Siroky MB, Olsson CA, Krane RJ: The flow rate nomogram: I. Development. J Urol 122:665, 1979.)

2. *Capacitance dipsticks* measure the drop in capacitance as the urine level rises in a vessel containing a metal strip capacitor. Electronic differentiation gives the rate of change in volume and hence the flow rate.

3. *Spinning disc flowmeters* measure the increase in power necessary to maintain the revolution of a disc at constant speed against the inertia of urine slowing it. The power required is proportional to the urine flow rate, and electronic integration allows calculation of the voided volume.

Radioactivity counts, drop spectrometry of the

urine stream, and momentum flux recording are regarded as research methods of uroflowmetry at present.

Patients should be allowed to void in privacy and in the normal position (seated for women). At least one flow rate measurement should be performed when the bladder has been filled physiologically and the patient has a normal desire to void. The patient should be asked to attend the study with a comfortably full bladder. A record should be made of any deviation from this norm, such as the method of filling or the presence of a catheter, since this may affect the result.

Parameters of Uroflowmetry

The most commonly measured flow parameters are shown in Figure 9–2. These are maximum flow rate, average flow rate, total voiding time, and time to maximum flow. Each is of some value in assessing the flow curve, but the maximum flow rate is undoubtedly the most important.

Maximum flow rate (Q$_{max}$) is the highest instantaneous flow recorded during a single void. Normally, Q$_{max}$ ranges from 15 to 30 ml/second depending on sex, age, and urine volume. As mentioned before, the dependence of Q$_{max}$ on initial bladder volume is even greater than its dependence on the voided volume. It has been suggested that when there is considerable residual urine, the use of flow rate nomograms based on the voided volume rather than the initial bladder volume may grossly overestimate the adequacy of the patient's flow.[2]

Normal women have a higher Q$_{max}$ than normal men, usually on the order of 5 ml/second for a given volume.[5, 6] Drach and associates have demonstrated that there is a greater increase in Q$_{max}$ per unit volume in women than in men. They also found a decrease in Q$_{max}$ with advancing age in men (a fall in Q$_{max}$ by 2 ml/second for every 10 years of age) but not in women.[6]

Average flow rate (Q$_{ave}$) is derived by dividing the voided volume by the total voiding time. However, because it is often difficult to determine the precise end of micturition, Q$_{ave}$ is beset with technical difficulties. Patients with an interrupted urine stream or terminal dribbling have no clearly definable voiding time, and for this reason Q$_{ave}$ cannot be accurately determined. To overcome these obstacles it has been suggested that Q$_{ave}$ be based on a certain percentage of the voided volume. For example, one might define Q$_{ave}$ as 90% of voided volume divided by the time taken to void that volume of urine.[7] Average flow varies from approximately 6 to 25 ml/second, depending on voided volume.

Total voiding time refers to the total time of urine flow. In patients with intermittent flow curves, it may be extremely difficult to measure this time accurately. When accurate measurements are possible, it has been determined that voiding time bears a linear relation to voided volume. Total voiding time varies from approximately 10 to 20 seconds for a voided volume of 100 ml to 25 to 35 seconds for a volume of 400 ml.[8]

Time to maximum flow (T$_{max}$) refers to the time from onset of flow to the attainment of Q$_{max}$ and bears a linear relation to voided volume. It is normally about one-third of the total voiding time. This relation remains constant even in the presence of outflow obstruction because the increased total voiding time is due primarily to the prolonged descending limb of the uroflow curve.[8]

Errors and Pitfalls in Recording Uroflowmetric Measurements

To gain the optimal information from urinary flow measurements, the examiner must be aware of the potential pitfalls and sources of error in the study. These errors can be ascribed to either the equipment or the individual being examined.[7]

Instrumental errors may be related to the static accuracy and calibration of the uroflowmeter or to its dynamic characteristics, namely, damping of the flow signal and time lag. Time lag is the time elapsed from the moment the urine passes the external meatus to the moment it is recorded by the equipment; it is affected by the distance from the external urethral meatus to the measuring transducer and the velocity of the stream.[7]

As for subject-related errors, because the uroflow measurement should be a reliable representation of the individual's voiding pattern, it is important to note that several disturbing factors may lead to a nonrepresentative urinary flow pattern during micturition: (1) psychological inhibition due to nervousness, (2) excessive abdominal straining, (3) sup-

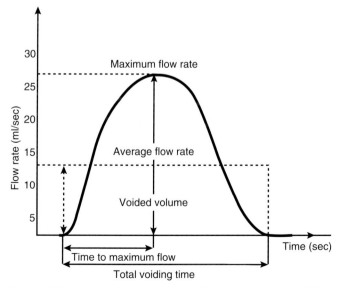

Figure 9-2 A normal flow curve, indicating the most widely measured uroflow parameters.

pression of the urge for bowel emptying, (4) rapid vertical movement of the stream alongside the funnel wall, resulting in a "wag-artifact," and (5) urethral instrumentation prior to micturition.[7]

In addition, the reliability of the urinary flow pattern may also be related to bladder physiology, such as the total voided volume and the degree of urge to urinate prior to the examination, as demonstrated by Rollema.[7]

Clinical Applications of Uroflowmetry

Urinary flow measurement can be an isolated test (free or noninvasive uroflowmetry), or it can be part of a more elaborate urodynamic investigation involving monitoring of intravesical and intra-abdominal pressures (pressure-flow study) and occasionally pelvic floor electromyography, depending on the type of disorder and the information required.

For a noninvasive uroflowmetric examination, the patient presents with a comfortably full bladder and simply voids into the flowmeter receptacle in utmost privacy. Most commercially available flowmeters provide a tracing of instantaneous flow versus time as well as a readout of values for (1) voided volume, (2) maximum flow rate, (3) average flow rate, (4) time to maximum flow, and (5) voided volume. The postvoid residual volume can be assessed by catheterization or sonography. The classic normal study, in which there is a voided volume of 150 to 400 ml, yields a smooth, uninterrupted, bell-shaped curve with a total voiding time of 10 to 35 seconds and a maximum flow rate of 25 to 30 ml/second (see Fig. 9–2). It should be noted, however, that a single office uroflowmetric measurement may not be sufficiently reliable to make a decision, especially a decision about the diagnosis of bladder outlet obstruction. The reason is that many patients are unable to relax and void in the normal fashion during uroflowmetry in the clinic. In addition, consecutive flow measurements are variable, specifically in regard to maximum flow rate.[9] This problem can be overcome by performing at least three consecutive office studies or by supplying the patient with an ambulatory home uroflowmetric device, which produces multiple flow measurements in the patient's own natural environment.[9]

It is well established that the maximum flow rate reflects bladder outlet obstruction better than any other uroflowmetric parameter.[10] Generally speaking, a maximum flow rate of over 15 ml/second excludes obstruction provided that the volume voided is at least 150 ml. A maximum flow rate of less than 10 ml/second suggests obstruction, and a rate of 10 to 15 ml/second is equivocal. As is apparent from the flow rate nomogram, a normal person voids with a low flow rate if the voided volume is small.

The actual shape of the uroflow curve is also informative. Prolonged voiding time suggests obstruction.

An intermittent curve in a male patient may suggest obstruction but may also result from voiding by abdominal straining. In female patients this is a normal variant that is seen frequently in the urodynamic laboratory setting and usually reflects habitual straining. However, abdominal straining in voiding may also originate from impaired detrusor contractility, and this can be diagnosed only by a synchronous pressure-flow study.

Synchronous pressure-flow measurements are very useful in the diagnosis of bladder outlet obstruction and in detecting detrusor contractility during voiding. They are carried out by recording detrusor pressure by means of a thin catheter (10 Fr or less), inserted either in the urethra or suprapubically, simultaneously with voiding. In a normal uroflow study, the measured detrusor pressure ranges from 20 to 50 cm of water, which is regarded as a normal pressure–normal flow relation (Fig. 9–3). In women who void with straining, this study helps to differentiate those who lack any detectable detrusor contractility and void by straining alone from those who have a normally functioning detrusor but are "habitual strainers" (Fig. 9–4).

In patients with compensated obstruction, generation of high intravesical pressure by strong detrusor contractions can overcome the obstruction to produce a normal or even elevated flow rate, yielding a high pressure–normal flow curve. With higher outlet resistance, the flow curve is obstructive despite a high voiding pressure, resulting in a high pressure–low flow curve. It must be recognized, however, that although a catheter of small diameter is used, even this small a catheter often causes a relative outlet obstruction and thus impedes flow.[11] Preliminary data suggest that even when flow is impaired by the presence of the catheter, useful diagnostic information can still be obtained. In fact, Griffiths and Scholtmeijer suggested that subtle bladder outlet obstruction may best be diagnosed by noting the effect of increasing catheter size on the pressure-flow curve.[12] They hypothesized that the obstructive effects of an intraurethral catheter would be more pronounced in patients with preexisting obstruction than in those without obstruction. Therefore, synchronous pressure-flow studies obtained with a transurethral catheter may be more sensitive than those obtained with a suprapubic one.

It should be remembered, however, that a low-flow and intermittent urinary stream may be secondary not to obstruction but to impaired detrusor contractility. In such a case a synchronous pressure-flow study will fail to detect any detrusor contractility, resulting in a low pressure–low flow curve. Pressure-flow relation is therefore the only way to differentiate bladder outlet obstruction from impaired detrusor contractility when a patient generates low maximum flow rates on uroflowmetry.

It is important to note that occasionally in women there is very little increase in recorded bladder pressure during voiding even when detrusor contractility is not impaired. The reason is that when the pelvic

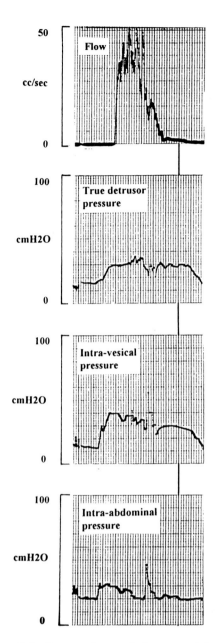

Figure 9-3 Pressure-flow study in a normal female.

gery may increase bladder outflow resistance. Patients with a small isometric rise (that is, a weak detrusor contraction) may have problems with voiding after such surgery.[4] If a patient cannot interrupt her own stream, it may be necessary to occlude the urethra physically during voiding to assess detrusor power. This can be done manually or by exerting traction on a small-caliber Foley catheter balloon left in the bladder during voiding.

Occasionally, an exaggerated rise in detrusor pressure can be detected at the termination of voiding, resulting in "postmicturition pressure" (Fig. 9–6). This is caused most probably by the detrusor contracting vigorously against tightening pelvic floor muscles and a closing bladder outlet.

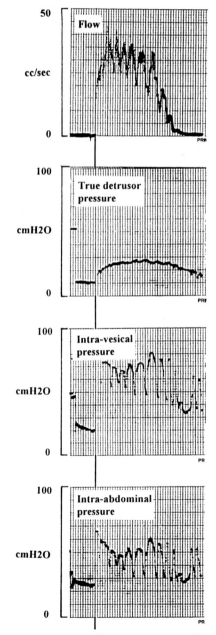

Figure 9-4 Pressure-flow study in a woman who is a "habitual strainer" and voids with straining, although her detrusor generates an adequate contraction.

floor relaxes, the bladder contracts, and the urethra opens wide, the flow of urine encounters little resistance, and the detrusor pressure required to maintain the flow is accordingly low. It is therefore not unusual to see excellent flow with no change in detrusor pressure. Normally, the patient should be capable of interrupting the flow of urine promptly on command by closing the urethra with pelvic floor contractions (stop-void test). Some women are able to achieve cessation of flow only by inhibiting detrusor contractions, which takes several seconds. When the urethra can be closed voluntarily, detrusor contractions become isovolumetric and increase to a maximum (P_{det} iso) (Fig. 9–5). This figure represents detrusor muscle power and is of paramount importance before surgery for stress incontinence because sur-

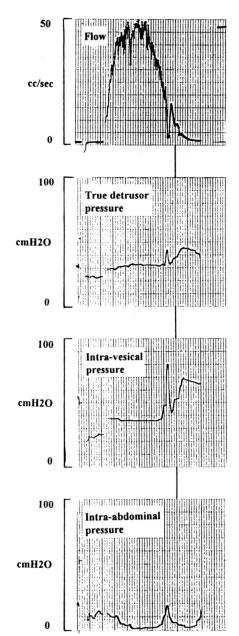

Figure 9-5 Pressure-flow study in a woman with stress incontinence, showing a normal flow pattern without any increase in true detrusor pressure. On closure of the urethra by sudden voluntary activation of the external sphincter (stop-void test), there is an isovolumetric bladder contraction that could not be detected while the urethra was open during micturition.

Uroflowmetry in Female Urology

Although most literature reports and clinical use of uroflowmetry involve male patients, the technique undoubtedly plays a major role in the assessment of female voiding disorders. It is used clinically in female urology to evaluate any impairment in the emptying phase of bladder function, namely, infravesical obstruction, incontinence, and neurogenic voiding dysfunction.

BLADDER OUTLET OBSTRUCTION

Bladder outlet obstruction in women is rare, and its cause is controversial and probably multifactorial. In addition to meatal stenosis, which is infrequent, it is thought that in some cases chronic inflammation leads to fibrosis, narrowing, and rigidity of the urethra.[13] Other investigators postulate that inflammation or urethral irritation by infection may lead to spasm of the external sphincter.[14] Neurologic disorders may cause nonrelaxation or dyssynergia of the external sphincter. Occasionally, voiding dysfunction can result from psychogenic causes. In some women who are very nervous and tense during the urodynamic evaluation, the pressure-flow study may demonstrate

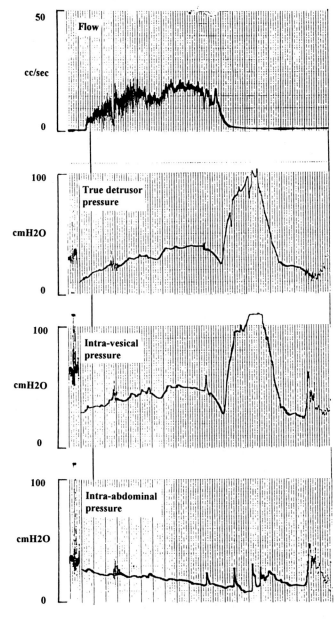

Figure 9-6 Exaggerated postmicturition pressure, reflecting a vigorous isovolumetric detrusor contraction against tightening pelvic floor muscles at the end of micturition.

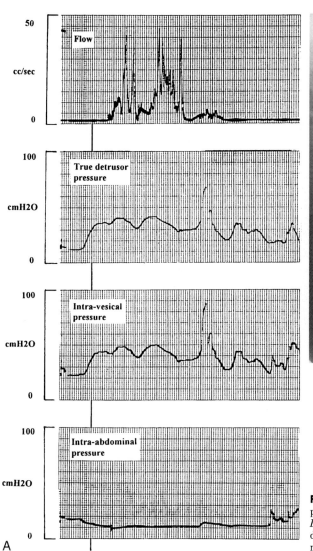

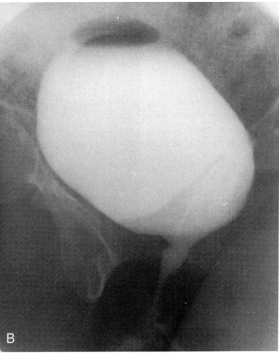

Figure 9-7 *A*, Obstructive pressure-flow study showing poor relaxation of the pelvic floor muscles during voiding. *B*, Simultaneous voiding cystography in the same patient, demonstrating the tight pelvic floor muscles and the external sphincter narrowing the urethral lumen.

an obstructive flow pattern because of nonrelaxation of the pelvic floor muscles (pseudodyssynergia) (Fig. 9–7).

In patients undergoing anti-incontinence surgery, misplaced sutures may also lead to infravesical obstruction, with secondary irritative voiding symptoms. Therefore, in women who present with urgency and urgency incontinence after surgery for stress incontinence, it is imperative to determine whether the irritative symptoms originate from bladder outlet obstruction. Complete urodynamic evaluation with synchronous pressure-flow studies is required before any further surgical intervention is undertaken.

Some patients who present with stress urinary incontinence may also have a large prolapsing cystocele. The anatomic configuration of the prolapsed bladder can create functional obstruction owing to kinking of the urethra at the bladder neck during voiding, resulting in a decreased urinary stream and incomplete emptying (Fig. 9–8). In such cases, bladder neck suspension and cystocele repair should resolve both the urine leakage during stress and the relative bladder outlet obstruction.

INCONTINENCE

The value of uroflowmetry in the investigation of women with incontinence has been neglected. In women with stress incontinence, a free uroflow examination may be important in appraising the quality of detrusor function and in detecting infravesical obstruction despite the fact that a differential diagnosis cannot be made accurately with uroflowmetry alone. As previously mentioned, although a considerable number of women void without any detectable change in detrusor pressure, this does not necessarily mean that detrusor contraction is absent and may well be due to a completely relaxed urethra. Thus, a supranormal urinary flow pattern (superflow) in a woman makes the existence of an infravesical obstruction unlikely. On the other hand, an abnormal uroflow pattern may imply either poor detrusor contractility or infravesical obstruction (organic or functional) and indicates a need for synchronous pressure-flow studies, particularly if an anti-incontinence procedure, which might increase outflow resistance, is contemplated.

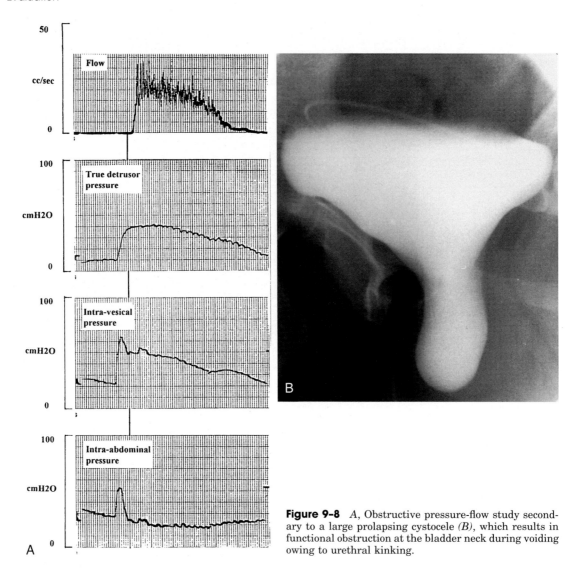

Figure 9-8 *A*, Obstructive pressure-flow study secondary to a large prolapsing cystocele *(B)*, which results in functional obstruction at the bladder neck during voiding owing to urethral kinking.

In addition, monitoring urine leakage by means of the uroflowmeter can be informative during urodynamic investigation of stress urinary incontinence. The pressure-flow study is an elegant method of detecting and quantifying urinary leakage caused by sudden increases in intra-abdominal pressure during the study with no concomitant change in true detrusor pressure.

NEUROGENIC VOIDING DYSFUNCTION

As for neurogenic voiding dysfunction, because neurologic disease (including spinal cord injury) may result in any combination of defects in the continence-voiding mechanism, it is necessary to gather all information possible to make a correct diagnosis. Nevertheless, it is still helpful to perform a free uroflow examination, provided the patient is able to void spontaneously, for the following reasons: (1) typical urinary flow patterns are associated with neurologic entities such as detrusor-sphincter dyssynergia, im-

paired or absent detrusor contractility leading to straining, detrusor hyperreflexia, and fluctuating contractions in the presence of detrusor decompensation; and (2) uroflowmetry appears to be very important in the follow-up of patients undergoing posterior pelvic exenteration or radical hysterectomy, who have a high incidence of postoperative voiding dysfunction due to interference with nerve and blood supply, because such dysfunction, as well as any signs of recovery on follow-up studies, can be easily detected by an abnormal urinary flow pattern.[7]

In summary, the measurement of urinary flow has an important role in the evaluation of lower urinary tract function. An understanding of the hydrodynamics of micturition is necessary to appreciate fully the clinical relevance of alterations in urinary flow pattern. Measurement of free urinary flow can be followed by synchronous pressure-flow studies as indicated and, when combined with residual urine evaluation, can help to define with reasonable accuracy and with no need for further testing which patients are urodynamically normal.

REFERENCES

1. Smith JC: Some theoretical aspects of urethral resistance. Invest Urol 1:447, 1964.
2. Siroky MB, Olsson CA, Krane RJ: The flow rate nomogram: I. Development. J Urol 122:665, 1979.
3. Ballanger EG, Elder OF, McDonald HP: Voiding distance decrease as important early symptom of prostatic obstruction. South Med J 25:863, 1932.
4. Massey A, Abrams P: Urodynamics of the female lower urinary tract. Urol Clin North Am 12(2):231, 1985.
5. Backman KA: Urinary flow during micturition in normal women. Acta Chir Scand 130:357, 1965.
6. Drach GW, Layton TN, Binard WJ: Male peak urinary flow rate: Relationship to volume voided and age. J Urol 122:210, 1979.
7. Rollema HJ: Uroflowmetry. *In* Krane RJ, Siroky MB (eds): Clinical Neurourology, 2nd ed. Boston, Little, Brown, 1991, p 201.
8. Siroky MB: Urinary flow rate: Diagnosis of bladder outflow obstruction. *In* Barrett DM, Wein AJ (eds): Controversies in Neuro-Urology. New York, Churchill Livingstone, 1984, p 145.
9. Golomb J, Lindner A, Siegel Y, et al: Variability and circadian changes in home uroflowmetry in patients with benign prostatic hyperplasia compared to normal controls. J Urol 147:1044, 1992.
10. Shoukry I, Susset JG, Elhilali M, et al: Role of uroflowmetry in the assessment of lower urinary tract obstruction in adult males. Br J Urol 47:559, 1975.
11. Ryall RL, Marshall VR: The effect of a urethral catheter on the measurement of maximum urinary flow rate. J Urol 128:429, 1982.
12. Griffiths DJ, Scholtmeijer RJ: Precise urodynamic assessment of meatal and distal urethral stenosis in girls. Neurourol Urodyn 1:89, 1982.
13. Susset JG, Shoukry I, Schlaeder G, et al: Stress incontinence and urethral obstruction in women: Value of uroflowmetry and voiding urethrography. J Urol 111:504, 1974.
14. Webster JR: Combined video-pressure-flow cystourethrography in female patients with voiding disturbances. Urology 5:209, 1975.

CHAPTER 10

Clinical Assessment of Urethral Sphincter and Conduit Function by Measurement of Abdominal and Detrusor Pressures Required to Induce Leakage

Edward J. McGuire, M.D.
E. Ann Gormley, M.D.

Leak Point Pressures

HISTORY OF LEAK POINT PRESSURE MEASUREMENTS

Use of leak point pressure measurements in urology began in children with myelodysplasia.[1] In these patients the bladder was filled slowly through a small catheter, resulting in a bladder pressure gain that ultimately produced urinary leakage visible at the urethral meatus. Because the children could not feel the instrumentation, accurate bladder pressures at the instant of leakage were easy to record. Data derived from these measurements demonstrated a relationship between the bladder pressure required to overcome urethral resistance and upper urinary tract integrity. That relationship appeared to exist whether the bladder pressure was the product of a reflex contraction or an "autonomous" myogenic or mural response to distention. When urethral resistance was high enough to require a bladder pressure of 40 cm H_2O to induce leakage, upper urinary tract deterioration was often present, or, if not present, it developed.[2] Other workers later noted that high leak point pressures were not synonymous with the existence of upper tract abnormalities. The observation that patients with high leak point pressures do not always have upper tract deterioration is perfectly accurate but misses the point. An untreated bladder, which over time faces a urethral sphincter that requires a bladder pressure of 40 cm H_2O or more to cause leakage, will ultimately lose compliance, lead-ing in time to radiographically visible upper tract abnormalities.[2–4]

Most of the children who were in the first groups studied had areflexic vesical dysfunction, although some had true reflex detrusor-sphincter dyssynergia, identical to that encountered in patients with suprasacral spinal cord injury.[1–4] When the bladder was areflexic, urethral resistance was invariably exerted solely by the distal part of the urethral sphincter mechanism. The proximal urethra from the bladder neck to the pelvic floor musculature was nonfunctional and always open. During bladder filling in these children the nonfunctional proximal urethra filled with contrast, and at the moment of leakage the radiographic picture of the lower urinary tract was identical to that associated with true detrusor-sphincter dyssynergia seen in patients with spinal cord injury (Fig. 10–1). These are not, despite the similar radiographic pictures, the same conditions, nor do they behave in a similar manner. Patients with true detrusor-sphincter dyssynergia can be effectively treated by intermittent catheterization and anticholinergic agents.[5–7] This treatment combination is associated with achievement of very high continence rates. On the other hand, myelodysplastic children with detrusor areflexia and a nonfunctional internal sphincter, despite function of the external sphincter and pelvic diaphragm, are frequently incontinent despite identical treatment.[8] These patients "fail" treatment with drugs and intermittent catheterization with respect to continence.

One of the reasons for the severity of the incontinence in myelodysplastic children with areflexic vesi-

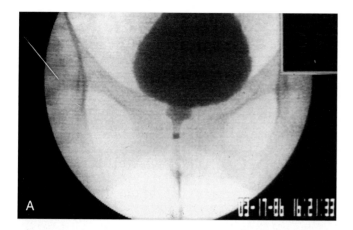

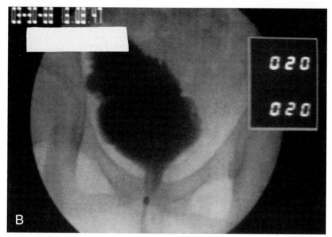

Figure 10-1 *A,* Detrusor sphincter dyssynergia recorded in a 28-year-old woman with a high spinal cord injury. Bladder pressure was 76 cm H$_2$O at the time the exposure was made. The bladder outlet and proximal urethra opened only when the bladder contracted. *B,* A bladder leak point pressure from a child with myelodysplasia. At a detrusor pressure of 20 cm H$_2$O leakage begins across a sphincter, which has a maximum pressure of 20 cm H$_2$O. The vesical outlet and proximal urethra were open from the beginning of the study, prior to any change in bladder pressure.

may be abetted by vesicoureteral reflux, but this is not required to institute the hydraulic effects on the kidney, which occur whether reflux can be demonstrated or not.[9] In fact, the pure radiographic demonstration of the presence or absence of reflux in children with areflexic vesical dysfunction is not very useful without some ancillary urodynamic data. If, for example, at a certain volume reflux occurred in a child studied during a "voiding cystourethrogram," observation of this abnormality is not the same as a determination that the same result would occur in this child in nonstudy circumstances. The observer does not have the pressure data that would enable him or her to assess the significance of the reflux or to plan appropriate treatment. If vesicoureteral reflux occurs during filling it could be termed low-pressure reflux because "voiding" did not occur at the time reflux was noted. However, in children and adults with neurogenic vesical dysfunction a bladder

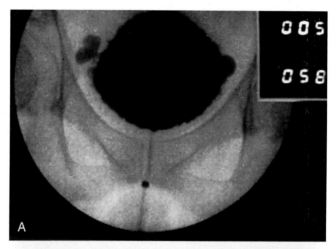

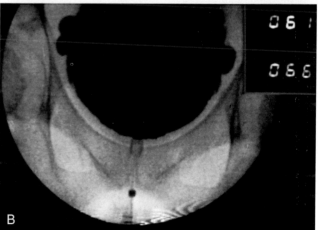

Figure 10-2 *A,* Early phase of a urodynamic study from a patient with a cauda equina lesion, an areflexive bladder, and functional internal and external sphincters. At this time bladder pressure is 5 cm H$_2$O, and maximum sphincter pressure is 58 cm H$_2$O. *B,* Later in the study at a volume of 300 ml a bladder pressure of 61 cm H$_2$O overcomes urethral resistance, maximum pressure is now 66 cm H$_2$O, and leakage occurs. Untreated, this situation leads to a steady-state constant urinary leakage at a pressure near 60 cm H$_2$O and bilateral hydroureteronephrosis. This condition must be treated.

cal dysfunction is the tendency of the bladder to gain pressure with incremental volume. This tendency imperils the fragile pressure advantage of the urethra over the bladder and results in steady-state urethral leakage. Once the pressure and volume in the bladder are sufficient to negate urethral resistance, continuous leakage occurs, and at that point ureteral peristalsis becomes the driving force behind the leakage. This situation in an untreated patient, or in a treated patient between intermittent catheterizations, is a mechanism for direct ureteral injury and creation of vesicoureteral reflux and renal damage. If urethral resistance is high enough (and we think a urethral closing pressure of 40 cm H$_2$O is high enough), the bladder pressure required to achieve steady-state leakage impedes continuous ureteral delivery of urine into the bladder. When this occurs, ureteral dilation develops, and the ureteral urine becomes a solid column of fluid. This produces a mechanism that transmits intravesical pressure directly to the renal papillae (Fig. 10–2). This process pressure gain associated with incremental volume may be enough to cause reflux, which is not "low pressure" even though it does not occur specifically during voiding.

Reflux that is visible radiographically *may* not be clinically significant. If the child has a low bladder leak point pressure, which is increased by the catheter used for filling, reflux may occur only during the study. If the child achieves a volume of 200 ml only during a "study," reflux that exists only at that volume may not be a clinical problem for that child (Fig. 10–3). Thus, the voiding cystourethrogram does not by itself provide enough information to be very useful.

Given the relationship between urethral resistance and bladder pressure and the relationship between bladder pressure and upper tract integrity, it should be apparent that when the detrusor is the force responsible for incontinence, treatment must be directed at the bladder. A urethral procedure that makes it more difficult for the bladder to induce leakage will do one of two things. Either the increase in urethral resistance will be overcome by higher detrusor pressures and the leakage will recur, or more effective urethral closure will permit the bladder to attain higher pressures, which results in transmission of those pressures to the ureters and kidneys. At sustained higher bladder pressures, compliance progressively deteriorates, and upper tract damage will occur at progressively smaller bladder volumes.[10]

ABDOMINAL PRESSURE AS AN EXPULSIVE FORCE

Using bladder pressure monitoring techniques over a period of many months in patients with myelodysplasia and spinal cord injury, it was sometimes difficult to reconcile low bladder pressures with reported incontinence. Despite the ability to predict the risk of upper tract deterioration by measuring bladder pressure and to prevent or reverse upper tract changes by lowering bladder pressure, some patients continue to be wet. This can occur despite frequent intermittent catheterization, adherence to medication regimens, and measured low bladder pressures. When these patients are studied with videourodynamic techniques, after a cystometrogram has demonstrated an absolutely flat bladder pressure-volume curve in relation to the volumes obtained by intermittent catheterization, leakage may be found to be driven by abdominal pressure. Urologists erred in assuming that intravesical pressure was the same force with respect to urethral continence whether it was generated by the detrusor or the abdomen. A study of spinal cord injury patients with absolutely flat bladder pressure-volume curves demonstrated that relatively low abdominal pressures could induce urethral leakage if proximal urethral function was poor.[7, 11] Studies of patients with myelodysplasia with a nonfunctional internal sphincter mechanism, women with type III stress incontinence, and men with postprostatectomy incontinence demonstrate that abdominal pressure is an expulsive force that induces leakage only in specific circumstances. The normally closed internal sphincter mechanism in men and women will not leak no matter how much abdominal pressure is attained. Abdominal pressure can be measured anywhere in the abdomen, but by convention it is usually measured intravesically. However, intravesical pressure produced by straining or the Valsalva maneuver is not the same, as far as the urethra is concerned, as intravesical pressure produced by contraction of the bladder. Bladder pressure resulting from detrusor contractility (or mural stretch) is directed right at the urethra and tends to force the urethra open. Abdominal pressure does not normally tend to force the urethra open—in fact, it tends to close it (Fig. 10–4).

Thus, if leakage occurs as a result of an increase in abdominal pressure, one of two things is wrong with the urethral sphincter mechanism. Either it moves from its position within the abdominal cavity, driven as it were by abdominal pressure, or the urethra from the bladder neck to the external sphincter is not normally closed. Patients with type III stress incontinence, postprostatectomy incontinence, and myelodysplasia all have an open nonfunctional internal sphincter mechanism and leak urine at relatively low abdominal pressures. Patients with urethral

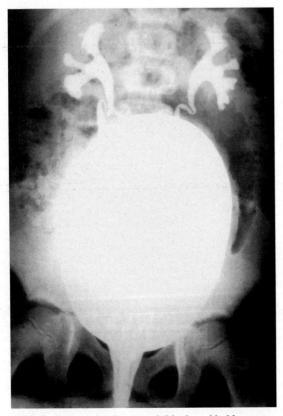

Figure 10-3 Bilateral reflux in a child whose bladder was grossly overfilled to induce voiding. Because of the overfilling, the significance of the bilateral reflux is questionable.

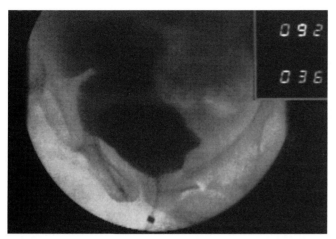

Figure 10-4 A vigorous Valsalva maneuver performed by an 18-year-old myelodysplastic man after collagen injection. This patient also had an augmentation cystoplasty and a very low reservoir pressure, but leakage occurred at a low abdominal pressure before collagen injection. The patient is dry, and no leakage occurred during this study. Abdominal pressure is 92 cm H_2O and maximum urethral pressure 36 cm H_2O (without leakage). Note the lack of relationship between urethral pressure and abdominal pressure. This satisfies the standard definition of stress incontinence because abdominal pressure here *exceeds* the maximum urethral closing pressure despite the lack of leakage. Obviously, something is wrong with the definition.

hypermobility and incontinence on that basis leak urine at considerably higher abdominal pressures.

CLINICAL CORRELATION

Bladder pressure has a constant linear hydraulic relationship with urethral resistance and also with ureteral function, whereas abdominal pressure does not. Bladder pressure must overcome the highest urethral resistance offered to it to induce leakage. Bladder pressure at the time of voiding is proportional to maximum urethral pressure and resistance. Bladder pressure can act against ureteral delivery of urine into the bladder. Abdominal pressure tends to abet internal sphincter function when that part of the urethral sphincter is normally closed and normally positioned. The abdominal pressure needed to cause leakage has no linear relationship to urethral closing pressure, and abdominal pressure has *no* effect on ureteral function.

Data gathered from the simultaneous measurement of abdominal and urethral pressures during repetitive coughing indicate that maximum urethral closing pressures are higher in normal patients without stress incontinence than in those with that condition, and further that the highest urethral closing pressures are invariably measured in the area of the external sphincter.[12] These observations, although absolutely accurate, do not prove that urethral pressures are equivalent to continence function vis-à-vis abdominal pressure, although we have assumed that to be the case. When a large group of incontinent patients was evaluated, we found no relationship

between the abdominal pressure required to cause leakage and the maximum urethral closing pressures. We measured both variables carefully at the time of leakage and at rest; leakage was determined precisely by a videourodynamic technique. This is not the same as the study of two groups of patients, one group of "normal women" and another group of women with stress urinary incontinence, in whom intravesical and intraurethral pressures are measured simultaneously but without making a determination of the precise pressure required to cause leakage (Fig. 10–5). When the latter is done, no relationship is found between the abdominal pressure needed to cause leakage and the urethral closing pressure measured in the high-pressure zone. Moreover, continent patients undergoing the same kind of videourodynamic study show that continence is maintained at the vesical outlet (the bladder neck or internal urethral sphincter) and not the midurethral high-pressure zone, where the highest pressures are measured. In short, the observations regarding urethral closing pressure and intravesical pressure are accurate, but the conclusions drawn from those data are not.

As a corollary, assumptions about urethral sphincter function and the "high-pressure zone" led to efforts to improve continence function by techniques that improved pelvic floor muscular contractility.[13, 14] The effects of electrical stimulation, various exercises, and physical therapeutic maneuvers on overall continence function have been documented, but the precise mechanism whereby these effects are exerted has not been conclusively proved, nor is it likely that such effects are a result of improvement in the external urethral sphincter and pelvic floor contractility, as that applies to urethral closing pressure.

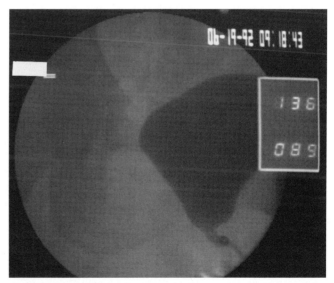

Figure 10-5 Lateral view of the bladder and urethra at the moment of leakage. Abdominal pressure is 136 cm H_2O and maximum urethral pressure 89 cm H_2O. The urethra and bladder base were first driven inferiorly and posteriorly by the straining maneuver; leakage then occurred at a relatively high abdominal pressure.

Measurement of the abdominal pressure required to cause leakage across an abnormal urethra is used chiefly to quantitate the defect in urethral sphincter function. A mobile urethra related to a lack of urethral support such as that encountered in women with typical stress incontinence will leak at pressures greater than 90 cm H_2O (see Fig. 10–5). A poorly closed urethra will leak at pressures of less than 60 cm H_2O (Fig. 10–6), and a urethra that is both poorly closed and mobile will leak at pressures between 40 and 90 cm H_2O (Fig. 10–7). Patients with low abdominal leak point pressures tend to fail to respond to standard suspension operations designed to cure incontinence related to urethral hypermobility. In most such patients leakage occurs without regard to physical activity—that is, leakage occurs more or less continuously. Leakage can result merely from assuming the upright position, gravity being a sufficient expulsive force to cause it (Fig. 10–8). These patients are not difficult to identify by the history, and their status is classified as grade III incontinence. Most urologists and gynecologists recognize that such patients are better treated by slings, injectable materials, or artificial sphincters than by standard suspension operations. More troublesome are those patients who leak urine with effort but who also have relatively poor urethral closing function. These patients are difficult to identify without leak point pressure measurements, but relatively high failure rates occur after standard suspension procedures.

Patients with abdominal leak point pressures of less than 60 cm H_2O are usually treated by sling procedures or, if no urethral mobility is present, by collagen injection. Slings raise the abdominal leak point pressure to infinity but change voiding pressure (bladder leak point pressure) only slightly. Collagen injection raises the abdominal leak point pressure significantly and can raise it to oppose abdominal pressures as high as 200 to 250 cm H_2O but does not raise voiding pressure.

These findings indicate the relative safety of slings and collagen injection procedures and their specificity for the internal urethral sphincter mechanism acting against abdominal pressure. They have no effect on the bladder pressure required to cause leakage and thus pose no danger to the upper urinary tract.[9, 10]

MECHANICS OF THE BLADDER LEAK POINT PRESSURE

We use a 10 Fr Bard triple-lumen urodynamic catheter, but any 8 or 10 Fr catheter will suffice. The study is done with the patient in the supine position if there is neural impairment. If obstructive uropathy is the working diagnosis, the upright position should be used for the examination. The bladder is filled at 50 ml/minute (less for children, 10 to 20 ml/minute) while the intravesical pressure is monitored constantly. If the urethra is visualized fluoroscopically 20% iodinated contrast material is used for filling. If simple visual observation of the external meatus is used to detect leakage, methylene blue can be added to the infusate for improved visibility.

In patients with neurologic disease the procedure is straightforward because leakage will occur at virtually identical pressures with repeat performance of the study regardless of whether leakage is a product of reflex detrusor activity or autonomous activity. The examination can be modified based on the clinical situation and the current method of management. If, for example, a patient is being managed by a combination of drugs and intermittent catheterization and reports no leakage, then the bladder need be filled only to the maximum volume ever obtained by intermittent catheterization to be certain that bladder pressures at that volume are in the "safe" range. Patients who are "voiding" into condom catheters must be studied to determine the pressure required to drive urine across the sphincter to be certain that that value is in the normal or safe range. Because no long-term prospective data on the upper limit of a "safe" range are available, this range is usually defined as 30 cm H_2O or less. This value is clearly conservative, and many paraplegic patients "void" at higher pressures for relatively short periods. Voiding pressures of less than 30 cm H_2O are, however, "normal" for males, and if pressures are kept at or below this value, upper urinary tract changes are not encountered in patients with neurogenic vesical dysfunction.

Leakage occurring between catheterizations may result from one of two conditions. Either bladder pressure is the driving force or there is some abnormality of urethral sphincteric function, or both conditions may exist simultaneously. The first step in evaluating such a patient is to prove that the bladder pressures obtained by intermittent catheterization at

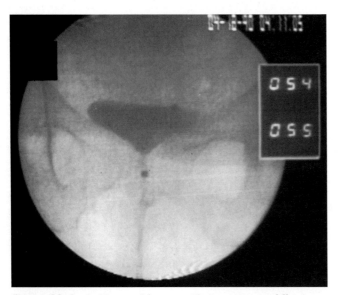

Figure 10–6 A 65-year-old man with incontinence following a radical prostatectomy leaks urine at an abdominal pressure of 54 cm H_2O.

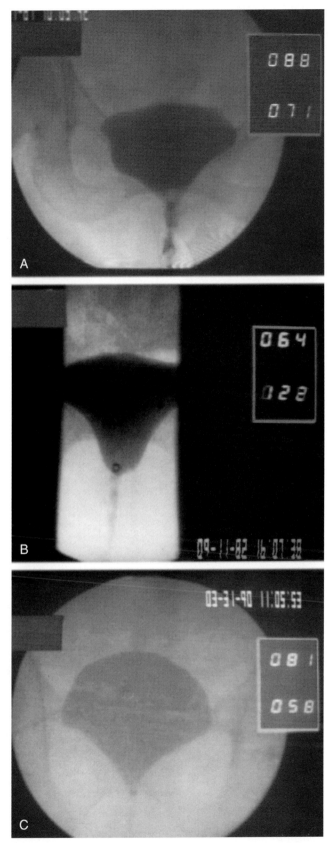

Figure 10-7   *A*, Leakage occurred at an abdominal pressure of 88 cm H_2O in a 54-year-old woman after two unsuccessful operations. There is considerable urethral mobility, but leakage occurs at a moderate pressure. Note the lack of bladder urethral pressure relationship. *B*, Leakage occurs at an abdominal pressure of 64 cm H_2O across a maximum urethral pressure of 122 cm H_2O. There is considerable motion but a relatively low leak point pressure. *C*, An elderly woman with leakage at an abdominal pressure of 81 cm H_2O and a maximum urethral pressure of 58 cm H_2O. There is some motion, and leakage occurs at a moderate pressure.

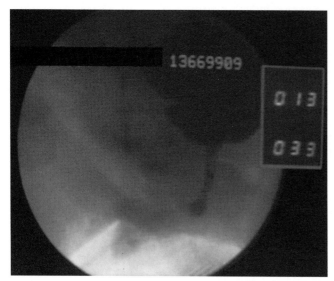

Figure 10–8 The upright position results in leakage at an abdominal pressure of 13 cm H_2O in this young boy with myelodysplasia despite a maximum urethral pressure of 33 cm H_2O.

the maximum volume are quite low, thus ruling out the bladder as a source of leakage. That determination then allows identification of any problem with urethral function. If any component of the leakage is driven by bladder pressure, that problem must be dealt with prior to or simultaneously with initiation of treatment for a coexisting urethral problem.

Assessment of bladder leak point pressure in patients in whom anatomic obstructive uropathy is suspected, for instance, patients with benign prostatic hypertrophy or women with obstructive symptoms following a urethral suspension operation, is somewhat more difficult than in patients with neurogenic vesical dysfunction. This difficulty exists because external sphincter activity results in an immediate increase in intravesical pressure, and it is difficult, using pressures alone, to be certain that external sphincter activity is not present during the urodynamic study. The best way to rule out sphincter activity is to use fluoroscopy (Fig. 10–9). Using a Bard triple-lumen urodynamic catheter, the urethral pressure-sensing aperture is localized within the external urethral sphincter. This structure must be demonstrated to be completely relaxed at the time bladder pressure is measured if bladder pressure is to be used as an index of the amount of urethral resistance remaining. The external urethral sphincter is the most powerful part of the urethral sphincter mechanism that acts against bladder pressure as an expulsive force. If the external sphincter contracts (volitionally or unconsciously) during measurement of the amount of bladder pressure required to drive urine across the sphincter, that measurement reflects resistance at the external sphincter rather than the proximal urethral sphincter mechanism. Bladder pressure cannot be used to indicate the relationship between the bladder and the internal sphincter, prostatic urethra, or bladder neck unless the external sphincter is completely relaxed. If the external sphincter is

relaxed, bladder pressure will reflect resistance at the bladder neck or prostatic urethra. Performing the study in this way gives the observer the advantage of being able to record a urethral pressure profile during flow, thus permitting determination of the amount of pressure drop across a putative "obstructive" area. If, for example, a voiding pressure of 78 cm H_2O is recorded in the bladder and this pressure drops across the bladder neck to a pressure of 12 cm H_2O in the urethra proximal to the external sphincter, one is dealing with a high-grade bladder neck obstruction.

DETERMINATION OF URETHRAL FUNCTION BY ABDOMINAL LEAKAGE PRESSURES

We use a 10 Fr Bard urodynamic catheter for these measurements, but this is not essential and any 8 or 10 Fr catheter will suffice. The bladder is filled to between 200 and 300 ml. With the patient in the upright position a progressively more vigorous Valsalva maneuver is done three or four times. Leakage is visualized fluoroscopically (or seen at the meatus), and the pressure required to induce it is recorded. The fluoroscopic mode is more precise, but the technique actually does not require great precision.

The critical feature is the demonstration of leakage at a low, high, or moderate abdominal pressure. Low abdominal pressure encompasses a range of 0 to 60 cm H_2O, moderate pressure is 60 to 90 cm H_2O, and high pressure is greater than 90 cm H_2O. These findings correlate with subjective continence grades. Individuals who are wet virtually continuously, without regard to activity (grade III incontinence), most often experience leakage at quite low pressures, and

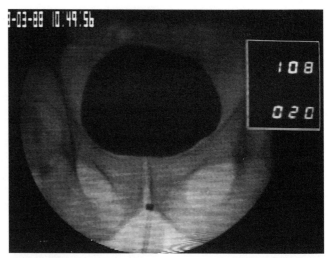

Figure 10–9 Voiding phase of a videourodynamic study from a 68-year-old man with high-grade prostatic obstruction of the bladder. External sphincter pressure is 20 cm H_2O (from a high of 148 cm H_2O). Bladder pressure is 108 cm H_2O, there is no flow, and the internal sphincter is not open. He cannot be straining, because that would increase the external sphincter pressure. At this point the bladder pressure, which is three times normal, reflects an abnormal outlet resistance at the bladder neck and prostate.

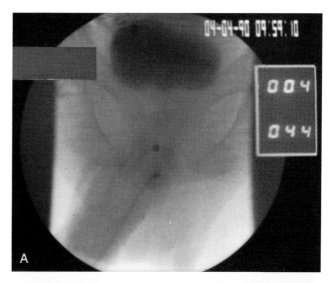

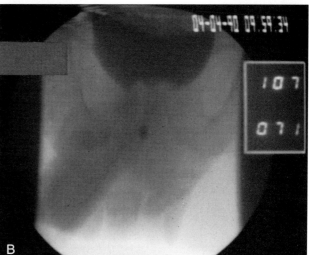

Figure 10-10 *A*, Abdominal pressure study in a 28-year-old patient with a T_{12} spinal cord injury. Maximum urethral pressure is 44 cm H_2O at rest. *B*, Valsalva-generated abdominal pressure of 107 cm H_2O measured in the bladder does not induce leakage. Maximum urethral pressure is 71 cm H_2O. Leakage occurred at 16 cm H_2O prior to collagen injection therapy, which was done three times to gain closure of the vesical outlet in this patient.

those who become wet only with vigorous exercise (jogging or aerobics) show leakage at higher pressures (grades I and II incontinence). Independent variables such as age and level of activity make blind assessment of the type of incontinence *only* by inference from subjective grading difficult and often inaccurate.

If leakage is not induced by repeated Valsalva maneuvers, a series of coughs can be used to attempt to induce leakage. Coughing results in very rapid pressure changes, and the fluid-filled external pressure transducer system has a relatively slow response time, so absolutely precise identification of the actual leak point pressure may require several measurements. Generally, when vigorous repeated coughing is required to induce leakage, the abdominal pressure required to accomplish this is high, well above 90 cm H_2O.

The other obvious use of "stress testing" by abdominal leak point pressure measurement is to rule out urethral dysfunction in patients complaining of incontinence. If a urethra can be demonstrated to withstand an abdominal pressure excursion of 200 cm H_2O, urethral function (at least against abdominal pressure) is probably normal, and the cause of the incontinence can be assumed to be other than urethral dysfunction. The other use of abdominal leak point pressure measurement is to quantify a change in the ability of the urethra to resist abdominal pressure conferred by a method of treatment, either medical or surgical (Fig. 10–10).

REFERENCES

1. McGuire EJ, Woodside JR, Borden TA, Weiss RM: Prognostic value of urodynamic testing in myelodysplastic patients. J Urol 126:205, 1981.
2. McGuire EJ, Woodside JR, Borden TA: Upper tract deterioration in patients with myelodysplasia and detrusor hypertonia: A follow-up study. J Urol 129:823, 1983.
3. Wang SC, McGuire EJ, Bloom DA: A bladder pressure management system for myelodysplasia: Clinical outcome. J Urol 140:1499, 1988.
4. Ghoneim GM, Bloom DA, McGuire EJ, Stewart KL: Bladder compliance in meningomyelocele children. J Urol 141:1404, 1989.
5. McGuire EJ, Savastano JA: Long term follow-up of spinal cord

injury patients managed by intermittent catheterization. J Urol 129:775, 1983.

6. McGuire EJ, Brady SM: Detrusor-sphincter dyssynergia. J Urol 121:774, 1979.

7. McGuire EJ, Savastano JA: Urodynamics and management of the neuropathic bladder in spinal cord injury patients. J Am Paraplegia Soc 8:28, 1985.

8. Purcell MH, Gregory JG: Intermittent catheterization: Evaluation of complete dryness and independence in children with myelomeningocele. J Urol 132:518, 1984.

9. McGuire EJ: The interaction of bladder filling behavior and urethral function. World J Urol 8:194, 1990.

10. McGuire EJ: Factors affecting bladder compliance. Dialogues Pediatr Urol 13:1, 1990.

11. Woodside JR, McGuire EJ: Urethral hypotonicity after suprasacral spinal cord injury. J Urol 121:783, 1979.

12. Constantinou CE: Resting and stress urethral pressures as a clinical guide to the mechanism of continence in the female patient. Urol Clin North Am 12:247, 1985.

13. Kegel AH: Progressive resistance exercise in the functional restoration of the perineal muscles. Am J Obstet Gynecol 56:238, 1948.

14. Wells TS: Pelvic (floor) muscle exercise. J Am Geriatr Soc 38:333, 1990.

CHAPTER 11

Urethral Pressures in the Study of Female Incontinence

C. E. Constantinou, Ph.D.
L. L. Christensen, M.D.

The International Continence Society (ICS) Committee on Standardization of Terminology defines urethral closure pressure as the subtraction of intravesical pressure from intraluminal urethral pressure.[1] In this ICS definition it is implicit that the intraluminal pressure in the urethra is considered in the context and terms of intravesical pressure. Intravesical pressure is evoked in this definition for convenience of measurement and as an approximation rather than an absolute pressure component that contributes to urethral closure. In anatomic terms, the urethra, as it traverses the symphysis and vagina, is under the influence of a number of paraurethral structures that exert different closure forces along its length. Closure forces produced by paraurethral structures can be passive or active and are not necessarily equal to intravesical pressure. What is common among paraurethral structures is that they are extrinsic to the urethra and invariably act in different directions. In addition to the extrinsic forces maintaining a closed urethra, there are the forces of the urethra itself, such as smooth muscle tone, sphincter, and blood supply, that constitute the intrinsic mechanism. The superimposition of extrinsic forces on intraluminal pressure is far more complex than can be encompassed by the simple subtraction of intravesical pressure, as the ICS definition suggests. For this reason, consideration of urethral pressures in the study of female incontinence should be focused on the totality of forces that act to maintain urethral closure. In view of the variety of structures involved and the degree of overlap between them, it is practically impossible to assess continence on the basis of urethral closure alone. There are no current diagnostic tests that are sufficiently sophisticated to assess the continence function of the urethra and localize the cause of leakage with precision.

One of the first diagnostic tests introduced into the field of urodynamics for the evaluation of urethral competence was the resting urethral pressure profile (UPP). The UPP is a topographic curve that is representative of pressures along the length of the urethra and is at best the most urostatic measurement in the field of urodynamics. As such, the UPP does not represent urethral function in many dynamic situations in which incontinence is likely to occur, and contrary to expectations, it has been of limited practical value in the consideration of continence. This is a predictable outcome, given the fact that the UPP includes so many variables in a single recording, which is often done under unrealistic clinical conditions. Indeed, appreciation of the anatomy of the pelvic floor and the associated paraurethral structures indicates that a primitive measurement such as the UPP alone could predictably provide only the most rudimentary measurements of urethral closure. On the other hand, if associated dynamic measurements are incorporated with the static measurements of the UPP, a better understanding of the mechanism of urethral forces emerges.

In this chapter, we describe the results of a number of recent basic and clinical investigations that will, it is hoped, place urethral pressures in their appropriate context. In so doing, we hope to provide a better understanding of the role of intrinsic and extrinsic urethral mechanisms in female continence. We first examine the anatomic support of the urethra and identify the known contributions of individual structures (extrinsic mechanisms). Visualizations obtained by MRI techniques are used to illustrate this material. We then consider such factors as the contribution of blood flow and the action of hormones on urethral closure and associated biomechanics (intrinsic mechanisms). These observations are integrated with recent reports of dynamic measurements of urethral function and their role in urinary continence.

Anatomic Considerations

RELATIONSHIP BETWEEN ANATOMY AND URETHRAL PRESSURE PROFILE

DeLancey considered the anatomic structures contributing to urethral closure and divided them into two main groups: structures forming the urethral sphincter, and its attachments.[2] The urethra possesses several different mechanisms composed of three elements that contribute approximately equally to its function: striated muscle, smooth muscle, and vascular elements.[3] The term urethral sphincter is used to define the striated intrinsic urethral sphincter; smooth muscle and vessels are included here because these structures participate in maintaining urethral closure pressure. Figure 11–1 illustrates the anatomic correlates of a UPP together with the terminology used to define significant parameters. The insert shows an MRI enhanced to identify the outline of the urethra with a catheter in its lumen. The striated muscle layer, forming the urethral sphincter, is located outside the smooth muscle and forms the position of the maximum urethral closing pressure (MUCP). The term urethral sphincter refers to the intrinsic external urethral sphincter, not the extrinsic periurethral musculature. The striated muscle fibers are thickest along the middle portion of the urethra, and in that area they completely surround the organ.[4] The portion between the urethra and the vagina is relatively thin. Striated muscle fibers extend into the anterior wall of the proximal and distal thirds of the urethra and are missing laterally and posteriorly at these levels.[5] At the level of the distal third, some of the striated muscle fibers leave the confines of the urethra and merge at its lateral aspect with striated muscle fibers originating near the pubic rami and the vaginal wall, respectively, forming a single muscle band that arches over the anterior part of the urethra.[4] The part of the muscle fibers originating near the pubic rami is referred to as the compressor urethra. The other part, originating from the vaginal wall, is named the urethrovaginal sphincter.

SPHINCTER MUSCLE AND FIBERS

Consideration of the type of muscle fibers present in the urethra was made by Gosling and colleagues,

FEMALE RESTING URETHRAL PRESSURE PROFILE

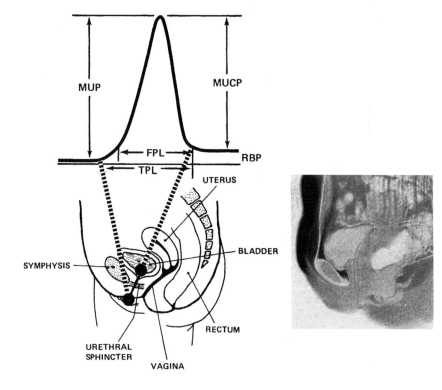

MUCP : MAXIMUM URETHRAL CLOSURE PRESSURE
MUP : MAXIMUM URETHRAL PRESSURE
FPL : FUNCTIONAL PROFILE LENGTH
TPL : TOTAL PROFILE LENGTH
RBP : RESTING BLADDER PRESSURE

Figure 11-1 Schematic diagram showing the relationship between resting urethral pressures and the anatomic correlates. The insert illustrates the position of the catheter within the urethra. This sagittal MR image was enhanced to show the relative position of the catheter with respect to the surrounding periurethral structures. The patient is placed supine, a position that is frequently used to produce a urethral pressure profile.

who divided them into two groups, type I (slow-twitch) fibers and type II (fast-twitch) fibers.[6] The two types contain different amounts of alkaline- and acid-stable myosin ATPase enzyme. These differences make it possible to separate the two types using enzyme-histochemical methods. Type I fibers are rich in mitochondria, in contrast to type II fibers, in which the concentration of mitochondria is low. These differences reflect the ability of type I fibers to contract slowly but sustain the contraction over a long period, whereas type II fibers contract quickly but maintain the contraction for only a short time. Muscle fibers in the striated urogenital sphincter are rich in acid-stable myosin ATPase and have a high mitochondrial content; they can be functionally classified as slow-twitch fibers, reflecting their ability to keep a lasting constant tone.[6] Studies of the periurethral portion of the striated levator ani muscle have shown that this muscle, in contrast to the external sphincter, consists of a mixture of large-diameter type I and type II fibers. It supports the theory that the levator ani assists the external urethral sphincter in urethral closure to ensure continence and also produces rapid occlusion during a rise in intra-abdominal pressure and voluntary contraction.[6] The major part of the smooth muscle is arranged longitudinally or obliquely surrounding the submucosa. It extends from the bladder neck to the external meatus. In the periphery of this smooth muscle layer a thin layer of muscle fibers is arranged circularly.

MACROSCOPIC SUPPORT

The urethra is also supported by paraurethral tissues, the basic element of the structures between the endopelvic fascia around the vagina and the proximal urethra, the arcus tendineus fascia pelvis and the levator ani muscle. An intimate connection exists between the anterior vaginal wall and the urethra. These structures are held together by connective tissue, called the endopelvic fascia, which surrounds both organs. The part of the endopelvic fascia between the proximal urethra and the vagina is attached laterally to the anterior part of the fibrous band, the arcus tendineus fascia pelvis, which runs from the pubic bone to the ischial spine. At the same level, the fascia surrounding the vagina is attached to the medial fibers of the levator ani muscle. These fascial and muscular attachments to the arcus tendineus and the levator ani are responsible for the position and mobility of the proximal urethra and the bladder neck. One of the best ways of visualizing the influence of pelvic floor contraction is through MRI, which shows the influence of voluntary activation of the skeletal musculature. Using subtracted MRI, the action of the pelvic floor muscles on the surrounding paraurethral structures can be seen. Figure 11–2 illustrates the displacement of the pelvic contents as a result of activation of the skeletal muscles in a series of sagittal images. These images contrast with the pelvic floor at rest, as illustrated in Figure 11–1.

The process of deriving these images is described in the legend for Figure 11–2.

In contrast to the intrinsic striated urethral sphincter with type I (slow-twitch) muscle fibers, the levator ani muscle consists primarily of type II (fast-twitch) muscle fibers except for part of the muscle adjacent to the proximal urethra and bladder neck.[7] In that region, the fibers are of the slow-twitch type, suggesting that the muscle in that region is specialized to maintain a constant tone. It has also been suggested that these structures ensure that any increase in intra-abdominal pressure can be transmitted to the urethra.[4] The levator muscle, under normal conditions, keeps a constant tone and relaxes only during voiding and defecation. These anatomic considerations focus on the fact that the female urethra is composed and supported by a complex framework of muscles and structures that contribute to the balance of forces that maintain closure. These structures are controlled, in addition, by somatic innervation. Somatic innervation of the urethra and periurethral muscles and pelvic floor is still under investigation, although it is generally accepted that the levator ani muscle is supplied by somatic fibers carried in the pudendal nerve.[8] These fibers originate from the second, third, and fourth sacral segments of the spinal cord. Innervation of the external intrinsic urethral striated sphincter is described in several different ways. One opinion is that branches of the pelvic (splanchnic) nerve carry some somatic motor fibers to the sphincter.[8] Juenemann and associates found that the pudendal nerve was responsible for innervation of both the levator ani muscle and the striated urethral sphincter, thereby implying that fibers from the pudendal nerve to the sphincter separate before the pudendal nerve becomes easily identifiable on dissection.[9]

In addition to somatic innervation, which serves primarily as a controlling mechanism for continence and reflex contraction, the autonomic nervous system is represented by both parasympathetic (cholinergic) and sympathetic (adrenergic) nerves to the bladder neck and urethral region. The bladder neck and urethral smooth muscles are richly innervated by cholinergic nerves. Gosling has shown that in the female there are very few adrenergic nerves. Finally, urethral closure is influenced directly by urethral blood flow.

The female urethra receives blood from the urethral artery coming from the internal pudendal arteries, which in turn are fed by the internal iliac arteries.[10] There is considerable individual variation in the vascular anatomy, and anastomoses are common. The urethra is lined with pseudostratified or stratified columnar epithelium. Below the epithelium is found the lamina propria, built up of connective tissue containing some very well developed venous plexus analogous to the male corpus spongiosum.[11] This similarity does not seem to be based directly on embryology because the part of the urogenital sinus that forms the entire female urethra develops in

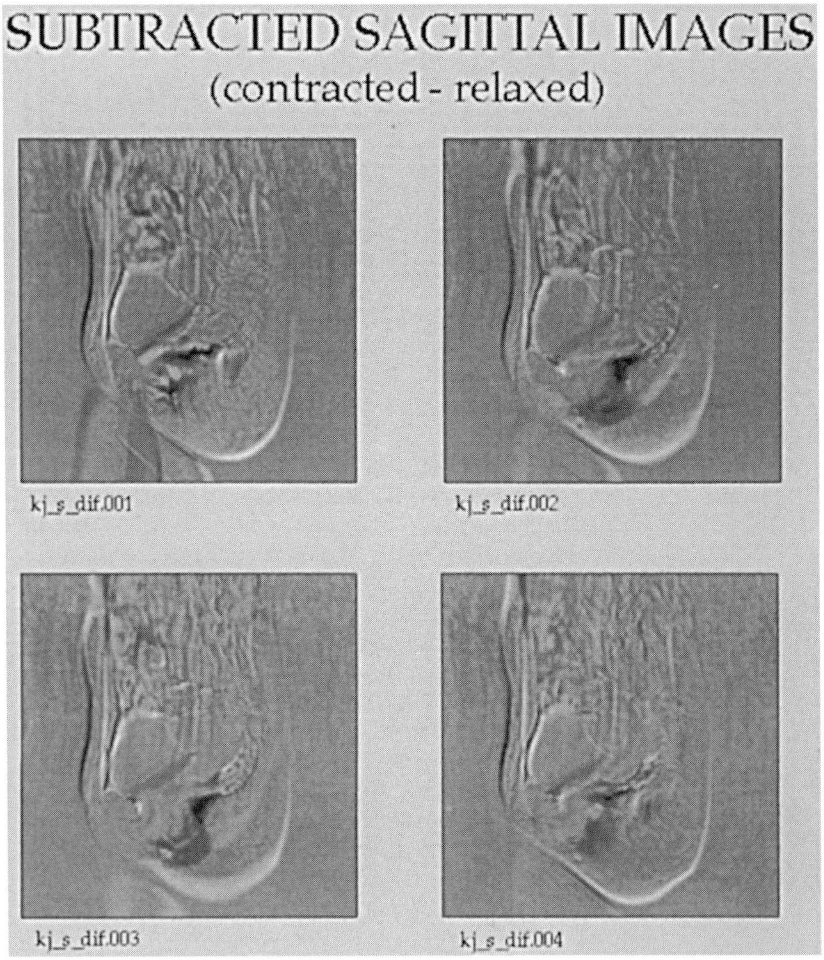

SUBTRACTED SAGITTAL IMAGES
(contracted - relaxed)

kj_s_dif.001

kj_s_dif.002

kj_s_dif.003

kj_s_dif.004

Figure 11-2 Sequence of subtracted sagittal MR images demonstrating the influence of voluntary pelvic floor contraction on the bladder and paraurethral structures. Clearly seen are the symphysis pubis, above which lies a distended bladder, the curve of the sacrum and coccyx, and the abdominal and gluteal fat. Pelvic floor movement is prominent. The black shades demonstrate contraction of the levator ani muscle with subsequent movement occurring superiorly and anteriorly. Associated structures, such as the anal canal and vagina, track this motion. The gluteal border has also moved markedly in the same direction. The difference images also indicate an anterior-superior movement of the entire bladder.

males as the supramontanal part of the prostatic urethra.[12]

The paraurethral muscles can be voluntarily activated, thereby compressing the region of the bladder neck. Figure 11–3 illustrates the dynamic changes typically visualized in transverse scans taken at the level of the symphysis pubis anteriorly and the ischial tuberosity posteriorly. In the difference image in Figure 11–3, a black V-shaped band is prominent as well as a C-shaped band that "caps" the V. These highlights represent anterior-directed movement of the levator ani on contraction. The vagina is compressed, which in turn compresses the bladder neck region. Note the absence of any highlights near the bony structures due to complete image subtraction, indicating very little movement.

Figure 11–4 further illustrates the influence of contraction on the paraurethral structures in the transverse plane. Black to deep shades represent maximum movements of the pelvic floor produced by contraction of the levator ani muscle. The darker shades, representing smaller movements, are located anteriorly. Movement is directed toward the symphysis pubis, which itself has not moved and hence has been subtracted from view.

Urodynamic Evaluation of the Urethra

RESTING URETHRAL PRESSURE PROFILE

The contribution of the sphincter and supporting structures of the urethra can be measured using the UPP. This test provides a graph that incorporates all closure forces that compress the urethral lumen. There are several methods of obtaining a profile of the urethral pressures. The intraurethral pressure is measured along the urethral length by pulling a pressure sensor from the bladder out through the urethra. Withdrawal of the catheter can be done manually in steps or mechanically at a fixed rate. Several types of catheter pressure systems have been used.[13] The pressure can be measured using either a fluid-filled system, which has a fluid column connected to an external transducer, or a catheter with a small microtip transducer mounted on the catheter itself. The side facing the measuring unit on a tip catheter provides information about directional differences in profilometry. Such information reflects the actions of the structures in different directions,

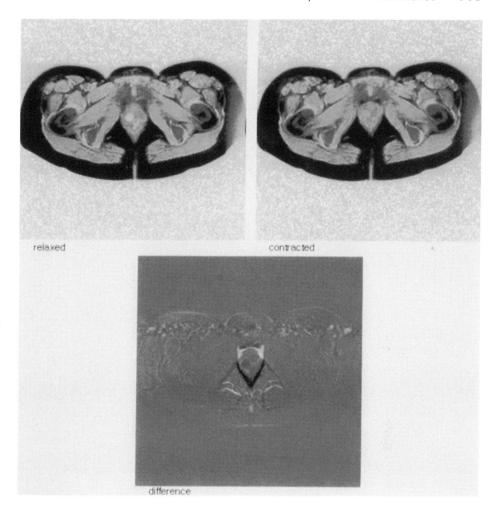

relaxed   contracted

difference

Figure 11–3 MR image taken at the level of the symphysis. The relaxed and contracted images of a single transverse level show the border of the levator ani muscle clearly demarcated against the fat of the ischiorectal fossa. Fat is dark in these digitally processed images. The digital subtraction of the contracted image from the relaxed gray scale image produces a new image that, when processed darker than the stationary structures, clearly identifies the regions where contraction has taken place.

thus, in the lateral plane the pressures are symmetrical.[14] In healthy female volunteers, the anterior and posterior oriented pressures were found to be equal, but the posterior functional length exceeded the anterior length.[15] The MUCP of women with incontinence originating in the detrusor but no urethral incontinence is given in Figure 11–5. Women with proven stress incontinence had significantly lower posterior pressures than anterior pressures. Figure 11–6 shows the relationship between the anterior and posterior MUCP in patients with stress incontinence. These differences may be due to forces acting on the urethra in this group of patients, or they may represent the bending of the structure in the presence of a catheter. This observation is supported by the fact that the differences are less pronounced when the measurements are made by a soft catheter than with a catheter made of a stiffer material.

ROLE OF VASCULAR, SKELETAL, AND SMOOTH MUSCLE COMPONENTS OF URETHRAL CLOSURE

A systematic study of the contribution of striated and smooth muscle within the urethra with special focus on the influence of systemic blood pressure was undertaken by Rud and colleagues.[3] In this study, UPP measurements were made before, during, and after curarization as well as clamping of the common iliac artery bilaterally. Figures 11–7 and 11–8 illustrate the response of the urethral closure pressure to these interventions. On the basis of such observations, it has been concluded that the striated muscle in the urethra, including the pelvic floor, is responsible for approximately one-third of the total intraurethral pressure exerted. Another third of the urethral closure pressure is contributed by blood flow, and the remaining third is contributed by connective and periurethral tissue.

Curarization causes a drop in maximum urethral pressure (MUP) of approximately 33% (Fig. 11–9). Clamping of the common iliac artery causes another 28% drop in MUP. Opening of the abdomen has a positive effect on MUP, even when the change in abdominal pressure and arterial blood pressure is taken into account. This effect is thought to be caused by direct nerve stimulation of the smooth muscles in the urethra because of an increased level of circulating catecholamines.

An effort to evaluate both passive and dynamic function of urethral pressure when the skeletal muscle is paralyzed was made more recently by Bump and coworkers.[16] Figure 11–10 shows the relative effect of paralyzed muscles on passive urethral func-

SUBTRACTED TRANSVERSE IMAGES
(contracted - relaxed)

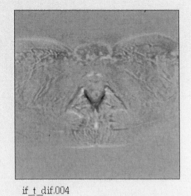

if_t_dif.004

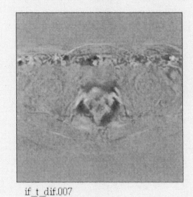

if_t_dif.005

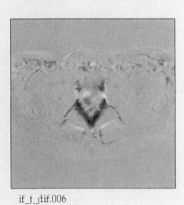

if_t_dif.006

if_t_dif.007

Figure 11-4 Four consecutive sections of subtracted images showing the influence of pelvic floor activation and compression of the urethra and vagina. A tampon in the vagina is clearly shown for reference. The lower scans show motion in or near the urogenital diaphragm internally and the gluteal region externally. The upper images demonstrate levator muscle motion.

tion in continent and incontinent patients. Analysis of the results shows that highly significant anesthetic effects influence all parameters, suggesting that the sphincter advantage is eliminated by skeletal paraly-

sis and loss of consciousness, particularly in spinal cord–injured patients. Thus, skeletal muscle activity occurring reflexively is important in closing the urethra. Passive urethral closure is less affected by loss

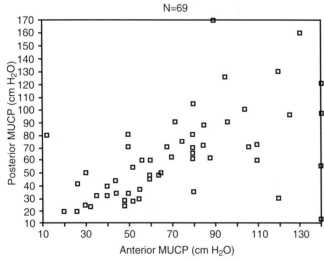

Figure 11-5 Relationship between anterior and posterior maximum urethral closure pressure (MUCP) in 69 women with detrusor incontinence. There is no demonstrable stress urinary incontinence.

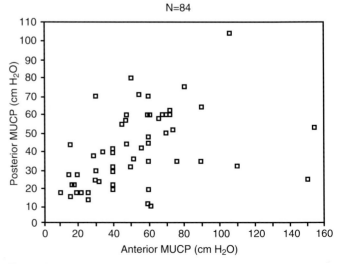

Figure 11-6 Relationship between anterior and posterior maximum urethral closure pressure (MUCP) in 84 women with stress urinary incontinence.

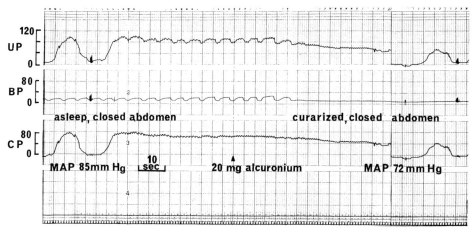

Figure 11-7 Urethral pressure recordings designed to identify the vascular, skeletal, and smooth muscle components contributing to intraurethral pressure. The figure shows a urethral pressure profile in a patient asleep but not curarized. The pressure variations seen in the bladder pressure (BP) tracing are synchronous with spontaneous respirations. After curarization *(arrow)* with 20 mg of curonium, the urethral pressure (UP) and closure pressure (CP) begin to decrease, whereas the BP remains constant. Urethral and bladder pressures are expressed in centimeters of water. Blood pressure is expressed in millimeters of mercury. Catheter withdrawal speed was 2.5 mm/sec. MAP, mean arterial pressure. (From Rud T, Andersson KE, Asmussen M, et al: Factors maintaining the intraurethral pressure in women. Invest Urol 17:343, 1980.)

of consciousness and paralysis. The data made available by Rud and colleagues and Bump and coworkers lends further credence to our observations of an active, anticipatory neuromuscular component.[17, 18] The location of this neuromuscular component and its mechanism of action have not been fully defined, although existing evidence suggests that it is extrinsic to the urethra and may indeed involve the pelvic floor and its attachment to the urethra.

ROLE OF HORMONES ON UPP

Estrogen has been found to increase the sensitivity of adrenergic receptors,[14, 19, 20] and specific estrogen

receptors have been demonstrated in the female urethra.[21] Progesterone facilitates beta-adrenergic sensitivity, and specific progesterone receptors have also been demonstrated.[22] The epithelium of the urethra is similar to that of the vagina, a nonkeratinized, squamous epithelium that is sensitive to hormonal stimulation. To act selectively on the tissue, female sex hormones can interact with receptors. The presence of specific estrogen receptors has been detected in the urinary bladder and urethra,[21] and only a few years ago histochemical evidence suggesting the presence of progesterone receptors in the same region was published.[22] Both receptor types are found in the vagina, which has the same embryologic origin as the urethra and trigone. Theoretically, gonadal hormones

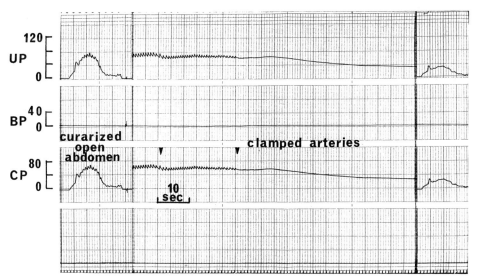

Figure 11-8 Continuation of recordings illustrated in Figure 11–7 with the same patient and same nomenclature. At the first arrow *(left)* the left common iliac artery is clamped; at the second arrow to the right it is also clamped. The urethral pressure profile is shown after both common iliac arteries have been clamped when the urethral pressure has been stabilized. (From Rud T, Andersson KE, Asmussen M, et al: Factors maintaining the intraepithelial pressure in women. Invest Urol 17:343, 1980.)

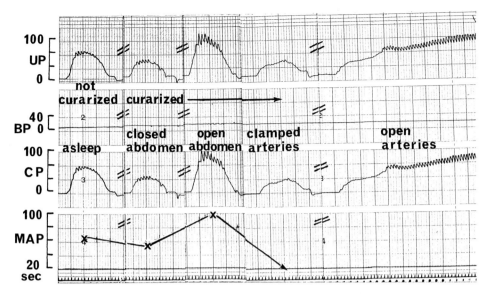

Figure 11-9 The influence of curarization of skeletal muscle and clamping of the common iliac arteries on urethral, bladder, and arterial pressures. Release of the left and right arteries is shown. Nomenclature is the same as that used in Figure 11–8. (From Rud T, Andersson KE, Asmussen M, et al: Factors maintaining the intraepithelial pressure in women. Invest Urol 17:343, 1980.)

can also influence the urinary tract by modifying the effect of adrenergic or cholinergic stimulation, as shown in animal studies.[23] As indicated in the studies of Rud and colleagues, the urethral vasculature affects urethral closure.[3] Because the vascularity of the urethra is also affected by estrogen, the magnitude of pulsations is greatest during periods of estrogen dominance and decreases with postmenopausal age.

In considering the role of hormones on the components of urethral closure, it should be borne in mind

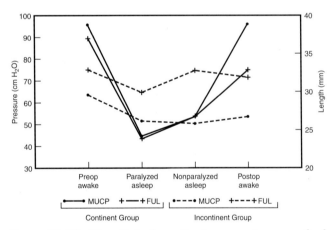

Figure 11-10 The effect of anesthesia on maximum urethral closure pressure (MUCP) and functional profile length (FUL) in continent and incontinent patients. Values in preoperative awake patients and asleep paralyzed subjects were compared. Paired analysis shows significant decreases from the awake preoperative state to the asleep paralyzed state for both MUCP and FUL. The differences between the awake preoperative and asleep nonparalyzed states are significant for FUL but not for MUCP. In the incontinent subgroup there were no significant differences in anesthetic states in either urethral closure or length. (From Bump RC, Huang KC, McClish DK, et al: Effect of narcotic anesthesia and skeletal muscle paralysis on passive and dynamic urethral function of stress continent and incontinent women. Neuroradiol Urodynamics 10:523, 1991. Reprinted by permission of John Wiley & Sons, Inc.)

that estrogen treatment improves transmission of intra-abdominal pressure to the urethra. Although there are few definitive controlled human studies identifying the role of sex hormones on urethral function, there are many recent experimental observations that merit consideration. Indeed, Iosif and associates have shown that estrogen deficiency could be the cause of incontinence.[21] Whether this estrogen effect is secondary to the reorganization (or up- or down-regulation) of urethral receptors remains to be seen. There is sufficient clinical evidence, however, from Sorensen's studies to show that symptomatic urodynamic changes occur in the urethra relative to age, menstrual cycle, and menopause.[24] In particular, sex hormones exert an additional influence on the pelvic floor, which indirectly affects urethral closure. The specific role of hormones on the female urinary tract has been examined by Miodrag and colleagues, who reviewed their role in relation to urethral mucosal changes, urethral blood supply, connective tissue, pelvic floor, and urethral smooth muscle.

Estrogen treatment has produced conflicting results in regard to the clinical effect (cure rates between 44 and 100%) and urethral pressure measurements.[25–29] Patients have reported subjective improvement in frequency, urgency, and detrusor incontinence after treatment, but attempts to show the improvement using more objective urodynamic methods have been inconclusive.[25] In one study the urethral pressure and functional and absolute urethral length increased after estrogen therapy, but there was no correlation between the improvement in these parameters and the subjective reports from the participating women.[26] The lack of correlation between high cure rates and the small changes in urodynamic parameters may be due to many different factors. The combination of estrogen and alpha-adrenoreceptor agonists (phenylpropanolamine) has shown promising results,[30, 31, 31a] which may be based on the ability of estrogen to increase the number of alpha-adrenergic receptors in the urethra.[19, 20] Treatment with progesterone[19] has produced no improvements in the parameters discussed previously.

Although the action of hormones on the urethra is beyond the scope of this chapter, it is emphasized that hormones do affect most of the components that constitute urethral closure. To summarize, then, female hormones affect the urethra in many ways: they interact with estrogen receptors, modify adrenergic receptor density and innervation, change the electrophysiologic properties of smooth muscle, inhibit extraneuronal uptake of catecholamine, modify cholinergic responses, and interact with prostaglandins.

It is clear that nervous control of the urethra depends not only on the distribution of nerves but also on the distribution of receptors. Much of the research has been focused in this field, which is beginning to reveal increasing complexity in the contribution of neurotransmitters such as adenosine triphosphate (ATP), vasoactive intestinal peptide (VIP), substance P, and leucine enkephalins in addition to the well-known acetylcholine and noradrenaline.

TRANSMISSION STUDIES

Transmission studies, defined as an increase in urethral pressure in proportion to the increase in bladder pressure, were conceived in an effort to develop a diagnostic test for the evaluation of urethral function in patients with stress urinary incontinence. Such tests attempt to emulate the dynamic conditions present when the patient coughs and urine leakage occurs. There are basically two ways of representing transmission studies. In one, the magnitude of pressure elevation from the baseline is measured in the urethra. This pressure rise is divided by the pressure rise in the bladder. This type of measurement is normally performed manually and ignores the resting urethral pressure. By making many such measurements when patients cough, a plot of transmission relative to the distance in the urethra can be constructed. The other form of transmission measurement is made by subtracting the abdominal or bladder pressure from the urethral pressure, thus representing the total intraluminal pressure. The results are plotted against urethral length by asking the subject to cough repeatedly. One of the most critical aspects of transmission studies is the ability to elicit sufficient coughing from the subject to allow a faithful mapping of the characteristics of the response. The most critical region in this respect is the vicinity of the external sphincter, particularly a region of about 7 mm from the sphincter to the external meatus. This can easily be missed by withdrawing the catheter. Enhörning was one of the first to use this method of monitoring the ability of the urethra to close under such conditions using a small balloon catheter.[32] Because of the size of the balloon, it was not possible to localize the rise in pressure accurately at different anatomic locations of the urethra. Enhörning showed, however, that a relationship existed between urethral and bladder

pressure rise, which became a model on which subsequent investigations were based. Careful examination of Enhörning's recordings, but not his conclusions, shows evidence of a rise in urethral pressure during coughing that is higher than the rise in abdominal pressure. This observation suggests that an external active component of compression of the recording balloon is involved. In other words, there is evidence of an active component of urethral closure. The fundamental disadvantage of the balloon was overcome by use of the perfusion method of Brown and Wickham.[13] The advantage of this method for this kind of monitoring is that resolution of measurement is much better than with the balloon, a few millimeters compared with a centimeter, and the measurement can be calibrated in hydrostatic terms. Using this method, a number of studies have been reported. We undertook a systematic study of the transmission of cough pressures along the length of the urethra in a variety of subjects. The results of cough pressure transmission measurements in young asymptomatic volunteers are illustrated in Figure 11–11.

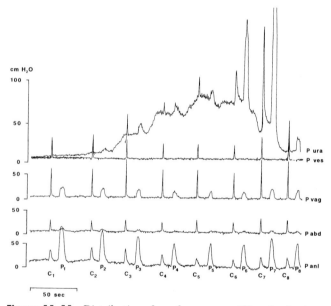

Figure 11-11 Distribution of cough pressures (C) and voluntary pelvic floor contractions (P) along the length of the urethra (P ura), bladder (P ves), vagina (P vag), abdomen (P abd), and anus (P anl). Urethral pressure measurement was performed with a perfused catheter with a single side hole oriented toward the symphysis pubis. The effect of eight coughs immediately followed by pelvic floor contractions is shown. As indicated, cough pressures are highest in the vagina, urethra, and abdomen and lowest in the anal sphincter. In the urethra, cough pressure rises variably, depending on location. The highest pressures occur in the distal third of the urethra; cough pressures there are 300 to 400% higher than in the proximal urethra. Consideration of pelvic floor contractions shows that the maximum increase in urethral closure also occurs in the distal urethra, where it is up to 600% higher than pressures in the vaginal or anal sphincter. Considering the relative rise of pelvic floor contraction pressures, there is no response in abdominal or vesical pressures. The anal and vaginal pressures rise most consistently in response to voluntary pelvic floor contraction. As with cough pressures, pelvic floor contractions produce the most effective closure in the distal segment of the urethra.

These transmission studies support evidence that active urethral closure pressures are higher than cough pressures. Transmitted pressures approach more than 100% of the cough pressure. The location of the maximum rise in pressure is distal to the region of MUCP[17, 18] in the resting UPP. Figure 11–12 shows a composite transmission-distance curve that summarizes the average response from a number of control volunteers.[17] Observations of more than a 100% rise in urethral pressures compared to abdominal pressures have been made using the perfusion methods of Brown and Wickham as well as microtip transducers.

Patients with demonstrable stress urinary incontinence observed during physical examination have qualitative transmission characteristics that are similar to those of controls,[32] although quantitatively the trend toward maximum developed pressures is evident in these patients. However, the magnitude of the closure pressure does not reach the values seen in controls. It is interesting that, following endoscopic bladder neck suspension, the characteristic

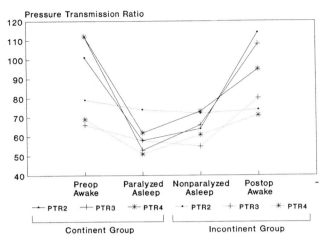

Figure 11-13 The effect of anesthesia on pressure transmission ratio (PTR) illustrating the dynamic response of the urethra. Significant transmission ratios are not seen in the proximal urethral segment but are evident in the mid and distal regions (PTR2 to PTR4). In incontinent women there was no significant increase in transmission along the entire urethral length. (From Bump RC, Huang KC, McClish DK, et al: Effect of narcotic anesthesia and skeletal muscle paralysis on passive and dynamic urethral function of stress continent and incontinent women. Neuroradiol Urodynamics 10:523, 1991. Reprinted by permission of John Wiley & Sons, Inc.)

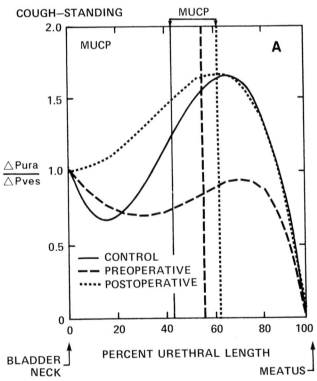

Figure 11-12 The ratio of change in bladder pressure during coughing. This ratio is shown as a function of urethral length starting at the bladder neck and descending to the meatus. The position of the maximal urethral closure pressure is shown. Controls are defined for the purposes of this study as normal, healthy volunteers with no symptoms of urinary incontinence. Preoperative indicates patients with demonstrable stress incontinence. Postoperative indicates the same patients following endoscopic bladder neck suspension. MUCP, maximum urethral closure pressure; $\triangle$Pura, change in urethral pressure; $\triangle$Pves, change in vesical pressure. (From Constantinou CE: Urethrometry: Considerations of static dynamic and stability characteristics of the female urethra. Neuroradiol Urodynamics 7:521, 1988. Reprinted by permission of John Wiley & Sons, Inc.)

trend seen in controls reappears immediately after surgery. This trend produces a maximum closure pressure that is again above 150% of the bladder pressure, suggesting that the urethra is brought within the region of muscle or ligamentous components. Figure 11–12 further illustrates the comparative transmission responses between controls, incontinent women preoperatively, and incontinent women postoperatively.

The relative influence of anesthesia on pressure transmission was also studied by Bump and coworkers, who analyzed the influence of skeletal muscle on urethral pressure transmission ratios.[16] Figure 11–13 illustrates the results. The role of the distal urethral compensatory mechanisms was reported in a careful study in a large number of patients by Versi and Cardozo, using stress urethral profiles.[33] In these studies, both transmission ratios and subtraction of urethral pressures from abdominal pressures are used to show the relationship between the bladder neck and the sphincter. Versi and Cardozo's observation suggests that female incontinence may be maintained in the presence of an incompetent bladder neck if the distal sphincter is competent. They have shown that bladder neck incompetence results in proximal shortening of the stress urethral profile while maintaining the stress functional length by decreasing the distal shortening of the stress profile. This observation is interpreted by Versi and Cardozo as a better use of the distal portion of the urethra by augmentation of the distal transmission ratio. In light of our visual observation and our own transmission studies, we interpret these results in a similar way; in addition, we suggest that the distal sphincter mechanism includes both the pelvic floor and other extrinsic forces as well as the intrinsic mechanisms of the urethra. On this basis and using different methods of measurement, transmission studies have shown that a competent bladder neck is not absolutely essential for the maintenance of continence because there is considerable redundancy with a competent pelvic floor and sphincteric function.

In recent years, the introduction of microtip transducers has provided a more convenient way of measuring pressure in the bladder and urethra. However, with the relative ease of use of the microtip transducer, a number of confounding considerations have emerged. Principal among these is the question of what is being measured and how the measurement is affected by local forces. In view of the fact that some of the earlier microtip transducers were mechanically rigid, an additional factor has been concern about the distortion of the urethra.[34-36] Furthermore, although hydrostatic pressure is used to calibrate the sensitivity of the microtip transducer ex vivo, the calibration inside a tube that is flexible, like the urethra, is subject to interpretation in terms of absolute pressure. On the other hand, the sensitivity of the microtip transducer to directional compression that may be extraurethral renders its use as a sensor of local forces useful as an exploratory research tool. Investigators using microtip transducers avoided the local confounding problems of anterior or posterior urethral measurements by orienting the transducer in the lateral plane. This orientation is less subject to variations and ostensibly more reproducible but may in fact mask important information. In the long run, when it is critically analyzed, the orientation of the transducer may provide the basis for a better understanding of the mechanisms involved in urethral closure and may prove to be useful in the diagnosis of urethral incontinence.

One of the most sophisticated systems for urethral pressure measurement was devised by Kauppila and colleagues, who used a No. 6 microtransducer catheter to evaluate the transmission of continent and incontinent patients.[37] The advantage of this system is that it obviates the need to move the transducer or catheter several times. By using single-cough urethrocystometry, Penttinen and coworkers observed significant improvements in transmission after surgery.[38] It is evident that more careful work needs to be done to clarify the mode of action of intra- and extraurethral structures before such measurements can be considered reliable.

PRESSURE VARIATIONS

As already shown, the intraurethral pressure is dynamic,[32] and the MUP decreases with increasing age, partly as a result of a decrease in the extent of vascularization.[39, 40] At the point of MUP, pressures can oscillate with pulsation of the vessels, and the amplitude of vascular pulsation also decreases with age. Because no large arteries are situated in the urethral wall, it is suggested that such pulsations may be caused by arterioles, capillaries, and cavernous tissue in the urethral submucosa. Variations also result from changes in abdominal pressure by pressure variations[41] such as an increase in the MUP and MUCP in the standing position compared to the supine position in normal volunteers. In younger individuals, the MUP is increased during bladder filling but remains unchanged in older women. The functional urethral length decreases,[39] although this decrease involves exclusively the upper part of the urethra, suggesting that these changes may be caused by the increased weight of the bladder. Before the initiation of voiding, intraurethral pressure is reduced, whereupon intravesical pressure increases and voiding begins.[42] Using combined urethrocystometric and urethrocystographic methods it has been shown that opening of the bladder neck and the premicturition pressure drop in the urethra occur simultaneously,[43] whereas during rest and sleep a significant decrease in MUP and MUCP has been observed.[44] Continuous long-term (1 hour) recordings of intraurethral pressures show variations in the MUCP.[24] These variations cover a broad spectrum of frequencies. During repeated examinations large inter- and intraindividual differences were found in both healthy fertile and postmenopausal women. Systematic studies of urethral pressure variations were carried out by Sorensen in a variety of incontinent women.[24] It was found that, in patients with detrusor incontinence, sudden pressure drops occurred that could not be distinguished from the pressure drop seen in normal individuals at the onset of micturition.[24] In addition, it was shown that no differences in pressure variations during long-term observation distinguished this group from normal fertile volunteers. The term urethral instability has been used to describe variations in urethral pressure greater than 15 cm H_2O (positive or negative).[45] Three types of urethral instability are recognized ranging from small fluctuations to marked variations in pressure. No significant differences in patients with pressure variations were found between stress incontinent and healthy postmenopausal women during long-term pressure recording.[24] It has been suggested that changing from the supine to the standing position seems to decrease MUCP because vesical pressure increases more than urethral pressure.[46]

NEW METHODS OF EVALUATION OF URETHRAL FUNCTION

The urethral pressure transmission studies described earlier have inherent limitations in terms of interpretation, artifacts, and precise definition of parameters. In recent years, new methods for the study of both the static and dynamic action of the urethra in maintaining continence have been introduced.[47-49] The purpose of such methods is to make possible a description of the mechanical properties of the urethra in terms of compliance, hysteresis, and power created by the urethral closure apparatus during voluntary contraction of the pelvic floor and coughing. Of particular interest is the attempt by Lose to measure the uninstrumented closure pressure using the field gradient method.[50] In static measurements made at rest in asymptomatic volunteers and patients with stress incontinence, he showed differences in the relationship between urethral pressure and the cross-sectional area at the bladder neck, midurethra, and distal urethra.[51, 52] In comparing these differences in stress incontinent patients and controls, he showed that, compared to compliance in normal women, compliance was significantly lower at the bladder neck in patients with stress incontinence, suggesting that the supporting structures around the bladder neck had been weakened. Although measurement of urethral function using the pressure-area methods described earlier has not been widely used, these methods have provided a reliable and quantitative way of diagnosis and have focused attention on the mechanism of continence and the role of the urethra. At first glance, it may be intuitively difficult to understand how the urethra can be evaluated by such tests, which are based on dilatation. Reflection on the process of micturition indicates that sudden urethral dilatation of the urethra occurs during coughing. Such dilatation simulates the entry of urine into the proximal urethra, thereby mimicking the conditions of incontinence. Finally, an emerging new methodology of measuring total urethral compliance in patients with stress incontinence has been described by Walter and colleagues based on measurements of bladder pressure and urine flow.[53] They showed that total urethral compliance increased in patients with stress incontinence, a finding that may be of diagnostic value. The principal advantage of this approach is that compliance can be used as an absolute physical quantity to compare patients with different voiding pressures.

Impact of Surgical Treatment of Urethra

OPERATIVE PROCEDURES

Transvaginal needle bladder neck suspension procedures for the treatment of stress incontinence exists in a large variety of different modifications of the first procedure described by Pereyra in 1959.[54] The main modifications used are the modified Pereyra procedure, the Stamey procedure,[55] and the Raz procedure.[56] The abdominal retropubic Burch colposuspension operation[57] and the operation developed by Marshall, Marchetti, and Krantz are also widely used. Also, the pubovaginal suspension of the bladder neck described by Gittes and Laughlin[58] and the modified Raz bladder neck suspension[59] should be mentioned. In the published literature only a few studies have reported specifically on the effect of surgery on urethral pressure in the context of other urodynamic parameters. In patients examined before and after the successful outcome of a Burch colposuspension the transmission ratio of abdominal pressure to the urethra during stress has been significantly increased in several studies.[15, 38] Although some studies reported significant increases in functional urethral length, this finding was not in agreement with the findings of other investigators.[60–62] Urodynamic parameters measured following the Pereyra bladder neck suspension were examined by Leach and colleagues, who observed that the transmission ratio of abdominal pressure to the proximal urethra during stress changed from negative to positive.[59, 63] Urethral resistance, MUP and MUCP, and functional urethral length remained unchanged. Stamey bladder neck suspension was shown to increase functional urethral length in the standing position (no significant change occurred in the sitting position), and the transmission ratio of abdominal pressure to the urethra was also significantly increased.[64, 65]

DETERMINANTS OF CURE

It is appropriate at this stage to consider in general terms the influence of procedures designed to cure incontinence. (This influence has been considered specifically in regard to establishing the determinants of cure by bladder neck suspension.[66]) In considering the cause of incontinence, there are basically two factors that are worth careful thought. (1) When urinary incontinence results from the breakdown of the physiologic function of the detrusor, such incontinence is termed detrusor incontinence. The degree of incontinence that occurs depends on the physiologic factors that are recruited to suppress the detrusor and close the urethra to prevent leakage. (2) Incontinence that occurs in the absence of bladder contraction but is due to pressures exerted outside the bladder depends on the competence of the urethral closure mechanisms. Incontinence that results from incompetence of the urethral structures is termed urethral incontinence. Some patients have both detrusor and urethral incontinence. Localization of the origin and extent of the incontinence (urethra or detrusor) is of crucial significance in deciding whether the course of treatment should be surgical or nonsurgical. In urethral, detrusor, and mixed incontinence, the stimulus precipitating the loss of urine may be intrinsic to the bladder or urethral structures or extrinsic (cough, sneeze, movement). Under such provocation, complex physiologic and anatomic mechanisms are brought into play. Their response then affects the forces acting directly on the bladder and urethra as well as those acting on the anatomic structures around them. Coughing, for example, results in a pressure pulse applied to the bladder and urethra from all directions. The reflexes involved (guarding) in turn activate the pelvic floor skeletal musculature to increase the closure pressure of the sphincters to counteract the elevation of abdominal pressure. As described earlier in this chapter, the urethra is influenced by activation of the surrounding structures such as the levator ani pubourethral ligaments, especially because of their anatomic juxtaposition to the symphysis pubis and pelvis and the position of the vesical neck.

Detrusor stability, urgency, and previous surgery are considered here as the principal determinants of cure. Analysis of these parameters is limited to the extent that stability is not readily quantified and urgency is also an unmeasurable quantity by urodynamic testing. Previous surgery encompasses a wide range of anatomic and functional changes. For these reasons, these parameters are referred to in the simplified form of their presence or absence with no effort to quantify their degree of severity.[66]

In patients in whom there is evidence (from urodynamic studies) of pure detrusor incontinence, a pharmacologic option is frequently considered first because the ability of the urethra to overcome a high-pressure bladder contraction is limited, particularly in older patients. Pharmacologic suppression of detrusor incontinence requires careful evaluation of each of the specific drugs frequently encountered, thereby limiting this mode of therapy.

ROLE OF DETRUSOR STABILITY IN CONTINENCE

In patients with mixed detrusor and urethral incontinence, the temptation is often overwhelming to treat urethral incontinence first, especially with surgery. There are some indications that under such conditions, detrusor incontinence is also suppressed. The distribution of detrusor relative to urethral incontinence has been systematically investigated.[67] Thus, urethral incontinence was demonstrated in 56% of 151 consecutive unselected patients complaining of incontinence. This indicates that incontinence in a large proportion of patients cannot be diagnosed by physical examination alone. Thus, physical examination by itself fails to localize and identify reliably the cause of the patient's complaints. Among these patients with urethral incontinence, urodynamic evaluation showed that approximately two-thirds had stable detrusor function while the remaining third had some evidence of instability, suggesting that a significant number of those with urethral incontinence may also have detrusor instability. In about half of the patients with stable bladder function, physical examination failed to identify the cause of incontinence. Thus, approximately half of the patients who demonstrate no incontinence on physical examination are likely to be incontinent owing to dysfunction of the bladder. One factor that should be considered in establishing detrusor stability in diagnostic tests such as filling cystometry is the inherent limitations of urodynamic methods of measurement. Because of these limitations, newer ambulatory monitoring techniques have been developed to uncover the presence of detrusor instability that can be elicited only in this way. Filling cystometry, in addition to profilometry, provides some basis on which patients with demonstrable stress inconti-

nence can be distinguished from those with instability of the detrusor. The most significant associated parameter that may be valuable in interpretation of the UPP is detrusor contraction during voiding because the pressure generated during voiding is partly dependent on the resistance of the urethra. Thus, a low-resistance urethra is not able to resist the contractility of the bladder, and flow is produced at lower pressures.

Urethral incompetence can be substantiated and verified by the UPP in most cases but not all. The posterior urethral closure pressure is significantly different in patients with and without demonstrable stress incontinence. Interpretation of urethral closure pressure requires correction for the patient's age before a decision on urethral competence can be made. However, even with uncorrected values, patients with urethral incontinence have significantly lower posterior urethral pressures, and hence the numerical values obtained from urodynamic recordings provide the physician with reliable information about the type of incontinence present in any particular patient.

IMPACT OF ENDOSCOPIC SUSPENSION ON THE URETHRA

As shown in Figure 11–12, transmission studies provide further useful information in the evaluation of continence. The advantage of transmission tests is that they evaluate the urethra at the very moment at which it is likely to fail. It is generally regarded that successful surgical correction of urethral incontinence in women depends on the relocation of the *proximal* urethra to a position that more completely transmits intra-abdominal pressures. However, it has been shown that this may not be the major factor involved. High transmission occurs *actively*, indicating the existence of a fast mechanism that closes the distal urethra. Patients with urethral incontinence do not have high transmission pressures, suggesting that the effectiveness of the distal active closure mechanism is reduced. After endoscopic bladder neck suspension, high transmission pressures are recorded, indicating that the relative position of the distal urethral mechanism to the levator ani or other periurethral structures has been realigned. As shown in Figure 11–2, the transmission of cough pressures is enhanced postoperatively both proximally and distally, which explains why pure urethral incontinence is readily corrected by endoscopic bladder neck suspension.

In addition to enhancement of transmission pressures on the urethra, endoscopic bladder neck suspension has an obstructive impact on the urethra. Obstructive pressures following endoscopic suspension approach those recorded on isometric tests in healthy subjects. Figure 11–14 provides a graphic comparison of voiding pressures obtained from controls with no symptoms and patients with stress urinary incontinence. In addition, the isometric test car-

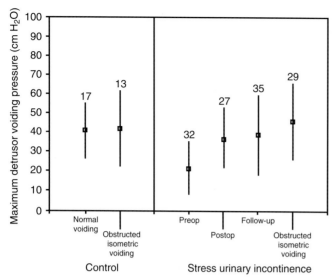

Figure 11-14 Comparison of maximum detrusor voiding pressures in controls and in patients with stress urinary incontinence before and following endoscopic bladder neck suspension. Isometric voiding pressures were compared as well. There is no significant difference between obstructed isometric voiding pressures and normal voiding in controls. Voiding in patients who have undergone operation occurs at pressures that approach the obstructive isometric values but are no higher. (From Constantinou CE, Stamey TA: Modification of urethral resistance and detrusor stability by endoscopic bladder neck suspension. Proceedings of Joint International Continence Society and Urodynamics Society Conference, October 1986.)

ried out using the methods described by Constantinou and colleagues[67] shows that urethral surgery increases voiding pressures to the values obtained by obstructive isometric tests.

In patients with mixed urethral and detrusor incontinence, detrusor stability is a parameter that determines the success or failure of incontinence therapy. If the bladder starts acting as a pump when it is in the reservoir phase, detrusor incontinence is likely to occur. Thus, evaluation of detrusor stability is crucial to any urodynamic study. Patients with detrusor instability were assessed with regard to the cure rate of endoscopic suspension of the bladder neck; the cure rate and the improvement rate were determined and are illustrated in Figure 11–15. The patients shown were from a group with demonstrable urethral incontinence on physical examination. Figure 11–15 clearly shows that the reported cure rate of patients with a stable bladder is almost double that of women with detrusor instability.

INFLUENCE OF PREVIOUS SURGERY AND URGENCY ON CURE RATE

Improvement was reported among patients with detrusor instability, although close examination of the surgical history of the patients shown in Figure 11–15 indicates that previous surgery is also an important factor in predicting the success rate of endoscopic suspension. Figure 11–16 shows the result of

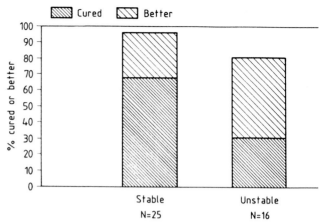

Figure 11-15 Comparison of the cure rate in patients with urethral incontinence before and after endoscopic bladder suspension. Patients with stable detrusor function report the highest rate of improvement. Patients with detrusor instability are significantly less likely to be cured. (From Constantinou CE: Determinants of cure by endoscopic suspension of the bladder-neck in the incontinent female patient. World J Urol 4:10–15, 1986.)

separating each of the two groups shown in Figure 11–15 into subgroups that had and had not had previous urethral operations; it is evident that patients with no previous surgery and with stable detrusor function were most likely to be cured of incontinence. The incidence of urgency incontinence is high among incontinent patients, although it is not related to urodynamically determined detrusor stability. There is some evidence from Sorensen that such urgency may originate from urethral instability on the basis of measurements of pressure variations.[24] However, there is no convincing clinical evidence to link detru-

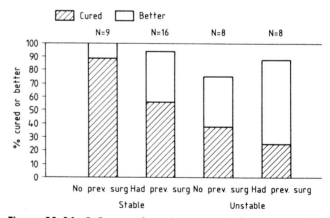

Figure 11-16 Influence of previous urogenital surgery and detrusor stability on cure rate. Patients with no previous surgery and a stable detrusor show the highest rate of cure or improvement. Previous surgery decreases the cure rate in patients with both stable and unstable detrusor function. The dominant predictor of cure rate is detrusor stability. Patients with no previous urogenital surgery who have a stable detrusor have a threefold higher cure rate than those who have had previous surgery and also have urodynamically proven detrusor instability. (From Constantinou CE: Determinants of cure by endoscopic suspension of the bladder-neck in the incontinent female patient. World J Urol 4:10–15, 1986.)

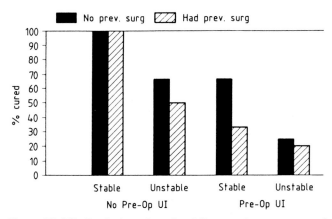

Figure 11-17 Predictive value of stability, previous surgery, and preoperative urgency in determining cure rate. Previous surgery affects the cure rate whether or not the detrusor is stable. Overall stability of the detrusor is more important than previous surgery in predicting cure.

sor instability with urgency.[68-75] If such a correlation could be made, the diagnostic value of this type of urethral pressure variation would be enhanced. Finally, the determinants of cure are shown in Figure 11–16, which compares the principal factors of stability and previous surgery.

As shown by Figure 11–17, detrusor stability, not urethral incompetence, is the primary factor that defines the characteristics of most patients cured by endoscopic bladder neck suspension. Indeed, a stable bladder with no evidence of preoperative urgency is likely to be 100% cured, whereas patients with an unstable bladder and urgency have the highest risk of encountering no cure with endoscopic bladder neck suspension.

Conclusions

This review provides some basic information on urethral function and the inevitable artifacts in its measurement. Central to this presentation is the functional contribution of the anatomy of the pelvic floor in relation to the urethra; it is evident that paraurethral structures contribute to the dynamics of the extrinsic mechanism of urethral pressures. In presenting some of the most recent imaging results, using MRI, we focused on the role of the striated pelvic floor musculature in modulating urethral closure. The anatomic contribution of the pelvic floor is most critical for an understanding of transmission studies in that the reflex activation of skeletal muscles is important in accomplishing the fast closure of the urethra in response to stress.

Bladder function is central in considering the ability of the urethra to maintain continence because an unstable bladder can so readily overpower the closure pressures of the urethra and induce urine loss. Associated with the issue of detrusor stability is urgency, a sensory aspect of urethral dysfunction that

is not readily amenable to urodynamic testing. Indeed, we have shown that the combination of urgency and detrusor instability, whether these are separate entities or not, is most likely to compromise the success rate of surgery. On the basis of our observations, we conclude that pelvic floor integrity, destrusor stability, and absence of urgency are the primary factors that determine continence. It is perhaps for these reasons that urethral pressures alone have not truly reflected the problems associated with achieving urethral continence.

REFERENCES

1. Abrams P, Blaivas JG, Stanton SL, et al: The standardization of terminology of lower urinary tract function. Scand J Urol Nephrol Supple 114:5, 1988.
2. DeLancey JOL: Structural aspects of the extrinsic continence mechanism. Obstet Gynecol 72:296, 1988.
3. Rud T, Anderson KE, Asmussen M, et al: Factors maintaining the intraurethral pressure in women. Invest Urol 17:343, 1980.
4. DeLancey JOL: Anatomy and physiology of the urinary continence. Clin Obstet Gynecol 33:298, 1990.
5. DeLancey JOL: Correlative study of paraurethral anatomy. Obstet Gynecol 68:91, 1986.
6. Gosling JA, Dixon JS, Critchley HOD, et al: A comparative study of the human external sphincter and periurethral levator ani muscles. Br J Urol 53:35, 1981.
7. Chritchley HOD, Dixon JS, Gosling JA: Comparative study of the periurethral and perianal parts of the levator ani muscle. Urol Int 35:226, 1980.
8. Gosling J: Structure of the bladder and urethra in relation to function. Urol Clin North Am 6:31, 1979.
9. Juenemann K-P, Lue TF, Schmidt RA, et al: Clinical significance of sacral and pudendal nerve anatomy. J Urol 139:74, 1988.
10. Ferner H, Staubesand J (eds): Sobotta Atlas of Human Anatomy, 10th ed. Munich/Baltimore, Urban & Schwartzenberg, 1982.
11. diFiore MSH: Atlas of Human Histology, 5th ed. Philadelphia, Lea & Febiger, 1981.
12. Langman J: Medical Embryology, 4th ed. Baltimore, Williams & Wilkins, 1981.
13. Brown M, Wickham JEA: The urethral pressure profile. Br J Urol 41:211, 1969.
14. Anderson RB, Shephert AM, Feneley RCL: Microtransducer urethral profile methodology: Variations caused by transducer orientation. J Urol 130:727, 1983.
15. Constantinou C: Resting and stress urethral pressures as a clinical guide to the mechanism of continence in the female patient. Urol Clin North Am 12:247, 1985.
16. Bump RC, Huang KC, McClish DK, et al: Effect of narcotic anesthesia and skeletal muscle paralysis on passive and dynamic urethral function of stress continent and incontinent women. Neurourol Urodyn 10:523, 1991.
17. Constantinou CE, Govan DE: Spatial distribution of transmitted and reflexly generated urethral pressures in healthy women. J Urol 127:964, 1982.
18. Constantinou CE: Urethrometry: Considerations of static dynamic and stability characteristics of the female urethra. Neurourol Urodyn 7:521, 1988.
19. Schreiter F, Fuchs P, Stockam K: Estrogenic sensitivity of alpha-receptors in the urethral musculature. Urol Int 31:13, 1976.
20. Caine M, Raz S: Some clinical implications of adrenergic receptors in the urinary tract. Arch Surg 110:247, 1975.
21. Iosif SC, Batra S, Ek A, et al: Estrogen receptors in the human female lower urinary tract. Am J Obstet Gynecol 141:817, 1981.
22. Gosling JA, Dixon JS, Lendon RG: The autonomic innervation

of the human male and female bladder neck and proximal urethra. J Urol 118:302, 1977.

23. Miodrag A, Castleden CE, Vallance TR: Sex hormones and the female urinary tract. Drugs 36:491, 1988.

24. Sorensen S: Urethral pressure variations in healthy and incontinent women (thesis). Neurourol Urodyn 11:549, 1992.

25. Walter S, Wolf H, Barlebo H, et al: Urinary incontinence in post-menopausal women treated with estrogens. A double blind clinical trial. Urol Int 33:135, 1978.

25. Wolf H, Wandt H, Jonat W: Immunohistochemical evidence of estrogen and progesterone receptors in the female lower urinary tract and comparison with the vagina. Gyncol Obstet Invest 32:227, 1991.

26. Rud T: The effect of estrogens and gestagens on the urethral pressure profile in urinary continent and stress incontinent women. Acta Obstet Gynecol Scand 59:265, 1980.

27. Schreiter F, Fuchs P, Stockamp K: Estrogen sensitivity of alpha-receptors in the urethra musculature. Urol Int 31:13, 1976.

28. Iosif CS: Effects of prorated administration of estriol on the lower genitourinary tract in postmenopausal women. Arch Gynecol Obstet 251:115, 1992.

29. Wilson PD, Faragher B, Butler B, et al: Treatment with oral piperazine oestrogene sulphate for genuine stress incontinence in postmenopausal women. Br J Urol 94:568, 1987.

30. Kinn AC, Lindskog M: Estrogens and phenylpropanolamine in combination for stress urinary incontinence in postmenopausal women. Urology 32:273, 1988.

31. Henriksson L, Ulmsten U, Andersson K-E: The effect of changes of posture on the urethral closure pressure in healthy women. Scand J Urol 11:201, 1977.

31a. Non-surgical treatment of stress incontinence (editorial). Lancet 340:643, 1992.

32. Enhörning G: Simultaneous recording of the intravesical and intraurethral pressure. Acta Chir Scand Suppl 276:1, 1961.

33. Versi E, Cardozo L: Distal urethral compensatory mechanisms in women with incompetent bladder neck who remain continent, and the effect of menopause. Neurourol Urodyn 90:574, 1990.

34. Plevnik S, Janez J, Vrtachk P, et al: Directional differences in urethral pressure recordings. Contributions from the stiffness and weight of the recording catheter. Neurourol Urodyn 5:117, 1984.

35. Schaffer W: Directional differences in urethral pressure recordings. Contributions from the stiffness and weight of the recording catheter (letter to the editor). Neurourol Urodyn 5:114, 1984.

36. Ulmsten U, Andersson K-E, Persson CGA: Diagnostic and therapeutic aspects of urge urinary incontinence in women. Urol Int 32:88, 1977.

37. Kauppila A, Pettinen J, Haggman V: Six-microtransducer catheter connected to computer evaluation of urethral closure function of women. Urology 23:159, 1989.

38. Penttinen J, Kaark K, Kauppila A: Effect of suprapubic operation on urethral closure—evaluation by single cough: urethrocystometry. Br J Urol 63:384, 1989.

39. Rud T: Urethral pressure profile in continent women from childhood to old age. Acta Obstet Gynecol Scand 59:331, 1980.

40. Henriksson L, Ulmsten U, Andersson K-E: The effect of changes of posture on the urethral closure pressure in healthy women. Scand Urol 11:201, 1977.

41. Ulmsten U, Andersson K-E, Persson CGA: Diagnostic and therapeutic aspects of urge urinary incontinence in women. Urol Int 32:88, 1977.

42. Rud T, Andersson K-E, Ulmsten U: Initiation of voiding in healthy and stress incontinent women. Acta Obstet Gynecol Scand 57:457, 1978.

43. Rud T, Ulmsten U, Westby M: Initiation of micturition: A study of combined urethrocystometry and urethrocystography in healthy and stress incontinent females. Scand J Urol Nephrol 13:259, 1979.

44. Politano VA, Small MP, Harper JM, et al: Periurethral Teflon injection for urinary incontinence. J Urol 111:180, 1974.

45. Ulmsten U, Henrikson L, Iosif S: The unstable female urethra. Am J Obstet Gynecol 144:93, 1982.

46. Henriksson L, Ulmsten U, Andersson K-E: The effect of changes of posture on the urethral closure pressure in stress-incontinent women. Scand J Urol Nephrol 11:207, 1977.

47. Colstrup H, Mortensen SO, Kristensen JK: A new method for investigation of closure function of resting female urethra. J Urol 130:507, 1988.

48. Reignier CH, Susset JG, Ghoniem GM, et al: A new catheter to measure urethral compliance in females: Normal values. J Urol 124:1060, 1989.

49. Harada T: Experimental study on measurements of compliance and cross-sectional area in the urethra through the field gradient principle. Jap J Urol 76:360, 1985.

50. Lose G: Mechanical properties of the urethra in healthy female volunteers. Static measurements in resting urethra. Neurourol Urodyn 8:451, 1989.

51. Blute ML, Tomera KM, Hellerstein DK, et al: Transurethral microwave thermotherapy for management of benign prostatic hyperplasia: Results of the United States Prostatron Cooperative Study. J Urol 150:1591, 1993.

52. Lose G: Simultaneous recording of pressure and cross-sectional area in female urethra: A study of urethral closure function in healthy and stress incontinent women. Neurourol Urodyn 11:550, 1992.

53. Walter JS, Wheeler JS, Morgan C, et al: Measurement of total urethral compliance in females with stress incontinence. Neurourol Urodyn 12:273, 1993.

54. Pereyra AJ: A simplified surgical procedure for the correction of stress incontinence in women. West J Surg 67:223, 1959.

55. Stamey TA: Endoscopic suspension of vesical neck for urinary incontinence. Surg Gynecol Obstet 136:547, 1973.

56. Raz S: Modified bladder neck suspension for female stress incontinence. Urology 17:82, 1981.

57. Burch JC: Urethrovaginal fixation to Cooper's ligament for correction of stress incontinence, cystocele, and prolapse. Am J Obstet Gynecol 81:281, 1961.

58. Gittes RF, Loughlin KR: No-incision pubovaginal suspension for stress incontinence. J Urol 138:568, 1987.

59. Bosman G, Vierhout ME, Huikeshoven FJM: A modified Raz bladder neck suspension operation. Results of a one to three year follow-up investigation. Acta Obstet Gynecol Scand 72:47, 1993.

60. Loughlin KR, Whitmore WF, Gittes RF, et al: Review of an 8-year experience with modifications of endoscopic suspension of the bladder neck for female stress urinary incontinence. J Urol 143:44, 1990.

61. Eriksen BC, Hagen B, Eik-Nes SH, et al: Long-term effectiveness of the Burch colposuspension in female urinary stress incontinence. Acta Obstet Gynecol Scand 69:45, 1990.

62. Penttinent J, Kaar K, Kauppila A: Effect of suprapubic operation on urethral closure. Evaluation by single cough urethrocystometry. Br J Urol 63:389, 1989.

63. Leach GE, Yip CM, Donovan BJ: Mechanism of continence after modified Pereyra bladder-neck suspension. Urology 24:328, 1987.

64. Constantinou CE, Faysal MH, Rother L, et al: The impact of bladder neck suspension on the mode of distribution of abdominal pressure along the female urethra. In Zinner NR, Sterling AM (eds): Female Incontinence. New York, Alan Liss, 1981, pp 121–132.

65. Stamey TA: Urinary incontinence in the female. In Walsh PC, Retik AB, Stamey TA, Vaughan ED (eds): Campbell's Urology, 6th ed. Philadelphia, W. B. Saunders, 1992.

66. Constantinou CE: Determinants of cure by endoscopic suspension of the bladder-neck in the incontinent female patient. World J Urol 4:10–15, 1986.

67. Constantinou CE, Djurhuus JC, Silverman DE, et al: Isometric detrusor pressure during bladder filling and its dependency on bladder volume and interruption to flow in control subjects. J Urol 131:86–90, 1984.

68. Park GS, Miller EJ: Surgical treatment of stress urinary incontinence: A comparison of the Kelly plication, Marchall-Marchetti-Krantz, and Pereyra procedures. Obstet Gynecol 71:575, 1988.

69. Raz S, Siegel AL, Short JL, et al: Vaginal wall sling. J Urol 141:43, 1989.

70. Penttinen J, Kaar K, Kauppila A: Colposuspension and transvaginal bladder neck suspension in the treatment of stress incontinence. Gynecol Obstet Invest 28:101, 1989.

71. Bathia NN, Bergman A, Karram M: Changes in urethral resistance after surgery for stress urinary incontinence. Urology 24:200, 1989.

72. Juma S, Little NA, Raz S: Basic evaluation of female urinary incontinence. Am J Kidney Dis 4:317, 1990.

73. Ramon J, Mekras J, Webster GD: Transvaginal needle suspension procedures for recurrent stress incontinence. Urology 38:519, 1991.

74. Kil PJM, Hoekstra JW, van der Meijden APM, et al: Transvaginal ultrasonography and urodynamic evaluation after suspension operations: Comparison among the Gittes, Stamey and Burch suspensions. J Urol 146:132, 1991.

75. Raz S, Sussman EM, Erickson DB, et al: The Raz bladder neck suspension: Results in 206 patients. J Urol 148:845, 1992.

CHAPTER 12

Micturition Profilometry

Maryrose P. Sullivan, Ph.D.
Subbarao V. Yalla, M.D.

Urethral pressure profilometry during urination— or micturitional urethral pressure profilometry (MUPP)—is a fundamental method of assessing the dynamic behavior of the lower urinary tract that is based on physical principles governing flow through collapsible tubes. The ability to trace the physical characteristics of the urinary stream through the urethra has improved our understanding of the relationship between the bladder and its outlet and has facilitated the clinical diagnosis of diverse voiding dysfunctions.

The rationale for the use of this technique is based on the theoretical pressure distribution of fluid in motion along a tube, as expressed by the Bernoulli principle. The total pressure at any point in the tube is the sum of the hydrostatic and dynamic (related to the velocity of the fluid) pressures. An end-hole catheter facing the oncoming stream will record the total pressure, whereas a catheter with a hole facing the lateral wall will measure static pressure. In this context, the word static refers to a specific component of the total pressure and is not meant to imply that measurement conditions are static. On the contrary, measurements are obtained under flow (dynamic) conditions.

The static pressure proximal to a urethral obstruction is elevated during flow. As the fluid passes through the constriction, the velocity of the stream is high, the dynamic pressure increases, and the static pressure decreases. Distal to the constriction, dynamic pressure decreases as urethral diameter increases, and, theoretically, static pressure may gradually increase.[1]

Micturition profilometry can be performed by measuring static or total pressure. Although both types of pressure are subject to measurement errors, static pressure profiles are more practical and clinically relevant. To evaluate total pressure profiles accurately using an end-hole catheter, percutaneous su-

prapubic vesical pressure monitoring is required. Furthermore, because the end-hole catheter is more likely to become displaced during urination, maintaining an accurate position during pressure recordings is more difficult. Because the catheter must be reinserted repeatedly through the proximal narrow urethral segment to ensure reproducibility, minor urethral trauma and discomfort to the patient are likely. With static pressure measurements, on the other hand, the catheter remains in the bladder throughout the study. Theoretically, total pressure represents only irreversible dissipative losses in the urethra, whereas changes in static pressure include the conversion of potential to kinetic energy as well as dissipative losses.[2] Thus, static pressure profiles may provide a more sensitive indication of the extent and location of an obstruction.

As with all catheter-based measurement systems, errors in urethral pressure measurement may be introduced by the partial occlusion of the lumen by the catheter, accelerative effects, wall friction, flow separation phenomena, radial flow components, and irregularities in the urethral wall. An accurate measurement of static urethral pressure during urination requires proper alignment of the catheter in the urine stream. To ensure that the pressure measured reflects only static pressure, the axis of the side hole should remain perpendicular to the direction of flow. Entrapment of the catheter against the urethral wall prevents contact of the side hole with the fluid layers, thus precluding the measurement of the true static pressure of the flowing fluid. To avoid artifactually high urethral pressure measurements due to compression of the pressure-sensing surface, the ideal catheter design should include circumferentially positioned lateral holes. The catheter should also be as small as possible to minimize hydrodynamic disturbances. Although experimental studies in animals have shown that catheter artifact is negligible, the precise amount of error created by the presence of a 5 or 10 Fr catheter in the obstructed urethra during flow has not been identified. In patients with a normal outlet and normal bladder contractility, this error is insignificant.[3]

Detrusor-Urethral Relationship During Micturition

A proper understanding of fluid mechanics and the pressure distributions occurring in the urethra during micturition requires a thorough appreciation of the events that occur during micturition. The relationship between the responses of the detrusor, the bladder neck, and the external sphincter, particularly during initiation of micturition, should be clarified. Studies by Tanagho and Miller have shown that a prevoid relaxation of the external sphincter occurs before the detrusor begins to contract.[4] Subsequent studies by Yalla and associates, however, suggest that this relationship is more complex and is related to the nature of the initiation of micturition.[5] Using a triple-transducer catheter (Fig. 12–1A) and radiologic monitoring, the interrelationships between the detrusor contraction and the responses of the bladder neck and external sphincter were examined. These responses depended on whether urination was initiated without a strong sense of desire or whether it was postponed until severe urgency developed.

In the former type of micturition (volitional voiding), both men and women showed synchronous detrusor contraction and striated sphincter relaxation (Fig. 12–1B, C). The bladder neck, however, did not open or relax; instead, pressure in the bladder neck region increased in parallel with the onset of detrusor contraction. Despite external sphincter relaxation, no fluid was observed in the proximal urethra. At a critical point during the initial phase of detrusor contraction (when detrusor pressure exceeded blad-

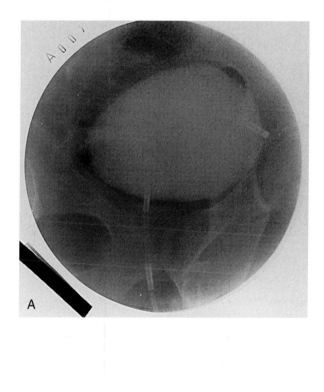

50 Cm
H₂O

10 s

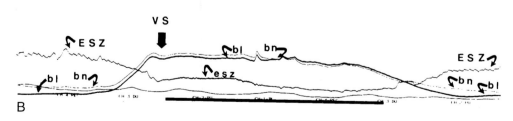

Figure 12-1 *A,* Radiograph showing a triple-transducer catheter in the bladder. One transducer can be seen inside the bladder, the second at the level of the bladder neck, and the third at the level of the external sphincter. *B,* Graphic representation of vesicourethral relationship during volitional urination in a normal male subject using a triple-transducer catheter showing bladder (bl) and bladder neck (bn) contractions with synchronous external sphincter (esz) relaxation. VS, voiding starts.

Illustration continued on following page

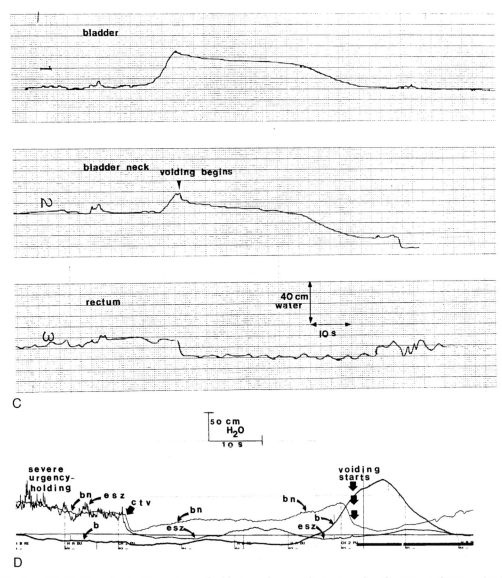

Figure 12-1 *Continued C,* Volitional urination using a double-transducer catheter in a female patient showing simultaneous bladder and bladder neck contractions prior to urination. *D,* Graphic representation of the bladder-urethral relationship during initiation of voiding using the catheter shown in *A.* Urgency voiding is characterized by release of the voluntary hold of the external sphincter zone (esz), shown by decrease in esz pressure on the left at command to void (ctv). Urination is preceded by contraction of bladder (b) and bladder neck (bn) and relaxation of the external sphincter zone.

der neck pressure), the bladder neck opened, and flow began through the already relaxed external sphincter.

The latter type of micturition (urgency voiding) was characterized by release of the voluntary hold on the external sphincter and thus elimination of reflex inhibition of the detrusor contraction. Subsequently, the onset of detrusor contractions occurred with simultaneous bladder neck contraction and reflex striated sphincter relaxation (Fig. 12–1*D*).

Some subjects with severe detrusor instability were unable to inhibit detrusor contractions despite vigorous attempts to prevent urination by contracting the external sphincter. In such conditions, the detrusor continued to contract, and the bladder neck opened appropriately. The urine was held in the posterior urethra only by mechanical closure of the ex-

ternal sphincter resulting from voluntary efforts. On the release of the voluntary hold of the external sphincter, flow occurred immediately. Changes in the bladder neck during initiation of urination may be obscured in patients with severe intravesical prostatic enlargement and in those who have had bladder neck resection or transurethral resection of the prostate.

Once urinary flow was established, the detrusor continued to contract in a sustained fashion, and the bladder neck and striated sphincter regions remained open, resulting in uninterrupted voiding except in patients with neuropathic dysfunctions such as striated sphincter dyssynergia. The terminal phase of micturition was characterized by a gradual elevation of striated sphincter pressure, diminished flow rate, and decreasing detrusor contraction pressure. The bladder neck gradually returned to its resting closure pressure.

To study the conduit properties of the outlet during urination, pressure profiles must be obtained during the midvoiding phase to avoid the transient responses of the bladder neck and external sphincter during the initiation and termination phases of the detrusor contraction.

The Technique of Micturitional Urethral Pressure Profilometry

A 10 Fr triple-lumen catheter with the characteristics described previously is used in these studies. The catheter is 30 cm long and has radiopaque markers that identify the sites of bladder and vesicourethral pressure measurements. Two of the lumens terminate with side openings at the catheter tip to allow bladder filling and measurement of detrusor pressure. Vesicourethral pressure is measured through the third lumen, which terminates 10 cm from the tip of the catheter in two lateral apertures. The catheter is graduated at 1-cm intervals. With this design, detrusor pressure, urethral pressure, and catheter position can be recorded simultaneously along the entire urethra in women and in the proximal 10 cm of the male urethra.[6] The Brown and Wickham infusion principle is used to record urethral closure pressure during the bladder filling phase.[7] Lidocaine (Xylocaine) jelly can be instilled in the urethra prior to introduction of the urodynamic catheter to minimize patient discomfort that may be associated with repeated catheter movement during the study. Because studies have shown that urethral closure pressure profiles (UCPPs) are unaffected by the use of anesthetic jelly,[8] full advantage of this simple step should be taken to prevent potential measurement artifacts due to patient anxiety. Rectal pressure should also be measured to distinguish bladder activity from changes in intra-abdominal pressure.

With both pressure ports initially located in the bladder, the catheter is withdrawn at a rate of 0.5 cm/second to obtain a UCPP while the bladder is at rest. Relevant landmarks such as the bladder neck, external sphincter region, bulbous urethra, and external meatus are identified in relation to the graduation marks on the catheter. These locations can be verified under fluoroscopy by visualization of the radiopaque markers. Although the UCPP provides important information about the functional and anatomic landmarks of the lower urinary tract, it must be stressed that neither the location nor the severity of an obstruction can be determined with this technique.

The catheter is then reinserted into the bladder, and the bladder is filled to capacity with dilute contrast solution. Patients are encouraged to relax the perineal muscles and urinate around the catheter. During steady urination, the catheter is pulled at a constant rate (0.5 cm/second), and each centimeter of

withdrawal is indicated by an event mark on the recording device.[6, 9] A mechanical puller can be used to maintain a constant withdrawal rate, but precautions must be taken to prevent the catheter from being expelled during urination.

Similar MUPP patterns can be obtained using antegrade or retrograde catheter motion and with or without perfusion of the urethral pressure port. The MUPP is usually performed in the supine position; however, for patients who cannot void in the supine position, the technique can easily be performed while the patient is inclined, sitting, or standing.

MUPP studies that were repeated using a 5 Fr catheter successfully reproduced the profile configurations obtained using the 10 Fr catheter. However, use of the 5 Fr catheter required suprapubic measurement of bladder pressure. The urodynamic diagnoses were essentially the same with either catheter. Although the 10 Fr catheter may be more obstructive than the 5 Fr catheter in certain patients, its advantages far outweigh those of the single-lumen 5 Fr catheter. The triple-lumen catheter allows simultaneous bladder filling and measurement of both bladder and urethral pressures, thereby eliminating the need for a more invasive percutaneous vesical pressure measurement.[3]

Experimental Validation

RIGID MODELS OF THE BLADDER-URETHRA

The technique for recording urethral pressure profiles during urinary flow was tested in a rigid bladder-urethra model to demonstrate its ability to evaluate accurately the location and significance of bladder outflow obstruction.[10] A glass reservoir that served as bladder pressure was connected to glass models of the urethra with or without strictures. The fluid-filled catheter that gave the most accurate recording of the static pressures in the model compared with the theoretically calculated pressure profiles was arranged so that the tip of the catheter did not leave the bladder until the measuring eye had passed the urethral segment of interest. The effective radius of the urethra and the flow rate did not change during the recording. Pressure profiles for urethral models with one or two obstructions closely resembled the theoretically calculated curves in which a prominent pressure drop registered at each stricture site in the model. Using an end-hole catheter to measure total pressure, a small pressure drop across the stricture was recorded, followed by a considerably greater pressure drop distal to the stricture. As the catheter passed through the stricture, the resistance in the stricture decreased and the flow rate increased, resulting in an "unplugging effect." In a urethral model with two strictures, the end-hole catheter did not register a pressure drop at the site of the first constriction. Although the results of this study are determined by rigid tube hydrodynamics, unlike the human urethra, which behaves like an elastic tube, these experiments provided important information about the characteristics of the ideal catheter and the anticipated pressure profiles of tubes with various configurations.

FLEXIBLE MODELS OF THE BLADDER-URETHRA

To examine some of the physical properties of the human urethra and determine the factors that govern the micturition process, a flexible model of the urethra was constructed.[11] A flexible tube was connected to a reservoir on one end and passed through a water tank that provided both a generalized (P_{eg}) and a localized (P_{el}) extrinsic pressure. The static pressure distribution during flow was measured by passing a small hollow stainless steel probe into the lumen. An analysis of the resulting profile revealed that a sudden fall of static pressure occurred at the distal end of P_{el} and again at the distal site of P_{eg} whenever P_{el} was greater than P_{eg}. If P_{el} was less than P_{eg}, or the static pressure at that point in the model, the presence of P_{el} could not be detected by the static pressure profile. These experiments clearly demonstrate that static pressure profilometry can be used to identify easily the precise location and severity of obstructions in flexible models of the urethra and suggest that this technique may provide a clinically useful method of evaluating the human lower urinary tract.

ANIMAL MODELS

To determine the potential sources of error involved in the measurement of total and static urethral pressures and to understand their clinical and scientific relevance, detailed studies were performed in dogs.[12] The canine bladder and urethra were entirely exposed, and two sets of cannulas were inserted transmurally to measure both total and static pressure in the proximal and distal urethra (Fig. 12–2A). A urethral constriction was created with an inflatable cuff. Flow through the urethra was achieved by infusing fluid through a large cannula inserted in the trigonal compartment of the bisected bladder.

The results of these studies confirmed that total and static urethral pressures increased in the proximal and distal segments as the infusion rate increased. In the presence of a midurethral constriction, proximal pressures (total and static) were higher at each flow rate (Fig. 12–2B). The total pressures were significantly higher than static pressures; however, the differences between these measurements were only 4 to 10% and were dependent on the infusion rate. These observations strongly emphasized the relevance of total and static urethral pressures in the clinical setting and suggest that these pressures are clinically reliable provided that the artifacts and limitations of the measurements are considered in the analysis. Studies in canines

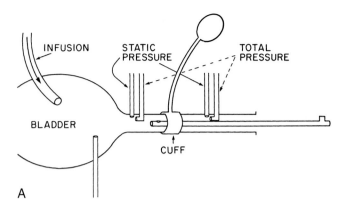

A

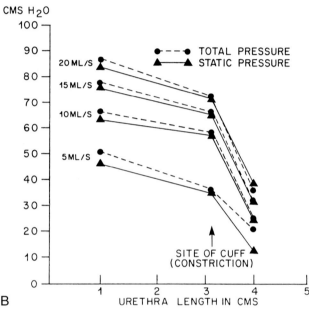

B

Figure 12-2 *A*, Schematic diagram of an experimental set-up for measuring bladder pressure as well as static and total pressures in the proximal and distal urethra with and without an obstruction created by the external cuff. *B*, Effects of elastic constriction on urethral pressures. Static and total urethral pressures increase with increasing infusion rates. Urethral pressures markedly increase proximal to the site of the constriction.

have also shown that the severity of the obstruction and the pressure drop across the constriction are interrelated; thus, the pressure disparity can potentially be incorporated in quantifiable measures of outlet obstruction.

Normal Micturitional Pressure Profiles

In men with no urinary tract symptoms and normal urinary flow rates, the supramembranous urethra is essentially isobaric with intravesical pressure. The urethral pressure drops precipitously across the membranous-bulbous urethral region and then decays gradually along the distal urethra. In these subjects, the physiologic pressure drop is determined by the narrowest portion of the urethra—the external sphincter zone (Fig. 12–3). This drop ranges from 20 to 30 cm H_2O for detrusor contraction pressures of 50 to 60 cm H_2O. The static pressure in the anterior urethra is typically 25 to 30 cm H_2O.

In normal women the bladder and nearly the entire urethra are isobaric except for the terminal 1 cm of the distal urethra where the physiologic pressure drop occurs[5] (Fig. 12–4). Similar profiles were obtained from women with stress urinary incontinence and no obstruction.[12] In these patients, the pressure drop reportedly occurred distal to the point of maximum urethral pressure (determined from UCPP) and proximal to the urethral meatus.

Urethral Obstruction in Women

In women with distal urethral obstruction, studies have shown that the site of obstruction can be identified by the drop in urethral pressure that occurs

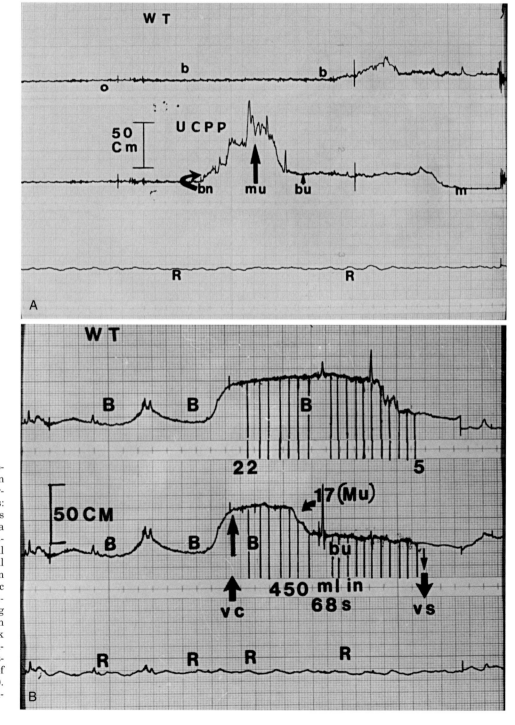

Figure 12-3 *A,* Urethral closure pressure profile (UCPP) in a normal male subject performed to identify landmarks: bladder neck (bn), membranous urethra (mu), bulbous urethra (bu). *Top tracing,* bladder pressure (b). *Bottom tracing,* rectal pressure (R). *B,* Micturitional urethral pressure profile from the same patient shows isobaric bladder neck and prostatic urethra *(middle tracing)* during sustained detrusor contraction *(top tracing).* Vertical lines mark each centimeter of catheter withdrawal. Physiologic drop in pressure can be seen in the region of the membranous urethra (Mu). vc, voiding commences; vs, voiding stops.

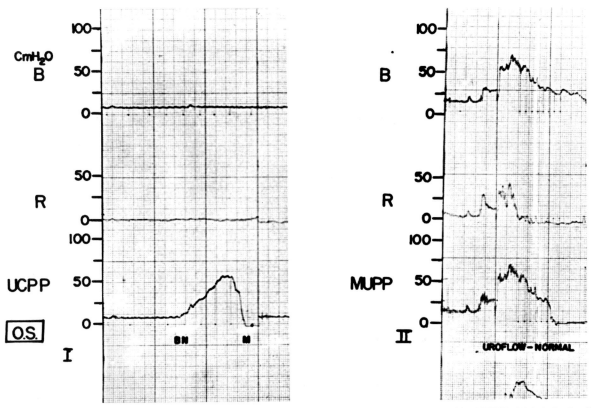

Figure 12–4   Urethral closure pressure profile (UCPP) *(left)* and micturitional urethral pressure profile (MUPP) *(right)* obtained from a normal female subject. Bladder pressure and pressure along the entire urethra are isobaric during voiding until the terminal 1-cm segment. BN, bladder neck; M, meatus; B, bladder pressure; R, rectal pressure.

proximal to the normal pressure drop observed in patients without obstruction.[13] This was confirmed by the presence of severe bladder trabeculation and elevated voiding detrusor pressures in these women. Although bladder neck obstructions in women are rare, distal urethral obstruction and meatal stenosis are more common. Typical MUPP patterns in women are shown schematically in Figure 12–5.

Benign Prostatic Hypertrophy

The diagnosis of urinary outlet obstruction in men is traditionally based on a clinical evaluation that may include a neurologic assessment, voiding history, uroflowmetry, rectal examination, and cystoscopy. Radiologic procedures—voiding cystourethrography and postvoid residual volume estimation—are occasionally added to confirm the diagnosis. Despite the use of objective methods of evaluation such as uroflowmetry and pressure-flow studies, the location and degree of obstruction may remain ambiguous, particularly in patients with low detrusor pressures associated with low urinary flow rates. The MUPP provides a more direct method of clinical evaluation.

MUPP patterns in patients with benign prostatic hypertrophy (BPH) are distinct from those of normal patients. Although the pressure profile depends on the anatomic distribution of the prostatic adenoma,

the pattern is typically characterized by a pressure drop in the vicinity of the vesicoprostatic junction (Fig. 12–6). After transurethral resection of the prostate or bladder neck incision, this supramembranous

Female Urinary Outlet Obstruction

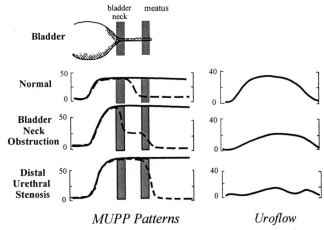

MUPP Patterns   *Uroflow*

Figure 12–5   Schematic diagram of micturitional urethral pressure profile (MUPP) patterns and corresponding flow patterns in women. Vertical shaded areas represent the bladder neck region and distal urethra. Sustained detrusor pressure *(solid line)* is superimposed on vesicourethral pressure *(dotted line)*. Note increased detrusor pressures and the drop in urethral pressure at the obstructed sites.

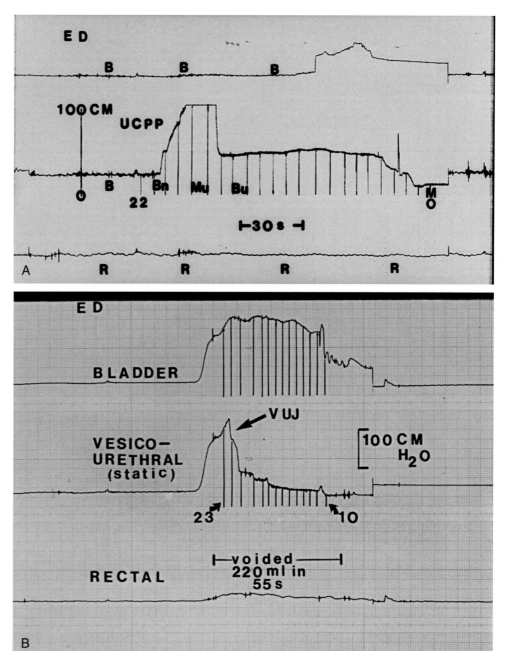

Figure 12-6 *A*, Urethral closure pressure profile (UCPP) and *B*, micturitional urethral pressure profile (MUPP) from same patient with prostatic obstruction. Detrusor contraction pressures are markedly elevated, and a precipitous drop of pressure occurs at the vesicourethral junction (VUJ). B, bladder pressure; Bn, bladder neck; Mu, membranous urethra; Bu, bulbous urethra; M, meatus; R, rectal pressure.

pressure drop is eliminated, and the profile essentially resembles a normal pattern. Detrusor contraction pressures are markedly diminished.

Using this technique to evaluate men with BPH, several interesting patterns have emerged relating the size of the prostate to the severity of the obstruction.[14] In this group of men, moderate to severe prostatic enlargement based on rectal and cystoscopic assessment was associated not only with severe obstruction (52%) but also with minimal or no obstruction (30%). Furthermore, severe obstructions were identified in patients with minimal or no prostatic enlargement (17%). Studies in this group of patients illustrate that prostatic urethral obstruction cannot be accurately determined by clinical and endoscopic assessment of the prostate. Using the MUPP, patients with symptoms of prostatism who have an obstruction can be separated from those without significant outlet obstruction.

Bladder Neck Obstruction in Men

Urodynamic findings in patients with mild bladder neck obstruction include a normal urinary flow rate, a normal or slightly increased detrusor contraction pressure, and a marked delay in bladder neck opening. During urination, a decrease in intraurethral static pressure in the bladder neck region may not be apparent.

In patients with moderate bladder neck obstruction, the urodynamic findings are characterized by an obstructed urinary flow rate, delayed bladder neck relaxation during detrusor contraction and external sphincter relaxation, a marked decrease in intraurethral static pressure in the bladder neck region, and a marked elevation of detrusor contraction pressure (Fig. 12–7).

The urodynamic catheter may completely occlude the already stenotic bladder neck in patients with severe bladder neck obstruction. Therefore, flow around the pressure-recording catheter may be prevented. In this situation, the intraurethral pressure in the bladder neck region and the proximal prostatic urethra represents the occlusion pressure of the stenotic segment, which is higher than the detrusor contraction pressure. Without urine flow, the urethral pressure measurement does not represent static pressure.

The MUPP technique can be used to identify various degrees of bladder neck obstruction. Relief of urinary symptoms coincident with markedly improved urinary flow rates after bladder neck surgery has provided evidence that the bladder neck alone was responsible for the clinical syndrome. Postoperative voiding profiles in these patients show a decrease in voiding pressures and an elimination of the pressure drop across the bladder neck area.[15]

Anterior Urethral Stricture

In patients with anterior urethral strictures, the urethral pressure proximal to the stricture is elevated, and a precipitous drop in pressure occurs in the distal urethra at the site of the stricture[16] (Fig. 12–8). Depending on the severity of the stricture, urethral pressures proximal to the stricture may appear isobaric with bladder pressure, thus concealing the physiologic pressure drop at the external sphincter region (Fig. 12–9). In cases of severe distal obstruction, the catheter may produce complete occlusion of the strictured area. During detrusor contraction and relaxation of the outlet, the fluid in the bladder is continuous with the fluid in the proximal anterior urethra, and thus the static pressure in this area is identical to that of the bladder because no fluid flows across the stenosis.

The MUPP in patients with both anterior and posterior urethral obstruction shows a drop in static pressure at the bladder neck and also at the site of the anterior urethral constriction.

Micturitional Urethral Pressure Profilometry and Pressure-Flow Studies

Urodynamic evaluation using pressure-flow (PQ) studies is currently recommended for the diagnosis of bladder outlet obstruction. However, these studies do not provide a direct assessment of the obstruction and are not practical in all patients, and the results are not always conclusive. Although prostatic obstruction is a common cause of symptoms of prostatism in elderly patients, other conditions, such as sphincter dysfunction (neurogenic or non-neurogenic) and anterior urethral strictures, can mimic prostatic obstruction. In these cases, PQ studies may indicate

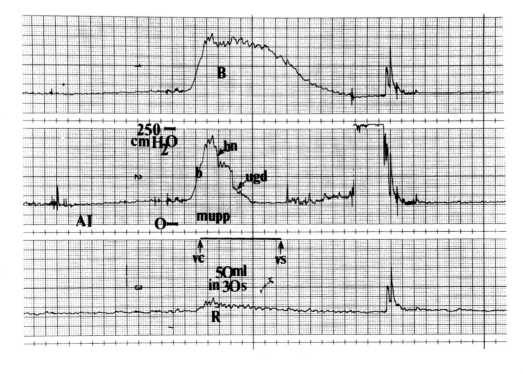

Figure 12-7 Micturitional urethral pressure profile (MUPP) obtained from a 57-year-old man who had had severe obstructive symptoms since the age of 30. Cystogram showed vesical diverticula and vesicoureteral reflux. Note the dramatic drop in pressure at the bladder neck and the high detrusor contraction pressure. B, bladder pressure; bn, bladder neck; vc, voiding commenced; vs, voiding stopped; ugd, urogenital diaphragm; R, rectal pressure.

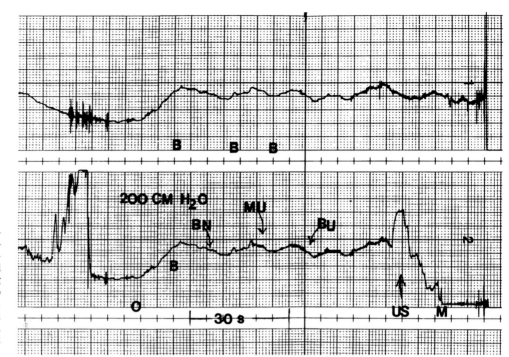

Figure 12-8 Micturitional urethral pressure profile from patient with severe urethral stricture. Bladder pressure *(top)* and urethral pressure *(bottom)* along the entire segment proximal to the stricture area are isobaric. B, bladder; BN, bladder neck; MU, membranous urethra; BU, bulbous urethra; US, urethral stricture; M, meatus.

that the outlet is obstructed, but the cause of the voiding dysfunction will remain obscure. Furthermore, PQ studies, which require patients to sit or stand to urinate, are impractical for bedridden patients, the elderly geriatric population, and patients with stroke or spinal cord injuries. For these reasons,

alternative methods of urodynamic evaluation such as the MUPP are essential.

The MUPP and standard PQ studies were performed in 39 patients with non-neuropathic urinary tract symptoms[17] to compare the effectiveness of these tests in the evaluation of bladder outlet ob-

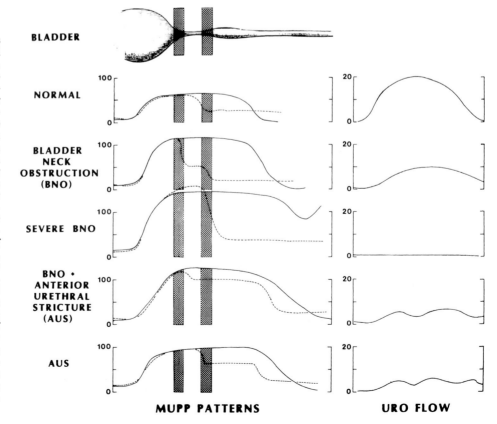

Figure 12-9 Schematic diagrams of various patterns of micturitional urethral pressure profile (MUPP). Vertical shaded areas represent regions of bladder neck and membranous urethra. Sustained detrusor pressure *(solid line)* is superimposed on vesicourethral pressure *(dotted line)*. In normal patients a pressure drop occurs in the region of the membranous urethra. With bladder neck obstruction, voiding pressures are elevated, and the pressure drop occurs at the bladder neck and at the membranous urethra. In cases of severe bladder neck obstruction, the entire supramontane urethra is in a state of contraction and no flow occurs. Double obstructions with bladder neck obstruction and anterior urethral stenosis cause an elevated voiding pressure, a drop in pressure at the bladder neck, and a second pressure drop at the distal site of obstruction. In cases of anterior urethral strictures, a decrease in pressure appears at the membranous urethra and at the site of the distal constriction. Corresponding flow patterns are illustrated on the right. Uro flow, urinary flow.

struction. Based on the results of the PQ studies, obstruction in 16 patients was identified. Using the MUPP, 15 of these were found to have an obstruction, and 1 patient was considered to have no obstruction because bladder and prostatic pressures were isobaric. Twelve patients were deemed to have no obstruction using both tests. In 11 patients, the results of the PQ studies were equivocal. Nine of these were found to be without obstruction, and two clearly had an obstruction using the MUPP.

Similar results have been obtained in our own experience with corresponding MUPP and PQ studies in patients with symptoms of prostatism. The MUPP appears to be as effective as, and perhaps more sensitive than, PQ studies in detecting patients with bladder outlet obstruction.[18]

Conclusion

The technique of pressure profilometry during urination has been used successfully in many urodynamic centers in the United States to assess patients with bladder outlet obstruction. Although analysis of the lower urinary tract using the MUPP requires some familiarity with concepts of basic fluid mechanics and experience with interpretation of the pressure profiles, this technique is simple to perform, highly reproducible, accurate, and clinically useful in detecting the presence of outlet obstruction, identifying its location, and assessing its severity. In addition, the MUPP offers practical advantages in evaluating elderly, nonambulatory patients or patients with severe detrusor instability as well as diagnostic advantages in the evaluation of patients with poor detrusor contractility or equivocal PQ studies. Therefore, the MUPP is an essential component of the urodynamic investigation of patients with voiding dysfunction. Patients with various types of voiding dysfunction have been studied extensively with this technique. Patterns of the vesicourethral pressure profile that are similar to those depicted here were described by Asklin and colleagues for normal subjects, patients with prostatic hyperplasia, bladder neck sclerosis, and urethral strictures.[19] These studies confirmed that the MUPP can be used to detect the presence of an obstruction, localize the site of the obstruction, differentiate between various types of obstruction, and, within limitations, estimate the diameter and resistance of the obstructed urethral segment.

REFERENCES

1. Smith JC: Urethral resistance to micturition. Br J Urol 40:125, 1968.
2. Updike OL: Information content of urodynamics. In Hinman F (ed): Benign Prostatic Hypertrophy. New York, Springer-Verlag, 1983, pp 559–565.
3. Yalla SV, Blute RD, Snyder H, et al: Isolated bladder neck obstruction of undetermined etiology (primary) in adult males. Urology 17:99, 1981.
4. Tanagho EA, Miller ER: Initiation of voiding. Br J Urol 42:175, 1970.
5. Yalla SV, Resnick N, Dyro FM: The responses of bladder neck and external sphincter regions during initiation of voiding. J Urol 131:167A, 1984.
6. Yalla SV, Sharma GVRK, Barsamian EM: Micturitional static urethral pressure profile: A method of recording urethral pressure profile during voiding and the implications. J Urol 124:649, 1980.
7. Brown M, Wickham JEA: The urethral pressure profile. Br J Urol 41:211, 1969.
8. Edwards L, Malvern J: The urethral pressure profile: Theoretical considerations and clinical application. Br J Urol 46:325, 1974.
9. Yalla SV, Resnick NM: Vesicourethral static pressure profile during voiding: Methodology and clinical utility. World J Urol 2:196, 1984.
10. Asklin B, Erlandson BE, Johansson G, Pettersson S: The urethral pressure profile during flow. Scand J Urol Nephrol 18:257, 1984.
11. Scott JES, Clayton CB, Dee PM, Simpson W: Dynamic and flexible models of the urethra. In Hinman F Jr (ed): Hydrodynamics of Micturition. Springfield, IL, Charles C Thomas, 1977, pp 124–132.
12. Yalla SV, Cravalho EG, Resnick NM, Chiang R: Experimental studies with total and static urethral pressures in canine urethra and their clinical significance. Neurourol Urodyn 6:439, 1988.
13. Woodside JR: Micturitional static urethral pressure profilometry in women. Neurourol Urodyn 1:149, 1982.
14. Yalla SV, Blute R, Waters WB, et al: Urodynamic evaluation of prostatic enlargements with micturitional vesicourethral static pressure profiles. J Urol 125:685, 1981.
15. Yalla SV, Waters WB, Snyder H, et al: Urodynamic localization of isolated bladder neck obstruction in men: Studies with micturitional vesicourethral static pressure profile. J Urol 125:677, 1981.
16. Yalla SV, Loughlin K: Urodynamic assessment of anterior urethral constrictions. Urology 29:106, 1982.
17. Desmond AD, Ramayya GR: Comparison of pressure flow studies with micturitional urethral pressure profiles in the diagnosis of urinary outflow obstruction. Br J Urol 61:224, 1988.
18. DuBeau CE, Sullivan MP, Cravalho EG, et al: Correlations between micturitional urethral pressure profile (MUPP) and pressure-flow criteria in bladder outlet obstruction. J Urol 154:498, 1995.
19. Asklin B, Erlandson BE, Johansson G, Pettersson S: The micturitional urethral pressure profile. Scand J Urol Nephrol 18:269, 1984.

CHAPTER 13

Endoscopic Evaluation of the Female Lower Urinary Tract

Carl G. Klutke, M.D.

More than a century has passed since the young Max Nitze first presented his newly developed instrument to the Gesellschaft der Ärzte in Vienna on March 9, 1879.[1] This first practical cystoscope—a marriage of the blossoming art of lenscraft and the newly developed light bulb—took the medical community into a new era wherein a disease process could be described, evaluated, and even treated within the body cavity. Technical refinements have led to a continual evolution of this early device to the point where clinicians today have at their disposal a simple, rapid, and safe procedure that can be used for evaluation and intervention. In the evaluation and treatment of genitourinary pathology, urethrocystoscopy has become one of the most useful tools for gathering information that allows proper treatment. Clearly, the greatest value of any diagnostic procedure comes from its integration with other means of assessment of the underlying abnormality, and when dealing with problems of the female lower genitourinary tract, the vitally important functional and anatomic information gained from urodynamic and radiologic evaluations must be included in the overall assessment. The urethrocystoscopic evaluation, however, allows the clinician to make a unique physical examination of the organ system in question and to gain direct access to it. It is therefore important for any clinician dealing with genitourinary pathology today to understand the indications, proper technique, and information gained from this procedure.

Indications

The indications for urethrocystoscopy are either absolute or relative. Absolute urologic indications include a history or urinalysis finding of hematuria or follow-up of a history of malignant bladder tumors.

Relative indications essentially include almost any situation in which direct visualization of the bladder and urethra can help the clinician to understand the problem and thus treat it more effectively. These situations may include the evaluation of such symptoms as urinary incontinence (both stress and urge), dysuria, recurrent urinary tract infections, voiding abnormalities, dyspareunia, and pelvic pain.[2] In this chapter, malignant pathology is purposely left out, and indications for this examination as well as the findings are confined to benign disease. The only true contraindication to urethrocystoscopic evaluation is an active urinary tract infection.

Technique

MATERIALS

The instrumentation available for urethrocystoscopy has evolved considerably since the development of Nitze's somewhat cumbersome device. Technical advances in lenses and fiberoptic illumination have made for great improvements in visibility, patient comfort, and ease of performance. The standard cystoscope today consists of a sheath surrounding a telescope held together by a bridge. This arrangement allows for a fluid medium to flow and working ports to be manipulated through the sheath external to the telescope. Furthermore, this arrangement gives the clinician the ability to vary the types of lenses used during the procedure as the situation demands. The cystoscope sheath has a fenestrated bill at its lower distal surface that allows the passage of ureteral catheters, biopsy forceps, electrodes, needles, and so on. Four telescopes are commonly available, all with a diameter of 4.0 mm. They are named by the angle of view offered (the angle between the optical axis of the lens and the axis of the probe). Thus, illumination and visualization of a field in the direct line of the scope are achieved with the 0-degree telescope (straight ahead); the 30-degree telescope gives a forward oblique view, the 70-degree a lateral view, and the 120-degree an almost retrograde view. Commonly, 0-, 30-, and 70-degree telescopes are used for complete visualization of urethral and bladder surfaces.

When the urethra alone is thought to be the site of pathology, as when a diverticulum or fistula at this site is suspected, a urethroscope may be used. This device differs from the standard cystoscope in that it has a sheath that lacks the distal bill, thus allowing the urethra to be distended by the infusing fluid medium for a more complete examination (Fig. 13–1).

In the past decade flexible cystoscopes have gained considerable popularity among practitioners. Their advantages over rigid cystoscopes, including ease of operation and patient comfort during the procedure, have made the flexible instrument extremely useful in the evaluation of male genitourinary pathology. In women, however, the flexible instrument inherently lacks the rigidity necessary to evaluate the bladder neck and proximal urethral mobility, which, in association with incontinence, is one of the more common indications for endoscopy.

Procedure

The initial step in performing a urethrocystoscopic evaluation is a discussion of the procedure with the patient. Clear understanding of the nature of the procedure, its potential risks and benefits, the events to be expected both during and after it, and reassurance often ease the patient's anxiety. Time spent in clarifying the procedure and correcting any misunderstandings the patient may have goes a long way toward relieving the uncertainty and anxiety that ultimately lead to most of the patient's discomfort. A sterile urine culture should be documented, and those patients known to have mitral valve prolapse should be pretreated with prophylactic antibiotics.

Anesthesia for the endoscopic procedure may be necessary to allow for complete evaluation without undue discomfort. Generally, older patients are less sensitive to urethral manipulation by the endoscope and therefore may require nothing more than lubricant alone over the tip of the instrument or application of a lubricant gel containing a local anesthetic. When parenteral sedation or analgesia is required either a short-acting benzodiazepam such as midazolam or a sedative such as propofol, together with a short-acting narcotic such as fentanyl, is useful. These agents must be closely monitored by an anesthetist using contemporary monitoring standards.[3]

The introitus is cleansed with an antiseptic solution. A fluid medium allows insufflation of the urethral and bladder lumen and thus ease of passage and more complete evaluation. Generally, physiologic saline at 50 to 70 cm gravity pressure is used for this purpose. The initial examination of the urethra is performed using the 0-degree lens to allow complete visualization of both the anterior and posterior surfaces. At the proximal urethra and bladder neck, note is made of the degree of movement occurring in association with the Valsalva maneuver and with coughing. The instrument is then passed into the bladder proper, and at this point, using the 30-degree and 70-degree lenses, complete visualization of the mucosal surface is achieved. When incontinence is being evaluated, it is often helpful to fill the bladder to a known volume (such as 200 ml) to look for leakage on coughing and straining after the cystoscope has been removed. The risk of infection from cystoscopy is very small. Antibiotic prophylaxis after the procedure is indicated only for patients who are at risk for significant morbidity from potential transient bacteremia such as those with cardiac valvular disorders or internal prosthetic devices.

Normal Anatomy of the Urethra

The normal female urethra is composed of a mucosal lining beneath which lies a thick submucosal layer. Luminal diameter ranges from 6.5 to 10 mm; however, owing to the submucosa with its rich vascular plexus and abundance of elastic and contractile fibers, the lumen remains in a closed or coapted state at rest. The initial impression of the endoscopist is the reddish appearance of the mucosa overlying the healthy vascular submucosa. With the 0-degree lens the entire urethral lumen can be clearly seen under the hydrostatic pressure of the flowing medium. If the fluid flow is interrupted, coaptation of the mucosal surface occurs rapidly. Distally, the ducts of the submucosal glands are most numerous and can on occasion be seen as small pits in the mucosal surface.[4] Some of these ducts may be visible at the perimeatal surface of the introitus, where they are referred to as Skene's glands. Within the distal urethra, the urethral gland ducts appear as small pinpoint openings in the mucosa and are most numerous between the 5 and 7 o'clock positions. In the midurethra, the surrounding pelvic diaphragm can be sensed by the slightly increased resistance to passage

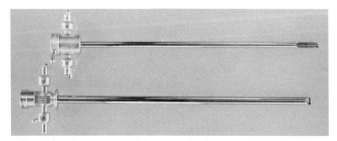

Figure 13-1 Cystoscope sheath *(top)*, with a fenestrated bill on its underside, and urethroscope *(bottom)*, with a distal bill absent to allow for complete urethral distention.

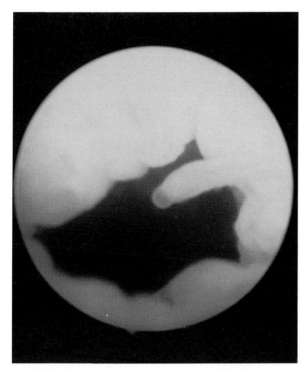

Figure 13-2   Pseudopolyps of the internal urethral meatus. Often confused by the inexperienced observer with transitional cell carcinoma, pseudopolyps at the internal urethral meatus appear as small mucosal projections with cystlike heads and have no pathologic significance.

of the instrument. The proximal urethra and bladder neck area is the site thought to be associated with passive continence in the female.[5–7] It is at this point that specialized fibers of the pubococcygeus muscle—the "urethropelvic ligaments"—surround the urethra and suspend it laterally on either side from the pelvic side wall via the tendinous arch of the obturator internus muscle. The urethropelvic ligaments, in patients with normal pelvic support, maintain the bladder neck and proximal urethra in a relatively fixed, high retropubic position that changes little with coughing or straining.[8] Therefore, in the proximal urethra–bladder neck region the endoscope must be angled upward to enter the bladder. At the bladder neck, pseudopolyps are frequently seen projecting into the lumen on mucosal stalks (Fig. 13–2).

Urethral Pathology

CHRONIC URETHRITIS

The term chronic urethritis generally refers to a set of symptoms in women thought to result from inflammation or infection within the periurethral glandular structures.[9] The best description of the anatomy of these structures comes from the work of Huffman, who performed serial sectioning of the female urethra and made wax reconstructions of its

glands.[4] So illustrated, the normal female urethra appears surrounded by a labyrinthine mass of paraurethral tubules, canaliculi, and glandular elements (Fig. 13–3). The glands themselves consist of complex mucin-secreting acini connected to the urethral lumen by ducts lined with low columnar epithelium. Functionally, the urethral glands by their mucus production are thought to act in defense of the bladder, slowing down or preventing the urethral ascent of bacteria.[10] When they are inflamed, various endoscopically apparent but nonspecific changes take place: Typically, the external urethral orifice is edematous and hyperemic, and there may be narrowing of the urethral lumen with inflammatory changes of the mucosa, including redness and exudate.[11, 12]

ATROPHIC URETHRITIS

As previously mentioned, the urethral submucosa is a thick, richly vascular structure that is important for proper luminal coaptation. This spongy tissue helps create the "washer effect" that is important in passive urinary continence as well as other urodynamic functions.[13] Estrogen appears to be important for proper maintenance of this submucosal sponge.[14] As many estrogen receptors are found in the urethra, bladder, trigone, and pubococcygeus muscle as in the vaginal epithelium.[15] Many investigators have noted the effect of estrogen administration on the urethral mucosa in cytologic studies, in which cellular maturational changes occur from the transitional to the intermediate squamous epithelium.[16, 17] Although urodynamic and urethral pressure studies have been misleading, several clinical trials have shown significant improvement in incontinent patients with estrogen usage, presumably on the basis of the changes just described.[18, 19]

With cessation of estrogen production during menopause or after surgical castration, atrophic changes in the urethra equivalent to those within the senile vagina can occur. Urethral mucosal cytologic characteristics change from the normal squamous epithelium to a predominantly transitional type. Urethral submucosal vascularity decreases, resulting in a reduction of its inherent coapting ability. Endoscopically, the urethral lining takes on a pale, even whitish hue owing to the decreased vascularity. Submucosal changes may be evidenced by poor luminal coaptation and a pronounced rigidity of the urethral walls. The urethra may be somewhat friable, and patients may have increased sensitivity during the procedure.

STRESS INCONTINENCE

Continence in women appears to be a result of a balance of forces. The urethral coapting ability, the bladder neck and proximal urethral anatomic location, reflex pelvic floor contractions at the time of cough and strain, the hormonal and neurologic milieu, as well as a host of less well understood factors

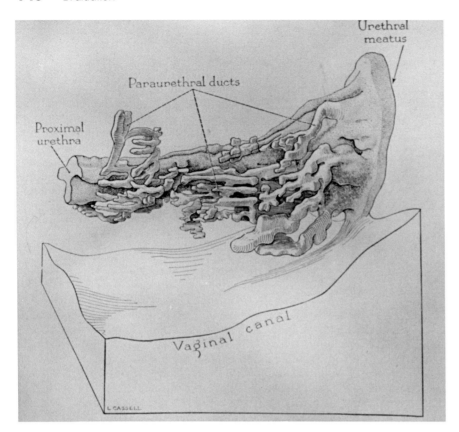

Figure 13-3 Labyrinthine mass of periurethral glands surrounding the female urethra. (From Huffman JW: The detailed anatomy of the paraurethral ducts in the adult human female. Am J Obstet Gynecol 55:86, 1948.)

all seem to play a role. Of these, only the anatomic support of the bladder neck and proximal urethra and the urethral coapting ability are responsive to surgical manipulation. Careful objective evaluation is required to determine which of these factors plays the major role in an individual patient's stress urinary loss. A different treatment plan will be applied in a patient with anatomic mobility of the bladder neck and proximal urethra than in a patient with an intrinsically dysfunctional proximal urethra. Endoscopy allows visual observation of the bladder neck and proximal urethra during coughing and straining, and this, following a thorough history and physical examination and aided by urodynamic and radiographic findings, helps the clinician categorize the pathology and thus decide on the most effective surgical therapy.

Anatomic Stress Incontinence

Anatomic incontinence is the most common type of stress urinary leakage. This situation results from inappropriate mobility of an otherwise normally functioning bladder neck and proximal urethra. Laxity of the supporting structures leads to a downward and outward movement of the sphincteric unit with coughing and straining and thus to improper through-transmission of intra-abdominal pressure.[20] Mobility of the bladder neck and proximal urethra can be observed endoscopically. Endoscopic evaluation is best performed after the bladder has been filled to a volume of roughly 200 ml to allow intra-abdominal forces to be effectively exerted against it. The endoscope with a 0-degree lens should be placed at the level of the bladder neck, at which point coughing and the Valsalva maneuver will reveal significant downward and outward movement of the sphincter.

Intrinsic Urethral Dysfunction

Proximal urethral coapting ability represents another important aspect of passive continence in women. Thought to be a result of expansile pressure of the submucosa inward toward the lumen by the surrounding smooth muscle, the resultant "washer effect" helps to maintain closure of the proximal urethra during sudden increases in intra-abdominal pressure.[21] Insults such as radiation, previous surgery, long-term indwelling catheters, and estrogen depletion can damage the fibrovascular submucosal sponge, whereupon stress incontinence of intrinsic urethral dysfunction may ensue.[22] Lack of neural tone to the urethral smooth muscle likewise can lead to lack of the mucosal seal. Often because of previous anti-incontinence surgery the bladder neck lies in a fixed, high retropubic position. Typical endoscopic findings include an open patulous proximal urethra at rest that may or may not be hypermobile with cough or Valsalva (Fig. 13–4). In severe cases, there may be a decrease in resilience of the submucosa secondary to scarring, leading to a rigid "pipe stem" urethra on endoscopy.

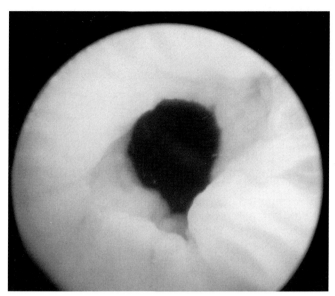

Figure 13-4 Open patulous fibrotic proximal urethra seen with severe intrinsic urethral dysfunction.

Bladder Pathology

URETEROCELE

A ureterocele is a cystic dilation of the terminal intravesical portion of the ureter, perhaps as a result of a stenotic opening in the bladder.[23] Two major types of ureteroceles are recognized: the simple orthotopic or intravesical ureterocele associated with a single ureter and situated wholly within the bladder, and the ectopic type, in which a portion may be situated at the bladder neck or in the urethra and is virtually always associated with the obstructed upper ureter of a duplex kidney.[24] The ectopic ureterocele is often detected on antenatal sonograms or in early life owing to urinary infection, urethral prolapse, or outlet obstruction. The simple orthotopic ureterocele, however, often remains asymptomatic in childhood and may be recognized in the adult either during routine evaluation for unrelated problems or for the symptoms it may eventually cause, generally urinary infection, although less commonly flank pain and recurrent hematuria may be present.[25] The urographic findings are pathognomonic of the condition; the cystogram reveals the so-called cobra head or spring onion deformity. On cystoscopic examination, the typical finding is a cystic swelling in the region of the ureteral orifice that can be seen to change in size with each efflux of urine (Fig. 13–5). Rarely is a simple intravesical ureterocele anything more than a cystoscopic or radiologic oddity in the adult woman. Indications for operative treatment of ureterocele include obstruction at the ureterovesical junction, ascending infection, secondary urolithiasis, and, less frequently, flank pain and recurrent hematuria.

URETERAL ECTOPY

Ureteral ectopy is present when a ureteral orifice opens at a site other than the posterolateral boundary of the trigone. More common in women than in men by a ratio of 6:1 or higher, an ectopic ureter is usually associated with ureteral duplication draining the upper of two kidney pelves.[26] The result of faulty development of the terminal wolffian duct, an ectopic ureter occurs when the ureteric bud originates considerably higher than normal and the migratory process that follows carries it too far distally. In women, unlike the situation in men, the final position of the ectopic ureteral orifice may be the intravesical or infrasphincteric urethra; thus only women with the anomaly may develop incontinence of urine.[27] Kjellberg and colleagues reported on the frequency of specific anatomic sites of ectopic ureters in their series of female children: vestibule, 38%; urethra, 32%; vagina, 27%; and uterus, 3%[28] (Fig. 13–6). Although the classically ectopic ureter causes symptoms of wetness or dribbling from childhood onward, at least half of ectopic ureters in women are not diagnosed until adult life, probably because the symptoms have been atypical or absent. Various nonspecific genitourinary problems such as vaginal discharge, pelvic or lower abdominal mass, urinary tract infection, and even late-onset stress incontinence may occur as the presenting sign of an ectopic ure-

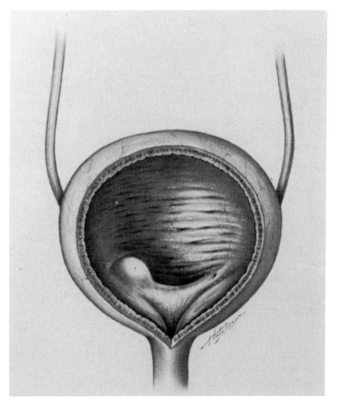

Figure 13-5 Simple orthotopic ureterocele. (From Kelalis PP: Anomalies of the urinary tract: Renal pelves and ureter. *In* Kelalis PP, King LR, Belman AB [eds]: Clinical Pediatric Urology, 2nd ed. Philadelphia, WB Saunders, 1985, pp 672–725.)

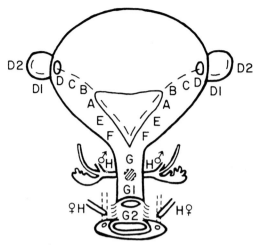

Figure 13–6 Schematic diagram of normal and ectopic orifice sites. A, normal position; B to D2, lateral ectopia; F to H, coital ectopia. (From Schwarz RD, Stevens FD, Cussen LJ: The pathogenesis of renal dysplasia. II. The significance of lateral and coital ectopy of the ureteric orifice. Invest Urol 19:97, 1981.)

ter.[29] Cystoscopy, urethroscopy, and occasionally vaginoscopy are necessary to make the diagnosis.[30] The ectopic orifice at times is very difficult to locate, and a careful search of the bladder, urethra, urethral meatus, and even the vagina may be required. At the time of endoscopy and visualization of the ectopic orifice, catheterization and retrograde pyelography should be considered to allow further evaluation of the associated upper tract.

TRIGONITIS

Trigonitis is a common finding on cystoscopy in the female bladder. First described by Heymann in 1905 as "trigonal cystitis,"[31] this condition has since been given a variety of names, including pseudomembranous trigonitis, urethrotrigonitis, granular trigonitis, and vaginal or squamous metaplasia of the trigonal epithelium.[31] The last term, squamous metaplasia, seems most appropriate because the histology typically includes partial or complete replacement of urothelium by mature nonkeratinized squamous epithelium. Controversy continues about why trigonitis develops in the first place and why only in some women and not all. One school of thought holds that this form of squamous metaplasia is an anatomic epithelial variant that develops under the influence of hormones because its incidence seems to be lowest in young girls and postmenopausal women.[32–34] Another widely held theory is that squamous metaplasia results from or is associated with repeated urinary infection.[35] Regardless of the cause, the condition is certainly common and in most cases has no associated symptoms or consequences.[36, 37]

Cystoscopically, the metaplasia tends to be localized to the midtrigone with tonguelike extensions toward the ureteral orifices. Its surface may appear quite rough and has a characteristic grayish white color with the appearance of a membrane (Fig. 13–7). Bleeding may occur when the area is scraped with the cystoscope. These whitish gray lesions confined to the trigone are not premalignant, and biopsy should be done only if significant doubt exists.

URETHRAL DIVERTICULA

Urethral diverticula are endothelium-lined urethral outpouchings. With an estimated incidence of 3 to 4.7% in women, urethral diverticula represent a not too uncommon cause of female genitourinary complaints.[38] The cause of this disorder is related to the structure of the female urethral glandular apparatus. The periurethral glands in women consist of a complex of mucin-secreting glands located mainly alongside the mid to distal urethra.[39] Considered the embryologic homologues of the male prostate, these glands seem to be important in inhibiting bacterial ascension into the bladder.[9] When infected, inflammatory ductal obstruction of the periurethral glands can lead to abscess formation and cystic enlargement. Urethral diverticula are presently thought to be endothelium-lined outpouchings resulting from the eventual rupture of these abscesses or cysts into the urethral lumen.[39] Typically, women with this disorder present with symptoms of chronic dysuria, dysparcunia, recurrent urinary tract infections, and, at times, postvoid dribbling. The following have been reported as possible risk factors for the development of female urethral diverticula: gonococcal urethritis, previous periurethral surgery, urethral instrumenta-

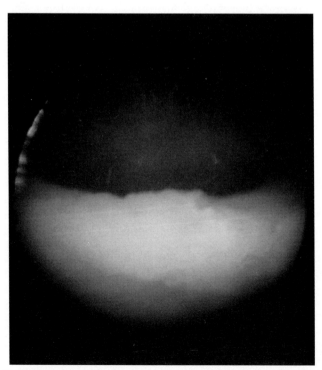

Figure 13–7 Squamous metaplasia with a characteristic whitish membrane located mainly over the right hemitrigone.

tion, and traumatic vaginal delivery.[40] Calculus formation can occur within the diverticulum and has been seen in up to 10% of all reported cases.[41, 42] Development of carcinoma within diverticula has been shown.[42–44]

Although cystoscopy remains an invaluable tool in the diagnosis and management of urethral diverticula, it appears to be less sensitive as a screening technique than urethrography.[45] Radiologic screening of patients in whom a urethral diverticulum is suspected is usually carried out with a voiding cystourethrogram with or without positive pressure urethrography. Urethroscopy is very helpful, however, in determining the location of the diverticulum along the urethra. Furthermore, notation of the number of openings into the diverticula is important because a significant percentage of patients have more than one and occasionally as many as three. Owing to the distribution of the periurethral glands, most diverticula develop along the posterolateral wall of the mid to distal urethra. Urethral diverticula are seen rarely on the anterior urethral wall (in a 9 to 3 o'clock position), in which case they are most likely of traumatic origin (e.g., traumatic catheterization). Use of the urethroscope, which lacks the distal bill of the cystoscope and thus allows more complete urethral distention, together with manual compression of the bladder neck, further increases urethral distention and thus diagnostic accuracy (Fig. 13–8). Note should be made of the size and number of diverticular openings and their location in relation to the bladder neck and urethral meatus. Finally, endoscopic evaluation of the competence of the bladder neck and degree of urethral hypermobility with stress should be performed to determine whether or not a suspension procedure should be combined with diverticulectomy.

INTERSTITIAL CYSTITIS

Interstitial cystitis is a chronic bladder inflammation of unknown cause presenting mostly in females with symptoms of urgency, frequency, nocturia, and varying degrees of suprapubic discomfort. First described by Nitze in 1907 as "cystitis parenchymatosa," the disease has had numerous synonyms including painful bladder disease, sensory bladder disease, and chronic abacterial cystitis. Not altogether rare, reported incidences range from 2 to 15 per 10,000 outpatient visits depending on the population studied.[46, 47] The estimated ratio of affected women to men is thought to be 10:1. Despite a great amount of attention focused recently on this disease, little objective progress concerning pathogenesis, histopathology, or treatment has been made.

Diagnosis of interstitial cystitis is currently made on the basis of exclusion of other disorders together with typical cystoscopic findings on bladder distention. Cystoscopy is best performed with the patient under general or spinal anesthesia because of the severe discomfort with bladder filling experienced by these patients. Anesthesia allows distention of the bladder to a volume greater than the patient's awake capacity. Care must be taken to avoid bladder perforation at these volumes; this can generally be avoided if the irrigating fluid is placed no higher than 80 cm above the ventral surface of the bladder.

Bladder findings are most evident on a second distention. Diffuse hemorrhagic spots called glomerulations are typically seen.[48] These spots often begin to ooze as the bladder is distended (which may discolor the irrigating fluid) and can be noted as a terminal bloody efflux on bladder emptying.[49] Although not pathognomonic, glomerulations strongly suggest a diagnosis of interstitial cystitis and are not seen in other types of bladder pathology. Two types of disease—"early" and "classic" interstitial cystitis—can be defined based on the cystoscopic findings and bladder capacity.[50] Early interstitial cystitis is typically associated with normal bladder capacity under anesthesia and reveals only the characteristic petechial bleeding (glomerulations) on second distention. Classic interstitial cystitis is associated with reduced bladder capacity, glomerulations, and ulcers. The ulcers of classic interstitial cystitis appear as pale scars surrounding a central hyperemic spot with small radiating vessels and are usually located on the dome or posterior wall of the bladder (Fig. 13–9).

Biopsy is usually performed in these patients to rule out malignancy and to supply further corroboration of the diagnosis.[51, 52] Samples should be taken from several areas of the bladder. Histologic examination of a bladder biopsy specimen taken from a patient with an interstitial cystitis can reveal a variety of changes; however, a nonspecific chronic inflammatory reaction in the deeper layers with or without significant mass cell infiltration is most commonly seen.

TRABECULATION

Trabeculation is a general term used to describe the endoscopic appearance of the bladder interior when

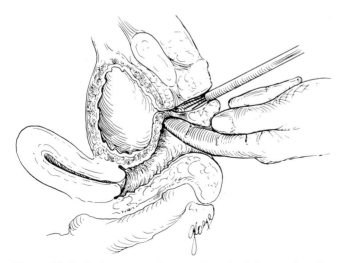

Figure 13-8 Endoscopic evaluation of urethral diverticula using the urethroscope with manual compression of the bladder neck.

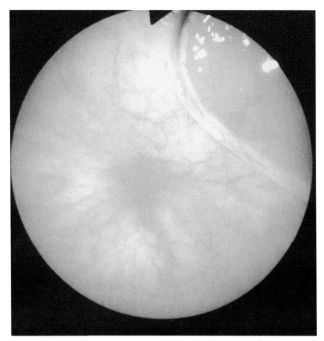

Figure 13-9 Hunner's ulcer located near the bladder dome with a characteristic white scar, central erythema, and surrounding hyperemic mucosa.

pronounced muscular ridges are visible. These ridges represent enlarged muscular bundles and are seen throughout the interior of the bladder but generally spare the region of the trigone. Trabeculation is commonly found in men with bladder outlet obstruction, and this relationship has been frequently applied to

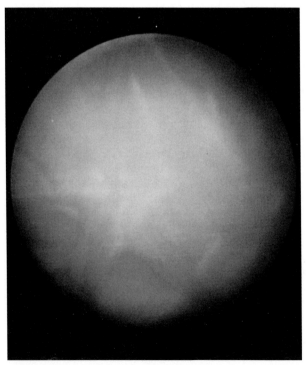

Figure 13-10 Endoscopic appearance of mild trabeculation.

the endoscopic findings in women as well. Outlet obstruction rarely occurs in women, however, and therefore it is important to question this interpretation of the appearance of bladder trabeculation in women.[53] Although trabeculation is an expression of increased muscular work, one very important cause is by detrusor instability, and this seems to be the most common reason for trabeculation in women.[54, 55] The cystoscopic finding of this entity alone in an otherwise normal woman has little functional or morphometric importance.

Trabeculation is best seen cystoscopically when the bladder is distended to a volume near the patient's capacity. As the bladder fills, muscular ridges begin to stand out in relief from the background bladder wall (Fig. 13-10). Mucosal changes are generally not apparent, and biopsy is not necessary. Trabeculation in the female bladder is common and most frequently represents an unstable bladder rather than outflow obstruction.

Fistulas

VESICOVAGINAL FISTULA

A vesicovaginal fistula, historically a complication of childbirth, is now most often a result of surgical trauma. Gynecologic surgery, usually total abdominal hysterectomy, presently accounts for the great majority of cases; a minority result from obstetric procedures, radiation, or trauma.[56, 57] Presenting signs are ususally noted soon after surgery; continuous day and night leakage usually points clearly to the diagnosis. Occasionally the leakage may be scant or intermittent, and further diagnostic aids such as the pyridium or methylene blue pad test or a cystogram are required.[58]

Following hysterectomy, vesicovaginal fistulas usually occur in the posterior bladder floor adjacent to the location of the closed vaginal cuff. In the early postoperative period the fistulous area may be edematous and inflamed, and suture material is still visibly present. The possibility of multiple holes should be entertained, and they should be carefully sought. Note should be made of the location of the fistula in relation to the ureteral orifice. Although most fistulas occur approximately 3 to 4 cm posterior to the trigone, occasionally they encroach on the trigonal region and consequently catheterization of the ureter at the time of fistula repair may be helpful.

Cystourethroscopy with concomitant vaginoscopy can be helpful in confirming the presence of the fistula and defining its location. The appearance of the vaginal mucosa surrounding the fistula (vascularity, amount of edema, presence of suture material, and inflammation or infection) gives further information that is important in timing the repair. Occasionally, vaginoscopy following instillation of methylene blue

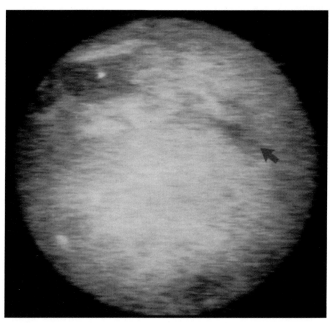

Figure 13-11 Vesicoenteric fistula located near the dome of the bladder with gas and debris bubbling out of the tract *(arrow)*.

VESICOENTERIC FISTULA

Fistulous tracts between the bowel and bladder occur much less frequently in women than in men, probably owing to the intermediate position of the uterus between these two structures.[59] When present, a fistula is usually the result of an inflammatory process or malignancy within the bowel. The vast majority involve the terminal ileum or sigmoid colon. These fistulas are by no means rare but are less frequently seen today owing to earlier diagnosis and treatment of the underlying intestinal disease.

Symptoms may be due to either the abnormal communication between the bowel and the bladder or the primary pathologic process. The latter presentation usually precedes the former by months or years depending on the nature of the disease. The pathognomonic bladder symptoms of vesicointestinal fistulas include terminal pneumaturia as well as the passage of fecal matter in the urine. Recurrent episodes of cystitis, often with mixed flora, is a common occurrence.

The patient's history, together with cystoscopy and bimanual pelvic examination under anesthesia is enough to make a firm diagnosis in the majority of cases. Indeed, in patients in whom a vesicoenteric fistula is suspected, cystoscopy may be the single most useful diagnostic test compared with radiographic studies such as barium enema or cystograms.[60] The cystoscopic appearance characteristically includes pus, fecal matter, or gas bubbles issuing from an area usually on the posterior bladder wall (Fig. 13-11). The "herald lesion," which appears on cystoscopy as a localized inflammatory polypoid lesion in the bladder mucosa on the posterior bladder wall, is typically located on the left side with vesicocolic fistulas and may be seen on the right side with vesicoileal fistulas.[61] The surrounding bladder mucosa is usually edematous and dusky red with a heaped-up polypoidal morphologic appearance resembling a malignancy. Biopsy of the surrounding irregular mucosa is important. When an actual fistulous tract is visualized, catheterization and fistulography should be performed.

RADIATION CYSTITIS

In recent years the dose of radiation utilized for treatment of gynecologic and pelvic malignancies has been diminished, resulting in a decrease in severity of bladder injury. Radiation effects on the bladder are still seen, however, generally becoming apparent long after radiation therapy has been given. The early reaction in the bladder to radiation consists of erythema, edema, hyperemia, and epithelial desquamation.[62] These early effects are noted 3 to 4 weeks after the treatment has been given and resolve within a short period of time. Urgency, frequency, and other initiative bladder symptoms accompany the early radiation reaction.

Late, or "tertiary," radiation reactions more commonly come to the attention of the urologist or gynecologist. These effects rarely appear earlier than a year after treatment and may not reveal themselves for over a decade. Tertiary effects are the result of obliterative endarteritis, and histologic examination reveals granulation tissue, blood vessel wall thickening, and various manifestations of inflammation.[63] The cystoscopic picture of tertiary radiation injury of the bladder mirrors this endarteritis, loss of vascularity of the submucosa producing an off-white color of the mucosa. Fibrosis and scarring of connective tissue result in contraction of the bladder, leading to loss of capacity and decreased bladder compliance. Ulceration can occur and appears as a white avascular area surrounded by a zone of dilated blood vessels. A radiation ulcer is usually located in the posterior third of the bladder base, almost always in the midline. In this location, ulceration not infrequently leads to vesicovaginal fistula formation, often associated with large tissue defects (Fig. 13-12).[64]

Photography

Photographs in this chapter were made using a Storz-Hopkins II, 0-degree enlarged-view, 4-mm × 30-cm telescope. The light source was a Storz-Xenon lamp with automatic flash and light. The camera was

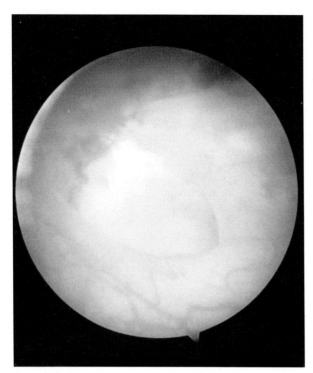

Figure 13-12 Vesicovaginal fistula associated with severe radiation cystitis.

a Nikon N5005 mirror flex with Storz special zoom lens 70 to 140 mm, including a Nikon sinc cable.

REFERENCES

1. Kneise O, Stolze M: Hand Atlas der Cystoskopie und Urethro Cystoskopie. Leipzig, G. Thieme, 1955, p 1.
2. Aldridge CW, Beaton JH, Nanzig RP: A review of office urethroscopy and cystometry. Am J Obstet Gynecol 131:432, 1978.
3. Fredrick KO: Management quality in anesthesia care. In Miller RD (ed): Anesthesia, 3rd ed, vol 2. New York, Churchill Livingstone, 1990, pg 2393.
4. Huffman JW: The detailed anatomy of the paraurethral ducts in the adult human female. Am J Obstet Gynecol 55:86, 1948.
5. Turner-Warwick R: Observations on the function and dysfunction of the sphincter and detrusor mechanism. Urol Clin North Am 6:13, 1979.
6. Golumb J, Klutke CG, Raz S: Surgery of female incontinence. In Drolle MJ (ed): Surgical Management of Urologic Disease and Anatomic Approach. St. Louis, Mosby-Year Book, 1992, pp 1055–1092.
7. Raz S, Little NA, Juma S: Female urology. In Walsh P, Retisk D, Stamey TA, Vaughan ED (eds): Campbell's Urology, 6th ed. Philadelphia, W. B. Saunders, 1992, pp 2782–2828.
8. Klutke CG, Golumb J, Barbaric Z, Raz S: The anatomy of stress incontinence: Magnetic resonance imaging of the female bladder neck and urethra. J Urol 143:563, 1990.
9. Scotti RJ, Ostergard DR: The urethral syndrome. Clin Obstet Gynecol 27:515, 1984.
10. Cox C: The urethra and its relationship to urinary tract infection: The flora of the normal urethra. South Med J 59:621, 1966.
11. Folsom IA: The female urethra, a clinical and pathological study. JAMA 97:1345, 1931.
12. Ormond JK: Non-purulent urethritis in women: Granular urethritis-cystalgia. J Urol 33:483, 1935.
13. Staskin DR, Zimmern PE, Hadley HR, Raz S: The pathophysiology of stress incontinence. Urol Clin North Am 12:271, 1985.
14. Krantz KE: The anatomy of the urethra and anterior vaginal wall. Am J Obstet Gynecol 62:374, 1957.
15. Iosif CS, Batra S, Ed A, et al: Estrogen receptors in the human female lower urinary tract. Am J Obstet Gynecol 141:817, 1981.
16. Smith P: Age changes in the female urethra. Br J Urol 44:667, 1977.
17. Bergman A, Karram MM, Bhatia NN: Changes in urethral cytology following estrogen administration. Gynecol Obstet Invest 29:211, 1990.
18. Fantl JA, Wyman JF, Anderson RL, et al: Post-menopausal urinary incontinence: Comparison between non-estrogen and estrogen supplanted women. Obstet Gynecol 71:823, 1988.
19. Hilton P, Stanton SL: The use of intravaginal oestrogen cream in genuine stress incontinence. Br J Obstet Gynecol 90:940, 1983.
20. Hodgkinson CP: Stress urinary incontinence in the female. Surg Gynecol Obstet 108:1141, 1970.
21. Hutch JA: A New Theory of the Anatomy and Physiology of the Bladder, Trigone and Urethra. New York, Appleton-Century-Crofts, 1972, p 78.
22. Blaivas JG, Olsson CA: Stress incontinence: Classification and surgical approach. J Urol 139:727, 1988.
23. Tanagho EA: Anatomy and management of ureteroceles. J Urol 107:729, 1972.
24. Glassberg KI, et al: Suggested terminology for duplex systems, ectopic ureters and ureteroceles. J Urol 132:1153, 1984.
25. Kelalis PP: Anomalies of the urinary tract: Renal pelves and ureter. In Kelalis PP, King LR, Belman AB (eds): Clinical Pediatric Urology, 2nd ed, vol 2. Philadelphia, W. B. Saunders, 1985, pp 672–725.
26. Schulman CC: Ureteroceles. In Glenn JF (ed): Urologic Surgery, 3rd ed. Philadelphia, J. B. Lippincott, 1983, pp 483–490.
27. Young DW, Lebowitz RL: Congenital abnormalities of the ureter. Sem Roentgenol 21:172, 1986.
28. Kjellberg SR, Ericsson NO, Rudhe U: The lower urinary tract in childhood: Some correlated clinical and roentgenologic observations. Chicago, Year Book, 1968.
29. Persky L, Noseworthy J: Adult ureteral ectopia. J Urol 116:156, 1976.
30. Brennan W, Henry HH: Ureteral ectopia: Report of 39 cases. J Urol 109:192, 1973.
31. Heymann A: Die Cystitis trigoni der Frau. Z Krankh Harn Sex Org. 16:422, 1905.
32. Henry L, Fox M: Histologic findings in pseudomembranous trigonitis. J Clin Pathol 24:605, 1971.
33. Tyler DE: Stratified squamous epithelium in the vesical trigone and urethra: Findings correlated with the menstrual cycle and age. Am J Anat 111:319, 1962.
34. Packham DA: The epithelial lining of the female trigone and urethra. Br J Urol 43:201, 1971.
35. Ney C, Ehrlich JC: Squamous epithelium of the trigone of the human female urinary bladder. J Urol 73:809, 1955.
36. Long ED, Shepherd RT: The incidence and significance of vaginal metaplasia of the bladder trigone in adult women. Br J Urol 55:189, 1983.
37. Wiener DP, Koss LG, Sabley B, Freed SZ: The prevalence and significance of Brunn's nests, cystitis cystica and squamous metaplasia in normal bladder. J Urol 122:317, 1979.
38. Widran J, Sanchez R, Gruhn J: Squamous metaplasia of the bladder: A study of 450 patients. J Urol 112:479, 1974.
39. Anderson MJF: The incidence of diverticula in the female urethra. J Urol 98:96, 1967.
40. Davis HJ, Telinde RW: Urethral diverticula: An assay of 121 cases. J Urol 80:34, 1958.
41. Leach GE, Bavendam TG: Female urethral diverticula. Urology 30:407, 1987.
42. Presman D, Rolnick D, Zumerchek J: Calculus formation within a diverticulum of the female urethra. J Urol 91:376, 1964.
43. Scrinivas V, Dow D: Transitional cell carcinoma in a urethral diverticulum with a calculus. J Urol 129:372, 1983.
44. Torres SA, Quattelbaum KB: Carcinoma in a urethral diverticulum. South Med J 65:1374, 1972.

45. Evans KJ, McCarthy MP, Sands JP: Adenocarcinoma of a female urethral diverticulum: A case report and review of the literature. J Urol 126:124, 1981.
46. Greenberg M, et al: Female urethral diverticula: Double balloon catheter study. AJR 136:259, 1981.
47. Oravisto KJ: Epidemiology of interstitial cystitis. Ann Chir Gynecol Fenn 64:75, 1975.
48. Leach GE, Raz S: Interstitial cystitis. *In* Raz S (ed): Female Urology. Philadelphia, W. B. Saunders, 1983, p 351.
49. Hand RJ: Interstitial cystitis. Report of 223 cases. J Urol 61:291, 1949.
50. Messing EM, Stamey TA: Interstitial cystitis. Urology 12:381, 1978.
51. Lam DL, Gittes RF: Inflammatory carcinoma of the bladder and interstitial cystitis. J Urol 117:49, 1977.
52. Utz PC, Zincke H: The masquerade of bladder cancer in situ as interstitial cystitis. J Urol 111:160, 1974.
53. Turner-Warwick R, et al: A urodynamic view of the clinical problems associated with bladder neck dysfunction and its treatment by endoscopic incision and trans-trigonal posterior prostatectomy. Br J Urol 45:44, 1973.
54. Shah PJR, Whiteside CG, Milroy EJG, Turner-Warwick R: Radiologic trabeculation of the male bladder—a clinical and urodynamic assessment. Br J Urol 53:567, 1981.
55. Bassi P, Artibani W, Pegovavo V, et al: Obstruction or no obstruction. Int Urol Nephrol 20:489, 1988.
56. Tancer ML: The past total hysterectomy (vault) vesicovaginal fistula. J Urol 123:839, 1980.
57. Lee RA, Symmonds RE, Williams TJ: Current status of genitourinary fistula. Obstet Gynecol 72:3313, 1988.
58. Labasky RF, Leach GE: Prevention and management of urovaginal fistulas. Clin Obstet Gynecol 33:382, 1990.
59. Nauclér J, Risberg B: Diagnosis and treatment of colovesical fistulas. Acta Chir Scand 147:435, 1981.
60. Carson CC, Malek RS, Remine WH: Urologic aspects of vesicoenteric fistulas. J Urol 119:744, 1978.
61. Nielsen K, Orholm M, Andersen SP, Kraup T: Herald lesion of the urinary bladder. Scand J Urol Nephrol 18:173, 1984.
62. Dean AL: Injury of the urinary bladder following irradiation of the uterus. J Urol 29:559, 1933.
63. Gowing NFC: Pathologic changes in the bladder following irradiation. Br J Radiol 33:484, 1960.
64. Boronow RC: Repair of the radiation-induced vaginal fistula utilizing the Martius technique. World J Surg 10:237, 1986.

CHAPTER 14

Female Uroradiology

Zoran L. Barbaric, M.D.

Did anybody build an upright MRI?

Dr. Shlomo Raz

Review of Imaging Methods

PROJECTIONAL RADIOGRAPHY

Projectional radiography depends on differences in attenuation of an x-ray beam as it passes through the body. The intensity of the attenuated beam is captured on film. Bone detail, calcifications, gas, and metal are well seen. Soft tissue contrast is limited because there is very little difference in x-ray attenuation between different soft tissues and water. Pelvic organs are somewhat visible mainly because they are outlined by relatively radiolucent fat.

To increase soft tissue attenuation, radiographic contrast material is instilled in retrograde manner (retrograde urethrogram, cystogram, pyelogram, loopogram), in an antegrade manner (nephrostogram, suprapubic cystogram), or by intravascular injection (intravenous pyelogram, renal arteriogram). Static radiographs obtained by such a procedure usually reflect gross pathologic processes accurately.

FLUOROSCOPY

Unlike static projectional radiography, fluoroscopy displays real-time images during the procedure. Resolution and tissue contrast are much less pronounced compared with those of projectional radiography, so that use of radiographic contrast material is almost always necessary.

In female uroradiology fluoroscopy is used often in several forms. It may be used during voiding cystourethrography (VCUG) to obtain a permanent ra-

diograph ("spot film") at just the right time. Or a real-time sequence may be recorded on videotape or other magnetic media and reviewed at leisure after the examination. From such a tape, a low-resolution permanent image can be recorded on film. Finally, simultaneous fluoroscopy and urodynamic recording is now a common procedure known as videourodynamic evaluation (Fig. 14–1).

A state license may be required to perform fluoroscopy without a radiologist in the room.

COMPUTED TOMOGRAPHY

Computed tomography (CT) has been the most revolutionary development in radiology. Its most important quality is that it can discern minute differ-

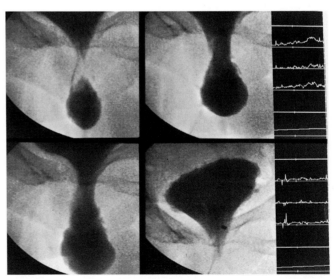

Figure 14-1 Spot films obtained during videourodynamic evaluation in a patient with moderate cystourethrocele. The graph represents true detrusor pressure when the spot film was obtained during fluoroscopy.

ences in the soft tissue attenuation of x-rays. It is possible to differentiate urine from bladder wall, acute hemorrhage from other fluid collections, and a cyst from a solid tumor. It is important also for its capability of showing slice-by-slice axial display without the overlapping densities that are so confusing on projectional radiography.

Radiographic contrast materials are still used in CT, usually by the intravenous route, to further amplify soft tissue contrast differences. Various tissues are "enhanced" according to their vascularity.

SONOGRAPHY

Although all methods using x-rays expose the patient to some radiation, diagnostic ultrasound, by all accounts, is free from any harmful energy deposition into the body. Although it is very useful in obstetric and gynecologic imaging, sonography has been only modestly useful in female uroradiologic imaging. It is most commonly used to check the kidneys for hydronephrosis and the bladder for postvoid residual urine and to search for intra-abdominal or pelvic fluid collections, such as abscesses or lymphoceles.

Other uses are being investigated. These include transperineal, transvaginal, and intraluminal imaging of the urethra, transvaginal imaging of distal ureteral obstruction, color flow imaging of ureteral jets, and possible imaging in urodynamic evaluation.

MAGNETIC RESONANCE IMAGING

In magnetic resonance imaging (MRI), radio waves from hydrogen nuclei in the body are detected, measured, and recorded. This process resolves the relative hydrogen distribution, concentration, and environment in which hydrogen atoms are bonded. For instance, urine, which has a large amount of hydrogen in the form of free water, emits radio waves in a radically different way than the hydrogen included in the body's fat or muscle. The beneficial result is

an exceptional differentiation of soft tissues on the resulting image. For instance, it is now possible to discriminate urethral muscular wall from urethral submucosa and to see the bladder, urethra, vagina, rectum, and levator muscles as separate organs without radiation or the use of contrast media.

To be sure, enticing hydrogen nuclei to become small radio stations is an expensive proposition. It requires a strong encompassing external magnet and repetitive jolts with an external radio wave by which the nuclei are made to resonate and emit at their own frequency. It is even more difficult to decipher exactly where in the body these signals are coming from and to map their intensity accurately in the form of images.

By changing certain parameters while listening for the radio signal from the patient or while inputting a radio signal into the patient, the received signal changes dramatically. These are known as T1-weighted (T1W) or T2-weighted (T2W) sequences. In the simplest possible terms, for example, urine is dark on T1W and bright on T2W sequences (Figs. 14–2 and 14–3). Many more sequences are already available or are being developed. Most likely MRI will be the dominant imaging modality in the next century (Fig. 14–4).

Just as iodinated contrast media enhance normal anatomic structures and many tumors on CT, paramagnetic contrast material enhances many lesions on MRI. The compound most commonly used is Gd-DTPA. Unlike iodinated contrast media, it does not harm the kidneys and can be used in patients with mild to moderate renal failure. Because it depends on glomerular filtration for excretion, it should not be used in patients with severe renal failure.

NUCLEAR MEDICINE

Except for voiding scintigraphy used specifically to search for vesicoureteral reflux, nuclear medicine has not found a niche in female uroradiology. Of course the usefulness of technetium-99m DTPA, techne-

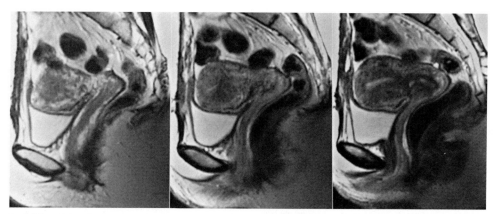

Figure 14–2 Sagittal T2-weighted sequences in the sagittal and parasagittal planes. The image on the far right shows the bladder with a dark (low-signal) wall and bright (high-signal) urine. The dome of the bladder is tented and adherent to the anterior abdominal wall because of scarring from an old cesarean section. The course of the urethra, vagina, and rectum is easily recognized. The rectum contains gas that is dark (low signal on practically all MR sequences). The uterus is anteflexed in the normal position.

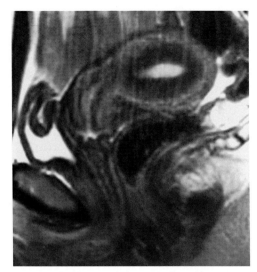

Figure 14-3 On this T2-weighted sagittal sequence the uterus is retroverted. The cervix is much more anterior compared with the uterus seen in Figure 14-2. This explains the unusual configuration of the partially filled bladder.

tium-99m DMSA, and technetium-99m MAG₃ in general urology should not be overlooked.

Bladder Imaging

BLADDER WALL THICKNESS

In the past 20 years giant leaps have been made in two medical disciplines. The first is genetics, and the second, without a doubt, is soft tissue imaging.

On most anatomic drawings, the urinary bladder is thick-walled compared with what is seen on CT or MRI. It is true that an empty bladder looks thick-walled, but this changes when even a modest amount of urine is present. A diffusely thick bladder wall implies hypertrophy, edema, or infiltration. Local wall thickening is almost always due to transitional cell carcinoma. Other neoplasms and leukoplakia are much less common.

There are two important reasons to consider bladder wall thickness. First, there is a need to try to stage early bladder carcinoma, that is, determine the depth of wall invasion. Because the bladder wall is very dark on T2W sequences, it is well contrasted with a relatively bright cancer on the same sequence.[1, 2] With contrast enhancement and improvement in resolution, it may be possible to stage such tumors as accurately as with transurethral resection (TUR).[3, 4] Histologic grading, however, is not possible with imaging alone, and it is unlikely that TUR will ever be replaced. Higher stages of cancer, particularly those involving perivesical fat infiltration, are already staged fairly accurately by MRI.

Second, the differentiation between edema or infiltration and fibrotic changes on MRI is highly accurate, although not as accurate as biopsy. On T2W sequences, fibrosis is dark while edema is bright.

DIVERTICULA

Bladder diverticula have a very thin wall because there is no muscular layer. Transitional cell carcinoma and calculi may originate or form within the diverticulum. At times, a good look into the diverticulum may be impossible or difficult at cystoscopy, and in such cases imaging can help. A simple suprapubic sonogram may determine whether there are filling defects in the diverticulum and can characterize it as soft tissue or a calculus. Otherwise, a cystogram or CT is usually sufficient to show the absence of filling defects in the bladder or to demonstrate a transitional cell carcinoma if one is present (Fig. 14-5).[5]

Spontaneous rupture of a bladder diverticulum has been described. Diagnosis can be made on cystography, CT, or sonography.[6]

A diverticulum close to the ureterovesical orifice can weaken the detrusor and promote vesicoureteral reflux. Such an entity is known as Hutch's diverticulum.[7]

INFECTIONS

A thickened bladder wall is the most common sign of infection. The other common finding is gas in the

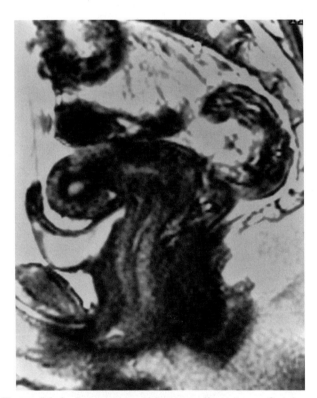

Figure 14-4 Some newer techniques allow a very fast image acquisition. For example, this snapshot of the uterus was obtained in one 20-second breath-held exposure. Although the image is somewhat noisier compared to those shown in Figures 14-2 and 14-3, the anatomic detail is truly remarkable. Indeed, it is anticipated that future generations of MR imagers will be able to obtain a full set of data from a volume of tissue in a matter of seconds and will be able to reconstruct the images in any plane desired.

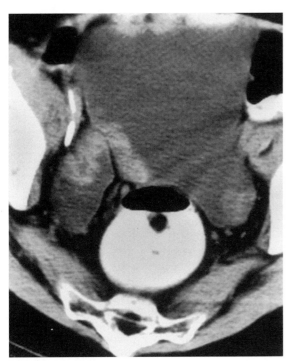

Figure 14-5 CT of the bladder and bladder diverticulum. Radiographic contrast medium has been introduced into the rectum. Bladder occupies most of the image and is fluid-filled, without contrast. Along the right posterior bladder wall there is a soft tissue density that represents transitional cell carcinoma of the bladder. In addition, a bladder diverticulum extends posteriorly and also contains transitional cell carcinoma. The diverticulum and its tumor content were not suspected or diagnosed on cystoscopy because the diverticular orifice was hidden from view by the bulky carcinoma. Multicentric transitional cell carcinoma was also found in the posterolateral bladder.

bladder, bladder wall, or even the perivesical areas, an entity known as emphysematous cystitis. As expected, bladder wall thickening and gas are best seen on CT (Fig. 14–6).[8] On sonography the bladder is

hyperechoic because gas bubbles cause a diffuse increase in acoustic impedance.[9, 10] It is common knowledge that several bacteria may cause emphysematous cystitis. It is less well known that strains of *Candida albicans* can also produce intraluminal gas in addition to fungus balls.[11]

FISTULA

Vesicovaginal fistula is best seen on a lateral view on cystography or voiding cystourethrography (VCUG). It is not absolutely necessary that a cystogram be obtained in the upright position, but it is necessary to obtain films *before* the voiding phase. Some retrograde vaginal filling is common during voiding, and there should be no confusion about where the contrast in the vagina came from. Vesicovaginal fistula can also be demonstrated on CT (Fig. 14–7).

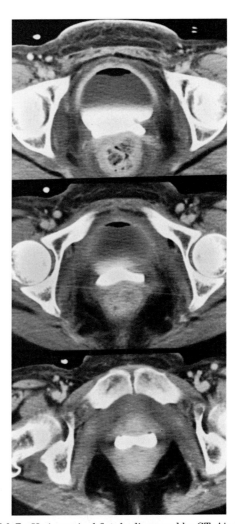

Figure 14-7 Vesicovaginal fistula diagnosed by CT. Air-fluid and fluid-fluid levels (urine and contrast) are seen in the bladder. In the absence of any bladder instrumentation or infection, the presence of intraluminal gas is diagnostic of a fistula. More caudally, the vagina is filled with contrast trickling through the fistulous tract from the bladder on this contrast-enhanced CT image. Note that no bladder catheter is in place.

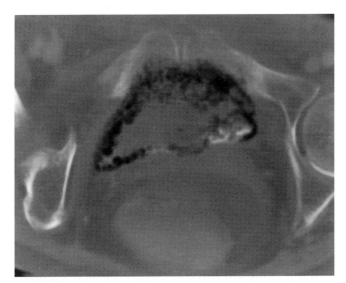

Figure 14-6 Emphysematous cystitis seen on CT. Multiple bubbles of gas are present in the bladder wall. The bubbles are radiolucent, or, in CT terminology, "hypodense."

Urethrovaginal fistula is less common and more difficult to diagnose precisely because of retrograde vaginal filling. Exceptionally good films must be obtained, usually in the upright projection, during the act of voiding. This is no small task because the true lateral projection usually turns out underexposed. The best projection is an upright steep oblique. At times an occlusive double-balloon catheter must be used to demonstrate the fistula and exclude vesicovaginal fistula (Fig. 14–8).

Vesicorectal fistula is rare. It is usually a complication of gynecologic surgery, made worse by radiation therapy or pelvic abscess. This type of fistula is difficult to image. Gas in the bladder (best seen on CT) is suggestive provided that the bladder has not been instrumented in the recent past. The traditional study is a cystogram followed by a contrast enema if the cystogram is inconclusive. Cystography could be performed in the CT scanner because a minute amount of contrast material, which may find its way into the rectum, is that much better seen.

Perineal fistulas complicating ileal loop or other diversionary procedures are usually easy to diagnose. These fistulas are usually the result of loop necrosis due to radiation therapy. A loopogram or a pouchogram in an oblique projection is sufficient and shows extravasation of contrast agent extending from the loop to the perineum. These patients are usually not candidates for surgery, and percutaneous diversion is necessary to dry the perineum. Percutaneous nephrostomy alone may not be sufficient. Some practitioners have proposed ureteral fulguration through the nephrostomy tract. The ureter will become fibrosed and close off within a day or two. When the fistula closes and the patient becomes a surgical candidate again, revision of the ileal loop and a new ureteral anastomosis can be considered.

FILLING DEFECTS

The traditional "big three" filling defects are bladder calculi, blood clots, and tumors. Less common are ureteroceles, fungus balls, and sloughed papilla. Calculi are easy to detect on sonography because they are markedly hyperechoic and produce extensive "shadowing." They are also easily detected on precontrast CT owing to the exceptional contrast resolution of this modality. Calculi are not easy to see on plain radiographs. Many are missed because of superimposed intestinal gas and osseous structures, which often obscure a rather poorly calcified bladder stone.

On precontrast CT acute blood clots have a higher density than other soft tissues, such as muscle.

Urethral Imaging

NORMAL ANATOMY

Until very recently only the urethral lumen could be rendered visible on cystourethrography or double-balloon retrograde urethrography. This modality alone provided important information about the relative position of the urethra, urethral strictures, urethral displacement (by tumor or periurethral abscesses), and urethral diverticula. Now, however, it is possible to examine the urethra in much greater detail. On T2W MRI sequences the dark outer muscular ring encloses and coapts the abundant and relatively bright submucosa. The soft tissues surrounding the urethra are also seen well on MRI. It is possible to discern layers of endopelvic fascia, periurethral fat, and retropubic space and to examine the position of the urethra in relation to the osseous structures in any plane. To a lesser extent this is also possible using an intraluminal ultrasound probe.

PROLAPSE

The relation of the bladder base and urethra to the pubosacral line determines whether urethral prolapse exists. Radiographically, this relationship is determined during upright voiding cystourethrography, often in conjunction with videourodynamic evaluation. Relaxed and strained images, preferably taken in a true lateral projection, show urethral mobility, the degree of urethral prolapse, and the presence of cystocele, rectocele, or enterocele (Fig. 14–9).

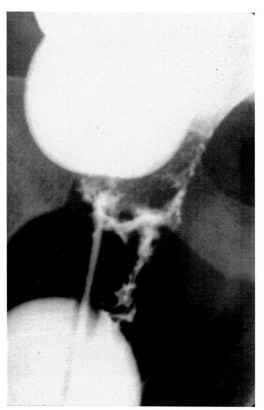

Figure 14-8 Urethrovaginal fistula. The origin of the fistula is demonstrated on a double balloon retrograde urethrogram. The fistulous tract rises very high, almost to the bladder neck, and extends posterolaterally to the vagina.

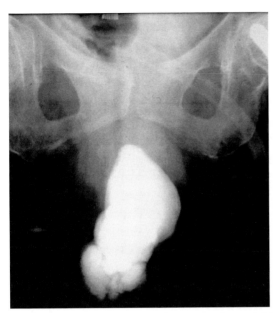

Figure 14-9 Total bladder prolapse is seen on the upright post-voiding radiograph taken as a part of a cystogram. Such a massive prolapse is almost always associated with large postvoiding residual urine.

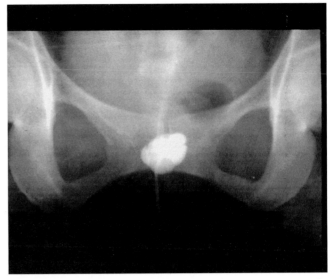

Figure 14-10 Urethral diverticulum arising from the mid-urethra. Radiographic contrast was injected directly into the diverticulum at the time of ureteroscopy.

Recently an attempt has been made to demonstrate prolapse and urethral mobility on sagittal MRI sequences obtained at varying degrees of straining and during a 20-second breath-hold. The resultant images can be looped electronically into a ciné format and replayed on the cathode ray tube (CRT) viewing station. A number of additional relative measurements are possible with this method, such as the relationship of the proximal and distal vagina, rectal ampulla, anus, and uterus to the pubosacral line. Aside from cost, the main disadvantages of this method are that the patient is in the supine position (stress incontinence is associated with an upright stance) and many elderly patients are unable to strain and hold the breath for as long as 20 seconds.

URETHRAL DIVERTICULA

Most urethral diverticula are filled with contrast and can be seen distinctly on a good VCUG film; they are also frequently detected on postvoiding films obtained during an intravenous pyelogram (Fig. 14–10). The need for double-balloon retrograde urethrography occurs very rarely.[12] High-resolution imaging of the urethra, using either MRI or intraluminal urethral sonography or endovaginal or transperineal sonography, may also be used.[13, 14] MRI has been recommended for imaging difficult diverticula (Figs. 14–11 and 14–12).[15]

On VCUG and double-balloon urethrography the diverticulum is usually visible posteriorly at the midurethra and may be slightly off center. At times it may be septated and may contain intraluminal filling defects such as a radiopaque stone, blood clot, or, rarely, a tumor. The diverticula are usually not very large. Occasionally, however, a large diverticulum may elevate the bladder base, producing an appearance very similar to that of an enlarged prostate in a male.

At the distal end of the urethra, abscessed Skene's glands may also assume diverticular shape.

PERIURETHRAL ABSCESSES

Both MRI and endovaginal or intraluminal urethral sonography can depict abnormal periurethral fluid collections. These patients are usually symptomatic

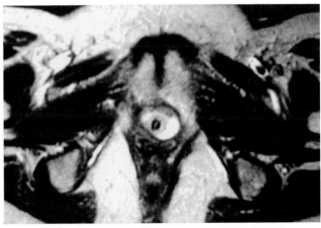

Figure 14-11 Urethral diverticulum. Axial T2-weighted sequence shows the urethral catheter (dark area) surrounded by submucosa (gray area). Fluid in the diverticulum (bright) is found predominantly toward the right but also partially encircles the submucosa. The peculiar finding is that the muscular sphincter, which normally is a dark ring encapsulating the mucosa, is seen surrounding the diverticulum. This suggests that the urethral diverticulum may in fact be contained within the muscular sphincter.

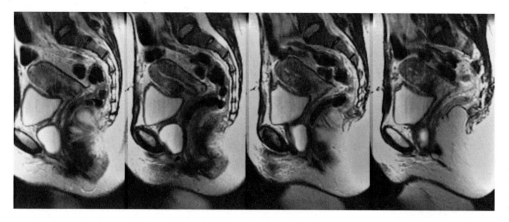

Figure 14-12 Urethral diverticulum. Composite of several sagittal and parasagittal images from a T2-weighted sequence. To find the midline cut it is best to look for the symphysis pubis. The symphysis is dark *(third image from the left)* in this sequence, as opposed to the pubic bones with their high-signal, bright bone marrow. A large diverticulum is present posterior and to one side of the urethra.

and may not be comfortable undergoing endoluminal sonography (Fig. 14–13).

INTRAURETHRAL INJECTIONS

Collagen, Teflon, and autologous fat have been injected into the urethral submucosa to increase resistance in the treatment of some types of urinary incontinence (Fig. 14–14).

Vaginal Imaging

ANATOMY

It was only with the introduction of MRI that vaginal anatomy became better understood. Unlike classic anatomic drawings, the vagina has a moderate midangulation such that it assumes a boomerang shape in the sagittal plane. In the axial plane the distal vagina has an H shape, whereas the more proximal

vagina with its fornices assumes an inverted U shape.

GARTNER'S DUCT CYST

Gartner's duct cysts are remnants of the wolffian duct and are found in the broad ligaments and vaginal wall, where they are usually small and asymptomatic.

Uterine Imaging

Because uterine or ovarian tumors may affect the bladder and interfere with normal voiding function, a brief survey of the current imaging methods of the pelvic organs is important.[16] Sonography remains the mainstay of gynecologic imaging. However, in the past several years MRI has provided superb detailed soft tissue differentiation of the uterus, particularly on T2-weighted sequences. The uterine cavity is bright (high signal) and is surrounded by grayish-

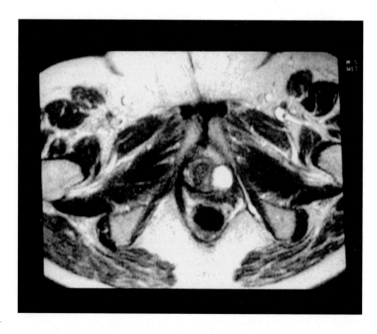

Figure 14-13 Periurethral abscess is seen as a bright collection of fluid to the left of the urethra. Unlike the diverticulum shown in Figure 14–11, the abscess is definitely outside of the muscular sphincter. This patient also had had periurethral injections of Teflon, which is not visible by MR imaging.

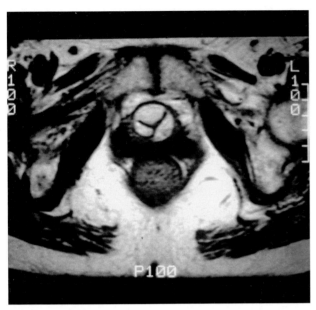

Figure 14-14 Submucosal injection of autologous fat has been tried in a group of patients with urinary incontinence. The fat is bright on a T2-weighted sequence. Seen here in detail is the new shape of the coapted urethral lumen. Instead of autologous fat, the current technique uses injections of collagen.

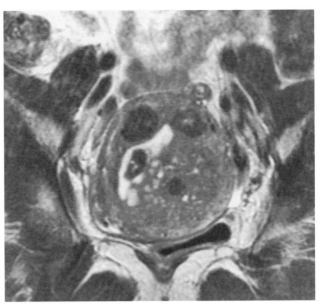

Figure 14-15 Leiomyoma and adenomyosis. On this T2-weighted coronal section through the uterus one can see a distorted endometrial cavity (bright area). The distortion is caused by a heterogeneous mass without clearly demarcated borders containing small bright areas that are probably hemorrhagic islands. This is typical of adenomyosis. Anterior to the endometrial cavity there is a well-demarcated, dark (low signal), small, 2-cm leiomyoma. Several other small leiomyomas may also be present—one in particular is probably subserosal because it protrudes into the endometrial cavity. Note how the rectum (low signal) is compressed between the mass and left levator ani muscle.

appearing myometrium. The innermost layer of myometrium is distinctly dark (low signal) and is referred to as the junctional zone.

Leiomyoma is the most common tumor of the uterus and, depending on its location, may interfere with pregnancy. Large tumors may impinge on the bladder or may be a source of pelvic pain. Because of its high fibrous tissue content the tumor appears dark on T2W sequences and is always well encapsulated. At times a bright rim is present, probably reflecting edema and enlarged lymphatic channels.[17] Large tumors may also degenerate or hemorrhage. These areas cause a dramatic change in signal intensity and appear heterogeneous and usually bright.[18]

Adenomyosis is also very common and may present as a uterine mass. The islands of endometrial tissues embedded in the myometrium respond to cyclical hormonal changes. Intermittent hemorrhage appears bright on T2W sequences, but in addition overgrowth and condensation of the smooth muscle occur as a response. These areas appear dark, and, unlike leiomyoma, there is no sharp demarcation between normal myometrium and the tumor mass.[19] MRI has become the imaging modality of choice in differentiating these two lesions, superseding even sonography (Fig. 14–15).[20]

ENDOMETRIOSIS

Common sites of ectopic endometrial implants outside the uterus are the ovary, the serosal surface of the uterus, the uterosacral ligament, and the cul-de-sac. These surface implants are not well imaged by any method short of laparoscopy. The response to

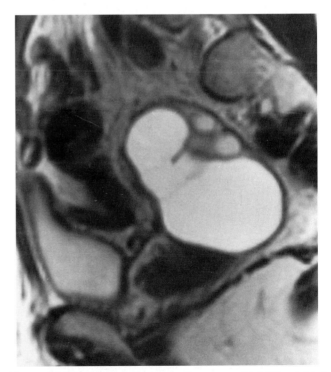

Figure 14-16 Endometrioma. On the parasagittal T2-weighted sequence the bladder is seen just above the pubic bone. A large endometrioma is typically bright (high signal) and is surrounded by dense fibrotic tissues.

cyclic hemorrhage may be a massive fibrotic reaction, which produces large adherent masses or encapsulated hemorrhagic cysts (endometrioma). Fibrotic masses and old hemorrhagic cysts are easily differentiated as such by MRI.[21, 22] Old hemorrhage is typically bright (high signal) on both T1W and T2W sequences (Fig. 14–16).

A similar reaction at the less common implantation sites may produce symptoms related to the urinary tract. For example, ureteral endometriosis may produce obstruction and hydronephrosis. Bladder endometriosis may interfere with normal bladder function or may mimic interstitial cystitis (Fig. 14–17).[23, 24]

Pelvic Inflammatory Disease

Of 1 million patients treated yearly for acute salpingitis, some 8.5% develop tubo-ovarian abscess (TOA).[25] Pelvic inflammatory disease and TOA are characterized by symptoms of abdominal pain, fever, and leukocytosis.

Sonography is usually the first imaging modality used and shows varying amounts of pelvic fluid or endometrial fluid. Hydrosalpinx and pyosalpinx are recognized as cystic structures with internal echoes producing adnexal distortion.[26]

TOA appears as one or more cystic or solid masses by any imaging modality. The lesion may be several centimeters in size and may be bilateral.[27]

Pelvic abscesses that do not respond to antimicrobial therapy may be percutaneously drained. A variety of percutaneous approaches are used, including anterior abdominal wall, transgluteal, transvaginal, and paracoccygeal approaches.[28, 29]

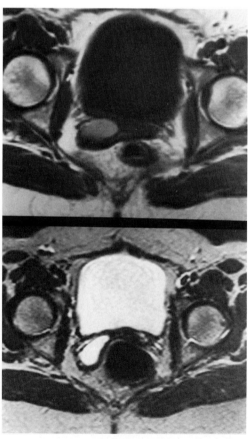

Figure 14–17 Bladder endometrioma. A mass at the posterior wall of the bladder is relatively bright on a T1-weighted sequence *(upper image)* and on a T2-weighted sequence *(lower image)*. The bladder behaves differently because on a T1-weighted sequence, in contrast to an endometrioma, it is typically of low signal intensity.

REFERENCES

1. Fisher MR, Hricak H, Tanagho EA: Urinary bladder MR imaging. Part II. Neoplasm. Radiology 157:471–477, 1985.
2. Rholl SK, Lee JKT, Heiken JP, et al: Primary bladder carcinoma: Evaluation with MR imaging. Radiology 163:117–121, 1987.
3. Neuerburg JM, Bohndorf K, Sohn M, et al: Urinary bladder neoplasms: Evaluation with contrast-enhanced MR imaging. Radiology 172:739–743, 1989.
4. Tanimoto A, Yuasa Y, Imai Y, et al: Bladder tumor staging: Comparison of conventional and gadolinium-enhanced dynamic MR imaging and CT. Radiology 185:741–747, 1992.
5. Dondalski M, White EM, Ghahremani GG, Patel SK: Carcinoma arising in urinary bladder diverticula: Imaging findings in six patients. AJR 161:817–820, 1993.
6. Itoh N, Kounami T: Spontaneous rupture of a bladder diverticulum: Ultrasonographic diagnosis. J Urol 152:1206–1207, 1994.
7. Hutch JH: Vesico-ureteral reflux in the paraplegic. Cause and correction. J Urol 68:457–465, 1952.
8. Bohlman ME, Fishman EK, Oesterling JE, Goldman SM: CT findings in emphysematous cystitis. Urology 32:63–64, 1988.
9. Kauzlaric D, Barmeir E: Sonography of emphysematous cystitis. J Ultrasound Med 4:319, 1985.
10. Quint HJ, Drach GW, Rappaport WD, Hoffmann CJ: Emphysematous cystitis: A review of the spectrum of disease. J Urol 147:134–137, 1992.
11. Bartkowski DP, Lanesky JR: Emphysematous prostatitis and cystitis secondary to *Candida albicans*. J Urol 139:1063–1065, 1988.
12. Greenberg M, Stone D, Cochran ST, et al: Female urethral diverticula: Double balloon catheter study. AJR 136:259–264, 1981.
13. Keefe B, Warshauer DM, Tucker SM, Mittelstaedt CA: Diverticula of the female urethra: Diagnosis by endovaginal and transperineal sonography. AJR 156:1195–1197, 1991.
14. Chang TS, Böhm-Vélez M, Mendelson EB: Nongynecologic applications of transvaginal sonography. AJR 160:87–93, 1993.
15. Kim B, Hricak H, Tanagho EA: Diagnosis of urethral diverticula in women: Value of MR imaging. AJR 161:809–815, 1993.
16. Langer R, Golan A, Neuman M, et al: The effect of large uterine fibroids on urinary bladder function and symptoms. Am J Obstet Gynecol 163:1139–1141, 1990.
17. Mittl RL, Yeh IT, Kressel HY: High-signal-intensity rim surrounding uterine leiomyomas on MR images: Pathologic correlation. Radiology 180:81–83, 1991.
18. Okizuka H, Sugimura K, Takemori M, et al: MR detection of degenerating uterine leiomyoma. J Comput Assist Tomogr 17:760–766, 1993.
19. Mark AS, Hricak H, Heinrichs LW, et al: Adenomyosis and leiomyoma: Differential diagnosis with MR imaging. Radiology 163:527–529, 1987.
20. Ascher SM, Arnold LL, Patt RH, et al: Adenomyosis: Prospective comparison of MR imaging and transvaginal sonography. Radiology 190:803–806, 1994.
21. Togashi K, Nishimura K, Kimura I, et al: Endometrial cysts: Diagnosis with MR imaging. Radiology 180:73–78, 1991.

22. Siegelman ES, Outwater E, Wang T, Mitchell DG: Solid pelvic masses caused by endometriosis: MR imaging features. AJR 163:357–361, 1994.
23. Sircus SI, Sant GR, Ucci AA Jr: Bladder detrusor endometriosis mimicking interstitial cystitis. Urology 32:339–342, 1988.
24. Shook TE, Nyberg LM: Endometriosis of the urinary tract. Urology 31:1–6, 1988.
25. Casola, G, vanSonnenberg E, D'Agostino HB, et al: Percutaneous drainage of tubo-ovarian abscesses. Radiology 182:399–402, 1992.
26. Bulas DI, Ahlstrom PA, Sivit CJ, et al: Pelvic inflammatory disease in the adolescent: Comparison of transabdominal and transvaginal sonographic evaluation. Radiology 183:435–439, 1992.
27. Wilbur AC, Aizenstein RI, Napp TE: CT findings in tubo-ovarian abscess. AJR 158:575–579, 1992.
28. Tyrell RT, Murphy FB, Bernardino ME: Tubo-ovarian abscesses: CT-guided percutaneous drainage. Radiology 175:87–89, 1990.
29. Longo JM, Bilbao JI, deVilla VH, et al: CT-Guided paracoccygeal drainage of pelvic abscesses. J Comput Assist Tomogr 17:909–914, 1993.

PART III

Voiding Dysfunction

CHAPTER 15

Interstitial Cystitis

C. Lowell Parsons, M.D.
J. Kellogg Parsons

Interstitial cystitis (IC) is a syndrome. It is a severe and debilitating disorder of the bladder characterized by severe urinary frequency, urgency, and/or lower abdominal or perineal pain. In all likelihood, several pathologic mechanisms produce the IC symptom complex. Patient histories obtained from individuals afflicted with a severe form of this bladder dysfunction reveal that in most cases it typically has a gradual onset and an insidious progression. One could pose the question, "What is the diagnosis for an individual with an early phase of IC?" To define the IC syndrome, it is important to consider this question, especially because the early (mild) phase of this disorder may be known by many names—urethral syndrome, trigonitis, urgency-frequency syndrome, or pseudomembranous trigonitis. All descriptions reduce to one common complaint: urinary urgency, frequency, or bladder pain in the absence of bacterial infection (or other definable pathology). The milder form of the urgency-frequency syndrome is present in perhaps 20% of individuals in whom recurrent urinary tract infection is initially diagnosed but who in fact have negative urinary cultures. These are the people whose symptoms persist despite antibiotic therapy and despite a negative culture. Physicians repeatedly tell such patients that they have a bladder infection and that symptoms will resolve spontaneously after several weeks or months. Consequently, the disorder in many such patients remains undiagnosed because they have no major clinical problem (or they learn to "live with their symptoms"). Without a clear-cut pathologic marker, it is difficult to put a distinct label on these patients. They are unlikely to be deemed to have IC, but in fact they may have a mild form of this disorder.

This presentation approach is adopted from the broader viewpoint that IC is a relatively heterogeneous disorder in which the severity of symptoms has a Poisson distribution. Patients at the extreme end of the bell-shaped curve have traditionally been assigned this diagnosis, but in fact most patients belong in the middle with mild and moderate symptoms that may be intermittent in nature. In addition to the diagnostic dilemma it poses, this disorder has been frustrating for the physician to treat because its cause (probably multifaceted) is unknown, and therapy consequently is not only limited but also different for the various subsets of patients. Fortunately, some advances have been made in pathogenesis, diagnosis, and treatment in recent years. These are reviewed in this chapter.

There are many misconceptions about IC. Confusion exists about normal bladder capacity under anesthesia, the appearance of a Hunner's ulcer, the existence of glomerulations, the definition of an abnormal voiding pattern, and what pathologic changes are found. These problems are also reviewed, first to help clarify them, second to provide some findings that may establish a clinical diagnosis, and third to promote better understanding of the different mechanisms involved in the pathogenesis and therapies of IC.

Definition

Because IC is a clinical syndrome rather than a pathologic diagnosis, its definition has undergone significant changes in recent years consequent to the marked interest in studying this disease. Expansion of the definition is controversial, but as clinical and epidemiologic data accumulate, this has been the steady trend. Historically, it has been widely accepted that patients with an extremely small bladder capacity who have the Hunner's ulcer (patch)[1, 2] and who also complain of severe bladder pain and urinary urgency represent the syndrome. Problems arise, however, when one attempts to diagnose a patient who has a relatively short history (perhaps 5 to 7 months) of urinary urgency and frequency and perhaps some bladder-associated pain. In these individuals urgency-frequency syndrome (UFS), urethral syndrome, urethrotrigonitis, or other related disorders may be diagnosed. There is, however, a growing tendency to consider such symptoms as a mild form of IC. IC is a good term for this symptom complex because it suggests involvement of layers deeper than the bladder epithelium, which is probably true because the sensory nerves that provide awareness of symptoms are in the interstitium.

This review uses the broad definition of IC and includes patients who have urinary urgency and frequency or bladder pain in the absence of any demonstrable infection or other pathologic entity (e.g., radiation cystitis or cancer) that might induce such symptoms. Furthermore, this review also assumes that the cause of this syndrome is probably not singular; rather, the syndrome represents several potential causes with a common result. In this sense, it is important to realize that IC is a "syndrome"—that is, there may be many stimuli that provoke the bladder and initiate IC symptoms. The bladder reacts to each of these stimuli with urgency, frequency, or pain—essentially its only possible response to noxious stimuli.

Another reason for using a broad definition of the syndrome is that the disorder is, in all probability, underdiagnosed. Many patients with milder forms of the disease could readily benefit from therapy if the diagnosis were considered. Treatment may be withheld and the patient's condition subsequently made worse if the physician reserves the diagnosis of IC for the more severe and "classic" symptoms.

Pathogenesis

Since the original description of the "elusive ulcer" of Hunner approximately 75 years ago,[1, 2] there has been slow progress in defining the cause of this disorder. In part, this is because the severe form is relatively rare, making access to large numbers of patients for studies difficult. Many causes of IC have been suggested. Explanations include problems with the lymphatic system; chronic infection; neurologic, psychologic, or autoimmune disorders; and vasculitis.[3–11] Most of the proposed causes are hypothetical and are supported by few data to define the role of these mechanisms. For example, Oravisto[10] has suggested that IC patients have increased levels of antinuclear antibodies. It is difficult to know what this means, however, because there is no obvious association with systemic autoimmune phenomena in these patients. In addition, modest rises in such antibodies may occur nonspecifically in any chronic disease.

Currently, several factors seem to play a causative role in IC. One of the more popular theories is that a defective bladder epithelium causes loss of the "blood-urine" barrier, resulting in a leaky membrane.[12, 13] Many of the symptoms associated with the complex could result from an epithelium that is permeable to small molecules. Chronic leak of small molecules could induce sensory nerves to depolarize, resulting in urgency-frequency.[14, 15] Diffusion of potassium across the membrane, for instance, could trigger the sensory nerve endings.[16] This ion permeability concept is attractive, particularly because most patients do not demonstrate any significant signs of inflammatory response in the bladder muscle or serum.[46] Moreover, no more than one-third of the patients have mast cells, the degranulation of which might otherwise account for the sensory-urgency symptoms.[9, 17–19]

EPITHELIAL LEAK

The more popular theory concerning pathogenesis today, as noted earlier, is that of an epithelial leak. Prior to 1986 there had been few data to support the concept that such a leak existed.[12] Studies were unable to confirm the initial observation that ruthenium red penetration in tight junctions is similar in normals and IC patients. Recently, however, a well-controlled study in 56 patients has provided data supporting the hypothesis that the bladder surface in many patients with IC may indeed leak.[13] These investigators, who have developed an extremely sensitive leak assay, believe that about 70% of patients with IC have a "leaky epithelium" and 30% do not.[90] They propose that those who do not experience leakage have some other problem, such as a neurologic abnormality or inflammation. They emphasize the fact that these findings support the concept that the urgency-frequency syndrome has several causes and that it may now be possible to stratify patients by etiology (leakers versus nonleakers).

GLYCOSAMINOGLYCANS: THE BLOOD-URINE BARRIER

Control of epithelial permeability in the bladder has traditionally been ascribed to tight junctions unique to the bladder epithelium and ion pumps.[12, 20–26] However, recent studies have provided physiologic data suggesting that bladder surface proteoglycans or glycosaminoglycans (GAG) may actually be the principal mechanism by which the epithelium maintains a barrier between the bladder wall and urine, the so-called blood-urine barrier.[13–15]

Surface proteoglycans (GAG, mucus) appear to have multiple protective roles in the bladder including antiadherence and regulation of transepithelial solute movement.[15, 27–29] The external surface glycosaminoglycans of the transitional cell are capable of preventing the adherence of bacteria, crystals, proteins, and ions. This function is lost when the GAG layer is removed by a dilute acid or detergent[27–30] but restored when it is replaced by exogenous polysaccharides such as heparin or pentosanpolysulfate (PPS).[27, 31, 32] The oxygen atom present on the sulfated polysaccharides is negatively charged and has a high tendency to bond ionically with water. This results in exclusion of urinary ionic solutes by the Donnan effect.[33] When GAG is present on a surface (the bladder), it will in effect bind water molecules tightly to the oxygen of the sulfate groups in preference to calcium, barium, and even hydrogen ions.[34–36] Water molecules are trapped and interposed at the boundary between the cell surface (bladder) and the environment (urine) (Fig. 15–1). This bound molecular layer of water acts as a physical barrier to urinary solutes like urea and calcium.[15, 27] Such substances are unable to reach the underlying cell membrane, adhere to it, or move across it.

Quaternary amines, on the other hand, demonstrate a high affinity for sulfated polysaccharides and displace the water bound to the oxygen groups.[33, 37, 38] This concept is supported by the fact that when GAG reacts chemically with quaternary amines, the result is an increased entropy reflecting the loss of water ordering around the sulfate groups.[33, 39] This interaction is the basis for the clinical use of protamine sulfate (a quaternary amine) to precipitate and inactivate the anticoagulant effects of heparin. It has been demonstrated in both animal and human models that protamine sulfate inactivates native cell surface polysaccharides and results in increased epithelial permeability. Such damage to the transitional cells can be reversed by the addition of glycosaminoglycans such as heparin.[14, 15]

Based on these concepts, Parsons and colleagues proposed that the surface polysaccharide is functionally defective (but not absent) in some patients with IC.[40–42] Possible causes for the deficiency include reduced sulfation of the polysaccharides, diminished density or thickness of material, or the presence of a

GAG layer–inactivating compound such as a urinary quaternary amine. It has been demonstrated that normal individuals in whom the bladder surface is challenged by the quaternary amine protamine lose the impermeability of the epithelium. Permeability to urea in normal individuals increases from 5 to 25%[14] (Fig. 15–2). When the blood-urine barrier is lost because of protamine treatment, all normal subjects experience urgency, frequency, and bladder pain (the same symptoms that characterize IC). These symptoms are reversed with subsequent treatment with heparin. These data are supported by the fact that a synthetic polysaccharide similar to heparin is effective in ameliorating the symptoms of IC.[40–42, 91, 92] To test the hypothesis that some patients with IC have a permeable transitional cell layer, Parsons and colleagues measured the permeability of the normal bladder epithelium to a concentrated solution of urea and compared it with the bladder epithelium in patients with IC.[13] Twenty-nine normal controls absorbed approximately 5% of the urea, whereas 56 patients with IC absorbed 25% (Fig. 15–3). Based on these observations, Parsons and colleagues proposed that some patients with IC do have a leaky epithelium. The leak, moreover, results in urgency, frequency, and other secondary changes seen in the subepithelial tissues. Probably about 70% of patients with IC have such leaks.

The role of mast cells in this disorder is not understood. Mast cells have been reported by a number of investigators to be present in IC bladders, yet other data suggest that they are also present in non-IC bladders.[9, 11, 18, 19] The central point of confusion is whether mast cells play a causative or a secondary role in IC. If their role is causative, the cells perhaps produce symptoms by degranulating. If it is secondary, on the other hand, they represent a response to whatever is causing IC (e.g., an epithelial leak). If

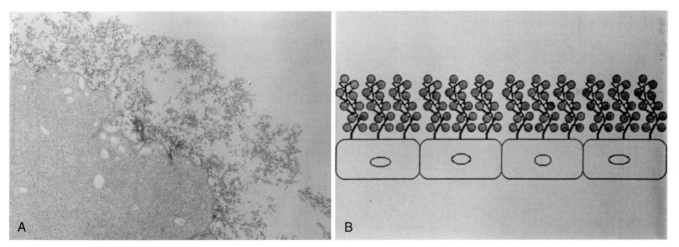

Figure 15–1 *A,* The electron microscopic photomicrograph supports the concept that the glycosaminoglycan hydrates the cell surface. The glycosaminoglycan is stained with ruthenium red. The spaces in the layer represent trapped (bound) water. *B,* The concept of a biofilm layer at the bladder surface is shown schematically and demonstrates the location of the trapped water at the surface. Circles represent bound water, and the wavy lines represent the protein backbone.

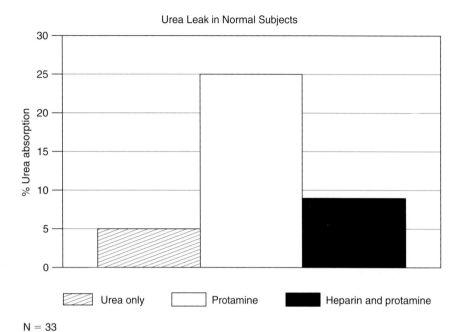

Figure 15-2 Results of urea movement across human epithelium. All subjects underwent three instillations of urea into the bladder. First, each person received urea; then, each was exposed to protamine (2.5 mg/ml for 15 minutes) and underwent a second urea test (protamine); next, each had a heparin treatment and underwent a third urea test (heparin). Protamine sulfate destroyed the permeability barrier (polysaccharide), as shown by increased urea absorption (25%). Heparin reduced the leak (9%).

the latter case is true, then the cells might be a type of defense mechanism that ultimately may even become part of the problem.

There have been attempts to quantify mast cells (granulated and degranulated) both in the mucosa and in the subepithelial tissues.[43–45] Some investigators believe that mast cells are involved in IC, whereas others believe that there is no increase in mast cells in IC compared with other patient groups. However, it is significant that most of the "controls" studied had bladder cancer and therefore were not normal.[43–45] Nonetheless, the presence of mast cells in one-third of patients may result in degranulation and aggravation of symptoms. Control of this degranulation (even though the cells may be a defense mechanism) may be helpful in some patients and will

be discussed later. It is important to reemphasize the potential for multiple causes of IC. The presence of mast cells in a subset of patients may turn out to be important for diagnosis and therapy in that select subset.

The role of inflammation and inflammatory mediators in IC is not known. Traditionally, there has been an assumption that inflammation is present in IC. However, this is probably not the case in most patients. First, almost no inflammation has been observed on biopsy specimens. Second, no systemic signs have been found—that is, no leukocytosis.[46] Third, no inflammatory mediators have been located in the urine of more than 90% of these patients.[47] Finally, patients with IC do not suffer from other generalized inflammatory diseases such as collagen

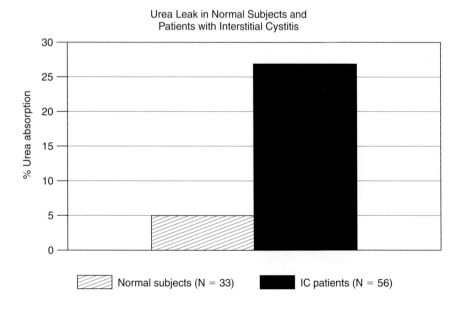

Figure 15-3 Absorption of a urea solution placed in the bladder of normal subjects was 5%, whereas it was 27% in subjects with interstitial cystitis (IC). In comparison, normal subjects whose mucus was destroyed by protamine absorbed 25% (see Fig. 15–2), similar to IC patients.

vascular disease.[3, 8] Still, there may be a significant interplay between mast cells and inflammatory cells (their mediators) that is yet to be determined in some subsets of patients.

It has been suggested that psychosomatic factors initiate IC, but this is rarely the case. On the other hand, most patients (especially those afflicted with chronic pain) are secondarily affected by their disease and, as a result, may show signs of mild or moderate chronic depression. Those suffering from severe nocturia show even more profound depression owing to sleep deprivation. In my experience, no one has ever been cured of IC by psychotherapy. Earlier researchers reported similar findings.[4] It is important to emphasize that treating depression can improve the overall sense of well-being of a patient and help him or her cope with the disease, but it will not cure IC or reduce the number of daily voids. It is true that acute stress causes flare-ups of IC symptoms and stress reduction improves them, but the patient still has IC. Thus, the physician should remember that IC is not a psychological disorder and should explicitly explain this to the patient.

Incidence and Epidemiology

Although IC was first identified in 1907 by Nitze, few epidemiologic studies have been reported.[48] Oravisto, in a Finnish study of 103 people with IC, estimated the annual incidence as 1.2 cases per 100,000 and the prevalence as about 10 to 11 per 100,000.[49]

The incidence in the United States has been estimated from two sources. Held and associates estimated the incidence as about 44,000 cases in the United States[50]; my estimate, extrapolated from San Diego County, is 40,000 to 60,000. Held and associates also estimated a worst-case incidence in the United States as 450,000.[51]

These studies reveal several risk factors in regard to demography. Sex, of course, is a risk factor; IC has a female-male ratio of about 9:1[50, 52–54] in all reports. Age is also a risk factor because incidence is generally limited to those over 18 years of age. Nevertheless, cases have been reported in younger people.[55–58] The median age at diagnosis is between 42 and 46 years in most series, but the disease appears several years earlier.[50, 52, 59] The average duration of symptoms is 3 to 4 years.[4, 59] Race and ethnicity appear to be risk factors because the disease occurs mostly in whites[60–62] but has also been reported in blacks.[63]

In a review of 300 cases at the University of California at San Diego, it was observed that patients without diabetes seem to be at a greater risk.[59] Finally, a 400% increased incidence was seen in Jewish people. All these findings are similar to those reported in patients with inflammatory bowel diseases.[52, 64–69]

Pathology

One of the main diagnostic problems with IC is the lack of pathologic findings that can be readily identified and quantified. Various descriptions have been proposed, but unfortunately there is nothing pathognomonic of IC in bladder biopsy specimens. The mast cell controversy has already been reviewed; approximately one-third of these patients have increased mast cell infiltration of the bladder wall and mucosa. The significance of this, as noted earlier, is unknown. Light microscopy generally reveals a urothelium that is thinned, readily detached, and nearly absent in many areas.

Unlike the normal epithelium, which is six or seven layers thick, the mucosa is frequently only two to four cell layers thick. These changes are consistent with a dysfunctional epithelium.[13] A generalized pancystitis[70–73] with infiltration of the lamina propria by mononuclear and chronic inflammatory cells is observed. However, these changes are also consistent with the effects of hydrodilation. Most physicians in fact, perform biopsy after the distention; thus, many of these changes may be artifacts.

The distribution of collagen within the bladder wall is controversial.[74] One hypothesis is that as the disorder progresses, a fibrotic small end-stage type of bladder develops. There are few or no data to support this theory. I believe that this is untrue; instead, I suggest that frequent low-volume voiding leads to a thinned epithelium with atrophic muscle bundles and a small bladder as a net result. Furthermore, the only scarring present in the bladder wall is probably iatrogenic and stems from prior biopsies because many of these patients undergo multiple biopsies over a period of years.[74] As the entire bladder shrinks from frequent low-volume voiding, this scar tissue assumes a disproportionate and artifactually enlarged total volume of the bladder wall. In my experience (over 500 biopsies), scarring in fact is not identified when biopsy specimens are obtained from an area of the bladder that has not previously undergone biopsy. At my institution, 27 patients have had cystectomy performed for IC. Seventy percent of these patients have a bladder composed of only epithelium and a few blood vessels and muscle bundles. There is also severe wasting of perivesical fat. Perhaps the urinary solutes leak through the thin (perhaps 3 to 4 mm) bladder wall, and the perivesical fat atrophies. This may help to explain the increasingly diffuse lower abdominal pain experienced by these patients. The medial thigh pain may represent provocation of the obturator nerves.

Bladder biopsy is useless in IC because it is not diagnostic. There is no way to diagnose or rule out this disorder by pathologic examination of bladder tissue. Some of the changes, as mentioned earlier, however, are associated with IC. Although it is rare for these patients to be confused with those having carcinoma in situ of the bladder, biopsy may be necessary to rule out cancer.[75] A combination of cytologic evaluation of the urine and bladder washings plus the biopsy is necessary to exclude malignancy. In more than 800 patients evaluated by the author, no cancers have been diagnosed.

Signs and Symptoms

The primary symptom of IC is the presence of abnormal sensory urgency. Sensory urgency leads to urinary frequency. In addition, most patients have associated bladder pain. A recent study[59] showed that of the patients presenting with IC, approximately 15% have little or no bladder pain whereas 85% had significant pain. It is important to determine whether the pain is of bladder origin. Pursuant to this, the physician should ask the patient whether the pain (despite being constantly present) becomes worse if the bladder is not emptied and diminishes (not disappears) with voiding. The bladder pain of IC is experienced suprapubically, in the perineum, vaginally, in the low back, or even medially in the thighs.[4] Two-thirds of patients do not experience dysuria.

Nocturia is variable. In general, however, 90% of patients complain of voiding at least one or two times per night.[59] Nocturia increases with the severity and duration of the disorder. The average patient voids approximately 16 times per day; a minimum for diagnostic purposes is considered to be eight voids per day.[76] The average voided volume is 75 ml. The ranges of average daily volumes and voids are shown in Figures 15–4 and 15–5.

Between 85 and 90% of individuals with IC are women. Of those who are sexually active, the majority (75%) complain of exacerbation of symptoms with sexual intercourse.[59] The increase in symptoms may be felt during sexual activity, immediately afterward, or within 24 hours. In addition, most women who are still menstruating complain of a flare of symptoms at the time of menstruation.[4, 59]

Evaluation

Physicians have struggled to establish a diagnosis of IC primarily because no objective "blood test" exists.

Evaluation of large numbers of patients with the urgency-frequency syndrome has revealed historical and clinical findings that can help to establish the diagnosis.

In August, 1987 a group of investigators and patients interested in IC met at the National Institutes of Health and defined the NIDDKD (National Institute of Diabetes and Digestive and Kidney Diseases) criteria to establish the diagnosis for research purposes.[76] These criteria were a practical attempt to quantify the findings in IC. In part they were based on a study reported by Parsons and colleagues in which the symptoms of more than 200 IC patients were measured and analyzed.[59] From Parsons' data each variable was examined; the point at which 90% of patients were included was the number taken for the NIDDKD criteria. For example, 90% of IC patients were found to void at least one to two times at night, reported eight or more voidings during the day, and had moderate urinary urgency. The presence of bladder pain was optional. The data on which these criteria were based are listed in Table 15–1. It is important to note that these criteria were developed to provide uniform criteria for researchers investigating IC. They were never meant to be a gold standard for diagnosis. Patients meeting these criteria have advanced disease. Many patients with IC (perhaps most) do not meet these criteria but nevertheless have the disease and will benefit from therapy.

A more accurate assessment of the number of daily voidings and the average volume can be determined from a 3-day voiding log for which each voiding is measured and recorded by the patient at home. From these data it was found that the average patient voids 16 times per day and has a bladder capacity of 73 ml (see Figs. 15–4 and 15–5). The voiding profile is a useful method that can help to establish the diagnosis of IC and may also be used subsequently to create a therapeutic plan and determine progress

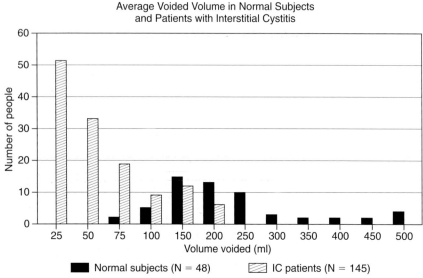

Average Voided Volume in Normal Subjects and Patients with Interstitial Cystitis

■ Normal subjects (N = 48) ▨ IC patients (N = 145)

Normal: average = 270 ml   IC: average = 73 ml

Figure 15–4 The average voided volume is about 75 ml, with a range as shown.

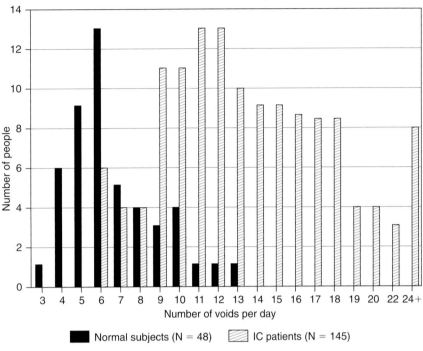

**Voids Per Day in Normal Subjects
and Patients with Interstitial Cystitis**

Figure 15-5 Average daily number of voids is approximately 16, with a range of 8 to 24+.

Normal subjects (N = 48)   IC patients (N = 145)

Normal: average = 6.5 ml   IC: average = 16.5 ml

in therapy. As might be anticipated, patients with a longer history of disease have a smaller functional bladder capacity, as reflected in the average voided volume and the number of daily voidings (see Table 15–1).

Duration of symptoms helps to distinguish patients with IC from those with urgency-frequency syndrome. A diagnosis of IC is more likely if the individual has had continuous symptoms for at least 6 months. To separate IC clinically from the urgency-frequency syndrome is worthwhile because the latter may need little or no therapy, and the prognosis for the patient is good.

PHYSICAL EXAMINATION

There is one important part of the physical examination that helps to confirm a diagnosis of IC. On exam-

ination more than 95% of patients complain of a tender bladder base during the pelvic examination. This discomfort is easily demonstrated by palpating the anterior vaginal wall.

Urine analysis of voided specimens is not useful in these patients because their low voided volumes make midstream collection impossible. One sees only vaginal secretions unless a catheterized specimen is obtained. A catheterized specimen examined under the microscope should show no bacteria, and most show no red or white blood cells. Urine should be sent for cytologic evaluation to rule out the possibility of carcinoma, but in actuality positive cytologic findings have never been seen at our center.

Urodynamics

The cystometrogram (CMG) is a valuable study in patients with this syndrome because a normal result essentially excludes a diagnosis of IC. Because all patients complain of significant urinary urgency, this can usually be documented with cystometry. If gas is employed, the patient will have a sensation of significant urgency at less than 125 ml; with water the sensation occurs with less than 150 ml. If this portion of the CMG is normal, the patient may not have IC or may have only a mild form of it. In 75 patients undergoing cystometrograms reported by Parsons, the average bladder capacity was 220 ml, and over 90% of patients had a functional volume of less than 350 ml[59] (Table 15–2). Patients should

TABLE 15–1

Comparison of Voided Volumes in Patients with a Short Disease History with Those with a Longer History

	Average at 1 Year[a]	Average at >7 Years[b]
No. patients	34	42
Voids	15.2	17.3
Voided volume	128 ml	105 ml
Anesthetic capacity	711 ml	518 ml

[a]Represents patients with symptoms for 1 year.
[b]Represents patients with symptoms for >7 years.

TABLE 15–2
Results of Cystometrograms in 75 Patients[a]

Average capacity	220 ml ± 68
90% cut-off level	<350 ml
Postvoid residual 750 ml	5/75
Number with increased sensory urgency[b]	71/75 (95%)
Patients with uninhibited contractions	4/75 (5%)
Detrusor myopathy	11/225[c]

[a]Listed are the average capacities and the 90% cut-off levels. All patients with uninhibited contractions did not respond to anticholinergic therapy.
[b]Patients with urgency at <100 ml. All had urgency at <125 ml.
[c]Detrusor myopathy is described by Holm-Bentzen and colleagues,[77] and all patients in whom it was suspected had cystometrograms. They had increased sensory urgency, postvoid residual urine of >50 ml, and poor detrusor contractions. Detrusor volume was >750 ml.

experience the same bladder discomfort with CMG that they normally have. However, there is an important caveat relative to maximum bladder capacity. A small group of patients (about 5%) with significant IC develop detrusor myopathy.[59, 77] Individuals with this complication have large atonic bladders in which little muscle is present. They have moderate to severe sensory urgency, have a large bladder capacity (>1000 ml), and usually carry residual urine (>100 ml). Detrusor function is poor or absent. Because most of these patients are women, they are able to void but do so primarily by using a Valsalva maneuver. Men with detrusor myopathy may require a program of intermittent catheterization (ICP) as part of

their treatment. In fact, because of the generalized atrophy of bladder muscle that occurs with this disease, men with low voiding pressures may require ICP.

CYSTOSCOPIC EVALUATION

Cystoscopic evaluation of the bladder under anesthesia is an important diagnostic and therapeutic maneuver. Examination under local anesthesia is to be discouraged because it offers little help in diagnosis and causes the patient severe discomfort. It is recommended that a cystoscopic examination be performed under anesthesia when IC is suspected, but not all patients need cystoscopy. Probably half the patients do not need this examination unless severe symptoms are present. It is best to omit cystoscopy in patients with milder disease and proceed with the other therapies listed subsequently.

Cystoscopy under anesthesia is performed for both diagnosis and treatment. Diagnosis depends on discovering one of two findings: a Hunner's ulcer or the presence of glomerulations or petechial hemorrhages. However, not all patients show these changes, so their absence does not exclude the diagnosis.

POTASSIUM CHLORIDE TEST

A simple method has been devised by Parsons (the Parsons test) to measure epithelial permeability. The test is based on the hypothesis that a solution of

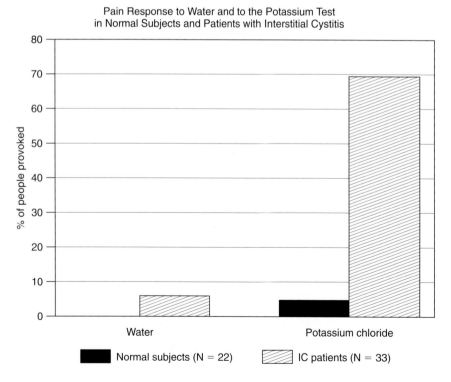

Pain Response to Water and to the Potassium Test in Normal Subjects and Patients with Interstitial Cystitis

Figure 15–6 Effect of water versus potassium chloride on the bladder in normal and IC subjects. Water provoked only 7% of IC subjects and no normal subjects, whereas potassium provoked 70% of IC patients but almost no normal subjects.

TABLE 15–3
Grading Scale for Symptoms

	None	Mild		Moderate		Severe
Pain	0	1	2	3	4	5
	None	Mild		Moderate		Severe
Urgency	0	1	2	3	4	5

NOTE: All subjects were told to consider the symptoms at the start as a baseline of 0. When a solution was added, they were asked to grade the symptoms it provoked (pain or urgency) on a scale of 0 to 5.

potassium chloride instilled into a normal bladder provokes no symptoms of urgency or pain. On the other hand, if such a solution is placed in a bladder in which the mechanism maintaining the impermeable epithelium is impaired, the potassium will diffuse across the transitional cells to stimulate the sensory nerves, causing urgency or pain.

To perform the test, two solutions are placed in the bladder for 5 minutes. The first solution is sterile water and the second contains 400 mEq/liter of KCl. The volume used is 45 ml to reduce stimulation due to volume.

After the solution has been instilled, the patient is asked to grade the symptoms it provokes on a scale of 1 to 5 (Table 15–3). If the patient does not respond to water and states that the KCl solution causes the symptoms to increase by a score of 2 or more, the test is considered positive. In a recent study, 70% of patients (23) experienced provocation of symptoms, whereas only 4% (1 of 22) of normals responded (Fig. 15–6). This is a useful test for separating leakers from nonleakers and is also good for testing an abnormal permeability barrier.

Cystoscopy

Cystoscopy should be performed in two phases. Phase one is the initial inspection. In this phase the physician should obtain specimens for cytology and urine for regular and tuberculosis culture (the latter is optional because it is almost never diagnosed). Visual examination of the bladder may reveal a true Hunner's ulcer (patch). This patch is a velvety red area (Fig. 15–7) that is present in only 6 to 8% of patients[59] and is very similar in appearance to carcinoma in situ. However, it is not actually a true ulcer, only a red patch. No biopsy is performed during this part of the cystoscopic examination. Prior biopsy site scars that are frequently mistaken for ulcers may also be seen.[74] Bladders with IC appear to heal poorly, and biopsy scars are frequently large but can be recognized by the wheel-spoke–type blood vessels that radiate from the central scarred portion (Fig. 15–8). These scars frequently tear and bleed after

they are distended and account for most so-called epithelial disruptions. Parsons reported that as many as 75% of ulcers described at previous cystoscopy by other urologists were actually biopsy site scars.[59]

The second phase of the cystoscopic procedure is the hydrodistention portion, which is done to demonstrate glomerulations. Hydrodistention also induces a disease remission in 60% of patients. Hydrodistention is performed by filling the bladder slowly using a maximum of 80 to 100 cm H_2O. The urethra of the female should be manually compressed over the

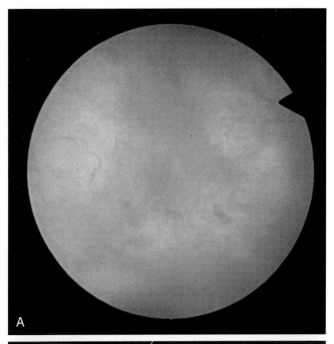

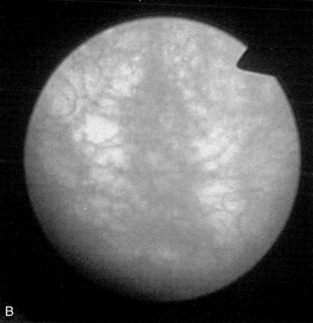

Figure 15–7 *A* and *B*, A classic Hunner's ulcer (patch, not a true ulcer), a velvety red patch resembling carcinoma-in-situ.

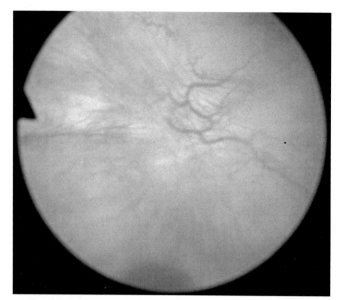

Figure 15-8 Prior biopsy site scar is recognized by the presence of neovascularity with blood vessels radiating in a wheel-spoke fashion.

cystoscope to prevent leakage of fluid. After several minutes, the bladder is emptied, and the volume is measured and recorded. The last part of the effluent is usually bloody if glomerulations or ulcers are present. When the bladder is reexamined, the glomerulations should be demonstrated. They are diffusely located around the bladder, with at least 10 to 20 per field of vision (Fig. 15–9). Hemorrhages on the trigone or posterior bladder wall are irrelevant and do not constitute a positive finding because they probably represent cystoscopic trauma.

What constitutes an abnormal bladder capacity under anesthesia may be surprising to many physicians. A normal female bladder holds well over 1000 ml. The IC bladder usually holds less than 850 ml.[59] The average capacity under anesthesia in IC patients is between 550 and 650 ml (Fig. 15–10). Patients with a longer history of symptoms have smaller bladder capacities, suggesting that the disease is slowly progressive.[59] This conclusion is also supported by the fact that patients with Hunner's ulcers have the worst symptoms, the smallest bladder capacity, and the greatest problem with loss of epithelial impermeability.[13, 59]

BIOPSY

The last part of the cystoscopic procedure should be the biopsy. One should *never* biopsy before hydrodistention is performed because the bladder could tear at the biopsy site, possibly leading to a significant bladder rupture. If a caustic agent is used for therapy, the biopsy is never done before the solution is placed in the bladder. Should the solution extravasate through the biopsy site, severe tissue damage could occur.

The biopsy itself is not diagnostic for IC but can rule out other diseases such as carcinoma in situ. The findings on pathologic examination include the presence of mast cells (demonstrated by toluidine blue staining),[43, 45] inflammatory cells, and a thinned mucosa. A normal biopsy *does not* exclude IC and should not be so used in diagnosis. Conversely, no pathologic findings specifically make a diagnosis of IC.

Although diagnosis of IC depends in part on abnormal cystoscopic findings, one cannot arbitrarily rule out the disease solely by the endoscopic findings. Many patients who have IC without such findings will benefit from therapy. The physician must remember that this disease complex is still primarily manifested by significant urinary urgency or frequency and perhaps few or no other findings.

At the end of the cystoscopic procedure, 10 ml of 2% viscous lidocaine (Xylocaine) jelly is placed in the bladder. This aids in pain control during the recovery period from anesthesia.

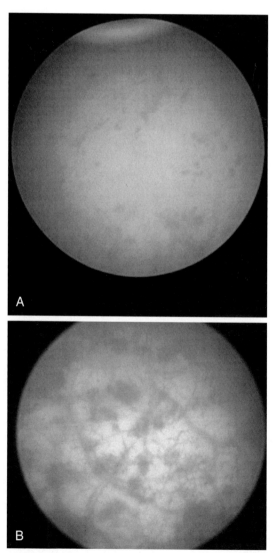

Figure 15-9 Glomerulations, moderate to severe *(A)* and severe *(B),* that occur after distending a bladder with water in a patient with interstitial cystitis.

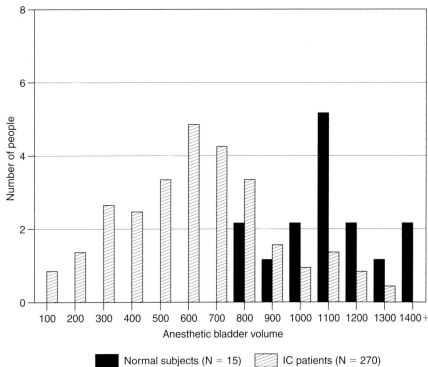

Anesthetic Bladder Capacity in Normal Subjects
and Patients with Interstitial Cystitis

Figure 15-10 These data show the range of bladder capacity under anesthesia in normal and IC subjects. Capacities are much larger for both groups than is generally believed.

■ Normal subjects (N = 15)   ▨ IC patients (N = 270)

Normal: average = 1115 ml   IC: average = 575 ml

Therapy

Until recently, few advances had been made in therapy for IC. Most medications were employed empirically, and all results were studied without controls. Drugs used for IC included anticholinergics, antihistamines, analgesics, and anti-inflammatories. Future drug efficacy studies should include controls to demonstrate whether therapy has been effective. Traditional and newer therapies that should aid the physician treating patients with IC are reviewed here.

When discussing therapy with the patient, it is important for the physician to emphasize that if the symptoms have been present for more than a year, no particular therapy is likely to be curative. Although the patient may have a significant remission of symptoms, in all probability relapse will occur. If patients are prepared for this eventuality, they are much less distressed when symptoms return and cope better with the disease. The physician-patient relationship is strengthened if this subject is addressed prior to initiation of treatment. Patients readily accept this explanation and appear to adjust better to their disorder when their outlook is realistic.

ANTIDEPRESSANT THERAPY

Chronic pain and sleep loss cause depression; thus, it is effective to place most IC patients on antidepres-

sant medications. If tricyclic antidepressants are used, low doses are used to start with (25 mg of imipramine 1 hour before bedtime), and patients are warned that they will be tired in the morning for the first 2 to 3 weeks of therapy. Once they become tolerant of this side effect, the dosage can be increased slowly if needed. Usually 25 mg is a sufficient dose. Imipramine or amitriptyline can be prescribed in doses beginning at 25 mg 1 hour before bedtime (aids in inducing sleep and reduces the tiring effect of the medication). If fluoxetine (Prozac) is selected, a dose of 20 mg/day is used and increased if necessary to 40 mg/day.

Antidepressant therapy is an important adjunct to treatment. It does not cure IC, but patients cope much better with their disabling symptoms if they are not depressed. In essence, they "feel better" even if they still void 20 times per day. It is important to emphasize to patients that antidepressants do not cure the disease, or they will assume that the physician is suggesting that the problem is "in their heads" and will not take the drug.

HYDRODISTENTION OF THE BLADDER UNDER ANESTHESIA

The report by Bumpus in 1930 that bladder hydrodistention diminished the symptoms of IC resulted in this procedure's becoming a mainstay of therapy.[78] Few question the activity of hydrodistention in ameliorating the symptoms in 60% of IC patients. The procedure must be performed under anesthesia because it is not possible to dilate a painful bladder without it. The procedure for hydrodistention has been described earlier under diagnosis. Pressure dilation of the bladder using a syringe should not be done because it can result in bladder rupture; a maximum pressure of 80 to 100 cm H_2O is recommended.

The mechanism by which hydrodistention improves symptoms is unknown; several theories have been postulated. Neurapraxis induced by mechanical trauma may occur in some individuals. However, few patients awaken with decreased pain, which would support the neurapraxis concept. Rather, most patients (90%) awaken from anesthesia with significantly worse pain that slowly improves over 2 to 3 weeks. This pain usually requires narcotic analgesia. Remission occurs over a period of several weeks. Because of the increased pain, it is recommended that all patients receive belladonna and opium rectal suppositories immediately in the recovery room. Better yet, 10 ml of 2% viscous lidocaine can be instilled into the bladder at the end of hydrodistention. In addition, patients should be discharged with medication (narcotic) to control the increased pain.

Because most patients' symptoms are exacerbated by hydrodistention, we believe that this is due to epithelial damage resulting from the mechanical trauma. The disruption in the integrity of the mucosal cells increases the epithelial leak, causing symptoms to flare. Healing may occur during the next several weeks, which correlates with the time of clinical remission. Perhaps the epithelium regenerates and for a period of time is "healthy" and impermeable. Then whatever events initiate the disease continue, and relapse occurs.

Remission may persist for 4 to 12 months. Hydrodistention may be repeated as needed. If no remission is obtained, the dilation is repeated at least two more times because frequently in our experience patients respond to a subsequent dilation.

DIMETHYLSULFOXIDE

Dimethylsulfoxide (DMSO) was approved for use in IC in 1977.[79] Although no controlled clinical trials were ever conducted with DMSO, it does appear to induce remission in 34 to 40% of patients. The difficulty with DMSO is that although it may induce an excellent remission in the first one to three cycles of therapy, as relapses occur and the patient requires subsequent treatment, progressive resistance to its beneficial effects is seen.

For treatment, 50 ml of 50% dimethylsulfoxide is instilled into the bladder for 5 to 10 minutes. Longer periods are unnecessary because DMSO is rapidly absorbed into the blood stream. Instillation is performed on an outpatient basis, or patients can be taught to perform it themselves. We recommend that patients receive six to eight weekly treatments to determine whether a therapeutic response is

achieved. If the symptoms are moderate or worse, the therapy is continued for an additional 4 to 6 months once every other week. One should remember that once DMSO therapy is stopped, the patient is likely to become resistant to its use. Some patients will experience a flare of symptoms when DMSO is placed in the bladder. This phenomenon may be related to DMSO's ability to degranulate mast cells and may occur primarily in patients who have significant bladder mastocytosis. Nonetheless, DMSO may be very effective in treating these patients. Should the patient experience pain with DMSO, it is recommended that he or she receive 10 ml of 2% viscous lidocaine jelly intravesically 15 minutes before DMSO is placed in the bladder. If this is not successful, an injectable narcotic or Toradol 60 mg intramuscularly is used before the intravesical instillation. The flare of symptoms associated with DMSO usually disappears over 24 hours. As these patients receive subsequent treatments, the pain tends to diminish.

Patients may also receive therapy with DMSO indefinitely. As originally reported by Stewart and colleagues, patients have used DMSO weekly for several years without problems.[79] DMSO has been associated with cataracts in animals; however, this complication has not been reported in humans. Therefore, for patients receiving chronic therapy, a slit-lamp evaluation at 3- to 6-month intervals is recommended.

AMITRIPTYLINE

In an uncontrolled trial, amitriptyline was reported by Hanno and associates to ameliorate the symptoms of IC.[80] The patients were treated with 25 mg of amitriptyline 1 hour before bedtime for 1 week; the dose was then increased weekly by 25 mg to a 75-mg dose. Fifty percent of patients responded to this medication. The exact mechanism of action is unknown, although it may block H_1 histamine receptors and perhaps mast cell degranulation. More likely, the drug raises pain tolerance owing to its antidepressant activity. Details of antidepressant therapy were described earlier.

ANTIHISTAMINES

Antihistamines have been tried in IC but without controlled studies. Antihistamines were chosen because of the possible role of mast cells.[70, 72, 81, 82] In our experience, though, antihistamines are of little use in the management of IC. However, some patients do respond to these medications (e.g., diphenhydramine [Benadryl] or terfenadine [Seldane]), especially if they have a history of allergies and tend to have symptom flares during allergy seasons.

STEROIDS

Because of the assumption that inflammation plays a role in this disorder, some patients have received steroids. Badenoch reported significant improvement in 19 of 25 patients treated with prednisone.[83] However, all of these patients were treated after hydrodistention under anesthesia, which may have been responsible for most of the benefit. In our experience, steroids do not ameliorate the symptoms of this complex. As with most drugs, no controlled clinical trials have been conducted on the efficacy of steroids in patients with IC.

INTRAVESICAL SILVER NITRATE

The use of intravesical silver nitrate was first reported in 1926 by Dodson.[84] Pool fashioned a treatment regimen in which bladder irrigations were begun under anesthesia using a 1:5000 concentration of this drug.[60] This was followed by gradual increases in the concentration on a daily basis, ultimately employing a 1% solution. Again, this drug regimen was used in an uncontrolled setting in patients who had had dilation of the bladder under anesthesia. Pool reported good results in 89% of his patients. There have been other uncontrolled studies reporting that this compound is helpful; nevertheless, it is not very widely used today. One caution in the use of silver nitrate should be noted: it should never be instilled into the bladder after biopsy. If there is a perforation and this solution is placed in the bladder, intraperitoneal and extraperitoneal extravasation could occur, resulting in major tissue damage.

INTRAVESICAL SODIUM OXYCHLOROSENE (CLORPACTIN WCS-90)

Clorpactin is a highly reactive chemical compound that is a modified derivative of hypochlorous acid in a buffered base. Its activity depends on the liberation of hypochlorous acid and its resulting oxidizing effects and detergency.[85] Its use was reported by Wishard and colleagues, who treated 20 patients with five weekly instillations of 0.2% clorpactin WCS-90 under local anesthesia.[85] Improvement was reported in 14 of the 20 patients, and follow-up was brief. Messing and Stamey, treating 38 patients with 0.4% Clorpactin, reported significant improvement in 72%.[54] Ureteral reflux is a contraindication to the use of Clorpactin. It is recommended that the compound usually be used under anesthesia.

HEPARIN

Heparin, given by injection, has been reported to alleviate the symptoms of IC.[86] Again, this recommendation has not been subjected to a controlled study. Chronic systemic heparin therapy cannot be used in most people because it results in osteoporosis in 100% of patients who use it for 26 weeks. In our experience, intravesical heparin shows significant activity in approximately 50% of patients. Here, too,

the data were obtained in an uncontrolled investigation. Previous controlled studies conducted by us demonstrated a placebo effect of approximately 20%, suggesting possible activity of heparin.[41] In this technique 10,000 units of heparin in 10 ml of sterile water are instilled intravesically three times per week. If there is no effect after 3 months, the frequency is increased to daily instillation. This treatment can be continued indefinitely. It takes 2 to 4 months to see improvements, but therapy should be encouraged and pursued for at least 6 months before it is abandoned. The best improvements are noted after 1 to 2 years. Long-term therapy is recommended for patients with moderate or worse disease who respond to its use. Serum prothrombin time and partial thromboplastin time are monitored for several weeks after therapy begins to rule out the formation of an unusual antibody to heparin or systemic absorption (heparin is not absorbed across the bladder mucosa). Patients are instructed in self-catheterization, so this therapy can be performed at home.

PENTOSANPOLYSULFATE

Parsons and colleagues first reported that pentosanpolysulfate was active in ameliorating the symptoms of IC.[40–42] Because pentosanpolysulfate (Elmiron) is a sulfated polysaccharide, theoretically it may augment the bladder surface defense mechanisms or detoxify agents in urine that have a capacity to attack the bladder surface (e.g., quaternary amines). In a controlled clinical study symptoms were improved in 42% of patients versus 20% for placebo.[41] This result has been borne out in several subsequent studies including a five-center trial in which 28% of patients improved versus 13% on placebo.[42] In a seven-center study of 150 patients improvement occurred in 32% of patients versus 15% on placebo.[93] Additionally, an English-Danish study also found a significant reduction of pain in patients taking the drug compared with placebo.[19] Elmiron is not currently approved for use in the United States, but it may be available soon and should be checked on. It is currently manufactured by Baker Norton Pharmaceuticals Inc. in Miami, Florida. It is used in an oral dose of 100 mg three times per day. In patients with moderate disease, it appears to have activity in about 40 to 50% of patients. In the controlled clinical trials encompassing patients with severe disease, its activity was lower. Continued use of Elmiron for several years leads to long-term disease control in most of the drug responders. This result has not previously occurred in any other therapy. Response to therapy first appears after 6 to 10 weeks. Patients do better after 6 to 12 months of therapy.

SURGERY

Approximately 3% of patients presenting with IC to the University of California at San Diego Medical

Center ultimately undergo some type of surgery for disease that is severe and refractory to all treatment. The question is which type of surgery to perform.

Cystolysis

Attempts to ablate the bladder innervation surgically by cystolysis are to be discouraged because it will fail in most patients, who will develop a neurogenic bladder with significant urinary pain and frequency, perhaps requiring intermittent catheterization.

Bladder Augmentation

A concept exists that these patients have small bladders and thus void frequently. Actually, the reverse is true. They have sensory urgency, void frequently, and subsequently develop a small bladder. Hence, attempts to augment the bladder with a patch of bowel are likely to fail. Patients will then have a bladder capacity that is perhaps large, but they will have more difficulty in emptying it (usually requiring intermittent catheterization) and still retain all their sensory urgency and pain.[87]

Urinary Diversion Alone

There are no controlled studies evaluating diversion alone, but studies suggest that it is not effective.[88] However, we have taken out two bladders in patients who had urinary diversions alone with persistent pelvic pain. The pain was eliminated by removing the bladder. In counseling, one should tell the patient that diversion alone may not be sufficient to control the pain and he or she may subsequently require a cystectomy. The patient can then decide whether to accept the risk of more than one operation. It is our experience that almost no one elects the potential of two surgical procedures.

Cystectomy and Diversion

This is the mainstay of therapy for patients with "end-stage bladder." It is successful, especially in today's environment of performing continent diversions. Pelvic pain occurs after the procedure in 5% of patients (Table 15–4). In general, if the patient has classic bladder pain associated with filling that is relieved or partially relieved by emptying and also has urinary frequency and urgency and the usual stigmata of IC under anesthesia, he or she is likely to obtain relief of symptoms with cystectomy. Those individuals who have severe pelvic pain not associated with classic parameters of IC and particularly *not* exacerbated by bladder filling are unlikely to experience pain relief (see Table 15–4).

BLADDER TRAINING

Whatever therapy is successful at alleviating the pain and sensory urgency of IC, the individual afflicted with the chronic form of the disorder has a small-capacity bladder that is based in part on sensory urgency and in part on frequent low-volume voiding. In controlled clinical trials it has been reported that even with good remission of pain and urgency, the patient experiences almost no change in urinary frequency during a 12-week period.[41, 42, 93] This issue must be addressed to obtain a functional recovery of the bladder. Persistent urinary frequency in a patient with a small bladder can be reversed after therapy has controlled urgency and pain. This is accomplished by training the patient to undergo a program of progressively holding his or her urine to increase bladder capacity.[89] This therapy can be directed by a urologic nurse. To begin this treatment, a 3-day voiding profile is obtained from the patient (which should include time of voiding and measurement of volume). The average time interval between voids is determined, and this interval is gradually increased monthly. For example, if the patient voids every hour, it is recommended that he or she attempt to void every hour and a quarter and then at the end of 1 month increase that interval to an hour and a half. The patient should never progress too quickly because she may become discouraged and drop out. It takes 3 to 5 months of this protocol to start to see results. At the end of 3 to 4 months, the bladder capacity will have increased approximately $2\frac{1}{2}$ times, and there will be a corresponding reduction in urgency and the number of voidings per day.[89]

We also discovered that in patients in whom minimal or no pain is associated with urinary frequency, bladder training may be the only therapy required to produce improvement, and in fact this is the only therapy that is effective. For more details about the use of this protocol, the reader is referred elsewhere.[89]

In summary, IC is a syndrome that is undergoing rapid change in regard to our understanding of the pathogenesis and development of therapy owing to a significant increase in research activity. These investigations are helping the clinician to quantify the symptoms and clinical findings to better diagnose the syndrome and are simultaneously leading to new therapies (hydrodistention, DMSO, Elmiron, or heparin) that will result in symptom reduction. In addition, bladder training methods can further rehabili-

TABLE 15–4
Surgery for Interstitial Cystitis[a]

Treatment	Persistent Pain	No Pain
Cystectomy	1/25	24/25 (96%)

[a]Twenty-five patients underwent cystectomy for interstitial cystitis at the University of California at San Diego. After 6 months only one patient had persistent pelvic pain. That patient did not have classic bladder pain that increases with bladder filling, but rather pelvic pain unrelated to voiding.

tate the patient with an IC bladder. As reviewed herein, perhaps 75 to 85% of patients with moderate to severe IC can experience significant indefinite remissions with conservative therapy and avoid the need for extirpative surgery.

REFERENCES

1. Hunner GL: A rare type of bladder ulcer in women. Report of cases. Boston Med Surg J 172:600, 1915.
2. Hunner GL: Elusive ulcer of the bladder: Further notes on a rare type of bladder ulcer with a report of 25 cases. Am J Obstet 78:374, 1918.
3. Oravisto KJ, Alfthan OS, Jokinen EJ: Interstitial cystitis. Clinical and immunological findings. Scand J Urol Nephrol 4:37, 1970.
4. Hand JR: Interstitial cystitis, a report of 223 cases. J Urol 61:291, 1949.
5. Hanash KA, Pool TL: Interstitial and hemorrhagic cystitis: Viral, bacterial and fungal studies. J Urol 104:705, 1970.
6. Oravisto KJ, Alfthan OS: Treatment of interstitial cystitis with immunosuppression and chloroquine derivatives. Eur Urol 2:82, 1976.
7. Gordon HL, Rosen RD, Hersh EM, Yium JJ: Immunologic aspects of interstitial cystitis. J Urol 109:228, 1973.
8. Silk MR: Bladder antibodies in interstitial cystitis. J Urol 103:307, 1970.
9. Holm-Bentzen M, Lose G: Pathology and pathogenesis of interstitial cystitis. Urology 29 (Suppl 4):8, 1987.
10. Oravisto KJ: Interstitial cystitis as an autoimmune disease. A review. Eur Urol 6:10, 1990.
11. Weaver RG, Dougherty TF, Natoli C: Recent concepts of interstitial cystitis. J Urol 89:377, 1963.
12. Eldrup J, Thorup J, Nielsen SL, et al: Permeability and ultrastructure of human bladder epithelium. Br J Urol 55:488, 1983.
13. Parsons CL, Lilly JD, Stein P: Epithelial dysfunction in nonbacterial cystitis (interstitial cystitis). J Urol 145:732, 1991.
14. Lilly JD, Parsons CL: Bladder surface glycosaminoglycans: A human epithelial permeability barrier. Surg Gynecol Obstet 171:493, 1990.
15. Parsons CL, Boychuk D, Jones S, et al: Bladder surface glycosaminoglycans: An epithelial permeability barrier. J Urol 143:139, 1990.
16. Hohlbrugger G, Lentsch P: Intravesical ions, osmolality and pH influence the volume pressure response in the normal rat bladder, and this is more pronounced after DMSO exposure. Eur Urol 11:127, 1985.
17. Lynes WL, Flynn SD, Shortliffe LD, et al: Mast cell involvement in interstitial cystitis. J Urol 138:746, 1987.
18. Hanno P, Levin RM, Monson FC, et al: Diagnosis of interstitial cystitis. J Urol 143:278, 1990.
19. Holm-Bentzen M, Jacobsen F, Nerstrom B, et al: Painful bladder disease: Clinical and pathoanatomical differences in 115 patients. J Urol 138:500, 1987.
20. Englund SE: Observation on the migration of some labeled substances between the urinary bladder and blood in rabbits. Acta Radiol Suppl 135:9, 1956.
21. Kerr WK, Barkin M, D'Aloisio J, Merczyk Z: Observations on the movement of ions and water across the wall of the human bladder and ureter. J Urol 89:812, 1963.
22. Lewis SA, Diamond JM: Active sodium transport by mammalian urinary bladder. Nature 253:747, 1975.
23. Fellows GJ, Marshall DH: The permeability of human bladder epithelium to water and sodium. Invest Urol 9:339, 1972.
24. Hicks RM: The permeability of rat transitional epithelium. J Cell Biol 28:21, 1966.
25. Hicks RM, Ketterer B, Warren RC: The ultrastructure and chemistry of the luminal plasma membrane of the mammalian urinary bladder: A structure with low permeability to water and ions. Phil Trans R Soc Lond (B) 268:23, 1974.
26. Staehelin LA, Chlapowski FJ, Bonneville MA: Luminal plasma membrane of the urinary bladder. J Cell Biol 53:73, 1972.
27. Parsons CL, Stauffer C, Schmidt J: Bladder surface glycosaminoglycans: An efficient mechanism of environmental adaptation. Science 208:605, 1980.
28. Parsons CL, Greenspan C, Mulholland SG: The primary antibacterial defense mechanism of the bladder. Invest Urol 13:72, 1975.
29. Parsons CL, Greenspan, C, Moore SW, Mulholland SG: Role of surface mucin in primary antibacterial defense of bladder. Urology 9:48, 1979.
30. Gill WB, Jones KW, Ruggiero KJ: Protective effects of heparin and other sulfated glycosaminoglycans on crystal adhesion to urothelium. J Urol 127:152, 1982.
31. Hanno PM, Parsons CL, Shrom SH, et al: The protective effect of heparin in experimental bladder infection. J Surg Res 25:324, 1978.
32. Parsons CL, Mulholland S, Anwar H: Antibacterial activity of bladder surface mucin duplicated by exogenous glycosaminoglycan (heparin). Infect Immun 24:552, 1979.
33. Menter JM, Hurst RE, Nakamura N, West SS: Thermodynamics of mucopolysaccharide-dye binding. III. Thermodynamic and cooperatively parameters of acridine orange-heparin system. Biopolymers 18:493, 1979.
34. Gryte CC, Gregor HP: Poly-(styrene solfonic acid)-poly-(vinylidene fluoride) interpolymer ion-exchange membranes. J Polymer Sci 14:1938, 1976.
35. Gregor HP: Anticoagulant activity of sulfonate polymers and copolymers. In Gregor HP (ed): Polymer Science and Technology, vol 5. New York, Plenum Press, 1975, p 51.
36. Gregor HP: Fixed charge ultrafiltration membranes. In Selegny E (ed): Charged Gels and Membranes, Part I. Dordrecht, Holland, D Reidel, 1976, p 235.
37. Hurst RE, Rhodes SW, Adamson PB, et al: Functional and structural characteristics of the glycosaminoglycans of the bladder luminal surface. J Urol 138:433, 1987.
38. Bekturov EA, Bakauova K (eds): Synthetic Water-Soluble Polymers in Solution. Basel, Hüthig & Wepf Verlag, 1986, p 38.
39. Hurst RE: Thermodynamics of the partition of chondroitin sulfate-hexadecylpyridinium complexes in butanol/aqueous salt biphasic solutions. Biopolymers 17:2601, 1978.
40. Parsons CL, Schmidt J, Pollen J: Successful treatment of interstitial cystitis with sodium pentosanpolysulfate. J Urol 130:51, 1983.
41. Parsons CL, Mulholland S: Successful therapy of interstitial cystitis with pentosanpolysulfate. J Urol 138:513, 1987.
42. Mulholland SG, Hanno P, Parsons CL, et al: Pentosan polysulfate sodium for therapy of interstitial cystitis: A double-blind placebo-controlled clinical study. Urology 35(6):552, 1990.
43. Theoharides TC, Sant GR: Bladder mast cell activation in interstitial cystitis. Semin Urol 9:74, 1991.
44. Lynes WL, Flynn SD, Shortliffe LD, et al: Mast cell involvement in interstitial cystitis. J Urol 138:746, 1987.
45. Larsen S, Thompson SA, Hald T, et al: Mast cells in interstitial cystitis. Br J Urol 54:283, 1982.
46. MacDermott JP, Miller CH, Levy N, Stone AR: Cellular immunity in interstitial cystitis. J Urol 145:274, 1991.
47. Felsen D, Frye S, Bavendam T, et al: Interleukin-6 activity in the urine of interstitial cystitis (IC) patients. J Urol 147:460A, 1992.
48. Nitze M: Lerbuch der Kystoscopie: Ihre Technik und Klinische Bedeutung. Berlin, J.E. Bergman, 1907, p 410.
49. Oravisto KJ: Epidemiology of interstitial cystitis: 1. In Hanno PM, Staskin DR, Krane RJ, et al (eds): Interstitial Cystitis. London, Springer-Verlag. 1990, p 25.
50. Held PJ, Hanno PM, Pauly MV, et al: Epidemiology of interstitial cystitis: 2. In Hanno PM, Staskin DR, Krane RJ, et al (eds): Interstitial Cystitis. London, Springer-Verlag, 1990, p 29.
51. American Foundation for Urologic Diseases: Research Progress and Promises. Baltimore, American Foundation for Urologic Diseases, 1980.
52. Oravisto KJ: Epidemiology of interstitial cystitis. Ann Chir Gynaecol Fenn 64:75, 1975.

53. Walsh A: Interstitial cystitis. *In* Harrison JH, Gittes RF, Perlmutter AD, et al (eds): Campbell's Urology, 4th ed. Philadelphia, W.B. Saunders, 1978.

54. Messing EM, Stamey TA: Interstitial cystitis: Early diagnosis, pathology, and treatment. Urology 12:381, 1978.

55. Farkas A, Waisman J, Goodwin WE: Interstitial cystitis in adolescent girls. J Urol 118:837, 1977.

56. Bowers JE, Lattimer JK: Interstitial cystitis. Surg Gynecol Obstet 105:313, 1957.

57. McDonald HP, Upchirch WE, Artime M: Bladder dysfunction in children caused by interstitial cystitis. J Urol 80:354, 1958.

58. Lapides J: Observations on interstitial cystitis. Urology 5:610, 1975.

59. Parsons CL: Interstitial cystitis: Clinical manifestations and diagnostic criteria in over 200 cases. Neurourol Urodyn 9(3):241, 1990.

60. Pool TL: Interstitial cystitis: Clinical considerations and treatment. Clin Obstet Gynecol 10:185, 1967.

61. de Juana CP, Everett JC: Interstitial cystitis: Experience and review of recent literature. Urology 10:325, 1977.

62. Hanno P, Wein A: Interstitial cystitis, Parts I and II. AUA Update Series, vol 1, no 9. Baltimore, American Urological Association, 1987.

63. Smith BH, Dehner LP: Chronic ulcerating interstitial cystitis (Hunner's ulcer). Arch Pathol 93:76, 1972.

64. Bures J, Fixa B, Komarkova O, et al: Nonsmoking: A feature of ulcerative colitis. Br Med J 285:440, 1982.

65. Calkins B, Lilienfeld AM, Mendeloff AI, et al: Smoking factors in ulcerative colitis and Crohn's disease in Baltimore. Am J Epidemiol 122:498, 1984.

66. Cope GF, Heatley RV, Kelleher J, Lee PN: Cigarette smoking and inflammatory bowel disease: A review. Human Toxicol 6:189, 1987.

67. Paulley JW: Ulcerative colitis: A study of 173 cases. Gastroenterology 16:566, 1950.

68. National Center for Health Statistics: Health and Nutrition Examination Survey, Cycle II, 1976–1980. Washington, DC, U.S. Government Printing Office, 1985.

69. Lilienfeld AM, Lilienfeld DE: Foundations of Epidemiology, 2nd ed. New York, Oxford University Press, 1980.

70. Larsen S, et al: Mast cells in interstitial cystitis. Br J Urol 54:283, 1982.

71. Fall M, Johansson SL, Vahlne A: A clinicopathological and virological study of interstitial cystitis. J Urol 133:771, 1985.

72. Smith B, Dehner LP: Chronic ulcerating interstitial cystitis. A study of 28 cases. Arch Pathol 93:76, 1972.

73. Jacobo E, Stamler FW, Culp DA: Interstitial cystitis followed by total cystectomy. Urology 3:481, 1974.

74. Johansson SL, Fall M: Clinical features and spectrum of light microscopic changes in interstitial cystitis. J Urol 143:1118, 1990.

75. Burford HE, Burford CE: Hunner ulcer of the bladder: A report of 187 cases. J Urol 79:952, 1958.

76. Gillenwater JY, Wein AJ: Summary of the National Institute of Arthritis, Diabetes, Digestive and Kidney Diseases Workshop on Interstitial Cystitis, National Institutes of Health, Bethesda, Maryland, August 28–29, 1987. J Urol 140(1):203, 1988.

77. Holm-Bentzen M, Larsen S, Hainau B, Hald T: Non-obstructive detrusor myopathy in a group of patients with chronic bacterial cystitis. Scand J Urol Nephrol 19(1):21, 1985.

78. Bumpus HC: Interstitial cystitis. Med Clin North Am 13:1495, 1930.

79. Stewart BH, Persky L, Kiser WS: The use of dimethylsulfoxide (DMSO) in the treatment of interstitial cystitis. J Urol 98:671, 1968.

80. Hanno PM, Buehler J, Wein AJ: Use of amitriptyline in the treatment of interstitial cystitis. J Urol 141:846, 1989.

81. Bohne AW, Hodson JM, Rebuck JW, Reinhard RE: An abnormal leukocyte response in interstitial cystitis. J Urol 88:387, 1962.

82. Simmons JL: Interstitial cystitis: An explanation for the beneficial effect of an antihistamine. J Urol 85:149, 1961.

83. Badenoch AW: Chronic interstitial cystitis. Br J Urol 43:718, 1971.

84. Dodson AI: Hunner's ulcer of the bladder: A report of 10 cases. Virginia Med Monthly 53:305, 1926.

85. Wishard WN, Nourse MH, Mertz JHO: Use of Clorpactin WCS-90 for relief of symptoms due to interstitial cystitis. J Urol 77:420, 1957.

86. Lose G, Frandsen B, Hojensgard JC, et al: Chronic interstitial cystitis: Increased levels of eosinophil cationic protein in serum and urine and an ameliorating effect of subcutaneous heparin. Scand J Urol Nephrol 17(2):159, 1983.

87. Nielsen KK, Kromann-Andersen B, Steven K, Hald T: Failure of combined supratrigonal cystectomy and Mainz ileocecocystoplasty in intractable interstitial cystitis: Is histology and mast cell count a reliable predictor for the outcome of surgery? J Urol 144 (2 Pt 1):255, 1990.

88. Eigner EG, Freiha FS: The fate of the remaining bladder following supravesical diversion. J Urol 144:31, 1990.

89. Parsons CL, Koprowski P: Interstitial cystitis: Successful management by a pattern of increasing urinary voiding interval. Urology 37:207, 1991.

90. Parsons CL, Stein PC, Bidair M, Lebow D: Abnormal sensitivity to intravesical potassium in interstitial cystitis and radiation cystitis. Neurourol Urodyn 13:515, 1994.

91. Fritjofsson A, Fall M, Juhlin R, et al: Treatment of ulcer and nonulcer interstitial cystitis with sodium pentosanpolysulfate: A multicenter trial. J Urol 138:508, 1987.

92. Holm-Bentzen M, Jacobsen F, Nerstrom B, et al: A prospective double-blind clinically controlled multicenter trial of sodium pentosanpolysulfate in the treatment of interstitial cystitis and related painful bladder disease. J Urol 138:503, 1987.

93. Parsons CL, Benson G, Childs SJ, et al: A quantitatively controlled method to prospectively study interstitial cystitis and demonstrate the efficacy of pentosanpolysulfate. J Urol 150:845, 1993.

CHAPTER 16

Urinary Tract Infections

David S. Grapey, M.D.
Anthony J. Schaeffer, M.D.

At least 30% of all women experience a urinary tract infection during their lifetime.[1] In addition to the discomfort, morbidity, and lost productivity, more than 1 billion dollars is spent annually on an estimated 500 million outpatient visits.[2, 3] The last 30 years have brought major insights into the pathogenesis, diagnosis, and treatment of urinary tract infections, which have added substantially to our ability to manage these patients successfully. These major contributions have been reviewed[4, 5] and are summarized here:

1. Appreciation that the classic diagnostic criteria for urinary tract infections, requiring a quantitative urine culture showing 100,000 colony-forming units (CFUs) or more per milliliter, has serious limitations and underdiagnoses as many as 50% of young women with acute bacterial cystitis.
2. Recognition that bacteria infecting the urinary tract arise from the fecal flora and that the susceptibility of women to recurrent urinary tract infection is largely a result of an abnormally high carriage of these potentially pathogenic bacteria on the vaginal and urethral mucosa.
3. Realization that most recurrent urinary tract infections in women are reinfections of the urinary tract from the fecal flora.
4. Introduction of new antimicrobial agents with an increased spectrum of activity against uropathogens and limited effects on the resident vaginal and fecal flora.
5. Documentation that low-dosage, prophylactic antimicrobial therapy with drugs that have minimal or no adverse effects on the resident fecal flora is safe and effective for preventing the majority of recurrent urinary tract infections in women.
6. Better understanding of the natural history of bacteriuria, including single and recurrent infections in women of all ages.

By understanding the basic principles underlying urinary tract infections, the clinician today should be able to approach the majority of patients in a medically sound and cost-efficient manner.

Classification

Urinary tract infections encompass an entire spectrum of clinical syndromes, each with a unique epidemiology, criteria for diagnosis, treatment considerations and prognosis. Numerous classification schemes have grouped patients on the basis of (1) the site of infection, (2) the presence or absence of symptoms, (3) the frequency of infection, and (4) complicating factors. Unfortunately, these categories often have overlapping criteria that make accurate patient assignment difficult. It is clinically useful to divide infections of the urinary tract into the following simple categories:[6]

1. Sporadic infection
2. Unresolved infection
3. Recurrent infection
   A. Reinfection
   B. Bacterial persistence

SPORADIC INFECTION

Sporadic or isolated infection is defined as an infection not preceded by an infection within the past 6 months or not more than two infections in the preceding year.

UNRESOLVED INFECTION

Unresolved infection implies that the initial therapy has been inadequate. This problem may go unrecog-

TABLE 16–1
Causes of Unresolved Bacteriuria

Bacterial resistance to chosen antimicrobial agent
Development of resistance from initially susceptible bacteria
Bacteriuria caused by two different bacterial species with
   mutually exclusive susceptibilities
Azotemia
Papillary necrosis
Giant staghorn calculi

Modified from Dairiki-Shortliffe LM, Stamey TA: Infections of the urinary tract: Introduction and general principles. *In* Walsh PC, Gittes RE, Perlmutter AD, et al (eds): Campbell's Urology, 5th ed. Philadelphia, WB Saunders, 1986, p 742.

nized because follow-up cultures are often not obtained, or, when they are, low colony counts may be misinterpreted as representing contamination. The most common cause of unresolved bacteriuria during treatment is the presence of resistant bacteria (Table 16–1). This usually occurs after treatment with antimicrobial agents that produce resistant organisms among the fecal flora, which subsequently infect the urinary tract. Furthermore, through plasmid-mediated resistance, a single course of recent treatment with any of several types of drugs (sulfonamides, penicillins, and cephalosporins) may produce bacteria that are simultaneously resistant to several other agents.

RECURRENT INFECTION

Recurrent urinary tract infections imply resolution of the initial bacteriuria followed by another infection. This term is reserved for patients with at least two infections within 6 months or three or more infections in 1 year. It is important to distinguish reinfections resulting from bacteria reentering the urinary tract after successful therapy from those due to bacterial persistence within the urinary tract.

Complicated Infection

Urinary tract infections should be considered complicated when host conditions exist that promote the development or persistence of infection (Table 16–2). When complicating factors are present, antimicrobial resistance is more prevelant, response to therapy is often poor, and complications occur frequently.[7–9]

TABLE 16–2
Factors Complicating Urinary Tract Infections

Functional or structural abnormalities of the urinary tract
Recent urinary tract instrumentation
Diabetes mellitus
Immunosuppression
Pregnancy
Hospital-acquired infection
Recent antimicrobial use

Overview of Bacteriuria in Women

Bacteriuria signifies the presence of bacteria in the urine that are not contaminants from the vagina or prepuce. The prevalence of bacteriuria is about 1% in school-age adolescent girls[10] and increases to 4 to 5% by young adulthood.[6] An increased prevalence associated with initiation of sexual activity is supported by numerous epidemiologic studies.[11–13] Kunin and McCormack showed that middle-aged nuns have a prevalence of bacteriuria similar to that of young school-age girls.[14] Other studies have shown that 75 to 85% of urinary tract infections occur within 24 hours of intercourse.[11, 15] It is presumed that sexual intercourse provides a mechanical effect, transferring colonized bacteria from the urethral mucosa to the urinary bladder.[16] The effectiveness of postcoital prophylactic antimicrobial regimens[17] lends further support to this relationship. With advancing age, the prevalence of bacteriuria slowly rises by about 1 to 2% per decade of life and has been reported to be as high as 50% in certain groups of institutionalized elderly women.[9, 18]

NATURAL HISTORY OF BACTERIURIA

Little is known about the natural history of untreated bacteriuria. Most studies comparing antimicrobials to placebo have shown that in 50 to 80% of patients taking a placebo the infection clears spontaneously.[19, 20] Mabeck found that of 53 bacteriuric women, the bacteriuria had cleared without treatment in 32 within a month and had cleared in 43 within 5 months.[19] Whether bacteriuria is symptomatic or asymptomatic is probably not an important distinction for prognosis. Asscher and colleagues reported that more than one-third of women with asymptomatic bacteriuria who were followed for 1 year developed a symptomatic infection, usually with the same strain.[21] Conversely, Mabeck followed 23 untreated women with acute symptomatic cystitis, and 21 were asymptomatic after 4 weeks but before the bacteriuria resolved. The term asymptomatic bacteriuria is misleading, given the dynamic nature of this entity. Some investigators feel that bacteriuria found under these clinical circumstances should simply be referred to as screening bacteriuria.[6]

The normal adult kidney appears to be astonishingly resistant to damage by bacteria in the absence of stones, obstruction, or papillary damage.[22] Numerous studies have failed to link uncomplicated urinary tract infection with progressive renal impairment in normal adults.[21, 23] A relationship between bacteriuria and hypertension has been found in some cross-sectional studies,[14, 24] but no prospective study has demonstrated that asymptomatic bacteriuria or uncomplicated urinary tract infection leads to hypertension.[25] Thus, the risk of asymptomatic bacteriuria as well as uncomplicated symptomatic urinary tract infections is essentially one of symptomatic morbidity. The clinician should focus on the diagnosis and treatment of symptomatic episodes rather than screening and treating asymptomatic populations with bacteriuria. One should be aware, however, that there are a number of host factors that significantly increase the risk of serious morbidity from bacteriuria[4] (Table 16–3).

NATURAL HISTORY OF RECURRENT URINARY TRACT INFECTIONS

Among the 20 to 30% of women who experience a urinary tract infection during their lifetime, some will have multiple recurrences.[26] Among women presenting with their first infection, 28% experienced a recurrence during the following 18 months compared with 83% who had previously had a documented urinary tract infection.[27] Stamey and colleagues followed 23 female patients who had histories of recurrent urinary tract infections (two or more infections during the previous 12 months) with monthly cultures.[28] They found that the average attack rate was approximately 2.0 infections per patient year. Ninety-four percent of all bacteriuric episodes had associated symptoms, and 73% of symptomatic events had associated bacteriuria. Among individual patients, long periods of remission were punctuated by clusters of infections. Stamm and colleagues reported an average rate of 2.6 infections per patient year (range, 0.3 to 7.6 episodes per patient year) among 51 women with a documented history of recurrent urinary tract infections.[26] Each woman developed infections at a relatively constant annual rate during 5 years of follow-up. Stamm and colleagues also noted definite clustering of infections in many individuals separated by periods of clinical remission.

THE BIOLOGY OF URINARY TRACT INFECTIONS

Landmark studies of the biology of recurrent bacteriuria clearly demonstrate that colonization of the vag-

TABLE 16–3
Conditions Associated with an Increased Risk of Severe Morbidity or Renal Scarring from Bacteriuria

Severe ureteral reflux
Infections caused by urea-splitting bacteria, which may cause struvite stones
Congenital urinary tract anomalies that become secondarily infected
Infections in the presence of acute or chronic urinary tract obstruction
Renal papillary necrosis
Diabetes mellitus
Spinal cord injury with high intravesical pressure
Pregnancy

Modified from Stamey TA: Recurrent urinary tract infections in female patients: An overview of management and treatment. Rev Inf Dis 9 (Suppl 2):S195, 1987.

inal and urethral mucosa with fecal bacteria precedes the occurrence of bacteriuria.[6, 28] Because the fecal bacterial reservoir is similar in all women, the variability in colonization of the vaginal introitus with Enterobacteriaceae species may determine susceptibility to infection. A significantly higher prevalence of enterobacterial colonization of the vaginal introitus is found in susceptible women compared with those who never have urinary tract infections.[29] Susceptible women were also reported to have larger numbers of pathogenic bacteria colonizing the mucosal surfaces and persisting through consecutive cultures for longer periods of time. A single vaginal culture, however, is often devoid of fecal bacteria, even in patients with frequent infections, indicating that colonization is a dynamic process.

BACTERIAL ADHERENCE

Colonization and ascent into the urinary tract require adherence of bacteria to the epithelial surfaces.[30] The host and bacterial factors that influence adherence to mucosal surfaces ultimately determine susceptiblity to urinary tract infection. Uropathogenic *Escherichia coli* strains adhere to vaginal and uroepithelial cells more avidly in women with a history of recurrent urinary tract infections.[31] Buccal cells from women with recurrent urinary tract infections also show increased bacterial adherence, suggesting the presence of a genetically programmed generalized alteration in epithelial cell surface characteristics in susceptible patients.[32] Among the possible genotypic determinants of susceptibility are the Lewis blood group antigens.[33] The secretor phenotype (Lewis a−, b+), associated with expression of specific blood group carbohydrates on the epithelial cell surface, has been correlated with a diminished susceptibility to recurrent urinary tract infection. It has been suggested that these carbohydrate structures may mask the receptors for uropathogenic bacteria. Because adherence of bacteria to vaginal and uroepithelial cells varies with the days of the menstrual cycle, the hormonal milieu may also modulate adherence characteristics.[34]

The bacterial complement to epithelial cell receptivity is the surface structures collectively termed adhesins, which bind to the putative receptors expressed on the host uroepithelial cells. The most important of these adhesins are the bacterial fimbriae or pili, which are long, filamentous protein appendages.[35] *E. coli* may produce a number of antigenically and functionally different types of pili on the same cell; others may produce a single type, and, in some isolates, no pili are seen.[36] Pili are classified functionally by their ability to mediate hemagglutination of specific types of erythrocytes. The best-described are the type 1 and P pili. Type 1 pili are frequently expressed on both nonpathogenic and pathogenic *E. coli* and appear to facilitate bacterial colonization of the vaginal mucosa.[37] P pili appear to be an important virulence factor in ascending infections of the kidneys.[30, 38] Most (>90%) pyelonephritic strains of *E. coli* express these pili, whereas P pili are found in a minority (<20%) of fecal strains.[39] Bacterial pilus expression is subject to rapid phase variation, and the occurrence of phase variation may contribute to pathogenesis.[40, 41] Initial expression may facilitate adherence and colonization, and subsequent nonproduction may inhibit phagocytic engulfment.[42] These observations support the concept that specific strains of bacteria possess virulence factors that facilitate colonization and infection of the urinary tract. These virulence factors are less critical in patients with an abnormal urinary tract and more important in those with healthy systems and normal defense mechanisms.

Diagnosis

CULTURES

Although urinary tract infections in women are often diagnosed clinically and treated empirically, confirmation requires urine culture. The traditional definition of significant bacteriuria of 100,000 CFUs/ml or more was originally published by Kass and Finland[43]; most bacteria allowed to incubate for several hours in urine will reach colony counts of this level. This discriminatory cut-off point, however, has an unacceptably low sensitivity among young and middle-aged women.[44] In patients with symptomatic infections, 20 to 50% present with bacteria counts of less than 100,000 CFUs/ml.[45] Stamm and colleagues compared midstream bladder cultures with those obtained via suprapubic aspiration or catheter placement.[46] They demonstrated that as few as 100 CFUs/ml were related to irritative voiding symptoms and represented true bacterial cystitis. Thus, in dysuric women, an appropriate threshold value for defining significant bacteriuria is 100 CFUs/ml or more, thereby increasing the sensitivity of urine cultures to about 95%.[46]

The overdiagnosis of urinary tract infection also remains problematic. Women who are susceptible to infection often carry large numbers of pathogenic bacteria on the perineum that can contaminate otherwise sterile bladder urine. Diagnostic accuracy can be maximized by using proper collection techniques coupled with a detailed history and a carefully performed urinalysis. The proper urine collection method is a midstream clean-catch performed with the labia held apart and preceded by gentle washing of the introitus with water. Diagnostic accuracy can be improved by suprapubic aspiration of bladder urine,[47] or, in women, a catheter can be used to obtain the urine sample.

The traditional quantitative culture technique used by most microbiology laboratories is the direct surface plating of a measured amount of urine on split-agar plates. Half is usually blood agar, which grows both gram-positive and gram-negative bacteria, and the other half is eosin-methylene blue or MacConkey agar, which selects for growth of gram-negative bacteria. The dip-slide culture (Uricult) is a simpler and less expensive but also less accurate technique. This method relies on slides coated with an agar medium on each side that are attached to screw-top caps. The slide is dipped into the urine and replaced in its sterile container, and subsequent growth is compared with a visual standard. A number of rapid automated methods have also been developed that detect bacterial growth in less than a quarter of the time needed for standard cultures.[48] These systems have sensitivities of over 95% when 100,000 or more CFUs/ml of urine is used as the standard of comparison. These tests are, however, significantly less sensitive for lower counts of bacteria, and their clinical usefulness is, therefore, currently limited.[49]

URINALYSIS

All components of a carefully performed urinalysis provide ancillary and confirmatory data for the diagnosis of urinary tract infection, but the most important assessment is that for the presence or absence of significant pyuria.[50] The absence of pyuria should raise doubt about the diagnosis of urinary tract infection. Significant pyuria can be simply and reliably determined by using a hemocytometer to count the number of white blood cells (WBCs) in the urine. A measurement of more than 10 WBCs/mm^3 of urine correlates well with the presence of bacteriuria and is rarely seen in nonbacteriuric patients.[51] Despite the accuracy and simplicity inherent in this technique it has not received wide acceptance, and most clinicians rely on the determination of WBCs per high-power field (hpf) in centrifuged urine. This is a much less precise method for evaluating pyuria, and as many as 50% of patients with proven urinary tract infections do not have 5 or more WBCs/hpf.[52]

RAPID SCREENING ASSAYS

Rapid screening assays have also been developed to determine quickly and inexpensively the presence of significant bacteriuria or pyuria. These tests detect either leukocyte esterase activity (LE test) or bacterial nitrite production (nitrite test) in the voided urine. In a study comparing traditional urine cultures with these "chem-strip" tests, the combined LE-nitrite test (either test positive) had a sensitivity of 71% and a specificity of 83% compared with the presence of 1000 or more CFUs/ml in culture.[53] Several investigators,[54, 55] however, have noted substantial variability in the sensitivity and specificity of the test results, which appear to be markedly influenced by the types of patients chosen to be evaluated by the tests. This spectrum bias was illustrated by a study that reported differences in the sensitivity of reagent strip testing ranging from 56 to 92% merely by changing the groups of patients included in the analysis.[56] Although false-positive results are relatively uncommon, the borderline sensitivity of these tests, especially among patients with less characteristic symptoms of urinary tract infection, does not allow these inexpensive tests to replace a careful microscopic urinalysis.

LOCALIZATION

It is often necessary to localize the source of infection to either the upper tract or the urinary bladder, especially in cases of apparent bacterial persistence. Localization is most precise when careful sampling of the bladder urine is coupled with upper tract specimens obtained by endoscopically placed ureteral catheters.[6] The antibody-coated bacteria (ACB) test is a less accurate but noninvasive method of localization. It relies on the observation that renal infection usually triggers a local immune response, resulting in antibody coating the surface of bacteria, which can be detected by fluorescein-labeled antihuman immunoglobulin.[57] The combined results of many different studies using this technique noted agreement in 88% of patients with upper tract infection and in 76% of those with infection confined to the bladder, compared with direct localization.[58] This method has uncovered unrecognized infection of the upper tract in up to a third of patients with symptoms of acute cystitis.[59] Historical features associated with an increased risk of occult renal infection include prolonged symptomatology (7 days or more), diabetes mellitus, immunosuppression, pregnancy, and a history of frequent urinary tract infections or pyelonephritis.[60]

INDICATIONS FOR EVALUATION

The initial evaluation in all women should include a voiding history and a sexual history. The relationship of symptoms to intercourse and the method of contraception used must be addressed. The urethra should be palpated to rule out the presence of a diverticulum. A patient with recurrent infections should be assessed for the presence of significant postvoid residual urine and the urethra should be calibrated. Additional urologic evaluation is unnecessary in the majority of women with genitourinary infections.[61, 62] Fowler and Pulaski prospectively performed excretory urography, cystoscopy, and cystography in women with documented recurrent urinary tract infections.[62] No abnormalities influencing treatment were found among the 104 intravenous pyelograms; 75 cystograms and 74 cystoscopic examinations produced only three cases of urethral diverticuli, which altered the patients' management. The low yield of investigative studies in women with recurrent urinary tract infections should not be surprising. The great majority of women with sporadic and recurrent urinary tract infections have entirely normal urinary tracts. The difficult task is identifying the subset of women in whom structural or functional abnormalities do exist. Clearly, any urinary tract infection associated with possible urinary tract obstruction must be evaluated. Further evaluation is indicated in patients whose pattern of recurrent urinary tract infection suggests bacterial persistence (recurrent infections with the same strain at short intervals). In a study of 186 women with recurrent urinary tract infections prospectively targeted for urologic evaluation based on certain selection criteria, 21% had significant abnormalities detected during urologic investigation, and approximately half of these required surgical intervention. The conclusion was that cystoscopy and upper tract evaluation do play a role in the management of a selected group of women with recurrent urinary tract infections. Indications included gross hematuria at presentation, persistent microscopic hematuria between infections, pyelonephritis, and an atypical presentation (obstructive symptoms, infection with urea-splitting bacteria, or urinary calculi).[63]

Treatment

GENERAL CONCEPTS

In addition to definitive therapy, initial management should include counseling to help prevent further occurrences. All women should be encouraged to maintain an adequate fluid intake and to void regularly and completely. This is especially important prior to and after sexual intercourse. Diaphragms and spermicides have been associated with an increased risk of urinary tract infection.[64] Alternative contraceptive choices should, therefore, be considered in patients with recurrent infections.

ANTIMICROBIAL AGENTS

Therapy for urinary tract infections must ultimately eliminate bacterial growth in the urine; this can occur within hours if the proper antimicrobial agent is used.[6] The efficacy of treatment is critically dependent on the level of the antimicrobial in the urine and the amount of time this level remains above the minimum inhibitory concentration of the infecting organism.[64] In the selection of the antimicrobial and the duration of therapy the physician must consider whether the infection is complicated or not, the spectrum of activity of the drug against the most probable pathogens, the potential adverse effects, and cost. An often underemphasized but important characteristic is the drug's impact on the resident fecal and vaginal flora. Finally, bacterial susceptibility and antimicrobial costs vary dramatically among inpatient and outpatient settings. It is imperative that each clinician keep abreast of changes that affect antimicrobial usage patterns.

The aminopenicillins (ampicillin and amoxicillin) have been used frequently in the past for the treatment of urinary tract infections, but the emergence of resistance in up to 30% of common urinary isolates has lessened the usefulness of these drugs.[64] The effects of these agents on the normal fecal and vaginal flora can predispose to reinfection with resistant strains and frequently leads to candidal vaginitis.[65] The addition of the beta-lactamase inhibitor clavulanate to amoxicillin (Augmentin) greatly improves its activity against certain bacteria that are resistant to amoxicillin alone[66]; however, its high cost and effects on the normal flora argue against its routine use. Generally, aminopenicillins should not be used for first-line therapy of urinary tract infections.[60]

The combination of trimethoprim-sulfamethoxazole (TMP-SMX) has been the most widely used antimicrobial for the treatment of acute urinary tract infection. TMP alone is as effective as the combination for most uncomplicated infections and may be associated with fewer side effects.[60] The addition of SMX, however, increases its efficacy in the treatment of upper tract infection via a synergistic bactericidal effect and may diminish the emergence of resistance.[67] TMP alone or in combination with SMX is effective against most common urinary pathogens with the notable exception of *Enterococcus* and *Pseudomonas* species. The TMP-SMX-based drugs are inexpensive, and their only disadvantages are relatively frequent adverse effects, consisting primarily of skin rashes and gastrointestinal complaints.[68]

All three generations of cephalosporins have oral preparations that have been used for the treatment of acute urinary tract infections.[69] In general, first-generation cephalosporins have greater activity against gram-positive organisms, whereas second- and third-generation drugs have greater activity against gram-negative bacteria. As a group, activity is high against Enterobacteriaceae species, but not against *Pseudomonas* species. Activity against enterococci is generally poor.[69] Cephalosporins produce less resistance among fecal bacteria than the aminopenicillins, but the incidence of candidal vaginitis is nearly the same.[65] Nitrofurantoin is also effective against most uropathogens including enterococci, but not *Pseudomonas* or *Proteus* species.[65]

Nitrofurantoin is rapidly excreted into the urine but does not achieve therapeutic levels in most body tissues; it is not useful, therefore, for upper urinary tract or complicated infections.[69] It has minimal effects on the resident fecal and vaginal flora and has been used effectively in prophylactic regimens.[4]

The fluoroquinolones share a common predecessor in nalidixic acid and inhibit DNA gyrase, a bacterial enzyme integral to replication. Bacterial resistance appeared initially to be uncommon but is now being reported at an increasing rate owing to the indiscriminate use of these agents.[70] The fluoroquinolones have a spectrum of activity that makes them ideal for the treatment of urinary tract infections. They

are highly active against *Enterobacteriaceae* species as well as *P. aeruginosa*. Activity is also high against *Staphylococcus aureus* and *S. saprophyticus*, but in general antistreptococcal coverage is marginal. Most anaerobic bacteria are resistant to these drugs, and therefore much of the normal vaginal and fecal flora is not altered.[70]

These drugs are not nephrotoxic, but renal insufficiency prolongs the serum half-life, requiring adjusted dosing in patients with creatinine clearances of less than 30 ml/minute. Adverse reactions are uncommon; gastrointestinal disturbances are the most frequent. Hypersensitivity, skin reactions, mild central and peripheral nervous system reactions, and even acute renal failure have been reported but are uncommon.[71] Administration of the fluoroquinolones to immature animals has caused damage to developing cartilage. It is unclear whether this occurs in humans, but these agents are currently contraindicated in children, adolescents, and pregnant or nursing women.[72] Important drug interactions are associated with the fluoroquinolones. Antacids containing magnesium or aluminum interfere with absorption of these drugs.[73] Certain fluoroquinolones (enoxacin and ciprofloxacin) elevate plasma levels of theophylline and prolong its half-life.[70] There are two distinct disadvantages of the fluoroquinolones: cost and acquired resistance. For most uncomplicated urinary tract infections, the fluoroquinolones are not significantly more effective than other less-expensive drugs. The fluoroquinolones have distinct advantages in the treatment of complicated urinary tract infections due to host factors, resistant organisms, or difficult-to-treat pathogens such as *P. aeruginosa*.[74]

Physicians have a large armamentarium of effective agents for use in the treatment of urinary tract infections. Comparative antimicrobial trials have, however, tended to be of low quality.[75] The reasons for this are numerous and have been reviewed.[76] Guidelines have been published for the design of antimicrobial trials,[77, 78] but until these recommendations are more universally accepted, final conclusions must be viewed skeptically.

Sporadic Infection

UNCOMPLICATED LOWER URINARY TRACT INFECTION

Afebrile women with the typical symptoms of an acute urinary tract infection, not overtly involving the upper tracts and with a corroborating urinalysis, can be treated presumptively without pretherapy urine cultures. Treatment decisions are usually made and therapy nearly completed before the culture and sensitivity results are available, adding significantly to the cost of management yet infrequently decreasing the duration of symptoms.[79, 80] Patients must be carefully selected for this type of approach. For individuals with evidence of a complicated urinary tract infection or a noncharacteristic clinical history or urinalysis, cultures must be obtained prior to initiation of antimicrobial therapy.

Until recently, acute urinary tract infections in women were treated with a 7- to 10-day course of a suitable oral antimicrobial agent. The literature is now, however, replete with clinical trials touting the efficacy of much shorter courses of therapy. The real and potential advantages include improved compliance, reduced cost, diminished emergence of resistance, and lower incidence of adverse reactions. Norrby has provided an excellent review of 28 separate clinical trials of short-term (single dose or 3-day) courses of antimicrobials for the treatment of uncomplicated cystitis in women.[81] He concluded that regardless of the antimicrobial used, single-dose therapy was not as effective as 3 days of treatment. This difference was less pronounced for the TMP-SMX combinations than for the beta-lactam antimicrobials. For the TMP-SMX combinations, courses longer than 3 days significantly increased the incidence of adverse effects without improving efficacy, leading to the conclusion that 3 days of therapy with these drugs is optimal. The ideal treatment duration for the beta-lactam agents is not clear; treatment for 5 days or longer is more effective but is also more likely to yield adverse reactions.

The fluoroquinolones have proved very effective in the treatment of acute cystitis. A number of studies have reported that 3-day fluoroquinolone courses are equivalent in therapeutic efficacy and are tolerated as well as or better than longer courses of TMP-SMX combinations.[82, 83] Considering the information given previously, the most cost-effective (Table 16–4) approach to uncomplicated acute cystitis is a 3-day course of TMP-SMX as a first-line empirical therapy.[64] The best alternative regimens are a 3-day course of nitrofurantoin or trimethoprim alone. Cephalosporins are also effective but probably require a 5-day course to obtain equivalent cure rates. The fluoroquinolones should be reserved for more problematic infections because of their cost and concern about the impact of indiscriminate use on resistance.

TABLE 16–4
Cost of Common Oral Antimicrobial Regimens Used for Acute Uncomplicated Cystitis

Regimen	Cost for 3 Days of Treatment[a]
TMP-SMX (160/800 mg bid)	$ 3.95 (generic)
Trimethoprim (100 mg bid)	$ 4.25 (generic)
Amoxicillin (500 mg tid)	$ 4.60
Nitrofurantoin (100 mg qid)	$ 7.95
Cephalexin (500 mg qid)	$ 9.15 (generic)
Ciprofloxin (500 mg bid)	$23.60
Ofloxacin (400 mg bid)	$27.10
Amoxicillin/clavulanate (500 mg tid)	$27.55

[a]Costs are based on current Northwestern Hospital outpatient pharmacy charges (personal communication, 1993).

Post-therapy cultures are generally not necessary and should be reserved for patients whose symptoms have not abated at the time of follow-up (3 to 5 days after therapy). This recommendation is based on the following arguments: (1) The great majority of women with uncomplicated cystitis are cured with proper therapy. (2) A large number of cultures would, therefore, have to be obtained to detect a few cases of persistent asymptomatic bacteriuria. (3) The presence of continued asymptomatic bacteriuria poses no significant risk to the healthy nonpregnant woman.

UNCOMPLICATED ACUTE PYELONEPHRITIS

The traditional treatment of acute pyelonephritis has been hospitalization and parenteral administration of antimicrobials either initially or for the entire course of therapy. The success of outpatient regimens[84] argues that the initial management decision should involve stratification of patients into those requiring hospitalization and those who can be safely managed as outpatients. Indications for hospitalization include an inability to take oral medication, dehydration, significant pain, evidence of toxemia, or the presence of host factors suggesting complicated infection. In a large retrospective study of women with acute pyelonephritis, Safrin and associates concluded that outpatient treatment with properly chosen oral antimicrobials is a safe and effective alternative for nonpregnant and immunocompetent women at less than 15% of the cost of inpatient care.[85] Most outpatients were treated with TMP-SMX combinations for 10 to 14 days, with approximately 90% success. Seven outpatients had a suboptimal outcome, but only two required hospitalization. No incidents of serious morbidity or mortality occurred. The combination of TMP-SMX has been the most studied and used regimen for outpatient therapy and should be considered the antimicrobial of choice.[64] Acute pyelonephritis can also be effectively treated with oral fluoroquinolones,[86, 87] although these agents should be reserved for patients who are intolerant of TMP-SMX.

In patients who require hospitalization, parenteral therapy should achieve acceptable tissue and urinary levels directed against enterococci and gram-negative bacilli. The combination of ampicillin and an aminoglycoside is the most frequently used empirical antimicrobial regimen. Other acceptable parenteral regimens include an aminoglycoside alone, TMP-SMX, second- or third-generation cephalosporins, fluoroquinolones, and some broad-spectrum penicillins. Urine cultures must be obtained prior to initiation of therapy, and treatment should be adjusted based on the results. Parenteral therapy should be continued until the patient has been afebrile for at least 24 hours, at which time an oral antimicrobial can be prescribed for the duration of therapy. Fourteen days of antimicrobial therapy is as effective as longer courses; side effects and reinfections with resistant organisms do not occur as frequently.[84] Repeat urine cultures should be performed 5 to 7 days after initiation of therapy and then 4 to 6 weeks later to ensure that the urinary tract remains free of infection.

COMPLICATED URINARY TRACT INFECTION

Complicated infections encompass a wide spectrum of disorders and a diversity of subjects, and therapy for such infections is difficult to summarize. The failure to recognize complicating factors at the initial presentation is the biggest obstacle to successful management. Although pregnancy or recent urinary tract instrumentation, for example, is easily identified, other abnormalities such as diverticuli are unlikely to be diagnosed until therapy fails or complications occur. The most important aspect of therapy should be a logical approach to identifying and correcting the abnormalities that exist. The increased incidence of certain pathogens, such as *P. aeruginosa* and enterococci, makes the usual oral antimicrobials much less efficacious; the fluoroquinolones have proved to be more effective for this type of infection.[86, 88] The ideal duration of therapy has not been established, but it should extend for at least 7 to 10 days. The high incidence of resistant organisms and treatment failures in these patients necessitates performing pretherapy and post-treatment cultures.

Unresolved Infections

In patients who remain symptomatic after 3 days of antimicrobial therapy, cultures should be done and the drug empirically switched to a fluoroquinolone antimicrobial. If the culture and sensitivity results demonstrate bacteria that are resistant to the original drug, no further evaluation or therapy is indicated. If, however, the bacteria are sensitive to the original drug, a directed evaluation should ensue. Specifically, one must look for a nidus of continued bacteriuria such as a large calculus. It is also possible that adequate urine antimicrobial levels were not achieved because of severe renal impairment or, more commonly, noncompliance with the regimen.

Recurrent Urinary Tract Infections

REINFECTIONS

Landmark studies on the biology and natural history of recurrent urinary tract infections have proved that almost all are due to reinfection rather than to occult bacterial persistence.[6] This critical observation underlies the basis for the successful management of these patients—prophylaxis against infection rather than intermittent treatment with increasingly powerful antimicrobial agents.[4] Recurrences in healthy women with normal urinary tracts do not indicate

treatment failure but are a result of mucosal colonization and subsequent ascending infection in susceptible patients.

Many effective prophylactic regimens have been established; they all rely on antimicrobials that have little impact on the anaerobic fecal flora and are given at a minimally effective dose. The mechanism of prophylaxis differs among the antimicrobials.[4] The fluoroquinolones and TMP-SMX eradicate much of the aerobic gut flora and are secreted in the vaginal fluid. These agents, therefore, eliminate carriage of Enterobacteriaceae on the vaginal and urethral mucosa. Nitrofurantoin does not have this effect; it probably works by intermittently sterilizing the urine. Management strategies have included continuous prophylaxis with either daily or thrice-weekly antimicrobial dosing, postcoital prophylaxis, or intermittent self-start therapy. Appropriate prophylactic regimens can be expected to reduce the frequency of recurrent infection by at least 90% in almost all patients[17, 26, 89–92] (Table 16–5).

Prophylaxis should be considered in anyone with at least two infections during a 6-month period or three or more infections during the previous year. An existing infection should be eradicated before initiating the prophylactic regimen. Most authorities recommend a 6-month trial of prophylaxis followed by observation and reassessment. Rates of infection returning to the baseline level are, however, usually observed after cessation of prophylaxis.[26] Stamm and colleagues studied various long-term prophylactic protocols and found that trimethoprim, TMP-SMX, and nitrofurantoin were all equally effective.[26] When the results were evaluated by year of prophylaxis, there was no apparent decrease in the effectiveness of prophylaxis even after 5 years. There was no significant increase in infections with antimicrobial-resistant strains as the duration of prophylaxis lengthened. Adverse reactions were also rare. These authors concluded that long-term regimens were safe and effective.

The disadvantages of continuous prophylaxis are cost, inconvenience, and adverse reactions. These can be partially mitigated by using postcoital prophylaxis in selected patients. In a randomized double-blind, placebo-controlled study, TMP-SMX (40/200 mg) administered after intercourse was very effective in preventing recurrent urinary tract infections[17] (see Table 16–5). Efficacy did not vary significantly compared with the frequency of intercourse. This type of approach is most appropriate for women who relate their recurrent infections temporally with intercourse or are hesitant to take daily antimicrobials.

Self-start therapy is an alternative to prophylactic regimens.[93] Reliable patients can be given a 3-day course of an empirical full-dose antimicrobial to use when typical symptoms of acute cystitis occur. Although not essential, patients can obtain their own dip-slide cultures prior to therapy. Cultures should be performed when symptoms do not abate promptly. A postinfection evaluation, including a urinalysis, should be performed approximately 1 week after

TABLE 16–5
**Recurrent Urinary Tract Infections in Women:
Prophylactic Management Regimens**

Investigator	Regimen	Infections per Patient-Year
Harding and Ronald (1974)[89]	1. Sulfamethoxazole 500 mg daily 2. TMP/SMX 40/200 mg daily 3. No drug	2.5 0.1 3.6
Harding et al (1982)[90]	TMP/SMX 40/200 mg 3 times weekly	0.14
Martinez et al (1985)[91]	Cephalexin 250 mg daily	0.18
Stapleton et al (1990)[17]	1. TMP/SMX 40/200 mg postcoital and placebo daily 2. Placebo postcoital and daily	0.30 3.60
Raz and Boger (1991)[92]	1. Norfloxacin 200 mg daily 2. Nitrofurantoin 50 mg daily	0.07 0.34
Stamm et al (1991)[26]	1. Nitrofurantoin 100 mg daily 2. Trimethoprim 100 mg daily 3. TMP/SMX 40/200 mg daily 4. No drug	0.1 0.03 0.6 1.9

Adapted from Nicolle LE, Ronald AR: Recurrent urinary tract infection in adult women: Diagnosis and treatment. Infect Dis Clin North Am 1:793, 1987.

completing therapy. At this time, the patient can be provided with another 3-day supply of antimicrobials and a dip-slide culture. This technique is particularly attractive for reliable patients who have less frequent infections and are willing to play an active role in diagnosis and management.

BACTERIAL PERSISTENCE

Despite adequate therapy and documented resolution of bacteriuria, recurrent infection can arise from the same organism sequestered in a site that escaped the action of the antimicrobial agent. Recurrent infections with the same strain of bacteria at close intervals often signal bacterial persistence. Many women with typical recurrences (reinfections), however, have vaginal colonization with the same pathogen over long periods of time, and these reinfections can cluster over short intervals.[6, 26] A suspicion of bacterial persistence should lead to a logical search for an identifiable abnormality that is allowing the bacteria to persist (Table 16–6). Causes may be subtle, requiring cystoscopic localization of the infection with ureteral catheters to define the focus of bacterial persistence.

Bacteriuria in Pregnancy

NATURAL HISTORY

Although the prevalence of bacteriuria does not change appreciably during pregnancy, the anatomic and physiologic changes induced by the gravid state significantly alter its natural history.[94] Although asymptomatic bacteriuria in nonpregnant patients often clears, pregnant women become symptomatic more frequently and tend to remain bacteriuric.[95]

Pyelonephritis develops in 1 to 4% of all pregnant women, an event that rarely occurs in nonpregnant women with uncomplicated urinary tract infections.[96] In a review, Sweet reported an average incidence of pyelonephritis of 28% in pregnant women with untreated bacteriuria; less than 2% of pregnant women with no bacteriuria on initial screening developed this complication.[97] By treating asymptomatic bacteriuria found early in pregnancy, the prevalence of subsequent acute pyelonephritis dropped from 28% to less than 3%.

SIGNIFICANCE OF BACTERIURIA

In the preantibiotic era, a high rate of infant prematurity and mortality occurred in pregnant women with bacterial pyelonephritis.[98] It is controversial whether women who have been treated for pyelone-

TABLE 16–6
Correctable Urologic Abnormalities That Cause Bacterial Persistence and Recurrent Urinary Tract Infection

Infection calculi
Unilateral infected atrophic kidneys
Vesicovaginal and vesicointestinal fistulas
Ureteral duplication and ectopic ureters
Foreign bodies
Urethral diverticula
Infected paraurethral glands
Unilateral infected medullary sponge kidneys
Infected urachal cysts
Infected communicating cysts of the renal calyces
Papillary necrosis

Modified from Dairiki-Shortliffe LM, Stamey TA: Infections of the urinary tract: Introduction and general principles. *In* Walsh PC, Gittes RE, Perlmutter AD, et al (eds): Campbell's Urology, 5th ed. Philadelphia, WB Saunders, 1986, p 743.

phritis or asymptomatic bacteriuria during pregnancy still have an increased risk of infant prematurity and perinatal mortality. Gilstrap and colleagues found no difference in pregnancy outcome among patients treated for either asymptomatic bacteriuria or acute pyelonephritis and nonbacteriuric controls.[98] Other studies found an association between pyelonephritis and preterm labor.[99] Whether clinical pyelonephritis during pregnancy causes an increased risk of prematurity and low birth weight is unclear, but bacteriuria in the symptomatic or asymptomatic pregnant woman should definitely be treated.

MANAGEMENT

An initial screening culture should be performed in all pregnant women during the first trimester.[99] Repeat cultures are generally unnecessary because patients in whom sterile urine is documented early in pregnancy are unlikely to develop bacteriuria late.[100] Special consideration must be given to the selection of antimicrobial agents to avoid fetal toxicity. The aminopenicillins and cephalosporins are considered safe and generally effective throughout pregnancy. In patients with penicillin allergies, nitrofurantoin is a reasonable alternative.[99] Given the lower efficacy of short-course beta-lactam therapy in nonpregnant women, it is prudent to prescribe a full 7-day course of therapy in pregnant women. Follow-up cultures should be obtained to document the desired response. Pregnant women with acute pyelonephritis should be hospitalized and treated initially with parenteral antimicrobials. An appropriate oral agent should then be chosen to complete therapy for at least 14 days.[101] These patients must be followed very closely for the remainder of their pregnancy, and consideration should be given to initiation of a prophylactic regimen. In patients with a history of frequent recurrent urinary tract infections or pyelonephritis prior to pregnancy, the initiation or continuation of an appropriate prophylactic strategy is an option. The efficacy of postcoital prophylaxis with either cephalexin (250 mg) or nitrofurantoin (50 mg) has been reported.[102]

Bacteriuria in the Elderly

Urinary tract infections in the elderly are common and are an expanding health problem.[103] The prevalence of bacteriuria in elderly women increases with age, institutionalization, and concurrent disease, often exceeding 50% in select groups.[104, 105] Longitudinal studies have helped clarify the dynamic aspects of bacteriuria in the elderly. The incidence of asymptomatic bacteriuria is much more common than is apparent from a single survey, implying that the majority of elderly women eventually have an episode of bacteriuria.[106]

PATHOGENESIS

The pathophysiology of increased susceptibility is multifactorial and poorly understood. Age-related changes include a decline in cell-mediated immunity, neurogenic bladder dysfunction, increased perineal soiling due to fecal and urinary incontinence, increased incidence of urethral catheter placement, and possible changes in the vaginal environment.[105] The bacteriologic features of infection in the elderly differ from those in younger women.[107] E. coli remains the most common uropathogen, but there is a significant increase in the incidence of *Proteus, Klebsiella, Enterobacter, Serratia,* and *Pseudomonas* species as well as enterococci. *Staphylococcus saprophyticus* is not seen in this population. Polymicrobial bacteriuria is also more common among the elderly.[108]

DIAGNOSIS

The diagnosis of urinary tract infections in the elderly can be difficult; symptoms are often absent or vague and concomitant diseases can mask or mimic urinary infection. Even severe upper tract infections may not be associated with fever or leukocytosis.[107] Therefore, a high index of suspicion is warranted, and diagnosis should rely on the results of a carefully obtained urinalysis and culture. The presence of 100,000 CFUs of bacteria or more per milliliter of urine remains the standard for diagnosis in these patients. Pyuria alone is not a good predictor of bacteriuria in this population. Boscia and colleagues reported that more than 60% of women in whom pyuria (≥ 10 WBCs/mm^3 of urine) was noted in midstream specimens did not have concurrent bacteriuria.[109] The absence of pyuria, however, was a good predictor of the absence of bacteriuria. Because urinary tract abnormalities can frequently complicate and predispose to bacteriuria in the elderly, a thorough urologic evaluation should be considered.

SIGNIFICANCE OF SCREENING BACTERIURIA

The significance of asymptomatic bacteriuria in the elderly is unclear.[105] There is no documented relationship between uncomplicated urinary tract infections and worsening renal function in this population. The treatment of asymptomatic bacteriuria to improve incontinence has not been justified.[107] Although studies have demonstrated decreased survival in bacteriuric patients compared with nonbacteriuric controls, it is unclear whether increased mortality and bacteriuria are causally related.[107] Nicolle and associates randomized institutionalized women with bacteriuria to treatment or observation and followed these patients over a 1-year period.[108] Treatment did not result in improved survival but was associated with a number of adverse effects.

MANAGEMENT

The exceedingly high prevalence and recurrence rates of bacteriuria in this population, concern over adverse reactions, and the emergence of resistance associated with antimicrobial use make a universal recommendation to treat asymptomatic bacteriuria in the elderly unwarranted. When treating symptomatic infections, antimicrobial selection should take into account the potential for impaired metabolism and excretion of these drugs as well as the greater likelihood of drug interactions in this population.

Catheter-Associated Bacteriuria

NATURAL HISTORY

Between 15 and 25% of patients in acute care hospitals have an indwelling urinary catheter at some time during their hospitalization.[110] It is not surprising, therefore, that catheter-associated urinary tract infections are the most commonly reported nosocomial infection.[111] With long-term catheterization, the development of bacteriuria is inevitable. Catheter insertion itself has been associated with rates of bacteriuria of less than 1% in healthy individuals to 15% in elderly hospitalized patients.[112] For each day the catheter remains indwelling the incidence of bacteriuria increases 5 to 10%, even with closed drainage systems.[113] The most important risk factors associated with an increased likelihood of developing catheter-associated bacteriuria are the duration of catheterization, female gender, absence of systemic antimicrobials, and catheter care violations.[111] The majority of catheter-associated urinary tract infections are asymptomatic. In patients with short-term catheter placement only 10 to 30% of bacteriuric episodes produce typical symptoms of acute infection.[110, 114] Similarly, although all patients with long-term catheters are bacteriuric, the incidence of febrile episodes occurs at a rate of only one per 100 days of catheterization.[115]

PATHOGENESIS

Bacteriuria can develop in catheterized patients in several possible ways. Bacteria can be introduced at the time of initial catheter placement by either mechanical insertion of urethral bacteria or contamination from poor technique. More commonly, bacteria subsequently gain access through a periurethral or intraluminal route.[111] In women, periurethral entry is most prevalent. Daifuku and Stamm found that among 18 women who developed catheter-associated bacteriuria, 12 had antecedent urethral colonization with the infecting strain.[116] Urinary catheters provide a unique environment that allows two distinct populations of bacteria: those that grow within the urine and those that grow on the catheter surfaces, termed biofilm growth. The biofilm represents a microenvironment of bacteria embedded in an extracellular matrix of bacterial products and host proteins that often leads to catheter encrustation.[111] Certain bacteria, particularly the *Pseudomonas* and *Proteus* species, are adept at biofilm growth, which may explain their higher incidence in this clinical setting.[117] The uropathogens isolated from the catheterized urinary tract often differ from those found in noncatheterized, ambulatory patients. There is a much higher incidence of *Pseudomonas, Proteus,* and enterococcal species.[115] In patients with long-term catheterization (>30 days), the bacteriuria is usually polymicrobial, and the presence of four or five pathogens is not uncommon.[118] Although certain species may persist for long periods of time, the bacterial populations in these patients tend to be dynamic.[118]

MANAGEMENT

Although symptomatic urinary tract infections can be treated successfully in patients with indwelling catheters, the source of bacteriuria will never be eradicated until the catheter is removed. Much of the research on catheter-associated bacteriuria has been directed toward preventing or retarding the development of bacteriuria in these patients. Unfortunately, many of these approaches, although logical, have failed in clinical practice. Periurethral care regimens have generally been unsuccessful.[111] Silver oxide, which is bactericidal and nontoxic, when incorporated into catheters has been reported to decrease the incidence of bacteriuria in some studies[119] but not in others.[111] Concurrent administration of systemic antimicrobials clearly decreases the incidence of bacteriuria associated with short-term catheterization,[119] but the cost, risk of adverse effects, and concern about the emergence of resistant organisms have limited this approach.[111] For patients requiring long-term or lifelong catheterization, bacteriuria is unpreventable. Attempts should be made to institute intermittent catheterization when this is clinically feasible.

In patients undergoing short-term catheterization it makes little sense to obtain screening cultures as long as the catheter remains indwelling. A reasonable approach to the asymptomatic patient is to begin empirical antimicrobial therapy on the day of catheter removal. Cultures can be obtained prior to the start of treatment but are probably unnecessary. In most situations a 3-day course of an antimicrobial such as TMP-SMX should suffice. We recommend that post-therapy cultures be obtained in this clinical setting to confirm the eradication of the bacteriuria. In patients with chronic indwelling catheters, asymptomatic bacteriuria should never be treated. When bacteriuria is symptomatic, cultures and sensitivity testing are necessary to guide effective therapy. Because of catheter encrustation that can theoretically shelter bacteria from the antimicrobial agent, the catheter should be changed at the initiation of therapy.

REFERENCES

1. Kunin CM: Detection, Prevention and Management of Urinary Tract Infections, 4th ed. Philadelphia, Lea & Febiger, 1987, pp 12, 82.
2. National Center for Health Statistics: National Hospital Discharge Survey. National Center for Health Statistics, 1989.
3. Johnson JR, Stamm WE: Diagnosis and treatment of acute urinary tract infections. Infect Dis Clin North Am 1:773, 1987.
4. Stamey TA: Recurrent urinary tract infections in female patients: An overview of management and treatment. Rev Infect Dis 9 (Suppl 2):S195, 1987.
5. Schaeffer AJ: Infections of the urinary tract. In Walsh PC, Retik AB, Stamey TA, et al (eds): Campbell's Urology, 6th ed. Philadelphia, WB Saunders, 1992, pp 731–806.
6. Stamey TA: Pathogenesis and Treatment of Urinary Tract Infections. Baltimore, Williams & Wilkins, 1980, pp 43–46.
7. Cattell WR: Urinary tract infections in adults. Postgrad Med 61:907, 1985.
8. Anderson RU: Urinary tract infections in adults. Urol Clin North Am 13:727, 1986.
9. Preheim LC: Complicated urinary tract infections. Am J Med 79:62, 1985.
10. Kass EH: Horatio at the orifice: The significance of bacteriuria. J Infect Dis 138:546, 1978.
11. Nicolle LE, Harding GKM, Preiksaitis J, et al: The association of urinary tract infection with sexual intercourse. J Infect Dis 146:579, 1982.
12. Remis RS, Gurwith MJ, Gurwith D, et al: Risk factors for urinary tract infection. Am J Epidemiol 126:685, 1987.
13. Leibovici L, Alpert G, Kalter-Leibovici O, et al: Urinary tract infections and sexual activity in young women. Arch Intern Med 147:345, 1987.
14. Kunin CM, McCormack RC: An epidemiologic study of bacteriuria and blood pressure among nuns and working women. N Engl J Med 278:635, 1968.
15. Pfau A, Sacks TG, Englestein D: Recurrent urinary tract infection in premenopausal women: Prophylaxis based on an understanding of the pathogenesis. J Urol 139:1250, 1983.
16. Bran JL, Levison ME, Kaye D: Entrance of bacteria into the female urinary bladder. N Engl J Med 286:626, 1972.
17. Stapleton A, Latham RH, Johnson C, et al: Postcoital antimicrobial prophylaxis for recurrent urinary tract infection: A randomized, double-blind, placebo-controlled trial. JAMA 264:703, 1990.
18. Baldassarre JS, Kaye D: Special problems of urinary tract infection in the elderly. Med Clin North Am 75:375, 1991.
19. Mabeck CE: Treatment of uncomplicated urinary tract infection in nonpregnant women. Postgrad Med 48:69, 1972.
20. Guttmann D: Follow-up of urinary tract infection in domiciliary patients. In Brumfitt W, Asscher AW (eds): Urinary Tract Infection. London, Oxford University Press, 1973, p 62.
21. Asscher AW, Sussman M, Waters WE, et al: Asymptomatic significant bacteriuria in the non-pregnant woman. II. Response to treatment and follow-up. BMJ 1:804, 1969.
22. Tencer J: Asymptomatic bacteriuria—a long-term study. Scand J Urol Nephrol 22:31, 1988.
23. Freedman LR: Natural history of urinary tract infection in adults. Kidney Int 8 (Suppl):S96, 1975.
24. Maill WE, Kass EH, Ling J, et al: Factors influencing arterial pressure in the general population of Jamaica. Br Med J 25 (2):497, 1962.
25. Ronald AR, Pattullo ALS: The natural history of urinary infection in adults. Med Clin North Am 75:299, 1991.
26. Stamm WE, McKevitt M, Roberts PL, et al: Natural history of recurrent urinary tract infections in women. Rev Infect Dis 13:77, 1991.
27. Harrison WO, Holmes KK, Belding ME, et al: A prospective evaluation of recurrent urinary tract infection in women. Clin Res 22:125A, 1974.
28. Stamey TA, Timothy M, Millar M, et al: Recurrent urinary infections in adult women. The role of introital enterobacteria. Calif Med 115:1, 1971.
29. Stamey TA, Sexton CC: The role of vaginal colonization with Enterobacteriaceae in recurrent urinary infections. J Urol 113:214, 1975.
30. Reid G, Sobel JD: Bacterial adherence in the pathogenesis of urinary tract infection: A review. Rev Infect Dis 9:470, 1987.
31. Fowler JE Jr, Stamey TA: Studies of introital colonization in women with recurrent urinary infections. VII. The role of bacterial adherence. J Urol 117:472, 1977.
32. Schaeffer AJ, Jones JM, Dunn JK: Association of in vitro Escherichia coli adherence to vaginal and buccal epithelial cells with susceptibility of women to recurrent urinary tract infections. N Engl J Med 304:1062, 1981.
33. Sheinfeld J, Schaeffer AJ, Cordon-Cardo C, et al: Association of the Lewis blood-group phenotype with recurrent urinary tract infections in women. N Engl J Med 320:773, 1989.
34. Schaeffer AJ, Amundsen SK, Schmidt LN: Adherence of Escherichia coli to human urinary tract epithelial cells. Infect Immun 24:753, 1979.
35. Briton CC Jr: Non-flagellar appendages of bacteria. Nature 183:782, 1959.
36. Klemm P: Fimbrial adhesins of Escherichia coli. Rev Infect Dis 7:321, 1985.
37. Sobel JD: Bacterial etiologic agents in the pathogenesis of urinary tract infection. Med Clin North Am 75:253, 1991.
38. Svenson SB, Kallenius G, Korhonen TK, et al: Initiation of clinical pyelonephritis—the role of P-fimbriae-mediated bacterial adhesin. Contrib Nephrol 39:252, 1984.
39. Kallenius G, Mollby R, Svensson SB, et al: Occurrence of P-fimbriated Escherichia coli in urinary tract infections. Lancet 2:1369, 1981.
40. Hultgren SJ, Schwan WR, Schaeffer AJ, et al: Regulation of production of type 1 pili among urinary tract isolates of Escherichia coli. Infect Immun 54:613, 1986.
41. Eisenstein BI: Phase variation of type-1 fimbriae in Escherichia coli is under transcriptional control. Science 214:337, 1981.
42. Silverblatt FJ, Dreyer JS, Schauer S: Effect of pili on susceptibility of Escherichia coli to phagocytes. Infect Immun 24:218, 1979.
43. Kass EH, Finland M: Asymptomatic infections of the urinary tract. Trans Assoc Am Physicians 69:56, 1956.
44. Kraft JK, Stamey TA: The natural history of symptomatic recurrent bacteriuria in women. Medicine 56:55, 1977.
45. Gallagher DJA, Montgomerie JZ, North JDK: Acute infections of the urinary tract and the urethral syndrome in general practice. Br Med J 1:622, 1965.
46. Stamm WE, Counts GW, Running KR, et al: Diagnosis of coliform infection in acutely dysuric women. N Engl J Med 307:463, 1982.
47. Stamey TA, Govan DE, Palmer JM: The localization and treatment of urinary tract infections: The role of bactericidal urine levels as opposed to serum levels. Medicine 44:1, 1965.
48. Pezzlo MT: Automated methods for detection of bacteriuria. Am J Med 75 (Suppl 1):71, 1983.
49. Pappas PG: Laboratory in the diagnosis and management of urinary tract infections. Med Clin North Am 75:313, 1991.
50. Stamm WE: Measurement of pyuria and its relation to bacteriuria. Am J Med 75 (Suppl):53, 1983.
51. Stamm WE, Running K, McKevitt M, et al: Treatment of the acute urethral syndrome. N Engl J Med 304:956, 1981.
52. Stamm WE: Criteria for the diagnosis of urinary tract infection and for the assessment of therapeutic effectiveness. Infection 20 (Suppl 3):S151, 1992.
53. Pfaller MA, Koontz FP: Laboratory evaluation of leukocyte esterase and nitrite tests for the detection of bacteriuria. J Clin Microbiol 21:840, 1985.
54. Pels RJ, Bor DH, Woolhandler S, et al: Dipstick urinalysis screening of asymptomatic adults for urinary tract disorders. JAMA 262:1220, 1989.
55. Hurlbut TA 3d, Littenberg B: The diagnostic accuracy of rapid dipstick tests to predict urinary tract infection. Am J Clin Pathol 96:582, 1991.
56. Lachs MS, Nachamkin I, Edelstein PH, et al: Spectrum bias in the evaluation of diagnostic tests: Lessons from the rapid dipstick test for urinary tract infection. Ann Intern Med 117:135, 1992.

57. Thomas VL: Antibody-coated bacteria in urinary tract infections. Kidney Int 21:1, 1982.
58. Schaeffer AJ: Renal infection. In Gillenwater JY, Grayhack JT, Howards SS, et al (eds): Adult and Pediatric Urology, 2nd ed. St. Louis, Mosby Year Book, 1991, pp 745–787.
59. Jones SR, Smith JW, Sanford JP: Localization of urinary tract infections by detection of antibody-coated bacteria in urine sediment. N Engl J Med 290:591, 1974.
60. Johnson JR, Stamm WE: Urinary tract infections in women: Diagnosis and treatment Ann Intern Med 111:906, 1989.
61. Fair WR, McClennan BL, Jost RG: Are excretory urograms necessary in evaluating women with urinary tract infection? J Urol 121:313, 1979.
62. Fowler JE Jr, Pulaski ET: Excretory urography, cystography, and cystoscopy in the evaluation of women with urinary-tract infection: A prospective study. N Engl J Med 304:462, 1981.
63. Nickel JC, Wilson J, Morales A, et al: Value of urologic investigation in a targeted group of women with recurrent urinary tract infections. Can J Surg 34:591, 1991.
64. Hooton TM, Stamm WE: Management of acute uncomplicated urinary tract infection in adults. Med Clin North Am 75:339, 1991.
65. Iravani A: Advances in the understanding and treatment of urinary tract infections in young women. Urology 37:503, 1991.
66. Amoxicillin-clavulanic acid. Med Lett Drugs Ther 26:99, 1984.
67. Burman LG: Significance of the sulfonamide component for the clinical efficacy of trimethoprim-sulfonamide combinations. Scand J Infect Dis 18:89, 1986.
68. Cockerill FR, Edson RS: Trimethoprim-sulfamethoxazole. Mayo Clin Proc 66:1249, 1991.
69. Wilhelm MP, Edson RS: Antimicrobial agents in urinary tract infections. Mayo Clin Proc 62:1025, 1991.
70. Wright AJ, Walker RC, Barrett DM: The fluoroquinolones and their appropriate use in treatment of genitourinary tract infections. In Ball TP, Novicki DE (eds): AUA Update Series. Houston, American Urologic Association, 1993, pp 50–55.
71. Hootkins R, Fenzer AZ, Stephens MK: Acute renal failure secondary to oral ciprofloxacin therapy: A presentation of three cases and a review of the literature. Clin Nephrol 32:75, 1989.
72. Christ W, Lehnert T, Ulbrich B: Specific toxicologic aspects of the quinolones. Rev Infect Dis 10:141, 1988.
73. Davies BI, Maesen FPV: Drug interactions with quinolones. Rev Infect Dis 11 (Suppl 5):1083, 1989.
74. Dalkin BL, Schaeffer AJ: Fluoroquinolone antimicrobial agents: Use in the treatment of urinary tract infections and clinical urologic practice. Probl Urol 2:476, 1988.
75. Norrby R: Quality of antibiotic clinical trials. J Antimicrob Chemother 14:205, 1984.
76. Norrby SR: Design of clinical trials in patients with urinary tract infections. Infection 20 (Suppl 3):S181, 1992.
77. Rubin RH, Shapiro ED, Andriole VT, et al: Evaluation of new anti-infective drugs for the treatment of urinary tract infection. Clin Infect Dis 15 (Suppl 1):S216, 1992.
78. Beam TR Jr, Gilbert DN, Kunin CM: General guidelines for the clinical evaluation of anti-infective drug products. Clin Infect Dis 15 (Suppl 1):S5, 1992.
79. Komaroff AL: Urinalysis and urine culture in women with dysuria. Ann Intern Med 104:212, 1986.
80. Carlson KJ, Mulley AG: Management of acute dysuria: A decision-analysis model of alternative strategies. Ann Intern Med 102:244, 1985.
81. Norrby SR: Short-term treatment of uncomplicated lower urinary tract infections in women. Rev Infect Dis 12:458, 1990.
82. Stein GE, Mummaur N, Goldstein EJC, et al: A multicenter comparative trial of three-day norfloxacin vs ten-day sulfamethoxazole and trimethoprim for the treatment of uncomplicated urinary tract infections. Arch Intern Med 147:1760, 1987.
83. Cox CE, Serfer HS, Mena HR, et al: Ofloxacin versus trimethoprim/sulfamethoxazole in the treatment of uncomplicated urinary tract infection. Clin Ther 14:446, 1992.
84. Stamm WE, McKevitt M, Counts GW: Acute renal infection in women: Treatment with trimethoprim-sulfamethoxazole or ampicillin for two or six weeks. A randomized trial. Ann Intern Med 106:341, 1987.
85. Safrin S, Siegel D, Black D: Pyelonephritis in adult women: Inpatient versus outpatient therapy. Am J Med 85:793, 1988.
86. Wolfson JS, Hoopern DC: Treatment of genitourinary tract infections with fluoroquinolones: Activity in vitro, pharmacokinetics and clinical efficacy in urinary tract infections and prostatitis. Antimicrob Agents Chemother 33:1655, 1989.
87. Ludwig G, Pauthner H: Clinical experience with ofloxacin in upper and lower urinary tract infections: A comparison with co-trimoxazole and nitrofurantoin. Drugs 34 (Suppl 1):95, 1987.
88. Cox CE: A comparison of the safety and efficacy of lomefloxacin and ciprofloxacin in the treatment of complicated or recurrent urinary tract infections. Am J Med 92 (4A):82S, 1992.
89. Harding GKM, Ronald AR: A control study of antimicrobial prophylaxis of recurrent urinary tract infection in women. N Engl J Med 291:597, 1974.
90. Harding GKM, Ronald AR, Nicolle LE, et al: Long-term antimicrobial prophylaxis for recurrent urinary tract infection in women. Rev Infect Dis 4:438, 1982.
91. Martinez FC, Kendrachuk RW, Thomas E, et al: Effect of prophylactic, low dose cephalexin on fecal and vaginal bacteria. J Urol 133:994, 1985.
92. Raz R, Boger S: Long-term prophylaxis with norfloxacin versus nitrofurantoin in women with recurrent urinary tract infection. Antimicrob Agents Chemother 35:1241, 1991.
93. Wong ES, McKevitt M, Running K, et al: Management of recurrent urinary tract infections with patient-administered single-dose therapy. Ann Intern Med 102:302, 1985.
94. Patterson TF, Andriole VT: Bacteriuria in pregnancy. Infect Dis Clin North Am 1:807, 1987.
95. Elder HA, Santamarina BAG, Smith S, et al: The natural history of asymptomatic bacteriuria during pregnancy: The effect of tetracycline on the clinical course and the outcome of pregnancy. Am J Obstet Gynecol 111:441, 1971.
96. Kass EH: The role of unsuspected infection in the etiology of prematurity. Clin Obstet Gynecol 16:134, 1973.
97. Sweet RL: Bacteriuria and pyelonephritis during pregnancy. Semin Perinatol 1:25, 1977.
98. Gilstrap LC, Leveno KJ, Cunningham FG, et al: Renal infection and pregnancy outcome. Am J Obstet Gynecol 141:709, 1981.
99. Androile VT, Patterson TF: Epidemiology, natural history, and management of urinary tract infections in pregnancy. Med Clin North Am 75:359, 1991.
100. McFadyen IR, Eykyn SJ, Gardner NHN, et al: Bacteriuria in pregnancy. J Obstet Gynaecol Br Commonw 80:385, 1973.
101. Faro S, Pastorek JG, Plauche WC: Short-course parental antibiotic therapy for pyelonephritis in pregnancy. South Med J 77:455, 1984.
102. Pfau A, Sacks TG: Effective prophylaxis for recurrent urinary tract infections during pregnancy. Clin Infect Dis 14:810, 1992.
103. Kaye D: Urinary tract infections in the elderly. Bull NY Acad Med 56:209, 1980.
104. Boscia JA, Kaye D: Asymptomatic bacteriuria in the elderly. Infect Dis Clin North Am 1:839, 1987.
105. Schaeffer AJ: Urinary tract infections in the elderly. Eur Urol 19 (Suppl 1):2, 1991.
106. Boscia JA, Kobasa WD, Knight RA, et al: Epidemiology of bacteriuria in an elderly ambulatory population. Am J Med 80:208, 1986.
107. Baldassarre JS, Kaye D: Special problems of urinary tract infection in the elderly. Med Clin North Am 75:375, 1991.
108. Nicolle LE, Mayhew WJ, Bryan L: Prospective, randomized comparison of therapy and no therapy for asymptomatic bacteriuria in institutionalized elderly women. Am J Med 83:27, 1987.
109. Boscia JA, Abrutyn E, Levison ME, et al: Pyuria and asymptomatic bacteriuria in elderly ambulatory women. Ann Intern Med 110:404, 1989.

110. Haley RW, Hooton TM, Culver DH, et al: Nosocomial infections in U.S. hospitals, 1975–1976: Estimated frequency by selected characteristics of patients. Am J Med 70:947, 1981.

111. Stamm WE: Catheter-associated urinary tract infections: Epidemiology, pathogenesis, and prevention. Am J Med 91 (Suppl 3B):65S, 1991.

112. Turck M, Goffe B, Petersdorf R: The urethral catheter and urinary tract infection. J Urol 88:834, 1962.

113. Van Der Wall E, Verkooyen RP, Mintjes-De Groot J, et al: Prophylactic ciprofloxacin for catheter-associated urinary-tract infection. Lancet 339:946, 1992.

114. Hartstein AI, Garber SB, Ward TT, et al: Nosocomial urinary tract infection: A prospective evaluation of 108 catheterized patients. Infect Control 2:380, 1981.

115. Warren JW: The catheter and urinary tract infection. Med Clin North Am 75:481, 1991.

116. Daifuku R, Stamm W: Bacterial adherence to bladder uroepithelial cells in catheter-associated urinary tract infections. N Engl J Med 314:1208, 1986.

117. Mobley HLT, Warren JW: Urease-positive bacteriuria and obstruction of long-term urinary catheters. J Clin Microbiol 25:2216, 1987.

118. Warren JW, Tenney JH, Hoopes JM, et al: A prospective microbiologic study of bacteriuria in patients with chronic indwelling urethral catheters. J Infect Dis 146:719, 1982.

119. Schaeffer AJ, Stony KO, Johnson SM: Effect of silver oxide/trichloroisocyanuric acid antimicrobial urinary drainage system on catheter-associated bacteriuria. J Urol 139:69, 1988.

CHAPTER 17

Urinary Retention

Victor W. Nitti, M.D.
Shlomo Raz, M.D.

Urinary retention, or incomplete bladder emptying, in women is probably more common than is diagnosed. This may be because retention in women tends to be insidious. Acute urinary retention is not a common presentation, and when it does occur, it has been associated with psychogenic factors.[1] The causes of chronic incomplete bladder emptying in women are just as numerous and varied as in men; however, their presumed infrequency and difficulty in diagnosis probably account for the lesser attention given to them. Although neurogenic causes of urinary retention are diagnosed as frequently in women as in men because of the obvious underlying etiology, obstructive processes are often overlooked. Therefore, it is the purpose of this chapter to familiarize the reader with the significant causes of urinary retention in women and their diagnosis and treatment.

It is difficult to define urinary retention as a specific volume of postvoid residual (PVR). No one would argue that the patient who cannot void at all or who is having overflow incontinence is in urinary retention. However, more frequently women present with varying degrees of incomplete bladder emptying. The clinical significance of incomplete emptying depends on several factors unique to each patient. For example, recurrent urinary tract infections, obstructive or irritative voiding symptoms, abdominal discomfort, and incontinence are important in the symptomatic patient. Significant parameters in the asymptomatic patient are often determined by ancillary procedures such as urodynamic examinations and upper tract imaging. These include bladder pressures during filling and storage, detrusor decompensation, and hydronephrosis. Thus, rather than treating a specific volume of PVR, we prefer to treat the effect of the residual. As in most voiding dysfunctions, diagnostic work-up is directed toward determining the underlying causes. Management is based on the relief of symptoms and treatment or on the prevention of dangerous sequelae of urinary retention and high-pressure storage.

In this chapter we do not attempt to describe all causes of urinary retention in women but rather focus on those that are unique to women or are particularly challenging to diagnose in the female population. In the sections that follow we will try to familiarize the reader with a simple classification system for urinary retention in women, discuss the pathophysiology and diagnostic evaluation, and finally describe some important specific causes of female retention along with suggested treatments. At the end of the chapter is a discussion of clean intermittent catheterization, a treatment modality that is useful for retention of almost any cause.

Classification of Female Urinary Retention

Urinary retention can be classified in a variety of ways. The first broad classification involves the differentiation of transient from established urinary retention. This is important because transient retention is usually acute and its cause is obvious, for example, institution of a new medication with anticholinergic effects or severe constipation. Timely treatment of the underlying cause usually results in a prompt return to normal voiding, obviating the need for any involved work-up. Common causes of transient retention are listed in Table 17–1. Established urinary retention may be caused by abnormalities in the bladder outlet (i.e., obstruction) or problems with the detrusor itself in the form of decreased or absent contractility. Both obstructive processes and impaired contractility have neurologic and nonneurologic causes (Table 17–2). In most cases established retention requires a detailed urologic evalua-

TABLE 17–1
Causes of Transient Urinary Retention

Immobility (especially postoperative)	Psychological problems
Fecal impaction	Endocrine abnormalities
Medications	Delirium
Urinary tract infection	

tion to determine its causes. Unless otherwise stated, we will concentrate on established retention for the rest of this chapter.

Pathophysiology of Incomplete Emptying

To understand the mechanisms of urinary retention a knowledge of more than just the classification schemes previously described is important. Although it is true that urinary retention secondary to "neurogenic bladder" can usually be explained on the basis of the level of the lesion and the specific nerves injured, most causes of incomplete emptying do not have an obvious neurologic origin. Bladder outlet obstruction may cause urinary retention, but why do many obstructed patients empty their bladders completely? It is known that bladder outlet obstruction may exist with normal or decreased contractility and with a stable or unstable bladder. But why? Elbadawi and colleagues have suggested that alterations in bladder structure are responsible for alterations in bladder function.[2] They performed a series of elegant studies correlating urodynamic findings with ultrastructural changes.[2-5] The concepts introduced by these authors, although described in elderly patients, give great insight into the pathogenesis of voiding dysfunction on a structural level. Previously, studies examining the effect of aging on the bladder have described only changes such as trabeculation, thinning, increased collagen content, atrophy of muscle cells, and decreased cholinergic innervation.[6-8]

Normally, the bladder stores urine at low pressures and voluntarily empties itself completely. On a struc-

TABLE 17–2
Urinary Retention in Females

I. Obstruction
  A. Non-neurogenic
    1. Anatomic obstruction
      a. Primary bladder neck obstruction
      b. Inflamatory processes
        (1) Bladder neck fibrosis
        (2) Urethral stricture
        (3) Meatal stenosis
        (4) Urethral caruncle
        (5) Skene's gland cyst/abscess
        (6) Urethral diverticulum
      c. Pelvic prolapse
        (1) Uterine prolapse
        (2) Cystocele
        (3) Enterocele
        (4) Rectocele
      d. Neoplastic
        (1) Urethral carcinoma
      e. Gynecologic (extrinsic compression)
        (1) Retroverted uterus
        (2) Vaginal carcinoma
        (3) Cervical carcinoma
        (4) Ovarian mass
      f. Iatrogenic obstruction
        (1) Anti-incontinence procedures
        (2) Multiple urethral dilatations
        (3) Urethral excision or reconstruction
      g. Miscellaneous
        (1) Urethral valves
        (2) Ectopic ureterocele
        (3) Bladder calculi
        (4) Atrophic vaginitis and urethritis
    2. Functional
      a. Dysfunctional voiding
      b. External sphincter spasticity
  B. Neurogenic
    a. Detrusor sphincter dyssynergia
      (1) Spinal cord injury (upper motor neuron)
      (2) Myelitis
      (3) Multiple sclerosis
    b. Parkinson's disease

II. Decreased Bladder Contractility
  A. Non-neurogenic
    1. Hypotonia or atony
      a. Chronic obstruction
      b. Radiation cystitis
      c. Tuberculosis
    2. Detrusor hyperactivity with impaired contractility
    3. Psychogenic retention
    4. Infrequent voiders syndrome
  B. Neurogenic
    1. Lower motor neuron lesion
      a. Cauda equina injury
        (1) Distal spinal cord
        (2) Intervertebral disc protrusion
        (3) Myelodysplasia
        (4) Primary and metastatic neoplasms
        (5) Vascular malformations
      b. Pelvic plexus injury
      c. Peripheral neuropathy
        (1) Diabetes mellitus
        (2) Pernicious anemia
        (3) Alcoholic neuropathy
        (4) Tabes dorsalis
        (5) Herpes zoster
        (6) Guillain-Barré syndrome
        (7) Shy-Drager syndrome
      d. Multiple sclerosis

tural level three components are responsible for this: smooth muscle, interstitium, and intrinsic nerves.[2] During filling, muscle cells and interstitium are responsible for compliance and interstitial nerves and smooth muscle for stability. For complete emptying to occur, a strong, speedy contraction must be initiated, summated throughout the detrusor and sustained. This is achieved by all three of the aforementioned components—the intrinsic nerves initiate a contraction generated by muscle cells that the interstitium converts into a unitary contraction by ensuring that it involves the entire detrusor.[3] Structural abnormalities at any of the three levels could account for impaired emptying.

Elbadawi and associates evaluated 35 patients (24 women) with geriatric voiding dysfunction.[2–5] Urodynamically, the patients were classified into four groups: detrusor overactivity, bladder outlet obstruction, bladder outlet obstruction and detrusor overactivity, and no obstruction with no detrusor overactivity. Each group had two subgroups composed of those with normal or impaired contractility. The authors were able to correlate ultrastructural changes (patterns) seen on electron microscopy with each of the four groups and subgroups without exception.[2–5] The "dense band pattern," which is characterized by muscle cell membranes dominated by dense bands, represents the ultrastructural pattern typical of the normal aging bladder (in the absence of obstruction or overactivity). Superimposed on this in patients with decreased contractility only, widespread degeneration of muscle cells may be seen.[3] Bladder overactivity is characterized by a "dysjunctional pattern" in which there are widened intracellular spaces, decreased intermediate cell junctions (which are responsible for mechanical coupling), and a predominance of two types of cell junctions with very close contact. This pattern may produce an increase in electrical coupling and urodynamically measurable uninhibited contractions. Again, cellular degeneration is superimposed on this dysjunctional pattern when decreased contractility accompanies bladder overactivity.[4] Obstructed bladders are characterized by the "myohypertrophy pattern," in which there are a wide separation of muscle cells with reduced intermediate cell junctions, abundant collagen deposition between cells, sometimes with elastin fibers, and enlarged hypertrophic cells. When detrusor overactivity coexists with obstruction, both the myohypertrophy and dysjunctional patterns are present. Again, cellular degeneration may be superimposed on these patterns in cases of concurrent decreased contractility.[5] Features of the myohypertrophy pattern help to explain why the obstructed detrusor is often unable to empty properly despite hypertrophy of individual cells: (1) The cells are often twisted and contorted; (2) there is a loss of intermediate cell junctions, which inhibits mechanical coupling and propagation of a contraction; (3) excessive intracellular collagen dissipates mechanical force; and (4) widespread cellular degeneration often exists in the obstructed bladder.[5]

The work of Elbadawi and colleagues goes a long way toward explaining the pathophysiology of voiding dysfunction on a structural basis. These theories can also explain the coexistence of multiple factors that all contribute to voiding dysfunction (e.g., obstruction plus overactivity plus decreased contractility). On a practical level, the coexistence of muscle cell degeneration with obstruction may explain why some patients with obstruction have urinary retention while others can empty the bladder completely. We must remember that these studies were done in elderly patients, and it is not known whether similar ultrastructural changes are present in younger patients with the same urodynamic findings. Continued research in this area will ideally produce more answers in the future.

As mentioned previously, urinary retention and incomplete bladder emptying can also be explained on the basis of neurologic disease. Normal bladder emptying requires a coordinated contraction by the detrusor of adequate magnitude and a concomitant lowering of resistance at the smooth and striated sphincters with an absence of obstruction.[9] The organizational center for this process is the pontine micturition center, which regulates the ascending and descending spinal cord pathways as well as inhibitory and stimulatory influences from other parts of the brain. Parasympathetic innervation of the bladder is provided by sacral nerves (S2, S3, S4) via the pelvic nerve. Individual nerves distal to the parasympathetic ganglia supplied by the pelvic nerve innervate the detrusor. The smooth muscle of the bladder neck (proximal sphincter) is innervated by sympathetic nerves of the lower thoracic and upper lumbar spinal cord, and the distal urethral sphincter is neurologically controlled by the somatic nerves of the sacral cord via the pudendal nerve. Lesions at various levels of the central and peripheral nervous system cause characteristic lower tract dysfunction, which leads to incomplete bladder emptying either by reducing bladder contractility or by causing a neurologically mediated obstruction (e.g., failure of sphincter relaxation during a bladder contraction).

A complete review of all neurologic diseases affecting bladder emptying is beyond the scope of this chapter, and the reader is referred elsewhere.[9–11] There are, however, consistent characteristics of various diseases that affect particular levels of the central and peripheral nervous systems. For example, suprasacral spinal cord lesions, whether caused by trauma, infection, neoplasm, or demyelinating diseases such as multiple sclerosis, tend to produce detrusor hyperreflexia. These become a greater problem when they are coupled with detrusor-sphincter dyssynergia (DSD), which may occur depending on the level and completeness of the lesion. DSD results in an obstructive process in which the uninhibited contraction is unable to empty the bladder effectively. Untreated patients are often incontinent and in retention. On the other hand, neurologic disease involving the lower motor neurons tends to cause an acontractile bladder with a loss of sensation. In the middle are sacral arc lesions, which produce a typical areflexic, poorly compliant bladder with high-pressure storage and incomplete emptying due to high outlet resistance at the distal sphincteric level. A summary of common neurologic causes of urinary retention is found in Table 17–2.

Evaluation

The evaluation of urinary retention in women starts with a thorough history. This should focus on the patient's voiding habits over time and the duration of the retention. A complete medical, surgical, obstetric-gynecologic, neurologic, and urologic history may uncover possible causes of the patient's voiding dysfunction. If retention is acute and there is an obvious cause (e.g., medication, recent surgery), then treatment should be directed toward alleviating the obvious cause (discontinuing medication, promoting ambulation and bowel movements for the postoperative patient). If there is no prior history of retention or voiding dysfunction, an extensive work-up can be postponed until after empirical treatment has failed. Thus, evaluation of transient retention is often limited. It is best to start treatment with clean intermittent catheterization (CIC) if possible while waiting for the retention to resolve. Once the patient has been given a reasonable chance to resume normal voiding, continued retention may prompt further testing. We generally prefer to wait until the patient is in her normal environment and living as nearly normal a life as possible. Urodynamic testing in the "bedridden" patient is of little value if the patient is expected to be ambulatory soon after. In summary, transient urinary retention is best treated by addressing the underlying cause and facilitating emptying with CIC or an indwelling catheter. Nothing more than a thorough history and physical examination are needed initially.

A systematic examination of the vagina and pelvis constitutes the next part of the evaluation. We like to use the posterior blade of a small vaginal speculum to retract the posterior vaginal wall to view the anterior wall. One should first inspect the mucosa for atrophic changes as well as signs of previous surgery. Also, the position of the urethra, bladder neck, and bladder can be observed at rest and with straining to determine hypermobility and degree of cystocele. The patient should also be assessed for stress urinary incontinence (SUI) because this can coexist with retention owing to urethral hypermobility, intrinsic sphincter dysfunction, or overflow. After examination of the anterior vaginal wall is completed, the blade of the speculum is rotated, and the posterior wall and vaginal vault are inspected. Careful vaginal examination may reveal evidence of pelvic prolapse in the form of rectocele, enterocele, or uterine prolapse, which may cause or contribute to urinary retention. When the vaginal examination is completed, a neurologic examination is performed. Attention should be paid to the sensory and motor functions of the sacral nerves including anal sphincter tone, perineal sensation, bulbocavernosus reflex, strength of the lower extremities, and deep tendon reflexes. A careful neurologic examination may help to confirm suspected disease or uncover an unknown lesion.

Urodynamic testing is an important part of the evaluation of female voiding dysfunction; however, it must always be kept in mind that it is only part of the evaluation and is used in conjunction with the rest of the assessment. Urodynamic findings that are inconsistent with patient symptoms, and events occurring during testing that are uncharacteristic of patients during normal activity outside the urodynamics laboratory, should be interpreted with caution. A simple noninvasive uroflow test and measurement of the postvoid residual give a good idea of how well the patient empties the bladder. More invasive testing is required, however, to determine *why* incomplete emptying or poor flow is present. Multichannel urodynamic testing with simultaneous measurement of vesical and abdominal pressure and "subtracted" detrusor pressure during filling (cystometry) can be used to determine the ability of the bladder to store urine effectively by assessing bladder stability, compliance, and capacity. Pressure-flow analysis during voiding allows the physician to look at bladder contractility and bladder outlet resistance. Electromyography may be added to assess the pelvic floor musculature and external sphincter. One must guard against making a diagnosis of bladder outlet obstruction in women based on pressure-flow analysis alone. Although it may be true that women who void with high pressure and low flow have bladder obstruction, those who void with normal or even very low pressures may also be obstructed. This may be due in part to the fact that some women void by pelvic relaxation or abdominal straining without generating significant detrusor pressures. Normally, sufficient emptying takes place in these women, but if some degree of obstruction is superimposed on this, emptying does not take place. Much of what we have learned about this process has come from treating patients with obstruction following anti-incontinence procedures and has been confirmed by other authors (see later discussion). Videourodynamics can be particularly helpful in confirming and localizing anatomic or functional obstruction. The addition of simultaneous fluoroscopy of the bladder outlet often reveals an obstruction that would not have been discovered on the basis of multichannel urodynamics alone.

When videourodynamics are not available, radiographic evaluation may still be useful in evaluating incomplete emptying. A standing cystogram in the anteroposterior, oblique, and lateral positions, with and without straining, assesses the degree of bladder and urethral prolapse and displacement or distortion of the bladder. It is a sort of "physical examination in the standing position." A voiding cystourethrogram shows the bladder, bladder neck, and urethra during voiding and is important in uncovering anatomic abnormalities.

The final component of the evaluation is cystourethroscopy, when indicated. A careful evaluation of the female urethra is facilitated by the use of a 0-degree lens and a cystoscope that has no beak. This allows for complete distention of the urethra. Scarring, kinking, or deviation of the urethra, especially after previous surgery, may be responsible for incomplete emptying. Rarely, a urethral lesion responsible for obstruction may be found. Examination of the bladder may uncover a lesion such as a tumor or stone and also may identify some of the changes associated with obstruction or retention.

Specific Causes and Treatment of Urinary Retention in Women

In this section we discuss several causes of incomplete bladder emptying in women, including both obstructive and nonobstructive causes. As mentioned previously, we focus on causes that are unique to women or are particularly challenging to diagnose in the female population. It is hoped that the reader will take the information supplied and apply it to causes of urinary retention that are not specifically covered here. We first discuss urinary retention caused by bladder outlet obstruction, beginning with non-neurologic causes and ending with neurologic processes. This is followed by a section on impaired contractility, again starting with non-neurologic causes. In the treatment section of each diagnosis emphasis is placed on restoring normal spontaneous emptying. If this cannot be achieved, either because of the disease itself or because of contraindications to specific treatments, other forms of bladder drainage such as CIC or indwelling catheters must be employed. The technique of CIC is described in general terms at the end of this section, and can be applied to any of the many underlying causes of urinary retention.

BLADDER OUTLET OBSTRUCTION

In women with bladder outlet obstruction, classic obstructive symptoms (e.g., poor flow, hesitancy, stranguria) are less common than in men. This is probably due in part to the fact that women are frequently poor historians with respect to the force of their urinary stream because they void in private and have little opportunity to compare their voiding with that of other women.[12] They more commonly present with urinary frequency, urgency, urge incontinence, and recurrent urinary tract infections. In addition, bladder outlet obstruction in women is less clearly defined than in men. There is some controversy in the literature about a standardized definition of outlet

obstruction in women. Some authors have attempted to define obstruction in women based on pressure-flow analysis. Massey and Abrams proposed that two or more of the following four parameters be included: flow rate of less than 12 ml/second, detrusor pressure at peak flow more than 50 cm H_2O, urethral resistance (P_{det} at Q_{max}/Q_{max}^2) of more than 0.2, or significant residual urine in the presence of high pressure or resistance. In a series of 5948 women who presented for urodynamic evaluation for a variety of complaints, the incidence of obstruction was found to be 2.74%. The urethral pressure profile was not helpful in diagnosing obstruction because it was abnormal in only one patient.[13] Farrar and associates used only flow rates to diagnose obstruction because they thought that low flow in the presence of normal or low detrusor pressures could be an indication of "relative" obstruction.[14] This was defined as a maximum flow rate of less than 15 ml/second with a volume of 200 ml or more.[14] In both of these series, irritative symptoms predominated. Bass and Leach stated that the presence of a peak flow of more than 15 ml/second with a voided volume of more than 100 ml, a normal uroflow curve configuration, and no significant residual usually excludes outlet obstruction.[12] In a small series of women with primary bladder neck obstruction, Axelrod and Blaivas defined vesical neck obstruction as a sustained detrusor contraction of at least 20 cm H_2O with a flow rate of less than 12 ml/minute.[15]

Based on our own experience and review of patients who had outlet obstruction after anti-incontinence procedures, we have found it difficult if not impossible to define outlet obstruction in women in terms of detrusor pressure or urinary flow rate, either independently or together.[16] Patients who had had urethrolysis for presumed outlet obstruction did equally well in achieving normal voiding and emptying regardless of urodynamic findings.[16] This includes patients with very low pressure and "acontractile" detrusors. Others have reported a similar experience.[17–18] These findings may be due in part to the fact that some women void by pelvic relaxation or abdominal straining without generating significant detrusor pressures. A small degree of outlet resistance may be enough to disrupt voiding, particularly in the elderly.

The studies performed on patients who had had urethrolysis have led us to rethink the concept of bladder outlet obstruction in women. We no longer rely strictly on urodynamic criteria but rather rely on an evaluation that includes urodynamic, radiologic, and endoscopic components. This evaluation can be applied to all causes of bladder outlet obstruction. Videourodynamics can be particularly helpful in confirming the diagnosis as well as localizing the site of obstruction. The addition of simultaneous fluoroscopy of the bladder outlet often uncovers an obstruction that would not have been seen on the basis of multichannel urodynamics alone. Videourodynamics is the single most useful test for the diagnosis of bladder outlet obstruction in women. Figure 17–1

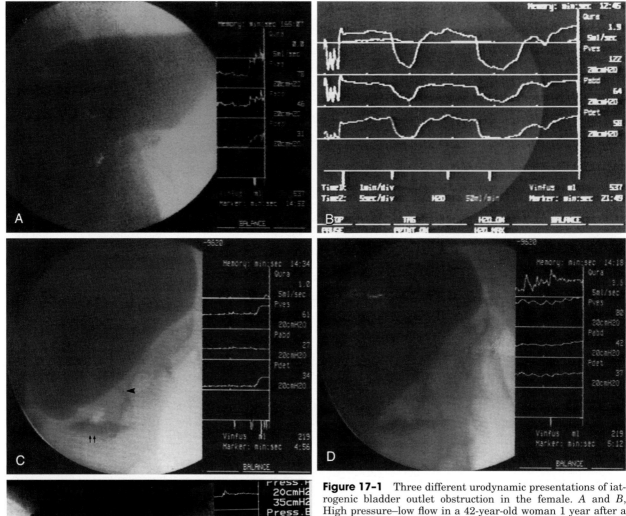

Figure 17-1 Three different urodynamic presentations of iatrogenic bladder outlet obstruction in the female. *A* and *B*, High pressure–low flow in a 42-year-old woman 1 year after a Marshall-Marchetti-Krantz procedure. Patient had recurrent urinary tract infection and severe obstructive and irritative voiding symptoms. *A*, Initiation of voluntary contraction with no opening of the bladder neck and a small cystocele (P_{det} = 31 cm H_2O). *B*, Later during voiding with high detrusor pressures and augmentation of voiding with abdominal straining. *C* and *D*, Normal pressure and low flow in a 72-year-old woman 2 years after transvaginal needle suspension who complained of obstructive and irritative voiding symptoms. *C*, Initiation of voiding with poor funneling of the bladder neck and extremely narrow urethra *(arrowhead)*. There is also voiding into the vagina *(double arrows)*. *D*, Later during voiding with "normal" detrusor pressure of 42 cm H_2O, a decreased flow rate, and abnormal flow curve pattern. The patient underwent transvaginal urethrolysis and resuspension of the bladder neck and had a successful outcome. *E*, Low pressure and no flow in an 85-year-old woman 3 years after excision of a urethral caruncle, which placed her in total urinary retention and on clean intermittent catheterization. Although there is only a low pressure detrusor contraction (15 cm H_2O), it is sustained, and there is an obvious distal urethral obstruction. At surgery the patient's true urethra was found to be closed off, and the catheter extended through a false passage above the true urethra. After urethral reconstruction, the patient voided spontaneously without residual.

shows three examples of bladder outlet obstruction with varied pressure-flow characteristics.

Iatrogenic Causes of Bladder Outlet Obstruction

OBSTRUCTION FOLLOWING ANTI-INCONTINENCE PROCEDURES
Surgical correction of SUI is the most common cause of iatrogenic bladder outlet obstruction in women and is probably the most common cause overall. The surgery can be done in a variety of ways including retropubic cystourethropexy and colposuspension procedures as well as a number of transvaginal procedures designed to reposition and support the bladder neck and proximal urethra.[19–25] A potential complication of all these procedures that surgically alter the anatomy is iatrogenic outlet obstruction leading to voiding dysfunction. This may result in obstructive symptoms with partial or total urinary

retention, recurrent urinary tract infections, or severe irritative symptoms such as frequency, urgency, and urge incontinence. The true incidence of iatrogenic obstruction and voiding dysfunction after anti-incontinence procedures is not known, but it has been estimated at 2.5 to 24% for different procedures.[26–30] We believe that it is often underestimated because irritative and obstructive symptoms tend to be overlooked in the presence of normal emptying. However, as in men with long-standing bladder outlet obstruction, detrusor decompensation and chronic urinary retention may result.

As previously mentioned, there is no fixed definition of bladder outlet obstruction in women. When one attempts to define obstruction after anti-incontinence procedures in a standard fashion, it becomes even more difficult, especially when preoperative voiding parameters are not available. Many women void by pelvic floor relaxation or abdominal straining, and even a mild elevation in outlet resistance can cause a "relative obstruction" producing significant voiding dysfunction. This concept is evident in data published by Juma and Sdrales, who performed preoperative urodynamic studies in 77 women undergoing Raz bladder neck suspension.[26] Twenty of these patients had a "noncontractile" bladder preoperatively. Twelve of these (60%) had significant PVR 3 months postoperatively. The noncontractile group also accounted for 86% of patients with residuals. The actual incidence of true obstruction caused by the surgery was 2.5%.[26]

The issue of whether a procedure causes an obstruction is largely based on technical factors, most specifically suture placement. Sutures placed too medially, close to the urethra, can cause urethral deviation or periurethral scarring, whereas sutures placed too distally can cause kinking, resulting in obstruction and continued SUI as the bladder neck and proximal urethra have not been adequately supported. In addition, sutures that are tied too tightly may result in overcorrection and "hypersuspension" of the bladder neck, kinking it shut. Certain procedures are more likely to cause obstruction than others. For example, the original description of the Marshall-Marchetti-Krantz urethropexy included placement of sutures in the proximal urethral wall.[19] Sutures placed here are likely to cause obstruction. This technique was later modified to avoid suture placement in the wall of the urethra.[31] Other suspension procedures such as the Raz bladder neck suspension rely on suture placement in supporting structures far lateral to the urethra at the level of the bladder neck and should result in a lower incidence of obstruction providing that these sutures are placed properly.[23] Other causes of iatrogenic obstruction following these procedures include periurethral scarring due to sutures placed through the urethral lumen with subsequent extravasation of urine, and fibrosis and scarring caused by the surgical dissection itself.[12] Even when properly performed, certain procedures designed to correct anatomic incontinence cause an increase in urethral resistance. In a prospective interval analysis of patients undergoing endoscopic bladder neck suspension, Pope and colleagues showed a threefold increase in urethral resistance 12 months after suspension. Voiding pressures were also more than twice the baseline values.[32]

Diagnosis of obstruction after anti-incontinence procedures cannot be made on the basis of urodynamic criteria alone. In fact, a history of normal voiding and emptying prior to the procedure is one of the most important factors used in deciding on treatment. Several studies, including our own, have failed to show any correlation between urodynamic findings and the likelihood of successful voiding after urethrolysis.[16–18] Even patients who failed to demonstrate contractility or who have very low detrusor pressures with poor flow seem to have success equal to those with the classic high-pressure, low-flow voiding characteristics of urodynamic obstruction. Table 17–3 summarizes our results in 41 patients who underwent urethrolysis for obstruction caused by an anti-incontinence procedure. We concluded that patients should not be excluded from urethrolysis based on urodynamic findings of hypocontractility or acontractility providing that they had normal voiding prior to anti-incontinence surgery.[16] When the patient's prior voiding history is not known, the diagnosis of obstruction is made, albeit without certainty at times, using a combination of urodynamic, radiologic, endoscopic, and physical examination findings as described previously.

Technique of Urethrolysis When a patient suffers from prolonged obstruction following anti-incontinence surgery, we prefer to perform a complete urethrolysis to provide the greatest chance of facilitating voiding. Several techniques have been described for the performance of urethrolysis to relieve urethral obstruction after pelvic surgery. We prefer the transvaginal technique originally described by Leach and Raz.[33] An inverted U incision is made in the anterior vaginal wall with the apex halfway between the bladder neck and the urethral meatus. Lateral dissection is performed along the glistening surface of the periurethral fascia to the pubic bone. The urethropelvic ligament is sharply perforated at its attachment to the obturator fascia, and the retropubic space is entered next (Fig. 17–2A). Sharp and blunt dissection

TABLE 17–3
Preoperative Voiding Dynamics and Outcome of Urethrolysis

Pressure-Flow	Number	Success
$Pdet_{max} \geq 30$, $Q_{max} \leq 12$	23 (56%)	16 (70%)
$Pdet_{max} \geq 30$, $Q_{max} > 12$	7 (17%)	4 (57%)
$Pdet_{max} < 30$, $Q_{max} \leq 12$	5 (12%)	3 (60%)
$Pdet_{max} < 30$, $Q_{max} > 12$	2 (5%)	2 (100%)
Acontractile	4 (10%)	4 (100%)

From Nitti VW, Raz S: Obstruction following anti-incontinence procedures: Diagnosis and treatment with transvaginal urethrolysis. J Urol 152:93, 1994.

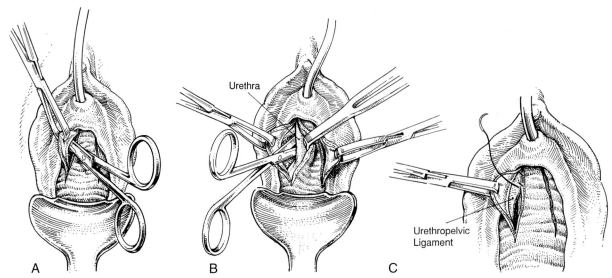

A   B   C

Figure 17-2 Transvaginal urethrolysis. *A,* Inverted U incision in the anterior vaginal wall and entrance into the retropubic space. *B,* The urethra is sharply dissected off the undersurface of the pubic bone. The urethropelvic ligament, periurethral fascia, and vaginal wall are retracted medially to expose the urethra in the retropubic space. *C,* Resuspension of the bladder neck by the Raz technique. (From Nitti VW, Raz S: Obstruction following anti-incontinence procedures: Diagnosis and treatment with transvaginal urethrolysis. J Urol 152:93, 1994.)

is done to open this space completely on each side. Next, urethrolysis is performed by sharply and bluntly dissecting the urethra off the undersurface of the pubic bone (Fig. 17–2*B*). The urethra should be completely freed anterior to the bladder neck so that the index finger can be placed between the urethra and the symphysis pubis. Resuspension of the bladder neck by the Raz technique is then performed as previously described (Fig. 17–2*C*).[23]

We prefer the transvaginal technique because of its ease and the reduced morbidity achieved by avoiding an abdominal procedure. The transvaginal technique allows safe and direct exposure of the urethra. In certain instances of very dense or recurrent scarring, a Martius flap may be interposed between the symphysis and the urethra to prevent readherence of these structures. Because a major abdominal operation is avoided, hospital and recovery time are kept to a minimum. In addition, any other vaginal pathology such as cystocele, enterocele, or rectocele can be repaired at the same time. In our series 15 patients (38%) underwent a simultaneous rectocele or enterocele repair.[16]

When a vaginal approach is not feasible owing to the patient's anatomy, or if the surgeon prefers, urethrolysis can be performed through a retropubic approach. This has been described by Webster and Kreder.[18] They reported excellent results with a retropubic takedown in which all adhesions from the prior cystourethropexy are sharply incised, and complete mobility of the anterior vaginal wall is restored. The procedure is completed by performing an obturator shelf repair to prevent rotational descent and placing an omental pedical to fill the retropubic dead space and prevent further scarring.[18] Regardless of the technique chosen, we recommend a complete free-

ing of the urethra in the retropubic space because it is often quite adherent to the pubic bone (Fig. 17–3). Because of the extensive urethrolysis performed, we believe that resuspension to restore support is very important to prevent recurrent SUI. Others have had no problems with recurrent SUI using this technique without routine resuspension.[17, 34] Although it may be argued that resuspension may contribute to persistent or recurrent obstruction, we believe that carefully placed sutures laterally in the urethropelvic ligament should not cause this result, and therefore we do this routinely.

Urethrolysis may also be performed by making a small, gently curved inverted U incision above the urethral meatus and dissecting the urethra dorsally. This is usually done without any other major dissection or resuspension. Large series using this technique have not been recently reported.

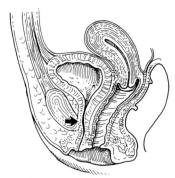

Figure 17-3 Sagittal view showing the urethra fixed to the undersurface of the pubic bone *(arrow).* The urethra is completely freed following urethrolysis. (From Nitti VW, Raz S: Obstruction following anti-incontinence procedures: Diagnosis and treatment with transvaginal urethrolysis. J Urol 152:93, 1994.)

Reported success rates for urethrolysis for obstruction following anti-incontinence procedures—that is, resumption of normal voiding with little or no irritative symptoms—range from 65 to 93%.[16–18, 35] In those patients who failed to void satisfactorily after urethrolysis, repeat urodynamic examination did not give conclusive information about the cause of the failure.[16] Possible explanations for failures include contractility insufficient to overcome even the reduced outlet resistance, and persistent obstruction. We believe that in some patients this continued obstruction is the result of intrinsic damage to the urethra resulting from surgery and is not due to periurethral fibrosis and scarring. In this case, urethrolysis will not relieve the obstruction. It is also possible that some failures result from "reobstruction" after a complete urethrolysis.

URETHRAL DILATATION Urethral dilatation has been used for many years as a treatment for recurrent cystitis, pelvic or bladder pain, and nonspecific voiding dysfunction in women. Although this procedure often results in temporary symptomatic relief, over time it may result in bladder outlet obstruction. The obstruction is caused by periurethral fibrosis and scarring of the urethral wall that results from multiple episodes of postdilatation bleeding or extravasation of urine into the periurethral tissue.[12] This can result in rigidity of the urethral wall and narrowing of the urethral lumen. The diagnosis is best made by videourodynamics, which should be able to localize the point of obstruction. Urethroscopy may be unremarkable.[12]

The management of posturethral dilatation obstruction can be challenging. The goal is to allow adequate emptying but avoid the complication of urinary incontinence. Conservative treatment with intermittent catheterization is an option. Curative therapy involves transurethral resection or incision of the involved area. Bass and Leach recommend a conservative resection or incision limited to 0.5 to 1 cm with additional incisions in separate sessions if obstruction persists.[12]

POSTSURGICAL STRICTURE AND STENOSIS True urethral stricture is rare in women but can occur as a result of urethral surgery such as urethral diverticulectomy or reconstruction. In these cases the narrowing is usually easily visualized endoscopically. We have also seen complete urethral obstruction following excision of a urethral caruncle (Fig. 17–1D). This probably occurred when the true mucosal edge of the distal urethra was lost after excision of the lesion. Postsurgical strictures can be treated with periodic self-catheterization or permanent CIC, transurethral incision, or urethral reconstruction. When reconstruction is needed, we prefer to excise the scarred portion of the ventral urethra and retubularize the urethra over a 12 Fr catheter approximating healthy mucosa. The urethra can be exposed by an inverted U flap incision of the anterior vagina as described for urethral diverticulectomy.[36] Where there is a long circumferential stricture, excision followed by reconstruction with vaginal wall may be necessary.[37]

Primary Bladder Neck Obstruction

Primary bladder neck obstruction may be defined as a failure of the bladder neck to open properly in the presence of a detrusor contraction of normal or increased amplitude and duration. It was originally described in a male patient by Marion in 1933.[38] Because there was no visible lesion on endoscopy, it was a diagnosis of exclusion. Today, with the use of videourodynamic testing, the diagnosis of primary bladder neck obstruction can be made accurately in both men and women.

Primary bladder neck obstruction in women is reported to be extremely rare. Farrar and colleagues reported four urodynamically proven cases in 2500 women, whereas Massey and Abrams reported no cases in a review of 5948 patients.[13, 14] In selected women undergoing videourodynamic examination, we found the disease to be somewhat more common but still relatively rare. The exact cause of primary bladder neck obstruction is unknown. One theory is that it is caused by smooth muscle hypertrophy or an increase in collagen deposition at the bladder neck.[39] Another is that a continual high tonus in the smooth muscle of the posterior urethra causes rigidity of the bladder neck.[40] An increased number of alpha-adrenergic receptors resulting in nonrelaxation during voiding has also been suggested.[39, 41] Women with primary bladder neck obstruction typically present initially with irritative voiding symptoms and are often treated with anticholinergics or antispasmodics for bladder hyperactivity.[42] The condition may then progress to periodic urinary retention or to a high PVR. Recurrent urinary tract infections are also common.[42]

The hallmark of primary bladder neck obstruction is incomplete opening or funneling of the bladder neck in the presence of a sustained detrusor contraction of normal or high amplitude with resultant poor or nonexistent flow (Fig. 17–4). Axelrod and Blaivas and Diokno and colleagues have each described small series of three patients with videourodynamically documented primary bladder neck obstruction.[15, 43] Patients presented initially with either irritative symptoms of frequency, urgency, and nocturia or obstructive symptoms of straining and poor flow or both. Half progressed to urinary retention before definitive treatment of bladder neck obstruction was performed. Two patients had recurrent urinary tract infections. Axelrod and Blaivas defined the entity as a sustained detrusor contraction of at least 20 cm H_2O, a flow rate of less than 12 ml/second, and radiographic evidence of obstruction at the bladder neck.[15] In this series electromyography of the external urethral sphincter was normal. In the series reported by Diokno and colleagues, all three patients had a detrusor voiding pressure of at least 60 cm H_2O.[43] Cystourethroscopy may show bladder changes consistent with chronic outlet obstruction, but the bladder neck usually appears normal.[15, 41] The largest series was reported from Denmark by Gronbaek and associates in 1992.[40] They described 38 women with blad-

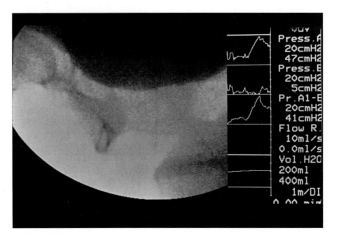

Figure 17-4 Primary bladder neck obstruction in a 35-year-old woman with a history of progressive obstructive voiding symptoms leading to complete urinary retention. During this voluntary attempt to void, note the sustained detrusor contraction (>40 cm H$_2$O) with a totally closed bladder neck. This patient had an excellent response after transurethral incision of the bladder neck. The third tracing from the top is subtracted detrusor pressure.

der neck obstruction. In this series simultaneous pressure-flow analysis and cystourethrography were not performed, and the diagnosis was made by evaluating each study separately. They also found a "rigid, elevated bladder neck," which was thought to be pathologic in 92% of their patients.[40]

TREATMENT Surgical treatment of primary bladder neck obstruction consists of transurethral bladder neck incision or Y-V bladder neck plasty. Axelrod and Blaivas reported excellent results in three patients treated with transurethral incision. They described two incisions, at 5 and 7 o'clock, beginning just inside the bladder neck and extending distally for 1 to 2 cm at a depth of 0.5 to 1 cm. No patients suffered incontinence.[15] Gronbaek and associates used a similar method, incising at 4 or 8 o'clock beginning midway between the ureteral orifices and the bladder neck.[40] To avoid potential incontinence, they made only one incision and made a second only if the bladder neck did not open widely or if the procedure did not succeed. They reported a 98% success rate at 4 weeks and a long-term success rate of 76% with a mean of 55 months follow-up. Incontinence occurred in only one patient (3%), who also had a cystourethrocele.[40] Bladder neck incision at the 12 o'clock position has also been described to avoid the potential complication of vesicovaginal fistula.[44] Diokno and associates treated two patients successfully with a Y-V plasty of the bladder neck. Although this appears to be efficacious, endoscopic incision seems easier.

We have recently treated three women with videourodynamically proven disease with terazosin, an alpha-1-adrenergic blocker. All three have been maintained on a dose of 5 or 10 mg at bedtime. All have experienced subjective improvement, with mean maximum and average flow rates increasing from 14.4 and 3.0 ml/second to 16.6 and 7.3 ml/second, respectively, and mean PVRs decreasing from 175 ml to 35 ml. One patient underwent a repeat videourodynamic evaluation that showed normal opening and funneling of the bladder neck during voiding. Although treatment with terazosin appears promising, it may require a lifetime of therapy.

Pelvic Prolapse

Cystoceles may cause bladder outlet obstruction and urinary retention. Patients often present with incomplete emptying and recurrent urinary tract infections with or without stress incontinence. Sometimes the patient may need to position herself in a certain way (e.g., leaning backward or squatting) or may need to reduce the cystocele in order to void. The obstruction occurs in the proximal to midurethra as a result of kinking of the urethra or urethrovesical junction. In a prospective study of 62 patients with cystoceles Gardy and associates found that 42% of patients had a PVR of at least 80 ml, and 3% were in retention on intermittent catheterization. Residual urine of 80 ml or more was more common in patients with larger cystoceles, grade III to IV (55%), than in those with smaller ones, grade I to II (28%).[45] In patients with very large cystoceles, the ureters may also prolapse outside of the pelvis, leading to ureteral obstruction and hydronephrosis. When severe, this condition may lead to olgiuria or anuria.[46] In addition to cystocele, prolapse of other pelvic organs, either independently or in conjunction with bladder prolapse, can lead to urinary retention. A large rectocele can compress the urethra and bladder neck from below, causing an obstruction. This may be aggravated by constipation. Enteroceles and uterine prolapse may cause urinary retention by external compression or by pulling and distorting the bladder neck and urethra. In patients with impaired detrusor contractility, especially elderly patients, less compression or distortion is needed to cause emptying problems.

Treatment of symptomatic pelvic prolapse is usually surgical and includes repair of all the prolapsing components. The ultimate goal of surgery should be to restore normal voiding, vaginal axis, and depth.[47, 48] Techniques of cystocele repair depend on the size and type of defect and are usually combined with bladder neck suspension to prevent anatomic incontinence.[49, 50] Enteroceles may be repaired by a transvaginal or abdominal approach.[48, 51–53] We prefer the transvaginal approach because it facilitates correction of all anomalies. Rectocele repair is easily accomplished either in conjunction with other procedures or by itself.[54]

Urethral Lesions

Lesions within the urethra or at the urethral meatus are an infrequent cause of outlet obstruction and urinary retention in women. Urethral diverticula occasionally present as urinary retention, usually as a result of a large proximally located diverticulum that impinges on the bladder neck or a stricture formation caused by recurrent infections. Treatment is excision of the diverticulum with urethral reconstruction when necessary.

Urethral valves are an extremely rare cause of obstruction and retention in women.[55, 56] The diagnosis is made endoscopically and radiographically. Voiding cystourethrograms may reveal a dilated proximal urethra, a small voided stream, and an intervening shadow representing the valve itself.[55] Cherrie and associates described the endoscopic appearance as a posterior-based sail-like structure extending from the mid to the proximal urethra.[55] Treatment of these valves is either transurethral incision or resection. Prolapsing ectopic ureteroceles can be a cause of urinary retention in girls but are usually diagnosed and treated before adulthood.

Inflammatory or infectious lesions such as urethral caruncle or Skene's gland abscess may cause retention either by anatomic obstruction caused by the lesion itself or by external sphincter spasticity due to pain or inflammation (see later discussion). Skene's gland abscesses may be given a trial of antibiotic therapy, but if this fails excision may be necessary. Symptomatic urethral caruncles are treated with local excision.

Urethral carcinoma is a rare lesion in women, accounting for less than 0.2% of all genital cancers in women.[57] It is, however, the only urologic malignancy found more frequently in women than in men. Women most commonly present with bleeding followed by irritative and obstructive symptoms. Treatment ranges from local excision for distal lesions to anterior exenteration.[57] Radiation therapy has also been used.

Obstetric and Gynecologic Causes of Bladder Outlet Obstruction

Obstetric and gynecologic causes of bladder outlet obstruction are primarily related to extrinsic compression of the involved organ or lesion on the bladder neck or urethra. Pelvic masses such as large uterine fibroids and ovarian cysts or tumors may cause such obstruction.[58–61] Malignant lesions such as carcinoma of the cervix, vagina, or vulva may rarely cause problems with urinary retention by either extrinsic compression or direct invasion into the urethra. In all cases treatment is directed toward the primary lesion.[12]

Acute urinary retention may occur during the first trimester of pregnancy because of a retroverted impacted uterus.[62–64] Retention results when the portio of the cervix becomes firmly applied to the anterior vaginal wall at the vesicourethral junction. In the literature this has been reported at between 10 and 16 weeks of gestation. This phenomenon generally does not occur after the first trimester because the position of the growing cervix changes to anteversion, and the cervix moves backward.[63] Treatment consists of manually dislodging the uterus from the true pelvis, which may require a general anesthetic.[62, 64] Some practitioners have used a pessary in con-

junction with replacement of the uterus or short-term catheterization until spontaneous voiding resumes.[63] Goldberg and Kwart reported a case of urinary retention at 10 weeks gestation in a patient with uterine prolapse and fibroids.[65] The patient was treated with a pessary, which restored voiding, for 2 weeks until uterine enlargement and ascent occurred. After this the pessary was no longer needed.

Incomplete Pelvic Floor Relaxation

DYSFUNCTIONAL VOIDING The concept of dysfunctional voiding, or dyscoordination between the detrusor and the activity of the pelvic floor–external sphincter complex in neurologically normally individuals, was first introduced in 1973 by Hinman and Baumann.[66] Much of the literature describes this phenomenon, also known as the non-neurogenic neurogenic bladder or the Hinman syndrome, as occurring in children and adolescents.[67–69] Patients typically present with enuresis, recurrent urinary tract infections, and sometimes hydronephrosis. However, dysfunctional voiding is also seen in adults and is occasionally a cause of incomplete emptying, recurrent urinary tract infections, and incontinence in these patients.[70, 71]

Urodynamically, dysfunctional voiding is characterized by a normal onset of micturition with relaxation of the pelvic floor and initiation of a detrusor contraction. However, after voiding starts there are frequent episodes of intermittent increases in pelvic floor electromyographic (EMG) activity accompanied by a decrease in flow and an increase in detrusor pressure.[70] During filling detrusor instability is frequently noted as EMG activity increases with the involuntary increase in bladder pressure.[69] Videourodynamically, the urethra is usually dilated to the level of the external sphincter ("spinning top urethra") both during unstable detrusor contractions and intermittently during voiding. The pelvic floor–external sphincter complex can be observed fluoroscopically to contract and relax with increases and decreases in detrusor pressure, causing interruption of normal flow.

Various theories have been proposed to explain the cause of dysfunctional voiding. The one that best explains this condition in adults is that of McGuire and Savastano.[71] They believe that the primary abnormality is detrusor instability and that the detrusor sphincter dysynergia that occurs develops as a result of sudden unanticipated detrusor contractility.[71] Contraction of the pelvic floor–external sphincter complex is a normal response to control urgent urination and results in a reflex inhibition of the detrusor. When this becomes habitual over a period of time the abnormal incoordination carries over to voluntary voiding, resulting in an intermittent urinary stream and residual urine.[69]

Theoretically, the treatment of dysfunctional voiding can be directed toward the bladder, the sphincter, or both. McGuire and Savastano recommend treatment with anticholinergic medication since they believe that the problem is primarily related to a hyperactive detrusor. Timed voiding and biofeedback have been used in patients in whom medical therapy has failed.[71] Kaplan and associates have had success using low-dose diazepam, which eliminated the characteristic DSD flow curve.[72] Baclofen, a muscle relaxant and antispasmodic used with some success to treat true DSD of neurologic origin, has not been successful in patients with dysfunctional voiding.[70] Our approach is to use a combination of biofeedback, behavioral modification (timed voiding, fluid restriction), and anticholinergics. After the diagnosis has been made, it is explained in detail to the patient. In a separate session EMG patch electrodes are placed and the bladder is filled using a small (5 Fr or smaller) catheter. When the patient feels the desire to void, she voids with her attention on the EMG monitor or audio. The bladder is then refilled. The purpose of the initial session is to teach the patient what she is doing and to start to retrain her to relax the pelvic floor and maintain a steady urinary stream during voiding. This process is practiced at home. In adults, two or three sessions are all that is usually required. Follow-up is maintained with periodic uroflow tests and PVRs. Anticholinergics help to control urgency and detrusor instability between voiding. This technique has been uniformly successful in reducing PVRs and symptoms in all adult women treated. In patients with complete urinary retention clean intermittent catheterization can be used until normal voiding returns.

External Sphincter Spasticity

Increased tone of the pelvic floor–external sphincter complex has been described as a cause of urinary retention and recurrent cystitis in women.[73, 74] It has been suggested that the syndrome of "external sphincter spasticity" may result from introital or vaginal infections, urethritis, Skene's gland abscesses, anorectal disease, or adnexal disease.[73] In a study of a group of women with unexplained partial or complete urinary retention, all had high urethral closure pressures as measured by urethral pressure profiles.[73] They responded to pudendal nerve block, and therefore the condition was attributed to "spasticity of the external sphincter and pelvic floor." The high tonic pressure in the urethra may lead to a reflex inhibition of detrusor function and urinary retention. Local factors such as pain, infectious or inflammatory processes, or traumatic intercourse may cause a high tonus of the pelvic floor and subsequent detrusor inhibition. Webster also described a group of women with recurrent urinary tract infections who had an apparent obstruction at the external sphincter on videourodynamic evaluation.[74] Again, spasticity in response to recurrent cystitis was proposed as the cause of the obstruction.[74]

Treatment of this condition should first be directed toward the suspected underlying painful or inflam-matory lesion. If this fails, or if the cause cannot be identified, some authors have suggested pharmacologic therapy with muscle relaxants such as diazepam.[12] Treatment with alpha-adrenergic blockers has been recommended to both relax the bladder neck and urethra and facilitate detrusor contraction by enhancing pelvic ganglionic transmission.[73] Alpha blockers may also be beneficial in treating urinary retention due to transient spasticity caused by acute pain or inflammation.

Detrusor Sphincter Dyssynergia

True DSD results from a suprasacral spinal cord lesion. Normal voiding consists of external sphincter–pelvic floor relaxation during a sustained voluntary detrusor contraction. Patients with DSD have detrusor hyperreflexia with an increase rather than a decrease in external sphincter activity during voiding. Several different patterns have been described.[75] The result is a detrusor contraction against a closed or partially closed outlet that may lead to urinary retention and damage to the upper urinary tract. DSD is often seen in patients with complete spinal cord injuries but may also be present in those with other neurologic conditions that affect the central nervous system. Multiple sclerosis is a neurologic disease that commonly causes voiding dysfunction including urinary retention in women. The usual cause of retention in patients with multiple sclerosis is DSD, although an acontractile bladder may also be responsible. Sirls and associates recently described urodynamic findings in 113 patients with multiple sclerosis and found that 70% had detrusor hyperreflexia, 28% had DSD, and 15% had detrusor acontractility.[76]

The ideal treatment for DSD is use of anticholinergic medications to induce complete urinary retention coupled with CIC. However, in some cases this is impossible, and chronic catheter drainage must be instituted instead.

IMPAIRED DETRUSOR CONTRACTILITY

Impaired detrusor contractility may lead to acute or chronic urinary retention. The decompensated detrusor may gradually empty less effectively, or an acute event such as fecal impaction, medication, or a mild degree of superimposed obstruction can result in retention of urine. This is especially true in women with poor contractility who empty the bladder primarily by pelvic floor relaxation or the aid of abdominal straining. Detrusor hypocontractility or acontractility may have a variety of causes including neurogenic, postobstructive, and idiopathic conditions. In addition, decreases in contractility are frequently associated with aging as the detrusor muscle cells degenerate.[2, 3] In this section we describe several causes of impaired detrusor contractility that are particularly common in women. Treatment of all entities, even those not mentioned specifically here, is similar. It is imperative that adequate bladder emptying and low-pressure storage be achieved. Ideally, this should occur naturally without the need for continuous or intermittent catheterization; however, this is often not possible. Treatment or removal of any coexisting problems that might induce retention in the presence of impaired contractility (e.g., medications, relative obstruction) may be necessary to avoid catheterization.

The widespread acceptance of CIC for the treatment of incomplete bladder emptying due to almost any cause but especially to poor contractility has been a major factor in the treatment of such patients. The history and details of CIC are described later. Another and somewhat more controversial treatment for bladder hypocontractility is the use of bethanechol chloride. This cholinergic agonist gained popularity in the 1960s and 1970s despite little evidence from controlled studies in favor of its efficacy. However, in the late 1970s and early 1980s several investigators questioned the effectiveness of bethanechol chloride in the treatment of non-neurogenic voiding dysfunction, particularly with respect to high residual urine. These investigators found no significant improvement in voiding function or residuals with either oral or subcutaneous administration of this drug.[77–80] It has been shown that bethanechol does affect the lower urinary tract, but this does not necessarily correspond to "improved voiding function." Bethanechol chloride can lower the volume needed to produce a severe urge to void, and it decreases bladder compliance and capacity.[77–81] Bethanechol chloride has also been advocated for the treatment of neurogenic voiding dysfunction. Again, much of this recommendation has been based on uncontrolled studies.[82–84] One thing is clear, however. For bethanechol chloride to work at all, an intact sacral micturition reflex arc must be present. Therefore, this medication is best suited for patients with partial lower motor neuron lesions.[82–84] It is ineffective in patients with complete lower motor neuron lesions or spinal shock. Awad and associates have suggested that the subcutaneous form of the drug is indeed effective in partial lower motor neuron lesions, but this effect is often not sustained when drug administration is changed to the oral form.[83] The literature does not give a clear definition of the therapeutic role of bethanechol chloride. Much of its early popularity was based on anecdotal experiences. However, one must be careful in assuming that because voiding function improves while on a pharmacologic agent it is necessarily because of that agent.[85] There are usually a multitude of other factors to consider. Based on the best controlled studies, it appears that the role of bethanechol chloride is limited. The ineffectiveness of the oral form is probably due to unpredictable absorption, and the subcutaneous form has severe limiting side effects (sweating, hot flashes, palpitations, and malaise).[84] For these reasons, we caution against the indiscriminate use of bethanechol chloride.

Detrusor Hyperactivity with Impaired Contractility

Recently, Resnick and Yalla described the syndrome of detrusor hyperactivity with impaired contractility (DHIC),[86, 87] which was discovered while studying a group of elderly institutionalized, incontinent patients to determine the cause of incontinence. They noted that 30% of these patients had an alteration in bladder reflex and contractile function in an opposite fashion such that uninhibited contractions emptied less than half the bladder volume despite the absence of obstruction (inadequate sphincter relaxation, DSD, or other bladder outlet obstruction). It was discovered that impaired emptying was not due to a low peak detrusor pressure, a contraction of shorter duration, or smaller voided volume. Only the speed of the contraction correlated with emptying. The authors concluded that in this group of patients, which constituted approximately half of all those studied who had detrusor hyperactivity, detrusor contractile function was impaired. Augmentation of voiding with abdominal straining was a frequent finding. Patients with DHIC voided an average of 37% of bladder volume and had average residuals of 95 ml.[86] By design of the study, none of the patients were in urinary retention; however, it was suggested that DHIC could result in progressive retention, and this occurred in two patients a year after diagnosis.[86] DHIC may result from a deterioration of detrusor function in patients with detrusor hyperactivity; however, this is not clear. Decreased contractility may be due to impaired neuromuscular transmission at the level of the detrusor or a myopathic process such as cellular degeneration.[4, 86]

Resnick and colleagues stressed the importance of videourodynamic evaluation in the diagnosis of DHIC. In their experience the addition of fluoroscopically monitored synchronous cystosphincterometry was invaluable in ruling out conditions such as stress urinary incontinence, outlet obstruction, sensory urgency, detrusor underactivity, and urethral instability.[87] Patients with DHIC who are not in urinary retention may be predisposed to develop retention in response to an added insult such as fecal impaction or medication.[86] Therefore, it is important to diagnose DHIC prior to embarking on therapy intended to treat incontinence because impaired emptying may be exacerbated. Ideally, DHIC may be treated with anticholinergics to control incontinence and some form of catheterization (e.g., CIC) to treat the impaired emptying.

Psychogenic Urinary Retention

Urinary retention sometimes develops with no evidence of organic disease. It may develop secondary to centrally mediated, subconscious inhibition of a detrusor contraction or sphincteric relaxation. This condition has been referred to as psychogenic retention.[88] It may occur after severe psychological trauma or sometimes with no identifiable cause. In Barrett's series 11 of 12 patients with psychogenic retention were women.[88] Cystometry and pelvic floor electromyography are normal except for a delayed sensation and a large-capacity bladder in some patients. The condition is usually temporary and responds well to supportive management, which should consist of psychiatric support when indicated as well as the use of CIC until normal voiding resumes. In Barrett's series 75% of patients were managed on an outpatient basis. Eighty-three percent of patients voided normally, although half of these used supplemental CIC to reduce residual volumes. Severe detrusor degeneration occurred in 17%, and these patients were dependent on CIC to empty the bladder.[88]

Pelvic Plexus Injury

Injury to the pelvic plexus may occur following major pelvic ablative surgery. In women such surgery is usually radical hysterectomy; however abdominoperineal resection, proctocolectomy, and low anterior resection for the treatment of colorectal malignancies may also be responsible. The incidence of voiding dysfunction following such major surgery has been reported to occur in 16 to 80% of cases.[89–95] Iatrogenic voiding dysfunction after pelvic surgery is the result of injury to the pelvic, hypogastric, and pudendal nerves. Also, the pelvic plexus may become involved in the malignant process itself by direct extension.[91, 96] The typical pelvic plexus injury is usually thought to produce the classic "flaccid bladder." However, careful clinical, urodynamic, and radiologic evaluation reveals that the nature of the neurologic lesion and its consequences may be variable owing to the complex assortment of partial or complete injuries to the parasympathetic, sympathetic, and somatic nervous systems.[97] Typically, parasympathetic injury produces a hypocontractile or acontractile bladder with decreased sensation. Sympathetic nerve injury can result in a bladder with decreased compliance and high storage pressures due to beta-adrenergic denervation. In addition, sympathetic denervation may cause bladder neck incompetence and incontinence. Sympathetic nerve injury has been reported to occur in about half of patients who have parasympathetic denervation resulting from pelvic plexus injury.[97]

With respect to hysterectomy, it is thought that bladder dysfunction results from parasympathetic damage due to extensive dissection inferolateral to the cervix.[90] Sympathetic nerve damage may occur secondary to hypogastric plexus injury at the pelvic brim (medial to the ureters), in the area lateral to the rectum, and in proximity to the cardinal ligaments.[97, 98] Extensive dissection in the region of the cardinal ligaments may account for the reported 50% incidence of combined sympathetic-parasympathetic denervation.[97, 98] From a clinical standpoint, Seski and Diokno feel that pelvic plexus injury after radical hysterectomy results primarily in a bladder with diminished contractile force and a decreased

ability to sense fullness.[92] The hypertonic phase tends to be transient and of less clinical significance.

The most common manifestation of pelvic plexus injury is urinary retention, although urinary incontinence may result from sympathetic or somatic damage. In most cases, symptoms resolve within several months but may persist in up to a third of patients. It is not fair to evaluate postoperative voiding dysfunction after major pelvic surgery until patients are ambulatory and relatively pain free. If urinary retention persists, management should focus on providing adequate bladder drainage. We prefer CIC as the method of choice. While the patient is on CIC spontaneous return of voiding can easily be assessed. In certain patients chronic indwelling catheter drainage may be necessary. Others have suggested using a suprapubic catheter connected to gravity drainage.[99, 100] In patients who do not desire an external collection device, the suprapubic catheter may be plugged and then opened periodically at the same intervals at which one would perform CIC. Some investigators favor supplementing CIC with oral bethanechol chloride in the hope of stimulating bladder function.[82, 92]

Diabetic Cystopathy

Women with long-term diabetes mellitus may suffer urologic manifestations of the disease. Classically, the clinical and urodynamic manifestations include decreased bladder sensation, increased bladder capacity, and impaired contractility, which may lead to urinary retention. Although one cannot argue that this presentation is common, a recent study suggested that detrusor instability may be even more common than impaired contractility or detrusor areflexia, at least in symptomatic patients.[101] Nevertheless, so-called diabetic cystopathy is a frequent cause of incomplete emptying of the bladder. Its onset is characterized by an insidious loss or impairment of bladder sensation followed by progressive increases in bladder volume and PVRs of urine and detrusor hypocontractility.[102–105] It is thought that impairment of the bladder muscle sensory reflex affects detrusor reflex generation.[106]

Classic diabetic cystopathy is frequently associated with peripheral neuropathy in the insulin-dependent diabetic.[102] It has been shown that in the autonomic nervous system, neuropathy is similar to that in the somatic nervous system—that is, segmental demyelination and axonal degeneration.[107, 108] Changes probably begin well before symptoms and even urodynamic changes are seen. Andersen and Bradley showed that segmental innervation of the bladder was affected by diabetes mellitus. They recorded spinal reflex-evoked potentials in diabetic patients and showed a slowing of conduction velocities even in the presence of a normal cystometrogram.[109]

The treatment of the diabetic bladder depends on the stage at which intervention is sought. Efforts are concentrated on achieving adequate bladder emptying. If the condition is diagnosed early enough and the patient is educated properly, the patient may respond well to timed voiding (e.g., every 3 to 4 hours whether or not sensation is present) as well as to double and triple voiding and Credé voiding to prevent overdistention. In advanced cases in which detrusor contractility is severely impaired owing to chronic overdistention, catheter drainage may be necessary. CIC is always the preferred mode of catheter drainage if it is possible. Some authors advocate the use of parasympathomimetic agents such as bethanechol chloride to facilitate emptying.[103, 105] Others have rarely found these to be effective.[110] Some investigators have suggested surgery in the form of transurethral resection or incision of the bladder neck in women who continue to have high residuals despite conservative management. The idea is to reduce the resistance at the bladder neck significantly so that the decreased pressure generated by the hypocontractile bladder is sufficient for emptying. This mode of treatment has not been particularly popular in the United States.[103, 105]

CLEAN INTERMITTENT CATHETERIZATION

The goal of intermittent catheterization is to facilitate emptying of the bladder while preserving renal function and reducing the rate of urinary tract infection. Intermittent catheterization is ideally performed by the patient herself (self-catheterization), but it may in certain circumstances be done by a caretaker. The concept was first recommended by Guttman as an aseptic technique.[111] However, pioneering work by Lapides and colleagues introduced the concept of CIC.[112–114] Its ease, safety, and low cost have made it the procedure of choice for chronic bladder drainage. Long-term acceptance (more than 10 years) of CIC has been demonstrated.[115] In addition, it has been shown to be a viable therapy in the elderly as well as in patients with spinal cord injuries.[116, 117]

The feasibility of unsterile catheterization is based on the theory proposed by Lapides and coworkers that clinical infection is the result of invading microorganisms and host resistance, the latter being more important.[112, 113] Their studies suggested that the most common cause of increased susceptibility to bacterial invasion is decreased blood flow to the tissues. This can occur with increased bladder pressure or overdistention. These authors believe that maintenance of a good blood supply to the urinary tract by the avoidance of high intraluminal pressures and overdistention is the key to preventing infection. Furthermore, they think that if these criteria are met, bacterial contamination may be disregarded.[112–114] Emphasis should be placed on frequency of catheterization and not sterility. It has been recommended that catheterization volumes be kept below 350 to 400 ml to prevent clinical infection.[117, 118]

TECHNIQUE OF CLEAN INTERMITTENT CATHETERIZATION Initially, patients must be taught to catheterize themselves. Although there is often resistance on the part of the patient, once she sees that the procedure is not difficult or painful, learning proceeds at a rapid rate and can usually be completed in a single session. We follow the method proposed by Lapides and colleagues.[114] Women should be taught initially sitting on an examining table with the feet on the table and the legs flexed and knees held apart. A mirror is placed at the foot of the table to allow the patient to visualize her perineum, vagina, and urethral meatus. The labia are separated and with the aid of the mirror, the patient is shown the urethral meatus, clitoris, and vaginal introitus. Next the patient directs the catheter (either a 14 Fr rubber Robinson or short plastic catheter) into the urethra and bladder under vision. One hand (usually the dominant) is used to direct the catheter and the other to separate the labia. The catheter should be held $\frac{1}{2}$ to 1 inch from its tip with the second and fourth fingers while the middle finger palpates and elevates the urethral meatus. After the bladder is emptied, the patient is instructed to gently advance and withdraw the catheter several times to make sure complete emptying has been achieved. In a short time most patients learn to identify the urethral meatus by palpation and the mirror is no longer necessary. Catheterization can be performed on a regular toilet seat or in the standing position in front of the toilet. The patient is instructed to wash her hands and the catheter with soap and water before each use. The catheter may be stored in a small plastic bag. Gloves, topical antiseptic preparations, and lubricating jelly are not necessary. Ease and convenience should be stressed so that the patient performs catheterization frequently.

REFERENCES

1. Blaivas JG, Labib KB: Acute urinary retention in women. Complete urodynamic evaluation. Urology 4:383, 1978.
2. Elbadawi A, Yalla SV, Resnick NM: Structural basis of geriatric voiding dysfunction. I. Methods of a prospective ultrastructural/urodynamic study and an overview of the findings. J Urol 150:1650, 1993.
3. Elbadawi A, Yalla SV, Resnick NM: Structural basis of geriatric voiding dysfunction. II. Aging detrusor: Normal versus impaired contractility. J Urol 150:1657, 1993.
4. Elbadawi A, Yalla SV, Resnick NM: Structural basis of geriatric voiding dysfunction. III. Detrusor overactivity. J Urol 150:1668, 1993.
5. Elbadawi A, Yalla SV, Resnick NM: Structural basis of geriatric voiding dysfunction. IV. Bladder outlet obstruction. J Urol 150:1681, 1993.
6. Susset JG, Servot-Viguier D, Lamy F, et al: Collagen in 155 human bladders. Invest Urol 16:204, 1978.
7. Gilpin SA, Gilpin CJ, Dixon JS, et al: The effect of age on the autonomic innervation of the urinary bladder. Br J Urol 58:378, 1986.
8. Levy BJ, Wight TN: Structural changes in the aging submucosa: New morphologic criteria for the evaluation of the unstable human bladder. J Urol 144:1044, 1990.
9. Wein AJ, Levin RM, Barrett DM: Voiding function and dysfunction. Voiding function relevant to anatomy, physiology and pharmacology. In Gillenwater JY, Grayhack JT, Howards SS, Duckett JW (eds): Adult and Pediatric Urology, 2nd ed, vol I. St. Louis, Mosby–Year Book, 1991, p 933.
10. Barrett DM, Wein AJ: Voiding dysfunction: Diagnosis, classi-

fication, and management. In Gillenwater JY, Grayhack JT, Howards SS, Duckett JW (eds): Adult and Pediatric Urology, 2nd ed, vol I. St. Louis, Mosby–Year Book, 1991, p 1001.

11. Krane RJ, Siroky MB (eds): Clinical Neuro-Urology, 2nd ed. Boston, Little Brown, 1991.

12. Bass JS, Leach GE: Bladder outlet obstruction in women. Prob Urol 5:141, 1991.

13. Massey JA, Abrams PA: Obstructed voiding in the female. Br J Urol 61:36, 1988.

14. Farrar DJ, Osborne JL, Stephenson TP, et al: A urodynamic view of bladder outflow obstruction in the female: Factors influencing the results of treatment. Br J Urol 47:815, 1976.

15. Axelrod SL, Blaivas JG: Bladder neck obstruction in women. J Urol 137:497, 1987.

16. Nitti VW, Raz S: Obstruction following anti-incontinence procedures: Diagnosis and treatment with transvaginal urethrolysis. J Urol 152:93, 1994.

17. Foster HE, McGuire EJ: Management of urethral obstruction with transvaginal urethrolysis. J Urol 150:1448, 1993.

18. Webster GD, Kreder KJ: Voiding dysfunction following cystourethropexy: Its evaluation and management. J Urol 144:670, 1990.

19. Marshall VF, Marchetti AA, Krantz KE: The correction of stress incontinence by simple vesicourethral suspension. Surg Gynecol Obstet 88:509, 1949.

20. Burch JC: Urethrovaginal fixation to Cooper's ligament for correction of stress incontinence, cystocele and prolapse. Am J Obstet Gynecol 81:281, 1961.

21. Shull BL, Baden WF: A six-year experience with paravaginal defect repair for stress urinary incontinence. Am J Obstet Gynecol 160:1432, 1989.

22. Pereyra AJ: Simplified surgical procedure for the correction of stress incontinence in women. West J Surg 67:223, 1959.

23. Raz S, Sussman EM, Erikson DE, et al: The Raz bladder neck suspension: Results in 206 patients. J Urol 148:845, 1992.

24. Stamey TA: Endoscopic suspension of the vesical neck for urinary incontinence in females: Report on 203 consecutive patients. Ann Surg 192:465, 1980.

25. Gittes RF, Loughlin KR: No-incision pubovaginal suspension for stress incontinence. J Urol 138:568, 1987.

26. Juma S, Sdrales L: Etiology of urinary retention after bladder neck suspension (abstract). J Urol 149:400A, 1993.

27. Spencer JR, O'Conor VJ Jr, Schaeffer AJ: Comparison of endoscopic suspension of the vesical neck with suprapubic vesicourethropexy for treatment of stress urinary incontinence. J Urol 137:411, 1987.

28. Rost A, Fiedler U, Fester C: Comparative analysis of the results of suspension-urethroplasty according to Marshall-Marchetti-Krantz and of urethrovesicopexy with adhesive. Urol Int 34:167, 1979.

29. Mundy AR: A trial comparing the Stamey bladder neck suspension with colposuspension for the treatment of stress incontinence. Br J Urol 55:687, 1983.

30. Cardoza LD, Stanton SL, Williams JE: Detrusor instability following surgery for genuine stress incontinence. Br J Urol 51:204, 1979.

31. Marchetti AA, Marshall VM, Shultis LD: Simple vesicourethral suspension; A survey. Am J Obstet Gynecol 74:57, 1957.

32. Pope AJ, Shaw PJR, Coptcoat MJ, et al: Changes in bladder function following a surgical alteration in outflow resistance. Neurourol Urodyn 9:503, 1990.

33. Leach GE, Raz S: Modified Pereya bladder neck suspension after previously failed anti-incontinence surgery. Urology 23:359, 1984.

34. McGuire EJ, Letson W, Wang S: Transvaginal urethrolysis after obstructive urethral suspension procedures. J Urol 142:1037, 1989.

35. Zimmern PE, Hadley HR, Leach GE, et al: Female urethral obstruction after Marshall-Marchetti-Krantz operation. J Urol 138:517, 1987.

36. Leach GE, Schmidbauer CP, Hadley HR, et al: Surgical treatment of female urethral diverticulum. Sem Urol 4:33, 1986.

37. Raz S: Transvaginal reconstruction of the female urethra. In Raz S (ed): Atlas of Transvaginal Surgery. Philadelphia, WB Saunders, 1992, p 181.

38. Marion G: Surgery of the neck of the bladder. Br J Urol 5:351, 1933.

39. Mayo ME: Primary bladder neck obstruction. Surg Rounds 5:66, 1982.

40. Gronbaek K, Struckmann JR, Frimodt-Moller C: The treatment of female bladder neck dysfunction. Scand J Urol Nephrol 26:113, 1992.

41. Norgaard JP, Swartz-Sorenson S, Djurhuus JC: Functional bladder neck obstruction in women. Urol Int 39:207, 1984.

42. Diokno AC: Bladder neck obstruction in women. Neurourol Urodyn 5:325, 1986.

43. Diokno AC, Hollander JB, Bennett CJ: Bladder neck obstruction in women: A real entity. J Urol 132:294, 1984.

44. Delaere KPJ, Debruyne FMJ, Moonen WA: Bladder neck incision in the female: A hazardous procedure? Br J Urol 55:283, 1983.

45. Gardy M, Kozminski M, DeLancy J, et al: Stress incontinence and cystoceles. J Urol 145:1211, 1991.

46. Nichols DH: Vaginal prolapse affecting bladder function. Urol Clin North Am 12:329, 1985.

47. Nichols DH, Milley PS, Randall CL: Significance of restoration of normal vaginal depth and axis. Obstet Gynecol 36:251, 1970.

48. Raz S, Nitti VW, Bregg KJ: Transvaginal repair of enterocele. J Urol 149:724, 1993.

49. Raz S, Klutke CG, Golub J: Four-corner bladder and urethral suspension for moderate cystocele. J Urol 142:712, 1989.

50. Raz S, Little NA, Juma S, et al: Repair of severe anterior vaginal wall prolapse (grade IV cystourethrocele). J Urol 146:988, 1991.

51. Nitti VW: Transvaginal repair of enterocele, with variations. Contemp Urol 6(4):50, 1994.

52. Nichols DH: Sacrospinous fixation for massive eversion of the vagina. Am J Obstet Gynecol 142:901, 1982.

53. Moschcowitz AV: The pathogenesis, anatomy and cure of prolapse of the rectum. Surg Gynecol Obstet 15:7, 1912.

54. Raz S: Vaginal prolapse. In Raz S: Atlas of Transvaginal Surgery. Philadelphia, WB Saunders, 1992, p 103.

55. Cherrie RJ, Leach GE, Raz S: Obstructing urethral valve in a woman: A case report. J Urol 129:1051, 1983.

56. Nesbit RM, McDonald HP Jr, Busby S: Obstructing valves in the female urethra. J Urol 91:79, 1964.

57. Sardosky MF: Urethral carcinoma. AUA Update Series, vol 6, no 13. Houston, American Urological Association, 1987.

58. Ward JN, Lavengood RW Jr, Draper JW: Pseudo bladder neck syndrome in women. J Urol 99:65, 1968.

59. Carvell JE, Stubbs SM: Acute retention of urine in a woman due to an exoenteric leiomyoma. Br J Urol 49:50, 1977.

60. Kingsnorth AN: Urinary retention due to ovarian cyst. Br J Urol 56:439, 1984.

61. Doran J, Roberts M: Acute urinary retention in the female. Br J Urol 47:793, 1976.

62. Silva PD, Berberich W: Retroverted impacted gravid uterus with acute urinary retention: Report on two cases and review of the literature. Obstet Gynecol 68:121, 1986.

63. Hansen JH, Asmussen M: Acute urinary retention in the first trimester of pregnancy. Acta Obstet Gynecol Scand 64:279, 1985.

64. Burdon S, Maurer JE, Lich R: Acute retention in pregnancy. J Urol 65:578, 1951.

65. Goldberg KA, Kwart AM: Intermittent urinary retention in first trimester of pregnancy. Urology 17:270, 1981.

66. Hinman F, Baumann FW: Vesical and ureteral damage from voiding dysfunction in boys without neurologic or obstructive disease. J Urol 109:727, 1973.

67. Allen TD: The non-neurogenic neurogenic bladder. J Urol 117:232, 1977.

68. Allen TD, Bright TC III: Urodynamic patterns in children with dysfunctional voiding problems. J Urol 119:247, 1978.

69. Hinman F Jr: Nonneurogenic neurogenic bladder (the Hinman syndrome)—15 years later. J Urol 136:769, 1986.

70. Jorgensen TM, Djurhuus JC, Schroder HD: Idiopathic detrusor sphincter dysnergia in neurologically normally patients with voiding abnormalities. Eur Urol 8:107, 1982.

71. McGuire EJ, Savastano JA: Urodynamic studies in enuresis and the nonneurogenic neurogenic bladder. J Urol 132:299, 1984.

72. Kaplan WE, Firlit CR, Schoenberg HW: The female urethral syndrome: External sphincter spasticity as an etiology. J Urol 124:43, 1980.

73. Raz S, Smith RB: External sphincter spasticity syndrome in female patients. J Urol 115:443, 1976.

74. Webster JR: Combined video/pressure/flow cystourethrography in female patients with voiding disturbances. Urology 5:209, 1975.

75. McGuire E: Electromyographic evaluation of sphincter function and dysfunction. Urol Clin North Am 6:21, 1979.

76. Sirls LT, Zimmern PE, Leach GE: Role of limited evaluation and aggressive medical management in multiple sclerosis: A review of 113 patients. J Urol 151:946, 1994.

77. Barrett DM: The effect of oral bethanechol chloride on voiding in female patients with excessive residual urine: A randomized double-blind study. J Urol 126:640, 1981.

78. Wein AJ, Malloy TR, Shofer F, Raezer DM: The effects of bethanechol chloride on urodynamic parameters in normal women and in women with significant residual urine volumes. J Urol 124:397, 1980.

79. Wein AJ, Raezer DM, Malloy TR: Failure of the bethanechol supersensitivity test to predict improved voiding after subcutaneous bethanechol administration. J Urol 123:202, 1980.

80. Wein AJ, Hanno PM, Dixon DO, et al: The effect of oral bethanechol chloride on the cystometrogram of the normal male adult. J Urol 120:330, 1978.

81. Blaivas JG: If you currently prescribe bethanechol chloride for urinary retention, please raise your hand. Neurourol Urodyn 3:209, 1984.

82. Diokno AC, Koppenhoefer R: Bethanechol chloride in neurogenic bladder dysfunction. Urology 8:455, 1976.

83. Awad SA, McGinnis RH, Downie JW: The effectiveness of bethanechol chloride in lower motor neuron lesions: The importance of mode of administration. Neurourol Urodyn 3:173, 1984.

84. Downie JW: Bethanechol chloride in urology—a discussion of issues. Neurourol Urodyn 3:211, 1984.

85. Wein AJ: Editorial comment. J Urol 126:642, 1981.

86. Resnick NM, Yalla SV: Detrusor hyperactivity with impaired contractile function—an unrecognized but common cause of incontinence in elderly patients. JAMA 257:3076, 1987.

87. Resnick NM, Yalla SV, Laurino E: The pathophysiology of urinary incontinence among institutionalized elderly persons. N Engl J Med 320:1, 1989.

88. Barrett DM: Evaluation of psychogenic urinary retention. J Urol 120:191, 1978.

89. Kirkergaad P, Hjortrup A, Sanders S: Bladder dysfunction after low anterior resection for mid-rectal cancer. Am J Surg 141:266, 1981.

90. Forney JP: The effect of radical hysterectomy on bladder function. Am J Obstet Gynecol 138:374, 1980.

91. Fowler JW, Brenner DN, Moffat LEF: The incidence and consequences of damage to the parasympathetic nerve supply to the bladder after abdominoperineal resection of the rectum for carcinoma. Br J Urol 50:95, 1978.

92. Seski JC, Diokno AC: Bladder dysfunction after radical abdominal hysterectomy. Am J Obstet Gynecol 128:643, 1977.

93. Eickenberg HU, et al.: Urologic complications following abdominoperineal resection. J Urol 115:180, 1976.

94. Smith PH, Ballantyne B: The neuroanatomical basis for denervation of the urinary bladder following major pelvic surgery. Br J Surg 55:929, 1968.

95. Marshall VF, Pollack RS, Miller C: Observations on urinary dysfunction after excision of the rectum. J Urol 55:409, 1946.

96. Woodside JR, Crawford ED: Urodynamic features in pelvic plexus injury. J Urol 124:657, 1980.

97. Yalla SV, Andriole G: Vesicourethral dysfunction following pelvic visceral ablative surgery. J Urol 132:503, 1984.

98. Pavlakis AJ: Cauda equina and pelvic plexus injury. In Krane RJ, Siroky MB (eds): Clinical Neuro-Urology, 2nd ed. Boston, Little Brown, 1991, p 333.

99. Buchsbaum HJ: Discussion. Am J Obstet Gynecol 128:649, 1977.

100. Giustini FG: Discussion. Am J Obstet Gynecol 128:650, 1977.

101. Kaplan SA, Te AE, Blaivas JG: Urodynamic findings in patients with diabetic cystopathy. J Urol 153:342, 1995.

102. Frimodt-Moller C: Diabetic cystopathy: Epidemiology and related disorders. Ann Intern Med 92:318, 1980.

103. Ellenberg M: Development of urinary bladder dysfunction in diabetes mellitus. Ann Intern Med 92:321, 1980.

104. Bradley WE: Diagnosis of urinary bladder dysfunction in diabetes mellitus. Ann Intern Med 92:323, 1980.

105. Frimodt-Moller C, Mortensen S: Treatment of diabetic cystopathy. Ann Intern Med 92:327, 1980.

106. Bradley WE, Timm GW, Scott FB: Cystometry V sensation. Urology 6:654, 1975.

107. Ewing DJ, Clarke BF: Diabetic autonomic neuropathy: Present insights and future prospects. Diabetes Care 9:648, 1986.

108. Van Poppel H, Stessens R, Van Damme B, et al: Diabetic cystopathy: Neuropathological examination of urinary bladder biopsies. Eur Urol 15:128, 1988.

109. Andersen JT, Bradley WE: Early detection of diabetic visceral neuropathy. An electrophysiologic study of bladder and urethral innervation. Diabetes 25:1100, 1976.

110. Mundy AR, Blaivas JG: Nontraumatic neurological disorders. In Mundy AR, Stephenson TP, Wein AJ (eds): Urodynamic Principles, Practices and Application. Edinburgh, Churchill Livingstone, 1984, p 278.

111. Guttman L: Initial treatment of traumatic paraplegia. Proc R Soc Med 47:1103, 1954.

112. Lapides J, Costello RT, Zierdt DK, et al: Primary cause and treatment of recurrent urinary infection in women: Preliminary report. J Urol 100:552, 1968.

113. Lapides J, Diokno AC, Silber SJ, et al: Clean, intermittent self-catheterization in the treatment of urinary tract disease. J Urol 107:458, 1972.

114. Lapides J, Diokno AC, Gould FR, et al: Further observations on self-catheterization. J Urol 116:169, 1976.

115. Diokno AC, Sonda LP, Hollander JB, et al: Fate of patients started on clean intermittent self-catheterization therapy 10 years ago. J Urol 129:1120, 1983.

116. Bennett CJ, Diokno AC: Clean intermittent self-catheterization in the elderly. Urology 24:43, 1984.

117. Maynard FM, Diokno AC: Clean intermittent catheterization for spinal cord injury patients. J Urol 128:477, 1982.

118. Bakke A, Vollset SE: Risk factors for bacteremia and clinical urinary tract infection in patients treated with clean intermittent catheterization. J Urol 149:527, 1993.

CHAPTER 18

Bladder Dysfunction After Radiation and Radical Pelvic Surgery

Philippe E. Zimmern, M.D., F.A.C.S.

*It is only with the heart that one can see rightly;
what is essential is invisible to the eye.*

Antoine de Saint-Exupéry
Le Petit Prince

The link between a bladder insult, as occurs with pelvic radiation therapy for cervical carcinoma or extensive pelvic surgery for rectal cancer, and various clinical degrees of bladder dysfunction has long been recognized. What is new, however, is a better understanding of the exact mechanisms underlying this bladder dysfunction, leading therefore to the availability of valuable preventive measures. In addition, more reliable diagnosis based on urodynamic studies can now be achieved, and from it more appropriate therapy can be derived.

This chapter will focus predominantly on (1) how radiation therapy affects the bladder, (2) how the pelvic plexus can be injured during surgery, (3) the current evaluation methods recommended to assess the type and severity of the resulting bladder dysfunction, and (4) what therapeutic alternatives are available.

Bladder Dysfunction After Radiation Therapy

ETIOLOGY AND INCIDENCE

Radiation therapy can affect the bladder when it is used primarily to treat bladder cancer. In this instance, radiation damage to the cancer cells becomes the goal and as such is not considered in this chapter.

The most commonly cited example of secondary damage to the bladder due to radiation therapy is the damage resulting from treatment of cervical cancer. Although less frequent, bladder compromise secondary to radiation has also been reported after irradiation for uterine cancer and colorectal carcinoma.

Overall, the incidence of serious radiation damage to the bladder resulting from treatment of pelvic neoplasms is 10%.[1] This percentage varies depending on the denominator used in the series and whether the denominator was the initial number of patients in the early stages of cancer (who have an expected better long-term prognosis) or the survivors in the more advanced stages of cancer.

Another variable requiring consideration is the definition of serious radiation damage. In this chapter serious radiation damage means irreversible bladder damage necessitating a surgical procedure (Table 18–1). The operative criteria, although the most objective index of severity, have unfortunately not been universally adopted.[2] Many grading systems now exist in which a high degree of subjectivity is

TABLE 18–1
Simplified Staging System for Urinary Tract Injuries Following Radiation Therapy for Cervical Carcinoma

Complete recovery following symptoms such as dysuria, hematuria, and hydroureter
Incomplete recovery from hematuria, edematous bladder mucosa, persistent hydroureter, requiring continuous medication
Severe injury requiring surgical intervention: bladder augmentation, cystectomy, urinary diversion, ureteral reimplantation, nephrectomy

Modified from Kagan AR, Nussbaum H, Gilbert H, et al: A new staging system for irradiation injuries following treatment for cancer of the cervix. Gynecol Oncol 7:166, 1979.

incorporated, resulting in ambiguous data and therefore unreliable conclusions.

IMPACT OF RADIATION DELIVERY TO THE BLADDER

The degree of radiation damage incurred is linked to technical details of delivering the radiation such as mode of delivery and total dose delivered.[1, 2] Cervical cancer, for example, is usually treated with a combination of intracavitary curietherapy (isotopes implanted interstitially) and external irradiation. Because the difference between permanent injury and reversible damage to the bladder can be as little as 500 rads, small variations in the patient's position during curietherapy, number of intracavitary applications, type of applicator, and use of a midline shield can have tremendous dosing repercussions. All these technical details would be less significant if the amount of radiation delivered to the bladder could be reliably recorded. But none of the current techniques such as radiography, intracavitary markers, and even CT-assisted delineation of bladder boundaries can provide precise dosing information.[3] In the field of radiation therapy for cervical carcinoma, most authors currently agree that a combined dose of 6500 to 7000 rads is safe, although irreversible bladder injury can still occur sporadically. Above 7500 rads, a predictable injury rate of 20% or more can be expected.

HISTOPATHOLOGY

The response of the bladder to radiation therapy is classically divided into two stages: early response and late response (Table 18–2). The early stage reflects cellular damage, whereas the late stage is characterized by reparation processes involving connective tissue and blood vessels. Each step has been extensively studied both in animals and humans.

TABLE 18–2
Impact of Radiation Therapy on the Bladder

Factor	Early Reaction	Late Reaction
Incidence	>70%	5–20%
Time	<6 weeks	6 months to 10 years or more
Symptoms	Dysuria, frequency	Frequency, urge, urge incontinence, hematuria, fistula, recurrent bacteriuria
Cystoscopy	Erythemas Bullous edema	Pale and thin mucosa Hemorrhagic pancystitis
Bladder capacity	Normal	Reduced with high pressure
Histology	Capillary dilatation Edema of submucosa Superficial ulcers	Epithelial denudation Ulceration, telangiectasia Fibrosis Obliterative endarteritis

Stewart and colleagues studied the effect of radiation therapy (1000 to 3000 rads) in the bladder of radiosensitive strains of mice.[4] Histologic changes and functional parameters (urinary frequency and cystometric bladder capacity under general anesthesia) were assessed. The early damage occurred in the first 3 weeks, lasted for 1 week, and consisted mostly of increased frequency (twice the control levels) and reduced bladder volume (volume was reduced by half in 20 to 40% of the mice). At 2 weeks there was no histologic difference between control and irradiated bladders.

However, late bladder damage appeared between 4 and 10 months after irradiation, was more intense and frequent with higher doses of irradiation, and was irreversible. Histologically, radiation damage was noted in all layers, with epithelial denudation and ulceration on the surface and fibrosis with muscle atrophy underneath it. Similar findings have been described in dogs[5] and in various radiosensitive mouse strains.[6]

In humans, Antonakopoulos and colleagues examined 30 bladder biopsy specimens obtained during follow-up cystoscopy of 25 patients treated with radiation therapy for bladder cancer, cervical cancer, or prostatic cancer.[7] The time interval after completion of radiation therapy ranged from 1 month to 22 years. Five normal controls were incorporated in the study. Seventeen specimens contained urothelium as well as muscular layers. Under electron microscopy, cytoplasmic vacuolization and numerous lysosomes were observed in all cell layers. In addition, vessel alterations, damage to the smooth muscle layers, and extensive fibrosis were also noted. Although the bladder appears to be fairly radioresistant initially or when low radiation doses are used, the early onset of radiation damage at the ultrastructural level is clearly demonstrated in this detailed study.[7]

CLINICAL PRESENTATION

As little as 5 to 8% of patients receiving radiation therapy for cervical carcinoma experience some of the early symptoms of acute radiation cystitis: frequency, urgency, suprapubic pain, dysuria, and occasionally gross hematuria.[8, 9] In general, these symptoms disappear after completion of radiation therapy. In fact, in one prospective study of 33 patients undergoing radiation therapy for cervical carcinoma, the presence of short-term urinary symptoms did not result in a higher risk of permanent bladder damage.[10]

Chronic radiation cystitis from pelvic irradiation, on the other hand, is neither transient nor temporary. This permanent bladder damage is best identified in series that have 5 to 10 years long-term follow-up. Few series, however, separate the urologic complications due to radiation from those due to recurrence or persistence of the tumor.[11] Whenever this separation is documented, an eight- to tenfold higher ratio for urologic complications due to tumor invasion and damage locally (20 to 25%) than for radiation damage alone (2 to 4%) is usually observed.[1, 11, 12] Symptoms of chronic radiation cystitis include irritative symptoms such as frequency, urgency, urge incontinence, and nocturia. Parkin and associates sent postal questionnaires to 97 patients 5 to 11 years after they had received radiotherapy for cervical carcinoma.[13] Among the 70% who replied, 26% had severe symptoms, with urge and urge incontinence being the most common (45%). Voiding problems, conversely, were uncommon.[13]

In addition to radiation cystitis (see Table 18–2), the long-term manifestations of radiation injury to the bladder include recurrent hematuria, vesicovaginal fistula, and decreased bladder compliance.[9] Changes in bladder compliance, defined by the International Continence Society (ICS) as the change in volume for a given change in pressure (calculated by dividing the volume change by the change in detrusor pressure),[14] were noted in one study for external radiation doses of over 3000 rads.[10] When presenting with incontinence, patients who have had pelvic radiation exposure must undergo a thorough work-up to investigate not only possible urethral damage (type III or intrinsic urethral dysfunction) but also bladder instability or reduced bladder compliance, or even a vesicovaginal or urethrovaginal fistula. Upper tract evaluation must be incorporated systematically because changes in bladder compliance or distal radiation ureteritis can affect one or both kidneys.[11]

DIAGNOSIS

Routine laboratory evaluation includes urinalysis, urine culture, urine cytology, and renal function tests (blood urea nitrogen, serum creatinine). Urinalysis and urine culture are important to document urinary tract infection and detect microscopic hematuria. Detection of multiple microorganisms on culture should raise the suspicion of a urointestinal fistula. Recognition of tumor persistence or recurrence by urine cytologic evaluation can be difficult because the radiation-induced cell changes can be mistaken for altered tumor cells. Renal function must be assessed routinely after pelvic radiotherapy. An increase in blood urea nitrogen or serum creatinine requires investigation with functional (renal scan) and anatomic (intravenous pyelography, ultrasound, retrograde pyelography) studies. Baseline studies obtained prior to radiotherapy are extremely useful for comparison.

Cystoscopy is an essential part of the work-up in a patient with sterile urine. Changes in bladder mucosa (see Table 18–2), bladder capacity, fistula openings, invading tumor, and residual urine are assessed. When indicated (by the presence of tumor or fistula), a bladder biopsy and eventually a retrograde pyelogram are performed under general anesthesia. Biopsies must remain superficial ("cold" cup biopsies) to avoid perforation or fistula formation that can easily result from the combination of poor vascularity due to radiation damage and a thermal or destructive tissue effect.

Finally, urodynamic testing, including videourodynamic monitoring when type III stress incontinence is suspected, is indicated in incontinent patients to distinguish between bladder and urethral dysfunction. Urge incontinence due to bladder instability or reduced bladder compliance can be documented during a filling cystometrogram. In patients who are severely incontinent owing to low urethral resistance, impaired bladder compliance can be masked by insufficient bladder filling. Occlusion of the bladder neck with a Foley balloon permits adequate bladder filling, thereby assessing the detrusor response.[15] Lack of reflux during filling and emptying, voiding pattern, and amount of postvoid residual can be accurately determined as well.

MANAGEMENT

Bladder irritative symptoms are initially treated with anticholinergic drugs. Anticholinergic medications, however, are less efficient in controlling chronic radiation cystitis caused by bladder wall fibrosis. Bacterial infections can be controlled by antimicrobials or topical antibiotics.[8]

The bladder with a small capacity owing to reduced bladder compliance that does not respond to anticholinergic therapy offers a significant therapeutic challenge. Treatment by bladder distention under anesthesia has been proposed, but its limited symptomatic impact combined with the risk of bladder rupture is a strong deterrent. Bladder augmentation or supravesical urinary diversion may be necessary in patients with debilitating urinary symptoms. During surgical exploration, the severity of radiation damage to the pelvis and small intestine often precludes performance of a simple ileocystoplasty. In this situation, a transverse colon urinary diversion may become the safest long-term alternative.[9]

Bladder Dysfunction After Radical Pelvic Surgery

RADICAL PELVIC SURGERY AND BLADDER FUNCTION

Many reports have shown that bladder dysfunction is a common sequel of abdominoperineal resection of the rectum (APR) or radical hysterectomy (RH).[16–18] How does damage to the nerve supply of the bladder occur during these procedures? Studies of the pelvic parasympathetic, sympathetic, and pudendal nerves in cadavers by Mundy suggested two mechanisms: first, a direct injury of the pelvic plexus during dissection of the anterolateral aspect of the rectum (inferior hypogastric plexus containing both parasympathetic and sympathetic postganglionic fibers) or dissection in the area of the pelvic brim medial to the ureters (superior hypogastric plexus containing sympathetic fibers) (Fig. 18–1), and second, an indirect injury caused by traction ("tenting effect") during mobilization of the lower rectum.[19] During radical hysterectomy the risk of damage is highest when the dissection is carried below the cardinal ligament where most of the pelvic nerves and plexuses lie.[20]

Histologically, parasympathetic denervation of the human bladder resulted in an increase in cholinergic innervation in bladder biopsies of patients studied 10 months after APR. In this same group, however, no changes were detected in bladder biopsies performed 7 weeks postoperatively or in biopsies from a control group of patients of similar age.[21] In this study, however, no increase in the density of adrenergic nerves was noted, suggesting that partial regeneration of the autonomic nerves occurred in the long term. These findings demonstrate one extremely important clinical point in that voiding dysfunction after radical pelvic surgery may change markedly over time and may eventually resolve, thereby justifying an initially conservative therapeutic approach.[22]

CLINICAL EVALUATION

Postoperative vesical dysfunction varies with the extent of the primary cancer (preexisting damage from infiltrative cancer or previous surgery), the extent of dissection during the procedure, and the interval after the surgery (early, late, or delayed changes).

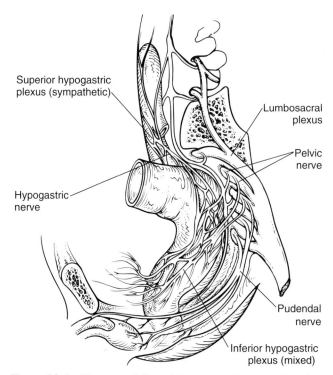

Figure 18–1 Diagram of the pelvic autonomic innervation demonstrating the close relationship of the inferior and superior hypogastric plexus to the rectum. (From Yalla SV, Andriole GL: Vesicourethral dysfunction following pelvic visceral ablative surgery. 132:509, 1984. © American Urological Association.)

Labels on figure:
Superior hypogastric plexus (sympathetic)
Hypogastric nerve
Lumbosacral plexus
Pelvic nerve
Pudendal nerve
Inferior hypogastric plexus (mixed)

Early changes (1 week to 3 to 6 months), usually transient, consist of (1) reduced bladder capacity, presumably due to surgical trauma and edema to the bladder and surrounding structures or possibly damage to the sympathetic system[23]; or (2) detrusor hypoactivity and diminished bladder sensation, manifested by urinary retention or overflow incontinence and presumably linked to damage to the bladder parasympathetic innervation.[16, 18] Incontinence may also result from bladder neck or urethral incompetence.

Changes that persist 6 to 12 months postoperatively are usually studied urodynamically.[24, 25] Emptying difficulties are generally due to a persistent acontractile bladder. Irritative symptoms with frequency, urgency, and urge incontinence are secondary to a small-capacity bladder due to reduced bladder compliance or detrusor instability. The cause of the reduction in bladder compliance has been linked to the effect of persistent parasympathetic motor denervation (neurologic factors) and to bladder wall changes (fibrosis or detrusor hypertrophy) resulting from chronic urinary tract infection or overdistention (physical factors).[16, 24, 25] A recent study of the long-term outcome of urinary dysfunction after RH, with or without subsequent radiation therapy, showed no improvement in urodynamic parameters between the initial (average, 15 months postoperative) and follow-up (average, 35 months) assessment in 16 symptomatic patients.[26]

Delayed onset of voiding dysfunction may indicate local cancer recurrence. Leach reported two patients with local pelvic cancer recurrence after APR; the first presenting symptoms were urgency and urge incontinence in one, and incomplete bladder emptying in the other.[27]

TREATMENT

During the early phase of voiding dysfunction after APR or RH, treatment is conservative and symptomatic. Urinary retention is managed by intermittent catheterization, and irritative symptoms such as urge and urge incontinence are controlled by anticholinergic medications, fluid restrictions, and timed voiding. Once voiding resumes, intermittent catheterization can be discontinued when postvoid residuals drop to less than 100 ml repetitively. For example, most studies report a mean duration of postoperative catheter drainage of 1 month after RH.[28, 29]

An augmentation cystoplasty may be indicated in small, contracted, noncompliant bladders that do not respond to anticholinergic therapy once the durability of the symptoms has been clearly established. Upper tract involvement resulting from sustained high intravesical pressure or urethral incompetence may dictate additional treatment not covered under the scope of this review.

REFERENCES

1. Kagan AR: Bladder, testicle, and prostate irradiation injury. *In* Vaeth JM, Meyer JL (eds): Radiation tolerance of normal tissues. Front Radiat Ther Oncol 23:323–337, 1989.
2. Kagan AR, Nussbaum H, Gilbert H, et al: A new staging system for irradiation injuries following treatment for cancer of the cervix. Gynecol Oncol 7:166, 1979.
3. Stuecklschweiger GF, Arian-Schad KS, Poier E, et al: Bladder and rectal dose of gynecologic high-dose-rate implants: Comparison of orthogonal and radiographic measurements with in vivo and CT-assisted measurements. Radiology 181:889, 1991.
4. Stewart FA, Lundbeck F, Oussoren Y, et al: Acute and late radiation damage in mouse bladder: A comparison of urination frequency and cystometry. Int J Radiation Oncol Biol Phys 21:1211, 1991.
5. Kinsella TJ, Sindelar WF, DeLuca AM, et al: Tolerance of the canine bladder to intraoperative radiation therapy: An experimental study. Int J Radiat Oncol Biol Phys 14:939, 1988.
6. Lundbeck F, Ulso N, Overgaard J: Acute changes in the bladder reservoir function after irradiation alone or in combination with chemotherapy: A matter of mouse strain. Scand J Urol Nephrol Suppl 125:141, 1989.
7. Antonakopoulos GN, Hicks RM, Berry RJ: The subcellular basis of damage to the human urinary bladder induced by irradiation. J Pathol 143:103, 1984.
8. Buschbaum HJ, Schmidt JD, Platz C, et al: Radiation cystitis, fistula and fibrosis. *In* Buschbaum HJ, Schmidt JD (eds): Gynecologic and Obstetric Urology. Philadelphia, W. B. Saunders, 1982, p 422.
9. Green TH: Urological complications of radical pelvic surgery and radiation therapy. *In* Coppleson M (ed): Gynaecologic Oncology: Fundamental Principles and Clinical Practice, vol 2. Edinburgh, Churchill Livingstone, 1982, pp 979–1000.
10. Farquharson DIM, Shingleton HM, Sanford SP, et al: The short-term effect of pelvic irradiation for gynecologic malignancies on bladder function. Obstet Gynecol 70:81, 1987.
11. Dean RJ, Lytton B: Urologic complications of pelvic irradiation. J Urol 119:64, 1978.
12. Zoubek J, McGuire EJ, Noll F, et al: The late occurrence of urinary tract damage in patients successfully treated by radiotherapy for cervical carcinoma. J Urol 141:1347, 1989.
13. Parkin DE, Davis JA, Symonds RP: Long-term bladder symptomatology following radiotherapy for cervical carcinoma. Radiother Oncol 9:195, 1987.
14. Bates CP, Bradley WE, Glen ES, et al: Fourth report on the standardisation of terminology of lower urinary tract function. Br J Urol 53:333, 1981.
15. Woodside JR, McGuire EJ: Technique for detection of detrusor hypertonia in the presence of urethral sphincteric incompetence. J Urol 127:740, 1982.
16. McGuire EJ: Neurovesical dysfunction after abdominoperineal resection. Surg Clin North Am 60:1207, 1980.
17. Blaivas JG, Barbalias GA: Characteristics of neural injury after abdominoperineal resection. J Urol 129:84, 1983.
18. Lapides J, Tank ST: Urinary complications following abdominal perineal resection. Cancer 28:230, 1971.
19. Mundy AR: An anatomical explanation for bladder dysfunction following rectal and uterine surgery. Br J Urol 54:501, 1982.
20. Twombly GH, Landers D: The innervation of the bladder with reference to radical hysterectomy. Am J Obstet Gynecol 71:1291, 1956.
21. Neal DE, Bogue PR, Williams RE: Histological appearances of the nerves of the bladder in patients with denervation of the bladder after excision of the rectum. Br J Urol 54:658, 1982.
22. Yalla SV, Andriole GL: Vesicourethral dysfunction following pelvic visceral ablative surgery. J Urol 132:503, 1984.
23. Seski JC, Diokno AC: Bladder dysfunction after radical abdominal hysterectomy. Am J Obstet Gynecol 128:643, 1977.
24. Chang PL, Fan HA: Urodynamic studies before and/or after abdominoperineal resection of the rectum for carcinoma. J Urol 130:948, 1983.
25. Gerstenberg TC, Nielsen ML, Clausen S, et al: Bladder function after abdomino-perineal resection of the rectum for anorectal cancer. Urodynamic investigation before and after operation in a consecutive series. Ann Surg 191:8, 1980.
26. Dwyer PL, O'Callaghan D: Urinary dysfunction following radical hysterectomy: Is there spontaneous improvement with time? Neurourol Urodyn 12:429, Abstract 72, 1993.
27. Leach GE, Yip CM: Delayed bladder dysfunction after abdominoperineal resection: An indicator of local recurrence. Urology 29:99, 1987.
28. Barclay DL, Roman-Lopez JJ: Bladder dysfunction after Schauta hysterectomy. One year follow-up. Am J Obstet Gynecol 123:519, 1975.
29. Jones CR, Woodhouse CR, Hendry WF: Urological problems following treatment of carcinoma of the cervix. Br J Urol 56:609, 1984.

CHAPTER 19

Lower Urinary Tract Disorders in the Elderly Female

Joseph G. Ouslander, M.D.

Aging is a continuous and inevitable process that affects everyone. It occurs at varying rates in different individuals and in different organ systems within the same individual. The individual organism's responses to the aging process are diverse and depend on many complex factors.

The lower urinary tract, as much as any other organ system, is greatly influenced by the interactive and additive effects of age-related changes and the accumulation of multiple pathologic entities with increasing age. Symptoms of lower urinary tract dysfunction are exceedingly common in elderly women. This chapter focuses on the age-related and age-associated changes that underlie lower urinary tract dysfunction in this population and reviews in some detail the two most common disorders of the lower urinary tract in elderly women—urinary incontinence and urinary tract infection.

Aging and the Female Lower Urinary Tract

When considering the effects of increasing age on any organ system, a crucial distinction must be made: that of true age-related changes that occur in everyone versus age-associated changes resulting from the accumulation of multiple pathologic conditions that do not occur in everyone. Table 19–1 lists age-related changes and age-associated factors that can influence lower urinary tract function and symptoms in elderly women. Because determining true age-related changes in the female lower urinary tract would involve invasive procedures (such as catheterization for urodynamic studies and cystoscopy) in continent elderly women without urinary symptoms, this type of information is rarely sought. Despite these difficulties, several types of age-related changes are known to have a prominent influence on lower urinary tract function.

One of the most important age-related changes affecting the female lower urinary tract is the postmenopausal decline in estrogen. The bladder, urethra, and genital tract have a common embryologic origin, and the epithelium of all of these tissues responds to hormonal changes. When estrogen influence declines, the epithelium and supporting tissues of the pelvic area atrophy, resulting in a friable mucosa and a tendency toward prolapse. The lower glycogen content in the vaginal epithelium results in less lactic acid metabolism by Doderlein's bacilli and an increase in the pH of vaginal secretions that may increase susceptibility to infection. Changes occur in the concentration of certain neurotransmitters in various locations in the central nervous system with increasing age. Given the important influence of the central nervous system on human bladder function, these age-related changes in central neurotransmitters may play a role in disorders of micturition in the elderly. Alterations in immune function also occur with increasing age. Although to date these changes have been noted mainly in cellular immunity, age-related changes in immune function, especially local immune activity in the lower urinary tract, could potentially play an important role in susceptibility to bacteriuria and symptomatic urinary tract infection in older women.

Certain functional changes appear to occur in the bladder and urethra with increasing age. In a study carried out almost 30 years ago, abnormal cystometrograms were found in 15 of 24 continent elderly women who were free of neurologic disease.[1] Twelve of these 15 showed uninhibited contractions; 10 had a bladder capacity of less than 250 ml. Other more recent studies have shown prevalence rates of 5 to 11% of abnormalities in continent older women.[2, 3]

TABLE 19-1
Aging and the Female Lower Urinary Tract

Age-Related Changes

Change	Potential Effects
A. Altered cell function	Altered interstitial tissues and mucosal surfaces Increased likelihood of pelvic prolapse and urinary infection
B. Decreased estrogen	Thinner and more friable mucosa and interstitial tissues Increased likelihood of pelvic prolapse, urinary symptoms, and infection
C. Altered concentrations of central nervous system neurotransmitters; altered nerve conduction	Increased likelihood of bladder and urethral dysfunction
D. Altered immune function	Increased susceptibility to infection

E. Altered bladder function
  1. Decreased capacity
  2. Increased uninhibited contractions
  3. Increased residual volume
	Increased likelihood of urinary symptoms, incontinence, and infection

F. Lower urethral pressure	Increased likelihood of incontinence

Age-Associated Factors

Factor	Potential Effects
Increased incidence of: A. Congitive and sensory impairment	Decreased ability to relate symptoms

B. Locomotor disturbances and immobility
  1. Stroke
  2. Hip fracture
  3. Peripheral vascular disease
  4. Parkinson's disease
	More difficulty getting to a toilet; increased likelihood of fecal impaction and incontinence

C. Poor fluid intake	Increased likelihood of fecal impaction and bacteriuria

D. Central nervous system diseases affecting bladder function
  1. Stroke
  2. Dementia
  3. Parkinson's disease
	Increased likelihood of incontinence

E. Other diseases affecting bladder function
  1. Malignancy
  2. Atherosclerotic vascular disease
	Increased likelihood of bladder dysfunction

F. Drug usage (see Table 19–2)	Increased likelihood of bladder or urethral dysfunction
G. Asymptomatic bacteriuria	Increased likelihood of symptomatic urinary infection

Maximal urethral pressure and functional urethral length are decreased in continent elderly women.[4, 5] In one study the maximal urethral pressure in continent women fell from a mean of 87 cm H_2O in the third decade to 42 cm H_2O in the seventh decade, a value that overlapped that of younger women with stress incontinence.[4] Such age-related changes in lower urinary tract function should be considered when evaluating urodynamic findings in elderly women. One postmortem study of 25 bladders from women aged 74 to 102 revealed marked trabeculation, diverticula, and cellular formation.[6] Histologic section of the bladder outlet showed a high incidence of chronic inflammation, edema, and fibrosis, presumed to be related to chronically infected residual urine. The trabeculation in these bladders was thought to be the result of loss of elastic tissue and coalescence of muscle fiber and of muscle hypertrophy secondary to either or a combination of bladder outlet obstruction and frequent uninhibited bladder contractions against a closed sphincter. Other investigators have reported that the bladder in elderly women is more often decompensated and thin-walled and that hypertrophy does not occur with uninhibited contractions.[7] Further research on the anatomic changes that occur in the aging lower urinary tract will help to clarify these issues.

Several age-associated factors, listed in Table 19–1, can have an important influence on lower urinary tract function and symptoms in elderly women. Although most elderly individuals are generally active and healthy, the incidence of several disorders does increase with age. Impairments of cognitive and sensory function are more common in the elderly than in younger populations. These impairments may make it difficult for the elderly to interpret and relate symptoms of lower urinary tract dysfunction accurately. Poor nutritional and fluid intake can predispose the elderly to fecal impaction and urinary infection. The prevalence of asymptomatic bacteriuria increases with age (see later discussion), and this situation also predisposes to symptomatic urinary infection. Locomotor disturbances are extremely common in the elderly. The incidence of stroke, arthritis, osteoporosis with resultant hip fractures, peripheral vascular disease with claudication or resultant amputations, Parkinson's disease, and other gait disorders increase with age. These disorders can make it difficult for the elderly to reach a toilet, especially in the presence of urinary frequency and urgency. Impaired mobility, therefore, may play a prominent role in the development of incontinence in elderly women (see later discussion). Diseases of the central nervous system, such as stroke, dementia, and Parkinson's disease, increase in incidence with age. Given the important role of higher centers in the control of micturition, these diseases are frequently involved in urinary dysfunction in the elderly. An associated problem is that as a result of the high prevalence of so many diseases among the elderly, they are also likely to be taking a wide variety of drugs (often several different agents in complex dosage schedules), many of which can affect lower urinary tract function (Table 19–2). Thus, an important component of the assessment of older women with lower urinary tract symptoms is evaluation of the potential role of medications in causing or contributing to their symptoms.

TABLE 19–2
Medications That Can Potentially Affect Continence

Type of Medication	Potential Effects on Continence
Diuretics	Polyuria, frequency, urgency
Anticholinergics	Urinary retention, overflow incontinence, impaction
Psychotropics	
Antidepressants	Anticholinergic actions, sedation
Antipsychotics	Anticholinergic actions, sedation, rigidity, immobility
Sedatives and hypnotics	Sedation, delirium, immobility, muscle relaxation
Narcotic analgesics	Urinary retention, fecal impaction, sedation, delirium
α-Adrenergic blockers	Urethral relaxation
α-Adrenergic agonists	Urinary retention
β-Adrenergic agonists	Urinary retention
Calcium channel blockers	Urinary retention
Alcohol	Polyuria, frequency, urgency, sedation, delirium, immobility

Urinary Tract Infection in Elderly Women

Asymptomatic and symptomatic urinary tract infections are common in the elderly. The prevalence of bacteriuria increases with age; it is more common in elderly women than in men, and in patients in nursing homes and hospitals than in elderly people residing at home. Table 19–3 summarizes several studies of the prevalence of bacteriuria in the elderly.[8–18] Longitudinal studies of bacteriuria among older women have documented that the organisms change over time and that bacteriuria resolves and returns spontaneously in many women.[12, 16–18] Several factors have been implicated in the increased prevalence of bacteriuria in the elderly, including atrophic mucosal changes as a result of estrogen deficiency, increased residual urine, immobility, the prevalence of fecal and urinary incontinence, and the relatively common use of catheters.[19] Symptoms common in elderly women that are usually associated with urinary tract infection, such as frequency, urgency, dysuria, and incontinence, do not reliably predict whether the urine is actually infected.[9, 10, 11, 13] In addition, midstream urine specimens in elderly women are highly unreliable in predicting true bladder infection. Not only do white blood cells on urinalysis correlate poorly with bladder infection,[6, 10] but there is also at least a 17% incidence of false-positive cultures when midstream urine specimens are repeated or compared with suprapubic aspirates.[12, 20] Growth of between 10^3 and 10^5 colonies/ml and contaminated specimens are also more common with midstream specimens. Taking two consecutive midstream specimens increases the reliability substantially. These factors can make the accurate diagnosis of true bladder infection difficult in elderly women.

Asymptomatic bacteriuria is generally considered a benign condition in the elderly who are free of catheters. Studies have, however, shown a substantial incidence of potentially correctable lower urinary tract disease that can contribute to bacteriuria in asymptomatic elderly patients.[14] One study found that bacteriuric elderly nursing home residents had a 30 to 50% lower survival (deaths being from a variety of causes) when followed for 10 years compared with nonbacteriuric residents matched for age, blood pressure, smoking habits, hematocrit, and blood cholesterol.[21] A second study of community-dwelling elderly also showed an association between bacteriuria and mortality,[22] but a cause-and-effect relationship has not been documented. Two studies of treated asymptomatic bacteriuria in older institutionalized[23] and ambulatory[24] women have not documented substantial effects on mortality. Thus, most experts do not recommend treating asymptomatic bacteriuria in older women.

Symptomatic infections in elderly women should be treated with an antimicrobial that achieves a high concentration in the urine, such as ampicillin, a tetracycline, a sulfonamide, a cephalosporin, nitrofurantoin, or a quinoline. Antimicrobial selection should be based on such factors as allergy, renal function, cost, and bacterial sensitivities (especially when infections are recurrent). Although age-related changes do occur in the kidney's ability to eliminate these drugs, dosage adjustments are generally not necessary unless the serum creatinine is above 2. Courses of treatment of 1 to 3 days may cure lower tract infections in younger women, but 10- to 14-day courses are recommended for older women because of the high failure rate reported with short courses of therapy. Compliance with drug regimens may be a problem in many elderly patients and should be kept in mind as a potential cause of treatment failure. Recurrent infections in elderly women are usually due to reinfection with a different organism. Relapse to the same organism should prompt a search for a structural abnormality in the lower urinary tract. When relapse occurs in the absence of a structural abnormality, a 3- to 6-week course of drug therapy should be given. Infrequent symptomatic reinfections should be treated as separate episodes; frequent symptomatic infections can be managed by long-term prophylaxis. Nitrofurantoin (100 mg/day) and trimethoprim-sulfamethoxazole (one single-strength tablet/day) have been shown to prevent recurrent symptomatic infections[25] and appear to be cost-effec-

TABLE 19–3
Prevalence of Bacteriuria in Elderly Women

Location	Percentage
Community	11–17
Nursing home	23–27
Hospital	32–50

tive, especially in women who have three or more symptomatic infections per year.[26]

Urinary Incontinence in Elderly Women

SCOPE OF THE PROBLEM

Incontinence is a common, disruptive, and potentially disabling condition in the elderly. The prevalence of urinary incontinence is illustrated in Table 19–4. Incontinence is a heterogeneous condition among older women, ranging in severity from occasional episodes of dribbling small amounts of urine to continuous urinary incontinence with concomitant fecal incontinence. Not all incontinent elderly women are severely demented, bedridden, and in nursing homes. Many, both in institutions and in the community, are ambulatory and have good mental function. Physical health, psychological well-being, social status, and the costs of health care can all be adversely affected by incontinence. Physical consequences can include skin breakdown, urinary tract infection, and even fractures, which may result if patients fall when they are forced to get up in the middle of the night to urinate. The psychosocial effects can be even more devastating; many elderly patients may suffer intense embarrassment, loss of self-esteem, feelings of helplessness, depression, and anxiety, resulting in a withdrawal from vital social contacts or, at the very least, a reluctance to go places or engage in activities that are not in close proximity to toilet facilities.[30] The financial impact of incontinence is also significant; it has been estimated that the cost of managing incontinence in elderly nursing home residents alone is close to $3 billion per year.[31] Urinary incontinence is curable in many elderly patients, especially those who have adequate mobility and mental function. Even when not curable, incontinence can always be managed in a manner that will keep patients comfortable, make life easier for caregivers, and minimize the cost of caring for the condition and its complications.

TABLE 19–4
Prevalence of Urinary Incontinence Among Older Women

Setting	Percentage
Community	Approximately 33%: any incontinence[a] 4–6%: severe incontinence[b]
Acute care hospital	Approximately 40%
Nursing home	50–70%

[a]Positive response to questioning about any uncontrolled urine loss in past year.
[b]Incontinence that occurs more than once a week or requires the use of pads.

ACUTE (REVERSIBLE) VERSUS PERSISTENT INCONTINENCE

The distinction between acute, reversible forms of incontinence and persistent incontinence is clinically important in older women because incontinence is often caused or contributed to by factors outside the lower urinary tract in this population. Acute incontinence refers to situations in which the incontinence is of sudden onset, usually related to an acute illness or an iatrogenic problem, and subsides once the illness or medication problem has been resolved. Persistent incontinence refers to incontinence that is unrelated to an acute illness and persists over time. The causes of acute and reversible forms of urinary incontinence can be remembered by the acronym DRIP (Table 19–5). It is important to recognize that many of the reversible factors listed in this table can also play a role in patients with persistent forms of incontinence. Thus, a search for these factors should be undertaken in all incontinent geriatric patients.

Persistent forms of incontinence can be classified clinically into four basic types in the geriatric population: stress, urge, overflow, and functional. These types can overlap each other, and an individual patient may have more than one type simultaneously. Although this classification does not include all of the neurophysiologic abnormalities associated with incontinence (such as reflex or "unconscious" incontinence), it is helpful in approaching the clinical assessment and treatment of incontinence in the elderly.[32]

Stress incontinence is the most common type among women younger than age 75, especially in ambulatory clinic settings.[33–35] It may be infrequent and involve very small amounts of urine and may need no specific treatment in women who are not bothered by it. On the other hand, it may be so severe or bothersome that it requires surgical correction. It is most often associated with weakened supporting tissues and consequent hypermobility of the bladder outlet and urethra caused by lack of estrogen or previous vaginal deliveries or surgery. Obesity and chronic coughing can also contribute. Many older women also develop stress incontinence owing to intrinsic urethral dysfunction after one or more lower urinary tract surgical procedures.

Urge incontinence is the most common symptomatic and urodynamic type of incontinence in women older than age 75, especially those in institutions.[36–38] Urge incontinence can be caused by a variety of lower genitourinary and neurologic disorders. It is most often, but not always, associated with detrusor motor instability or detrusor hyperreflexia. Some patients have a poorly compliant bladder without involuntary contractions (e.g., due to radiation or interstitial cystitis, both of which are unusual conditions in older women). Other patients have symptoms of urge incontinence but do not exhibit detrusor motor instability on urodynamic testing. This is generally termed sensory instability or hypersensitive bladder; it is likely that some of these patients do have detrusor

TABLE 19–5
Reversible Factors That May Contribute to Urinary Incontinence ("DRIP")

Acronym	Definition	Description
D	Delirium	New-onset urinary incontinence (UI) may be associated with delirium because of acute underlying conditions requiring diagnosis and treatment
R	Restricted mobility	Acute conditions causing immobility may precipitate UI; environmental manipulation and scheduled toileting are appropriate unitl condition resolves
	Retention	Urinary retention may be precipitated by many drugs (see Table 19–2) or may occur acutely because of anatomic obstruction; immobility and large fecal impactions may also contribute
I	Infection	Acute cystitis may precipitate urge UI
		Otherwise asymptomatic bacteriuria may contribute to urinary frequency and should be eradicated before any urodynamic evaluations are carried out
	Inflammation	Atrophic vaginitis and urethritis can cause irritative voiding symptoms including UI
	Impaction	Fecal impaction as well as fecal incontinence may be associated with UI
P	Polyuria	Poorly controlled diabetes with glucosuria can contribute to urinary frequency and UI
		Edema due to congestive heart failure or venous insufficiency can cause nocturia and exacerbate nocturnal UI
	Pharmaceuticals	See Table 19–2

motor instabiity in everyday life that is not documented at the time of the urodynamic study. On the other hand, some patients with neurologic disorders do have detrusor hyperreflexia on urodynamic testing but may not have urgency and are incontinent without any warning symptoms ("unconscious incontinence"). These patients are generally treated as if they have urge incontinence if they can empty the bladder and do not have other correctable genitourinary pathology (see later). Recently, a subgroup of very elderly incontinent patients with detrusor hyperreflexia has been described who also have impaired bladder contractility; they empty less than a third of the bladder volume with involuntary contractions on urodynamic testing.[37, 39] The implications of this urodynamic finding for the pathophysiology and treatment of incontinence in the elderly are unclear and are currently under investigation.

Urinary retention with overflow incontinence is relatively unusual among older women and can result from anatomic or neurogenic outflow obstruction, a hypotonic or acontractile bladder, or both (Table 19–6). Several types of drugs can also contribute to this type of incontinence (see Table 19–2).

Stress, urge, and overflow incontinence can occur in combination. About one-third of older women with stress incontinence also have symptoms of urge incontinence and detrusor instability. Similarly, about one-third of women with urge incontinence also have symptoms or signs of stress incontinence.[33–35, 40] These mixed types of incontinence can have important therapeutic implications, especially in decisions about surgery for stress incontinence.

Functional incontinence results when an elderly person is unable or unwilling to reach a toilet on time. Distinguishing this type of incontinence from other types of persistent incontinence is critical to appropriate management. Factors that cause func-

tional incontinence (such as inaccessible toilets and psychological disorders) can also exacerbate other types of persistent incontinence. Patients with incontinence that appears to be predominantly related to functional factors may also have abnormalities of the lower genitourinary tract such as detrusor hyperreflexia. In some patients it can be very difficult to determine whether the functional factors or the genitourinary factors predominate without a trial of specific types of treatment. It is therefore appropriate to consider functional incontinence as a diagnosis of exclusion among older patients. Thus, cognitive impairment or impaired mobility should not preclude

TABLE 19–6
Causes of Urinary Retention in Elderly Women

A. Bladder outlet obstruction
  1. Mechanical compression
    Gynecologic malignancy
    Uterine fibroids
    Ovarian cyst
    Fecal impaction
  2. Fibrosis of bladder outlet (uncommon) secondary to chronic inflammation
B. Urethral obstruction
  1. Stricture
  2. Prolapse and urethral distortion
C. Hypotonic bladder
  1. Peripheral neuropathy
    Diabetes
    Alcoholism
  2. Mechanical interruption of motor innervation
    Tumor
    Herniated disc
    Trauma
  3. Overdistention injuries
D. Detrusor-sphincter dyssynergy
E. Drug-induced retention (see Table 19–2)

a trial of specific treatment for incontinence when indicated.

EVALUATION

In patients with a sudden onset of incontinence (especially one associated with an acute medical condition and hospitalization), the possible causes (see Table 19–5) can be determined by a brief history, physical examination, and basic laboratory studies (urinalysis, culture, serum glucose or calcium).

Table 19–7 lists the basic components of the evaluation of persistent urinary incontinence. All patients should have a focused history, targeted physical examination, urinalysis, and a determination of postvoid residual. The history should focus on the characteristics of the incontinence, current medical problems and medications, and the impact of incontinence on the patient and caregivers. Bladder records or voiding diaries are often helpful. Physical examination should focus on abdominal, rectal, and genital examinations and on evaluation of lumbosacral innervation. During the history and physical examination, special attention should be paid to factors such as mobility, mental status, medications, and accesibility of toilets that may be either causing incontinence or interacting with urologic and neurologic disorders to make the condition worse. A clean urine sample should be collected for urinalysis to exclude glucosuria, pyuria, bacteriuria, and hematuria. Persistent sterile microscopic hematuria (>5 red blood cells/high-power field) is an indication for further evaluation to exclude a tumor or other urinary tract abnormality.

TABLE 19–7
Components of the Diagnostic Evaluation of Urinary Incontinence in Older Women

All Patients
Focused history
Targeted physical examination
Urinalysis
Postvoid residual determination

Selected Patients
Simple urodynamic test
Complex urodynamic tests
    Dual-channel cystometrogram
    Pressure-flow study
    Urethral pressure profilometry
    Sphincter electromyography
    Videourodynamic evaluation
Laboratory studies
    Urine culture
    Renal function tests
    Blood glucose
    Serum calcium
    Urine cytology
Radiologic studies
    Renal ultrasound
    Voiding cystourethrography
Urologic or gynecologic evaluation
    Cystourethroscopy

A series of simple tests of lower urinary tract function can be carried out in a clinic, hospital, nursing home, or even at home. They include observation of voiding, a pad test for stress incontinence, and simple cystometry.[41] These simple tests are not necessary in all patients (see later discussion). Like other diagnostic tests, they should be performed only if the results will change the patient's management. When they are performed, they must be carried out and interpreted carefully in light of other information from the history and physical examination. Bladder capacity and stability as determined by simple cystometry have been shown to be highly correlated with results of formal multichannel cystometrograms.[42] Simple cystometry may be unnecessary to make a reasonable treatment plan in many elderly patients, such as those who have sterile urine and no atrophic vaginitis, meet none of the criteria given in Table 19–8, and (1) reliably give a history of stress incontinence without irritative or obstructive voiding symptoms, leak with stress maneuvers, and can empty the bladder completely (they can be treated for stress-type incontinence), or (2) reliably give a history of urge incontinence without symptoms of stress incontinence or voiding difficulty and can empty the bladder completely (they can be treated for urge-type incontinence). These simple tests are also not essential for patients who are going to be treated initially with behavioral therapy alone, which can be used for stress, urge, mixed, and functional incontinence. The criteria for referral for further evaluation given in Table 19–8 have been shown to be reasonably sensitive but not very specific for identifying patients who require further evaluation for appropriate treatment.[36]

MANAGEMENT

Several therapeutic modalities are used in managing incontinent older women. Special attention should be paid to the management of acute forms of incontinence, which are most common in elderly patients in acute care hospitals. These forms of incontinence are often transient if managed appropriately; on the other hand, inappropriate management may lead to a permanent problem. The most common treatment for incontinent elderly patients in acute care hospitals is indwelling catheterization. In some instances this therapy is justified by the necessity for accurate measurement of urine output during the acute phase of an illness. In many instances, however, it is unnecessary and poses a substantial and unwarranted risk of catheter-induced infection. Although it may be more difficult and time-consuming for caregivers, making toilets and toilet substitutes accessible combined with some form of scheduled toileting is probably a more appropriate approach to the treatment of patients who do not require indwelling catheters. Newer launderable or disposable and highly absorbent bed pads and undergarments may also be helpful in managing these patients. These products may

TABLE 19–8
Criteria for Referral of Elderly Incontinent Women for Urologic, Gynecologic, or Urodynamic Evaluation

Criteria	Definition	Rationale
History		
1. Recent history of lower urinary tract or pelvic surgery or irradiation	Surgery or irradiation involving the pelvic area or lower urinary tract within the past 6 months	A structural abnormality relating to the recent procedure should be sought
2. Relapse or rapid recurrence of a symptomatic urinary tract infection	Onset of dysuria, new or worse irritative voiding symptoms, fever, suprapubic or flank pain associated with growth of $>10^5$ colony-forming units of a urinary pathogen; symptoms and bacteriuria that return within 4 weeks of treatment	A structural abnormality or pathologic condition in the urinary tract predisposing to infection should be excluded
Physical Examination		
1. Marked pelvic prolapse[a]	Pronounced uterine descent to or through the introitus, or a prominent cystocele that descends the entire height of the vaginal vault with coughing during speculum examination	Anatomic abnormality may underlie the pathophysiology of the incontinence and may require surgical repair
2. Severe stress incontinence[a]	Prominent, bothersome stress incontinence that has failed to respond to adequate trials of nonsurgical therapy	Bladder neck suspension procedures are generally well tolerated and successful in properly selected elderly women who have stress incontinence that responds poorly to more conservative measures
3. Severe hesitancy, straining, or interrupted urinary stream	Straining to begin voiding and a dribbling or intermittent stream when the patient's bladder feels full	Signs suggest obstruction or poor bladder contractility
Postvoid Residual		
1. Difficulty in passing a 14 Fr straight catheter	Catheter passage is impossible or requires considerable force or a larger and more rigid catheter	Anatomic blockage of the urethra or bladder neck may be present
2. Postvoid residual volume >200 ml[b]	Volume of urine remaining in the bladder within 5 to 10 minutes after the patient voids spontaneously in as normal a fashion as possible	Anatomic or neurogenic obstruction or poor bladder contractility may be present
Urinalysis		
1. Hematuria (sterile)	Greater than 5 red blood cells/high-power field on microscopic examination in the absence of infection	A pathologic condition in the urinary tract should be excluded
Uncertain Diagnosis	After the history, physical examination, simple tests of lower urinary tract function, and urinalysis, none of the other referral criteria are met, and the results are not consistent with predominantly functional, urge, or stress incontinence	A formal urodynamic evaluation may help to better define and reproduce the symptoms associated with the patient's incontinence and target treatment

[a]If medical conditions preclude surgery, or if the patient is adamantly opposed to considering surgical intervention, the patient should not be referred.
[b]Some patients with lesser degrees of urinary retention may also require evaluation depending on other findings.

be more costly than catheters but probably result in less morbidity (and therefore a lower overall cost) in the long run. Specially designed incontinence undergarments and pads can be very helpful in many nonhospitalized patients but must be used appropriately. They are now being marketed on television and are readily available in retail stores. Although they can be effective, several caveats should be mentioned: (1) garments and pads are a nonspecific treatment. They should not be used as a first response to incontinence or before some type of diagnostic evaluation is done; (2) many patients are curable if treated with specific therapies, and some have potentially serious factors underlying their incontinence that must be diag-

nosed and treated; and (3) pants and pads can interfere with attempts at certain types of behaviorally oriented therapies (see later discussion).

Supportive measures are critical in managing all forms of incontinence and should be used in conjunction with other more specific treatment modalities. A positive attitude, education, environmental manipulations, appropriate use of toilet substitutes, avoidance of iatrogenic contributions to incontinence, modifications of diuretic and fluid intake patterns, and good skin care are all important.

To a large extent the optimal treatment of persistent incontinence depends on identifying the types of incontinence that exists. Table 19–9 outlines the

TABLE 19–9
Primary Treatments for Different Types of Urinary Incontinence in Elderly Women

Type of Incontinence	Primary Treatment
Stress	Pelvic muscle (Kegel) exercises
	α-Adrenergic agonists
	Estrogen
	Biofeedback, bladder training
	Surgical intervention
Urge	Bladder relaxants
	Estrogen (if vaginal atrophy is present)
	Behavioral intervention (e.g., bladder training, biofeedback)
	Surgical removal of pathologic lesions
Overflow	Surgical removal of obstruction
	Intermittent catheterization (if practical)
	Indwelling catheterization
Functional	Behavioral therapies (e.g., prompted voiding, habit training)
	Environmental manipulations
	Incontinence undergarments and pads
	External collection devices
	Bladder relaxants (selected patients)[a]
	Indwelling catheters (selected patients)[b]

[a]Many patients with functional incontinence also have detrusor hyperreflexia, and some may benefit from bladder relaxant drug therapy (see text).
[b]See Table 19–11.

primary treatments used for the basic types of persistent incontinence found among older incontinent women. Each treatment modality is briefly discussed in the following sections.

DRUG TREATMENT

The efficacy of drug treatment has not been as well studied in the elderly as in younger populations,[42, 43] but for many patients, especially those with urge or stress incontinence, drug treatment may be very effective. Drug treatment can be prescribed in conjunction with one or more of the behavioral interventions discussed in the following section. There are no data on the relative efficacy of drug versus behavioral versus combination treatment in the elderly. Thus, until the results of controlled trials are available, treatment decisions should be made on an individual basis and depend in a large part on the characteristics and preferences of the patient and the physician.

For urge incontinence, drugs with anticholinergic and bladder smooth muscle–relaxing properties are used. All of them may cause bothersome systemic anticholinergic side effects in the elderly, especially dry mouth, and they can precipitate urinary retention in some patients. Patients with Alzheimer's disease must be followed for the development of drug-induced delirium, which is unusual. Oxybutynin, starting at half the usual recommended dose (i.e., 2.5 mg three times per day), may offer some advantage over other drugs with more pronounced systemic an-

ticholinergic side effects,[44] and it does not have the potentially serious effects on blood pressure and cardiac conduction characteristic of imipramine. Calcium channel blockers have been used for urge incontinence in Europe but have not yet been approved for this indication in the United States. Several studies suggest that cognitive and physical functional impairments are associated with poor responses to bladder relaxant drug therapy.[45–47] The results of these studies should not, however, preclude a treatment trial in this patient population. Some patients may respond, especially in conjunction with scheduled toileting or prompted voiding (see next section). The goal of treatment in these patients may not be to cure the incontinence but to reduce its severity and prevent discomfort and complications.

For stress incontinence, drug treatment involves a combination of an alpha-adrenergic agonist and estrogen. Drug treatment is appropriate for motivated patients who (1) have mild to moderate degrees of stress incontinence, (2) do not have a major anatomic abnormality (e.g., large cystocele), and (3) do not have any contraindications to these drugs. These patients may also respond to behavioral treatments (see next section), and some data suggest that the two treatment modalities are roughly equivalent, with about three-quarters of patients reporting improvement.[48] A combination of these modalities would also be a reasonable approach for some patients. Estrogen alone is not as effective as it is in combination with an alpha agonist for stress incontinence. If either oral or vaginal estrogen is used for a prolonged period of time (more than a few months), cyclic administration and the addition of a progestational agent should be considered. Estrogen is also used, either chronically or intermittently (i.e., 1- to 2-month courses), for the treatment of irritative voiding symptoms and urge incontinence in women with atrophic vaginitis and urethritis.

Drug treatment for chronic overflow incontinence using a cholinergic agonist or an alpha-adrenergic antagonist is usually not effective. Bethanechol may be helpful when given for a brief period subcutaneously in patients with persistent bladder contractility problems after an overdistention injury but is generally not effective when given orally over the long term.[49]

Symptomatically and urodynamically, many elderly women have a combination of both urge and stress incontinence. A combination of estrogen and imipramine would, at least in theory, be appropriate for these patients because imipramine has both anticholinergic and alpha-adrenergic effects. If urge incontinence is the predominant symptom, a combination of estrogen and oxybutynin would be appropriate. Behavioral interventions are also a reasonable approach to women with mixed incontinence (see following section).

BEHAVIORAL INTERVENTIONS

Many types of behavioral procedures have been described for the management of urinary incontinence.[50, 51] The nosology of these procedures has been somewhat confusing, and in much of the literature the term bladder training is used to encompass a wide variety of techniques. It is important to distinguish between procedures that are patient-dependent (i.e., require adequate function and motivation of the patient), in which the goal is to restore a normal pattern of voiding and continence, and procedures that are caregiver-dependent and can be used for functionally disabled patients, in which the goal is to keep the patient and environment dry (Table 19–10).

Pelvic muscle (Kegel) exercises consist of repetitive contractions of the pelvic floor muscles. This procedure is taught by having the patient interrupt voiding to get a sense of the muscles used or by asking the patient to squeeze the examiner's fingers during a vaginal examination (without doing a Valsalva maneuver, which is the opposite of the intended effect). One exercise consists of a several-second squeeze and a several-second relaxation. Once learned, the exercises should be practiced many times throughout the day (up to 40 exercises per day) and, importantly, should be used in everyday life during situations (e.g., coughing, running water) that might precipitate incontinence. Pelvic muscle exercises may be taught in conjunction with biofeedback procedures and can be especially helpful for women who bear down (increasing intra-abdominal pressure) when they attempt to contract the pelvic floor muscles. Vaginal cones (weights) are also useful adjuncts to pelvic muscle exercises in some patients.

Biofeedback procedures involve the use of bladder, rectal, or vaginal pressure or electrical activity recordings to train patients to contract the pelvic floor muscles and relax the bladder. Studies have shown that these techniques can be very effective for managing both stress and urge incontinence, even in the elderly.[52] The use of biofeedback techniques may be limited by requirements for equipment and trained personnel; in addition, some of these techniques are relatively invasive and require the use of bladder or rectal catheters, or both. Some newer biofeedback techniques use surface electrodes and are less invasive. Electrical stimulation, either vaginally or rectally, has also been used in the management of both stress and urge incontinence. Electrical stimulation techniques are not acceptable to many patients and

TABLE 19–10
Examples of Behavioral Interventions for Urinary Incontinence Among Elderly Women

Procedure	Definition	Types of Incontinence	Comments
Patient-Dependent			
Pelvic muscle (Kegel) exercises	Repetitive contraction of pelvic floor muscles	Stress	Requires adequate function and motivation
Biofeedback	Use of bladder, rectal, or vaginal pressure recordings to train patients to contract pelvic floor muscles and relax bladder	Stress and urge	Requires equipment and trained personnel
Bladder training	Use of educational components of biofeedback, bladder records, pelvic muscle, and other behavioral exercises	Stress and urge	Requires trained therapist, adequate cognitive and physical functioning, and patient motivation
Bladder retraining	Progressive lengthening or shortening of intervoiding interval, with adjunctive techniques[a] Intermittent catheterization used in patients recovering from overdistention injuries with persistent retention	Acute (e.g., postcatheterization, with urge or overflow, poststroke)	Goal is to restore normal pattern of voiding and continence; requires adequate cognitive and physical function and patient motivation
Caregiver-Dependent[a]			
Scheduled toileting	Fixed toileting schedule	Urge and functional	Goal is to prevent wetting episodes
Prompted voiding	Regular opportunities to toilet with behavioral reinforcement		Can be used in patients with impaired cognitive or physical functioning
Habit training	Toileting based on established individual pattern with behavioral reinforcement		Requires staff or caregiver availability and patient motivation

[a]Techniques to trigger voiding (running water, stroking thigh, suprapubic tapping), completely empty bladder (bending forward, suprapubic pressure), and alterations of fluid or diuretic intake patterns may be helpful in some patients.

have been not well studied or used to any great degree in the elderly in this country.

Other forms of patient-dependent training procedures include various forms of bladder training and bladder retraining. Bladder training procedures generally involve the educational components taught during biofeedback but not the use of biofeedback equipment. Patients are taught how to do pelvic muscle exercises, strategies for managing urgency, and to regularly use bladder records. These techniques are highly effective in selected community-dwelling patients, especially women.[53]

The goal of caregiver-dependent behavioral interventions such as prompted voiding and habit training is to prevent incontinence episodes rather than restore the normal pattern of voiding and complete continence. Such procedures have been shown to be effective in reducing incontinence in selected nursing home residents. In its simplest form, scheduled toileting involves toileting the patient at regular intervals, usually every 2 hours during the day and every 4 hours during the evening and night. Habit training involves a schedule of toiletings or prompted voidings that is modified according to the patient's pattern of continent voids and incontinence episodes as demonstrated by a monitoring record. Positive reinforcement is offered for continent voids, and neutral reinforcement when incontinence occurs. Adjunctive techniques to prompt voiding (e.g., running tap water, stroking the inner thigh, or suprapubic tapping) and to help empty the bladder completely (e.g., bending forward after completion of voiding) may be helpful in some patients. Prompted voiding has been the best studied of these procedures. It is a simple behavioral procedure that combines several of the elements mentioned earlier.[57] The success of these procedures is largely dependent on the knowledge and motivation of the caregivers implementing them, rather than on the physical functional and mental status of the incontinent patient. These techniques are not feasible in home settings without available caregivers. For these types of procedures to be feasible and cost-effective in the nursing home setting, the amount of time generally spent by the nursing staff in changing patients after incontinence episodes should not be exceeded by the time and effort needed to implement such training procedures. Targeting these procedures to selected patients, such as those with less frequent voiding and larger bladder capacities or voided volumes may enhance their cost-effectiveness.[57] Quality assurance methods, based on principles of statistical quality control used in industry, have been shown to be helpful in maintaining the effectiveness of prompted voiding in nursing homes.[58]

SURGERY

Surgical interventions are described in detail in other chapters in this text. Surgery should be considered for elderly women with stress incontinence that continues to be bothersome after attempts at nonsurgi-cal treatment have been made and in women with a significant degree of pelvic prolapse or intrinsic urethral dysfunction. As with many other surgical procedures, patient selection and the experience of the surgeon are critical to success. All women being considered for surgical therapy should have a thorough evaluation, including urodynamic tests, before undergoing the procedure. Women with mixed stress incontinence and detrusor motor instability may also benefit from surgery, especially if the clinical history and urodynamic findings suggest that stress incontinence is the predominant problem. New modified techniques of bladder neck suspension can be done with minimal risk and are highly successful in achieving continence, even in the elderly. Urinary retention can occur after surgery, but it is usually transient and can be managed by intermittent catheterization. Periurethral injection of collagen and other materials should be available in the near future and may offer some patients an alternative to major surgery.

CATHETERS AND CATHETER CARE

Three basic types of catheters and catheterization procedures are used for the management of urinary incontinence: external catheters, intermittent straight catheterization, and chronic indwelling catheterization. An external catheter for use in women is now commercially available, but its safety and effectiveness have not been well documented in the elderly. Intermittent catheterization can help in the management of patients with urinary retention and overflow incontinence. The procedure can be carried out by either the patient or a caregiver and involves straight catheterization two to four times daily depending on residual urine volume. In the home the catheter should be kept clean (but not necessarily sterile). Studies conducted largely among younger paraplegics have shown that this technique is practical and reduces the risk of symptomatic infection compared with chronic catheterization. Self-intermittent catheterization has also been shown to be feasible for elderly women outpatients who are functional and are willing and able to catheterize themselves.[59] However, studies carried out in young paraplegics and elderly female outpatients cannot automatically be extrapolated to frail elderly women or the institutionalized population. The technique may be useful in certain patients in acute care hospitals or nursing homes, such as those who have undergone bladder neck suspension, or in certain situations, such as following removal of an indwelling catheter in a bladder retraining protocol. Nursing home residents, however, may be difficult to catheterize, and the anatomic abnormalities commonly found in elderly patients' lower urinary tracts may increase the risk of infection because of repeated straight catheterizations. In addition, use of this technique in an institutional setting (which may have an abundance of organisms that are relatively resistant to many

TABLE 19–11
Indications for and Principles of Chronic Indwelling Catheter Use

A. Indications
  1. Urinary retention that
     a. Is causing persistent overflow incontinence, symptomatic infections, or renal dysfunction
     b. Cannot be corrected surgically or medically
     c. Cannot be managed practically with intermittent catheterization
  2. Skin wounds, pressure sores, or irritations that are being contaminated by incontinent urine
  3. Care of terminally ill or severely impaired patients for whom bed and clothing changes are uncomfortable or disruptive
  4. Preference of patient or caregiver when patient has failed to respond to more specific treatments
B. Catheter care
  1. Maintain sterile, closed, gravity drainage system; change catheter every 4 to 8 weeks
  2. Avoid breaking the closed system
  3. Use clean techniques in emptying and changing the drainage system; wash hands between patients in institutionalized setting
  4. Secure the catheter to the upper thigh or lower abdomen to avoid perineal contamination and urethral irritation due to movement of the catheter
  5. Avoid frequent and vigorous cleaning of the catheter entry site; washing with soapy water once per day is sufficient
  6. Do not irrigate routinely
  7. If bypassing occurs in the absence of obstruction, consider the possibility of a bladder spasm, which can be treated with a bladder relaxant
  8. If catheter obstruction occurs frequently, increase the patient's fluid intake and acidify the urine if possible
  9. Do not routinely use prophylactic or suppressive urinary antiseptics or antimicrobials
  10. Do not perform routine surveillance cultures to guide management of individual patients because all chronically catheterized patients have bacteriuria (which is often polymicrobial), and the organisms change frequently
  11. Do not treat infection unless the patient develops symptoms; symptoms may be nonspecific, and other possible sources of infection should be carefully excluded before attributing symptoms to the urinary tract
  12. If a patient develops frequent symptomatic urinary tract infections, a genitourinary evaluation should be considered to rule out pathology such as stones, periurethral or prostatic abscesses, or chronic pyelonephritis

commonly used antimicrobial agents) may yield an unacceptable risk of nosocomial infections, and the use of sterile catheter trays for these procedures would be very expensive; thus, it may be extremely difficult to implement such a program in a typical nursing home setting.

Chronic indwelling catheterization is overused in some settings, and when used for periods of up to 10 years it has been shown to increase the incidence of a number of other complications, including chronic bacteriuria, bladder stones, periurethral abscesses, and even bladder cancer. Elderly female nursing home residents managed by this technique are at relatively high risk of developing symptomatic infections.[60] Given these risks, it seems appropriate to recommend limiting the use of chronic indwelling catheters to certain specific situations and to follow sound principles of catheter care when using indwelling catheterization to attempt to minimize complications (Table 19–11).

REFERENCES

1. Brocklehurst JC, Dillane JB: Studies of the female bladder in old age I. Cystometrograms in non-incontinent women. Geront Clin 8:285, 1966A.
2. Jones KW, Schoenberg HW: Comparison of the incidence of bladder hyperreflexia in patients with benign prostatic hypertrophy and age-matched female controls. J Urol 133:425, 1985.
3. Diokno AC, Brown MB, Brock BM, et al: Clinical and cystometric characteristics of continent and incontinent non-institutionalized elderly. J Urol 140:567, 1988.
4. Edwards L, Malvern J: The urethral pressure profile: Theoretic considerations and clinical application. Br J Urol 46:325, 1974.
5. Henriksson L, Anderson KL, Ulmsten U: The urethral pressure profiles of continent and stress incontinent women. Scand J Urol Nephrol 13:5, 1979.
6. Brocklehurst JC: The bladder. In Brocklehurst J (ed): Textbook of Geriatric Medicine and Gerontology. New York, Churchill Livingstone, 1992, pp 629–646.
7. McGuire EJ: Urinary dysfunction in the aged: Neurological considerations. Bull NY Acad Med 56:275, 1980.
8. Romano JM, Kaye D: UTI in the elderly: Common yet atypical. Geriatrics 36:113, 1981.
9. Akhtar AJ, Andrews GR, Cairo FI, et al: Urinary tract infection in the elderly: A population study. Age Ageing 1:48, 1972.
10. Brocklehurst JC, Dillane JB, Griffiths L, et al: The prevalence and symptomatology of urinary infection in an aged population. Geront Clin 10:242, 1968.
11. Brocklehurst JC, Fry J, Griffiths LL, Calton G: Dysuria in old age. J Am Geriat Soc 19:582, 1971.
12. Brocklehurst JC, Bee P, Jones D, et al: Bacteriuria in geriatric hospital patients—its correlates and management. Age Ageing 6:240, 1977.
13. Garibaldi RA, Brodine S, Matsumiya S: Infections among patients in nursing homes—policies, prevalence and problems. N Engl J Med 305:731, 1981.
14. Gladstone JL, Friedman SA: Bacteriuria in the aged: A study of its prevalence and predisposing lesions in a chronically ill population. J Urol 106:745, 1971.
15. Jewett MAS, Fernie GR, Holliday PJ, et al: Urinary dysfunction in a geriatric long-term care population: Prevalence and patterns. J Am Geriatr Soc 29:211, 1981.
16. Sourander LB, Kasanen A: A 5-year follow-up of bacteriuria in the aged. Geront Clin 14:274, 1972.
17. Boscia JA, Kobasa WD, Knight RA, et al: Epidemiology of bacteriuria in an elderly ambulatory population. Am J Med 80:208, 1986.
18. Abrutyn E, Mossey J, Levison M, et al: Epidemiology of asymptomatic bacteriuria in elderly women. J Am Geriatr Soc 39:388, 1991.
19. Sobel JD, Kaye D: Host factors in the pathogenesis of urinary tract infections. Am J Med 76(Suppl 5A):122, 1984.
20. Moore-Smith B: Bacteriuria in elderly women (Letter to the editor). Lancet 2:827, 1972.

21. Dontas AS, Kashi-Charvati P, Papanyiotou PC, et al: Bacteriuria and survival in old age. N Engl J Med 304:939, 1981.

22. Nordenstam GR, Brandberg CA, Oden AS, et al: Bacteriuria and mortality in an elderly population. N Engl J Med 314:1152, 1986.

23. Nicolle LE, Mayhew JW, Bryan L: Prospective randomized comparison of therapy and no therapy for asymptomatic bacteriuria in institutionalized elderly women. Am J Med 83:27, 1987.

24. Boscia JA, Kobasa WD, Knight RA, et al: Therapy vs. no therapy for bacteriuria in elderly ambulatory nonhospitalized women. JAMA 257:1067, 1987.

25. Stamey TA, Condy M, Minara G: Prophylactic efficacy of nitrofurantoin macrocrystals and trimethoprim-sulfamethoxazole in urinary infection. N Engl J Med 296:780, 1977.

26. Stamm WE, McKevitt M, Counts GW, et al: Is antimicrobial prophylaxis of urinary tract infections cost effective? Ann Intern Med 94:251, 1981.

27. Herzog AR, Fultz NH: Prevalence and incidence of urinary incontinence in community-dwelling populations. J Am Geriatr Soc 38:273, 1990.

28. Sier H, Ouslander JG, Orzeck S: Urinary incontinence among geriatric patients in an acute-care hospital. JAMA 257:1767, 1987.

29. Ouslander JG, Kane RL, Abrass IB: Urinary incontinence in elderly nursing home patients. JAMA 248:1194, 1982.

30. Ouslander JG, Abelson S: Perceptions of urinary incontinence among elderly outpatients. Gerontologist 30:369, 1990.

31. Hu T-W: Impact of urinary incontinence on health-care costs. J Am Geriatr Soc 38:292, 1990.

32. Ouslander JG: Geriatric urinary incontinence. Dis Mon 2:67, 1992.

33. Ouslander JG, Raz S, Hepps K, Su HL: Genitourinary dysfunction in a geriatric outpatient population. J Am Geriatr Soc 34:507, 1986.

34. Wells TJ, Brink CA, Diokno AC: Urinary incontinence in elderly women: Clinical findings. J Am Geriatr Soc 35:933, 1987.

35. Diokno AC, Wells TJ, Brink CA: Urinary incontinence in elderly women: Urodynamic evaluation. J Am Geriatr Soc 35:940, 1987.

36. Ouslander JG, Leach G, Staskin D, et al: Prospective evaluation of an assessment strategy for geriatric urinary incontinence. J Am Geriatr Soc 37:715, 1989.

37. Resnick NM, Yalla SV, Laurino E: The pathophysiology of urinary incontinence among institutionalized elderly persons. N Engl J Med 320:1, 1989.

38. Pannill FC, Williams TF, Davis R: Evaluation and treatment of urinary incontinence in long term care. J Am Geriatr Soc 36:902, 1988.

39. Resnick NM, Yalla SV: Detrusor hyperactivity with impaired contractile function: An unrecognized but common cause of incontinence in elderly patients. JAMA 257:3076, 1987.

40. Fantl JA, Wyman JF, McClish DK, Bump RC: Urinary incontinence in community-dwelling women: Clinical, urodynamic, and severity characteristics. Am J Obstet Gynecol 162:946, 1990.

41. Ouslander JG, Leach G, Staskin D: Simplified tests of lower urinary tract function in the evaluation of geriatric urinary incontinence. J Am Geriatr Soc 37:706, 1989.

42. Ouslander JG, Sier HC: Drug therapy for geriatric incontinence. Geriatr Clin 2:789, 1986.

43. Agency for Health Care Policy and Research, Urinary Incontinence Guidelines Panel: Urinary Incontinence in Adults: Clinical Practice Guideline. AHCPR Pub. No. 92–0038. Rockville, MD, Agency for Health Care Policy and Research, Public Health Service, U.S. Department of Health and Human Services, 1992.

44. Ouslander JG, Blaustein J, Connor A, et al: Pharmacokinetics and clinical effects of oxybutynin in geriatric patients. J Urol 140:47, 1988.

45. Castleden CM, Duffin HM, Asher MJ, Yeomanson CW: Factors influencing outcome in elderly patients with urinary incontinence and detrusor instability. Age Ageing 14:303, 1985.

46. Zorzitto ML, Jewett MAS, Fernie GR, et al: Effectiveness of propantheline bromide in the treatment of geriatric patients with detrusor instability. Neurol Urodyn 5:133, 1986.

47. Tobin GW, Brocklehurst JC: The management of urinary incontinence in local authority residential homes for the elderly. Age Ageing 15:292, 1986.

48. Wells TJ, Brink CA, Diokno AC, et al: Pelvic muscle exercise for stress urinary incontinence in elderly women. J Am Geriatr Soc 39:785, 1991.

49. Finkbeiner AE: Is bethanechol chloride clinically effective in promoting bladder emptying? A literature review. J Urol 134:443, 1985.

50. Burgio KL, Burgio LD: Behavior therapies for urinary incontinence in the elderly. Geriatr Clin 2:809, 1986.

51. Hadley BJ: Bladder training and related therapies for urinary incontinence in older people. JAMA 256:372, 1986.

52. Burgio KL, Whitehead WE, Engel BT: Urinary incontinence in elderly—Bladder-sphincter biofeedback and toileting skill training. Ann Intern Med 104:507, 1985.

53. Fantl JA, Wyman JF, McClish DK, et al: Efficacy of bladder training in older women with urinary incontinence. JAMA 265:609, 1991.

54. Schnelle JF: Treatment of urinary incontinence in nursing home patients by prompted voiding. J Am Geriatr Soc 38:356, 1990.

55. Hu T-W, Igou JF, Kaltreider DL, et al: A clinical trial of a behavioral therapy to reduce urinary incontinence in nursing homes. JAMA 261:2656, 1989.

56. Colling J, Ouslander JG, Hadley BJ, et al: The effects of patterned urge-response toileting (PURT) on urinary incontinence among nursing home residents. J Am Geriatr Soc 40:135, 1992.

57. Schnelle JF: Managing Urinary Incontinence in the Elderly. New York, Springer-Verlag, 1991.

58. Schnelle JF, Newman D, White W, et al: Maintaining continence in nursing home residents through the application of industrial quality control. Gerontologist 33:114, 1992.

59. Bennett CJ, Diokno AC: Clean, intermittent self-catheterization in the elderly. Urology 24(1):43, 1984.

60. Warren JW, Damron D, Tenney JH, et al: Fever bacteremia and death as complications of bacteriuria in women with long-term urethral catheters. J Infect Dis 155:1151, 1987.

Detrusor Hyperactivity

Stephen D. Mark, M.B., F.R.A.C.S.
George D. Webster, M.B., F.R.C.S.

Detrusor hyperactivity is a common cause of urinary incontinence, especially in the elderly. A profusion of labels have been applied to this condition, and the International Continence Society (ICS) has standardized the nomenclature and has drafted terminology related to lower urinary tract dysfunction.[1] Both *the unstable bladder*, a term first coined by Bates in 1970, and *detrusor hyperreflexia* will be discussed in this chapter. By definition, the unstable bladder occurs in the non-neuropathic patient and has been shown objectively to contract during the filling or storage phase of cystometry while the patient attempts to inhibit micturition. Detrusor hyperreflexia represents a similar urodynamic picture that is seen in patients with clinically relevant neuropathy. Previously, 15 cm H_2O or less of bladder pressure was arbitrarily set as the highest pressure rise that was accepted as being within normal limits; however, more recent classifications state that any rise in bladder pressure associated with a sensation of urgency is considered abnormal.

Patients who have symptoms that suggest bladder hyperactivity but have a normal cystometrogram are classified as having *sensory urgency*. These patients may be divided into two separate groups: (1) those whose desire to void arises primarily from the need to relieve pain, subclassified as the "painful bladder syndrome," incorporating interstitial cystitis and other inflammatory conditions of the bladder, and (2) those whose desire to void arises from the wish to prevent urinary leakage, subclassified as "sensory bladder instability." A careful history should be able to differentiate these two conditions, and the painful bladder syndromes are covered elsewhere in this text (see Chapter 8).

Bladder hyperactivity is common, being found in 10 to 15% of asymptomatic men and women between the ages of 10 and 50 years.[2] There is an increased incidence of detrusor hyperactivity with increasing age. The cause of detrusor instability remains unknown; however, there appear to be three etiologic groups, a congenital group, a group associated with bladder outlet obstruction and stress urinary incontinence, and an age-related group.

Clinically, patients with an unstable bladder may present with a symptom complex of frequency, nocturia, urgency, and urge incontinence, known collectively as the "urge syndrome." After ruling out inflammatory, infective, and malignant conditions, the diagnosis is made based on abnormal provocative cystometric evaluation.

There are many facets of management of the hyperactive bladder, but overall they incorporate a reduction in detrusor activity and regular bladder emptying, especially in the neuropathic patient. Four main categories of management are discussed in this chapter—behavioral, pharmacologic, electrical stimulation, and surgical methods. Management should proceed in a stepwise fashion commencing with conservative reversible therapies. Behavioral modification (bladder drill) and pharmacotherapy succeed in improving symptoms to a tolerable level that interferes minimally with lifestyle in about 80% of cases.[3] Only when these and other conservative measures fail should one resort to surgical management, of which the most effective and commonly performed procedure is the "clam" augmentation enterocystoplasty. Unfortunately, augmentation cystoplasty is not without morbidity, including occasional voiding difficulties that require intermittent catheterization, metabolic repercussions from reabsorption of some urinary constituents, and concern about malignancy in the long term. This procedure should therefore be considered a last resort.

Terminology

To standardize the terminology of lower urinary tract dysfunction, the ICS used urodynamic criteria to classify the hyperactive bladder. Originally the ICS made the following statement about detrusor hyperactivity:

> The presence of contractions exceeding 15 cm of water clearly indicates an uninhibited detrusor contraction, when the patient has been asked to inhibit micturition.

The arbitrary selection of 15 cm H_2O was subsequently removed from the definition. In 1988 the updated definition stated:

> Detrusor contractions are noted during the filling phase, which may be involuntary and provoked and which the patient cannot completely suppress.

These contractions may be provoked during cystometry by rapid filling, changes in posture, coughing, walking, jumping, handwashing, and other triggering procedures. The presence of these contractions does not necessarily imply a neurologic cause.

A profusion of other labels has also been applied to the hyperactive bladder, including uninhibited, irritable, spastic, reflex, overfacilitated, systolic, and hypertonic. These labels should no longer be used and should be replaced by the term detrusor instability when the cause remains unknown and detrusor hyperreflexia when there is objective evidence of a relevant neurologic disorder.

Using this terminology, patients who present with symptoms suggestive of bladder hyperactivity and do not demonstrate involuntary bladder contractions on provocative cystometry would be defined as stable. However, we believe that these patients have sensory detrusor instability. This contention is reinforced by the results of ambulatory urodynamic studies, which show an increased incidence of motor instability when this group of patients is studied under more physiologic conditions and for longer periods of time.[4]

Poor compliance, defined as elevated bladder pressure with an increased filling volume (dv/dp), is separate from detrusor instability and may reflect not only the filling rate of the bladder during cystometry but also the shape and thickness of the bladder wall, mainly the noncontractile elements.

Incidence and Epidemiology

The true incidence of bladder hyperactivity remains unknown. Accurate figures are difficult to obtain because urinary incontinence is underreported owing not only to patient embarrassment but also to medical inattention.

Age does appear to be associated with the incidence of hyperactive bladder. In the very young, bladder hyperactivity is physiologic, and the success of toilet training is probably due to the achievement of volitional control of the detrusor reflex and maturation of the neurologic pathways involved.[5, 6] As stated

before, Turner-Warwick estimates the incidence of bladder hyperactivity to be 10% of the general population, and this figure increases with age. In a unique study of noninstitutionalized elderly people, Diokno and colleagues performed cystometrograms on 169 randomly selected women and found that approximately 8% had detrusor instability.[7] This figure probably represents our best estimate of the overall prevalence of the hyperactive bladder in the community-dwelling elderly, a prevalence that goes up dramatically in the institutionalized elderly.

Considering women who present for evaluation of incontinence as a group, the presence of instability ranges from 9 to 55%.[8] Arnold and coworkers found that detrusor instability was a contributing factor to incontinence in 73 of 133 female patients referred for evaluation, a figure similar to those in others' reports.[9, 10] Among incontinent women, Sand and colleagues found that 38% had mixed instability and stress incontinence and 16.5% had detrusor instability alone as the cause of the incontinence.[11] As stated before, although genuine stress incontinence is probably the most common cause of urinary incontinence in women, the incidence and prevalence of detrusor hyperactivity increase with age.[12] In women with recurrent urinary incontinence following a failed repair, the incidence of instability is far higher, 76% as reported by Arnold and colleagues.[9]

Detrusor hyperactivity is also associated with bladder outlet obstruction, most commonly due to prostatic obstruction in men; it is rare in women. In men presenting with symptoms suggestive of bladder outlet obstruction, as many as 50 to 80% have detrusor instability, which disappears after successful treatment in approximately 60%.[13, 14] In women, bladder outlet obstruction may result from cystourethropexy, and such patients generally develop de novo symptoms of detrusor hyperactivity.[15] Following surgical revision, most patients experience relief from their symptoms.

Etiology and Pathophysiology

The neurologic regulation of the lower urinary tract is complex and is still being elucidated. It is apparent, however, that an intact neurologic axis from the cerebral cortex through the brain stem and spinal cord to the sacral micturition center and peripheral nerves innervating the bladder is crucial for normal bladder function of storage and complete elimination of urine. Disease at any level of this complex neurologic network can adversely affect bladder function. In patients with detrusor instability spinal infiltration with local anesthetic, which blocks the micturition reflex, abolishes detrusor instability, and therefore detrusor instability represents a hyperexcitable micturition reflex. A variety of diverse factors have been implicated in the etiology of detrusor hyperactivity as outlined in Table 20–1.

TABLE 20–1
Suggested Etiologic Factors in the Hyperactive Bladder

Neurologic disease
Bladder instability
  Congenital factors
  Bladder outlet obstruction
  Urethral instability
  Psychosomatic factors
  Aging

NEUROLOGIC DISEASE

Control of the bladder and sphincter depends on an intact cerebral cortex and peripheral nervous system. Bradley and coworkers, among others, explored the neuroanatomic basis of micturition control and identified the function of four distinct neuroanatomic circuits, the integration of which provides coordination of detrusor and sphincter activity during bladder storage and elimination.[16] Loops I and II are concerned with detrusor control, whereas loops III and IV dictate sphincter function and its coordination with the detrusor. Loop I includes connections from the frontal cortex to the micturition center in the pontine mesencephalic reticular formation, with added contributions from the thalamic nuclei, basal ganglia, and cerebellum. Loop II includes efferent axons from this center that travel down the spinal cord in the reticulospinal tract to the detrusor motor nucleus (Onuf's nucleus) in the sacral spinal cord.

A wide variety of neurologic diseases may interfere with these pathways, contributing to detrusor hyperreflexia. Pathologic events above the pontine center such as cerebrovascular accidents (CVA), ischemia, brain tumor, head injury, multiple sclerosis, or Parkinson's disease may cause disruptions of loop I. These result in a coordinated hyperreflexic detrusor contraction. Spinal cord trauma is the most frequent cause of interruption of the loop II fibers in the reticulospinal tract. The completeness and level of the lesion determine the severity of detrusor hyperreflexia and whether or not bladder contractions are coordinated with sphincter relaxation.

Whether or not the hyperreflexic contractions result in urgency or urge incontinence depends on the intactness of the sensory pathway and also on whether volitional control of the external striated sphincter remains intact. If sensory pathways are intact, as they generally are in loop I lesions, the patient will recognize the uninhibited contraction as a sudden urge to void and may be able to prevent incontinence by voluntary contraction of the external sphincter. With more extensive neurologic lesions in which the sensory pathways are also involved, recognition of hyperreflexic contractions will not occur, and reflex urinary incontinence will develop. Lesions below loop II will cause an areflexic bladder that is generally unable to empty. It is beyond the scope of this text to discuss the various ramifications of further neurologic bladder dysfunction. The interested reader is referred to more specific literature on this subject.[17]

CAUSES OF DETRUSOR INSTABILITY

In patients without neurologic disease, the origins of detrusor instability remain unclear. Undoubtedly idiopathic detrusor instability represents a complex web of many contributing causes, including those discussed in the following sections.

Congenital Causes

As previously noted, bladder instability is physiologic in the very young. Children with persistent day and night incontinence have a greater incidence of instability than those who have either type of incontinence alone. In reviewing 50 male and female patients with isolated primary nocturnal enuresis persisting after the age of 6, Whiteside and Arnold found that only 15% of patients had unstable bladders.[18] However, the incidence rose to 97% in patients who had both diurnal and nocturnal enuresis.[18] In adult women presenting with enuresis alone, abnormal cystometrograms suggestive of detrusor instability have been reported in 61% of patients.[19] Although nocturnal enuresis may be associated with detrusor instability, urodynamic evaluation is not advocated in the investigation of pediatric patients in whom enuresis occurs alone. Patients with congenital instability are likely to have a lifelong history of frequency and to be late bedwetters.

Aging

The incidence of detrusor hyperactivity increases with age independent of clinical neurologic disease. It is probably the most frequent cause of incontinence in the elderly population, and in women is usually associated with increasing urethral incompetence. In a study focusing on cerebral perfusion by SPECT scanning in elderly patients with detrusor instability, reduced perfusion to the frontal lobes was shown, particularly the right lobe, suggesting that a subclinical neuropathic cause may exist.[20]

Bladder Outlet Obstruction

Outflow obstruction is believed to result in detrusor instability, an observation supported by its prevalence in men with prostatic obstruction and its relief after surgical treatment.[14] Men with a greater degree of obstruction by urodynamic criteria also appear to have a greater incidence of instability.[21]

These clinical findings are also reflected in women with bladder outlet obstruction. Although not common in women, as previously noted, this situation may occur following an overcorrected cystourethropexy, in which scenario the majority of patients present with postoperative voiding difficulties and new-onset symptoms of bladder instability. Cardoza and colleagues reported that 17 of 92 women developed new-onset bladder instability symptoms following successful colposuspension, a procedure that may be related to obstruction.[22] In a reported series of surgical revisions of obstructive cystourethropexies resolution of symptoms of instability occurred in more than 90%.[15]

Human and animal detrusor muscle has been subjected to extensive laboratory-based in vitro muscle strip studies. In comparison of obstructed stable and obstructed unstable bladders, cholinergic supersensitivity was seen in the latter.[23] This postjunctional supersensitivity to acetylcholine appears to result from a partial parasympathetic denervation from associated neuroanatomic studies of similar bladder biopsies.[24] Furthermore, in the animal model there was evidence that on relief of obstruction, the detrusor was capable of returning to normal behavior and undergoing reinnervation.[25] These combined results suggest a subclinical neuropathic cause of instability associated with bladder outlet obstruction.

Urethral Instability

In physiologic voiding, a drop in urethral pressure immediately precedes an elevation in bladder pressure, implicating urethral relaxation as the first part of the micturition reflex. Pathologic fluctuations in urethral pressure, called urethral instability, may therefore be implicated as a cause of detrusor instability.[26, 27] This theory is not yet proved; if, however, instability originates in the urethra, which appears probable, targeting treatment to the urethra would be a more rational alternative.

These theories of detrusor instability are similar to the suggestion that urine in the posterior urethra may result in the urge to void and thus to an involuntary bladder contraction. This has been the subject of considerable controversy. However, studies of bladder pressure during injection of saline into the proximal urethra have not shown any provocation of bladder contraction.[28] Clinically, bladder instability has been associated with stress urinary incontinence, especially in the elderly. It is known that urethral competence, as measured by urethral profilometry, decreases linearly with age.[29] It is recognized that detrusor instability and genuine stress incontinence may coexist; however, currently there is no evidence that one necessarily precipitates the other.

Psychologic Causes

Because idiopathic instability implies no known cause, some investigators contend that psychogenic instability is a better term.[30] Frewen argues that once structural, organic, and infective causes have been excluded, the cause of 80% of unstable bladders is psychosomatic.[30] This is not a widely held hypothesis, and most investigators would call this type of instability idiopathic.

Patient Evaluation

The symptoms of bladder instability, frequency, nocturia, urgency, and urge incontinence are collectively known as the urge syndrome. Clearly, however, these symptoms are not exclusive to instability, and any bladder irritative state such as acute urinary tract infection, urethral syndrome, interstitial cystitis, or carcinoma in situ, may be responsible. Diagnosis of bladder instability requires ruling out such disorders by urine microscopy and culture, urine cytology and cystoscopy when warranted, and objective testing through urodynamic evaluation.

HISTORY

Farrah and colleagues published an interesting study of 570 women with micturition disorders in which the presenting symptoms were correlated with the function of the bladder on urodynamic testing.[31] They noted that patients with frequency of micturition without urgency or urge incontinence rarely had bladder instability, whereas those with urgency or nocturia had bladder instability more frequently. Cantor and Bates suggested that the symptoms of nocturia, urge incontinence, and nocturnal enuresis were important in the diagnosis of detrusor instability.[32] In their group of 214 incontinent women, if one of these symptoms was present, 64% had an unstable bladder on cystometry; if two were present, this figure rose to 76%; and if all three symptoms were present, 81% of patients had detrusor instability. Of course, 19% of patients with all three symptoms did not have motor detrusor instability and would therefore be classified as having sensory urgency. Among patients presenting with pure stress urinary incontinence, bladder instability has been diagnosed on cystometry in up to 30%.[8] In Farrar and colleagues' series, if frequency and nocturia were present in addition to stress leakage, the incidence of an unstable detrusor was appreciable, and if urgency and episodes of urge incontinence accompanied stress leakage, the bladder was unstable in 80% of cases. The incidence of instability was 80% in patients who complained of "always being wet" regardless of associated symptoms.

Cardoza and Stanton also presented a clinical and urodynamic review of 200 incontinent women in which they identified the different symptomatology in 100 women shown objectively to have genuine stress incontinence and 100 shown to have an unstable bladder.[33] Their results suggest that a definitive diagnosis cannot be made on the history alone (Table 20–2).

Symptomatic evaluation is more unreliable in the

TABLE 20–2
**Incidence of Symptoms Associated with Genuine Stress Incontinence vs.
Detrusor Instability**

	Genuine Stress Incontinence (%)	Detrusor Instability (%)
Stress incontinence	89	49
Urge incontinence	55	38
Mixed urge-stress incontinence and frequency-nocturia	19	26
Present enuresis	14	13
Past enuresis	13	24
Wet on standing up	45	31
Diurnal frequency	57	79
Nocturnal frequency	38	69
Diurnal and nocturnal frequency	28	56
Difficulty voiding	6	9
Sensation of prolapse	42	18

elderly owing to their failing mental acuity and disorientation associated with the transient medical problems seen in this age group that may lead to incontinence.[34]

In any age group, in addition to obtaining the urologic history, it is important to inquire about the patient's personal, family, social, and environmental history. Frewen lays great emphasis on this general evaluation, believing that the stimulus for abnormal bladder activity is not a local one but may be central in origin and may be influenced by psychosocial and environmental factors.[30]

The phenomenon of "giggle incontinence" is also unreliably correlated with detrusor instability. This condition should not be confused with genuine stress incontinence during laughter; rather, it refers to a sudden involuntary, uncontrollable, and often complete emptying of the bladder while laughing in a person who is otherwise fully continent.[35] The cause of this condition remains unclear, and urodynamic evaluation is usually unrewarding, but occasionally detrusor instability may be demonstrated.[36] This condition is probably more common than reported and most likely involves triggering of the micturition reflex through an unknown mechanism.

PHYSICAL EXAMINATION

General physical examination should include a screening neurologic examination with inspection of the lower back, gait assessment, ankle reflexes, perineal sensation, and bulbocavernosus reflex. In patients with overt neurologic disease and in those with neurologic symptoms and signs a neurologic opinion should be obtained. Pelvic and vaginal speculum examinations are performed to identify local irritative factors, and the presence or absence of stress incontinence should be elucidated. The patient should be examined with a moderately full bladder in both the erect and supine positions; if there is stress urinary leakage, note should be made of whether the leakage

is transient and occurs simultaneously with a cough (in which case it is likely to be due to sphincter weakness), or whether it occurs momentarily after the cough and is more prolonged, which may be due to an involuntary bladder contraction precipitated by either the stress or the cough. If incontinence cannot be precipitated during supine testing, the patient should be examined erect. If a Marshall-Bonny test is performed, care should be taken in both performance and interpretation of the test because a false-positive result may be obtained if the urethra is inadvertently compressed by the elevating fingers.

The occurrence of a cystocele does not correlate well with the presence of either detrusor instability or genuine stress incontinence. When radiographic techniques were used to identify anatomic changes, 85% of patients with genuine stress incontinence showed significant descent of the urethrovesical junction on straining, but 65% of patients with detrusor instability did so also.[33] The most important reason for recognizing and categorizing prolapse in the incontinent patient is not to determine the cause of the incontinence but to enable the surgeon to select the most appropriate surgical procedure.

URINE EXAMINATION

Because the symptoms of bladder instability may be mimicked by an acute infection or other bladder irritative phenomena, urinalysis, microscopy and culture of urine, and cytologic evaluation of urine are important. Microscopic hematuria raises the suspicion of malignancy, prompting performance of urine cytology and cystourethroscopy. Pyuria and microscopic hematuria may also occur in patients with inflammatory disorders of the lower urinary tract such as interstitial cystitis and the urethral syndrome, or they may be due to bladder calculi, and therefore cystoscopic and appropriate radiographic studies of the upper tract may be necessary.

RADIOGRAPHIC STUDIES

Excretory urography or renal ultrasound has a place in the routine screening of patients with neurogenic bladder disease. The patient with neurologic disease may be unable to perceive symptoms, and deterioration of the upper tract may be recognizable only by radiologic studies. An abdominal scout film may identify unsuspected spinal anomalies, suggesting an underlying neurologic cause for the bladder dysfunction, but the role of excretory urography in the patient with idiopathic instability is not as clear. The adult with an unstable bladder usually has coordinated sphincter function and therefore is at little risk of upper tract deterioration. Hence, it may be acceptable to reserve intravenous urography for those who have symptoms or signs requiring further elucidation, and certainly the upper tracts can be screened by ultrasound. Voiding cystourethrography is performed in patients in whom the upper tracts are abnormal. It is best performed with fluoroscopic visualization, and even more interpretable results are obtained when the study is combined with a simultaneous pressure-flow urodynamic study (video-urodynamics).

ENDOSCOPY

Cystourethroscopy is necessary in the patient with microscopic hematuria and may also assist in the diagnosis of other bladder irritative phenomena. The patient with the urethral syndrome frequently exhibits no endoscopic changes, and the correlation of findings of pseudomembranous urethrotrigonitis with bladder irritative symptoms is poorly established. Endoscopy may be useful in the diagnosis of interstitial cystitis; however, the characteristic diagnostic features are seen only after distention under anesthesia.

Trabeculation of the bladder wall is a frequent finding in men with bladder outlet obstruction or detrusor instability. However, in women, fine trabeculation is common to the point of normality and rarely has an obstructive or functional cause.[37]

Gross incompetence of the sphincter mechanism and scarring or atrophy of the urethra may be seen on urethroscopy, but functional disturbances of the sphincter mechanism are difficult to diagnose. Urethral diverticulum should be sought in women with bladder irritative symptoms, particularly those with voiding discomfort.

URODYNAMICS

Because the bladder is such a poor witness, and symptoms of bladder instability are common in a variety of other conditions, objective identification of detrusor dysfunction is the only accurate way to make the diagnosis. The bladder normally stores urine at low pressure and then empties to completion at a socially acceptable time and place. The filling cystometrogram is an attempt to better define the storage phase of this cycle. To evaluate only this aspect of bladder function may be inadequate, however, because sphincter dysfunction, outlet obstruction, and voiding problems frequently coexist and should be identified to aid in therapy. For these reasons, cystometry may be complemented by the performance of simultaneous sphincter electromyography to evaluate the striated sphincter; by urethral pressure studies to measure the urethral response during filling, storage, and voiding; and by micturition studies to monitor the detrusor pressure and urine flow rate during voiding.[38] Performance of all these studies, particularly if done in conjunction with intermittent simultaneous cystourethrography during the filling, storing, and voiding phases of the micturition cycle, gives the most objective information about micturition function (Table 20–3).[39]

Cystometry

Cystometry is the mainstay of investigation of bladder storage function. The bladder is an intra-abdominal organ, and therefore total bladder pressure is the summation of intrinsic detrusor pressure and the surrounding intra-abdominal pressure. Because measurement of bladder pressure alone is inadequate, detrusor pressure (P_{det}) is evaluated by electronically subtracting abdominal pressure (P_{abd}, rectal or vaginal) from bladder pressure.[40] Cystometry may be described as conventional fluid fill, gas fill, or ambulatory (physiologic) fill. All pressures are zeroed at atmospheric pressure at the level of the pubic symphysis at the start of each study.

Conventional fluid fill cystometry is usually performed at either a slow fill rate (≤ 10 ml/minute), which may be appropriate in evaluation of the neuropathic bladder, medium fill rate (10 to 100 ml/minute), or fast fill rate (>100 ml/minute), which is more provocative. During filling, cystometry provides information about detrusor sensation, capacity, activity, and compliance.

There is still some debate about the most appropriate medium to be used for cystometry. Carbon dioxide cystometry, commonly used in the office, is clean and economical but is certainly unphysiologic. It is easy to infuse at a constant rate, and because it is soluble in blood, there is little risk of embolus. However, because gas is compressible, low-pressure involuntary contractions may be missed and leaks

TABLE 20–3
Urodynamic Studies in the Investigation of Bladder Instability

Provocative cystometry
Micturition studies
Videourodynamics
Sphincter electromyography
Urethral pressure studies

cannot be easily detected. Because abdominal pressure is not routinely used during carbon dioxide cystometry, calculation of detrusor pressure is not done. Pressure-flow micturition study and videourodynamics are also not possible. Thus, water and saline are the best filling media, although they are more time-consuming and expensive. They facilitate simultaneous measurement of bladder and abdominal pressure, allowing determination of detrusor pressure. They facilitate pressure-flow micturition studies, and, if a radiographic contrast agent is used, one can simultaneously visualize the lower urinary tract during the study by using intermittent fluoroscopy (videourodynamics).[41]

Bladder instability may exhibit a number of different patterns on cystometry. Unstable detrusor contractions may be spontaneous or unprovoked or may occur on provocation such as a cough or posture change. Because supine and erect filling alone will not identify all unstable bladders, provocative maneuvers such as rapid fill, cold fill, heel jouncing, squatting, handwashing, and so on should be used in patients in whom there is a high index of suspicion.

At the end of bladder filling, a period of approximately a 1 to 2 minutes for pressure normalization is useful for determining the true maximum resting detrusor pressure. During this resting period provocative maneuvers should be done frequently in an attempt to unmask unstable contractions. According to reports, about 44% of unstable bladders are discovered during simple supine filling, and the remainder develop contractions in response to cough (17%), posture change (22%), erect fill (10%), and catheter removal (7%).[41–43]

A further pattern of abnormal detrusor activity is a steep rising curve of a cystometrogram without obvious contractions. This is defined as poor compliance (dv/dp), represented as ml/cm H_2O pressure; it is variably dependent on a number of factors including rate of fill and the shape and thickness of the bladder wall, but generally it reflects noncontractile factors such as the connective tissues or inflammatory changes within the bladder wall.

MICTURITION STUDIES

Pressure-flow studies evaluate the second or voiding phase of the bladder cycle. The urethral filling catheter is removed when cystometry has been completed and maximum cystometric capacity has been reached; continuous pressure and flow are monitored simultaneously while voiding proceeds. This provides information on bladder contractility as well as outlet resistance factors.

These studies are indicated in patients who have voiding difficulty by the history, uroflowmetry, or identification of a significant postvoid residual. Bladder contractility can be further examined by using the "stop test." This is a measure of maximum isometric pressure and is the pressure achieved when the patient interrupts flow in midvoiding by voluntary sphincter contraction. This volume-dependent and relatively nonphysiologic test is used infrequently in clinical practice.

AMBULATORY URODYNAMIC STUDIES

Conventional urodynamic studies remain unphysiologic, and recently ambulatory studies have been introduced in an attempt to address this problem. Studies are performed using a small-caliber urethral and rectal catheter, and the data are stored by means of either magnetic tape or microprocessor solid-state memory.

The appropriate role for ambulatory urodynamics has not yet been defined, but it is useful in the investigation of patients whose symptoms are not confirmed by conventional studies. Comparative studies of conventional and ambulatory urodynamics in the same patients show a higher voiding pressure and lower flow rate in the ambulatory group.[44] This result may be due to minimal lower urinary tract obstruction caused by mild urethral obstruction, which in turn is due to catheter irritation and edema. McInerney and colleagues reported instability not documented by conventional studies in 5 of 12 patients with the urge syndrome and enuresis using ambulatory studies.[45]

VIDEOURODYNAMICS

If radiographic contrast agent is used as the filling medium during conventional urodynamics the bladder and outlet may be visualized by intermittent fluoroscopy at the same time that electronic pressure and flow data are recorded. This videourodynamic evaluation represents the most comprehensive form of functional investigation of the lower urinary tract, especially if it is performed with sphincter electromyographic (EMG) and urethral pressure profilometry.[39] It is particularly useful for determining the site of obstruction in patients with voiding dysfunction and the degree of bladder neck competence and urethrovesical anatomy in patients with stress urinary incontinence. The healthy bladder neck is cough and strain competent and opens only when the bladder contracts, either voluntarily or involuntarily; incompetence of the female bladder neck in the absence of a detrusor contraction implies that there is proximal urethral sphincter deficiency. In the absence of simultaneous bladder pressure measurement, an open bladder neck on fluoroscopy may be due to either sphincter weakness or an involuntary contraction. Mixed stress and urge incontinence is common, and patients with this problem are still candidates for surgical correction of the stress component by bladder neck suspension, any persistent symptoms of bladder instability being managed subsequently by pharmacologic or other methods. In the patient with only an unstable bladder, the bladder neck will remain competent until the detrusor contracts, when it will open and the proximal urethra will fill down to the external sphincter level. The patient, perceiving an urgent desire to void, actively contracts the external sphincter and maintains continence at this level. If the uninhibited bladder contraction is suppressed, urine in the proximal urethra will be "milked back," and the bladder neck will close. Should the unstable contraction continue, ultimately the external sphincter will tire, and leakage will occur.

Videourodynamic study provides an opportunity to evaluate the outflow tract radiographically under conditions of stress that approach those under which leakage normally occurs in an incontinent woman. Lateral cystourethrographic screening may demonstrate hypermobility of the bladder base and urethra, with significant descent and alteration in the urethral axis. Such anatomic changes do not invariably predict that incontinence, if present, is of the stress variety; however, interpreted intelligently, video studies may help in the selection of the most appropriate surgical procedure for the incontinent woman and may help predict the likelihood of surgical success.[46]

Computer-aided image analysis systems in combination with software manipulation of pressure-flow data obtained from the urodynamic equipment measurements are under development.[47]

URETHRAL PRESSURE PROFILE

There is considerable controversy about the clinical value of urethral pressure profile measurement. Classically, perfusion profilometry was used; however, this has been replaced in part by microtip transducer techniques. In these techniques, however, care must be taken to interpret the data appropriately because of the technical limitations of pressure reference and artifact and the limited measurement angle.[48] Another form of urethral pressure measurement performed in evaluation of incontinent women is the urethral pressure transmission test. This study has many advocates, particularly among gynecologists, who suggest that it helps to determine whether the proximal urethra is adequately supported in an intra-abdominal position.[48]

Sorenson has demonstrated that urethral pressure profiles decrease linearly with age in otherwise healthy women, and this may explain the increasing incidence of stress urinary incontinence in direct relationship to age.[29] It has also been shown that significant reductions in the urethral pressure measurement occur immediately prior to the onset of unstable bladder contractions. This supports the theory that the hyperexcitable micturition reflex required for detrusor instability has its origin within the urethra.

SPHINCTER ELECTROMYOGRAPHY

EMG studies are indicated only in the evaluation of patients with and those suspected of having neuropa-

thy. The information obtained relates to the function of the distal striated sphincter (intrinsic and extrinsic) and does not provide information on proximal sphincter function. EMG has a dual role—first, using simple instrumentation, it provides information about the coordination between the sphincter and the bladder, and second, using more sophisticated technology, including an oscilloscope and concentric needle electrode or single-fiber techniques, it may provide objective evidence about the innervation of these muscles and may be used to diagnose occult neuropathy. Recently, a standardization report has been published.[1]

Treatment

The object of treatment is to effect improvement in the symptoms of frequency, nocturia, urgency, and urgency incontinence, and a number of therapeutic alternatives exist, including behavioral management, pharmacologic therapy, electrical stimulation, and surgery (Table 20–4). We will explore these methods and try to identify their relative merits and indications.

BEHAVIORAL MODIFICATION

A number of studies attest to the efficacy of various forms of behavioral intervention in treating detrusor hyperactivity; however, few have reported long-term follow-up of symptom improvement or objective change in bladder behavior by repeat cystometry. The success of behavioral intervention in the treatment of urge incontinence probably lies in the reestablishment of cortical control over the hyperexcitable micturition reflex. Caution must, however, be required in evaluating studies because of the success of placebo in this condition.

Biofeedback training is a form of learning or reeducation in which the patient receives feedback or information about one or more of her normally unconscious physiologic processes, this information being made available as a visual, auditory, or tactile signal.[49, 50] *Bladder retraining* (bladder drill) was pioneered by Frewen.[51] A voided volume chart is used

TABLE 20–4
Treatment Options in Detrusor Hyperactivity

Behavioral	Bladder drill
	Reduced fluid intake
	Biofeedback
Pharmacologic	Anticholinergic drugs
	Spasmolytic agents
	Tricyclic antidepressants
Electrical stimulation	
Surgical	Augmentation
	Diversion

to establish the patient's customary voiding frequency. The patient is then instructed to gradually increase the voiding interval, using the voided volume chart to reinforce the program and to give an objective assessment of response. This approach has been used in both men and women, although it is used more often in women with idiopathic detrusor instability, sensory urgency, and bladder hypersensitivity symptoms. An 85% subjective and a 50% objective response has been achieved. In the long term, however, 43% of patients with symptoms of instability relapsed after initial improvement.[51, 52] Frewen, however, in a 6-year follow-up of 50 patients, noted an overall subjective cure rate of 86%, his patients being initially managed as inpatients.[53, 54] It appears that urge incontinence, due either to detrusor instability or sensory urgency, can be effectively treated by intensive bladder drill on either an inpatient or an outpatient basis; what is clearly important is enthusiastic patient contact, reassurance, and good long-term support and follow-up. The single most important factor predictive of success in this kind of treatment is patient compliance with the treatment regimen.

PSYCHOTHERAPY

In addition to bladder drill, several other related behavioral interventions have been tried in the management of detrusor instability. Haffner and associates reported on a group of 26 patients with bladder instability treated with six 1-hour sessions of group psychotherapy; one-third benefited considerably, one-third showed minimal or no improvement, and one-third either refused or dropped out prematurely.[55] Further studies have confirmed that the efficacy of psychotherapy is less than that of bladder drill.[56] Hypnosis has been reported to produce a subjective cure in 58% and improvement in 28%, with 50% showing a cystometric conversion to stability.[57] The efficacy of both psychotherapy and biofeedback treatment reinforces the belief that psychosocial factors are important not only in the cause but also in the treatment of detrusor instability. Although these methods are effective, they are very time consuming and labor intensive; also symptoms may recur according to variations in the patient's psychological condition.

ACUPUNCTURE

Acupuncture is a novel and minimally invasive treatment modality that has shown promising early results.[58] Philip and colleagues treated 17 patients with detrusor instability in weekly acupuncture sessions for 10 to 12 weeks; they reported that 77% of patients with diurnal symptoms showed significant improvement and 63% of patients with incontinence became dry.[58]

PHARMACOTHERAPY

When the measures described previously fail, pharmacologic therapy should be instituted. A comprehensive review of the physiology and pharmacology of the lower urinary tract is beyond the scope of this chapter, and for further information a number of excellent reviews are available.[59-61] If the mechanisms of drug actions are to be understood, however, some general remarks on the neuropharmacology of the bladder and urethral outlet are in order.

The detrusor muscle has both sympathetic and parasympathetic innervation. The neurotransmitter providing nerve-mediated detrusor contraction in humans is primarily acetylcholine, and cholinergic receptors are present throughout the bladder.[62] Alpha-adrenergic sympathetic innervation is virtually absent in the bladder dome, this location having a preponderance of beta-adrenergic receptors. Alpha-adrenergic receptors predominate in the bladder neck and proximal urethra. The density of cholinergic receptors is reportedly decreased and that of adrenergic receptors increased in patients with detrusor hyperreflexia compared with normal controls.[63] Recently, nonadrenergic noncholinergic (NANC) or purinergic nerves have been demonstrated in the human detrusor muscle, and these are hypothesized to act as neuromodulators rather than by direct muscle stimulation.[64] Modification of both cholinergic and adrenergic nerve function with medication combined with direct muscle inhibition reflects the majority of drug-mediated attempts to treat the overactive bladder. An excellent in-depth review of the pharmacotherapy used to facilitate bladder storage has been written by Wein.[65]

ANTICHOLINERGIC MEDICATIONS   Because the major neurohumoral stimulus for physiologic bladder contraction is cholinergic, anticholinergic medications are predominantly used to treat bladder hyperactivity whether of idiopathic or neurogenic origin. In such patients the effect of this medication is to increase the bladder volume at which involuntary contractions occur and to decrease the amplitude of these contractions. The net result is to increase overall bladder capacity and reduce symptoms.[66] The majority of patients experience typical anticholinergic side effects, which include dry mouth, constipation, blurred vision, and increased heart rate; the patient should be counseled to expect these before therapy is initiated.

In general, these are safe drugs; however, they should be used cautiously in patients with significant cardiac arrhythmias or narrow angle glaucoma.[67] The most widely used anticholinergic agent is probanthine bromide, which is prescribed in a dose of 15 to 30 mg every 4 to 6 hours in adults. Poor gastrointestinal absorption leads to low bioavailability after oral administration, and it should therefore be taken on an empty stomach. Few controlled clinical trials of this drug are available, and reported clinical response is not impressive.

MUSCULOTROPIC RELAXANTS   These agents depress smooth muscle activity by acting directly at a site distal to the cholinergic receptor mechanism and also have variable anticholinergic and local anesthetic properties. Oxybutynin chloride (Ditropan) is the medication most commonly used for the treatment of detrusor instability; it is a moderately potent anticholinergic with a strong independent direct muscle relaxant activity. The customary adult dose is 5 mg three to four times per day, and the side effects are the same as those reported for anticholinergics. This drug has been successfully used to depress bladder hyperactivity resulting from both neurogenic and idiopathic causes.[68] As intermittent catheterization has become more acceptable and more frequently used in the management particularly of neurogenic bladder hyperactivity, intravesical or topical application of oxybutynin has been used with it and may give better results with reduced side effects.[69] Flavoxate hydrochloride (Urispas) is used in a dose of 100 to 200 mg three to four times per day, and few anticholinergic side effects have been described. The clinical efficacy of this drug has not been confirmed by controlled trials, but it continues to be widely prescribed.[70]

CALCIUM ANTAGONISTS   Calcium antagonists have been shown to inhibit detrusor muscle contractility effectively in vitro and in clinical trials.[71] Terodoline, the most effective agent, has now been withdrawn from the market because of the development of potentially fatal cardiac arrhythmias; however, other agents are under development.

BETA-ADRENERGIC AGONISTS   The predominance of beta-adrenergic receptors within the bladder muscle has prompted studies of beta agonist activity in the treatment of detrusor overactivity. Terbutaline given orally in a dose of 5 mg three times a day has been reported to produce a clinical effect in some patients with bladder hyperactivity.[72]

TRICYCLIC ANTIDEPRESSANTS   Urologic interst in this heterologous group of compounds stems from their effectiveness in the treatment of nocturnal enuresis in children. Their mode of action has not been fully elucidated, but they appear to possess at least three major pharmacologic actions: (1) a central and peripheral anticholinergic effect, (2) a central sedative effect, and (3) an alpha-adrenergic agonist effect. Clinically, therefore, the medication should decrease bladder contractility and increase outlet resistance.[73]

Imipramine hydrochloride is the most commonly used drug in this category. The usual adult dose is 25 mg three to four times daily. Side effects consist of systemic anticholinergic effects, although allergic reactions such as skin rash and obstructive jaundice and agranulocytosis may rarely occur. Fatigue, postural hypotension, tremor, and altered mental states have also been reported. Cardiotoxicity has been reported in animal studies but has not been confirmed in vivo, and this problem is rarely clinically significant, particularly because the dose used for detrusor dysfunction is much lower than that used in depression.[74]

In elderly patients the use of imipramine has produced continence in 60% of patients with detrusor instability.[75] Imipramine may also be used in conjunction with anticholinergic medications for additive effectiveness.

OTHER AGENTS   DDAVP (exogenous antidiuretic hormone [ADH]) may be used to resorb water from urine in the collecting system, thereby reducing urine production. Studies have shown that children with enuresis are relatively deficient in ADH production overnight.[75] In patients with bladder hyperactivity, a reduction in urine production may be used effectively to combat symptoms of nocturia with a single nighttime dose. Caution should, however, be used in prescribing this drug for the elderly, especially those with congestive heart failure, or for children under the age of 5, in whom water intoxication may occur.

ELECTRICAL STIMULATION

There is experimental and clinical evidence that local (vaginal and anal) electrical stimulation activates the musculature of the urethra to increase outlet resistance and also inhibits the detrusor muscle, reducing detrusor hyperactivity.[76] Stimulation may be given in the form of low-intensity, subthreshold continuous electrical waves or as intermittent maximal stimulation. Because high-amplitude maximal stimulation appears to produce more pronounced bladder inhibition, intermittent maximal stimulation is the modality used primarily for the treatment of bladder hyperactivity.[77] Erickson and colleagues reported a trial of 48 women with detrusor instability, each of whom received 20 minutes of simultaneous vaginal and anal stimulation for an average of seven treatments.[77] Initial clinical and urodynamic cures occurred in 50% of patients, and a further 33% reported improvement; at 1 year a durable therapeutic effect was seen in 77%. Others, however, have not reported such successes.[78, 79] The placebo effect of electrical stimulation is difficult to quantify, and the overall results of this method therefore remain incompletely defined. More work is required in this area to determine the role of electrical stimulation in the unstable bladder.

Direct neurostimulation has been used in the treatment of the neurogenic bladder. Implantable electrodes are placed either intradurally or extradurally to produce intermittent controlled electrical stimulation of the sacral nerve roots, leading to a volitionally controlled detrusor contraction. This technique may improve the efficiency of bladder emptying in patients with a neurogenic bladder; however, in patients with incomplete lesions radiation of pain to the peripheral nerve roots currently precludes its use.

INTERMITTENT CATHETERIZATION

Intermittent catheterization plays little role in the management of patients with idiopathic detrusor instability; however, its use remains pivotal in the management of neurogenic hyperreflexia, particularly when functional obstruction due to a dyssynergic sphincter exists. As originally popularized by Lapides and colleagues, clean intermittent catheterization has proved to be a safe way to produce bladder emptying, reducing both symptomatic infections and upper tract deterioration.[80] It is most commonly used in conjunction with anticholinergic medications in patients with neurogenic detrusor hyperactivity.

Surgical Management

Surgery is reserved for the uncommon patient in whom intractable symptoms of detrusor hyperactivity persist despite use of the conservative measures previously discussed. A number of procedures have been reported in the past, many of which now have only historic interest, and the current mainstay of surgical management is bladder augmentation by enterocystoplasty.

BLADDER DISTENTION

Bladder distention has been shown to cause degeneration of unmyelinated nerve fibers in the bladder wall, which may result in reduced bladder sensory and motor function.[81] Results of this procedure suggest a 70% symptomatic and 60% objective response rate; however, there are few long-term successes. Pengalley and colleagues reported only a 9% success rate after 6 months.[82] Even though this procedure is simple and can be repeated if it is effective, it is not without risks, and bladder rupture has been reported in 7 of 128 cases.[83]

PERIPHERAL DENERVATION PROCEDURES

Several treatment modalities have been directed toward dividing the sacral nerves in an attempt to inhibit the micturition reflex. Cystolysis, popularized by Turner-Warwick for the management of interstitial cystitis, attempted to denervate the bladder peripherally by separating it from all of its attachments above the trigone via an abdominal surgical dissection.[84] Encouraging results were reported in patients with detrusor hyperreflexia; however, its place in the management of detrusor instability is not clear, and its use has not stood the test of time. Transvaginal denervation procedures have also been described; they are performed after an initial therapeutic trial by lidocaine (Xylocaine) injection into the bladder base to determine whether contractions can be abolished. Studies have shown a cure rate of over 50% with a mean follow-up of 1 year.[85] Bladder transection using a circumferential bladder incision was also reported to achieve a 75% success rate.[86] More recent reports, however, have failed to replicate these results, and the procedures have fallen into disrepute.[87]

SUBTRIGONAL PHENOL

Denervation of the detrusor may be achieved by infiltration of the pelvic plexus immediately behind the trigone with a 6% aqueous solution of phenol. Initial reports using this procedure were promising; however, recently long-term results have not supported its efficacy.[88] The procedure may be associated with significant morbidity and has been complicated by fistula, ureteral injury, and neural injury; it is therefore not recommended.

AUGMENTATION "CLAM" CYSTOPLASTY

Currently, augmentation enterocystoplasty is the most successful surgical intervention for detrusor hyperactivity. In this procedure the bladder is subtotally transected in either the coronal or the sagittal plane, and a strip of detubularized bowel is interposed into the defect, effectively enlarging the bladder capacity and dissipating the high-pressure contractions. In 1982 Bramble reported that cures were achieved by this method in 13 of 15 adult enuretics who had failed to respond to conservative nonsurgical treatment.[89] Subsequently, reports confirmed this high success rate in patients with both detrusor instability and neuropathic hyperreflexia.[90, 91]

Preoperative assessment of patients considered for augmentation cystoplasty ideally includes complete videourodynamic evaluation looking specifically at bladder capacity and compliance, voiding dysfunction, outlet competence, and the presence or absence of reflux. These findings determine the surgical technique used and provide valuable information useful in preoperative patient counseling. If associated outlet incompetence is suggested by the video study and by a low leak pressure, the surgery may have to be enhanced to increase urethral resistance by using cystourethropexy, placement of an artificial urinary sphincter, or injection of a periurethral bulking agent. However, if outlet resistance is increased at the time of augmentation cystoplasty, there is a high risk of postoperative voiding problems that may require use of self clean intermittent catheterization.

Surgical Technique

In summary, the bladder is subtotally transected in the coronal or sagittal plane to within 2 cm of the bladder neck. A segment of terminal ileum (approximately 25 cm) or other bowel segment is isolated on its mesentery and opened along its antimesenteric border to create an open plate. The length of bowel isolated equals the length of the incision in the bladder unless the bladder is thick walled and of small volume, in which case a longer segment of bowel is used and folded to create a larger intestinal plate. The isolated segment is then anastomosed into the bladder defect, effectively increasing its capacity by the desired amount. Postoperatively, urodynamic studies have shown an increased functional bladder capacity, increased compliance, and a reduction in unstable contractions.[89] Voiding dysfunction may occur postoperatively; however, few patients with idiopathic bladder instability who do not also undergo an outlet procedure require intermittent catheterization. Other problems include metabolic disturbances due to absorption of urinary metabolites and leading to hyperchloremic metabolic acidosis, especially in patients with renal impairment. Mucus is produced in the urinary tract following augmentation cystoplasty; however, apart from children (particularly young boys), this is rarely a problem. More recently, concern has been raised about the possibility of an increased risk of malignancy in augmented bladders.

URINARY DIVERSION

Despite the array of treatments described, there do remain occasional patients with disabling incontinence in whom a urinary diversion is appropriate. In women in whom external collecting devices are particularly unsuccessful and in whom chronic indwelling catheter drainage has attendant risks of infection, painful bladder spasm, and pericatheter leakage, a continent catheterizable diversion will considerably improve the quality of life.

REFERENCES

1. Abrams PH, Blaivas JG, Stanton SL, Anderson JT: Standardization of terminology of lower urinary tract function. Neurourol Urodyn 7:403–428, 1988.
2. Turner-Warwick RT: Observation on the function and dysfunction of the sphincter and detrusor mechanism. Urol Clin North Am 6:13, 1979.
3. Frewen WK: Urge and stress incontinence: Fact and fiction. Br J Obstet Gynecol 77:932, 1970.
4. Webb RJ, Ramsden PD, Neal DE: Ambulatory monitoring and electronic measurement of urinary leakage in the diagnosis of detrusor instability and incontinence. Br J Urol 68:148–152, 1991.
5. Yeates WK: Bladder function in normal micturition. Clin Develop Med 48/49:28–38, 1973.
6. Muellner SR: Development of urinary control in children. JAMA 172:1256, 1960.
7. Diokno AC, Brown MB, Brock BM, et al: Clinical and cystometric characteristics of continent and incontinent noninstitutionalized elderly. J Urol 145:567, 1988.
8. Webster GD, Sihelnik SA, Stone AR: Female urinary incontinence: The incidence, identification and characteristics of detrusor instability. Neurourol Urodyn 3:235, 1984.
9. Arnold EP, Webster JR, Luc H, et al: Urodynamics of female incontinence: Factors influence the results of surgery. Am J Obstet Gynecol 17:805, 1973.
10. Nordling J, Myhoff H, Anderson JT, et al: Urinary incontinence in the female. The value of detrusor reflex activation procedures. Br J Urol 51:110, 1979.
11. Sand PK, Hill RC, Ostegard DO: Supine urethroscopic and standing cystometry as screening methods for the detection of detrusor instability. Obstet Gynecol 70:57, 1987.
12. Bates CP: The unstable bladder. Clin Obstet Gynecol 5:109, 1978.
13. Abrams P, Farrar DJ, Turner-Warwick RT, et al: The results of prostatectomy: A symptomatic and urodynamic analysis of 152 patients. J Urol 121:640, 1979.
14. Abrams P: Detrusor instability and bladder outlet obstruction. Neurourol Urodyn 4:317, 1985.
15. Webster GD, Kreder KJ: Voiding dysfunction following cystourethropexy: Its evaluation and management. J Urol 144:670–673, 1990.
16. Bradley WE, Timm GW, Scott FB: Innervation of the detrusor muscle and urethra. Urol Clin North Am 1:3, 1974.
17. Webster GD, Mark SD: Neurourology. In Wilkins RH, Rengachary SS (eds): Neurosurgery, 2nd ed. New York, McGraw Hill, 1993.
18. Whiteside CG, Arnold EP: Persistent primary enuresis: A urodynamic assessment. Br Med J 1:364, 1975.
19. Torrens MJ, Collins CD: The urodynamic assessment of adult enuresis. Br J Urol 47:433, 1975.
20. Griffiths DN, McCracken PN, Moore K: Location of cerebrolesions responsible for geriatric urge incontinence. ICS Abstract, Proceedings of the International Continence Society, Neurourol Urodyn 11:422–423, 1992.
21. Cucchi A: Detrusor instability and bladder outflow obstruction. Evidence for a correlation between the severity of obstruction and the presence of instability. Br J Urol 61:420, 1988.
22. Cardoza LD, Stanton SL, Williams JE: Detrusor instability following surgery for genuine stress incontinence. Br J Urol 51:204, 1979.
23. Harrison CW, Hunnam GR, Furman P, et al: Bladder instability and denervation in patients with bladder outflow obstruction. Br J Urol 65:19, 1987.
24. Speakman MJ, Brading AF, Guilpin CJ, et al: Bladder outflow obstruction: A cause of denervation supersensitivity. J Urol 138:1461–1466, 1987.
25. Mundy AR: Detrusor instability. Br J Urol 62:393–397, 1988.
26. Cardoza L: Urethral instability in normal postmenopausal patients. In Proceedings of the 22nd Meeting of the International Continence Society, Halifax, September, 1992, p 103.
27. Sorenson S, Norgard JP, Djurhuus JC: Continuous urethral pressure measurement in healthy female volunteers. Neurourol Urodyn 5:525, 1986.
28. Suthhurst JR, Brown M: The effect on the bladder pressure of sudden entry of fluid into the posterior urethra. Br J Urol 50:400, 1978.
29. Sorenson S: Urethral pressure variations in healthy and incontinent women. Neurourol Urodyn 6:549–591, 1992.
30. Frewen WK: An objective assessment of the unstable bladder of psychosomatic origin. Br J Urol 50:246, 1978.
31. Farrah DJ, Whiteside CG, Osbourne JL, et al: A urodynamic analysis of micturition symptoms in the female. Surg Gynecol Obstet 141:875, 1975.
32. Cantor TJ, Bates CB: A comparative study of symptoms and objective urodynamic findings in 214 incontinent women. Br J Obstet Gynecol 87:889, 1980.
33. Cardoza L, Stanton SL: Genuine stress incontinence and detrusor instability: A clinical and urodynamic review of 200 cases. Br J Obstet Gynecol 87:184, 1980.
34. Helton P, Stanton SL: Algorhythmic method for assessing urinary incontinence in elderly women. Br Med J 282:940, 1981.
35. Cooper CE: Giggle micturition. In Colvin I, McKeith RC, Meadow RS (eds): Bladder Control and Enuresis. Clinical Developmental Medicine, No. 48 & 49. London, William Heinneman Medical Books, 1973, pp 61–65.
36. Rogers MD, Gittes RF, Dawson DM, et al: Giggle incontinence. JAMA 247:1446, 1982.
37. Turner-Warwick R, Milroy E: A reappraisal of the value of routine urologic procedures and the assessment of urodynamic function. Urol Clin North Am 6:63, 1979.
38. Webster GD: Urodynamic studies. In Resnick MI, Older RA, (eds): Diagnosis of Genitourinary Disease. New York, Thieme Stratton, 1982, p 173.
39. Webster GD, Older RA: Videourodynamics. Urology 16:106, 1980.
40. Bartia NM, Bergman A: Urodynamic appraisal of vaginal vs. rectal pressure recordings as indication of intraabdominal pressure changes. Urology 57:482, 1986.
41. Bates CP, Whiteside CG, Turner-Warwick R: Synchronous

cine/pressure/flow cystourethrography with special reference to stress and urge incontinence. Br J Urol 42:714, 1970.

42. Anderson JT, Bradley WE: Postural detrusor hyperreflexia. J Urol 116:228, 1976.

43. Turner-Warwick RT: Observation on the function and dysfunction of the sphincter and detrusor mechanism. Urol Clin North Am 6:13, 1979.

44. Webb RJ, Griffiths CJ, Ramsden PD, et al: Measurement of voiding pressures on ambulatory monitoring: Comparison with conventional cystometry. Br J Urol 65:152–154, 1990.

45. McInerney PD, Vanner TF, Harris AB, Stephenson TP: Ambulatory urodynamics. Br J Urol 67:272–274, 1991.

46. Webster GD: Urinary incontinence. *In* Resnick MK, Older RA (eds): Diagnosis of Genitourinary Disease. New York, Thieme Stratton, 1982, p 517.

47. Jonas U, Kramer AEJL: Trends in future urodynamics: Computer support data base digitized imaging. Urol Int 47 (Suppl 1):9–15, 1991.

48. Esk P, Hawk B: Pressure measurement techniques in urodynamic investigation. Neurourol Urodyn 9:1–15, 1990.

49. Stroebel CF, Glueck BC: Biofeedback treatment in medicine and psychiatry: An ultimate placebo? Semin Psych 5:379, 1973.

50. Cardoza LD, Abrams PD, Stanton SL, Finelly RCL: Idiopathic bladder instability treated by biofeedback. Br J Urol 50:521, 1978.

51. Frewen WK: Role of bladder training in the treatment of the unstable bladder in the female. Urol Clin North Am 6:273, 1979.

52. Holmes DM, Stone AR, Berry PR: Bladder training. Three years on. Br J Urol 55:660–664, 1983.

53. Frewen WK: The significance of the psychosomatic factor in urge incontinence. Br J Urol 56:313, 1984.

54. Elder DD, Stephenson TP, Berry TR: An assessment of the Frewen regimen in the treatment of detrusor dysfunction in females. *In* Zinner NR, Sterling AM (eds): Female Incontinence. New York, Alan R. Liss, 1982, pp 321–328.

55. Haffner RJ, Stanton SL, Guy J: Psychiatric study of women with urgency and urge incontinence. Br J Urol 49:211, 1977.

56. McCauley AJ, Stern RS, Holmes DM, et al: Micturition and the mind: Psychologic factors in the etiology and treatment of urinary symptoms in women. Br Med J 294:540, 1987.

57. Freeman RM, Baxby K: Hypnotherapy for incontinence caused by the unstable bladder. Br Med J 284:1831, 1982.

58. Philip T, Shore TJR, Worth PHL: Acupuncture and the treatment of bladder instability. Br J Urol 61:419, 1988.

59. Elbadawi A: Neuromuscular mechanisms of micturition. *In* Yalla SV, McGuire EJ, Elbadawi A (eds): Neurourology and Urodynamics. New York, Macmillan, 1988, pp 3–35.

60. Gosling JA, Dixon JS, Humphryson JR: Functional Anatomy of the Urinary Tract. London, Gower Medical, 1983.

61. Wein AJ, Barrett DM: Voiding Function and Dysfunction: A Logical and Practical Approach. Chicago, Year Book, 1988.

62. Benson GS, Wein AJ, Raezer DM, et al: Adrenergic and cholinergic stimulation and blockade of the human bladder base. J Urol 116:174, 1976.

63. Restorek JM, Mundy AR: The density of cholinergic and alpha and beta adrenergic receptors into the normal and hyperreflexic human detrusor. Br J Urol 63:32, 1989.

64. Mundy AR: Neuropeptides in lower urinary tract function. World J Urol 2:211, 1984.

65. Wein AJ: Nonsurgical management of bladder dysfunction. *In* Webster GD, Kirby R, Goldwasser B, King LR (eds): Reconstructive Urology. Boston, Blackwell Scientific, 1993, p 403.

66. Jensen D Jr: Pharmacological studies of the uninhibited neurogenic bladder. Acta Neurol Scand 64:175, 1981.

67. Weiner N: Atropine scopalamine and related antimuscuritic drugs. *In* Gilman AG, Goodman LS, Raul TW, et al (eds): Goodman and Gilman's Pharmacologic Basis of Therapeutics, 7th ed. New York, Macmillan, 1985, pp 130–144.

68. Wein AJ: Drug treatment of voiding dysfunction. AUA Update Series, vol. 7, nos. 14, 15. Houston, American Urological Association, 1988, pp 106–109.

69. Nadzebaker H, Jil G: Control of detrusor hyperreflexia by the intravesical instillation of oxybutynine hydrochloride. Paraplegia 19:84, 1991.

70. Kholer R, Morales P: Cystometric evaluation of flavoxate hydrochloride in normal and neurogenic bladders. J Urol 100:79, 1968.

71. Peters D, Multicenter Study Group: Terodtoline in the treatment of urinary frequency and motor urge incontinence. A controlled multicenter trial. Scand J Urol Nephrol 87 (Suppl):21, 1984.

72. Lindholm P, Luc G: Terbutaline (Bricanyl) in the treatment of female urge incontinence. Urol Int 41:158, 1986.

73. Raezer DM, Benson GS, Wein AJ, Duckett W: The functional approach to the management of the pediatric neuropathic bladder. J Urol 117:649, 1977.

74. Burgess C, Turner T: Cardiotoxicity of antidepressant drugs. Neuropharmacology 19:115, 1980.

75. Castleden C, George C, Redwick A: Imipramine: A possible alternative to current therapy for urinary incontinence in the elderly. J Urol 125:218, 1981.

76. Rittig S, Knudsen UB, Norgaard SP, et al: Abnormal diurnal rhythm of plasma vasopressin and urinary output in patients with enuresis. Am J Physiol 256:664, 1989.

77. Erickson BC, Bergman S, Eik-nes SH: Maximal electrostimulation of the pelvic floor in female idiopathic detrusor instability and urge incontinence. Neurourol Urodyn 8:219, 1989.

78. Ohlsson BL, Fall M, Frankenberg-Sommar S: Effects of external and direct pudendal nerve maximal electrical stimulation in the treatment of the uninhibited overactive bladder. Br J Urol 64:374, 1989.

79. Plevnik S, Jenes J, et al: Short term electrical stimulation: Home treatment for urinary incontinence. World J Urol 4:24, 1986.

80. Lapides J, Diokno AL, Silber SJ, Lowe BS: Clean intermittent self-catheterization in the treatment of urinary disease. J Urol 107:458–461, 1972.

81. Seen JT: Anatomic effect of distension therapy on unstable bladders: A new approach. Urology 11(6):581, 1978.

82. Pengelly AW, Stephenson TP, Milroy EJ, et al: Results of prolonged bladder distension as treatment for detrusor instability. Br J Urol 50:243, 1978.

83. Higson RH, Smith JC, Whelin P: Bladder rupture: An acceptable complication of distension therapy? Br J Urol 55:299, 1978.

84. Turner-Warwick R, Ashken MA: The functional result of partial, subtotal and total cystoplasty with special reference to ureterocecoplasty, selective sphincterotomy and cystocystoplasty. Br J Urol 39:3–12, 1967.

85. Hodgkinson CP, Drucker BH: Intravesical nerve resection for detrusor dyssynergia. Acta Obstet Gynecol Scand 56:41, 1977.

86. Parsons KF, Oboil PJ, Gibbon NOK: A further assessment of bladder transection in the management of adult enuresis and allied conditions. Br J Urol 49:509–514, 1977.

87. Mundy AR: Long term results of bladder transection for urge incontinence. Br J Urol 55:642–644, 1983.

88. Chapple C: Subtrigonal phenol injection. How safe and effective is it? Br J Urol 68:483, 1991.

89. Bramble FJ: The treatment of adult enuresis and urge incontinence by enterocystoplasty. Br J Urol 54:693, 1982.

90. Mundy AR, Stephenson TP: "Clam" ileocystoplasty for the treatment of refractory urge incontinence. Br J Urol 57:641, 1985.

91. McRae P, Murray KAH, Nurse DHE, et al: Clam enterocystoplasty in the neuropathic bladder. Br J Urol 65:23, 1987.

92. Webster GD: The unstable bladder. *In* Raz S (ed): Female Urology. Philadelphia, W. B. Saunders, 1983, pp 139–160.

CHAPTER 21

Bladder Training in the Management of Urinary Incontinence in Community-Dwelling Women

Denise M. Elser, M.D.
J. Andrew Fantl, M.D.

Voluntary control over bladder function is learned in early childhood. Therefore, continence combines normal physiologic function with a learned social behavior. An adult woman with a "normal" bladder is able to suppress detrusor contractions until the time and place are appropriate for voiding. Besides maintaining continence, the absence of involuntary contractions enables the bladder to accommodate a reasonable volume of urine before the sensation of bladder filling and the urge to urinate are experienced.

Behavioral interventions have become popular in the management of dysfunctions of the lower urinary tract. They are helpful in the treatment of incontinence due to urethral sphincter or detrusor dysfunction as well as idiopathic sensory syndromes (urgency-frequency). Bladder training, a form of behavioral therapy, is appealing as a first-line treatment because of its relatively low cost, absent risk of morbidity, and preservation of other treatment options such as pharmacologic or surgical interventions.

Bladder training is based on the principles of operant learning.[1] Accordingly, new behaviors are learned by gradually changing old behaviors toward the desired goal. The final objective is achieved by using intermediate steps and positive reinforcement. The intermediate goals in bladder training are gradually increased interval times between voluntary voiding episodes. If this is effective, the positive reinforcement is represented by decreased incontinence, decreased urinary urgency, and praise from the therapist. Most behavioral interventions focus on dysfunction of the storage phase. A classification of different lower urinary tract dysfunctions is presented in Table 21–1.[2] Several different types of behavioral therapies are presently used. In those therapies us-

ing training based on the principle of operant learning, the following types were described in the recent Clinical Guidelines published by the Agency for Health Care Policy and Research Guidelines for Urinary Incontinence in Adults[3] (Table 21–2).

Bladder training or bladder retraining essentially consists of three primary components: education, scheduled voiding, and positive reinforcement. Patients are educated about the physiology and pathophysiology of continence and incontinence. The voiding schedule requires a gradual increase in the time elapsed between voluntary micturition. The patient is taught to employ distraction or relaxation techniques if an urge to urinate occurs prior to the sched-

TABLE 21–1
The ICS Classification of Lower Urinary Tract Dysfunction

The Storage Phase	The Voiding Phase
Bladder function during storage	Detrusor function during voiding
1. Detrusor activity	voiding
a. Normal	1. Normal
b. Overactive	2. Underactive
2. Bladder sensation	3. Acontractile
a. Normal	Urethral function during
b. Increased (hypersensitive)	voiding
c. Reduced (hyposensitive)	1. Normal
d. Absent	2. Obstructive
3. Bladder capacity	a. Overactive
4. Bladder compliance	b. Mechanical
Urethral function during storage	
1. Normal	
2. Incompetent	

From Walters MD: Mechanisms of continence and voiding, with International Continence Society classification of dysfunction. Obstet Gynecol Clin North Am 16(4):773–786, 1989.

247

TABLE 21–2
**Scheduling Regimens Used as Behavioral Interventions for Urinary
Incontinence**

Regimen	Interval Between Micturitions	Characteristics	Clinical Base
Bladder training	Increased	Intervals are progressively increased; increments may be mandatory or self-adjusted	Mostly used in functionally and mentally intact subjects
Habit retraining	Increased or decreased	Schedule is adjusted to the patient's natural pattern, but patient then tries to increase the interval	Same
Timed voiding	Unchanged or fixed	Typically every 2 hours	Mostly used in nursing home residents or patients with neurogenic dysfunctions
Prompted voiding	Voidings are prompted and schedules are variable	—	Used in institutionalized subjects with cognitive and mobility impairment

Modified from Hadley EC: Bladder training and related therapies for urinary incontinence in older people. JAMA 256:372–379, 1986. Copyright 1986, American Medical Association.

uled voiding episode. The patient is praised for achieving an increase in time between voids or a decrease in incontinent episodes.

Habit training or timed voiding involves setting a schedule for a patient to toilet on a planned basis. The schedule for each patient is individualized and attempts to match the patient's own voiding schedule. No special effort is made to delay voiding or to resist urge.

Prompted voiding has mainly been useful in treating cognitively impaired nursing home patients. Prompted voiding has three main components. The first is monitoring, with which the patient is checked on a regular basis and asked to report if she is wet or dry. The second component is prompting, with which the patient is asked to use the toilet and is given assistance if necessary. Finally, the patient is praised both for keeping dry and for trying to toilet. In some programs the patient is also praised for correctly reporting whether she is wet or dry.

Behavioral therapies can also be categorized as (1) *self-management strategies*, which are used in ambulatory, cognitively intact adults (i.e., bladder training), and (2) *environmental or external strategies*, which are used in physically or cognitively impaired adults living in institutional settings (i.e., prompted voiding).

History and Evolution of Bladder Training

This intervention has been used in both inpatient and outpatient programs.

INPATIENT PROGRAMS

Jeffcoate and Francis originally introduced bladder training for the treatment of urgency incontinence in women approximately 30 years ago.[4] They observed that women with urinary urgency, who voided frequently during the day, for the most part did not do so at night. They concluded that frequent voiding in these patients was a bad habit and that there was

no evidence of intrinsic bladder pathology. They also noted that the peak age range of these patients was 40 to 60 years, which led them to correlate these lower urinary tract dysfunctions to situational life stresses characteristic of such an age group. These authors believed that retraining programs would help in acquiring good bladder habits in addition to providing psychological support.

In their original work, Jeffcoate and Francis reported 300 women with "urge incontinence." These patients had been admitted to the hospital for evaluation and treatment. Organic causes of urgency, such as cystitis or bladder tumor, were ruled out and an intensive inpatient routine of bladder discipline was started. Education of the patient and participation in her own care was stressed. Jeffcoate and Francis noted that "the essential treatment in all cases consists of making the woman aware of the nature of her problem, and in teaching her to correct what has become a bad habit of voiding frequently and to regain voluntary control of the bladder reflex."

Each patient was instructed to void every 1 or 2 hours by the clock. The time interval depended on the severity of the particular case. "Under no circumstances" was the patient allowed to void before the instructed time. When a woman was able to void comfortably by the schedule, usually in a few days, the time interval was then increased by half an hour. After an average of $2\frac{1}{2}$ weeks, the patient was able to void only every $3\frac{1}{2}$ to 4 hours. Hospital admission was considered necessary to maintain adequate discipline by a "firm but sympathetic nursing staff" and to remove the patient from "causal environmental factors." A patient was discharged home only after she was voiding comfortably every $3\frac{1}{2}$ hours and had developed confidence that she had her bladder under control. Bladder training is now performed in an outpatient setting, but otherwise not much has changed since this original description.

OUTPATIENT PROGRAMS

Frewen popularized the use of bladder training.[5] He analyzed the results of outpatient bladder training in 90 patients with urgency and frequency, with or without urinary incontinence. This intervention did not make use of adjuvant pharmacologic management. Patients recorded the frequency of their voids on a chart. The improved voiding pattern on the bladder diary was considered to be strong positive feedback. Education about the storage function of the bladder was stressed. A patient was considered cured if her voiding chart was free from abnormal symptoms and if voids were no closer than every 3 hours. After 3 months, 86.6% patients were considered cured. In 82 patients who had undergone pretreatment cystometry, the symptomatic cure rate was not related to the persistence or disappearance of abnormal cystometric findings of detrusor instability. This led Frewen to believe that "detrusor instability" is the end product of urgency-frequency syndromes and not the cause.

Pengelly and Booth observed that three factors were found to correlate with poor success in using bladder training: (1) a history of nocturnal enuresis at any time after age 10; (2) a strong (above 100 cm H_2O) isometric contraction during voluntary interruption of micturition; and (3) failure to show improvement within the first 2 weeks of treatment.[6] The third observation seems to be shared with most investigators of this technique, including ourselves.

Sensory Syndromes (Urgency-Frequency) and Bladder Training

By 1981, bladder drill was widely considered the first-line treatment for frequency, nocturia, urgency, and incontinence associated with an unstable bladder.[7] The use of bladder drill has been extended to treat patients with primary vesical sensory urgency. Essentially, this diagnosis is applied to patients with complaints of urgency and frequency whose only abnormal cystometric finding is a first sensation of a need to void at 75 ml or less, or a maximum bladder capacity of less than 500 ml. Jarvis treated 33 women with primary vesical sensory urgency as inpatients using bladder drill.

The first urge to void and the maximum cystometric capacity increased from 40 ml and 279 ml prior to treatment to 93 ml and 463 ml, respectively. Sixty-one percent of the women were subjectively cured of urgency 6 months after the treatment period.

Anticholinergic Therapy

Jeffcoate and Francis treated all their patients on bladder training with anticholinergic medications during their entire inpatient stay and for several weeks after they returned home.[4] They believed that the medications were of great psychological benefit to the patients in their attempt to gain control of bladder function.

Mahady and Begg treated 78 women with subjective urge incontinence using bladder "reeducation."[8] They also employed psychotherapy, daily micturition charts, and voiding schedules. These authors believed that anxiety about waiting until the next scheduled void time acted as negative feedback. The improvement in voiding frequency as evidenced by the notations in the bladder diary was considered positive biofeedback. Mahady and Begg also included pharmacologic treatment in the intervention. All patients were initially treated with emepronium bromide 200 mg three times a day and 400 mg at night, as well as chlordiazepoxide 10 mg three times a day. As soon as the patients were continent between voids, the drugs were rapidly withdrawn. No controlled studies were done to determine the benefits of bladder training with and without the addition of pharmacologic therapy.

In a review of 92 patients with a urodynamically proven diagnosis of idiopathic detrusor instability, Fantl and colleagues ascertained that the success rate of bladder drills was not improved by the concomitant use of anticholinergic drugs.[9]

Bladder Training in Older Women

Fantl and colleagues studied the efficacy of bladder training in community-dwelling women 55 years of age or older.[10] One hundred and twenty-three such women underwent urodynamic testing. They were classified as having either pure genuine stress incontinence (GSI) or detrusor instability either alone or with GSI. All patients were randomly placed into a treatment group of 6 weeks of bladder training or into the control group. Those in the control group were asked to return after 6 weeks without intervention. At the end of this period, the controls also underwent 6 weeks of bladder training. After completion of bladder training, there was a significant decrease in the number of incontinent episodes in the treatment group (9 per week vs. 21 per week previously). There was no significant change for the control group.

An unexpected finding in this study was that the specific urodynamic diagnosis, pure GSI or detrusor instability with or without GSI, did not affect the results of bladder training. Previously, bladder training had been used only to treat women with detrusor dysfunction as opposed to those with sphincteric problems, which were always considered "anatomic disorders." These observations cannot yet be fully explained. Possible mechanisms of action of this type of intervention include changes in the physiologic mechanism of continence such as striated muscle contraction (voluntary or involuntary) as well as detrusor inhibition. It is also likely that the patient may adopt continence-promoting behaviors such as emptying the bladder prior to exercise or avoidance of situations leading to incontinent episodes.[11] Table 21–3 contains a summary of previous reports of the

TABLE 21–3
Previous Reports of the Use of Bladder Training in Urinary Incontinent Women

Authors	Design	No. Subjects and Ages	Urodynamic Category	Outcome Criteria	Cure Rates[a] (%)	Follow-up Period
Svigos and Matthews[12]	Series	n = 28 age not stated	DI	Subjective	50	6–12 months
Frewen[13]	Series	n = 50 age 15–77	DI	Subjective stable detrusor	82	3 months
Pengelly and Booth[6]	Series	n = 27 age 10–70	DI	NA	44	3 months
Elder and Stephenson[14]	Series	n = 21 age 12–59	Urge incontinence, DI, reduced compliance, SI	NA	52–86	3 months
Mahady and Begg[8]	Series	n = 48 age 22–82	DI, reduced compliance, reduced capacity	Subjective	75–90	6–48 months
Jarvis and Millar[15]	Randomized with untreated controls	n = 60 age 27–78	DI	NA	86–90	6 months
Fantl et al[9]	Series	n = 92 age 35–55	DI	Subjective	72	6 months
Jarvis[16]	Randomized with drug-treated controls	n = 50 age 33–61	DI	NA	47–64	1–4 to 12 weeks
Jarvis[7]	Series	n = 33 age 44	Sensory urgency without DI	Subjective urilos test	61–65	6 months
Frewen[5]	Series	n = 33 age 5–75	DI	Subjective	66–97	3 months
Fantl et al[18]	Randomized clinical trial	n = 131 age 55–90	GSI, DI, DI ± GSI	Subjective and objective	57	6 months

Abbreviations: DI, detrusor instability; NA, not applicable; GSI, genuine stress incontinence
[a]Definitions vary widely among studies
Modified from Hadley EC: Bladder training and related therapies for urinary incontinence in older people. JAMA 256:372–379, 1986. Copyright 1986, American Medical Association.

TABLE 21–4
Bladder Training Instructions

The Bladder Training Program is expected to help you regain bladder control. The program works by assisting you to reestablish a normal pattern. (Remember, **voiding** is the term used to describe voluntary emptying of the bladder.) You will do this by practicing voiding on a specified schedule. Initially the schedule time between voidings will be brief. However, this time period will gradually be lengthened over the course of the program until you achieve a normal voiding pattern.
It is important for you to follow the directions exactly as they are described. **The success of the program depends on careful and consistent following of the voiding schedule.**

Instructions
1. Begin the bladder training program tomorrow morning.
2. Immediately upon arising, go to the toilet and empty your bladder as completely as you can.
3. Follow the assigned voiding schedule as listed below: Voiding schedule _____
   This means you should go to the toilet and try to empty your bladder as completely as you can every _____ during waking hours.
4. Begin your schedule every morning upon getting out of bed, and make every effort to wait until your assigned time.
5. If you feel the need to empty your bladder prior to your scheduled voiding, make every effort to wait until your assigned time.
   A suggestion which may help you push off this desire to void is to concentrate on a task which you need to complete. For example, think about preparations for the next meal, balancing the checkbook, or some other activity that requires a great deal of concentration. Another suggestion would be to sit down and take five slow deep breaths. Try to concentrate on your breathing and not your bladder sensation. Often times, the urge to empty your bladder will pass.
   If you have to interrupt your schedule, get back on schedule at the assigned time even if it has been only a few minutes.
6. Follow your voiding schedule as closely as you can. Even if **you do not feel the desire to void**, go to the toilet at the assigned time, and try to empty your bladder. Remember, the amount of urine in your bladder is not important; the important part is your effort to empty it. Whether you urinate a few drops or a pint, if really does not matter. The important thing is the effort.
7. Record each of your voidings on the Treatment Log. Use a new Treatment Log each day.
   a. Make a check ($\checkmark$) in the circle by the time on the clock face to show that you followed the schedule.
   b. If you miss voiding at the assigned time, leave the circle blank.
   c. If you interrupt your interval between a scheduled voiding, record the time you did so using the back side of the Treatment Log.
   d. Use the back side of the Treatment Log for all voidings off schedule including any incontinent or leaking episodes, and the times of your nighttime voiding.
8. If you missed one or more scheduled voidings, return to the schedule as soon as you remember.
9. Your Treatment Logs will be reviewed each week. If you have been able to control your bladder on this schedule without any problems, the voiding interval will be increased by 30 minutes. This pattern will gradually continue each week until you achieve a normal voiding schedule.
   If you have had difficulty controlling your bladder on this schedule, the time period between voidings may remain the same or be shortened. It will be adjusted to meet your needs.

From Wyman JF, Fantl JA: Bladder training in ambulatory care management of urinary incontinence. Urol Nurs 3:11–17, 1991.

use of bladder training in urinary incontinent women.

Current Bladder Training Program at The Medical College of Virginia

In our institution, the bladder training program involves a 6-week outpatient treatment period. Candidates for this behavioral therapy are women who suffer from incontinence or urgency and are mentally intact, motivated, and ambulatory. Poor candidates for bladder training are those considered physically or mentally unable to comply with a voiding schedule or to toilet with or without assistance. Patients with incontinence due to causes other than GSI or detrusor instability are not considered likely to benefit from this behavioral therapy. Our program is based on the teachings of behavioral modification and involves the following components: (1) a scheduled voiding protocol, (2) patient education, which includes strategies for controlling urgency, (3) self-monitoring of voiding behavior, and (4) reinforcement techniques with treatment compliance assessment.

SCHEDULED VOIDING PROTOCOL

Individuals are assigned a voiding schedule. They are asked to comply with this schedule during wak-

Instructions: Use this side to indicate all unscheduled voidings including interruptions in schedule, nighttime voidings, and incontinent episodes.

TIME	URINATE IN TOILET	LEAKING ACCIDENT	COMMENTS
12-1 AM			
1-2 AM			
2-3 AM			
3-4 AM			
4-5 AM			
5-6 AM			
6-7 AM			
7-8 AM			
8-9 AM			
9-10 AM			
10-11 AM			
11-12 NOON			
12-1 PM			
1-2 PM			
2-3 PM			
3-4 PM			
4-5 PM			
5-6 PM			
6-7 PM			
7-8 PM			
8-9 PM			
9-10 PM			
10-11 PM			
11-12 PM			

Awake Time _____ Bed Time _____ # of Pads Used _____

Figure 21-2 Treatment log 2 used in a continence program for women. (Used with permission from J.F. Wyman, Ph.D., R.N. [unpublished].)

ing hours. Usually the initial assignment is to void every hour, but lesser time intervals are considered when needed. The voiding interval is gradually increased by half an hour weekly until the goal of voiding every 3 to 4 hours is achieved.

PATIENT EDUCATION

All patients are provided with audiovisual, written, and verbal instructions on normal bladder control, the pathophysiology behind the patient's particular type of incontinence, and a description of the bladder training intervention. The importance of breaking old habits such as running to the toilet at the first urge is emphasized. Descriptions of distraction techniques are provided in Table 21–4.

Each patient monitors herself via a treatment log. The patient is given a log in the form of a clock face as shown in Figures 21–1 and 21–2. The assigned schedule is indicated by open circles placed at the appropriate number on the clock. The patient checks the circle if she is compliant and leaves it blank if she is not. On the back of each log the patient records incontinence episodes, symptoms of urgency, and nocturnal frequency. In the early part of treatment, weekly visits with a nurse specialist or physician provide positive feedback, encouragement, and a chance to ask questions.

Tuesday

Continence Program For Women
Treatment Log

Chart No. _____   Date ___ / ___ / ___

MIDNIGHT TO NOON   **NOON TO MIDNIGHT**

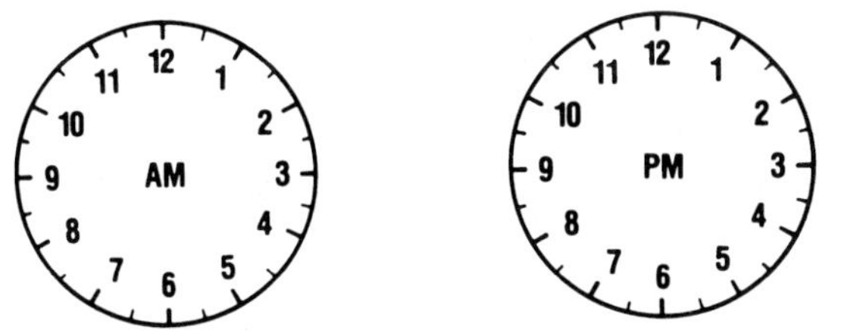

WEEKLY VOIDING INTERVAL _____

Treatment Number _____

No. of Scheduled Voidings _____

No. of Scheduled Voidings Missed _____

No. of Scheduled Voidings Interrupted _____

Nocturnal Frequency _____

Incontinent Episodes _____

Day Missed (Y/N) _____

Figure 21-1 Treatment log 1 used in a continence program for women. (Used with permission from J.F. Wyman, Ph.D., R.N. [unpublished].)

Conclusion

Behavioral therapy, specifically bladder training, is an effective means of treating genuine stress incontinence, detrusor instability, and mixed incontinence. Bladder training is also useful in the management of patients who suffer sensory urge but are not incontinent. Bladder training is inexpensive, has no side effects, is implemented in an outpatient setting, and requires no special equipment. In addition to these advantages, bladder training cures or effects significant improvement in many women who suffer from urinary incontinence.

REFERENCES

1. Wyman JF, Fantl JA: Bladder training in ambulatory care management of urinary incontinence. Urol Nurs September: 11–17, 1991.
2. Abrams P, Blaivas JG, Stanton SL, Andersen JT: The International Continence Society on Standardisation of Terminology. The standardisation of terminology of lower urinary tract function. Scand J Urol Nephrol (Suppl 114):5–19, 1988.
3. Agency for Health Care Policy and Research, Clinical Practice Guidelines: Urinary Incontinence in Adults. Rockville, MD, Agency for Health Care Policy and Research, Public Health Service, U.S. Department of Health and Human Services, 1992.
4. Jeffcoate TNA, Francis WJA: Urgency incontinence in the female. Am J Obstet Gynecol 94:604–618, 1966.
5. Frewen WK: A reassessment of bladder training in detrusor dysfunction in the female. Br J Urol 54:372–373, 1982.
6. Pengelly AW, Booth CM: A prospective trial of bladder training as treatment for detrusor instability. Br J Urol 52:463–466, 1980.
7. Jarvis GJ: The management of urinary incontinence due to primary vesical sensory urgency by bladder drill. Br J Urol 54:374–376, 1982.
8. Mahady IW, Begg BM: Long-term symptomatic and cystometric cure of the urge incontinence syndrome using a technique of bladder re-education. Br J Obstet Gynecol 88:1038–1043, 1981.
9. Fantl JA, Hurt WG, Dunn LJ: Detrusor instability syndrome: The use of bladder retraining drills with and without anticholinergics. Am J Obstet Gynecol 140:885–890, 1981.
10. Fantl JA, Wyman JF, McClish DK, et al: Efficacy of bladder training in older women with urinary incontinence. JAMA 265:609–613, 1991.
11. Hadley EC: Bladder training and related therapies for urinary incontinence in older people. JAMA 256:372–379, 1986.
12. Svigos JM, Matthews DC: Assessment and treatment of female urinary incontinence by cystometrogram and bladder retraining programs. Obstet Gynecol 50:9–12, 1977.
13. Frewen WK: Urgency incontinence. J Obstet Gynaecol Br Comm 79:77, 1972.
14. Elder DD, Stephenson TP: An assessment of the Frewen regime in the treatment of detrusor dysfunction in females. Br J Urol 52:467–471, 1980.
15. Jarvis GJ, Millar DR: Controlled trial of bladder drill for detrusor instability. Br Med J 281:1322–1323, 1980.
16. Jarvis GJ: A controlled trial of bladder drill and drug therapy in the management of detrusor instability. Br J Urol 53:565–566, 1981.
17. Fantl JA: Behavioral therapy for detrusor instability of idiopathic etiology. In Ostergard DR (ed): Gynecologic Urology and Urodynamics: Theory and Practice, 2nd ed. Baltimore, Williams & Wilkins, 1985.
18. Fantl JA, Wyman JF, McClish DK, et al: Efficacy of bladder training in older women with urinary incontinence. JAMA 265:609–613, 1991.

CHAPTER 22

Biofeedback Therapy

Pat D. O'Donnell, M.D.

There are many patients with symptoms of voiding dysfunction for whom a nonsurgical approach is the preferred treatment option based on either patient preference or the clinical situation. In addition, many patients who are treated nonsurgically with medication either fail to respond to this therapy or are unable to tolerate the side effects. When surgical treatment is not the preferred initial management option and pharmacologic therapy is not effective, behavioral therapy is an excellent treatment alternative. The results of behavioral therapy have been extremely successful in the management of many different types of voiding dysfunction affecting a wide age range of patients. For this reason, behavioral therapy has become the preferred initial treatment choice for many bladder-related symptoms because of its excellent therapeutic results and minimal side effects.

Of the different types of behavioral therapy commonly used in urology, biofeedback therapy is the most specific and has the greatest potential for producing the best results in the most patients. In addition to the excellent clinical results achieved in initial treatment of voiding dysfunction, behavioral therapy is also an excellent choice for treatment of symptoms that occasionally remain following surgical or pharmacologic therapy. Also, behavioral therapy can be used in combination with pharmacologic therapy for treatment of residual bladder symptoms following surgical procedures. Therefore, at any time in the course of management of voiding dysfunction, behavioral therapy can provide an excellent response with minimal side effects and can be used as either a primary treatment choice or secondarily to augment other treatment.

In clinical urology the management of voiding dysfunction in women represents a significant segment of any practice, and it is important to be able to offer biofeedback therapy as a choice. The results of biofeedback therapy have been excellent for almost all clinicians and investigators who have used the technique.[1–19] Currently, the attitude of women in our society is changing to one that is much more positive toward personal participation in the management of their own health problems. This is extremely important because the personal commitment of the patient is essential for the success of biofeedback therapy. Also, when the patient is personally involved in treatment, the option of biofeedback therapy is usually much more attractive to the patient.

Although setting up a biofeedback laboratory and successfully treating patients with voiding dysfunction are not complicated, there are many aspects of the use of biofeedback in the treatment of lower urinary tract disorders that must be understood by the clinician to ensure success. Like many treatment options, biofeedback has many advantages as well as some disadvantages. For both the patient and the clinician, behavioral therapy is very different from most medical or surgical treatment programs. For example, in treating a problem such as voiding dysfunction, biofeedback therapy is very different from taking a pill three times a day and evaluating the response. Very little patient involvement is required in swallowing a pill. However, changing the visceral responses of body organs using behavioral therapy is a very complex physiologic process. Although the results of biofeedback therapy for many disorders have been excellent, the mechanism by which these changes occur is not well understood. Although it is not possible to understand completely how biofeedback works, much information is available about it that can help the clinician in applying this treatment to specific problems of the lower urinary tract. It is important to recognize that these principles must be understood by the clinician to ensure the success of the treatment.

Instrumental Learning

In instrumental learning, also called operant conditioning or trial and error learning, a response is learned and performed depending on whether that response is followed by reinforcement.[20–22] Instrumental learning is more flexible than classic conditioning because it does not depend on an unconditioned stimulus that already elicits the response to be learned. In instrumental learning the responses that are reinforced are strengthened, and those that are not reinforced are weakened. For example, if a person is learning to shoot a basketball from the free throw line, the sight of the ball going through the hoop indicates success and through visual feedback serves as a reinforcement to repeat the same muscle activity, thus producing the same successful result. Likewise, seeing it miss the hoop indicates failure and shows that the effort that led to that result must be changed to produce a successful result. In this situation, the person will improve his or her shooting skills only if he has knowledge of the results of the performance. If the athlete were blindfolded to prevent any knowledge of where the basketball was in relation to the basket, he would not learn to shoot free throws successfully. The sight of the course of the basketball relative to the basket is the visual feedback of performance. This is a simple example of a method of learning voluntary motor skills that is very similar to the technique and concepts used in biofeedback therapy for urinary incontinence.

In the early experiments of Pavlov, the "unconditioned response" of salivation in dogs in response to the smell of meat was coupled with the sound of a bell that subsequently produced the "conditioned response" of salivation in response to the sound of the bell only. These early studies demonstrated that autonomically innervated reactions could be modified by conditioning. Because "classic conditioning" had shown that autonomic responses could be modified, the next question was whether autonomic responses could be modified by trial and error learning. Many excellent studies have clearly demonstrated that a large number of autonomic body functions can be modified by learning.[23–28] Of particular importance to urologists is the ability of a patient to modify bladder function through instrumental learning or operant conditioning. Because there is no unconditioned response in the environment that produces micturition such as occurs in dogs salivating in response to the smell of food, classic conditioning is not used in behavioral therapy for voiding dysfunction.

Modifying the physiologic basis of autonomic functions is an extremely complex physiologic process, and modifying control of bladder function is no exception. Modification of bladder function using biofeedback has had its most successful application in patients with disorders of bladder storage, particularly urinary incontinence and irritative bladder syndromes. Although normal voiding is a voluntary function, bladder storage is involuntary. For example, people do not constantly voluntarily inhibit the bladder or contract the external sphincter to prevent incontinence throughout the day during normal daily activities. People are normally unaware of their bladder status except when a need to void is perceived by

the brain. Therefore, the control of bladder storage normally occurs automatically. Between episodes of normal voiding, urinary leakage and distracting sensations such as an intense and inappropriate need to void do not occur in the normal individual. When either incontinence or distracting bladder symptoms occur, the automatic storage function of the bladder is abnormal. In these patients, the sensory-motor balance or facilitory-inhibitory balance of bladder control appears to be abnormal. The regulatory balance of bladder control and urethral function must be modified in these patients.

Effective functioning of any biologic system is contingent on the return of information about its performance to that system. All homeostatic mechanisms of the body depend on complicated interrelated feedback mechanisms that serve to stabilize the internal environment. In a similar way, all skill learning depends on a knowledge of results. In any biologic system under voluntary control, practice makes perfect only if the individual is aware of how well he or she performs.[29] The common element among all behavioral approaches to the treatment of urinary incontinence is the concept of applying learning theory to the acquisition of a clinical therapeutic skill.[1] In the application of biofeedback to the treatment of urinary incontinence, the concepts of neurophysiology of voiding and learning and conditioning are combined to accomplish the clinical objective of voluntary control of bladder function.

Early successful attempts to modify bladder control were made by Kegel.[30–32] He introduced a systematic schedule of voluntary contractions of the pelvic muscles for the treatment of urinary incontinence. In the original studies of Kegel, a perineometer was used to provide feedback to the patient to enhance the skill acquisition of voluntary contraction of the pubococcygeus muscle. Through the perineometer, the original Kegel exercises were based on the principles of instrumental learning.

Since the initial descriptions made by Kegel, pelvic muscle exercises have been used extensively to treat women with urinary incontinence. Considerable variation has occurred in the methods used in pelvic muscle exercise programs, called Kegel exercises, but the programs usually have little in common with the technique originally used by Kegel. Kegel focused the program on the acquisition of a skill involving a specific muscle group and provided feedback of performance to the patient. Most pelvic muscle exercise programs now use verbal instruction alone to train the patient. The use of verbal instructions alone to train patients to perform tasks involving pelvic muscle activity is similar to blindfolding a basketball player and then asking him to learn to shoot free throws—he has no feedback about his own performance and has been denied the basic principles of trial and error learning. In the absence of the basic principles of operant conditioning, which involve a reward for performance of the specific task, specific task-oriented learning cannot occur. In the case of the blindfolded basketball player, regardless of motivation, his poor performance will soon cause him to become discouraged and dislike the game because it is too difficult to play successfully. Similar attitudes are often encountered in patients who have participated in a verbal instruction pelvic muscle exercise program, and the subsequent clinical results have been less encouraging than Kegel's original program.

Biofeedback treatment programs target specific learning objectives with well-defined performance goals for each patient. For the clinician using biofeedback therapy for long-term treatment of incontinence in women, a well-structured biofeedback program that teaches the patient specific muscle exercises should be used, followed by a maintenance program that uses verbal instructions to explain pelvic muscle exercises, because the patient will then be aware of the specific task to be performed. Once specific muscle exercise skills have been learned during biofeedback, verbal instructions are appropriate because they primarily concern the schedule of exercises and are not part of skill acquisition.

Clinical Background

Biofeedback had its origins in basic laboratory research on human subjects, which began more than 25 years ago. Since then, a veritable explosion of potential practical applications of biofeedback has taken place, including applications to the training of many organ systems of the body. Biofeedback therapy has been applied to the urinary bladder, and subsequent research performed in behavioral treatment of bladder dysfunctions has included primarily studies of urinary incontinence. Unfortunately, the promise of biofeedback therapy for many applications has exceeded its actual performance. There are many reasons for this, one being the fact that basic laboratory investigation of biofeedback therapy and its underlying physiologic mechanisms has not kept pace with the growth of its applications. Not enough is known about how biofeedback actually works to provide a sufficient theoretical basis for the systematic development of effective practical applications. For example, in a clinical approach to biofeedback treatment of urinary bladder disorders, the complex neurophysiology and modulation of lower urinary tract function by the central nervous system has not been well integrated with theories of learning and behavioral modification. Ideally, biofeedback therapy should be focused on the acquisition of a specific skill that directly controls the physiologic process being modified. Most biofeedback programs for the treatment of urinary incontinence in women involve acquisition of the skill of voluntary contraction of the pelvic muscles—specifically, the pubococcygeus and levator ani complex or the external anal and urethral sphincters. Systematic contraction of these muscles has the treatment goal of modifying visceral control of the autonomic storage mechanisms of the urinary bladder and urethra. Therefore, the visceral response of

bladder control resulting from biofeedback in this case is not actually feedback from the specific physiologic mechanisms directly involved in bladder control. The desired involuntary visceral response appears to result at least in part from reflex mechanisms such as reflex inhibition of detrusor contractions in response to external sphincter contraction.

Because of the difficulty experienced by the patient in understanding the muscle contraction skill that is to be acquired in pelvic muscle exercise programs, biofeedback therapy has become recognized as a very specific skill training technique and has been used successfully to improve the efficacy of the pelvic muscle exercise concept. Although biofeedback therapy of urinary incontinence in women has many potential advantages, there are still many areas of this approach that need further study and more precise definition.

ANATOMY OF THE PELVIC MUSCLES

When the objective of a biofeedback program is the voluntary contraction of the pubococcygeus muscle, the location of the muscle must be identified by the clinician and the patient. Kegel described the location of the pubococcygeus muscle and the ease with which it can be palpated transvaginally. By placing the index finger inside the vagina along the lateral surface, the pubococcygeus can be palpated along the vaginal wall approximately 3 to 4 cm deep to the labia minora. The pubococcygeus is part of the levator ani complex. The perineometer used by Kegel measured the pressure generated by voluntary contraction of the pelvic muscles and provided feedback of the success of this contraction to the patient. The levator ani complex receives motor innervation from the S2 spinal cord level. Innervation occurs through the pudendal nerve, which innervates the deep pelvic floor muscles.

Superficial to the deep pelvic floor muscles are the external anal sphincter and the external urethral sphincter. These muscles also have been used in biofeedback training. Like the deep muscles of the pelvic floor, the superficial sphincteric muscles of the anus and urethra are innervated from the S2 spinal cord level through the pudendal nerve. Voluntary contraction of the external urethral sphincter is an activity that arises in the periurethral striated muscle area of the cortex[33] and travels through the corticospinal tract to the sacral motor area and subsequently through the pudendal nerve to the external urethral sphincter as voluntary motor activity. Voluntary contraction of the external urethral sphincter results in interruption of micturition or prevention of incontinence during an episode of urgency. Voluntary contraction of the external anal and urethral sphincters also results in reflex inhibition of the bladder.

The external urethral sphincter and external anal sphincter have similar electromyographic (EMG) activity except in some patients with neurologic disorders. Therefore, contraction of the external anal sphincter also results in contraction of the external urethral sphincter. Also, voluntary contraction of the pubococcygeus muscle results in contraction of the entire levator ani complex as well as the external anal and urethral sphincters. The pelvic muscles involved in biofeedback training programs include the levator ani complex and the external anal and urethral sphincter muscles, which are superficial to the levator ani. Because the activity of these muscles can be measured, this physiologic response is a commonly used signal source in biofeedback therapy of urinary bladder storage problems.

The exact mechanism of the improvement that occurs in bladder control following pelvic muscle exercise programs is unclear. It does not appear that pelvic muscle exercise programs or muscle-specific biofeedback training programs result in an increase in maximum urethral closing pressure.[6] Thus, the effect of pelvic muscle contractions on bladder control appears to be unrelated to any effect on resting urethral pressure. Contraction of the pelvic muscles does result in reflex inhibition of the bladder. Most women who have stress urinary incontinence also have a component of urgency, and many women with stress urinary incontinence have detrusor instability during urodynamic evaluation. It is possible that pelvic muscle exercises reflexly inhibit involuntary detrusor contractions that are sometimes associated with the urge component of incontinence. Urodynamic studies of patients with genuine stress incontinence before and after biofeedback therapy show no change in any parameter measured, although the objective measures of continence are significantly improved.[4] However, patients who have detrusor instability before biofeedback therapy show a significant reduction in unstable detrusor contractions following biofeedback therapy.[5, 12, 16] Although the clinical studies completed so far suggest that an improvement in stress urinary incontinence occurs with pelvic muscle exercises,[6, 11, 34] the mechanism of that improvement is unclear at the present time. However, it is clear that the response to biofeedback therapy in patients with symptoms of stress urinary incontinence has been excellent throughout the many clinical studies performed. Further studies on the physiologic effect of biofeedback programs on genuine stress incontinence and on the response to therapy stratified by the type of incontinence clearly need to be done.

Biofeedback Technique

As stated previously, the original studies of pelvic muscle exercises performed by Kegel involved the use of a perineometer that provided feedback to the patient. After many years of modification of pelvic muscle exercise techniques, the perineometer is no longer used by most clinicians; verbal instructions are used instead. Although pelvic muscle exercise programs using verbal instruction alone are often

called Kegel exercises, these training programs lack the essential element of feedback of patient performance to aid in skill acquisition. In a study by Bump and colleagues, it was found that verbal instructions alone are inadequate to allow the patient to acquire the skills required to achieve the treatment goal.[35] The lack of standardization of pelvic muscle exercise programs has led to discouraging results for some clinicians and patients.

Although biofeedback treatment of incontinence is well recognized as effective, many questions about its use in the management of urinary bladder problems remain. These questions include queries by clinicians about proper patient selection, the skill and supervision of the person administering biofeedback therapy, the capabilities of the equipment used, the signal source used for feedback to the patient, and comparison of the performance outcome with the clinical outcome for the patient. For example, the use of pelvic muscle activity as a signal source for feedback of performance to the patient results in a performance outcome measured by the patient's ability to achieve the goal of increasing pelvic muscle activity. The clinical objective is a reduction in urinary incontinence, and the outcome measures of this goal are the frequency and volume of incontinence episodes.[36–41] Thus, the clinical success of the program is determined by the patient's ability to reduce the frequency and volume of incontinence episodes, whereas the biofeedback performance goal is a measurable increase in voluntary control of pelvic muscle activity. However, an increase in voluntary control of pelvic muscle activity and a specific pelvic muscle exercise program will result in a significant reduction in the frequency and volume of incontinence episodes. Although the distinction between these two outcome measures may be clinically irrelevant, it is important for the clinician to be aware of the different treatment goals used in biofeedback to allow this extremely valuable treatment option to become better understood, more precisely defined as a treatment choice, and further modified to improve its efficacy.

BLADDER FILLING

Many technical issues in regard to biofeedback therapy must be evaluated.[1, 42, 43] Urinary incontinence in women usually occurs more commonly when the bladder is full than when it is empty. Therefore, a simple question such as whether the bladder should be filled during a biofeedback session remains unanswered. It may be important for voluntary contraction of the pelvic muscles during biofeedback sessions to be coupled with simultaneous filling of the bladder to associate the visceral response of bladder control with the somatic response of pelvic muscle contraction (see later discussion). Therefore, artificial filling of the bladder in the biofeedback laboratory would represent more accurately the conditions under which continence must be achieved during regular daily activities. Although this concept appears to be clinically relevant and represents one of the clinical conditions of our previous studies,[1] it is not known whether bladder filling during biofeedback sessions is a treatment advantage because comparative studies have not been done.

Filling of the bladder requires catheterization with its associated discomfort and risk. In biofeedback laboratories where small urethral catheters are commonly used, catheterization can be done with minimal discomfort to patients, and prophylactic antibiotic use is a common practice following these catheterizations. Thus, artificial filling of the bladder during biofeedback sessions is associated with minimal risk and discomfort to the patient. For this reason, when voluntary increase in external sphincter activity is the skill to be acquired, artificial filling of the bladder using a medium fill rate allows the patient to develop the skill under conditions of changing intravesical volume that simulate the actual circumstances under which urinary incontinence occurs. Again, comparative studies on this concept have not been performed, and standardization of biofeedback therapy techniques for the treatment of incontinence should be more precisely defined based on comparative studies.

SIGNAL SOURCE

Another important technical issue in biofeedback therapy is the signal source used for feedback of performance to the patient.[1, 43] If the signal source does not accurately reflect the physiologic activity of the skill to be acquired, there is no logical basis for the biofeedback program. Bladder pressure, anal sphincter pressure, and anal sphincter EMG have been used as signal sources for biofeedback therapy of urinary incontinence. EMG activity has evolved as the preferred signal source for many types of biofeedback therapy,[23–28] and EMG activity of pelvic muscle contractions has become one of the most commonly used signal sources for the treatment of urinary incontinence. In our clinical studies, we have used external anal sphincter EMG as the signal source because we can be sure that the signal is accurate and the feedback to the patient represents actual performance.[1] We recommend continuous oscilloscope monitoring of the EMG signal to be certain that there is no undetected signal interference and that electrode placement provides an appropriate EMG signal.[1, 44, 45] Surface electrodes can be used in the same way they are used in diagnostic sphincteric EMG.[45] Correct placement of surface electrodes is essential for an accurate signal. Measurement of conductance across the electrodes can be done to ensure that contact of the electrode with the skin is appropriate. Finally, oscilloscope monitoring of the signal source will ensure that there is no 60-cycle power source interference and that the signal accurately represents sphincteric activity. Without an accurate signal, performance feedback to the patient is incorrect. It would be similar to the basketball player shooting free throws while wearing glasses that distorted the actual location of the basket. Thus, the importance of an accurate signal and appropriate feedback of performance cannot be overemphasized because they represent the foundation of the concept of operant conditioning and the clinical basis of biofeedback therapy.

The most accurate EMG signal from any of the pelvic muscles is obtained by using a needle electrode. The disadvantages of needle electrodes include the discomfort of the patient and the fact that they are easily dislodged and frequently require replacement. Patients undergoing multiple sessions of biofeedback therapy requiring EMG signal monitoring find repeated placement of a needle electrode extremely unpleasant; patient compliance is therefore poor and the dropout rate is high. The techniques previously described for placement of surface electrodes provide an excellent signal source with minimal discomfort to the patient.[44, 45]

The three common signal sources used (bladder pressure, anal sphincter pressure, and sphincteric EMG) are significantly altered by increases in intraabdominal pressure. Therefore, simultaneous measurement of abdominal activity must be done with all biofeedback therapy techniques.[1] If abdominal activity is not monitored, the patient often learns to strain as a way of increasing sphincteric muscle activity and showing an apparent improvement in performance. We prefer to monitor EMG activity of the rectus abdominis muscle because of the easy access and simplicity of the technique. Because the signal from the rectus abdominis is strong, that signal can be connected directly to a standard EMG amplifier in the biofeedback unit without using oscilloscope monitoring.

EQUIPMENT

At the present time, biofeedback equipment has become extremely sophisticated and user friendly and has almost unlimited options for visual display of performance as well as simultaneous auditory feedback. Once the biofeedback training objectives have been defined and the appropriate signal source and methodology have been determined, the next step is to acquire a biofeedback system that has the desired display capabilities. One should select a unit with multiple choices for visual display of performance. The system should have adjustable target performance levels for the individual based on varying levels of skill. The unit should also have capabilities for simultaneous monitoring and display of abdominal EMG activity. Many currently available biofeedback systems in a moderate price range have all of these features with a wide selection of displays and circuits. It is important to be able to interface the unit with an existing diagnostic EMG system, should that be desired; this is rarely a problem with most current systems. Also, the limitations of the currently available electronics in biofeedback equipment are rarely a problem. Instead, the limiting factors are usually related to the methods and clinical experience of the individuals in the biofeedback environment.

In selecting a biofeedback unit for setting up a laboratory, the Self-regulation System (SRS) Orion unit shown in Figure 22–1 can be recommended as an example of a unit that has the capabilities and versatility to accommodate any biofeedback training requirements as well as any required changes in technique or environment for specific applications. The amplifiers are components that fit in slots in the back of the unit. Any combination of amplifiers can be selected according to the specific training application. The training program and type of display are contained in interchangeable cartridges as shown in Figure 22–1. The target performance level for any patient is adjustable, as are almost all aspects of the video display such as scale and time. The quadraplex cartridge shown in Figure 22–2A is the performance display that we use[1] because both sphincteric and abdominal EMG can be displayed simultaneously (Fig. 22–2B). The abdominal EMG display appears in a muted color near the bottom of the screen that is visible to the biofeedback technician and allows monitoring of abdominal straining. The upper line, which represents sphincteric activity, is a brighter color and is the focus of patient performance. A performance goal line added above the sphincteric EMG display line is the target performance for the patient and is adjusted for each session and each patient according to performance capabilities. The quadraplex display is easy for almost all patients to use and provides excellent reinforcement for performance of specific muscle contractions. Pitch-variable auditory feedback is also presented simultaneously. For the patient who requires a display that is more interesting, the animated tortoise and hare (Fig. 22–3A) will provide interesting reinforcement to almost any patient. The tortoise represents the performance of the patient, and the hare represents the performance goal (Fig. 22–3B).

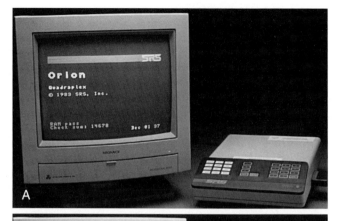

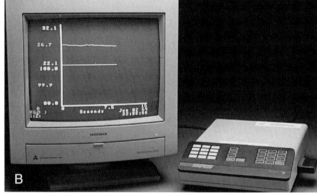

Figure 22-2 *A,* The display unit with the quadruple cartridge in place. *B,* The quadraplex cartridge produces a color line graph with adjustable scale and time. It is capable of producing multiple simultaneous displays. It can be used for simultaneous display of sphincteric electromyographic activity and abdominal muscle electromyographic activity.

The length of each session, the interval between sessions, and the total number of sessions that should be used have not been standardized. Sessions probably should last at least 30 minutes and should be held at least twice weekly for at least 1 month. This schedule will provide a general beginning program that can be modified according to the patient's needs and the clinical environment.

For long-term management of incontinence using biofeedback therapy, a maintenance program of some type is required. Once the initial biofeedback program has been completed, maintenance can be done using a pelvic muscle exercise program with verbal instruction or a home training biofeedback unit.

Other units that have less flexibility but have an advantage in convenience and are readily transferable from the office setting to the home training unit are the MyoDac2 (Fig. 22–4) and the MyoTrac (Fig. 22–5). The MyoTrac unit is a dedicated biofeedback unit for treatment of urinary incontinence and can be interfaced with a standard office microcomputer. The MyoDac2 is a home unit that provides a graphic display of performance to the patient and can be used for long-term maintenance by the patient at home, a considerable convenience. However, all of the technical problems associated with biofeedback therapy are much more likely to occur with the home units. Stud-

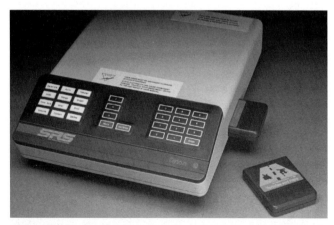

Figure 22-1 The hardware portion of a dedicated biofeedback unit that has the complete range of flexibility required for any application of biofeedback therapy to the treatment of urinary incontinence.

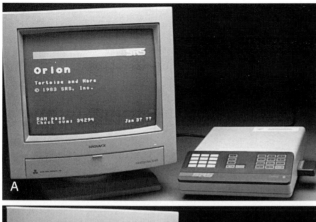

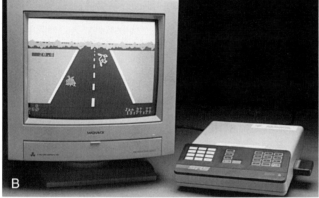

Figure 22-3 *A,* The graphic display for an animated graphic display of performance. *B,* An easily understood graphic display of performance that is presented to the patient. The patient performance is on the left and the performance goal on the right.

ies of use of home units for long-term maintenance treatment of urinary incontinence are not currently available. Therefore, at present a commonly used treatment program is one that involves office biofeedback with a verbal pelvic muscle exercise maintenance program.

The original use of the perineometer by Kegel was

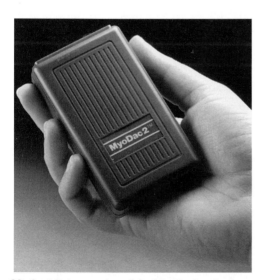

Figure 22-4 A home version of the MyoDac2 unit. On top of this unit is a lighted visual scale that displays patient performance.

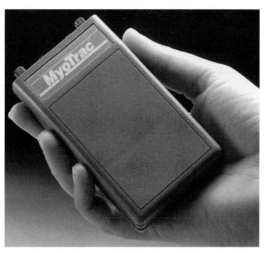

Figure 22-5 A dedicated biofeedback hardware unit (MyoTrac) that interfaces with a microcomputer to provide graphic display of performance to the patient.

an important beginning in the evolution of training women patients to learn how to perform pelvic muscle exercises. Biofeedback using a current sophisticated system with an appropriately selected signal source is considerably advanced compared with the original technique and represents the contemporary method of teaching the technique of pelvic muscle exercises. Once the technique of pelvic muscle exercises has been learned by the patient, it can be performed with a much greater degree of specific muscle contractions than any other training technique currently available. For this reason, biofeedback training programs are beginning to be used by some clinicians as preliminary programs to long-term pelvic muscle exercise training in the behavioral therapy of urinary incontinence in women. Again, further clinical investigation involving combination behavioral therapy is needed.

SELECTION OF PATIENTS

The low risk of behavioral therapy for the treatment of urinary incontinence makes this approach an extremely important treatment alternative for many patients who are not candidates for other treatment options. Biofeedback therapy has a low morbidity and a high response rate to treatment, although in general biofeedback therapy and pelvic muscle exercises are effective only as long as they are being performed. The selection of patients who are most likely to benefit from biofeedback therapy also is an area that needs further research. Many characteristics of patients such as mental status, attitude, motivation, and skill acquisition ability have not been well defined in regard to response to therapy. The pretreatment severity of incontinence represents another important influence on patient success. For example, it is more common for a woman who uses one pad a day to become completely continent than for a woman who uses four pads a day. If a patient who uses four pads a day improves to two pads a day following treatment, this change represents a significant improvement in the quality of her life, but it may not be perceived by her as a success if complete continence is the desired outcome.

SURGERY AS A CHOICE

Behavioral therapy techniques such as biofeedback and pelvic muscle exercises represent an important consideration in the initial therapy of urinary incontinence for women of all ages. However, the patient also needs to understand that there may be significant advantages to a surgical procedure as the initial treatment for correction of stress incontinence compared with behavioral therapy, especially in those with more severe incontinence. Surgery for genuine stress urinary incontinence will cure the problem in almost all patients with no drug side effects and no requirement for continued long-term therapy. In the small number of patients who are not completely cured following surgery or who have postoperative irritative bladder syndromes, biofeedback therapy and pelvic muscle exercises represent an excellent adjunctive treatment choice. Every surgeon who performs procedures for urinary incontinence in women should have access to a well-equipped biofeedback laboratory.

Urinary incontinence is an exceedingly distressing problem for a woman. Often, the progression of the condition has been relatively slow. Likewise, the psychological and social impact has progressed slowly, and its magnitude on the patient's quality of life is often not recognized until she no longer has to deal with the enormous inconvenience and severe restrictions that urinary incontinence entails. Many patients who could expect excellent results from surgery are often confused and unsure about what to do. They know that urinary incontinence is not fatal and does not represent an immediate threat to their health, but a decision to undergo a surgical procedure to enhance their personal convenience and improve their quality of life is often confusing because they know that they can just continue to live with incontinence. Biofeedback therapy can do many things for these patients. They can become involved in their own treatment and personally make a difference in something that has caused a loss of self-esteem and immense despair. With the improvement in symptoms that occurs following biofeedback therapy, the patient finally feels some control over the problem that has previously debilitated her. At that point she can better recognize the impact of incontinence on her quality of life and feels more in control of her decision. If she decides to have surgery to correct the problem, as she often will at some point, it is a decision made with the positive attitude of being in control of her own health care rather than one made in despair.

In general, women who have very mild urinary incontinence may become continent using behavioral therapy only and may postpone the need for surgical correction to a later time. However, in patients with more severe stress incontinence (use of three or more pads daily) significant improvement can be expected, but complete continence is more likely with surgery than with behavioral therapy alone. For this reason, the option of initial biofeedback therapy for the patient with mild incontinence (one pad daily) should be a consideration because such a patient has a reasonable likelihood of becoming continent. In patients who have significant preoperative irritative symptoms, the likelihood of postoperative irritative syndromes is higher,[46] and the possible need for supplemental postoperative therapy using biofeedback therapy may be higher also. Thus, an excellent supporting behavioral therapy laboratory is necessary for the surgeon handling more complicated cases to ensure the best long-term continence response rate.

BIOFEEDBACK IN ELDERLY PATIENTS

The clinician using biofeedback should be aware of some of the special problems with biofeedback therapy for incontinence in the elderly.[42, 43, 47–53] First, elderly women must have the mental capacity to comprehend the purpose of the program and to learn the required skills needed to perform the pelvic muscle exercises. In general, a Mini-Mental Status Evaluation (MMSE) score of greater than 23 indicates that a person is capable of performing the required tasks.[6] The MMSE can be given reasonably quickly and is an adequate evaluation of global mental status. Use of the MMSE is recommended in the elderly because demented patients are extremely frustrating and time-consuming to work with in the biofeedback laboratory.

Second, incontinence in elderly women is more complex than that in younger women. A complete evaluation of the type of incontinence is necessary. For example, intrinsic sphincteric deficiency (ISD) is more common in this group. Although a coexisting bladder disorder in the elderly woman may respond to biofeedback therapy, ISD will not.

REFERENCES

1. O'Donnell PD, Doyle R: Biofeedback therapy technique for treatment of urinary incontinence. Urology 37(5):432–436, 1991.
2. Middaugh SJ, Whitehead WE, Burgio KL, Engel BT: Biofeedback in treatment of urinary incontinence in stroke patients. Biofeedback Self-Regulation 14(1):3–19, 1989.
3. Burgio KL, Whitehead WE, Engel BT: Urinary incontinence in the elderly: Bladder-sphincter biofeedback and toileting skills training. Ann Intern Med 104:507–515, 1985.
4. Meyer S, Dhenin T, Schmidt N, De Grandi P: Subjective and objective effects of intravaginal electrical myostimulation and biofeedback in patients with genuine stress urinary incontinence. Br J Urol 69:584–588, 1992.
5. Cardozo L, Abrams PD, Stanton SL, Feneley RCL: Idiopathic bladder instability treated by biofeedback. Br J Urol 50:521–523, 1978.

6. Burns P, Pranikoff K, Nochajski T, et al: Treatment of stress incontinence with pelvic floor exercises and biofeedback. J Am Geriatr Soc 8:341–344, 1990.
7. Burgio KL, Stutzman RE, Engel BT: Behavioral training for post-prostatectomy urinary incontinence. J Urol 141: 303–306, 1989.
8. Holmes DM, Plevnick S, Stanton SL: Bladder neck electrical conductivity in the treatment of detrusor instability with biofeedback. Br J Obstret Gynaecol 96:821–826, 1989.
9. Burgio KL, Engel BT: Biofeedback-assisted behavioral training for elderly men and women. J Am Geriatr Soc 38:338–340, 1990.
10. Libo LM, Arnold GE, Woodside JR, et al: EMG biofeedback for functional bladder-sphincter dyssynergia: A case study. Biofeedback Self-Regulation, 8(2):243–253, 1983.
11. Burgio KL: Behavioral training for stress and urge incontinence in the community. Gerontology 36(Suppl 2):27–34, 1990.
12. Cardozo L, Stanton SL, Hafner J, Allan V: Biofeedback in the treatment of detrusor instability. Br J Urol 50:250–254, 1978.
13. Philips HC, Fenster HN, Samsom D: An effective treatment for functional urinary incoordination. J Behav Med 15:45–63, 1992.
14. Burton JR, Pearce KL, Burgio KL, et al: Behavioral training for urinary incontinence in elderly ambulatory patients. J Am Geriatr Soc 36:693–698, 1988.
15. Cardozo LD, Stanton SL: Biofeedback: A 5-year review. Br J Urol 56:220, 1984.
16. Millard RJ, Oldenburg BF: The symptomatic, urodynamic and psychodynamic results of bladder re-education programs. J Urol 130:715–719, 1983.
17. Engel BT, Burgio LD, McCormick KA, et al: Behavioral treatment of incontinence in the long-term care setting. J Am Geriatr Soc 38:361–363, 1990.
18. Oldenburg B, Millard RJ: Predictors of long term outcome following a bladder re-training programme. J Psychosom Res 30(6):691–698, 1986.
19. McDowell BJ, Burgio KL, Dombrowski M, et al: An interdisciplinary approach to the assessment and behavioral treatment of urinary incontinence in geriatric outpatients. J Am Geriatr Soc 40:370–374, 1992.
20. Miller NE: Need for evaluation and basic research. In Richter (ed): Biofeedback. North Holland, Elsevier, 1900.
21. Miller NE: Foundations for biofeedback as a part of behavioral medicine. In Basmajian JV (ed): Biofeedback. Baltimore, Williams & Wilkins, 1989.
22. Brenner JM: Psychological mechanisms in biofeedback. In White L, Tursky B (eds): Clinical Biofeedback: Efficacy and Mechanisms. New York, The Guilford Press, 1982.
23. King T: The use of electromyographic biofeedback in treating a client with tension headaches. Am J Occup Ther 1991.
24. Galegos X, Medina R, Espinoza E, Bustamante A: Electromyographic feedback in the treatment of bilateral facial paralysis: A case study. J Behav Med 15(5):533–539, 1992.
25. Gow ML, Ingham RJ: Modifying electroglottograph-identified intervals of phonation: The effect on stuttering. J Speech Hearing Res 35:495–511, 1992.
26. Turnball GK, Ritvo PG: Anal sphincter biofeedback relaxation treatment for women with intractable constipation symptoms. Supported by the Medical Research Council of Canada. Grant # MA-10371.
27. Peper E, Tibbetts V: Fifteen-month follow-up with asthmatics utilizing EMG incentive inspirometer feedback. Biofeedback Self-Regulation 17(2):143–151, 1992.
28. Schoenen J, Gerard P, DePasqua V, Juprelle M: EMG activity in pericranial muscles during postural variation and mental activity in healthy volunteers and patients with chronic tension type headache. Headache 31:321–324, 1991.
29. Orne MT: The efficacy of biofeedback therapy. Ann Rev Med 30:489–503, 1979.
30. Kegel AH: Progressive resistance exercise in the functional restoration of the perineal muscles. Am J Obstet Gynecol 56(2):238–248, 1948.
31. Kegel AH: Physiologic therapy for urinary stress incontinence. JAMA 146(10):915–917, 1951.
32. Kegel AH: Stress incontinence of urine in women: Physiologic treatment. J Int Coll Surg 25(4):487–499, 1956.
33. Bradley WE, Brantley Scott F: Physiology of the urinary bladder. In Harrison JH, Gittes RF, Perlmutter AD, et al (eds): Campbell's Urology, 4th ed, vol 1, Philadelphia, WB Saunders, 1978.
34. Burgio KL, Robinson JC, Engel BT: The role of biofeedback in Kegel exercise training for stress urinary incontinence. Am J Obstet Gynecol 154(1):58–64, 1986.
35. Bump RC, Hurt WG, Fantl JA, Wyman JF: Assessment of Kegel pelvic muscle exercise performance after brief verbal instruction. Am J Obstet Gynecol
36. O'Donnell PD, Sutton LE, Beck CE: Urinary incontinence detection in elderly inpatient men. Neurourol Urodyn 6(20):101–108, 1987.
37. O'Donnell PD, Marshall M: Telemetric ambulatory urinary incontinence detection in the elderly. J Ambul Monit 1(3):233–240, 1988.
38. O'Donnell PD, Beck CM, Finkbeiner AE: Urinary incontinence volume measurement in elderly male inpatients. Urology 35(6):499–503, 1990.
40. O'Donnell PD: Microcomputer-based incontinence data management system for elderly inpatients. Neurourol Urodyn 9:145–153, 1990.
41. O'Donnell PD, Calandro V: Incontinence management scale for elderly inpatient men. Urology 37(3):220–223, 1991.
42. O'Donnell PD: The management of urinary incontinence in the elderly. Rehab Aging Population 4(1):113–120, 1990.
43. O'Donnell PD: Behavioral therapy for incontinence. In O'Donnell PD (ed): Geriatric Urology. Boston, Little Brown, 1994.
44. O'Donnell PD, Beck C, Eubanks C: Surface electrodes in perineal electromyography. Urology 32(4):375–379, 1988.
45. O'Donnell PD: Pitfalls of urodynamic testing. Urol Clin North Am 18(2):257–268, 1991.
46. Karram MM, Bhatia NN: Management of coexistent stress and urge urinary incontinence. Obstet Gynecol 73(1):4–7, 1989.
47. O'Donnell PD: Geriatric issues in female incontinence. In Walters MD, Karram MM (eds): Clinical Urogynecology. Chicago, Mosby-Year Book, 1993.
48. O'Donnell PD: Surgical goals and mechanism of continence in treatment of stress incontinence. In McGuire EJ, Kursh E, (eds): Female Urology. Philadelphia, JB Lippincott, 1994.
49. O'Donnell PD: The pathophysiology of urinary incontinence in the elderly. Adv Urol 4:129–142, 1991.
50. O'Donnell PD, Hawkins WH: Effects of subcutaneous bethanechol on bladder sensation during cystometry. Urology 41(5):452–454, 1993.
51. O'Donnell PD: Pathophysiology of urinary incontinence in elderly men. In O'Donnell PD (ed): Geriatric Urology. Boston, Little Brown, 1994.
52. O'Donnell PD, Beck CM: Urinary incontinence volume patterns in elderly inpatient men. Urology 38(2):128–131, 1991.
53. O'Donnell PD, Walls RC: Residual urine volume following involuntary voiding in elderly inpatient men.

CHAPTER 23

Pelvic Floor Rehabilitation

Alain P. Bourcier, M.D.

In addition to surgery, which has been used for a number of years for treatment of pelvic floor disorders, new therapies that have been highly praised have been developed. The various forms of therapy used to avoid surgery or to maximize the results obtained after surgery are considered conservative treatment.

Pelvic floor exercises became widely known after A. H. Kegel developed the concept.[1] Kegel noted that some of his patients who had undergone surgery for urinary incontinence relapsed quickly, and he was surprised by the weakness of the perineal muscles in these women. He introduced an effective regimen of progressive resistance exercises for the pelvic floor muscles. Eventually, by according the pubococcygeus muscle the importance it deserved, he recommended exercises to strengthen the pelvic floor muscles instead of surgery.[2]

Data on pelvic floor exercises as a conservative treatment show an average improvement of 80% according to different series.[3, 4] Other authors have noted similar data with a relapse rate that is generally related to weakness of the pelvic floor. The variation in results may be explained by two different factors: (1) The protocol used for pelvic floor exercises and (2) whether these exercises are performed by patients at home or in hospital.

For some time there has been great interest in this method of treating incontinence, particularly among the elderly and in women following childbirth. In the past many physicians believed that these exercises did not usually work or that they helped only women with mild urinary incontinence. Further examination has revealed that failure with these exercises resulted from problems of understanding or motivation. New methods of muscular reeducation have been developed to improve the results of physical therapy by using electrical stimulation and the appropriate behavioral modifications (biofeedback). The popularity of these new methods is due to their ease of use, the comfort of the patient, and the total absence of side effects in most cases. The result is that the reeducation of the pelvic floor muscles and home exercises have become recognized treatments for women with urinary incontinence.

Aims of Pelvic Floor Reeducation

Physical therapy should aim to strengthen the pelvic floor musculature with emphasis on improving urinary and fecal continence. It therefore improves a woman's quality of life through recovery of normal physiologic function. The anatomic deterioration related to age and the resulting sexual disturbances demand physical therapy in the postmenopausal period and in elderly incontinent women.

Recent studies have suggested the importance of pelvic floor control after childbirth[5-7] and during activities of daily living.[8] Incontinence affects different women in different ways, and studies have shown that the prevalence of urinary incontinence varies according to age, the threshold of social or hygienic acceptability, and the type of leakage. Studies of stress incontinence among women show that its prevalence varies from 8.2 to 58% (Fig. 23–1). In a recent study, Diokno and colleagues found that 37.7% of noninstitutionalized women over age 60 suffered from urinary incontinence, but only 41% of these women had sought medical care.[9] So far this urinary disorder has been considered a problem that mostly affects the elderly and is a common cause of admission to geriatric units. However, many young women, in whom childbirth problems may be a factor, also complain of urinary incontinence[10-12] or pelvic relaxation syndrome, particularly when participating in sports or undertaking heavy physical activities.

Among the several factors postulated to be responsible for the onset of incontinence, the pelvic floor muscles and the suspensory mechanism are important in causing a weak or inefficient distal sphinc-

Prevalence of Pelvic Floor
Relaxation Syndrome

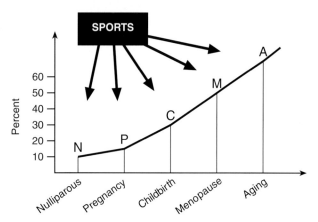

Figure 23-1 Prevalence of urinary incontinence and pelvic floor relaxation in women varies from 7 to 65% depending on age.

ter mechanism. More thorough study is necessary to determine whether bladder neck incompetence in these women makes them more likely to develop stress incontinence if the distal sphincter mechanism is damaged during a future delivery. The presence of stress incontinence and above all an enlarged vagina is a matter of concern in nongravid nulliparous women, particularly those who hope to become pregnant quickly.[12] A thorough examination including a urodynamic investigation is essential to help the physician formulate an appropriate plan of conservative treatment. Besides urinary incontinence, symptoms frequently occur after a long period of standing and increase as the day progresses; this represents the so-called pelvic relaxation syndrome (Table 23-1).

Recently a great deal of information about the problem of urinary incontinence in women has been discussed in newspaper and magazine articles and on television. In countries such as Sweden, Norway, France, and Belgium there has been an increase in women wishing to start a pelvic floor training program. There are several reasons for this interest: (1) women are being informed that physical therapy is available and that symptoms can be alleviated, if not eradicated, by this method; and (2) physicians are becoming increasingly aware of the importance of prevention and the benefits of physical therapy after childbirth.[13]

TABLE 23-1
Symptoms of Pelvic Relaxation Syndrome

Discomfort in the pelvic area
Heaviness or dropping feeling in the vaginal area
Low back pain
Embarrassing vaginal wind
Urinary or fecal incontinence
Sexual dysfunction

TABLE 23-2
Rehabilitation Techniques

Pelvic floor training
Biofeedback
Electrical stimulation
Behavioral modification
Voiding maneuvers

Stages in Pelvic Floor Reeducation

Rehabilitation techniques (Table 23-2) must be rationally selected,[14] and health care professionals must make their choices based on the patient's problem. Treatment of urogynecologic disorders by physical therapy requires the patient to pass through four different stages to achieve success (Table 23-3). The different stages are essential and are always carried out in current practice. The fourth stage represents the last goal of physical therapy, but it is not attainable by all patients and is not always achieved by those with pelvic floor disorders.[15] In fact, at the end of the awareness process, the patient must be conscious of a constant contraction of the levator ani during daily activities. The underlying goal is that every woman benefit from this muscular training to develop levator ani contractions before any increase in intra-abdominal pressure.

FIRST STAGE: INFORMATION

Considering the complexity of the principles discussed previously, health providers must make an effort to explain them to their patients. This information stage should not be neglected, because it represents the essential phase in reeducation (Table 23-4).

During the first interview the therapeutic plan must be explained. In order to emphasize the need for the patient to persevere in the exercise advocated, it must be pointed out that without treatment, deterioration will inevitably occur. To achieve this goal it is useful during the first interview to give a simple explanation of delivery. Risk factors (Table 23-5) are now better known, and patients should understand that damage to the pelvic floor muscles is due to vaginal delivery.[6, 7, 13, 16] Testing of the pelvic floor musculature is essential before any exercise program is started. Different women have different problems. When a woman has recently delivered a child, she

TABLE 23-3
Stages of Physical Therapy

Information given to the patient
Awareness of pelvic floor muscles
Strengthening of pelvic floor muscles
Achievement of perineal blockage before stress

TABLE 23–4
Reeducation of the Pelvic Floor Musculature

First Stage: Information

Improvement of public knowledge: Periodicals, magazines, radio interviews, TV programs
Development of professional awareness: Continence societies, meetings, and training programs

Second Stage: Awareness

Attainment of normal vaginal tension level
Improvement in voluntary perineal command
Avoidance of reversed perineal command

Third Stage: Strengthening

Periurethral striated sphincter: Improvement in occlusive action
Levator ani: Enhancement of vaginal support

Fourth Stage: Reflex Contraction

Women must be aware of constant contraction of pelvic floor because of activities of daily living

Fifth Stage: Perineal Blockage

Pelvic floor muscles must be contracted before any rise of intra-abdominal pressure such as coughing, lifting, or during sports

---

may have only minor problems and not be highly motivated to undertake an exercise program; on the other hand, there are elderly women in whom vaginal atresia makes perineal examination painful and quite frequently causes the cessation of sexual intercourse.

The duration of the information stage is variable. Confidence, gentleness, tact, and persuasion are necessary during the first session. If patients were better informed about the fact that many problems are caused by pelvic floor weakness, more of them would choose a conservative treatment such as physical therapy. For example, before undertaking voluntary contraction, it is essential that women who have been referred for physical therapy know exactly how to localize the intravaginal muscles, yet we constantly come across patients who are completely ignorant that these muscles exist and are unaware of the possibility of voluntary control. Because these muscles are not voluntarily contracted during daily activity and are anatomically hidden, most women are unable to contract the pelvic floor muscles even after receiving individual instruction. Bourcier and associates demonstrated that 248 among 316 women 1 year post partum failed to contract the pubococcygeus muscles properly.[17] In the same study of 316 patients with pelvic floor disorders, a digital assessment for testing the levator ani muscle showed that 22% had a normal score, 41% had a moderate score, and 37% had a low score. In another study, Bo and colleagues demonstrated that 19 of 60 women with urinary stress incontinence (32%) could not contract the pelvic floor muscles correctly.[18]

SECOND STAGE: AWARENESS OF PELVIC FLOOR MUSCULATURE

Attainment of Normal Vaginal Tension Level

Vaginal tonicity is important in the quality of sexual intercourse in women.[19] In addition to its other functions, the role of the pelvic floor muscles in sexuality must be emphasized. Support of the vagina, urethra, bladder, and rectum is provided by the pelvic diaphragm, composed mainly of the levator ani. The vagina undergoes marked physical changes in response to psychogenic and somatogenic erotic stimuli and during coitus presents different vaginal pressure areas. Pelvic floor tonus and strength have a major role in sexual function.

Among organic lesions leading to dyspareunia, some such as vulvar episiotomy scars could be treated by physical therapy. Introital laxity is another common problem that occurs after childbirth under certain obstetric conditions. Perineal risk factors are observed in the postnatal period 6 weeks after delivery. The main symptom is an enlarged vagina, which is responsible for embarrassing vaginal air during sexual intercourse or physical activity. The weakness or laxity of the muscles interferes with the orgasmic platform. A vagina with a narrow caliber requires relaxation techniques and biofeedback. This type of therapy could help women with dyspareunia related to tense pelvic muscles and an inability to relax the pelvic floor muscles properly.

Improvement of Voluntary Perineal Command

There is a difference between the sexes in regard to voluntary perineal commands. Whereas men can control the pelvic floor muscles and are able to stop the flow of urine, women have a problem controlling this musculature. They have a smaller sphincter muscle mass and thus a less effective closure of the bladder outlet than men. Another possible cause of this problem may be a sexually conditioned one. Because men stand to void, they have no difficulty in contracting the pelvic floor musculature on command to inhibit the urethral sphincter, whereas because women sit to void, they find this much harder to do. In countries where there is simply a hole in the floor, women must aim the urine stream accurately to avoid soiling their feet and thus have better control.

In addition to sex differences, the sphincter muscles and the motor neurons that innervate them are

TABLE 23–5
Risk Factors for Pelvic Floor Disorders

Congenital anatomic defects
Traumatic childbirth
Previous genitourinary surgery
Practice of sports with high risk level
Occupation involving heavy activities
Prolonged erect posture

also different. The dendritic bundles may be important in coordinating the activity of all sphincter motor neurons. These motor neurons of the sphincter muscles are a special group that are partly like automatic neurons and partly like traditional neurons.[20]

During evaluation of young female patients after childbirth for a pelvic floor training program, the response to the order "squeeze on the examining fingers" is sometimes wrong. A few patients, instead of squeezing, push down. Thus, the patient misunderstands and performs a "reversed perineal command"[8, 12, 13, 15] instead and is actually increasing the intra-abdominal pressure. This type of response is more frequent than we think. We estimate its frequency as more than 22% of the total number of postpartum patients; it decreases in women around menopause to about 12%. It is obvious that a patient who performs a reversed perineal command cannot be asked to practice Kegel's exercises at home on her own. At each contraction, she is going to push, thus increasing any potential vaginal wall descent, which later will create a vaginal prolapse.

Most often during rehabilitation sessions different patterns of response are obtained following the order to "squeeze" or "hold": (1) The patient performs a proper voluntary perineal contraction without contracting any other muscles, or (2) the patient performs a perineal contraction disturbed by the presence of synergic muscles—(a) abdominal (she contracts her abdominal wall); (b) adductors (she presses her knees); or (c) gluteal (she squeezes her buttocks).

THIRD STAGE: STRENGTHENING

The levator ani muscles hold the intrapelvic organs like a hammock, thus providing support as well as stabilization. Normally, when the woman is erect, the levator ani muscles, together with the respective fasciae, contribute to the support of the vaginal canal, the urethra, and the rectum. In patients with pelvic floor relaxation (Fig. 23–2), this normal muscular support is lost. The levator ani hiatus is now wider and the levator plate is weakened and relaxed.[21]

When the pubococcygeal portions of the levator ani sling contract, they shorten lengthwise, gaining thickness and lessening the pelvic floor aperture transversely, thus reducing the anteroposterior diameter considerably. These anatomic data are favorable to physical therapy as a first treatment of pelvic floor relaxation as well as vaginal prolapse such as cystocele grade 1.[13, 22]

A tonic contraction of the levator ani maintains a high position of the vesical neck and may contract during any increase in intra-abdominal pressure. Restoration of these muscles depends on different factors and differs in different races. The reasons for such anatomic differences are not clear but include genetic influence, living habits, obstetric conditions, pelvic nerve damage, and modern living conditions (environmental stress, increased emphasis on work-

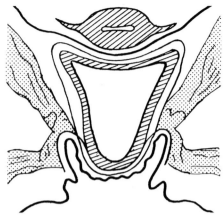

Figure 23–2 Pelvic floor relaxation with weakening and stretching of the levator ani.

ing outside the home, and increased emphasis on fitness and looks). Genital prolapse occurs less often in westernized Chinese women than in occidental women.[23] It might be hypothesized that the different incidence is related to a deterioration in pelvic floor function as a result of the new life style.

Once the awareness stage has been established, a pelvic floor training program can be proposed. Although many protocols and programs have been described and although programs may vary, it is always important to follow basic rules:

1. Patients should be selected according to grades of pelvic floor function.
2. A trained physical therapist, nurse, or midwife should be present to give proper instruction.
3. Attention should be concentrated on isolating specific muscle groups.
4. The number of daily contractions prescribed should be divided into several sessions.
5. The pelvic floor exercise regimen should be tailored to the individual.
6. Positions should be modified after several weeks of training.
7. The type of contractions should be alternated.

A knowledge of the musculature is as important in managing the physical therapy of pelvic floor disorders as it is in the reeducation stage. The strength of the levator ani muscles can be used as a therapeutic measure, and muscular factors are important in the etiology of pelvic relaxation leading to vaginal prolapse and urinary incontinence. The levator ani comprises a mixture of two types of muscle fiber: (1) slow-twitch (aerobic-oxidative) fibers, which are type I muscle fibers with a small diameter (45 μm); they are functionally adapted to maintain tone over long periods and may be of considerable importance in producing urethral closure and support of the pelvic viscera; and (2) fast-twitch (anaerobic-glycolytic) fibers, which are type II muscle fibers and have a larger diameter (59 μm); they are responsible for rapid forceful contractions and are actived as a short-term response to sudden increases in intra-abdominal pressure.[24]

It is very important to recruit fast-twitch fibers by fast contractions to develop strength and slow-twitch fibers by slow contractions to increase endurance.[25] To induce hypertrophy, both fast- and slow-twitch fibers should be contracted. To achieve these objectives, a successful pelvic floor muscle training program must include rapid forceful contractions, sustained maximal voluntary contractions, and fast contractions superimposed on the end of each prolonged contraction.

The only anatomic relationship between the levator ani and the other pelvic muscles is provided by the obturator internus. The pubococcygeal segment of the levator ani originates in the tendinous arch, a thickening of the obturator fascia; the iliococcygeus begins at a membranous insertion to the inner surface of the obturator internus at the tendinous arch of the levator ani.[26] This anatomic consideration of the voluntary or reflex contraction of the levator ani and obturator internus during increases in intra-abdominal pressure is important in setting up the protocol of a pelvic muscle training program. This endopelvic connection to the tendinous arch may assist the levator ani in support because it limits the descent of the pelvic organs during the stress of increases in intra-abdominal pressure when the levator ani are relaxed. Physiologic studies have demonstrated that at rest, in contrast to other skeletal muscles, there is constant activity in the anal sphincter and in the levator ani owing to the slow-twitch fibers (resting tone). It could be postulated that in patients with weakening and stretching of the levator ani, or even in those with partial denervation, some muscular components such as the obturator internus might be recruited in the early stages of pelvic exercises. If there is a major weakness of the pelvic floor, contraction of the gluteus maximus can also produce an overflow of activity into the levator ani.

Different exercises may be proposed to the patient.[27] The "flick contraction" exercise is performed by contracting and relaxing the levator ani as tightly as possible for 1 second; an average of 20 to 50 contractions per day is recommended. The "hold contraction" exercise is performed by lifting and pulling up the levator ani and then holding the contraction at least 6 seconds; as control improves, the time of this sustained pubococcygeal contraction can be extended to more than 12 seconds. The "intensive contraction" exercise involves the recruitment of levator ani muscles with other groups of muscles in different positions, contracting the levator ani in controlled increments to the point of maximum tension (Fig. 23–3).

FOURTH STAGE: PERINEAL BLOCKAGE BEFORE STRESS

In normal situations, with increased intra-abdominal pressure, the rectum, uterus, and upper vagina are pushed downward and backward. The levator plate tenses and rises owing to reflex muscular contraction. Sudden increases in intra-abdominal pressure

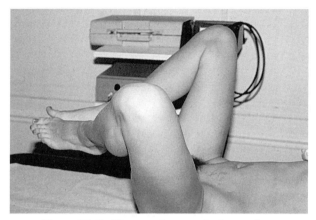

Figure 23-3 Therapeutic gynecologic exercises.

are transmitted to the urethra. It has been suggested that pressure rise in this area of the urethra is higher than the increase in intra-abdominal pressure and precedes the rise in intra-abdominal pressure, suggesting the presence of reflex muscle contraction. Sudden changes in abdominal pressure elicit a reflex contraction of the levator ani muscles. The intra-abdominal pressure in the standing position is two to three times greater than that in a normal situation.

It has been claimed that the downward pressure from the abdominal viscera has to be offset by the strength of the urogenital diaphragm, and the forward pressure of the visceral canals to the lowest level of the pelvic floor increases the tendency to visceral protusion.

In pelvic floor disorders female patients lose this reflex muscle contraction ability, and one of the goals of rehabilitation is to enable patients to relearn this reflex.[8, 13, 15] The teaching process aims to demonstrate how the levator ani muscles must be contracted before any increase in intra-abdominal pressure occurs (Figs. 23–4 and 23–5), particularly with strenuous effort during heavy physical activity. It is difficult to obtain perineal blockage before stress. Active perineal exercises have numerous advantages; however, they do not allow a distinction to be made between perineal and abdominal contractions.

Plevnik in 1985 described an innovative approach to augmenting pelvic floor muscle tone by the use of special exercises with intravaginal devices—weighted vaginal cones.[28] Tampon-like vaginal cones (Fig. 23–6) are inserted into the vagina by the patient and are held in place for about 15 to 30 minutes a

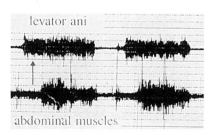

Figure 23-4 Perineal blockage before stress technique.

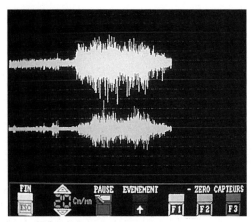

Figure 23–5 Perineal blockage before stress technique: The levator ani muscles are contracting before *(top)* any increase in intra-abdominal pressure occurs *(bottom)*.

day. A set of five cones in medical-grade plastic and weighing 20, 32.5, 45, 60, and 75 g is now available. When the cone is placed inside the vagina, the pelvic floor muscles have to contract to keep it in place. When the patient contracts these muscles to keep it from dropping out, she also contracts the urethral sphincter, increasing its activity.

This interesting method for testing and strengthening the pelvic floor muscles is effective and cost-effective.[29] Easy to use and involving a marked reduction in physical therapy time, it could be a primary method of treatment at home after a few sessions in the hospital or private office to train the patient properly before she uses the cones. Although it enhances the performance of patients practicing Kegel exercises, in patients with severe pelvic floor dysfunction it is not sufficient. If it is not successful after a trial of 4 weeks, patients must undergo pelvic floor therapy with electrical stimulation and biofeedback.

Classification of Pelvic Floor Abnormalities After Childbirth

Physical therapy is to be recommended more frequently to mothers after childbirth, when high-risk

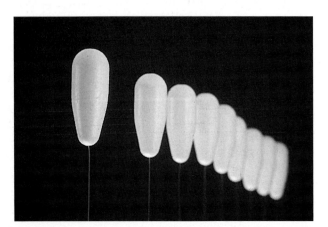

Figure 23–6 A set of vaginal cones. A cone in place is retained by the pelvic floor. Any increase in pressure will cause it to drop out.

factors for dysfunction of the pelvic floor exist (see Table 23–5). Vaginal delivery may cause stretching and tearing of the pelvic support tissue, and recent electrophysiologic evaluation of the muscles of the pelvic floor provide additional evidence of the importance of the pelvic floor musculature. Immediate postpartum abnormalities are most marked in multiparous women (Table 23–6).

Vaginal delivery with a prolonged second stage of labor and delivery of high-birth-weight babies is a risk factor for nerve damage (Table 23–6). This partial denervation and consequent weakening of the pelvic floor muscles[5, 6, 7, 16] lends support to the etiologic role of muscle damage in these conditions and provides an explanation for the loss of levator ani muscle tone. Pelvic and pudendal nerve damage caused by childbirth may result in urinary incontinence. Electromyographic (EMG) studies have shown a significant increase in motor unit duration and a delay in pudendal nerve conduction in women after childbirth. Similarly, it has been shown[30] that the pubococcygeus is partially denervated in women suffering from stress incontinence or presenting with genital prolapse. Physical therapy (see Tables 23–5 and 23–6) should be advised more frequently in young women as a preventive measure when they have high risk factors after delivery.[31, 32]

APPLIED BIOFEEDBACK

Rationale

Biofeedback (see Chapter 22) is defined as the use of monitoring equipment to measure internal physiologic events and various body conditions of which a person is unaware in order to develop conscious control over body processes. Physical therapy has always attempted to assist patients by increasing their physiologic self-regulation within their natural environment. Biofeedback has now gained several potential applications for urologic conditions.[33, 34] In recent years, biofeedback has been used successfully in pa-

TABLE 23–6
Classification of Postnatal Abnormalities

First Group: Cesarean Section or Normal Vaginal Delivery
History: No symptoms, no complaints
Physical examination: No pelvic prolapse, no leakage
Pelvic floor assessment: Normal

Second Group: Vaginal Delivery with Risk Factors
Prolonged labor
Baby weight >3700 g
Baby head size >35.5 cm
Tears and no episiotomy
Urinary problems during pregnancy
Vaginal prolapse

History: Symptoms, complaints
Physical examination: Pelvic relaxation, leakage
Pelvic floor assessment: Weakness

tients with urologic disorders such as detrusor instability, detrusor sphincter dyssynergia (DSD), and enuresis. Patients with these disorders are good candidates for biofeedback therapy because the primary objective is to enable them to acquire an increased sensory awareness of their voiding patterns or to train the skeletal muscles to either strengthen (SUI) or relax (DSD) the urethral sphincter.

Once movement occurs, the EMG-force relationship depends on the speed of muscle contraction and the length of the muscles involved. Functional activities rarely occur at either a constant speed or a constant muscle length; therefore, all biofeedback sessions include procedures in which the active functional movement velocity changes freely. Specific exercises help the patient to identify the pelvic floor muscles and strengthen them, thus enhancing the support of the pelvic viscera.

The levator ani muscle is a heterogeneous mixture of fast-twitch (type I) fibers and slow-twitch (type II) fibers. Functionally, type II fibers, which maintain static muscle tone, are responsible for maintaining the tone of the pelvic floor muscles.[35, 36] Type I fibers are activated mainly during events that increase intra-abdominal pressure. This morphology of the levator ani muscle is important in understanding the pelvic floor exercises assisted by biofeedback therapy. It has been demonstrated in recent studies[36] that the diameter of fast-twitch fibers varies in different women: those with fibers of larger diameter produce significantly higher urethral closure pressures during coughing. During stressful events, phasic fast-twitch fibers provide rapid forceful contractions.

Stress urinary incontinence is primarily related to erect posture. We may assume that erect posture and a constant increase in intra-abdominal pressure alter female urethrovesical function. In the vertical position the urethra leaves the bladder at the point of maximum combined intra-abdominal pressure and gravity force. On the basis of this concept we developed the applied biofeedback technique,[37] referring to electromyography of the levator ani combined with synergic-antagonist muscle activity in a standing position (Table 23–7). A certain relationship must therefore exist between the practice of sports or strenuous activity and the level of intra-abdominal pressure (Fig. 23–7). This could explain the fact that symptoms occur most of the time in patients involved in manual or agricultural labor or in sports.[38] Put another way, the evolution of women's professional

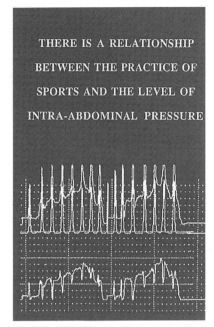

Figure 23–7 Relationship between the practice of sports and the level of intra-abdominal pressure.

and business activities and stressful environments, such as those involved in traveling, shopping, and housekeeping, represent high-risk factors for pelvic floor relaxation (see Table 23–1).

The goal of the exercise is to contract the levator ani properly, but the proprioceptive signals generated by the substituting muscles such as the abdominal, adductor, or gluteal muscles may easily be misinterpreted as originating from the pelvic floor rather than from these antagonist muscles. When the substituting muscles contract, their afferents can mask any low-intensity sensory signals that may be generated by the weakened pelvic floor muscles. To show the patient what is happening, abdominal or gluteal muscle contractions are measured by surface electrodes. A vaginal EMG probe is used to obtain a correlative measure of the levator ani. Multicomponent instrumental biofeedback allows the patient to acquire volitional control over skeletal muscle activity.

Practice of Applied Biofeedback

In our practice, we currently use a microcomputer-based system (Fig. 23–8) that has a wide range of parameters that allows us to tailor the treatment to the specific requirements of the patient, thus providing flexibility and accuracy in treatment. A new generation of perineal reeducation products is now available. Among these new types of office equipment, the PRS 9300 Professional Notebook System (Fig. 23–9) allows the therapist to use electrical stimulation and pressure or EMG biofeedback therapy to treat patients with pelvic floor muscle dysfunction. This device is available in a menu-driven unit that allows

TABLE 23–7
Advantages of Applied Biofeedback

More representative of pelvic floor dysfunction
Electromyographic training can be performed during selected events
Develops better control of the pelvic floor muscles on dominant patterns
Training can be given in everyday activities

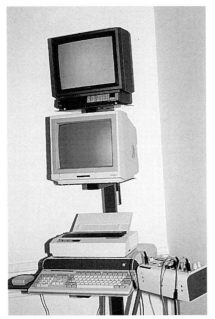

Figure 23-8 Equipment for applied biofeedback training with microcomputer base system and video system.

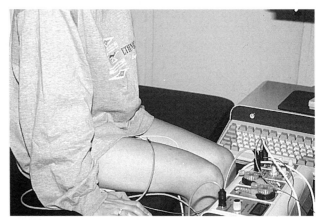

Figure 23-10 Patient involved in a pelvic training program in the sitting position.

the caregiver to concentrate on the patient during training sessions. This system is microprocessor-based, which means that it is versatile and expandable to meet the therapist's changing needs. In most types of equipment available, a remote color monitor provides the patient with clearly visible, colorful records of the therapy sessions and data analysis results. This separate color monitor allows the patient to concentrate on the training exercises.

These systems (1) facilitate patient awareness and learning processes, allowing faster development of physiologic self-regulation for selected patients; (2) increase the patient's interest in the therapy; and (3) improve patient care and efficiency by providing graphic representations of physiologic data and allowing the possibility of storage and statistical analyses.

If patients are required to assume specific positions such as sitting or standing to perform perineal blockage before stress (Fig. 23–10), some flexibility is useful. Feedback must be relevant to enhance learning and focus attention on agonist (pelvic floor) and antagonist (abdominal) muscles. Due to the participation of different muscles in different series of exercises and physical activities, we use multichannel biofeedback systems (Fig. 23–11). With these it is possible to propose a more attractive program using "templates." In such a protocol, the patient follows a series of drawings as she attempts to contract the pelvic floor muscles at the right time and at the proper strength (Fig. 23–12).

Use of Applied Biofeedback in Activities of Daily Living

Physical therapy has always attempted to assist patients by increasing their ability to regulate their own physiologic processes within their natural environment. Caregivers assist patients in changing their reactions by establishing goals and helping patients

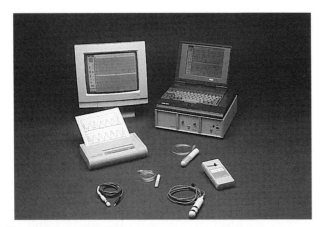

Figure 23-9 PRS 9300 Notebook system. (Permission to reproduce this copyrighted material has been granted by the owner, Hollister Incorporated.)

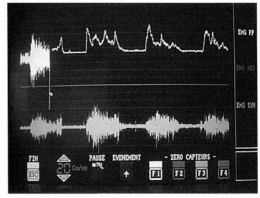

Figure 23-11 Recordings of both the levator ani muscles *(top)* and the abdominal muscles *(bottom)*. During the hold exercise the patient cannot sustain more than 3 seconds, instead of the usual 10 seconds.

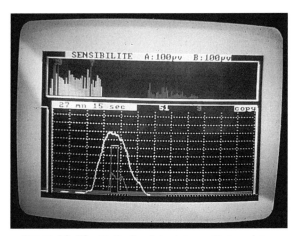

Figure 23-12 Biofeedback training with templates.

achieve a better response by developing new habits and modifying their physical activities. The simulation of daily activity is a very important stage in which selected "home stress" or a physical task is set to assess the patient's ability to perform a real-life activity. In general, caregivers should start with easy tasks and then progressively make the activities more difficult and more functional. It is especially helpful to have patients perform these activities while standing. When using biofeedback one must determine whether the final goal is predominantly strength or refined control. If the health professional is directing therapy to achieve control, improvement will be diminished if a denervation of the pelvic floor muscles exists. Successful restoration of daily activities is evident only if pelvic floor muscle strength is coupled with performance of the functional activity during the therapeutic process. People overlook the fact that recorded activity will be affected by the position of the patient, the dependence on gravity, and whether the pelvic floor musculature is slightly or greatly stretched.

Without a protocol developed for a standing position, especially with movement, neuromuscular reeducation is pointless. Applied biofeedback therapy is favored by a provocative technique triggered by a rise in intra-abdominal pressure such as occurs with standing or exercising. The therapy's ultimate aim is to gain strength and, most of all, refined control of pelvic floor function—that is, to achieve perineal blockage before stress. During the learning process, the levator ani must be contracted before any intra-abdominal pressure rise occurs, particularly with strenuous activity during work or sports.

The patient's history, initial test results, and professional activity can be relevant in choosing a particular approach. At this stage documentation and information about the patient's response to varied conditions and home tasks focus the patient's ability to achieve progressively more control over the pelvic floor musculature in home tasks. Each patient is asked to perform some activities at home. During these sessions she is instructed to perform specific movements such as coughing, rising, squatting, and lifting (Fig. 23–13).

Physical Activity, Sports, and the Pelvic Floor Muscles

Little attention has been paid to the problem of urinary stress incontinence associated with fitness and sports activities. Moreover, it has been generally believed that women who exercise regularly do not experience muscular weakness and may be "protected" against pelvic floor disorders. Despite the lack of any reliable studies, the prevalence of incontinence in physically active women is significantly higher than that in sedentary women. Almost one-third of young women who practice sports on a regular basis seek medical advice for urinary symptoms (Fig. 23–14).

Wolin reported a prevalence rate of SUI of 16% in young nulliparous female nurse students.[10] Bo and colleagues reported a prevalence rate of SUI symptoms of 26% in female physical education students.[11] Approximately one-third of female exercisers are incontinent of urine during exercise, and some of them give up exercise because of this problem. Bourcier,[12] in a study on sportswomen and stress,[39] studied the relationship between exercise and incontinence and found that 33% of women who exercised suffered from urinary incontinence during at least one type of exercise.

Conceptually, we can hypothesize a certain relationship between the pelvic floor support and the presence of intra-abdominal pressure.[12, 40] High-impact movements such as running and jumping can result in impact forces that are as much as three to four times higher than a person's body weight. The

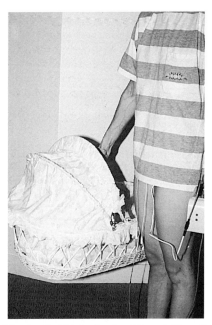

Figure 23-13 Applied biofeedback with activities of daily living.

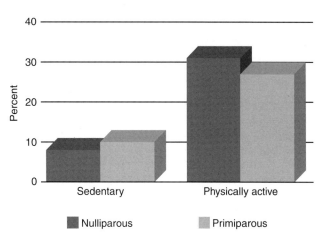

Prevalence of SUI In Young Women

■ Nulliparous   ■ Primiparous

Figure 23-14 Prevalence of urinary stress incontinence among physically active women.

practice of sports imposes a much higher intra-abdominal pressure, which must be compensated for by an equally high pelvic floor support. In the past, Nichols and Milley suggested that the suspensory mechanism (cardinal and uterosacral ligaments) and the support mechanism (pelvic floor musculature) could be damaged by chronic and repeated high intra-abdominal pressure.[41] A certain relationship must exist between the practice of sports and the level of intra-abdominal pressure (see Fig. 23-7).

However, one should clearly differentiate the risks specific to the type of sport practiced. There are numerous variables that have not been studied or evaluated. These include the presence of pelvic floor weakness (the quality of collagen or muscular function), the effects of childbirth, and the amount of stress placed on the pelvic floor specifically related to the practice of sports.

Table 23-8 shows that the type of sport practiced has a major impact on the risk of developing pelvic floor disorders. We have defined three groups based on the amount of intra-abdominal pressure generated on the pelvic floor.[12, 38, 42] Because of the onset of incontinence during high-impact aerobics, a number of women discontinue this activity. Perhaps low-impact aerobics can minimize the deleterious effects on the pelvic floor. It has been reported that some exercisers change the way they perform an exercise because of urinary incontinence.

The benefits of physical activity are so obvious that it would indeed be preferable to educate physical fitness instructors about pelvic floor dysfunction instead of advising incontinent women to give up exercise altogether. Emphasis must be placed on developing a specific training program for active women who develop SUI during sports. The MAB program practiced in our clinic uses mainly applied biofeedback, which is efficient and allows many women to exercise without incurring the troublesome symptoms of incontinence.

During the learning process, the levator ani muscles must be contracted before any intra-abdominal pressure rise occurs. The perineal blockage technique, carried out before an increase in intra-abdominal pressure, is efficient in providing feedback to the sportswoman during exercise. Different types of exercises involving progressively higher intra-abdominal pressures and the recruitment of different groups of muscles involved in sports are suggested (Table 23-9). As soon as the pelvic floor muscle contraction is effective, we ask the patient to contract the synergistic muscles and to vary the posture. All these exercises are performed using the perineal blockage technique.

The exercises performed by the patient include the use of different muscle groups:

1. Pelvic floor and abdominal muscles.
2. Pelvic floor and gluteal muscles.
3. Pelvic floor and adductor muscles.
4. Pelvic floor, abdominal, gluteal, and adductor muscles.

Another important point is to carry out these exercises in different positions: lying, sitting, and standing. We suggest, for example, a combined exercise: with the feet hooked under a bar, the patient rolls up into a sitting position and stays in this position for an increased period of time ranging from 6 to 30 seconds (Fig. 23-15). Figure 23-16 illustrates the computerized EMG measurements of the vaginal, abdominal, and adductor muscles during a training program of the pelvic floor muscles.

Using a treadmill we have defined a protocol of exercises[31] combining speed and endurance (Fig. 23-17). The underlying concept here is the fact that the mechanism of incontinence must be taken into account during biofeedback sessions to provoke a re-

TABLE 23-8
Classification of Risk Factors for Pelvic Floor Disorders in Sports

High Risk
  Athletics: Long jump, triple jump, high jump, hurdles
  Gymnastics: Floor exercises, parallel bars, trampoline
  Team games: Basketball, volleyball, handball
  Combat sports: Karate, judo
  Bodybuilding
  Horseback riding

Medium Risk
  Jogging, tennis, skiing, skating

No Risk
  Rowing, cycling, swimming

TABLE 23-9
Muscular Parameters in Physical Therapy Management

Pelvic floor activity	Strength and endurance of levator ani
Reflex activity	Reflex pelvic floor contractions
Volitional control	Perineal blockage before stress (PBBS)

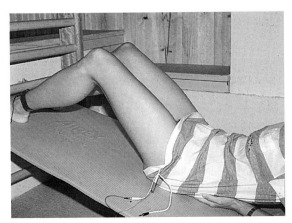

Figure 23-15 Physical activities, fitness, and pelvic floor muscles: exercises with the PBBS (perineal blockage before stress) technique.

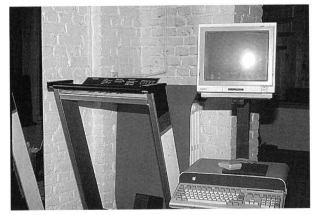

Figure 23-17 MAB program: Equipment with treadmill computer and monitor.

flex pelvic floor contraction in response to stress. This is the most efficient method of training the pelvic floor muscles for sportswomen. They must be aware of the reflex pelvic floor contraction in order to maintain it during walking, running, and jumping.

For the first stage of the MAB program, we prefer to use computerized measurements to provide accurate data to the patient. At least two separate EMG instrumentation channels are used. One set of electrodes is placed on the rectus abdominus muscle, and the other is an intravaginal tampon electrode. The purpose of the electrodes is to record the levator ani activity with a minimum of discomfort. The vaginal probes are designed to prevent dislodgment during pelvic exercises, especially when sitting and standing, without requiring that the patient hold the electrode in place.

The introduction of a rehabilitation treadmill in our program for sportswomen is the only way in a medical environment to allow the patient to perform real physical activities that affect the pelvic floor. With such a machine we can vary the speed from 2.5

to 5 mph and the grade from 5 to 15%. Accuracy of speed and grade is assumed for a precisely controlled workout (Fig. 23–18).

We have developed a 15-minute exercise program involving a workout that combines routines performed at 2.5 mph with a 15% grade, at 3.5 mph with a 10% grade, and at 5 mph with a 5% grade. Each of the exercises is continued for 5 minutes.

In the advanced program, the patient jogs while listening to instructions concerning levator ani contractions given by audible signals from a loudspeaker. While jogging, she attempts to contract the perineal muscles at different periods of time and controls the results by using the perineal blockage technique, which is reflected on a screen.

It is possible to combine the use of cones[28, 43] and the treadmill to train patients more quickly and less expensively in pelvic floor exercises.[40] In this case, we use the same method, asking the patient to hold one of the five available sizes of cone for a period of 15 minutes (5 minutes per exercise). Instead of electrodes, patients carry out the same protocol with

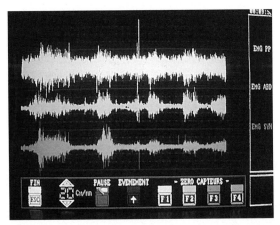

Figure 23-16 Recordings of levator ani muscle activity combined with abdominal and adductor muscle activity during exercises in a standing position.

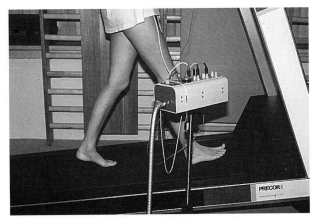

Figure 23-18 MAB program: Patient jogs for 15 minutes, and parameters are selected according to the type of exercise chosen, strength, or endurance.

cones. The proper use of the pelvic floor muscles is shown by preventing the loss of cones.

Sixty-eight young nulliparous women recruited from sports centers were divided into two groups, group one representing student athletes and group two representing students who practiced sports on a regular basis. Results (Table 23–10) showed that the group one athletes improved, but none demonstrated a complete cure. Patients in group two had excellent results as shown by a consistent and significant increase in the parameters measured, but they need to undergo a maintenance program to avoid relapse, which is always possible in these patients.[41]

We found that patients who learned the technique of perineal blockage before stress were more likely to benefit from such a therapeutic program. A particular advantage of this approach is the flexibility it allows to accommodate the patient's physical condition—for instance, women who are incontinent in physical activities can use a program specifically designed to suit their levator ani strength and endurance. This technique appears to be a very promising adjunctive modality for pelvic floor rehabilitation and can be used for active women who are incontinent mainly as a result of high-risk factors to the pelvic floor before or after surgery.

As sports have become a highly fashionable and social activity for women, the applied biofeedback MAB program[43] has proved to be a good solution to the management of incontinence in women athletes and appears to be a promising modality for pelvic floor rehabilitation in nulliparous women.

Functional Electrical Stimulation

Functional electrical stimulation (FES) has been used in medical practice and physical medicine in the form of functional (electrical) protheses developed to improve gait. We use the term functional stimulation to apply to control of micturition and continence. In the past, Bors described the influence of electrical stimulation on the pelvic floor,[45] and Caldwell and colleagues, using electrical stimulation, showed that it is possible to control different types of incontinence in 30 to 80% of cases.[46] Alexander and associates, using an electrical pessary,[47] and Suhel and coworkers, who introduced an integrated appliance,[48] have

provided new methods of nonimplantable perineal stimulation.

PHYSIOLOGIC BASIS OF ELECTRICAL STIMULATION

Perineal methods of electrical stimulation use the natural neural pathways and micturition reflexes. The therapeutic effects of FES depend on artificial neural activation. The stimulation intensity must be high enough to induce impulses in the nerves. Electrical stimulation induces a reflex contraction of the striated muscles. Based on animal experiments it appears that direct stimulation of efferent fibers is the most important mechanism in enhancing the reflex responses.

Urethral closure during FES has been determined to result from direct stimulation of the efferent pudendal nerves aided by activation of hypogastric fibers controlling the response of the smooth periurethral muscles.[49] Bladder inhibition is accomplished through two spinal reflex systems, which are activated during FES through stimulation of the pudendal nerves.[50] Detrusor relaxation results from a longlasting reflex discharge in the hypogastric efferents at low pressure and in the pelvic efferents at high pressure.

The threshold intensity varies inversely with fiber diameter. Any pulse configuration will serve for nerve activation, and a wide range of stimulation waveforms has been used to cause neural excitation. Different types are available in most stimulators: biphasic square pulses, alternating pulses, and monophasic capacitively coupled spike pulses. Short square-wave pulses (0.2 and 0.5 ms) are most effective. Very short pulses require very large amplitudes.

To minimize electrochemical reactions at the electrode-mucosa interface, biphasic or alternating pulses are recommended.[51] Small electrodes and high charge densities are desirable to avoid the risk of tissue damage and corrosion of the electrode (through generation of heat or formation of toxic products).

Effects on urethral closure and bladder inhibition are obtained at two different optimal frequencies. Urethral closure requires a frequency of 50 to 100 Hz, and inhibitory reflex systems operate at low frequencies of between 5 and 20 Hz. For many years it has been common to use these stimulation parameters. The most commonly used frequencies and pulse durations are 20 Hz and 0.75 ms for bladder inhibition and 50 Hz and 1 ms for urethral closure.

To compensate for the distance between the electrodes and the nerves being stimulated, the amplitude of the current must be increased. Electrical stimulators provide constant voltage or constant current that maintains the same current waveform regardless of changes in impedance. There are great individual variations in the stimulus that can be tolerated without incurring unpleasant sensations. This difference is related to the difference in impedance.

TABLE 23–10
Results in Sportswomen After MAB Program

	PF Grade (0-5)	Perineometer (cm H₂O)	Cones (gr)	Test (gr)	UPP (cm H₂O)
Group I	1.1	25.2	20	3.2	11.3
Group II	3.0[a]	46.7[a]	40[a]	5.4[a]	12.7[a]

Abbreviations: PF, pelvic floor, UPP, urethral pressure profile.
[a]$p < .05$

Another factor to be considered is muscle fatigue and the effect of stimulation on the striated muscles. At high frequencies, the muscle fatigues rapidly owing to neuromuscular transmission; at lower frequencies there is less fatigue. It has been suggested that chronic stimulation increases the relative number of slow-twitch fibers, probably by aiding the transformation of fast-twitch fibers to slow units, which can sustain the contraction longer.[52]

Long-term electrical stimulation induces an almost complete transformation of fast- to slow-twitch fibers that have a high energy capacity.[53] Frequencies in the range of 10 to 60 Hz induce such a transformation, which occurs after almost 30 days of stimulation. Most patients experience some relapse after a period of 30 days; this may be due to the reverse process associated with immobilization or inactivity. This observation is important and supports the concept of a maintenance program; continuous treatment is required, whereas permanent reeducation may be achieved after a period of 1 month of electrical stimulation.[54, 55]

To obtain a favorable effect on the urethral sphincter and bladder, total or partial peripheral innervation of the pelvic floor must be present. No effect can be expected in patients with complete lower motor neuron lesions. If the muscles have been completely denervated, physiotherapy is unlikely to be effective. However, any surviving muscle fibers will be hypertrophied. Therefore, electrical stimulation may improve reinnervation after partial denervation by enhancing sprouting of the surviving motor axons.[56]

STIMULATION MODALITIES

The best responses to electrical stimulation are obtained when the electrodes are positioned close to the pudendal nerves. Such placement produces effective excitation of the levator ani muscles. Stimulation allows excitation of the pudendal nerves only, without the participation of other nonrelevant groups of muscles. A good indication of the response to stimulus of the efferent pudendal nerves is achieved by visual assessment of contraction of the pelvic floor muscles. Visual assessment is also used to determine the proper position of the probes in the pelvic floor. The ideal placement of probes for stimulation is not necessarily related to the muscles themselves but rather to the nerve trunks that supply the muscles. We have noticed that different sites of stimulation lead to movement of the legs owing to triceps surae or obturator contractions (due to S_1 activation). The anal probe is better retained and does not vary much in positioning because the electrode is kept in place by the striated anal sphincter. Vaginal probes may involve problems of positioning: the shape, size, and diameter of the vagina are of the utmost importance for suitable response.

The position of the electrodes is fundamental, and the contact area must be as large as possible. Accuracy of electrode placement must be ensured regard-

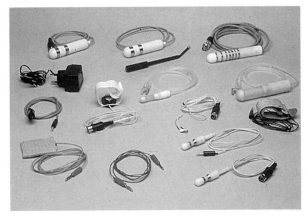

Figure 23-19 Set of probes used in functional electrical stimulation.

less of individual anatomic differences. Only electrodes that ensure perfect contact by means of their adaptation to the vagina are to be used in current practice. In every patient there is one combination of electrode and position that produces the most pronounced effect on the pelvic floor and thus enhances the urethral closure pressure. For this reason, a set of probes is necessary to achieve this ideal combination (Fig. 23–19). A set of probes consists of

1. A standard two-ring vaginal probe.
2. A tampon two-ring vaginal probe (Fig. 23–20).
3. A thin "elderly model" vaginal probe.
4. An inflatable (expandable) intravaginal probe (Fig. 23–21).
5. A monopolar intravaginal probe (Fig. 23–22).
6. An intra-anal probe (Fig. 23–23).

OFFICE THERAPY AND HOME CARE PERINEAL STIMULATION

Functional electrical stimulation has undergone extensive research in the past and is now a very common therapy in European countries; it has recently regained interest in North America. According to the

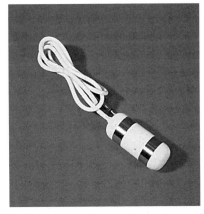

Figure 23-20 Tampon two-ring vaginal probe used in FES and electromyographic biofeedback.

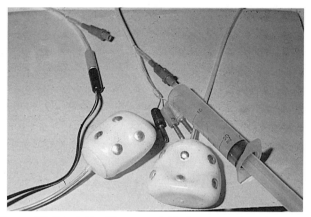

Figure 23-21 Inflatable, expandable intravaginal probe used in functional electrical stimulation.

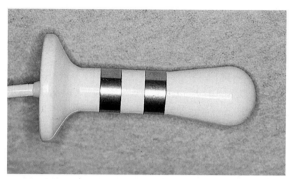

Figure 23-23 Intra-anal probe used in functional electrical stimulation and electromyographic biofeedback.

literature, most stimulators have become easy to use and are available at low cost for home treatment. On the other hand, a new line of products—more sophisticated but also more expensive—is now available for office therapy. It is difficult for health care professionals to understand clearly the different methods and techniques of therapeutic perineal electrostimulation: long-term (chronic) electrical stimulation; short-term (acute) electrical stimulation[59]; acute maximal functional electrical stimulation[60]; and maximum pelvic floor stimulation.[57–59] In practice, different types of stimulation may be proposed to patients. For a better understanding of the clinical approach, we have divided electrical stimulation therapy into two parts[60]: office therapy and a home treatment program.

Office Therapy (Also Called Outpatient Program or In-Clinic Treatment)

In this approach, a stationary device with a wide range of electrical parameters is used in the office or clinic under the control of a therapist. The system used is capable of being changed to fit the needs of

the patient. Microcomputers are used to allow prompt changes in optimal stimulation parameters, which are based on urodynamic data. The stimulation parameters (waveform, pulse width, frequency, pulse rise, and so on) are based directly on urodynamic measurements. Another advantage is the possibility of achieving the best combination of the various types of electrodes described previously (see Figs. 23–20 to 23–23). We would like to emphasize the role of electrodes in achieving a better response from the striated muscles. Individual anatomic conditions must always be considered before starting a stimulation protocol. These special conditions include

1. Vaginal size (4 to 12 cm in depth).
2. Vaginal shape (atresia or gaping vagina).
3. Vaginal angle (10 to 45 degrees).
4. Quality of the levator ani (thin or thick fibers).
5. Type or degree of prolapse (cystocele or uterus prolapse).

Accurate assessment of individual anatomic differences allows the therapist to select the best electrode for the most effective effect on the pelvic floor.

Home Treatment Program (Also Called Home Care)

The home treatment program is available for patients who have been previously instructed in how to use the stimulator devices.[61] Different types of stimulator units have been developed (Figs. 23–24 to 23–26). Most of them consist of a separate box containing the electronic parts and battery with a probe connected to it. Another type consists of a fully integrated unit with the electronic circuit and battery within the plug. Most devices on the market consist of a battery-powered stimulator that provides stimulus output.

For long-term treatment, nonimplantable stimulators consist of a battery-operated external pulse generator connected to vaginal or anal electrodes with wire. Short-term maximal stimulators consist of a one-channel battery-powered unit emitting either continuous or intermittent biphasic pulses from 10 Hz to 100 Hz and a width pulse of from 0.5 ms to 1

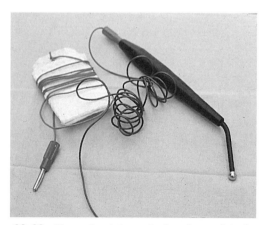

Figure 23-22 Monopolar intravaginal probe used in functional electrical stimulation.

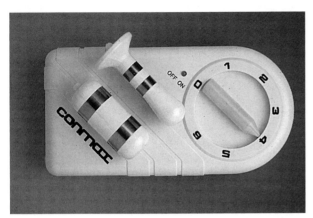

Figure 23-24 Short-term electrical stimulation with a home care device (Conmax).

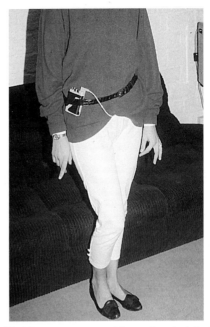

Figure 23-26 Home treatment with an electrical device (Innova) with two stimulation channels.

ms. Anal or vaginal probes are connected to these stimulators. Some stimulators now have adjustable frequencies, duty cycles, and timing controls. The stimulus can be adjusted to control the current intensity, and all these systems allow easy gradations in the intensity of the contractions.

PRACTICAL ASPECTS OF PERINEAL STIMULATION

Long-term or chronic electrical stimulation is characterized by daily applications (6 to 8 hours) of low-strength stimuli (below 12 volts) for a period of several (3 to 6) months. Either vaginal or anal application is available. The applied stimulation is so weak that it does not reach the sensory threshold. Many patients find the different devices uncomfortable to wear for a prolonged period.

Short-term electrical stimulation is more popular, for reasons of both time and practicality; it is prescribed in many countries. Patient selection, application time, and variation in electrical parameters may explain the wide variations seen in therapeutic effect and result. We think that these devices should be used after an interview and trial with a therapist.

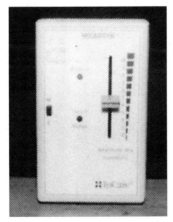

Figure 23-25 Home care with a personal short-term device (Microgyn).

We ask patients to contact the therapist in case of technical problems and propose to meet with him or her 2 weeks after the start of stimulation and then every month for 3 months.[60]

Acute maximal stimulation can be used in both methods of stimulation therapy, but according to the previous work of Kralj and colleagues[61] it is our opinion that this treatment should be exclusively part of the office therapy. The pelvic floor as a functional unit is stimulated simultaneously by three pairs of electrodes, which has the advantage of spatial summation. Three different kinds of electrodes are used: vaginal and anal plugs and needle electrodes applied to the levator ani. The mean values of currents and voltage are 45.7 mA for the vagina, 32.5 mA for the anal plug, and 15.8 mA for the needle electrodes.

The mechanism of acute maximal stimulation may be the facilitation of the supraspinal neuron or direct action on the lower motor neuron. Spatial summation improves bladder relaxation and urethral activation. If no improvement occurs after 1 month of functional electrical stimulation in home care or 20 sessions of office therapy, acute maximal stimulation of the pelvic floor may be a therapeutic alternative.[59] In our practice, in-clinic stationary equipment with a dual-channel system is used[62]; anal and vaginal probes can thus be operated either separately or together (Fig. 23–27). The strength of the stimulus is determined individually by the patient's level of pain tolerance. An average of 10 sessions lasting 20 minutes each given twice a week is recommended. The urethral closure pressure is increased and the bladder pressure is relaxed by using the following guidelines:

1. Vaginal probe: alternating pulses of 50 Hz with a duration of 1.5 ms; used intermittently with a 6-second duty cycle up to 90 mA.

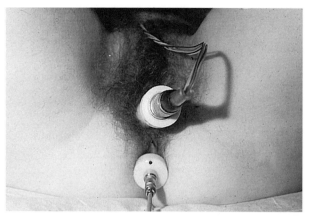

Figure 23-27 Acute functional maximal stimulation: Double stimulation, with one channel for vaginal and one channel for anal stimulation.

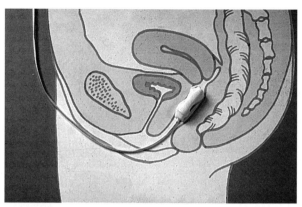

Figure 23-29 Electrical stimulation with inflatable probe in cases of vaginal prolapse: A cuff with six electrodes pointed posteriorly activates the levator ani fibers.

2. Anal probe: biphasic spike pulses of 20 Hz, 0.75 ms, used continuously up to 40 mA.

For safety, a remote control device enables the patient to decrease the level of stimulation in each channel and to stop the stimulation at any time during the session. The outpatient program facilitates patient compliance and better control and can be administered by specialized physical therapists and nurses after a training program has been completed by the patient.

In patients with vaginal prolapse who cannot retain a vaginal probe, we can improve muscular strength by using anal stimulation or a vaginal monopolar probe. This monopolar probe looks like a pen with a round metallic bulge of a very small diameter at the end. A grounded electrical connection with a wet sponge placed under the buttocks of the patient is mandatory for this type of stimulation. The patient is placed in the lithotomy position with one leg well supported; the therapist, after properly applying the monopolar probe (Fig. 23–28) into the vagina, stimulates the pubococcygeus on each side for 10 minutes. The reaction of the levator ani is excellent. This is the best method of stimulation in

patients with severe anatomic defects. Another form of stimulation in patients with cystocele or hysterocele is the use of the expandable probe (see Fig. 23–21). The vaginal inflatable cuff with four or six electrodes pointed posteriorly is inflated through a syringe to a comfortable size to push up the vaginal vault prolapse (Figs. 23–29 and 23–30). In this way, electrical current is delivered through the probe, which cannot fall out owing to a loose insertion into the vagina; this seems to be the only possible way of treating patients with urinary incontinence associated with vaginal prolapse.

INDICATIONS AND CONTRAINDICATIONS TO ELECTRICAL STIMULATION

Because of the second generation of removable devices in Europe and stationary systems in France, this therapeutic stimulation method is largely advocated for women suffering from urinary incontinence and, more recently, for those with pelvic floor dysfunction such as vaginal prolapse and sexual distur-

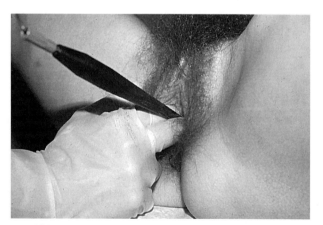

Figure 23-28 Monopolar intravaginal probe: Position of patient and therapist in order to stimulate one side of the pubococcygeal portion of the levator ani.

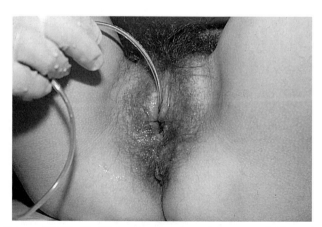

Figure 23-30 Position and retention of the expandable probe used for electrical stimulation in cases of vaginal prolapse (cystocele).

bances. We recommend it for patients who are incontinent but desire pregnancy; have a high operative risk; are on a waiting list for surgery; are reluctant to have surgery; or have an unstable bladder or urethral sphincter weakness.

When electrical stimulation is started, it may be performed in conjunction with a pelvic muscle training program or bladder drill. In certain circumstances, it may be necessary to add biofeedback therapy or behavioral therapy.

Electrical stimulation may be applied in the clinic at low cost; it has a potential curative effect and very few side effects and contraindications.[62, 63] Among the latter are (1) on-demand heart pacemakers, (2) pregnancy or the risk of pregnancy, (3) urine residuals of more than 100 ml, (4) urethral obstruction or high detrusor compliance, (5) bleeding (sessions are not held during menstrual periods), (6) urinary tract infection or vaginal infection, or (7) complete peripheral denervation of the pelvic floor.

Summary

Pelvic floor disorders can be improved by various methods of conservative treatment. Pelvic floor rehabilitation is an effective conservative therapy, but its success depends on a proper selection of patients (Fig. 23–31) to avoid unnecessary physical therapy sessions and to identify which patients are most likely to be cured while excluding those most likely to fail. This neuromuscular therapy requires an average of 2 months of an intensive exercise program (Table 23–11) comprising six sessions held twice weekly (office therapy) and 1 month of treatment with daily practice (home care).

Physical therapy should be recommended more frequently to mothers after childbirth when high-risk factors for pelvic floor relaxation exist. Urogynecologic rehabilitation should also be routinely prescribed during the months preceding some surgical procedures (Table 23–12).

Time is required before any change is noted, and the exercises must be continued for life if improvement or cure is to be maintained (maintenance program). Patients should be referred for therapy as early in the course of the disorder as possible so that treatment can be primarily preventive.

Based on my experience since 1977 in pelvic floor

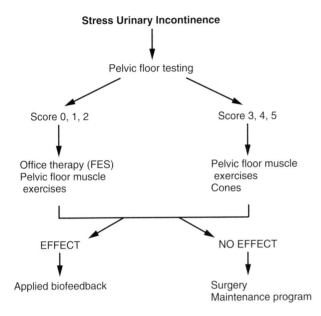

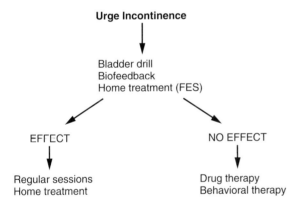

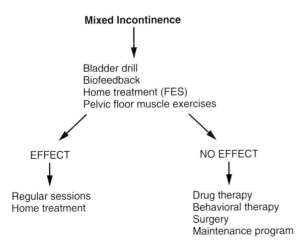

Figure 23-31 Algorithm for physical therapy management. FES, functional electrical stimulation.

TABLE 23–11
Steps in Physical Therapy Management of Pelvic Floor Disorders

Step	Method
Step One Avoid reverse perineal command Increase levator ani muscle activity	Home care
Step Two Develop perineal blockage at stress Adapt program to patient's requirements	Applied biofeedback
Step Three Develop new habits Train patients with realistic goals	Fitness program

TABLE 23–12
Postoperative Physical Therapy Management

Functional training depending on professional and physical activities

Rehabilitation through biofeedback training and low-impact aerobic exercise

Patient education about postoperative precautions and general instructions

rehabilitation, I suggest that this conservative treatment be offered to any incontinent patient before surgery. Patients who fail to achieve satisfactory results with this therapy should be referred for surgery after a 6-week trial. Physical therapy should be advised more frequently as a preventive measure in young women who have high risk factors (see Table 23–5). When physical therapy has been successful in preventing or delaying surgery, a maintenance program is necessary to avoid a relapse. It goes without saying that, to gain the best results, this treatment must be a lifetime endeavor.[44]

REFERENCES

1. Kegel AH: Progressive resistance exercise in the functional restoration of the perineal muscles. Am J Obstet Gynecol 56:238–248, 1948.
2. Kegel AH: Physiologic treatment of poor tone and function of the genital muscles and urinary stress incontinence. West J Surg 57:527–535, 1949.
3. Wilson PD, Sammarait AL, Deake M, et al: An objective assessment of physiotherapy for female genuine stress incontinence. Br J Obstet Gynecol 94:575–582, 1987.
4. Benvenuti C, Caputo GM, Bandanelli S, et al: Reeducative treatment of female genuine stress incontinence. Am J Phys Med 66:155–168, 1987.
5. Amarenco G: Explorations neurophysiologiques périnéales. Ed Techniques, Encycl. Med. Chir. Neurologie, 17030 C 10, 1991.
6. Sultan AH, Kamm MA, Bartram CL, Hudson CN: Perineal damage at delivery. Contemp Rev Obstet Gynecol 6:18–24, 1994.
7. Haadem K: The effects of parturition on pelvic floor anatomy and function. Curr Opin Obstet Gynecol 6(4):326–329, 1994.
8. Bourcier A: A new approach to biofeedback. In Proceedings of XIII Annual Meeting of the International Urogynecological Association, Riva del Garda, 1989.
9. Diokno AC, Brock BM, Brown MB, Herzog AR: Prevalence of urinary incontinence and other urological symptoms in non-institutionalized elderly. J Urol 136:1022, 1986.
10. Wolin JH: Stress incontinence in young healthy nulliparous female subjects. J Urol 101:545–549, 1969.
11. Bo K, Maelum S, Oseid S, Larsen S: Prevalence of stress urinary incontinence among physically active and sedentary female students. Scand J Sports Sci 11(3):113–116, 1989.
12. Bourcier A: La rééducation du plancher pelvien chez la femme sportive. In Proceedings of the IX Congrès Int. de la Méd. du Sport, Charleroi, 1989.
13. Bourcier A: Rééducation et urodynamique dans le post-partum. Dossiers Obstet 85:16–23, 1982.
14. Andersen JT, Blaivas JG, Cardozzo LD, Thuroff J: Lower urinary tract rehabilitation techniques: Seventh report on the standardization of terminology of lower urinary tract function. Int Urogynecol J 3:75–80, 1992.
15. Bourcier A: Pelvic floor rehabilitation. Int Urogynecol J 1:31–35, 1990.
16. Tapp A, Cardozzo LD, Versi E, et al: The effect of vaginal delivery on the urethral sphincter. Br J Obstet Gynaecol 95:142–146, 1988.
17. Bourcier A, Juras J: Conduite à tenir en obstétrique. In Urodynamique et Réadaptation en Urogynécologie. Paris, Vigot, 1986, pp 326–348.
18. Bo K, Oseid S, Kvarstein B, et al: Knowledge about and ability to correct pelvic floor muscle exercises in women with urinary stress incontinence. Neurol Urodyn 7(3):261–262, 1988.
19. Bourcier A: The influence of the pelvic floor dysfunction on sexuality. In Continence for All—A Global Perspective. Proceedings Association of Continence Advice, Bournemouth, April 1993, pp 24–26.
20. De Groat WC, Booth AM: Autonomic systems to the urinary bladder and sexual organs. In Dyck PJ, et al (eds): Peripheral Neuropathy. 2nd ed, vol 1. Philadelphia, WB Saunders, 1984.
21. Raz S: The anatomy of pelvic support and stress incontinence. In Raz S: Atlas of Transvaginal Surgery. Philadelphia, WB Saunders, 1992, pp 1–22.
22. Bourcier A, Juras J: Conduite à tenir devant un touble urogynécologique: Prolapsus génital. In: Urodynamique et Réadaptation en Urogynécologie. Paris, Vigot, 1986, pp 317–320.
23. Zaccharin RF: A Chinese anatomy: The pelvic supporting tissues of the Chinese and occidental female compared and contrasted. Aust NZ J Obstet Gynaecol 17:1–12, 1977.
24. Dixon JS, Gosling JA: The role of the pelvic floor in female urinary incontinence. Int Urogynaecol J 1:212–217, 1990.
25. Samples JT, Dougerthy MC, Abrams RM, Batich CD: The dynamic characteristics of the circumvaginal muscles. JOGNN, 17(3):194–201, 1988.
26. DeLandey JOL: Functional anatomy of the female lower urinary tract and pelvic floor. In Block G, Wheland J (eds): Neurobiology of Incontinence. London, John Wiley & Sons Ltd., 1990, pp 57–76.
27. Bourcier A, Juras J: Kinésithérapie pelvi-périnéale. In Urodynamique et Réadaptation en Urogynécologie. Paris, Vigot, 1986, pp 209–235.
28. Plevnik S: New method for testing and strengthening of pelvic floor muscles. In Proceedings of the 15th Annual Meeting of the International Continence Society, London, 1985, pp 267–268.
29. Peattie AB, Plevnik S, Stanton SL: Vaginal cones: A conservative method of treating genuine stress incontinence. Br J Gynecol 95:1049–1053, 1988.
30. Smith ARB, Hosker GL, Warrell DW: The role of pudendal nerve damage in the aetiology of genuine stress incontinence of urine. Br J Obstet Gynaecol 96:29–32, 1989.
31. Bourcier A, et al: Prevention et conseil d'hygiène de vie. In Le Plancher Pelvien, Exploration et Réadaptation. Paris, Vigot, 1989, pp 291–293.
32. Bourcier A: Prévention. In Proceedings of the First International Congress of Institut Français de Réadaptation Uro-Génitale—The Pelvic Floor: Investigations and Rehabilitation. Cannes, 1989, pp 21–23.
33. Burgio KL, Whitehead WE, Engel BT: Urinary incontinence in the elderly; bladder sphincter biofeedback and toiletting skills training. Ann Intern Med 103:507–515, 1985.
34. Cardozzo LD, Stanton SL: Biofeedback: A 5 year review Br J Urol 56:220, 1984.
35. Gosling JA, Dixon JS, Gritchley HOD, Thompson SA: A comparative study of the human external sphincter and periurthral levator ani muscles. Br J Urol 53:35–41, 1981.
36. Koelb H, Strassegger H, Riss PA, Gruber H: Morphologic and functional aspects of pelvic floor muscles in patients with pelvic relaxation and genuine stress incontinence. Obstet Gynecol 74:789–795, 1989.
37. Bourcier A: A new approach to biofeedback. In Proceedings of the XIII Annual Meeting of the International Urogynecological Association, Riva del Garda, 1989.
38. Bourcier A: Final general discussion. In Block G, Wheland J (eds): Neurobiology of Incontinence. London, John Wiley & Sons Ltd., 1990, pp 318–322.
39. Nygard IE, Delancey JOL: Exercise and incontinence. Obstet Gynecol 75:848–851, 1990.
40. Bourcier A, Pigne A: Le post partum des sportives. In Etre femme et sportive à Paris. Paris, Doin, 1991, pp 135–140.

41. Nichols DH, Milley PS: Functional pelvic anatomy: The soft tissue supports and spaces of the female pelvic organs. Reprod Med 2:21–37, 1978.

42. Bourcier A: Conservative treatment of stress incontinence in sportswomen. Proceedings of the Urodynamics Society. Neurol Urodyn 9:232, 1990.

43. Bourcier A: Périnée Féminin: Activités Physiques et Sport, Part I, Sisma Video, Time 52 Mn, Paris, Avril 1995.

44. Bourcier A, Juras J: Pelvic floor rehabilitation: A 7-year follow-up. *In* Proceedings of the 24th Annual Meeting of International Continence Society. Prague, 1994, p 43.

45. Bors E: Effect of electrical stimulation of the pudendal nerves on the vesical neck: Its significance for the function of cord bladders. J Urol 67:925, 1952.

46. Caldwell KPS, Cook PJ, Flack FC, James ED: Stress incontinence in females: Report on 31 cases of treated electrical implants. J Obstet Gynaecol Br Commonwlth 75:777, 1968.

47. Alexander S, Rowan D, Millar W, Scott R: Treatment of urinary incontinence by electric stimulation pessary. A report of 18 patients. Br J Urol 42:184, 1970.

48. Suhel P, Rakovec S, Godec C, et al: Functional electrical stimulation of the external urinary sphincter and fatigue of the sphincter. *In* Proceedings of the 4th International Symposium on External Control of Human Extremities. Dubrovnik, 1973, p 632.

49. Erlandson BE, Fall M, Carlsson CA, Linder LE: Mechanisms for closure of the human urethra during intravaginal electrical stimulation. Scand J Urol Nephrol 44(suppl):49–54, 1978.

50. Vodusek DB, Light JK, Libby JM: Detrusor inhibition induced by stimulation of pudendal nerve afferents. Neurourol Urodyn 5:381–389, 1986.

51. Plevnik S, Vodusek DB, Vrtacnik P: Optimatization of pulse duration in treatment of urinary incontinence. World J Urol 4:22–23, 1986.

52. Bazed MA, Thuroff JW, Schmidt RA: Effect of chronic electro-stimulation of the sacral roots on the striated urthral sphincter. J Urol 128:1357–1362, 1982.

53. Pette D: Activity induced fast to slow transitions in mammalian muscle. Med Sci Sports Exerc 16:517, 1984.

54. Fall M: Does electrostimulation cure urinary incontinence? J Urol 131:664–667, 1984.

55. Fall M, Lindstrom S: Functional electrical stimulation: physiological basis and clinical principles. Int Urogynecol J 5:296–304, 1994.

56. Fall M, Lindstrom S: Electrical stimulation. A physiologic approach to the treatment of urinary incontinence. Urol Clin North Am 18:1, 1991.

57. Ohlsson BL, Fall M, Sommar S: Effects of external stimulation and direct pudendal nerve maximal electrical stimulation in the treatment of the uninhibited overactive bladder. Br J Urol 64:374–380, 1989.

58. Bent AE, Sand PK, Ostergard DR: Transvaginal electrical stimulation in the treatment of genuine stress incontinence and detrusor instability. Int Urogynecol J 4:9–13, 1993.

59. Eriksen BC, Bergmann S, Erik-Nes SH: Maximum electrostimulation of the pelvic floor in female idiopathic detrusor instablity and urge incontinence. Neurourol Urodyn 8:219, 1989.

60. Bourcier A: Office therapy and home care perineal stimulation Urodinamica Neurourodynamics Continence 2(1):83–86, 1992.

61. Kralj B, Plevnik S, Janko M, Vrtacnik P: Urge incontinence and maximal electrical stimulation. *In* Proceedings of 7th Annual Meeting of International Continence Society. Protoroz, 1977, p 16.

62. Bourcier A, Juras J: Electrical stimulation for sphincter incompetence. J Urol 153(4), AUA Ninetieth Annual Meeting, Las Vegas, April 23–28, 1995.

63. Bourcier A, Juras J: Electrical stimulation: Home treatment versus office therapy. J Urol 161(5), AUA Eighty-ninth Annual Meeting, San Francisco, May 14–19, 1994.

CHAPTER 24

Principles of Pharmacologic Therapy: Practical Drug Treatment of Voiding Dysfunction in the Female

Alan J. Wein, M.D.

The lower urinary tract performs two basic functions: storage of urine and emptying of urine. The physiology and pharmacology of micturition have been described by many qualified authors, each of whom has reported his or her own particular concept of the neuroanatomy, neurophysiology, and neuropharmacology of the smooth and striated muscular structures involved; the peripheral, autonomic, and somatic neural factors; and the spinal and supraspinal influences that are necessary for normal function (see references 1 to 5 for summaries and references). Although there are significant disagreements about the finer details, it is important to realize that exact agreement about neuromorphology, neurophysiology, and neuropharmacology is *not necessary* for an understanding of the pharmacologic principles and applications involved in drug-induced alteration of voiding function and dysfunction. Despite disagreements about various details, all "experts" would doubtless agree that, for the purposes of description and teaching, one can succinctly summarize the two phases of micturition from a conceptual point of view. Bladder filling and urine storage require (1) accommodation of increasing volumes of urine at a low intravesical pressure and with appropriate sensation; (2) a bladder outlet that is closed at rest and remains so during increases in intra-abdominal pressure; and (3) absence of involuntary bladder contractions (detrusor instability or hyperreflexia). Bladder emptying requires (1) a coordinated contraction by the bladder smooth musculature of adequate magnitude and duration; (2) concomitant lowering of resistance at the level of the smooth sphincter (the smooth muscle of the bladder neck and proximal urethra) and of the striated sphincter (the periurethral and intramural urethral striated musculature); and (3) absence of anatomic obstruction.

This very simple but acceptable overview implies that any type of voiding dysfunction (i.e., of storage, emptying, or a combination of these must result from an abnormality of one or more of the factors listed previously. This description, with its implied subdivisions under each category, provides a logical framework for the discussion and classification of all types of voiding dysfunction. There are indeed some types of voiding dysfunction that represent combination of filling or storage and emptying abnormalities. Within this scheme, however, these become readily understandable, and their detection and treatment can be logically described. In addition, all aspects of urodynamic, radiologic, and videourodynamic evaluation can be conceptualized in regard to exactly what they evaluate in terms of either bladder or outlet activity during filling or storage or emptying within this scheme. Likewise, one can easily classify all known treatments for voiding dysfunction under the broad categories of facilitating either filling–storage or emptying, and achieving this by acting primarily on the bladder or on one or more of the components of the bladder outlet.

As a result of advances in the knowledge of the neuropharmacology and neurophysiology of the lower urinary tract, effective pharmacologic therapy does exist for the management of many types of voiding dysfunction. This chapter summarizes the treatments available for female voiding dysfunction within this functional classification (Tables 24–1 and 24–2). As an apology to others in the field whose works have not been specifically cited in this chapter, it should be noted that citations have generally been chosen primarily because of their review or informational content or sometimes their controversial nature, and not because of their originality or initial publication on a particular subject.

TABLE 24–1
Therapy Used to Facilitate Bladder Emptying

A. Increasing intravesical pressure or bladder contractility
　1. External compression, Valsalva maneuver
　2. Promotion or initiation of reflex contractions
　　a. Tigger zones or maneuvers
　　b. Bladder training, tidal drainage
　3. Pharmacologic therapy
　　a. Parasympathomimetic agents
　　b. Prostaglandins
　　c. Blockers of inhibition
　　　(1) Alpha-adrenergic antagonists
　　　(2) Opioid antagonists
　4. Electrical stimulation
　　a. Directly to the bladder or spinal cord
　　b. To the nerve roots
　　c. Transurethral intravesical electrotherapy
　5. Reduction cystoplasty
B. Decreasing outlet resistance
　1. At a site of anatomic obstruction
　　a. Prostatectomy, otomy (diathermy, laser, heat)
　　b. Balloon dilation
　　c. Intraurethral stent
　　d. Pharmacologic—decrease prostate size or tone
　　　(1) Luteinizing hormone–releasing hormone agonists
　　　(2) Antiandrogens
　　　(3) 5α-reductase inhibitors
　　　(4) Alpha-adrenergic antagonists
　　e. Urethral stricture repair or dilation
　2. At the level of the smooth sphincter
　　a. Pharmacologic therapy
　　　(1) Alpha-adrenergic antagonists
　　　(2) Beta-adrenergic agonists
　　b. Transurethral resection or incision of the bladder neck
　　c. Y-V plasty of the bladder neck
　3. At the level of the striated sphincter
　　a. Pharmacologic therapy
　　　(1) Skeletal muscle relaxants
　　　　(a) Benzodiazepines
　　　　(b) Baclofen
　　　　(c) Dantrolene
　　　(2) Alpha-adrenergic antagonists
　　b. Urethral overdilation
　　c. Surgical sphincterotomy, botulinum A toxin
　　d. Urethral stent
　　e. Pudendal nerve interruption
　　f. Psychotherapy, biofeedback
C. Circumventing the problem
　1. Intermittent catheterization
　2. Continuous catheterization
　3. Urinary diversion

Clinical Uropharmacology of the Lower Urinary Tract: Some Useful Concepts

Clinical uropharmacology of the lower urinary tract is based primarily on an appreciation of the innervation and receptor content of the bladder and its related anatomic structures. The drugs or classes of drugs used were, in general, developed originally for their actions on other organ systems whose functions are controlled or affected by innervation or drug-receptor interaction. The targets of pharmacologic intervention in the bladder body, base, or outlet include nerve terminals that alter the release of spe-

cific neurotransmitters, receptor subtypes, cellular second-messenger systems, and ion channels identified in the bladder and urethra. Peripheral nerves and ganglia, spinal cord, and supraspinal areas are also sites of action of some agents to be discussed. Because autonomic innervation and receptor content are ubiquitous throughout the human body's organ systems, there are no agents in clinical use that are purely selective for action on the lower urinary tract. The majority of side effects attributed to drugs facilitating bladder storage or emptying are collateral effects on organ systems that share some of the same neurophysiologic or neuropharmacologic characteristics as the bladder.

Principles of Pharmacotherapy: Evaluation of Drug Effects on Lower Urinary Tract Function

Most pharmacologic agents produce their effects by combining with specialized functional components of cells. The cell component directly involved in the initial action of a drug is known as its receptor. The drug–receptor interaction alters the function of the cell component involved and initiates the series of biochemical and physiologic changes that characterize the effects produced by the agent. Most of the agents that alter the urodynamics of the lower urinary tract affect the synthesis, transport, storage, and release of the neurotransmitter; the combination of the neurotransmitter with postjunctional receptors; or the inactivation, degradation, or reuptake of the neurotransmitter. Complex metabolic changes occur after receptor activation, and these mechanisms, which are "metabolically distal" to membrane receptor sites, are also potential sites of stimulation, inhibition, or modulation. The central nervous system, preganglionic and postganglionic autonomic nerves and their ganglia, and peripheral somatic nerves are also potential sites of drug action.

To use any drug intelligently, it is necessary to be familiar not only with its biochemical and physiologic effects and mechanisms of action but also with all the factors that determine concentration at its site of action. One must be thoroughly familiar with the literature on the use of a particular agent, but great caution should be exercised in drawing inferences from only laboratory results and assuming application of such inferences to human systems. We have found the following precepts useful in evaluating the literature used to support the use of certain drugs for voiding dysfunction.[1]

1. The bewildering array of experimental models must be carefully considered. A small change in one model may make the results of tests totally noncomparable to those obtained in another model.

2. Results in certain animal models do not necessarily imply exact similarity to humans or other spe-

TABLE 24–2
Therapy Used to Facilitate Urine Storage

A. Inhibiting bladder contractility, decreasing sensory input, or increasing bladder capacity
   1. Habit training (timed voiding); prompted voiding
   2. Bladder training (± biofeedback)
   3. Pharmacologic therapy
      a. Anticholinergic agents
      b. Musculotropic relaxants
      c. Calcium antagonists
      d. Potassium channel openers
      e. Prostaglandin inhibitors
      f. Beta-adrenergic agonists
      g. Tricyclic antidepressants
      h. Dimethyl sulfoxide (DMSO)
   4. Bladder overdistention
   5. Electrical stimulation (reflex inhibition)
   6. Acupuncture
   7. Interruption of innervation
      a. Central (subarachnoid block)
      b. Peripheral (sacral rhizotomy, selective sacral rhizotomy)
      c. Dorsal
      d. Perivesical (peripheral bladder denervation)
   8. Augmentation cystoplasty
B. Increasing outlet resistance
   1. Physiotherapy (± biofeedback)
   2. Electrical stimulation of the pelvic floor
   3. Pharmacologic therapy
      a. Alpha-adrenergic agonists
      b. Tricyclic antidepressants
      c. Beta-adrenergic antagonists
      d. Estrogens
      e. Beta-adrenergic agonists
   4. Vesicourethral suspension (SUI)
   5. Bladder outlet reconstruction
   6. Surgical mechanical compression
      a. Sling procedures
      b. Artificial urinary sphincter
   7. Nonsurgical mechanical compression
      a. Periurethral collagen, polytef, fat injection
      b. Occlusive devices
C. Circumventing the problem
   1. Antidiuretic hormone–like agents
   2. Intermittent catheterization
   3. Continuous catheterization
   4. Urinary diversion
   5. External collecting devices
   6. Absorbent products

cies. Results obtained in one type of tissue may not be equivalent to those from another, even if the tissues are from the same species, seem similar, and are adjacent anatomically.

3. Significant changes in pharmacologic action may be secondary to alterations induced by or related to age, sex, hormonal status, infection, denervation or decentralization, stretch, and the effects of certain drugs, including laboratory and clinical anesthetics. Additionally, long-term effects may be different from acute ones.

4. In vitro experimental results are not necessarily the same as in vivo experimental results, and neither of these are necessarily equivalent to "normal."

5. Receptors do not necessarily imply innervation or function. The effect produced by an agonist or antagonist does not necessarily impart physiologic significance to a particular neurotransmitter or component of the nervous system.

6. Pressure or tension generation by a whole organ model or muscle strip is not necessarily the same as contractility, and neither of these is necessarily translatable into assumptions about bladder storage or emptying ability, or outlet resistance.

7. A particular compound may act at multiple sites within a neural pathway or effector, and the net action on function may not be consistent with an individual laboratory experiment on one component of a system.

Although a number of clinical trials in the literature are of high quality, many have deficiencies in design, conduct, analysis, or presentation of results. This is especially true in studies of non-neuropathic voiding dysfunction, in which symptomatic and urodynamic correlates seem to be less constant from day to day than in patients with a fixed neurologic lesion. Criteria cited for an ideal clinical trial of a pharmacologic agent for treatment of a particular voiding dysfunction, generally modified from those in older editions of Goodman and Gilman,[2] are as follows:

1. Lack of bias
2. Inclusion of an adequate number of subjects
3. Use of appropriate and sensitive methods of evaluation
4. Double-blind conditions and a placebo
5. Statistical validation

Appropriate and sensitive methods of evaluation should include objective as well as subjective data. Ideally, these methods will yield objective urodynamic data that are easily subject to statistical analysis. Subjective data, usually in the form of symptoms, are generally difficult to quantify and analyze. A double-blind study refers to one in which the subject and the investigator are unaware of the identity of the treatment. Ideally, the drug under consideration is compared with a placebo. In protocols that use primarily subjective criteria for assessment, it has long been recognized that improvement in such criteria may occur in 35% of placebo-treated patients.[2] In general, the placebo effect can be boosted by a very positive and enthusiastic attitude on the part of the treating physician, by the length of time spent with the patient, and by an in-hospital type of regimen. Unfortunately, most, if not all, clinically useful pharmacologic agents have some side effects. It is virtually impossible to build into a placebo the potential side effects of a therapeutic agent under consideration without making it something other than an inert compound. Determination of changes of statistical significance and objective parameters does not usually present a problem, especially when dealing with a placebo-controlled study. Subjective variables are extremely difficult to quantify statistically. Many such variables are often graded according to severity, and the resultant changes in grade are subjected to analysis. Unless the changes are marked, this type of analysis has obvious potential shortcomings because adjacent categories may exhibit only shades of difference that are not clinically significant. The concept of *clinical significance*, as opposed to *statistical significance*, must always be kept in mind when reporting the results of a therapeutic trial. This is especially true when an investigator chooses to report results in terms of percentage changes rather than absolute changes. For instance, an increase in mean flow rate from 3 to 6 ml/second obviously represents a very statistically significant change, as does a decrease in residual urine from 300 to 200 ml, an increase in urodynamic bladder capacity from 100 to 150 ml, and a decrease in the number of daily incontinence episodes from six to four. One must always consider differences between such statistical improvements and what constitutes a truly clinically significant improvement. Finally, if a drug is found to be clinically effective it should be compared, over pharmacologic dose ranges, with an available and generally less expensive "reference drug" in terms of effectiveness, selectivity, and side effects.

Generally speaking, the simplest and least hazardous form of treatment should always be tried first. A combination of therapeutic maneuvers or pharmacologic agents can sometimes be used to achieve a particular effect, especially if their mechanisms of actions are different and their side effects are not synergistic. At the outset, it should be noted that in our experience, although great improvement often occurs with rational pharmacologic therapy, a perfect result (restoration to normal status) is seldom if ever achieved.

The Elderly Patient

In the aging patient many nonurinary pathologic, anatomic, and physiologic factors serve as comorbidities in the development of acute incontinence or the aggravation of chronic incontinence. Potentially reversible pathologies should be appreciated by the treating physician: infection, atrophic vaginitis and urethritis, fecal impaction, limited mobility, delirium, and hyperglycemia. Elderly patients are frequently taking many drugs, and iatrogenic incontinence (physician-induced) may result from the pharmacologic side effects of well-intentioned therapy. Sedative hypnotics and alcohol depress general behavior and sensorium; they may also depress bladder contractility and reduce attention to bladder cues. Diuretics produce polyuria and may be the source of complaints of urgency, frequency, and nocturia. Agents with anticholinergic properties may significantly decrease detrusor contractility; these include antihistamines, antidepressants, antipsychotics, opiates, gastrointestinal antispasmodics, and anti-Parkinsonian drugs. Alpha-adrenergic agonists (contained in many decongestants or cold remedies) can increase bladder neck tone and may promote urinary retention. Alpha-adrenergic antagonists may predispose to sphincteric

incontinence. Calcium channel blockers for hypertension or coronary artery disease are smooth muscle relaxants, can facilitate bladder storage, and may cause urinary retention and overflow incontinence.

Specific Methods of Pharmacologic Treatment

FACILITATION OF BLADDER EMPTYING

Absolute or relative failure to empty results from decreased bladder contractility, increased outlet resistance, or both.[6] Absolute or relative failure of adequate bladder contractility may result from temporary or permanent alteration in any one of the neuromuscular mechanisms necessary for initiating and maintaining a normal detrusor contraction. In a neurologically normal individual inhibition of the micturition reflex may also be secondary to painful stimuli, especially stimuli from the pelvic and perineal areas, or it may be psychogenic. Some types of drug therapy may also inhibit bladder contractility through either neurologic or myogenic mechanisms. Non-neurogenic causes include intrinsic impairment of bladder smooth muscle function, which may result from overdistention, severe infection, or fibrosis. Increased outlet resistance is generally secondary to anatomic obstruction but may be secondary to a failure of coordination of the smooth or striated sphincter during bladder contraction. Treatment of failure to empty generally consists of attempts to increase intravesical pressure or facilitate the micturition reflex, to decrease outlet resistance, or both.

Increasing Intravesical Pressure or Facilitating Bladder Contraction

PARASYMPATHOMIMETIC AGENTS   Because a major portion of the final common pathway in physiologic bladder contraction is stimulation of parasympathetic postganglionic muscarinic cholinergic receptor sites, agents that imitate the actions of acetylcholine (ACh) might be expected to be effective in treating patients who cannot empty because of inadequate bladder contractility. ACh itself cannot be used for therapeutic purposes because of its actions at central and ganglionic levels and because of its rapid hydrolysis by acetylcholinesterase and butyrylcholinesterase.[7] Many acetylcholinelike drugs exist, but only bethanechol chloride (BC) has a relatively selective in vitro action on the urinary bladder and gut with little or no nicotinic action.[7] BC is cholinesterase-resistant and causes an in vitro contraction of smooth muscle from all areas of the bladder.[8, 9]

Agents similar to BC have long been recommended[10] for the treatment of postoperative or postpartum urinary retention. In such cases, BC should be used only if the patient is awake and alert and if there is no outlet obstruction. The dose is 5 to 10 mg given subcutaneously. For more than 30 years BC has been recommended for the treatment of the atonic or hypotonic bladder,[11] and it has been reported to be effective in achieving "rehabilitation" of the chronically atonic or hypotonic detrusor.[12] Bethanechol has also been used to stimulate or facilitate the development of reflex bladder contractions in patients in spinal shock secondary to suprasacral spinal cord injury.[13]

Although BC has been reported to increase gastrointestinal motility and has been used in the treatment of gastroesophageal reflux, and although anecdotal success in specific patients with voiding dysfunction seems to occur, there is little or no evidence to support its success in facilitating bladder emptying in series of patients in which the drug was the only variable.[14] In one set of trials, a pharmacologically active subcutaneous dose (5 mg) did not demonstrate significant changes in flow parameters or residual urine volume in (1) a group of women with a residual urine volume equal to or greater than 20% of bladder capacity but no evidence of neurologic disease or outlet obstruction, (2) a group of 27 "normal" women of approximately the same age, or (3) a group of patients with a positive reaction to a bethanechol supersensitivity test.[15, 16] This dose did increase cystometric filling pressure and also decreased bladder capacity threshold, findings previously described by others.[12] Short-term studies in which the drug was the only variable have generally failed to demonstrate significant efficacy in terms of flow and residual urine volume data.[17] Farrell and colleagues conducted a double-blind randomized trial that looked at the effects of two catheter management protocols and the effect of BC on postoperative urinary retention following gynecologic incontinence surgery.[18] They concluded that BC was not helpful at all in this setting. Although BC is capable of eliciting an increase in bladder smooth muscle tension, as would be expected from in vitro studies, its ability to stimulate or facilitate a coordinated and sustained physiologic-like bladder contraction in patients with voiding dysfunction has been unimpressive.[14] Similar sentiments have been expressed by Andersson[7] and others.[9]

It is difficult to find reproducible urodynamic data that support recommendations for the usage of BC in any specific category of patients. Most, if not all, "long-term" reports in such patients are neither prospective nor double-blind and do not exclude the effects of other simultaneous regimens (such as treatment of urinary infection, bladder decompression, timed emptying, or other types of treatment affecting the bladder or outlet), an important observation to be considered when reporting such drug studies. Whether repeated doses of BC or any cholinergic agonist can achieve a clinical effect that a single dose cannot is speculative, as are suggestions that BC has a different mode of action or effect on atonic or decompensated bladder muscle than on normal tissue. BC, administered subcutaneously, does cause an increased awareness of a distended bladder.[19] This could facilitate more frequent emptying at lower volumes, thereby helping to avoid overdistention. In the laboratory, a functioning micturition reflex is an absolute requirement for the production of a sustained bladder contraction by a subcutaneous injection of the drug. Patients with incomplete lower motor neuron lesions constitute the most reasonable group for a trial of BC,[20] although subcutaneous administration may be required. It is generally agreed that, at least in a "denervated" bladder, an oral dose of 200 mg is required to produce the same urodynamic effects as a subcutaneous dose of 5 mg.[21]

O'Donnell and Hawkins administered 5 mg of BC subcutaneously to 10 neurologically intact men and made the following cystometric observations: Bladder volume at first desire to void decreased (220 ml to 85), maximum bladder capacity decreased 380 ml to 160), first desire to void occurred at a higher pressure (5 vs. 28 cm H_2O), and compliance was reduced.[22] They concluded that BC affects the ability of the bladder to accommodate volume. Patients were comfortable at a resting bladder pressure of 20 cm H_2O (uncommon in their population), and the pressures at maximum bladder capacity were considerably higher than those commonly seen under normal conditions. This suggested to these authors either that bladder pressure alone is not a significant factor in the perception of a sensation of first desire to void *or* that BC somehow alters the threshold at which perception of desire to void occurs (because these patients showed a tolerance for increased intravesical pressure prior to the first desire to void and at maximum bladder capacity).

Other methods of achieving a cholinergic effect are seldom used in the United States. Philp and coworkers reported that a 4-mg oral dose of carbachol, a cholinergic agonist that also possesses some ganglionic-stimulating properties, had a much more favorable effect on urodynamic parameters in patients with cholinergic supersensitivity than a 50-mg oral dose of BC, with no apparent increase in side effects.[23] Voided volumes were reduced, detrusor pressures increased, and the length of contraction shortened. Hedlund and Andersson treated patients with benign prostatic hyperplasia with 2 to 4 mg three times a day of carbachol.[24] Although gastrointestinal side effects were experienced, there were no changes in urodynamic variables. Taylor states that carbachol is "no longer available" because of its nicotinic action.[7] Anticholinesterase agents also have the net effect of producing or enhancing cholinergic stimulation. Philp and Thomas reported that parenteral but not oral distigmine improved voiding efficiency in patients with neurogenic bladder dysfunction with reflex detrusor activity.[25] Shah and associates, however, reported a double-blind study in which parenteral distigmine produced no statistically significant differences in voiding effectiveness after prostatectomy in patients with large preoperative residual urine volumes.[26]

No agreement exists about whether cholinergic

stimulation produces an increase in urethral resistance.[15, 16] It appears that pharmacologically active doses do in fact increase urethral closure pressure, at least in patients with detrusor hyperreflexia.[27] This would of course tend to inhibit bladder emptying. As to whether cholinergic agonists can be combined with agents to decrease outlet resistance to facilitate emptying and achieve an additive or synergistic effect, our own experience with such therapy, using even as much as 200 mg of oral BC daily, has been extremely disappointing. Certainly, most clinicians would agree that a total divided daily dose of 50 to 100 mg rarely affects any urodynamic parameter at all. The potential side effects of cholinomimetic drugs include flushing, nausea, vomiting, diarrhea, gastrointestinal cramps, bronchospasm, headache, salivation, sweating, and difficulty with visual accommodation.[7] Intramuscular and intravenous use can precipitate acute and severe side effects, resulting in acute circulatory failure and cardiac arrest, and is therefore prohibited. Contraindications to the use of this general category of drug include bronchial asthma, peptic ulcer, bowel obstruction, enteritis, recent gastrointestinal surgery, cardiac arrhythmia, hyperthyroidism, and any type of bladder outlet obstruction.

One potential avenue of increasing bladder contractility is cholinergic enhancement or augmentation. Such an action might be useful above or in combination with a parasympathomimetic agent. Metoclopramide (Reglan) is a dopamine antagonist with cholinergic properties. It has a central antiemetic effect in the chemoreceptor trigger zone and peripherally increases the tone of the lower esophageal sphincter, promoting gastric emptying. Its effects seem to be related to its ability to antagonize the inhibitory action of dopamine, to augment ACh release, and to sensitize the muscarinic receptors of gastrointestinal smooth muscle.[28] Some data in the dog suggest that this agent can increase detrusor contractility,[29] and there is one anecdotal case report of improved bladder function in a diabetic patient treated originally with this agent for gastroparesis.[30] Cisapride is a substituted synthetic benzamide that enhances the release of ACh in Auerbach's plexus (in the gastrointestinal tract). In 15 patients with complete spinal cord injury treated with 10 mg of cisapride three times a day for 3 days, Carone and associates noted earlier and higher amplitude reflex contractions in those with hyperactive bladders; in those with hypoactive bladders there was a significant decrease in compliance.[31] There was also increased activity and decreased compliance of the anorectal ampulla with no alteration in striated sphincter activity. In another study in paraplegic patients cisapride was found to decrease colonic transit time and maximal rectal capacity; an incidental decrease in residual urine was also noted (though only from 51.5 to 27.7 ml).[32]

PROSTAGLANDINS The reported use of prostaglandins (PG) to facilitate emptying is based on the hypothesis that these substances contribute to the maintenance of bladder tone and bladder contractile activity (see references 1 and 33 for a complete discussion). PGE_2 and $PGF_{2\alpha}$ cause in vitro and in vivo bladder contractile response. PGE_2 seems to cause a net decrease in urethral smooth muscle tone; $PGF_{2\alpha}$ causes an increase. Bultitude and colleagues reported that instillation of 0.5 mg PGE_2 into the bladders of women with varying degrees of urinary retention resulted in acute emptying and in improvement of longer-term emptying (several months) in two-thirds of the patients studied (n = 22).[34] In general, they reported a decrease in the volume at which voiding was initiated, an increase in bladder pressure, and a decrease in residual urine. Desmond and coworkers reported the results of intravesical use of 1.5 mg of this agent (diluted with 20 ml of 0.2% neomycin solution) in patients whose bladders exhibited no contractile activity or in whom bladder contractility was relatively impaired.[35] Twenty of 36 patients showed a strongly positive response, and six showed a weakly positive immediate response. Fourteen patients were reported to show prolonged beneficial effects, all but one of whom had shown a strongly positive immediate response. Stratification of the data revealed that an intact sacral reflex arc was a prerequisite for any type of positive response. The authors noted additionally that the effects of PGE_2 appeared to be additive or synergistic with cholinergic stimulation in some patients.

Vaidyanathan and colleagues reported that intravesical instillation of 7.5 mg of $PGF_{2\alpha}$ produced reflex voiding in some patients with incomplete suprasacral spinal cord lesions.[36] The favorable response to a single dose of drug, when present, lasted from 1.0 to 2.5 months. Tammela and associates reported that one intravesical administration of 10 mg of $PGF_{2\alpha}$ facilitated voiding in women who were in retention 3 days after surgery for stress urinary incontinence.[37] The drug was administered in 50 ml of saline as a single dose and retained for 2 hours. It should be noted, however, that in these "successfully" treated patients, the average maximum flow rate was 10.6 ml/second with a mean residual urine volume of 107 ml; also, the authors state that "bladder emptying deteriorated in most patients on the day after treatment." Jaschevatsky and colleagues reported that 16 mg of $PGF_{2\alpha}$ in 40 ml of saline given intravesically reduced the frequency of urinary retention in a group of women undergoing gynecologic surgery but, inexplicably, only in women undergoing vaginal hysterectomy with vaginal repair—not in those undergoing vaginal repair with urethral plication or vaginal repair alone.[38] Koonings and colleagues reported that daily intravesical doses of $PGF_{2\alpha}$ and intravaginal PGE_2 reduced the number of days required for catheterization after stress incontinence surgery compared to a control group receiving intravesical saline.[39] Other investigators, however, have reported conflicting (negative) results. Stanton and associates and Delaere and coworkers reported no success using intravesical PGE_2 in doses similar to those reported earlier[40, 41]; Delaere and coworkers similarly reported no success using $PGF_{2\alpha}$ in a group of women with emptying difficulties of various causes, although it should be noted that they used lower doses than those reported earlier.[41] Wagner and colleagues used PGE_2 in doses of 0.75 to 2.25 mg and reported no effect on urinary retention in a group of patients who had undergone anterior colporrhaphy.[42] Schubler reported that both intravesical PGE_2 and sulprostone (a derivative) caused a strong sensation of urgency in normal female volunteers, resulting in reduced bladder capacity and instability.[43] Both agents also decreased resting urethral closure pressure. PGE_2 increased detrusor pressure at opening and during maximum flow. Sulprostone slightly decreased these latter two parameters. All effects had disappeared 24 hours after administration. Prostaglandins have a relatively short half-life, and it is difficult to understand how any effects after a single application can last as long as several months. If such an effect does occur, it must be the result of a "triggering effect" on some as yet unknown physiologic or metabolic mechanism. Because of the number of conflicting positive and negative reports with various intravesical preparations, double-blind placebo-controlled studies would obviously be helpful to determine whether there are circumstances in which PG usage can reproducibly facilitate emptying or treat postoperative retention. Potential side effects of prostaglandin usage include vomiting, diarrhea, pyrexia, hypertension, and hypotension.[44]

BLOCKERS OF INHIBITION DeGroat and coworkers[1, 4, 45] have demonstrated a sympathetic reflex during bladder filling, that, at least in the cat, promotes urine storage partly by exerting an alpha-adrenergic inhibitory effect on pelvic parasympathetic ganglionic transmission. Some investigators have suggested that alpha-adrenergic blockade, in addition to decreasing outlet resistance, may in fact facilitate transmission through these ganglia and thereby enhance bladder contractility. On this basis, Raz and Smith first advocated a trial of an alpha-adrenergic blocking agent for the treatment of nonobstructive urinary retention.[47] Tammela reported that phenoxybenzamine (POB) was more effective in preventing recurrent retention after initial catheterization in a group of postoperative patients than was either carbachol or placebo.[48] Goldman and colleagues reported on a prospective randomized study of 102 patients over age 60 undergoing hernia repair.[49] Of the 44 control patients, 26 developed postoperative retention, whereas no treated patients (who were given POB 10 mg the night before and 2 hours before surgery, and twice a day for 3 days afterwards) did so. In 21 of 26 patients with urinary retention, the retention disappeared within 48 hours after POB administration (and bladder decompression). Although such an effect may be due solely to an alpha-adrenergic effect on the outlet (see next section, Decreasing Outlet Resistance), it may be that alpha-adrenergic blockade can under certain circumstances facilitate the detrusor reflex—through either a direct effect on parasympathetic ganglia or an indirect one (a mechanism associated with a decrease in urethral resistance).

OPIOID ANTAGONISTS Recent advances in neuropeptide physiology and pharmacology have provided new insights into lower urinary tract function and its potential pharmacologic alteration. It has been hypothesized that endogenous opioids may exert a tonic inhibitory effect on the micturition reflex at various levels,[1, 3] and agents such as narcotic antagonists therefore may offer possibilities for stimulating reflex bladder activity. Thor and associates were able to stimulate a micturition contraction with naloxone, an opiate antagonist, in unanesthetized cats with chronic spinal disease.[50] The effects, however, were transient, and tachyphylaxis developed. Vaidyanathan reported that an intravenous injection of 0.4 mg of naloxone enhanced detrusor reflex activity in five of seven patients with neuropathic bladder dysfunction caused by incomplete suprasacral spinal cord lesions.[51] The maximum effect occurred in 1 to 2 minutes after intravenous injection and was gone by 5 minutes. Murray and Feneley reported that in a group of patients with idiopathic detrusor instability, the same dose of naloxone caused an increase in detrusor pressure at zero volume and at first desire to void, a decrease in the maximum cystometric capacity, and a worsening of the degree of instability.[52] Galeano and coworkers reported that although naloxone increased bladder contractility in the cat with chronic spinal disease, it also aggravated striated sphincter dyssynergia and spasticity—a potential problem in the treatment of patients with emptying failure.[53] Wheeler and colleagues, however, noted no significant cystometric changes in a group of 15 patients with spinal cord injury following intravenous naloxone, and they noted that 11 showed decreased perineal electromyographic (EMG) activity.[54] Although this issue is intriguing, it is of little practical use at present.

Decreasing Outlet Resistance

At the Level of the Smooth Sphincter

ALPHA-ADRENERGIC ANTAGONISTS Whether or not one believes there is significant innervation of the bladder and proximal urethral smooth musculature by postganglionic fibers of the sympathetic nervous system, one must acknowledge the existence of alpha- and beta-adrenergic receptor sites in these areas.[1, 5] The smooth muscle of the bladder base and proximal urethra contains predominantly alpha-adrenergic receptors. The bladder body contains both varieties of adrenergic receptors, the beta variety being more common. The implication that alpha-adrenergic blockade could be useful in certain patients who cannot empty the bladder was actually first made by Kleeman in 1970.[55] Krane and Olsson were among the first to endorse the concept of a physiologic internal sphincter that is partially controlled by tonic sympathetic stimulation of contractile alpha-adrenergic receptors in the smooth musculature of the bladder neck and proximal urethra.[56, 57] Further, they hypothesized that some obstructions that occur at this level during detrusor contraction result from an inadequate opening of the bladder neck or an inadequate decrease in resistance in the area of the proximal urethra. They also theorized and presented evidence that alpha-adrenergic blockade could be useful in promoting bladder emptying in such a patient—one with an adequate detrusor contraction but without anatomic obstruction or detrusor–striated sphincter dyssynergia. Abel and colleagues called attention to the fact that such a functional obstruction, which they, too, presumed to be mediated by the sympathetic nervous system, could be maximal at a urethral rather than bladder neck level, and coined the term "neuropathic urethra."[58]

Many others have subsequently confirmed the utility of alpha-blockade in the treatment of what is now usually referred to as smooth sphincter or bladder neck dyssynergia or dysfunction (see reference 9 for other references). Successful results, usually defined as an increase in flow rate, a decrease in residual urine, and an improvement in upper tract appearance (when that is pathologic), can often be correlated with an objective decrease in urethral profile closure pressures. One would expect such success with alpha-adrenergic blockade in treating emptying failure to be least evident in patients with detrusor–striated sphincter dyssynergia, as reported by Hachen.[59] Although most would agree that alpha blockers exert their favorable effects on voiding dysfunction primarily by affecting the smooth muscle of the bladder neck and proximal urethra, some information suggests that they may affect (decrease) striated sphincter tone as well. Other data suggest that they may exert some effects on the symptoms of voiding dysfunction in certain circumstances by decreasing bladder contractility (see later discussion, Decreasing Bladder Contractility).

Much of the confusion relative to whether alpha blockers have a direct (as opposed to an indirect) inhibitory effect on the striated sphincter relates to the interpretation of observations about their effect on urethral pressure and periurethral striated muscle EMG activity in the region of the urogenital diaphragm. It is impossible to tell by pressure tracings alone whether a decrease in resistance in one area of the urethra is secondary to a decrease in smooth or striated muscle activity. Nanninga and colleagues found that EMG activity of the external sphincter decreased after phentolamine (Regitine) administration in three paraplegic patients[60]; they attributed this to direct inhibition of a sympathetic action on the striated sphincter. Nordling and colleagues demonstrated that clonidine and POB (Dibenzyline), both of which pass the blood–brain barrier, decreased urethral pressure and EMG activity from the area of the striated sphincter in five normal women; phentolamine, which does not pass the blood–brain barrier, also decreased urethral pressure in this area but had no effect on EMG activity.[61] They concluded (1) that the effect of phentolamine was due to smooth muscle relaxation

alone; (2) that the effect of clonidine and possibly POB was elicited mostly through centrally induced changes in striated urethral sphincter tonus; and (3) that these agents also had an effect on the smooth muscle component of urethral pressure. None of the three drugs, however, affected the reflex rise in either urethral pressure or EMG activity that was seen during bladder filling, and none decreased the urethral pressure or EMG activity response to voluntary contraction of the pelvic floor striated musculature.

Pedersen and associates showed that thymoxamine (an alpha-adrenergic antagonist that passes the blood–brain barrier) decreased peak urethral pressure and striated sphincter EMG activity in patients with spastic paraplegia and speculated that the drug acted on the striated sphincter on a central basis.[62] Gajewski and colleagues concluded that alpha blockers do not influence the pudendal nerve–dependent urethral response in the cat through a peripheral action, but that at least prazosin can significantly inhibit this response at a central level.[63] Thind and coworkers reported on the effects of prazosin on static urethral sphincter function in ten healthy women.[64] They found that function was diminished, predominantly in the midurethral area, and hypothesized that this response was due to a decrease in both smooth and striated sphincter muscle, the latter as a result of a reduced somatomotor output from the central nervous system.

Alpha-adrenergic blocking agents have also been used to treat both bladder and outlet abnormalities in patients with so-called autonomous bladders.[65] These include those with myelodysplasia, sacral or infrasacral spinal cord neural injury, and voiding dysfunction following radical pelvic surgery. Parasympathetic decentralization has been reported to lead to a marked increase in adrenergic innervation of the bladder, resulting in conversion of the usual beta (relaxant) bladder response to sympathetic stimulation to an alpha (contractile) response.[66] Although the alterations in innervation have been disputed, the alterations in receptor function have not. Koyanagi demonstrated urethral supersensitivity to alpha-adrenergic stimulation in a group of patients with autonomous neurogenic bladders, implying that a change had occurred in adrenergic receptor function in the urethra following parasympathetic decentralization.[67] Parsons and Turton observed the same phenomenon but ascribed the cause to adrenergic supersensitivity of the urethral smooth muscle caused by sympathetic decentralization.[68] Nordling and colleagues described a similar phenomenon in women who had undergone radical hysterectomy and ascribed this change to damage to the sympathetic innervation.[69] Decreased bladder compliance is often a clinical problem in such patients, and this, along with a fixed urethral sphincter tone, results in the paradoxical occurrence of both storage and emptying failure. Norlen has summarized the supporting evidence for the success of alpha-adrenolytic treatment in these patients.[65] POB is capable of increasing bladder compliance (increasing storage) and decreasing urethral resistance (facilitating emptying). Andersson and coworkers used prazosin (Minipress) in such patients and found that maximum urethral pressure during filling was decreased, whereas "autonomous waves" were reduced.[70] McGuire and Savastano reported that POB decreased filling cystometric pressure in the decentralized primate bladder.[71]

Alpha-adrenergic blockade can decrease bladder contractility in patients with voiding dysfunction by another mechanism as well. Jensen reported an increase in the "alpha-adrenergic effect" in bladders characterized as "uninhibited."[72–74] Short- and long-term prazosin administration increased bladder capacity and decreased the amplitude of contractions. Thomas and colleagues found that intravenous phentolamine produced a significant reduction in maximum voiding detrusor pressure, voiding volumes, and peak flow rates in patients with suprasacral spinal cord injury with no reduction of outflow obstruction.[75] Rohner and associates found that the normal beta response of canine bladder body smooth musculature was changed to an alpha response after bladder outlet obstruction.[76] Perlberg and Caine studied bladder dome muscle from patients with obstructive prostatic hypertrophy and found an alpha-adrenergic response to noradrenalin stimulation instead of the usual beta response in 23% of 47 patients.[77] They theorized that at least some of the symptomatic improvement in irritative symptoms that occurs in such patients treated with alpha-adrenergic antagonists is due to a direct effect on bladder muscle rather than on outflow resistance and hypothesized that the irritative symptoms of prostatism and this altered adrenergic response are related.

POB was the alpha-adrenolytic agent originally used for the treatment of voiding dysfunction. It and phentolamine have blocking properties at both alpha-1 and alpha-2 receptor sites. The initial adult dosage of this agent is 10 mg/day, and the usual daily dose for voiding dysfunction is 10 to 20 mg. Daily doses larger than 10 mg are generally divided and given every 8 to 12 hours. After the drug has been discontinued, the effects of administration may persist for days because the drug irreversibly inactivates alpha receptors, and the duration of effect depends on the rate of receptor resynthesis.[78] Potential side effects include orthostatic hypotension, reflex tachycardia, nasal congestion, diarrhea, miosis, sedation, nausea, and vomiting (secondary to local irritation). Those who still use POB for long-term therapy should be aware that it has mutagenic activity in the Ames test and that repeated administration to animals can cause peritoneal sarcomas and lung tumors.[78] Further, the manufacturer has reported a dose-related incidence in rats of gastrointestinal tumors,[79] the majority of which were in the nonglandular portion of the stomach. Although this agent has been in clinical use for some 30 years without clinically apparent oncologic associations, one must now consider the potential medicolegal ramifications of long-term therapy, especially in younger persons.

Prazosin hydrochloride (Minipress) is a potent selective alpha-1 antagonist,[78] and its clinical use to lower outlet resistance has already been mentioned. The duration of action is 4 to 6 hours; therapy is generally begun in doses of 2 to 3 mg/day, divided. The dose may be very gradually increased to a maximum of 20 mg daily, although seldom is more than 9 to 10 mg daily used for voiding dysfunction. The potential side effects of prazosin are a consequence of its alpha-1 blockade. Occasionally, there occurs a "first-dose" phenomenon, a symptom complex of faintness, dizziness, palpitations, and, infrequently, syncope, thought to be due to acute postural hypotension. The incidence of this phenomenon can be minimized by restricting the initial dose of the drug to 1 mg and administering this at bedtime. Other side effects associated with chronic prazosin therapy are generally mild and rarely necessitate withdrawal of the drug.

Terazosin (Hytrin) and doxazosin (Cardura) are two of the latest in the series of highly selective postsynaptic alpha-1 blocking drugs. They are readily absorbed and have a high bioavailability and a long plasma half-life, enabling their activity to be maintained over 24 hours following a single oral dose.[80, 81] Their use has been recently promoted for the treatment of voiding dysfunction secondary to benign prostatic hyperplasia (BPH) consequent to the alpha-1 receptor content of the prostatic stroma and capsule. Their side effects are similar to those of prazosin. Daily doses range from 1 to 10 mg given generally at bedtime, a convenient advantage over a three-times-daily dosage schedule. Terazosin is said to have the same affinity for alpha-1 receptors in genitourinary as in vascular tissue and a fourfold greater selectivity for alpha-1 receptors than doxazosin.[82] Alfluzosin is a new agent that is reported to be a selective and competitive antagonist of alpha-1 mediated contraction of the prostate capsule, bladder base, and proximal urethral smooth muscle. It is said to be more specific for such receptors in the genitourinary tract than in the vasculature, raising the possibility that voiding may be facilitated by doses that have minimal vasodilatory effects, thus minimizing postural hypotension.[83] The drug requires three-times-daily dosing (7.5 to 10 mg total).

Thus, agents with alpha-adrenergic blocking properties at various levels of the neural organization have been used in patients with very varied types of voiding dysfunction—functional outlet obstruction, urinary retention, decreased compliance, and detrusor instability or hyperreflexia. Our own experience suggests that a trial of such an agent is certainly worthwhile because its effect or noneffect will become obvious in a matter of days, and the pharmacologic side effects are of course reversible. However, our results with such therapy for non-BPH related voiding dysfunction have been somewhat less spectacular than those of at least some other investigators.

OTHER POTENTIAL NONSPECIFIC THERAPY Beta-adrenergic

stimulation has been shown experimentally to decrease the urethral pressure profile and, by inference, urethral resistance.[84] Vaidyanathan et al (1980) reported a decrease in urethral closure pressure after administration of terbutaline, a relatively specific beta-2 agonist.[85] Other investigators (see later section, Increasing Outlet Resistance) have reported that beta-2 agonists potentiate in vitro periurethral striated muscle contraction. It seems doubtful that a beta agonist will prove clinically useful in facilitating bladder emptying by decreasing outlet resistance. Progesterone has been suggested as a possible treatment for emptying abnormalities in women. In a study of normal women looking at the effects of estrogen alone (E) versus estrogen plus progesterone (E + P), maximum flow in the E only group increased from 26 to 28 ml/second, whereas in the E + P group it increased from 26 to 38 ml/second. A sphincteric effect was hypothesized.[86] Finally, nitric oxide (NO) has been suggested to be a mediator of nonadrenergic noncholinergic (NANC) relaxation of the smooth muscle of the bladder outlet that occurs with bladder contraction.[5] Whether this means that analogs or substances that release NO in vivo will prove useful in decreasing smooth muscle–related outlet resistance in humans remains to be seen. If so, one could envision a role for NO synthetase inhibitors to stabilize urethral pressure or increase outlet resistance as well. NO is a ubiquitous molecule, however, and exerts inhibitor effects on the detrusor body in vitro (see later section, Decreasing Bladder Contractility) as well. Opposite functional effects on the bladder and outlet (on contractility and resistance) could well frustrate any clinical application.

At the Level of the Striated Sphincter

There is no class of pharmacologic agent that selectively relaxes the striated musculature of the pelvic floor. Three different types of drugs have been used to treat voiding dysfunction secondary to outlet obstruction at the level of the striated sphincter: the benzodiazepines, dantrolene, and baclofen. All are characterized generally as antispasticity drugs.[87] Baclofen and diazepam act predominantly within the central nervous system, whereas dantrolene acts directly on skeletal muscle. Unfortunately, there is no completely satisfactory form of therapy for alleviation of skeletal muscle spasticity. Although these drugs are capable of providing variable relief in specific circumstances, their efficacy is far from complete, and troublesome muscle weakness, adverse effects on gait, and a variety of other side effects minimize their overall usefulness[87] as a treatment for spasticity. Glycine and gamma-aminobutyric acid (GABA) have been identified as the major inhibitory neurotransmitters in the spinal cord.[88] Evidence favors glycine as the mediator of intraspinal postsynaptic inhibition and the most likely inhibitory transmitter in the reticular formation. GABA appears to mediate presynaptic inhibition in the spinal cord and the inhibitory actions of local interneurons in the

brain. The specific substrate for spinal cord inhibition consists of the synapses located on the terminals of the primary afferent fibers. GABA is the transmitter secreted by these synapses and activates specific receptors, resulting in a decrease in the amount of excitatory transmitter released by impulses from primary afferent fibers, consequently reducing the amplitude of the excitatory postsynaptic potentials. The inhibitory action of GABA in the brain occurs through an increase in chloride conductance with hyperpolarization of the membrane.

BENZODIAZEPINES   The benzodiazepines potentiate the action of GABA at both presynaptic and postsynaptic sites in the brain and spinal cord.[89, 90] When GABA recognition sites are activated, increased chloride conductance across the neuronal membrane produces inhibitory effects. The benzodiazepines increase the affinity of the GABA receptor sites on central nervous system membranes, and the increased binding increases the frequency with which the chloride channels open in response to a given amount of GABA. Presynaptic inhibition is augmented, and it is thought that this reduces the release of excitatory transmitters from afferent fibers, thereby reducing the gain of the stretch and flexor reflexes in patients with bladder spasticity. This is a postulated mechanism of action of the muscle relaxant properties of at least diazepam.[89] Another benzodiazepine-binding site exists that is not linked to the GABA receptor. This is a peripheral receptor with different pharmacologic characteristics. The organ-specific densities and physiologic functions of this second class of benzodiazepine receptor remain incompletely clarified and have unknown relevance, if any, for the lower urinary tract.[91]

Benzodiazapines are extensively used for the treatment of anxiety and related disorders,[92] although pharmacologically they can also be classified as centrally acting muscle relaxants. The generalized anxiety disorder responsive to pharmacotherapy by these agents is characterized by unrealistic or excessive anxiety and worry about life circumstances. Specific symptoms can be related to motor tension, autonomic hyperactivity (frequent urination can be a manifestation of this, as well as nausea, vomiting, diarrhea, and abdominal distress), and excessive vigilance. Other common uses include treatment of insomnia, stress-related disorders, muscle spasm, epilepsy, and preoperative sedation.[90] Side effects include nonspecific central nervous system depression, manifested as sedation, lethargy, drowsiness, slowing of thought processes, ataxia, and decreased ability to acquire or store information.[92] Some authors believe that any muscle relaxant effect in clinically used doses is due to the central nervous system depressant effects and cite a lack of clinical studies showing any advantages of these agents over placebo or aspirin in this regard.[93] Effective total daily doses of diazepam (Valium and others), the most widely used agent of this group, range from 4 to 40 mg. Other benzodiazepine anxiolytic agents include chlordiazepoxide (Librium and others), clorazepate (Tranxene), prazepam (Centrax), halazepam (Paxipam), clonazepam (Klonopin), lorazepam (Ativan and others), oxazepam (Serax), and alprazolam (Xanax).

There are few available references that provide valuable data on the use of any of the benzodiazepines for treatment of functional obstruction at the level of the striated sphincter. Opinions, however, are commonly expressed, at least in regard to diazepam. In view of the information previously cited on the use of alpha-adrenergic blocking agents for treating or preventing postoperative urinary retention, it is interesting to note that one of the few articles that specifically mentions diazepam reports that it is more effective than oral POB, intravesical PGE$_2$, or oral BC in promoting spontaneous voiding after colposuspension surgery.[40] We have not found the recommended oral doses of diazepam effective in controlling the classic type of detrusor–striated sphincter dyssynergia secondary to neurologic disease. If the cause of incomplete emptying in a neurologically normal patient is obscure, and the patient has what appears urodynamically to be inadequate relaxation of the pelvic floor striated musculature (e.g., occult neuropathic bladder, the Hinman syndrome), a trial of such an agent may be worthwhile. The rationale for its use is that it relaxes the pelvic floor striated musculature during bladder contraction, or that such relaxation removes an inhibitory stimulus to reflex bladder activity. However, improvement under such circumstances may simply be due to the antianxiety effect of the drug or to the intensive explanation, encouragement, and modified biofeedback therapy that usually accompany such treatment in these patients.

BACLOFEN Baclofen (Lioresal) depresses monosynaptic and polysynaptic excitation of motor neurons and interneurons in the spinal cord and was originally thought to function as a GABA agonist.[87, 89] However, its electrophysiologic and pharmacologic profile is quite different from that of GABA. Although its effects superficially resemble those of GABA, some specific GABA inhibitors (e.g., bicuculline) do not antagonize the actions of baclofen. Baclofen does not cause depolarization of primary afferent nerve terminals, and there is no evidence that baclofen increases chloride conduction, the most prominent action of GABA. Because both GABA and baclofen can produce some effects that are insensitive to blockade by classic GABA antagonists, two classes of GABA receptors have been proposed, the a receptor (the classic receptor) and the b receptor. Baclofen does not bind strongly or specifically to classic GABA a receptors but does to b receptors in brain and spinal membranes. Currently, it is thought that activation of the GABA receptors by baclofen causes a decrease in the release of excitatory transmitters onto motor neurons by increasing the threshold for excitation of primary afferent terminals in the spinal cord. This may result from increasing potassium conductance or by inhibiting calcium influx. Baclofen's primary site of action is the spinal cord, but it is also reported to be active at more rostral sites in the central nervous system.

Milanov states that, like a GABA-b agonist, baclofen suppresses excitatory neurotransmitter release but also has direct GABAergic activity.[94] Its effect in reducing spasticity is caused primarily by normalizing interneuron activity and decreasing motor neuron activity (perhaps secondary to normalizing interneuron activity).[94]

Baclofen has been found useful for the treatment of skeletal spasticity due to a variety of causes (especially multiple sclerosis and traumatic spinal cord lesions).[87] Determination of the optimal dose in individual patients requires careful titration. Treatment is started at an initial dose of 5 mg twice a day and increased every 3 days up to a maximum daily dose of 20 mg four times a day. With reference to voiding dysfunction, Hachen and Krucker found that a daily oral dose of 75 mg was ineffective in patients with striated sphincter dyssynergia and traumatic paraplegia, whereas a daily intravenous dose of 20 mg was highly effective.[95] Florante and associates reported that 73% of their patients with voiding dysfunction secondary to acute and chronic spinal cord injury had lower striated sphincter responses and decreased residual urine volume following baclofen treatment but only with an average daily oral dose of 120 mg.[96] Potential side effects of baclofen include drowsiness, insomnia, rash, pruritus, dizziness, and weakness. It may impair the ability to walk or stand and is not recommended for the management of spasticity due to cerebral lesions or disease. Sudden withdrawal has been shown to provoke hallucinations, anxiety, and tachycardia; hallucinations during treatment have also been reported that have responded to reductions in dosage.[97]

Drug delivery often frustrates adequate pharmacologic treatment, and baclofen is a good example of this. GABA's hydrophilic properties prevent its crossing the blood–brain barrier in sufficient amounts to make it therapeutically useful. For oral use a more lipophilic analog, baclofen, was developed. However, its passage through the barrier is likewise limited, and it has proved to be a generally insufficient drug when given orally to treat severe somatic spasticity and micturition disorders secondary to neurogenic dysfunction.[98] Intrathecal infusion bypasses the blood–brain barrier. Cerebrospinal fluid (CSF) levels 10 times higher than those reached with oral administration are achieved with infusion amounts 100 times less than those taken orally.[99] Direct administration into the subarachnoid space by an implanted infusion pump has shown promising results not only for skeletal spasticity but for striated sphincter dyssynergia and bladder hyperactivity as well. Nanninga and colleagues reported on such administration to seven patients with intractable bladder spasticity.[100] All patients experienced a general decrease in spasticity, and the amount of striated sphincter activity during bladder contraction decreased; six showed an increase in bladder capacity. Four previously incontinent patients were able to stay dry with clean intermittent catheterization (CIC). The action of baclofen on bladder hyperactivity is not unexpected, given its spinal cord mechanism of action, and this inhibition of bladder contractility when the drug is administered intrathecally may in fact prove to be its most important benefit. Loubser and colleagues studied nine patients with spinal cord injury and refractory spasticity using an external pump to test the initial response.[101] Eight showed objective improvement in functional ability; three of seven studied urodynamically showed an increase in bladder capacity. Kums and Delhaas reported on nine men who were paraplegic or quadriplegic secondary to trauma or multiple sclerosis and also had intractable muscle spasticity; they were treated with intrathecal baclofen.[98] After a successful test period during which the drug was administered through an external catheter, a drug delivery system was implanted and connected to a spinal catheter. Doses ranged from 74 to 840 µg/24 hours. Patients were studied before and 4 to 6 weeks after initiation of therapy. Mean residual urine volume fell from 224 to 110 ml ($p = .01$), mean urodynamic bladder capacity rose from 162 to 263 ml ($p < .005$), and pelvic floor spasm decreased at both baseline and maximum bladder capacity ($p < .005$ and .025, respectively). Three subjects became continent. Additionally, CIC was no longer complicated by adductor spasm. Development of tolerance to intrathecal baclofen with a consequent requirement for increasing doses may prove to be a problem with long-term chronic use, and studies are under way to investigate this.

DANTROLENE Dantrolene (Dantrium) exerts its effects by direct peripheral action on skeletal muscle.[87, 89] It is thought to inhibit the excitation-induced release of calcium ions from the sarcoplasmic reticulum of striated muscle fibers, thereby inhibiting excitation-contraction coupling and diminishing the mechanical force of contraction. The blockade of calcium release is not complete, however, and contraction is not completely abolished. It reduces reflex more than voluntary contractions, probably because of a preferential action on fast-twitch rather than slow-twitch skeletal muscle fibers. It has been shown to have therapeutic benefits for chronic spasticity associated with central nervous system disorders. The drug improves voiding function in some patients with classic detrusor–striated sphincter dyssynergia and was initially reported to be very successful in doing so.[102] In adults the recommended starting dose is 25 mg daily, gradually increasing by increments of 25 mg every 4 to 7 days to a maximum oral dose of 400 mg given in four divided doses. Hackler and colleagues reported improvement in voiding function in approximately half of their patients treated with dantrolene but found that such improvement required oral doses of 600 mg daily.[103] Although no inhibitory effect on bladder smooth muscle seems to occur,[104] the generalized weakness that dantrolene can induce is often significant enough to compromise its therapeutic effects. Other potential side effects include euphoria, dizziness, diarrhea, and hepatotoxicity. Fatal hepatitis has been reported in approximately 0.1 to 0.2% of patients treated with the drug

for 60 days or longer, and symptomatic hepatitis may occur in 0.5% of patients treated for more than 60 days; chemical abnormalities of liver function are noted in up to 1%. The risk of hepatic injury is twofold greater in women.[105] One use of dantrolene for which agreement exists is the acute management of malignant hyperthermia, a rare hereditary syndrome characterized by vigorous contraction of skeletal muscle precipitated by excess release of calcium from the sarcoplasmic reticulum, generally in response to neuromuscular blocking agents or inhalational anesthetics. Virtually all hospital pharmacies stock parenteral dantrolene for this purpose.

OTHER AGENTS Beta-adrenergic agonists, especially those with prominent beta-2 characteristics, are able to produce relaxation of some skeletal muscles of the slow-twitch type.[106, 107] This action could be significant in view of the fact that the portion of the external urethral sphincter comprising the outermost urethral wall is said to consist exclusively of slow-twitch fibers,[108] whereas the striated muscle fibers of the levator ani contain both fast- and slow-twitch fibers, although the majority are of the slow-twitch type. This type of action may account at least in part for the decrease in urethral profile parameters seen with terbutaline (see earlier section, Decreasing Outlet Resistance at the Level of the Smooth Sphincter). This area of pharmacology and its clinical relevance is somewhat confusing at the moment because beta-2 adrenergic drugs have been reported to potentiate periurethral striated muscle contraction, albeit in a different in vitro system (see later section, Increasing Outlet Resistance). Botulinum toxin (an inhibitor of acetylcholine release at the neuromuscular junction of striated muscle) has been injected directly into the striated sphincter to dyssynergia.[109] Injections carried out weekly for 3 weeks can achieve a duration of effect averaging 2 months. The number of patients tested seems thus far to be small, and more information is needed about criteria for success and side effects. Fowler and colleagues used botulinum toxin injections in six women with difficult voiding or urinary retention secondary to abnormal myotonus-like EMG activity in the striated urethral sphincter.[110] Although voiding did not improve in any patient (attributed to the type of repetitive discharge activity present), three patients developed transient stress incontinence, indicating that the sphincter muscle had indeed been weakened.

FACILITATION OF URINE STORAGE

The pathophysiology of failure of the lower urinary tract to fill with or store urine adequately may be secondary to problems related to the bladder, the outlet, or both.[6] Hyperactivity of the bladder during filling can be expressed as discrete involuntary contractions (IVC) or as reduced compliance with or without phasic contraction. Involuntary contractions are most commonly associated with inflammatory or irritating processes in the bladder wall or with bladder outlet obstruction, or they may be idiopathic. Decreased compliance during filling may be secondary to the sequelae of neurologic injury or disease but may also result from any process that destroys the elastic or viscoelastic properties of the bladder wall. Purely sensory urgency may also account for storage failure; such urgency may result from inflammatory, infectious, neurologic, or psychologic factors, or it may be idiopathic. A fixed decrease in outlet resistance may result from damage to the innervation of or the structural elements of the smooth or striated sphincter or from neurologic disease or injury, surgical or other mechanical trauma, or aging. Classic stress urinary incontinence (SUI; also called genuine stress incontinence) in women implies a failure of the normal transmission of increases in intra-abdominal pressure to the area of the bladder neck and proximal urethra. This failure is acknowledged to be associated mainly with changes in the anatomic position of the vesicourethral junction and proximal urethra during increases in intra-abdominal pressure (hypermobility), and this in turn is thought to accompany pelvic floor weakness or relaxation, which may be secondary to a number of causes. The pathophysiology of SUI may also involve a decrease in the reflex striated sphincter contraction, which occurs with a number of maneuvers that increase intra-abdominal pressure. Treatment of abnormalities related to the filling or storage phase of micturition is directed toward inhibiting bladder contractility, increasing bladder capacity, or decreasing sensory input during filling or toward increasing outlet resistance, either continuously or only during abdominal straining.

Decreasing Bladder Contractility

ANTICHOLINERGIC AGENTS

General Discussion The major portion of the neurohumoral stimulus for physiologic bladder contraction is acetylcholine-induced stimulation of postganglionic parasympathetic muscarinic cholinergic receptor sites on bladder smooth muscle.[1, 5] Atropine and atropine-like agents therefore depress normal bladder contractions and IVC of any cause.[72, 111, 112] In such patients the bladder volume at the first IVC is generally increased, the amplitude of the IVC decreased, and maximum bladder capacity increased. However, although the volume and pressure thresholds at which an IVC is elicited may increase, the "warning time" (the time between the perception of an IVC about to occur and its occurrence) and the ability to suppress an IVC are not increased. Thus, urgency and incontinence still occur *unless* such therapy is combined with a regimen of timed voiding or toileting. Bladder compliance in normal individuals and in those with detrusor hyperreflexia in whom the initial slope of the filling curve on cystometry is normal prior to the involuntary contraction does not seem to be significantly altered.[72] McGuire and Savastano reported that atropine increased both the

compliance and the capacity of the neurologically decentralized primate bladder, and that both of these effects were additive to those produced by POB[71] (see previous discussion on inhibition of bladder contractility by alpha-adrenergic blocking agents). However, the effect of pure antimuscarinics in those who exhibit only decreased compliance has not been well studied. Outlet resistance, at least as reflected by urethral pressure measurements, does not seem to be clinically affected by anticholinergic therapy.[113]

Although antimuscarinic agents usually produce significant clinical improvement in patients with involuntary bladder contractions and associated symptoms, generally only partial inhibition results. In many animal models atropine only partially antagonizes the response of the whole bladder to pelvic nerve stimulation and of bladder strips to field stimulation, although it does completely inhibit the response of bladder smooth muscle to exogenous cholinergic stimulation. Of the theories proposed to explain this phenomenon, called "atropine resistance," the most attractive and most commonly cited is the idea that a major portion of the neurotransmission involved in the final common pathway of bladder contraction is nonadrenergic and noncholinergic— secondary to release of a transmitter other than acetylcholine or norepinephrine.[1, 2, 5] Although the existence of atropine resistance in human bladder muscle is by no means agreed on, this concept is the most common hypothesis invoked to explain clinical difficulty in abolishing IVC with anticholinergic agents alone, and it is also used to support the rationale of treatment of such types of bladder activity with agents that have different mechanisms of action.

Both Brading[114, 115] and Andersson[5] discuss the difficulty of evaluating apparently conflicting data in the literature with respect to atropine resistance. Brading[115] states that the size of the atropine-resistant component varies markedly among different species and also depends in a given preparation on the frequency of nerve stimulation. At frequencies producing maximum contractile responses, Brading cites studies showing that approximately 76% of the response is atropine resistant in the guinea pig and cat, 56% in the rabbit, 15% in the pig, and zero in strips from normal human detrusor. Andersson[5] states that "most probably normal human detrusor muscle exhibits little atropine resistance" but does not exclude its existence in morphologically or functionally abnormal bladders.

Receptor subtyping is a particularly relevant concept for drug development in general and for antimuscarinic compounds in particular. Subtyping can be based on functional assays, on radioligand-binding affinity, and on receptor cloning and expression. At least five different genetically established (by cloning) muscarinic subtypes exist (designated m_1 to m_5).[116] The nomenclature M_1 to M_3 describes the pharmacologically defined (using subtype selective agonists and antagonists) muscarinic subtypes.[5, 117] Pirenzepine (a selective muscarinic blocker) was originally used to subdivide muscarinic receptors into

M_1 and M_2 categories; using this subclassification, detrusor muscarinic receptors have been found to be the M_2 type.[5, 118, 119] On further analysis of the M_2 receptor population a small proportion of glandular M_2 receptors was found that could represent the pharmacologic type responsible for muscarinic agonist–induced contractions. This subtype is now called the M_3 receptor, and, although a systematic subclassification of human detrusor M receptors remains to be made, indirect evidence suggests that human detrusor also contains this subtype.[5, 117]

Some patients appear to become relatively refractory to anticholinergic drugs after a while. Such an effect could have many causes, but one pharmacologic fact that could contribute to such a phenomenon is a change in receptor density in response to certain stimuli (up- or down-regulation). Experimentally, at least, Levin and colleagues have shown that an increase in peripheral muscarinic receptor density occurs with chronic atropine administration (in the rat).[119] On the other hand, certain pathologic states may be associated with changes in receptor density, which may in turn affect the response to anticholinergic (and other) agents. Restorick and Mundy described a decrease in density of muscarinic cholinergic receptors and an increase in density of alpha-adrenergic receptors in bladder dome samples from humans with detrusor hyperreflexia; beta-adrenergic receptor density remained unchanged.[120] Lepor and associates described a similar decrease in cholinergic receptor density in bladder specimens from children and adults with voiding dysfunction due to myelomeningocele, spinal cord injury, or multiple sclerosis, all of whom had involuntary bladder contractions.[121] Proposed mechanisms include down-regulation due to hyperactivity, smooth muscle hypertrophy, and bladder wall fibrosis.

Specific Drugs Propantheline bromide (e.g., Pro-Banthine) is the classically described oral agent for producing an antimuscarinic effect in the lower urinary tract. The usual adult oral dose is 15 to 30 mg every 4 to 6 hours, although higher doses are often necessary. Propantheline is a quarternary ammonium compound, which is poorly absorbed after oral administration.[122] Oral administration in the fasting state rather than with or after meals is preferable from the standpoint of drug bioavailability.[123] There seems to be little difference between the antimuscarinic effects of propantheline on bladder smooth muscle and those of other antimuscarinic agents such as glycopyrrolate (Robinul), isopropamide (Darbid), anisotropine methylbromide (Valpin), methscopolamine (Pamine), and homatropine. Some of these agents, such as glycopyrrolate, have a more convenient dosage schedule (two to three times daily), but their clinical effects on the lower urinary tract are indistinguishable. Although there are obviously many other considerations in accounting for the activity of a given dose of drug at its site of action, there is no oral drug available whose direct in vitro antimuscarinic binding potential approximates that of atropine better than the long available and rela-

tively inexpensive propantheline bromide.[124, 125] There is a surprising lack of evaluable data on the effectiveness of propantheline for the treatment of bladder hyperactivity. As Andersson points out,[112] anticholinergic drugs in general have been reported to have both great and poor efficacy for this indication. To show the range of variation, Zorzitto and colleagues concluded that propantheline bromide administered orally in doses of 30 mg four times a day to a group of institutionalized incontinent geriatric patients had marginal benefits that were outweighed by the side effects.[126] Blaivas and colleagues, on the other hand, by increasing the dose of propantheline (up to 60 mg four times a day) until incontinence was eliminated or side effects precluded further use, obtained a complete response in 25 of 26 patients with involuntary bladder contractions.[111] Differences in bioavailability, selective drug delivery, receptor selectivity, receptor density, atropine resistance, pathophysiology, susceptibility to dose-limiting side effects, and mental status are all potential factors that could explain such disparate results. The Agency for Health Care Policy and Research (AHCPR) clinical practice guidelines[127] lists five randomized controlled trials for propantheline, in which 82% of the patients were women. Percent cures (all figures refer to percent *minus* percent on placebo) are listed as 0–5%, percent reduction in urge incontinence as 0–53%, percent side effects 0–50%, and percent dropouts 0–9%.

Atropine is reported to be available in a 0.5-μg tablet, although we have yet to find it. Atropine and all related belladonna alkaloids are well absorbed from the gastrointestinal tract. Atropine is said to have almost no detectable central nervous system effects at clinically used doses.[122] It has a half-life of about 4 hours. Scopolamine is another belladonna alkaloid marketed as a soluble salt. It has prominent central depressive effects at low doses, probably due to its greater penetration (compared with atropine) through the blood–brain barrier. Transdermal scopolamine has been used for treating involuntary bladder contractions.[128] The "patch" provides continuous delivery of 0.5 mg daily to the circulation for 3 days. Cornella and associates, however, reported poor results with this form of drug in treating ten patients with detrusor instability.[129] Only two patients showed a positive response, an additional one showed a slight improvement, and in eight of ten it had to be discontinued because of side effects. Side effects were related to the central nervous system (ataxia, dizziness) and included blurred vision and dry mouth as well. A double-blind placebo study on the effects of transdermal scopolamine in postsuprapubic prostatectomy patients was performed to investigate its use in the treatment or prevention of pain, involuntary bladder contractions, urgency, and bladder pressure rises of 15 cm H_2O. No statistical differences were found,[130] although the occurrence of involuntary bladder contractions was 33% in the treated group versus 54% in the placebo group. The percentage of patients requiring injectable analgesia on day 1 was similar in treated and control patients, but on day 2 it was statistically lower in the scopolamine group (4% vs. 31%). In our experience, in treating patients with involuntary bladder contractions with this method, results were very erratic and skin irritation with the patch was a problem for some patients. Caution should be exercised in the use of the patch in the elderly and young because of the fixed dose.

Hyoscyamine (Cystospaz) and hyoscyamine sulfate (Levsin, Levsinex, Cystospaz-M) are reported to have about the same general anticholinergic actions and side effects as the other belladonna alkaloids. Hyoscyamine sulfate is available as a sublingual formulation (Levsin SL), a theoretical advantage, but controlled studies of its effects on bladder hyperactivity are lacking. Glycopyrrolate (Robinul) is a synthetic quaternary ammonium compound that is a potent inhibitor of both M_1 and M_2 receptors but has a preference for the M_2 subtype.[131] It is available in both oral and parenteral preparations; the latter is commonly used as an antisialog during anesthesia.

An anticholinergic agent with a significant ganglionic-blocking action as well as such action at the peripheral receptor level might be more effective in suppressing bladder contractility. Although methantheline (Banthine) has a higher ratio of ganglionic-blocking to antimuscarinic activity than does propantheline, the latter drug seems to be at least as potent in each respect, clinical dose for dose. Methantheline does have similar effects on the lower urinary tract, and some clinicians still prefer it over other anticholinergic agents. Few real data are available regarding its efficacy.

A lack of selectivity is a major problem with all antimuscarinic compounds because they tend to affect parasympathetically innervated organs in the same order; generally larger doses are required to inhibit bladder activity than to affect salivary, bronchial, nasopharyngeal, and sweat secretions. The potential side effects of all antimuscarinic agents include inhibition of salivary secretions (dry mouth), blockade of the ciliary muscle of the lens to cholinergic stimulation (blurred vision for near objects), tachycardia, drowsiness, and inhibition of gut motility. Those agents that possess some ganglionic-blocking activity may also cause orthostatic hypotension and impotence at high doses (generally required for nicotinic activity to become manifest). Antimuscarinic agents are generally contraindicated in patients with narrow angle glaucoma and should be used with caution in patients with significant bladder outlet obstruction because complete urinary retention may be precipitated.

MUSCULOTROPIC RELAXANTS These agents fall under the general heading of direct-acting smooth muscle depressants, whose "antispasmodic" activity reportedly affects smooth muscle directly at a site that is metabolically distal to the cholinergic or other contractile receptor mechanism. Although all of the agents discussed in this section do relax smooth muscle in vitro by papavarine-like (direct) action, all have been found to possess variable anticholinergic and

local anesthetic properties in addition. There is still some uncertainty about how much of their clinical efficacy is due only to their atropine-like effect. If any of these agents does exert a clinically significant inhibitory effect that is independent of antimuscarinic action, a therapeutic rationale exists for combining them with a relatively pure anticholinergic agent.

Oxybutynin chloride (Ditropan) is a moderately potent anticholinergic agent that has strong independent musculotropic relaxant activity as well as local anesthetic activity. Comparatively higher concentrations in vitro are necessary to produce direct spasmolytic effects, which may be due to calcium channel blockade.[132, 133] The recommended oral adult dose is 5 mg three or four times a day; side effects are antimuscarinic and dose-related. Initial reports documented success in depressing detrusor hyperreflexia in patients with neurogenic bladder dysfunction,[134] and subsequent reports documented success in inhibiting other types of bladder hyperactivity as well.[112]

A randomized double-blind, placebo-controlled study comparing oxybutynin 5 mg three times a day with placebo in 30 patients with detrusor instability was carried out by Moisey and colleagues.[135] Seventeen of 23 patients who completed the study with oxybutynin had symptomatic improvement, and nine showed evidence of urodynamic improvement, mainly an increase in maximum bladder capacity. Hehir and Fitzpatrick reported that 16 of 24 patients with neuropathic voiding dysfunction secondary to myelomeningocele were cured or improved (17% dry, 50% improved) with oxybutynin treatment.[136] Average bladder capacity increased from 197 ml to 299 ml (with drug) versus 218 ml (with placebo). Maximum bladder filling pressure decreased from 47 to 37 cm H_2O (with drug) versus 45 cm H_2O (with placebo).

In a prospective randomized study of 34 patients with voiding dysfunction secondary to multiple sclerosis, Gajewski and Awad found that a dose of 5 mg three times a day of oral oxybutynin produced a good response more frequently than 15 mg of propantheline three times a day. They concluded that oxybutynin was more effective in the treatment of detrusor hyperreflexia secondary to multiple sclerosis.[137]

Holmes and associates compared the results of oxybutynin and propantheline in a small group of women with detrusor instability.[138] The experimental design was a randomized crossover trial with a patient-regulated variable dose regimen. This kind of dose titration study allows the patient to increase the drug dose to whatever he or she perceives to be the optimum ratio between clinical improvement and side effects—an interesting way of comparing two drugs while minimizing differences in oral absorption. Of the 23 women in the trial, 14 reported subjective improvement with oxybutynin as opposed to 11 with propantheline. Both drugs significantly increased the maximum cystometric capacity and reduced the maximum detrusor pressure on filling. The only significant objective difference was a greater increase in the maximum cystometric capacity with oxybutynin. The mean total daily dose of oxybutynin tolerated was 15 mg (range, 7.5 to 30), and that of propantheline was 90 mg (range, 45 to 145).

Thuroff and colleagues compared oxybutynin to propantheline and placebo in a group of patients with symptoms of instability and either detrusor instability or hyperreflexia.[139] Oxybutynin (5 mg three times a day) performed best, but propantheline was used at a relatively low dose—15 mg three times a day. The rate of side effects was higher for oxybutynin at just about the level of clinical and urodynamic improvement. The mean grade of improvement on a visual analog scale was higher for oxybutynin (58.2%) versus propantheline (44.7%) and placebo (43.4%). Urodynamic volume at the first involuntary bladder contraction increased more with oxybutynin (51 vs. 11.2 vs. 9.7 ml), as did the change in maximum cystometric capacity (80.1 vs. 48.9 vs. 22.5 ml). Residual urine volume also increased more (27.0 vs. 2.2 vs. 1.9 ml). The authors further subdivided their overall results into excellent (>75% improvement), good (50 to 74%), fair (25 to 49%), and poor (<25%). Percentages for treatment with oxybutynin were, respectively, 42%, 25%, 15%, and 18%. The authors compared their 67% rate of good or excellent results with those reported in seven other oxybutynin series in the literature (some admittedly poorer studies included) and concluded that their results compared favorably with the range of results calculated from these studies (61 to 86%). The results of propantheline treatment generally ranked between those of oxybutynin and placebo but did not reach significant levels over placebo in any variable. Subdivision of propantheline results into excellent, good, fair, and poor categories yielded percentages of 20%, 30%, 14%, and 36%, respectively. The authors compared their 50% ratio of good or excellent results with those achieved in six other propantheline studies reported in the literature (30 to 57%) and concluded that their results were consistent with these. Although this study is better than most in the literature, it does have drawbacks, and anyone using it in a meta-analysis would be well advised to read it and the other cited studies very carefully.

Zeegers and colleagues reported on a double-blind prospective crossover study comparing oxybutynin, flavoxate (see later in this section), emepronium, and placebo.[140] Although there was a high dropout rate (19 of 60 patients) and the entry criteria were vague (frequency, urgency, urge incontinence), the results were scored as 5 (excellent overall effect) to 1 (no improvement) by both patients and physicians, and the results were combined into a single number. The percentages of results in categories 3 to 5 for the agents used were oxybutynin 61%, placebo 41%, emepronium 34%, and flavoxate 31%. The results of the first treatment gave corresponding percentages of only 63%, 29%, 18% (probably reflecting eight dropouts due to side effects), and 44%. Ambulatory urodynamic monitoring and pad weighing were used to assess the effects of oxybutynin on detrusor hyperactivity by Von Doorn and Zwiers.[141] The 24-hour average frequency of involuntary bladder contractions decreased from 8.7 to 3.4, the maximum contraction amplitude decreased from 32 to 22 cm H_2O, and the duration of the average involuntary bladder contraction decreased from 90 to 60 seconds. However, the daily micturition frequency did not change (11 to 10), nor did the amount of urine lost—findings the authors try to minimize by pointing out that some patients had sphincteric incontinence also and that a higher fluid intake during treatment may have occurred. The AHCPR guideline[127] lists six randomized controlled trials for oxybutynin; 90% of patients were women. The percentage of cures (all figures refer to percentage *minus* percentage on placebo) is listed as 28% and 44%, percentage of reduction in urge incontinence is 9 to 56%, and the percentages of side effects and dropouts are 2 to 66% and 3 to 45%, respectively.

There are some negative reports on the efficacy of oxybutynin. Zorzitto and colleagues came to conclusions similar to those resulting from their study of propantheline (see earlier) in a double-blind, placebo-controlled trial conducted in 24 incontinent geriatric institutionalized patients; oxybutynin 5 mg twice a day was no more effective than placebo with scheduled toileting in treating incontinence in this type of population with detrusor hyperactivity.[142] An incontinence profile was used to assess results. The only significant difference noted was an increase in residual urine volume (159 vs. 92 ml). Ouslander and colleagues reported similar conclusions in a smaller study of geriatric patients and in an accompanying article (they concluded simply that the drug is safe for use in the elderly at doses of 2.5 to 5 mg three times a day).[143–144]

Topical application of oxybutynin and other agents to normal or intestinal bladders has been suggested and implemented.[145] This conceptually attractive form of alternative drug administration, delivered either by periodic intravesical instillation of liquid or by timed-released pellets, awaits further clinical trials and the development of preparations specifically formulated for this purpose. Madersbacher and Jilg reviewed such usage of oxybutynin and presented data on 13 patients with complete suprasacral cord lesions who were on CIC.[146] One 5-mg tablet was dissolved in 30 ml of distilled water, and the solution was instilled intravesically. Of the 10 patients who were incontinent, 9 remained dry for 6 hours. For the group the changes in bladder capacity and maximum detrusor pressure were statistically significant. Some of the more interesting data were given in a figure showing plasma oxybutynin levels in a group of patients in whom administration was intravesical or oral. The level following an oral dose rose to 7.3 mg/ml within 2 hours and then precipitously dropped to slightly less than 2 mg/ml at 4 hours. Following intravesical administration, the level rose gradually to a peak of about 6.2 mg/ml at 3.5 hours, but at 6 hours it was still greater than 4 mg/ml, and at 9 hours it was still between 3 and 4 mg/ml. Did the intravesically applied drug act locally or systemically? Weese and colleagues reported on a similar dose of oxybutynin (5 mg in 30 ml of sterile water) to treat 42 patients with involuntary bladder contractions who had either failed oral anticholinergic therapy (11 patients) or had intolerable side effects (31 patients).[147] Twenty had hyperreflexia, 19 had detrusor instability, and 3 had bowel or bladder hyperactivity after augmentation. The drug was instilled two or three times a day for 10 minutes by catheter. Twenty-one percent (nine patients) dropped out because they were unable to tolerate CIC or retain the solution properly, but there were no reported side effects. Fifty-five percent of patients (18 of 33) who were able to follow the protocol reported at least a moderate subjective improvement in incontinence and urgency. Nine patients became totally continent and experienced complete resolution of their symptoms; 18 patients improved and experienced a decrease of 2.5 pads per day. There were no urodynamic data. Follow-up ranged from 5 to 35 months (mean, 18.4 months). The lack of side effects prompted some speculation about the mechanism of drug action. One possibility suggested was simply a more prolonged rate of absorption. Another and more intriguing one was a decreased pass through the liver and therefore a decrease in metabolites, the hypothesis being that perhaps the metabolites and not the primary compound are responsible for the side effects.

With regard to the subject of hyperactivity in augmented or intestinal neo-bladders, for which there is no separate section in this chapter, Andersson and colleagues recently reviewed this phenomenon and its pharmacologic treatment.[148] They noted few instances of positive results with agents given systemically. Locally applied agents were thought to offer more promise. A list of possibilities and their assessments was included. Pure anticholinergics have produced no good results, either locally or systemically. Oxybutynin has shown poor results with systemic therapy but some good results with local therapy. Alpha agonists have produced no effect; beta agonists have shown no local effects and equivocal effects when administered subcutaneously, but the comment was made that such use will probably be limited by side effects. Other possibilities mentioned for future use included opioid agonists (diphenoxylate—a component of Lomotil—and loperamide), calcium antagonists, potassium channel openers, and NO donors.

Dicyclomine hydrochloride (Bentyl) is also reported to exert a direct relaxant effect on smooth muscle in addition to an antimuscarinic action.[149] An oral dose of 20 mg three times a day in adults has been reported to increase bladder capacity in patients with detrusor hyperreflexia.[150] Beck and coworkers compared the use of 10 mg dicyclomine, 15 mg propantheline, and placebo three times a day in patients with detrusor hyperactivity.[151] The cure or improved rates, respectively, were 62%, 73%, and 20%. Awad and associates reported that 20 mg of dicyclomine three times a day caused resolution or significant improvement in 24 of 27 patients with involuntary bladder contractions.[152]

Flavoxate hydrochloride (Urispas) has a direct inhibitory action on smooth muscle but very weak anticholinergic properties.[112, 153] Overall favorable clinical effects have been noted in some series of patients with frequency, urgency, and incontinence and in patients with urodynamically documented detrusor hyperreflexia.[154, 155] However, Briggs and colleagues reported that this drug had essentially no effect on detrusor hyperreflexia in an elderly population, an experience that coincides with the laboratory effects obtained by Benson and associates.[157] The recommended adult dosage is 100 to 200 mg three or four times a day. As with all agents in this group, a short clinical trial may be worthwhile. Reported side effects are few.

CALCIUM ANTAGONISTS The role of calcium as a messenger in linking extracellular stimuli to the intracellular environment is well established, including its involvement in excitation-contraction coupling in striated, cardiac, and smooth muscle.[1, 5] The dependence of contractile activity on changes in cytosolic calcium varies from tissue to tissue, as do the characteristics of the calcium channels involved, but interference with calcium inflow or intracellular release is a very potent potential mechanism for bladder smooth muscle relaxation.

Nifedipine has been shown to be an effective inhibitor of contraction induced by several mechanisms in human and guinea pig bladder muscle.[112, 158] It has also been shown to block completely the noncholinergic portion of the contraction produced by electrical field stimulation in rabbit bladder.[159] Nifedipine more effectively inhibited contractions induced by potassium than by carbachol in rabbit bladder strips, whereas terodiline, an agent with both calcium antagonistic and anticholinergic properties, had the opposite effect. However, terodiline did cause complete inhibition of the response of rabbit bladder to electrical field stimulation. At low concentrations terodiline has mainly an antimuscarinic action, whereas at higher concentrations a calcium antagonistic effect becomes evident. In vitro experiments appeared to show that these two effects were at least additive with regard to bladder contractility. Other experimental studies have confirmed the inhibitory effect of the calcium antagonists nifedipine, verapamil, and diltiazem on a variety of experimental models of the activity of spontaneous and induced bladder muscle strips and whole bladder preparations.[160, 161] Andersson and colleagues showed that nifedipine effectively and with some selectivity inhibited the nonmuscarinic portion of the contraction of rabbit detrusor strips, whereas verapamil, diltiazem, flunarizine, and lidoflazine caused a marked depression of both the total and the nonmuscarinic parts of contraction, suggesting that differences exist between various calcium channel blockers with respect to their effects on at least electrically induced bladder muscle contraction.[162] These results were used as support for the view that, even if "atropine resistant" contractions in rabbit and human bladder had different causes, combined muscarinic receptor and calcium channel blockade might offer a more effective way of treating bladder hyperactivity than the single-mechanism therapies presently available.

A number of clinical studies on the inhibitory action of terodiline on bladder hyperactivity have shown clinical effectiveness.[163] In a double-blind crossover study of 12 women with motor urge incontinence, Ekman and colleagues reported an increase in bladder capacity and the volume at which sensation of urgency was experienced in all but one of the patients treated with terodiline, whereas placebo treatment had no objective or subjective effect.[164]

Peters and associates reported the results of a multicenter study that ultimately included data from 89 patients (from an original 128) and compared terodiline and placebo in women with motor urge incontinence.[165] The daily dose in this study was 12.5 mg in the morning and 25 mg at night. The authors concluded that terodiline was more effective than placebo but noted that this improvement was much more apparent on subjective than on objective assessment of cystometric and micturition data. Sixty-three percent of patients preferred terodiline regardless of treatment sequence. Although statistically significant objective differences between terodiline and placebo were recorded, they were not very impressive. Frequency of voluntary micturition decreased from 9.6 to 8.9 in 24 hours on placebo, and from 9.9 to 7.3 on terodiline. Involuntary voidings decreased from 2.3 to 1.7 on placebo and from 2.5 to 1.5 on terodiline. Volume at first desire to void increased from 159 to 162 ml in those on placebo and from 151 to 198 ml in those on terodiline; bladder capacity increased from 312 to 318 ml on placebo and from 320 to 374 on terodiline.

Tapp and colleagues reported on a double-blind, placebo-controlled study, using a dose titration technique, that included 70 women with urodynamically proven detrusor instability and bladder capacities of less than 400 ml.[166] Sixty-two percent of the 34 women in the terodiline group considered themselves improved, and 38% were unchanged. Of the 36 women in the placebo group, 42% considered themselves improved, 47% unchanged, and 11% worse, a statistically significant response in favor of terodiline with regard to the improvement percentage. Micturition variables of daytime frequency, daytime incontinence episodes, number of pads used, and average voided volumes were statistically changed in favor of terodiline, but the absolute changes were relatively small (for instance, a change in daytime incontinence episodes in patients on placebo from 2.5 to 1.9 per day as opposed to 3.7 to 1.6 for those taking terodiline). Urodynamic data, while showing a trend in favor of terodiline in each parameter, showed no statistically significant differences in any category. Side effects were noted in a large number and with equal frequency in both groups after the dose titration phase. However, the incidence of anticholinergic side effects was higher in the drug group; 29% of the terodiline patients versus 11% of the placebo patients spontaneously complained of a dry mouth, and 20% of the terodiline patients but none of the placebo patients complained of blurred vision. The AHCPR guidelines[127] list seven randomized controlled trials for terodiline; 94% of patients were women. The percentage of cures (all figures refer to percentage *minus* percentage on placebo) is listed as 18% and 33%, percentage of reduction in urge incontinence is 14 to 83%, and the percentages of side effects and dropouts are 14 to 40% and 2 to 8%, respectively. Terodiline also exhibits an inhibitory effect on experimental hyperreflexia in the rabbit whole bladder model, suggesting a possible role for local administration as well.[167]

Terodiline is almost completely absorbed from the gastrointestinal tract and has a low serum clearance. The recommended dosage in adults is 25 mg twice a day, reduced to an initial dose of 12 mg twice a day in geriatric patients. The half-life is around 60 hours, and Abrams[163] logically proposes, on this basis, a once-daily dose but emphasizes the necessity of dose titration for each patient. The common side effects seen with calcium antagonists (hypotension, facial flushing, headache, dizziness, abdominal discomfort, constipation, nausea, rash, weakness, and palpitations) have not been reported in the larger initial clinical studies with terodiline, side effects consisting primarily of those consequent to its anticholinergic action. However, questions have been raised about the occurrence of a rare arrhythmia (torsades de pointes) in patients taking terodiline simultaneously with antidepressants or antiarrhythmic drugs.[168, 169] Stewart and colleagues reported a prolongation of QT and QTc intervals and a reduction in heart rate in elderly patients taking 12.5 mg twice a day of terodiline.[170] These effects were apparent after 1 week but not after 1 day of therapy. These investigators also reported polymorphic ventricular tachycardia in four patients (three over age 80) receiving the drug. They advised avoiding use of the drug by patients with cardiac disease requiring cardioactive drugs or those with hypokalemia, or in combination with other drugs that can prolong the QT interval such as tricyclic antidepressants or antipsychotics. After other reports of apparent cardiac toxicity, the drug was voluntarily withdrawn by the manufacturer pending the results of further safety studies. The studies conducted for approval by the Food and Drug Administration (FDA) were likewise voluntarily halted by the manufacturer; there is current activity directed toward their reinstitution.

Other calcium antagonist drugs have not been widely used to treat voiding dysfunction. Palmer and colleagues reported a double-blind, placebo-controlled trial with a single 20-mg daily dose of flunarizine in 14 women with detrusor instability and consequent symptoms.[171] A statistically significant decrease in urgency was produced in the drug-treated group, but there was no change in the frequency of micturition. Although a trend toward improvement of cystometric parameters occurred, it was not statistically significant ($p > .05$). Nifedipine is useful as prophylaxis against the development of autonomic hyperreflexia during endoscopic examination in patients with high spinal injury. A 10-mg dose given 30 minutes prior to the examination has been successful, and a sublingual dose of 10 mg has been effective in relieving an episode.[172]

POTASSIUM CHANNEL OPENERS Potassium channel openers efficiently relax various types of smooth muscle by increasing potassium efflux, resulting in membrane hyperpolarization.[173] Hyperpolarization reduces the opening probability of ion channels involved in membrane depolarization, and excitation is reduced. Andersson[33] summarized studies showing that, in isolated human and animal detrusor muscle, potassium channel openers reduce spontaneous contractions and contractions occurring in response to electrical stimulation, carbachol, and low (but not high) external potassium concentrations. There are some suggestions that bladder instability, at least that associated with infravesical obstruction and detrusor hypertrophy, may be secondary to supersensitivity to depolarizing stimuli. Theoretically, then, potassium channel openers might be an attractive alternative for the treatment of detrusor instability in such circumstances without inhibiting the normal voluntary contractions necessary for bladder emptying.[174] Pinacidil is a compound that, in a concentration-dependent fashion, inhibits not only spontaneous myogenic contractions but also contractile responses induced by electrical field stimulation and carbachol in isolated human detrusor[175] and in normal and hypertrophied rat detrusor. Unfortunately, a preliminary study of this agent in a double-blind crossover format produced no effects on symptoms in nine patients with detrusor instability and bladder outlet obstruction.[176] Nurse and associates reported on the use of cromakalim, another potassium channel opener, in 17 patients who had refractory detrusor instability or hyperreflexia or had stopped other drug therapy because of intolerable side effects.[177] Six of 16 (35%) patients who completed the study showed a decrease in frequency and an increase in voided volume. Long-term observation was not possible because the drug was withdrawn owing to reported adverse effects of high doses in animal toxicologic studies. Potassium channel openers are not at present very specific for the bladder and are more potent in relaxing other tissues—hence their potential utility in the treatment of hypertension, asthma, and angina. If tissue-selective potassium activator drugs can be developed, they may prove very useful for the treatment of detrusor instability, irritable bowel, and epilepsy.[178] Intravesical use has also been suggested.[179]

Side effects of pinacidil have been studied best; they include headache, peripheral edema (in 25 to 50% of patients and dose-related), weight gain, palpitations, dizziness, and rhinitis. Hypertrichosis and asymptomatic T-wave changes have also been reported (30%). Fewer data are available on cromakalim, which can produce dose-related headache but rarely edema.[33]

PROSTAGLANDIN INHIBITORS Prostaglandins (PG) are ubiquitous compounds that have a potential role in the excitatory neurotransmission to the bladder, the development of bladder contractility or tension occurring during filling, the emptying contractile response of bladder smooth muscle to neural stimulation, and even the maintenance of urethral tone during the storage phase of micturition as well as the release of this tone during the emptying phase (see references 1 and 5 for discussion and references). Downie and Karmazyn suggest a different type of contractile influence of PG on detrusor muscle.[180] They found that mechanical irritation of the epithelium of rabbit bladder increased basal tension and spontaneous activity in response to electrical stimulation, and that these responses, related to the intensity of the irritative trauma, were mimicked by prostaglandins. The effect was significantly reduced by pretreatment of the epithelium, but not the muscle, with PG synthetase inhibitors. Andersson suggests a possible sensitization of sensory afferent nerves by prostaglandins, increasing afferent input at a given degree of bladder filling and contributing to the triggering of involuntary bladder contractions at a small bladder volume.[112] Thus, there are many mechanisms whereby PG synthesis inhibitors might decrease bladder contractility in response to various stimuli. However, objective evidence that such can occur is scant.

Cardozo and colleagues reported a double-blind, placebo-controlled study on the effects of 3-times-daily administration of 50 mg of flurbiprofen, a PG synthetase inhibitor, on 30 women with detrusor instability.[181] They concluded that the drug did not abolish involuntary bladder contractions or abnormal bladder activity but did delay the intravesical pressure rise to a greater degree of distention. Forty-three percent of the patients experienced side effects, primarily nausea, vomiting, headache, indigestion, gastric distress, constipation, and rash. Cardozo and Stanton reported symptomatic improvement in patients with detrusor instability who were given indomethacin in doses of 50 to 200 mg daily, but this was a short-term study with no cystometric data, and the drug was compared only with bromocriptine.[182] The incidence of side effects was high (19 of 32 patients), although no patient had to stop treatment because of them. Numerous PG synthetase inhibitors exist, most of which belong in the category of nonsteroidal anti-inflammatory drugs, and every clinician has a favorite. It should be remembered that these drugs can interfere with platelet function and contribute to excess bleeding in surgical patients; some may have adverse renal effects as well.[183]

BETA-ADRENERGIC AGONISTS The presence of beta-adrenergic receptors in human bladder muscle has prompted attempts to increase bladder capacity with beta-adrenergic stimulation. Such stimulation can cause significant increases in the capacity of animal bladders, which contain a moderate density of beta-adrenergic receptors.[1] In vitro studies show a strong dose-related relaxant effect of beta-2 agonists on the bladder body of rabbits but little effect on the bladder base or proximal urethra. Terbutaline, in oral doses of 5 mg three times a day, has been reported to have a "good clinical effect" in some patients with urgency and urgency incontinence but no significant effect on the bladders of neurologically normal humans without voiding difficulty.[184] Although these results are compatible with those seen in other organ systems (beta-adrenergic stimulation causes no acute change in total lung capacity in normal humans but does favorably affect patients with bronchial asthma), there are few adequate studies of the effects of beta-adrenergic stimulation in patients with detrusor hyperactivity. Lindholm and Lose used 5 mg three times a day of terbutaline in eight women with motor and seven with sensory urge incontinence.[185] After 3 months of treatment, 14 patients claimed to have experienced beneficial effects, and 12 became subjectively continent. In six of eight cases, the detrusor became stable on cystometric examination. Interestingly, the volume at first desire to void increased in the patients with originally unstable bladders from a mean of 200 to 302 ml, but the maximum cystometric capacity did not change. Nine patients had transient side effects, including palpitations, tachycardia, or hand tremor, and in three of these, the side effects continued but were acceptable to the patient. In one patient the drug was discontinued because of severe adverse symptoms. Gruneberger, in a double-blind study, reported that clenbuterol had produced a good therapeutic effect in 15 of 20 patients with motor urge incontinence.[186] Unfavorable results of beta-agonist usage for bladder hyperactivity were published by Castleden and Morgan[187] and Naglo and associates.[188]

TRICYCLIC ANTIDEPRESSANTS Many clinicians have found that tricyclic antidepressants, particularly imipramine hydrochloride, are especially useful for facilitating urine storage, both by decreasing bladder contractility and by increasing outlet resistance.[9] These agents have been the subject of a voluminous and highly sophisticated pharmacologic investigation to determine the mechanisms of action responsible for their varied effects.[93, 189–190] Most data have been accumulated as a result of trying to explain the antidepressant properties of these agents and consequently involve primarily central nervous system tissue. The results, conclusions, and speculations based on the data are extremely interesting, but it should be emphasized that it is essentially unknown whether they apply to or have relevance for the lower urinary tract. In varying degrees, all of these agents have least three major pharmacologic actions. They have central and peripheral anticholinergic effects at some (but not all) sites; they block the active transport system in the presynaptic nerve ending that is responsible for the reuptake of the released amine neurotransmitters norepinephrine and serotonin; and they are sedatives, an action that occurs presumably on a central basis but is perhaps related to antihistaminic properties (at H_1 receptors, though they also antagonize H_2 receptors to some extent). There is also evidence that these agents desensitize at least some alpha-2 and some beta adrenoreceptors. Paradoxically, they also have been shown to block

some alpha and serotonin-1 receptors. Imipramine has prominent systemic anticholinergic effects but only a weak antimuscarinic effect on bladder smooth muscle.[191, 192] It does have a strong direct inhibitory effect on bladder smooth muscle, however, that is neither anticholinergic nor adrenergic.[157, 191, 193] This may be due to a local anestheticlike action at the nerve terminals in the adjacent effector membrane, an effect that seems to occur also in cardiac muscle,[194] or it may be due to an inhibition of the participation of calcium in the excitation-contraction coupling process.[191, 195] Akah has provided supportive evidence in the rat bladder that desipramine, the active metabolite of imipramine, depresses the response to electrical field stimulation by interfering with calcium movement (perhaps not only extracellular calcium movement but also internal translocation and binding).[196] Direct evidence suggesting that the effect of imipramine on norepinephrine reuptake occurs in lower urinary tract tissue as well as brain tissue has been provided by Foreman and McNulty in the rabbit.[197] In addition, they describe a significantly greater but similar effect of tomoxetine in the bladder and urethra in this model. Tomoxetine inhibits norepinephrine reuptake selectively, whereas imipramine has a nonselective effect. This fact suggests a potential new clinical approach to the use of more selective and potent reuptake inhibitors for the treatment of incontinence. In attempting to correlate clinical effects with mechanisms of action, one might also postulate a beta receptor–induced decrease in bladder body contractility if peripheral blockade of norepinephrine reuptake does occur there owing to the increased concentration of beta receptors compared with alpha-adrenergic receptors in that area. An enhanced alpha-adrenergic effect in the smooth muscle of the bladder base and proximal urethra, where alpha receptors outnumber beta receptors, is generally considered the mechanism whereby imipramine increases outlet resistance.

Clinically, imipramine (e.g., Tofranil) seems to be effective in decreasing bladder contractility and increasing outlet resistance.[198–202] Castleden and colleagues began therapy in elderly patients with detrusor instability with a single 25-mg nighttime dose of imipramine, which was increased every third day by 25 mg until the patient either was continent or had side effects, or a dose of 150 mg was reached.[202] Six of 10 patients became continent, and, in those who underwent repeated cystometry, bladder capacity increased by a mean of 105 ml and bladder pressure at capacity decreased by a mean of 18 cm H_2O. Maximum urethral pressure (MUP) increased by a mean of 30 cm H_2O. Although our subjective impression[200] was that the bladder effects became evident only after many days of treatment, some patients in the Castleden series became continent after only 3 to 5 days of therapy. Our usual adult dose for treatment of voiding dysfunction is 25 mg four times a day; less frequent administration is possible because of the drug's long half-life. Half that dose is given in elderly patients, in whom the drug half-life may be prolonged. In our experience, the effects of imipramine on the lower urinary tract are often additive to those of atropine-like agents; consequently a combination of imipramine and an antimuscarinic or an antispasmodic is sometimes especially useful for decreasing bladder contractility.[200] If imipramine is used in conjunction with an atropine-like agent, it should be noted that the anticholinergic side effects of the drugs may be additive. It has been known for many years that imipramine is relatively effective for the treatment of nocturnal enuresis in children. Doses for this condition range from 10 to 50 mg daily. Whether the mechanisms of drug action in this situation are the same as those for decreasing bladder contractility or increasing outlet resistance, or whether the antienuretic effect is more centrally mediated, is unknown. Korczyn and Kish have presented evidence that the antienuretic effect results from a different mechanism than the peripheral anticholinergic effect and the drug's antidepressant effect.[203] The antienuretic effect occurs soon after initial administration, whereas the antidepressant effects generally take 2 to 4 weeks to develop.

Doxepin (Sinequan) is another tricyclic antidepressant that has been found to be more potent, using in vitro rabbit bladder strips, than other tricyclic compounds with respect to antimuscarinic and musculotropic relaxant activity.[193] Lose and colleagues, in a randomized double-blind crossover study of women with involuntary bladder contractions and either frequency, urgency, or urge incontinence, found that this agent caused a significant decrease in control over nighttime frequency and incontinence episodes and a near-significant decrease in urine loss (by the pad weighing test) and in the cystometric parameters of first sensation and maximum bladder capacity.[204] The dose of doxepin used was either a single 50-mg bedtime dose or this dose plus an additional 25 mg in the morning. The number of daytime incontinence episodes decreased in both doxepin and placebo groups, and the difference was not statistically significant. Doxepin treatment was preferred by 14 patients, whereas 2 preferred placebo. Three patients had no preference. Of the 14 patients who stated a preference for doxepin, 12 claimed that they became continent during treatment, and 2 claimed improvement. The 2 patients who preferred placebo claimed improvement. The AHCPR guidelines[127] combine results for imipramine and doxepin, citing only three randomized controlled trials, with an unknown percentage of women patients. The percentage of cures (all figures refer to percentage *minus* the percentage on placebo) are listed as 31%, percentage of reduction in urge incontinence as 20 to 77%, and percentage of side effects as 0 to 70%).[127]

When used in the generally larger doses employed for antidepressant effects, the most frequent side effects of the tricyclic antidepressants are those attributable to their systemic anticholinergic activity.[93, 190] Allergic phenomena, including rash, hepatic dysfunction, obstructive jaundice, and agranulocytosis may also occur but are rare. Central nervous system side

effects may include weakness, fatigue, parkinsonian effect, fine tremors noted mostly in the upper extremities, a manic or schizophrenic picture, and sedation, probably from an antihistaminic effect. Postural hypotension may also be seen, presumably due to selective blockade (a paradoxical effect) of alpha-1 adrenergic receptors in some vascular smooth muscle. Tricyclic antidepressants may also cause excess sweating of obscure origin and a delay in orgasm or orgasmic impotence, whose cause is likewise unclear. They may also produce arrhythmias and can interact in deleterious ways with other drugs—thus, caution must be observed in using these drugs in patients with cardiac disease.[93] Whether cardiotoxicity will prove to be a legitimate concern in patients receiving the smaller doses (smaller than those used for treatment of depression) for lower urinary tract dysfunction remains to be seen but is a matter of potential concern. Consultation with a patient's internist or cardiologist is always helpful before such therapy is instituted in questionable situations. The use of imipramine is contraindicated in patients receiving monoamine oxidase inhibitors because severe central nervous system toxicity can be precipitated, including hyperpyrexia, seizures, and coma. Some potential side effects of antidepressants may be especially significant in the elderly, specifically weakness, fatigue, and postural hypotension. If imipramine or any of the tricyclic antidepressants is to be prescribed for the treatment of voiding dysfunction, the patient should be thoroughly informed about the fact that this is *not* the usual indication for this drug and that potential side effects exist. Reports of significant side effects (severe abdominal distress, nausea, vomiting, headache, lethargy, and irritability) following abrupt cessation of high doses of imipramine in children suggest that the drug should be discontinued gradually, especially in patients receiving high doses.

DIMETHYL SULFOXIDE (DMSO) DMSO is a relatively simple, naturally occurring organic compound that has been used as an industrial solvent for many years. It has multiple pharmacologic actions (membrane penetrant, anti-inflammatory, local analgesic, bacteriostatic, diuretic, cholinesterase inhibitor, collagen solvent, vasodilator) and has been used for the treatment of arthritis and other musculoskeletal disorders, generally in a 70% solution. The formulation for human intravesical use is a 50% solution. Sant has summarized the pharmacology and clinical usage of DMSO and has tabulated good to excellent results in 50 to 90% of collected series of patients treated with intravesical instillations for interstitial cystitis.[205] However, DMSO has not been shown to be useful in the treatment of detrusor hyperreflexia or instability or in any patient with urgency or frequency but without interstitial cystitis. The subject of interstitial cystitis and its treatment is considered in Chapter 15.

POLYSYNAPTIC INHIBITORS Baclofen has been discussed previously with agents that decrease outlet resistance secondary to striated sphincter dyssynergia. It is also capable of depressing detrusor hyperreflexia due to a spinal cord lesion.[206] Taylor and Bates, in a double-blind crossover study, reported that it was very effective in decreasing both day and night urinary frequency and incontinence in patients with idiopathic instability.[207] Cystometric changes were not recorded, however, and considerable improvement was also obtained in the placebo group. The intrathecal use of baclofen for treatment of detrusor hyperactivity is a potentially exciting area (see prior discussion), and further reports are awaited.

OTHER POTENTIAL AGENTS Nitric oxide (NO) is hypothesized to be a mediator of the nonadrenergic noncholinergic relaxation of the outlet smooth muscle that occurs with bladder contraction.[5] Evidence exists that it is also involved in relaxation of bladder body smooth muscle,[208] and this provides interesting fodder for speculation—is relaxation impaired in some types of hyperactivity and can NO analogs or synthetase stimulators be developed as agents to inhibit detrusor contractility? Glyceryl trinitrate releases NO in vivo and achieves its cardiovascular effects by relaxing vascular smooth muscle. A pilot study of 10 patients with instability given transdermal NO showed significant decreases in episodes (per 24 hours) of frequency (9.7 to 6.7), nocturia (1.84 to 1.09), and incontinence (0.61 to 0.36).[209] Although the ubiquity of NO might seem to mitigate its potential use in treating bladder hyperactivity (unless more organ-specific substrates or receptors are found), randomized controlled trials should be done.

Soulard and colleagues have described the effects of JO 1870 on bladder activity in the rat.[210] This nonanticholinergic probable opioid agonist increased bladder capacity and threshold pressure responsible for micturition in a dose-dependent fashion, raising the possibility of the use or development of opioid agonists with selectivity for receptors involved in the micturition reflex. Propiverine has been described by Haruno to inhibit spontaneous or agonist-induced bladder contractility in various preparations by either an anticholinergic or calcium channel blocking effect; it has relative selectivity (10 to 100 times) for bladder and ileum.[211] No clinical trials have been reported.

Constantinou described the effects of thiphenamil hydrochloride on the lower urinary tract of healthy female volunteers and those with detrusor incontinence.[212, 213] In a randomized controlled trial, based on diary records from 14 patients with instability, it was reported that voiding frequency per day decreased significantly (from 10.3 to 8.0 times), but placebo values were not given. Daily incontinence episodes decreased in nine analyzable patients from 2.3 to 1.6 (not significant, placebo values not given) with pad dryness (rated on a 0 to 4 scale) improving from 1.6 to 1.2 (significant, but no placebo data given). Objective urodynamic results (in 16 patients) showed no flowmetry changes, no changes in bladder capacity, some increase in first sensation of fullness, and a significant decrease in detrusor voiding pressure (46.1 to 31.9 cm H_2O) over placebo. The data and interpretation in this article are confusing to me,

especially because the study of healthy volunteers showed no urodynamic differences except an *increase* in detrusor pressure at maximum flow (from 36 to 49.5 cm H_2O) and an *increase* in maximum flow rate (from 16.9 to 27.7 ml/second) at a dose of 800 mg of drug. This drug was said to be a "synthetic antispasmodic." The most that can be said about the clinical use of thiphenamil is that, now that a question has been raised, it needs to be addressed by further "cleaner" studies with internally consistent results.

Increasing Bladder Capacity by Decreasing Sensory (Afferent) Input

Decreasing afferent input peripherally is the ideal treatment for both sensory urgency and instability or hyperreflexia in a bladder with relatively normal elastic or viscoelastic properties in which the sensory afferents constitute the first limb in the abnormal micturition reflex. Maggi has written extensively about this type of treatment, specifically with reference to the properties of capsaicin.[214–216] This drug is an irritant and algogenic compound obtained from hot red peppers that has highly selective effects on a subset of mammalian sensory neurons, including polymodal receptors and warm thermoreceptors.[217] Capsaicin produces pain by selectively activating polymodal nociceptive neurons by membrane depolarization and opening a cation-selective ion channel, which can be blocked by ruthenium red. Repeated administration induces desensitization and inactivation of sensory neurons by several mechanisms. Systemic and topical capsaicin produces a reversible antinociceptive and anti-inflammatory action after an initially undesirable algesic effect. Local or topical application blocks C-fiber conduction and inactivates neuropeptide release from peripheral nerve endings, accounting for local antinociception and reduction of neurogenic inflammation. Systemic capsaicin produces antinociception by activating specific receptors on afferent nerve terminals in the spinal cord, and spinal neurotransmission is subsequently blocked by a prolonged inactivation of sensory neurotransmitter release. With local administration (intravesical) the potential advantage of capsaicin is a lack of systemic side effects. The actions are highly specific when the drug is applied locally—the compound affects primarily small-diameter nociceptive afferents, leaving the sensations of touch and pressure unchanged, although heat (not cold) perception may be reduced. Motor fibers are not affected.[218] The effects are reversible, although it is not known whether initial levels of sensitivity are regained. Craft and Porreca list intravesical doses in the rat as 0.03 to 10.0 μM for 15 to 30 minutes and in humans a maximum of 1 to 2 mM.[218]

Maggi reviewed the therapeutic potential of capsaicinlike molecules.[216] Capsaicin-sensitive primary afferents (CSPA) innervate the human bladder, and intravesical instillation of capsaicin into human bladder produces a concentration-dependent decrease in first desire to void, decreased bladder capacity, and a warm burning sensation. Maggi used doses of 0.01, 1.0, and 10 μM, administered in ascending order at 10- to 15-minute intervals as constant infusions of 20 ml/minute until micturition occurred.[214] Five capsaicin-treated patients with "hypersensitive disorders" reported either a complete disappearance of symptoms (four patients) or marked attentuation of symptoms (one patient), beginning 2 to 3 days after administration and lasting 4 to 16 days. After that time the symptoms gradually reappeared but were no worse. Fowler and colleagues found that considerably higher doses (up to 1 to 2 mM for 30 minutes) were necessary to produce an effect in humans.[219] However, these investigators reported that bladder control improved within 2 days, and the improvement lasted for 3 to 6 months. Lower doses (0.1 to 100 μM) produced "no long lasting benefit." An *efferent* function of CSPA is the release of neurotransmitters from the peripheral endings of these sensory neurons, such as tachykinins and calcitonin gene-related peptide (CGRP).[216] These neurotransmitters can produce events collectively known as neurogenic inflammation, which can include all or some smooth muscle contractions, increased plasma protein extravasation, vasodilation, mast cell degranulation, facilitation of transmitter release from nerve terminals, recruitment of inflammatory cells, and so on. This is another reason why intravesical capsaicin could theoretically be useful in treating the pain and related problems of interstitial cystitis and certain types of bladder hyperactivity that originate in primary afferents.

The peripheral terminals of CSPA form a dense plexus just below the bladder urothelium, and fibers penetrating the urothelium come into contact with the lumen. This location, combined with the peculiar chemosensitivity of the CSPA, permits them to detect "backflow" of chemicals across the urothelium, which is thought to occur during conditions leading to breakdown of the "barrier function" of the urothelium.[216] If the "barrier" theory or "leaky urothelium" theory (see Chapter 15) of the pathogenesis of interstitial cystitis is true for some or many patients with this condition, the CSPA in such patients may be stimulated by urine constituents leaking back across the urothelium, and, under these circumstances, a local release of neuropeptides may well contribute in producing neurogenic inflammation. If this is so, as Maggi suggests,[216] a local treatment leading to desensitization of CSPA would be doubly advantageous. With capsaicin, however, excitation precedes desensitization, somewhat limiting the potential for therapy in humans. A preferable analog would produce the latter action while reducing or eliminating the former one. Last, Maggi discusses the possible long-term disadvantages of such therapy as related to the potential physiologic roles, trophic or protective, of CSPA and their secretions in response to stimulation.[216]

Increasing Outlet Resistance

ALPHA-ADRENERGIC AGONISTS The bladder neck and proximal urethra contain a preponderance of alpha-adrenergic receptor sites, which, when stimulated, produce smooth muscle contraction.[1, 2, 5] The static infusion urethral pressure profile is altered by such stimulation, producing an increase in maximum urethral pressure (MUP) and maximum urethral closure pressure (MUCP). Various orally administered pharmacologic agents producing alpha-adrenergic stimulation are available. Generally, outlet resistance is increased to a variable degree by such an action. The potential side effects of all these agents include blood pressure elevation, anxiety, and insomnia due to stimulation of the central nervous system, headache, tremor, weakness, palpitations, cardiac arrhythmias, and respiratory difficulties. All such agents should be used with caution in patients with hypertension, cardiovascular disease, or hyperthyroidism.[220]

The use of ephedrine to treat SUI was mentioned as early as 1948.[221] This is a noncatecholamine sympathomimetic agent that enhances release of norepinephrine from sympathetic neurons and directly stimulates both alpha- and beta-adrenergic receptors.[220] The oral adult dosage is 25 to 50 mg four times a day. Some tachyphylaxis develops in response to its peripheral actions, probably as a result of depletion of norepinephrine stores. Pseudoephedrine, a stereoisomer of ephedrine, is used for similar indications and carries similar precautions. The adult dosage is 30 to 60 mg four times a day, and the 30-mg-dose form is available in the United States without prescription. Diokno and Taub reported a "good to excellent" result in 27 of 38 patients with sphincteric incontinence treated with ephedrine sulfate.[222] Beneficial effects were most often achieved in those with minimal to moderate wetting; little benefit was achieved in patients with severe stress incontinence. A dose of 75 to 100 mg of norephedrine chloride has been shown to increase MUP and MUCP in women with urinary stress incontinence.[223] At a bladder volume of 300 ml, MUP rose from 82 to 110 cm H_2O, and MUCP rose from 63 to 93 cm H_2O. The functional profile length did not change significantly. Obrink and Bunne, however, noted that 100 mg of norephedrine chloride given twice a day did not improve severe stress incontinence sufficiently to offer it as an alternative to surgical treatment.[224] They further noted in their group of 10 such patients that the MUCP was not influenced at rest or with stress at low or moderate bladder volumes. Lose and Lindholm treated 20 women with stress incontinence with norfenefrine, an alpha agonist, given as a slow-release tablet.[225] Nineteen patients reported reduced urinary leakage; 10 reported no further stress incontinence. MUCP increased in 16 patients during treatment, the mean rise being 53 to 64 cm H_2O. It is interesting and perplexing that most patients reported an effect only after 14 days of treatment. This delay is difficult to explain on the basis of drug action, unless one postulates a change in the number or sensitivity of alpha receptors.

The group at Kolding Hospital in Denmark has published three other articles of note on the use of norfenefrine for sphincteric incontinence. The results are interesting. Forty-four patients with SUI were randomized to treatment with norfenefrine 15 to 30 mg three times a day versus placebo for 6 weeks.[226] Subjectively, 12 of 23 (52%) of the norfenefrine group reported improvement as opposed to 7 of 21 (33%) of the placebo group, a difference that was not statistically significant. Continence was reported by six (26%) norfenefrine patients and three (14%) placebo patients (not significant). Judged by a stress test, seven patients in each group became continent; 11 of 23 (48%) improved both subjectively and objectively in the norfenefrine group as opposed to 5 of 21 (24%) in the placebo group ($p = .09$). MUCP increased significantly (from 50 to 55 cm H_2O in the norfenefrine group, and from 55 to 65 cm H_2O) in the placebo group. Although the patients were said to have "genuine stress incontinence," 5 of 12 with "urge incontinence" were reported cured with norfenefrine, and 4 of 7 with placebo.

Diernoes and associates reported on the results of a 1-hour pad test in 33 women with either SUI or combined stress incontinence and urgency treated with 30 mg three times a day of norfenefrine.[227] Leakage of more than 10 g was required for entry into the study. Subjective improvement was reported by 10 patients (61%). Continence as shown by pad test was found in six patients (18%). Pad tests were graded on a scale of 1 to 4. At 12 weeks, 20 patients (61%) had improved by at least one grade ($p < .05$), but at 3 weeks the number was 13 (39%) (not significant).

Lose and colleagues studied 44 women scheduled for operation for SUI who were treated with 15 to 30 mg three times a day of norfenefrine versus placebo for 3 to 4.5 months and were then evaluated for outcome after a median observation period of 30 months.[228] The description and categorization of results were somewhat confusing, but the results (in my interpretation, at least) were interesting. Originally 23 patients were allocated to the norfenefrine group, and 21 to placebo. Results were categorized in the following way: cured or much improved with no further treatment wanted; underwent surgery for relief; wanted medical therapy reinstituted; uncertain about what kind of treatment they wanted; used pads or pelvic floor exercises. At the end of a 6-week initial treatment period and reevaluation, patients whose initial treatment had had no effect at all were crossed over to the other group. Categorization of results is shown in Table 24–3. It is obvious that a powerful placebo effect occurred, for which the reasons are unknown, and therefore caution must be exercised in the evaluation of *all* modalities of therapy for sphincteric (and detrusor) incontinence.

Phenylpropanolamine hydrochloride (PPA) shares the pharmacologic properties of ephedrine and is approximately equal in peripheral potency while causing less central stimulation.[220] It is available in 25- and 50-mg tablets and 75-mg timed release capsules and is a component of numerous proprietary mixtures marketed for the treatment of nasal and sinus congestion (usually in combination with an H_1 antihistamine) and as appetite suppressants. Using doses of 50 mg three times a day, Awad and associates found that 11 of 13 women and 6 of 7 men with stress incontinence were significantly improved after 4 weeks of therapy.[229] MUCP increased from a mean of 47 to 72 cm H_2O in patients with an empty bladder and from 43 to 58 cm H_2O in patients with a full bladder. Using a capsule (Ornade) containing 50 mg of PPA, 8 mg of chlorpheniramine (an antihistamine), and 2 mg of isopropamide (an antimuscarinic), Stewart and colleagues found that, of 77 women with SUI, 18 were completely cured with one sustained release capsule.[230] Twenty-eight patients were "much better," 6 were "slightly better," and 25 were no better. In 11 men with postprostatectomy stress incontinence, the numbers in the corresponding categories were 1, 2, 1, and 7. The formulation of Ornade has now been changed, and each capsule of drug contains 75 mg of PPA and 12 mg of chlorpheniramine. Collste and Lindskog reported on a group of 24 women with SUI

TABLE 24–3
Norfenefrine and Placebo in 44 Women Scheduled for Surgery for SUI[a]

Results	Patient Groups (n 44)[b]			
	Placebo Not Crossed Over (11)	Placebo Crossed Over to Norfenefrine (10)	Norfenefrine Not Crossed Over (13)	Norfenefrine Crossed Over to Placebo (10)
Cured or improved	6	2	3	3
Surgery	2	3	2	3
Wanted medical therapy reinstituted	0	3	7	1
Uncertain	2	0	1	3
Pad or pelvic floor exercises	1	2	0	0

[a]See text for further description.
[b]In the placebo group (21 patients), 10 crossed over to the norfenefrine group after 6 weeks. In the norfenefrine group (23 patients), 10 crossed over to placebo after 6 weeks.
Data based on study by Lose et al (1989).[228]

treated with PPA or placebo with a crossover after 2 weeks.[231] Severity of SUI was graded 1 (slight) or 2 (moderate). Average MUCP overall increased significantly with PPA compared with placebo (48 to 55 vs. 48 to 49 cm H_2O). This was a significant difference in grade 2 but not in grade 1 patients. The average number of leakage episodes per 48 hours was reduced significantly overall for PPA patients but not in placebo patients (five to two vs. five to six). This was significant for grade 1 but not for grade 2 patients. Subjectively 6 of 24 patients thought that both PPA and placebo were ineffective. Among the 18 patients (of 24) who reported a subjective preference, 14 preferred PPA and 4 placebo. Improvements were rated subjectively as good, moderately good, and slight. Improvements obtained with PPA were significant compared with those for placebo for the entire population and for both groups separately. The AHCPR guidelines[127] reported eight randomized controlled trials with PPA 50 mg twice a day for SUI in women. Percent cures (all figures refer to percent *minus* percent on placebo) are listed as $0-14$, percent reduction in incontinence as $19-60$, and percent side effects and percent dropouts as $5-33$ and $0-4.3$, respectively.

Some authors have emphasized the potential complications of phenylpropanolamine. Mueller reported on a group of 11 patients who had significant neurologic symptoms (acute headache, psychiatric symptoms, or seizures) after taking "look-alike pills" thought to contain amphetamines but actually containing PPA. Baggioni emphasized the possibility of blood pressure elevation, especially in patients with autonomic impairment.[233] Lasagna pointed out that prior reported blood pressure elevations occurred with a product that differed from American PPA and probably contained a different and much more potent isomer.[234] He noted that although a huge volume of PPA has been consumed in the form of decongestants and anorectic medications, the world literature has reported only a minimum number of possible toxic reactions, most of which involved excessively high doses in combination medications. Liebson found no cardiovascular or subjective adverse effects with doses of 25 mg three times a day or a 75-mg sustained-release preparation in a population of 150 healthy normal volunteers.[235] Blackburn, in a larger series of healthy subjects using many over-the-counter formulations, concluded that a statistically significant but clinically unimportant pressor effect existed during the first 6 hours after administration of PPA and that this was greater with sustained-release preparation.[236] Caution should still be exercised in individuals known to be significantly hypertensive and in elderly patients, in whom pharmacokinetic function may be altered.

Midodrine is a long-acting alpha-adrenergic agonist reported to be useful in the treatment of seminal emission and ejaculation disorders following retroperitoneal lymphadenectomy. Treatment with 5 mg twice a day for 4 weeks in 20 patients with stress incontinence produced a cure in 1 and improvement

in 14.[237] MUCP rose by 8.3%, and the planometric index of the continence area on profilometry increased by 9%. The actions of imipramine have already been discussed. On a theoretical basis, an increase in urethral resistance might be expected if indeed an enhanced alpha-adrenergic effect at this level resulted from an inhibition of norepinephrine reuptake. However, as mentioned previously, imipramine also causes alpha-adrenergic blocking effects, at least in vascular smooth muscle. Many clinicians have noted improvement in patients treated with imipramine primarily for bladder hyperactivity but who had in addition some component of sphincteric incontinence. Gilja and colleagues reported a study of 30 women with stress incontinence who were treated with 75 mg of imipramine daily for 4 weeks.[238] Twenty-one women subjectively reported continence. Mean MUCP for the group increased from 34.06 to 48.23 mmHg.

Although some clinicians have reported spectacular cure and improvement rates with alpha-adrenergic agonists and agents that produce an alpha-adrenergic effect in the outlet of patients with sphincteric urinary incontinence, our own experience coincides with those who report that such treatment often produces satisfactory or some improvement in mild cases but rarely total dryness in patients with severe or even moderate stress incontinence. A clinical trial, when possible, is certainly worthwhile, however, especially in conjunction with pelvic floor physiotherapy or biofeedback.

BETA-ADRENERGIC ANTAGONISTS AND AGONISTS Theoretically, beta-adrenergic blocking agents might be expected to "unmask" or potentiate an alpha-adrenergic effect, thereby increasing urethral resistance. Gleason and colleagues reported success in treating certain patients with SUI with propranolol, using oral doses of 10 mg four times a day.[239] The beneficial effect became manifest only after 4 to 10 weeks of treatment. Cardiac effects occur rather promptly after administration of this drug, but hypotensive effects do not usually appear as rapidly, although it is difficult to explain such a long delay in onset of the therapeutic effect on incontinence on this basis. Kaisary also reported success with propranolol in the treatment of stress incontinence.[240] Although such treatment has been suggested as an alternative to alpha agonists in patients with sphincteric incontinence and hypertension, few if any subsequent reports of such efficacy have appeared. Others have reported no significant changes in urethral profile pressures in normal women after beta-adrenergic blockade.[241] Although 10 mg four times a day is a relatively small dose of propranolol, it should be recalled that the major potential side effects of the drug are related to its therapeutic beta-blocking effects. Heart failure may develop, as well as an increase in airway resistance, and asthma is a contraindication to its use. Abrupt discontinuation may precipitate an exacerbation of anginal attacks and rebound hypertension.[220]

Beta-adrenergic stimulation is generally conceded

to decrease urethral pressure (see reference 5 for references), but beta-2 agonists have been reported to *increase* the contractility of fast-contracting striated muscle fibers (extensor digitorum longus) from guinea pigs and suppress that of slow-contracting fibers (soleus).[242] Clenbuterol, a selective beta-2 agonist, has been reported to potentiate, in a dose-dependent fashion, the field stimulation–induced contraction in isolated periurethral muscle preparation in the rabbit. The potentiation is greater than that produced by isoproterenol and is suppressed by propranolol.[243] The authors reported an increase in urethral pressure with clinical use of clenbuterol and speculated on its promise in the treatment of sphincteric incontinence. Although the differential effects on the smooth and striated musculature of the outlet and even on different fiber types on the striated sphincter may be functionally antagonistic, one should not ignore the possibility of an augmentative effect on outlet resistance by a drug like clenbuterol under certain physiologic conditions. Other beta-2 agonists are salbutamol and terbutaline.

ESTROGENS Although estrogens were recommended for the treatment of urinary incontinence in women as early as 1941,[244] there is still controversy over their use and benefit-risk ratio for this purpose. This subject is a good example of why it is sometimes difficult to obtain a consensus about the efficacy or nonefficacy of a particular category of drug for the treatment of incontinence. There is an impressive basic science literature on the effects of estrogen on the lower urinary tract but no strictly appropriate experimental model of either stress incontinence or detrusor hyperactivity or hypersensitivity. There are numerous clinical trials, some controlled and some not, some using estrogen alone and some using estrogen plus alpha agonists. There is little consistency in methodology, and the manner in which some authors have chosen to express their data and conclusions is confusing, at least to me. In some cases raw data seem to be ignored in favor of statistics, but, as always, there is no lack of opinions.

Much attention has been paid to the innervation, physiology, and pharmacology of the smooth muscle of the uterus. Estrogens have been found to affect many related properties including excitability, neuronal influences on the muscle, receptor density and sensitivity, and transmitter metabolism, especially in adrenergic nerves. The urethra (and trigone) are embryologically related to the uterus, and significant work has also been done on the effects of estrogenic hormones on the lower urinary tract. Hodgson and associates reported that the sensitivity of the rabbit urethra to alpha-adrenergic stimulation was estrogen-dependent[245]; castration caused decreased sensitivity, and treatment with low levels of estrogen reversed this. Levin and coworkers showed that parenteral estrogen administration can change the autonomic receptor content and the innervation of the lower urinary tract of immature female rabbits.[246, 247] A marked increase in response to alpha-adrenergic, muscarinic, and purinergic stimulation

occurred in the bladder body but not the base, and there was a significant increase in the number of alpha-adrenergic and muscarinic receptors in the bladder body but not the base. Other work[5] has shown a decrease in muscarinic receptor density following estradiol treatment of mature female rabbits, and either no change or a decreased detrusor response to cholinergic and electrical stimulation. Levin and coworkers concluded that pregnancy induced an increase in the purinergic and a decrease in the cholinergic responses of the rabbit bladder to field stimulation,[248] and Tong and colleagues reported a decrease in the alpha-adrenergic response of the midbladder and base of pregnant as opposed to virgin rabbits.[249] Larsson and associates reported that estrogen treatment of the isolated female rabbit urethra caused an increased sensitivity to norepinephrine.[250] The mechanism was postulated to be related to a more than twofold increase in the alpha-adrenergic receptor number. Callahan and Creed reported that pretreatment with estrogen of oophorectomized dogs and wallabies did increase sensitivity of urethral strips to alpha-adrenergic stimulation, but that this did not occur in the rabbit or guinea pig.[251] Bump and Friedman reported that sex hormone replacement with estrogen, but not testosterone, enhanced the urethral sphincter mechanism in the castrated female baboon by effects that were unrelated to skeletal muscle.[252] They added that these effects might not be related just to changes in the urethral smooth musculature, but to changes in the urethral mucosa, submucosal vascular plexus, and connective tissue.

Estrogen therapy certainly seems to be capable of facilitating urinary storage in some postmenopausal female patients. Whether this effect is related just to changes in the autonomic innervation, receptor content, or function of the smooth muscle or to changes in estrogen-binding sites[253] or changes in the vascular or connective tissue elements of the urethral wall has not been settled. Batra and colleagues have shown that low doses of estradiol and estratriol increased blood perfusion into the urethra (as well as the vagina and uterus) of oophorectomized mature female rabbits.[254] After menopause, urethral pressure parameters normally decrease somewhat,[255] and although this change is generally conceded to be related in some way to decreased estrogen levels, it is still largely a matter of speculation whether the actual changes occur in smooth muscle, blood circulation, supporting tissues, or the "mucosal seal mechanism." Versi and associates describe a positive correlation between skin collagen content, which does decline with declining estrogen status, and parameters of the urethral pressure profile, suggesting that the estrogen effect on the urethra may be predicted, at least in part, by changes in the collagen component.[256] Eika and colleagues reported that bladders from ovariectomized rats weighed less and had a higher collagen content and decreased atropine resistance than controls, and that estrogen substitution reversed these parameters.[257]

Raz and coworkers reported that progesterone enhanced the beta-adrenergic response of the dog urethra and ureter.[258] Progesterone receptors have been identified in the human urethra,[259] but Rud reported that treatment with gestagens had no effect on urethral profile parameters.[260] Raz reported that oral medroxyprogesterone acetate 20 mg daily exacerbated stress incontinence in 60% of women so treated, with corresponding changes in urethral pressures.[261]

Raz and associates found that a daily dose of 2.5 mg of Premarin (conjugated estrogens) improved stress incontinence and increased urethral pressure in 65% of postmenopausal patients, effects that the authors attributed to mucosal proliferation with a consequently improved "mucosal seal effect" and to enhancement of the alpha-adrenergic contractile response of urethral smooth muscle to endogenous catecholamines.[261] Schreiter and associates reported similar benefits after 10 days of treatment with daily divided doses of 6 mg of estriol.[262] They also presented evidence that the effects of estrogen and of exogenous alpha-adrenergic stimulation were additive. In one of the first studies that presented some quantitative data on estrogen, Rud reported the effects of 4-mg daily doses of estradiol and 8-mg daily doses of estriol on 30 women with an average age of 61, 24 of whom had SUI.[260] Small but statistically significant increases occurred in the MUP (59 to 63 cm H_2O), functional urethral length (25 to 28 mm), and actual urethral length (33 to 37 mm). No statistically significant change occurred in urethral closure pressure (37 to 39 cm H_2O). Eight of the 24 incontinent patients experienced subjective and objective improvement, nine experienced subjective improvement only, and seven experienced neither subjective nor objective improvement. There was no correlation between subjective or objective improvement and urodynamic parameters. However, of 18 patients in whom pressure transmission to the urethra was recorded during cough, seven improved. All of these reported subjective improvement, and five were shown objectively to be dry. Rud pointed out that it is hard to believe that the small changes in urodynamic measurements that occurred, although statistically significant, were directly related to resumption of continence and noted that the increased pressure transmission ratio might be due to factors outside the urethra—either in the striated musculature of the pelvic floor or in the periurethral vasculature or supporting tissues. Rud also studied profilometry during the menstrual cycle in six women.[255] There was no change in any profilometric value during the menstrual cycle and no correlation between estrogen levels and MUP. It may be, as suggested, that at physiologic levels estrogens have little influence on urodynamic measurements related to continence and that only pharmacologic doses cause urodynamically significant changes. Pharmacologic doses may also alter responses to other exogenous autonomic stimulation, particularly alpha-adrenergic stimulation, as laboratory experiments suggest.

Beisland and colleagues carried out a randomized,

open, comparative crossover trial in 20 postmenopausal women with urethral sphincteric insufficiency.[263] Both oral PPA, 50 mg twice a day, and estriol vaginal suppositories, 1 mg daily, significantly increased the MUCP and the continence area on profilometry. PPA was clinically more effective than estriol but not sufficiently so to obtain complete continence. However, with combined treatment, eight patients became completely continent, nine were considerably improved, and only one remained unchanged. Two patients dropped out of the study because of side effects. Bhatia and colleagues used 2 g daily of conjugated estrogen vaginal cream for 6 weeks in 11 postmenopausal women with SUI.[264] Six were cured or improved significantly. Favorable response was correlated with increased closure pressure and increased pressure transmission. In an accompanying article, Karram and associates reported that estrogen administration in six women with premature ovarian failure (but without lower urinary tract problems) did not produce any change in urethral pressure, functional length, or cystometric parameters.[265] However, a significant increase in the pressure transmission ratio to the proximal and midurethra (89 to 109% and 86 to 100%, respectively) was noted after vaginal estrogen but not after oral estrogen, although serum E-2 levels and cytologic changes were similar in the two modes of administration. Negative effects from estrogen alone on stress incontinence were reported by Walter and colleagues,[266] Hilton and Stanton,[267] and Samsioe and associates,[268] but in each of these studies urge symptomatology was favorably affected. In a review article, Cardozo concluded that "there is no conclusive evidence that estrogen even improves, let alone cures, stress incontinence," although it "apparently alleviates urgency, urge incontinence, frequency, nocturia and dysuria."[269]

Kinn and Lindskog described the results of treatment of 36 postmenopausal women with SUI with oral estriol and PPA, alone and in combination, in a double-blind trial after a 4-week run-in period with PPA.[270] Although some of the data are difficult to interpret, the authors concluded that PPA alone and PPA plus estriol raised the intraurethral pressure and reduced urinary loss by 35% (significant) in a standardized physical strain test. Leakage episodes and amounts were significantly reduced by estriol and PPA given separately (28%) or combined (40%). The authors found no evidence of a synergistic effect but did indicate that an additive effect was present. Walter and colleagues completed a complicated but logical study of 28 (out of 38 original subjects) postmenopausal women with SUI.[271] After 4 weeks of a placebo run-in, patients were randomized to oral estriol (E3) or PPA alone for 4 weeks and then to combined therapy for 4 weeks. In the group that sequentially received placebo, PPA and PPA/E3, the percentages reporting cure or improvement, respectively, were 0 and 13%, 13 and 20%, and 21 and 14%. In the group receiving placebo, E3, and E3/PPA, the corresponding percentages were 0 and 0%, 14 and

29%, and 64 and 7%. Objective parameters showed the following: The number of leak episodes per 24 hours in patients treated with PPA first showed a 31% decrease (~3 to 2) compared to placebo ($p <$ .003). For those treated with E3 first the change was not significant (~1.5 to 0.8). Combined treatment produced a mean decrease of 48% over placebo. There was a greater effect with E/PPA than with PPA/E. Pad weights (in grams in a 1-hour test) decreased significantly with PPA alone (~27 to 6 g), but there was no difference between PPA and PPA/E3. E3 alone significantly decreased pad weights (~47 to 15 g). Although E3/PPA was not significantly different, there was a further numerical loss from ~15 to 3 g. The overall conclusions were that E3 and PPA are each effective in treating SUI in postmenopausal women, and, based on subjective data, combined therapy is better than either drug alone. This conclusion was substantiated by a significant decrease in the number of leak episodes in the patients in whom E3 was given before PPA but was not confirmed statistically by pad-weighing tests.

Hilton and colleagues published the results of a double-blind study of 60 (originally) postmenopausal women with SUI who were treated for 4 weeks with oral and vaginal estrogen alone and in combination with PPA.[272] There were six groups in this study: vaginal estrogen (VE) and PPA; VE and oral placebo (OP); oral estrogen (OE) and PPA; OE and OP; vaginal placebo (VP) and PPA; and VP and OP. Subjective symptoms and reported pads per day decreased in all groups; the greatest reduction occurred in those treated with VE, although the reduction in groups 1, 2, 4, and 6 were all significant. Objective pad weight after exercise testing showed a slight decrease in all groups except the double placebo one. Reduction was maximal in the VE/PPA group (22 to 8 g), but the pretreatment values for pads per day and pad weight varied greatly (<0.5 to ~3.5 pads per day; <5 g to 22 g). There was no change in cystometric or urethral profilometric evaluation, either resting or stress.

Sessions and associates reviewed the benefits and risks of estrogen replacement therapy.[273] Improvements in vasomotor symptomatology and osteoporosis prevention are well established. There is also substantial evidence of a decreased risk of cardiovascular disease, perhaps because of an effect on the lipid profile. There is little question, however, that unopposed estrogen use in those with an intact uterus increases the risk of endometrial cancer. Progestin treatment exerts a protective effect, and daily administration of an estrogen and progestin provides an attractive alternative because of a lack of withdrawal bleeding (with sequential therapy) and consequent increased patient compliance. Whether progestin administration adversely affects the results of estrogen treatment of SUI is unknown but must be considered (see prior discussion of the effect of progestin on urethral responses and flowmetry). Progestins may also cause mastalgia, edema, and bloating. It is concluded, further, that there is no evidence for an increase in thromboembolism or hypertension

with estrogen replacement. Transdermal administration of estrogen avoids any theoretical problems associated with the first-pass effect through the liver with oral administration (alteration in clotting factors and increase in renin substrate). The evidence does suggest an association between breast cancer and estrogen replacement therapy but only for those who have received such therapy for more than 15 years. A preventive role of progestin in this regard is controversial, as is the dose of estrogen necessary to produce this effect. As to the preferred type of estrogen preparation, transdermal seems to be as effective as oral, and subcutaneous implants seem to produce physiologic serum levels. Percutaneous and intramuscular estrogen seem to produce variable serum levels. Vaginal creams are said to produce variable serum levels but physiologic E_2/E_1 ratios.[273] We agree that "hands on" application to the "affected area" may have a psychological benefit as well, as suggested by Murray.[274]

Circumventing the Problem

ANTIDIURETIC HORMONE–LIKE AGENTS   The synthetic antidiuretic hormone (ADH) peptide analog DDAVP (1-deamino-8-D-arginine vasopressin) has been used for the symptomatic relief of refractory nocturnal enuresis in both children and adults.[275, 276] The drug can be administered conveniently by intranasal spray at bedtime (in a dose of 10 to 40 μg) and effectively suppresses urine production for 7 to 10 hours. Its clinical long-term safety has been established by continued use in patients with diabetes insipidus. Normal water deprivation tests in the Rew and Rundle article[276] seem to indicate that long-term use does not cause depression of endogenous ADH secretion, at least in patients with nocturnal enuresis. Changes in diuresis during 2 months of treatment in an elderly group of 6 men and 12 women with increased nocturia and decreased ADH secretion were reported by Asplund and Oberg.[277] Nocturia decreased 20% (in milliliters) in men and 34% in women. However, the number of voids from 8 PM to 8 AM decreased from 4.3 to 4.5 in men and from 3.5 to 2.8 in women, but the drug was not given until 8 PM. At present, this novel circumventive approach to the treatment of urinary frequency and incontinence has been largely restricted to those with nocturnal enuresis and diabetes insipidus. The fact that the drug seems to be much more effective than simple fluid restriction alone for the former condition is perhaps explained by relatively recent reports suggesting a decreased nocturnal secretion of ADH by such patients.[275] Recently, suggestions have been made that DDAVP might be useful in patients with refractory nocturnal frequency and incontinence who do not belong in the category of primary nocturnal enuresis. Kinn and Larsson reported that micturition frequency "decreased significantly" in 13 patients with multiple sclerosis and urge incontinence who were treated with oral tablets or desmopressin and that less leakage occurred.[278] The actual approximate average change in the number of voids during the 6 hours after drug intake was 3.2 to 2.5. A similar circumventive approach is to give a rapidly acting loop diuretic 4 to 6 hours before bedtime. This, of course, assumes that the nocturia is not due to obstructive uropathy. A randomized double-blind crossover study of this approach using bumetanide in a group of 14 general practice patients was reported by Pedersen and Johansen.[279] Control nocturia episodes per week averaged 17.5; with placebo, this decreased to 12 (!), and with drug to 8. Bumetanide was preferred to placebo by 11 of 14 patients. It will be interesting to see whether any drug companies pursue this avenue of treatment for the large number of patients with refractory nocturnal bladder storage problems or for "spot" usage prior to some important event in patients with urgency and frequency with and without incontinence.

REFERENCES

1. Wein AJ, Levin RM, Barrett DM: Voiding function: Relevant anatomy, physiology, and pharmacology. *In* Gillenwater JY, Grayhack JT, Howards ST, Duckett JW (eds): Adult and Pediatric Urology, 2nd ed. St. Louis, Mosby-Year Book, 1991, pp 933–999.
2. Wein AJ, Van Arsdalen KN, Levin RM: Pharmacologic therapy. *In* Krane RJ, Siroky MB (eds): Clinical-Neuro-Urology. Boston, Little Brown, 1991, pp 523–558.
3. Steers WD: Physiology of the urinary bladder. *In* Walsh PC, Retik AB, Stamey TA, Vaughan ED Jr (eds): Campbell's Urology, 6th ed. Philadelphia, WB Saunders, 1992, pp 142–169.
4. DeGroat WC: Anatomy and physiology of the lower urinary tract. Urol Clin N Am 20:383–401, 1993.
5. Andersson KE: Pharmacology of lower urinary tract smooth muscles and penile erectile tissues. Pharmacol Rev 45:253, 1993.
6. Wein AJ: Neuromuscular dysfunction of the lower urinary tract. *In* Walsh PC, Retik AB, Stamey TA, Vaughan ED Jr (eds): Campbell's Urology, 6th ed. Philadelphia, WB Saunders, 1992, pp 573–642.
7. Taylor P: Cholinergic agonists. *In* Gilman AG, Rall TW, Nies AS, Taylor P (eds): Goodman and Gilman's The Pharmacological Basis of Therapeutics, 8th ed. New York, Pergamon Press, 1990, pp 122–130.
8. Raezer D, Wein A, Jacobowitz D, et al: Autonomic innervation of canine urinary bladder. Cholinergic and adrenergic contributions and interaction of sympathetic and parasympathetic systems in bladder function. Urology 2:211, 1973.
9. Barrett D, Wein AJ: Voiding dysfunction: Diagnosis, classification and management. *In* Gillenwater JY, Grayhack JT, Howards ST, Duckett JW (eds): Adult and Pediatric Urology, 2nd ed. St. Louis, Mosby-Year Book, 1991, pp 1001–1099.
10. Starr I, Ferguson CK: Beta methylcholine urethane. Its action in various normal and abnormal conditions, especially postoperative urinary retention. Am J Med Sci 200:372, 1940.
11. Lee L: The clinical use of urecholine in dysfunctions of the bladder. J Urol 62:300, 1949.
12. Sonda L, Gershon C, Diokno A: Further observations on the cystometric and uroflowmetric effects of bethanechol chloride on the human bladder. J Urol 122:775, 1979.
13. Perkash I: Intermittent catheterization and bladder rehabilitation in spinal cord injury patients. J Urol 114:230, 1975.
14. Finkbeiner AE: Is bethanechol chloride clinically effective in promoting bladder emptying? A literature review. J Urol 134:443, 1985.
15. Wein A, Malloy T, Shofer F, et al: The effects of bethanechol chloride on urodynamic parameters in normal women and in women with significant residual urine volumes. J Urol 124:397, 1980.
16. Wein A, Raezer D, Malloy T: Failure of the bethanechol supersensitivity test to predict improved voiding after subcutaneous bethanechol administration. J Urol 123:202, 1980.
17. Barrett DM: The effects of oral bethanechol chloride on voiding in female patients with excessive residual urine: A randomized double-blind study. J Urol 126:640, 1981.
18. Farrell SA, Webster RD, Higgins LM, Steeves RA: Duration of postoperative catheterization: A randomized double-blind trials comparing two catheter management protocols and the effect of bethanechol chloride. Int Urogynecol J 1:132, 1990.
19. Downie J: Bethanechol chloride in urology—a discussion of issues. Neurourol Urodyn 3:211, 1984.
20. Awad SA: Clinical use of bethanechol. J Urol 134:523, 1985.
21. Diokno AC, Lapides J: Action of oral and parenteral bethanechol on decompensated bladder. Urology 10:23, 1977.
22. O'Donnell P, Hawkins WH: Effects of subcutaneous bethanechol on bladder sensation during cystometry. Urology 41:452, 1993.
23. Philp N, Thomas D, Clarke S: Drug effects on the voiding cystometrogram: a comparison of oral bethanechol and carbachol. Br J Urol 52:484, 1980.
24. Hedlund H, Andersson KE: Effects of prazosin and carbachol in patients with benign prostatic obstruction. Scand J Urol Nephrol 22:19, 1988.
25. Philp NH, Thomas DG: The effect of distigmine bromide on voiding in male paraplegic patients with reflex micturition. Br J Urol 52:492, 1980.
26. Shah PJR, Abrams P, Choa R: Distigmine bromide and post prostatectomy voiding. Br J Urol 55:229, 1983.
27. Sporer A, Leyson J, Martin B: Effects of bethanechol chloride on the external urethral sphincter in spinal cord injury patients. J Urol 120:62, 1978.
28. Albibi R, McCallum RW: Metoclopramide: Pharmacology and clinical application. Ann Intern Med 98:86, 1983.
29. Mitchell WC, Venable DD: Effects of metoclopromide on detrusor function. J Urol 134:791, 1985.
30. Nestler JE, Stratton MA, Hakin CA: Effect of metoclopramide on diabetic neurogenic bladder. Clin Pharmacol 2:83, 1983.
31. Carone R, Vercella D, Bertapelli P: Effects of cisapride on anorectal and vesicourethral function in spinal cord injured patients. Paraplegia 31:125, 1993.
32. Binnie N, Creasey G, Edmond P, Smith A: The action of cisapride on the chronic constipation of paraplegia. Paraplegia 26:151, 1988.
33. Andersson KE: Clinical pharmacology of potassium channel openers. Pharmacol Toxicol 70:244, 1992.
34. Bultitude M, Hills N, Shuttleworth K: Clinical and experimental studies on the action of prostaglandins and their synthesis inhibitors on detrusor muscle in vitro and in vivo. Br J Urol 48:631, 1976.
35. Desmond A, Bultitude M, Hills N, Shuttleworth KED: Clinical experience with intravesical prostaglandin E_2: A prospective study of 36 patients. Br J Urol 53:357, 1980.
36. Vaidyanathan S, Rao M, Mapa M, et al: Study of instillation of 15(S)-15-methyl prostaglandin $F_{2\alpha}$ in patients with neurogenic bladder dysfunction. J Urol 126:81, 1981.
37. Tammela T, Kontturi M, Kaar K, Lukkarinen O: Intravesical prostaglandin F_2 for promoting bladder emptying after surgery for female stress incontinence. Br J Urol 60:43, 1987.
38. Jaschevatsky OE, Anderman S, Shalit A: Prostaglandin $F_{2\alpha}$ for prevention of urinary retention after vaginal hysterectomy. Obstet Gynecol 66:244, 1985.
39. Koonings P, Bergman A, Ballard CA: Prostaglandins for enhancing detrusor function after surgery for stress incontinence in women. J Reprod Med 35:1, 1990.
40. Stanton SL, Cardozo LD, Ken-Wilson R: Treatment of delayed onset of spontaneous voiding after surgery for incontinence. Urology 13:494, 1979.
41. Delaere KPJ, Thomas CMG, Moonen WA, Debruyne FMJ: The value of intravesical prostaglandin $F_{2\alpha}$ and E_2 in women

with abnormalities of bladder emptying. Br J Urol 53:306, 1981.

42. Wagner G, Husstein P, Enzelsberger H: Is prostaglandin E_2 really of therapeutic value for postoperative urinary retention? Results of a prospectively randomized double-blind study. Am J Obstet Gynecol 151:375, 1985.

43. Schubler B: Comparison of the mode of action of PGE_2 and sulprostone, a PGE_2 derivative, on the lower urinary tract in healthy women. Urol Res 18:349, 1990.

44. Rall TW: Oxytocin, prostaglandins, ergot alkaloids and other drugs; tocolytic agents. In Gilman AG, Rall TW, Nies AS, Taylor P (eds): Goodman and Gilman's The Pharmacological Basis of Therapeutics, 8th ed. New York, Pergamon Press, 1990, pp 933–953.

45. deGroat WC, Booth AM: Autonomic systems to the urinary bladder and sexual organs. In Dyck PJ, Thomas PK, Lambert EH, et al (eds): Peripheral Neuropathy. Philadelphia, WB Saunders, 1984, pp 285–299.

46. deGroat WC: Anatomy and physiology of the lower urinary tract. Urol Clin N Am 20:383–401, 1993.

47. Raz S, Smith RB: External sphincter spasticity syndrome in female patients. J Urol 115:443, 1976.

48. Tammela T: Prevention of prolonged voiding problems after unexpected postoperative urinary retention: Comparison of phenoxybenzamine and carbachol. J Urol 136:1254, 1986.

49. Goldman G, Levian A, Mazor A, et al: Alpha-adrenergic blocker for posthernioplasty urinary retention. Arch Surg 123:35, 1988.

50. Thor KB, Roppolo JR, deGroat WC: Naloxone-induced micturition in unanesthetized paraplegic cats. J Urol 129:202, 1983.

51. Vaidyanathan S, Rao M, Chary KSN, et al: Enhancement of detrusor reflex activity by naloxone in patients with chronic neurogenic bladder dysfunction. J Urol 126:500, 1981.

52. Murray KHA, Feneley RCL: Endorphins: A role in urinary tract function? The effect of opioid blockade on the detrusor and urethral sphincter mechanisms. Br J Urol 54:638, 1982.

53. Galeano C, Jubelin B, Biron L, Guenette L: Effect of naloxone on detrusor-sphincter dyssynergia in chronic spinal cat. Neurourol Urodyn 5:203, 1986.

54. Wheeler JS Jr, Robinson CJ, Culkin DJ, Nemchausky BA: Naloxone efficacy in bladder rehabilitation of spinal cord injury patients. J Urol 137:1202, 1987.

55. Kleeman FJ: The physiology of the internal urinary sphincter. J Urol 104:549, 1970.

56. Krane R, Olsson C: Phenoxybenzamine in neurogenic bladder dysfunction: I. Clinical considerations. J Urol 110:650, 1973.

57. Krane R, Olsson C: Phenoxybenzamine in neurogenic bladder dysfunction: II. Clinical considerations. J Urol 110:653, 1973.

58. Abel B, Gibbon N, Jameson R, et al: The neuropathic urethra. Lancet 2:1229, 1974.

59. Hachen H: Clinical and urodynamic assessment of alpha adrenolytic therapy in patients with neurogenic bladder function. Paraplegia 18:229, 1980.

60. Nanninga J, Kaplan P, Lal S: Effect of phentolamine on peripheral muscle EMG activity in paraplegia. Br J Urol 49:537, 1977.

61. Nordling J, Meyhoff H, Hald T: Sympatholytic effect on striated urethral sphincter. A peripheral or central nervous system effect? Scand J Urol Nephrol 15:173, 1981.

62. Pedersen E, Torring J, Kleman B: Effect of the alpha-adrenergic blocking agent thymoxamine on the neurogenic bladder and urethra. Acta Neurol Scand 61:107, 1980.

63. Gajewski J, Downie J, Awad S: Experimental evidence for a central nervous system site of action in the effect of alpha adrenergic blockers on the external urethral sphincter. J Urol 133:403, 1984.

64. Thind P, Lose G, Colatrue H, Andersson KE: The effect of alpha adrenoceptor stimulation and blockade on the static urethral sphincter function in healthy females. Scand J Urol Nephrol 26:219, 1992.

65. Norlen L: Influence of the sympathetic nervous system on the lower urinary tract and its clinical implications. Neurourol Urodyn 1:129, 1982.

66. Sundin T, Dahlstrom A, Norlen L, Svedmyr N: The sympathetic innervation and adrenoreceptor function of the human lower urinary tract in the normal state and after parasympathetic denervation. Invest Urol 14:322, 1977.

67. Koyanagi T: Further observation on the denervation supersensitivity of the urethra in patients with chronic neurogenic bladders. J Urol 122:348, 1979.

68. Parsons K, Turton M: Urethral supersensitivity and occult urethral neuropathy. Br J Urol 52:131, 1980.

69. Nordling J, Meyhoff H, Hald T: Urethral denervation supersensitivity to noradrenaline after radical hysterectomy. Scand J Urol Nephrol 15:21, 1981.

70. Andersson K, Ek A, Hedlund H, et al: Effects of prazosin on isolated human urethra and in patients with lower neuron lesions. Invest Urol 19:39, 1981.

71. McGuire E, Savastano J: Effect of alpha adrenergic blockade and anticholinergic agents on the decentralized primate bladder. Neurourol Urodyn 4:139, 1985.

72. Jensen D Jr: Pharmacological studies of the uninhibited neurogenic bladder. Acta Neurol Scand 64:175, 1981.

73. Jensen D Jr: Altered adrenergic innervation in the uninhibited neurogenic bladder. Scand J Urol Nephrol 60:61, 1981.

74. Jensen D Jr: Uninhibited neurogenic bladder treated with prazosin. Scand J Urol Nephrol 15:229, 1981.

75. Thomas DG, Philp NH, McDermott TE: The use of urodynamic studies to assess the effect of pharmacological agents with particular references to alpha adrenergic blockade. Paraplegia 22:162, 1984.

76. Rohner T, Hannigan J, Sanford E: Altered in vitro adrenergic responses of dog detrusor muscle after chronic bladder outlet obstruction. Urology 11:357, 1978.

77. Perlberg S, Caine M: Adrenergic response of bladder muscle in prostatic obstruction. Urology 10:524, 1982.

78. Hoffman BB, Lefkowitz RJ: Adrenergic receptor antagonists. In Gilman AG, Rall TW, Nies AS, Taylor P (eds): Goodman and Gilman's The Pharmacological Basis of Therapeutics, 8th ed. New York, Pergamon Press, 1990, pp 221–243.

79. Physicians Desk Reference. Oradell, NJ, Medical Economics Co, 1992.

80. Taylor SH: Clinical pharmacotherapeutics of doxazosin. Am J Med 87 (Suppl 2A):25, 1989.

81. Lepor H: Role of long acting selective alpha-1 blockers in the treatment of benign prostatic hyperplasia. Urol Clin N Am 17:651, 1990.

82. Wilde M, Fitton A, Sorkin E: Terazosin—a review of its pharmacodynamic and pharmacokinetic properties and therapeutic potential in BPH. Drugs Aging 3:258, 1993.

83. Wilde, M, Fitton A, McTavish D: Alfluzosin—a review of its pharmacodynamic and pharmacokinetic properties and its therapeutic potential in BPH. Drugs 45:410, 1993.

84. Raz S, Caine M: Adrenergic receptors in the female canine urethra. Invest Urol 9:319, 1971.

85. Vaidyanathan S, Rao M, Bapna B: Beta adrenergic activity in human proximal urethra. J Urol 124:869, 1980.

86. Burton G, Dobson C: Progesterone increases flow rates. A new treatment for voiding abnormalities? Neurourol Urodyn 12:398, 1993.

87. Cedarbaum JM, Schleifer LS: Drugs for Parkinson's disease, spasticity, and acute muscle spasms. In Gilman AG, Rall TW, Nies AS, Taylor P (eds). Goodman and Gilman's The Pharmacological Basis of Therapeutics, 8th ed. New York, Pergamon Press, 1990, pp 463–484.

88. Bloom FE: Neurohumoral transmission and the central nervous system. In Gilman AG, Rall TW, Nies AS, Taylor P (eds): Goodman and Gilman's The Pharmacological Basis of Therapeutics, 8th ed. New York, Pergamon Press, 1990, pp 244–268.

89. Davidoff RA: Antispasticity drugs: Mechanisms of action. Ann Neurol 17:107, 1985.

90. Lader M: Clinical pharmacology of benzodiazepines. Ann Rev Med 38:19, 1987.

91. Rampe D, Triggle DJ: Benzodiazepines and calcium channel function. Trends Pharmacol Sci November:461, 1986.

92. Shader RI, Greenblatt DJ: Use of benzodiazepines in anxiety disorders. N Engl J Med 328:1398, 1993.

93. Baldessarini RJ: Drugs and the treatment of psychiatric disorders. *In* Gilman AG, Rall TW, Nies AS, Taylor P (eds): Goodman and Gilman's The Pharmacological Basis of Therapeutics, 8th ed. New York, Pergamon Press, 1990, pp 383–435.

94. Milanov IG: Mechanisms of baclofen action on spasticity. Acta Neurol Scand 85:305, 1991.

95. Hachen H, Krucker V: Clinical and laboratory assessment of the efficacy of baclofen on urethral sphincter spasticity in patients with traumatic paraplegia. Eur Urol 3:237, 1977.

96. Florante J, Leyson J, Martin B, Sporer A: Baclofen in the treatment of detrusor sphincter dyssergy in spinal cord injury patients. J Urol 124:82, 1980.

97. Roy CW, Wakefield IR: Baclofen pseudopsychosis: Case report. Paraplegia 24:318, 1986.

98. Kums JJM, Delhaas EM: Intrathecal baclofen infusion in patients with spasticity and neurogenic bladder disease. World J Urol 9:99, 1991.

99. Penn RD, Savoy SM, Corcos D, et al: Intrathecal baclofen for severe spinal spasticity. N Engl J Med 320:1517, 1989.

100. Nanninga JB, Frost F, Penn R: Effect of intrathecal baclofen on bladder and sphincter function. J Urol 142:101, 1989.

101. Loubser PG, Narayan RK, Sadin KJ: Continuous infusion of intrathecal baclofen: Long term effects on spasticity in spinal cord injury. Paraplegia 29:48, 1991.

102. Murdock M, Sax D, Krane R: Use of dantrolene sodium in external sphincter spasm. Urology 8:133, 1976.

103. Hackler R, Broecker B, Klein F, Brady S: A clinical experience with dantrolene sodium for external urinary sphincter hypertonicity in spinal cord injured patients. J Urol 124:78, 1980.

104. Harris JD, Benson GS: Effect of dantrolene on canine bladder contractility. Urology 16:229, 1980.

105. Ward A, Chaffman MO, Sorkin EM: Dantrolene. A review of its pharmacodynamic and pharmacokinetic properties and therapeutic use in malignant hyperthermia, the neuroleptic syndrome and an update of its use in muscle spasticity. Drugs 32:130, 1986.

106. Olsson AT, Swanberg E, Svedinger I: Effects of beta adrenoceptor agonists on airway smooth muscle and on slow contracting skeletal muscle: In vitro and in vivo results compared. Acta Pharmacol Toxicol 44:272, 1979.

107. Holmberg E, Waldeck B: On the possible role of potassium ions on the action of terbutaline on skeletal muscle contractions. Acta Pharmacol Toxicol 46:141, 1980.

108. Gosling JA, Dixon JS, Critchley HOD, et al: A comparative study of the human external sphincter and periurethral levator ani muscles. Br J Urol 53:35, 1981.

109. Dykstra DD, Sidi AA: Treatment of detrusor-striated sphincter dyssynergia with botulinum A toxin. Arch Phys Med Rehabil 71:24, 1990.

110. Fowler CJ, Jewkes D, McDonald WI, et al: Intravesical capsaicin for neurogenic bladder dysfunction. Lancet 329:1239, 1992.

111. Blaivas J, Labib K, Michalik S, et al: Cystometric response to propantheline in detrusor hyperreflexia: Therapeutic implications. J Urol 124:259, 1980.

112. Andersson KE: Current concepts in the treatment of disorders of micturition. Drugs 35:477, 1988.

113. Ulmsten U, Andersson KE, Persson CGA: Diagnostic and therapeutic aspects of urge urinary incontinence in women. Urol Int 32:88, 1977.

114. Brading A: Physiology of bladder smooth muscle. *In* Torrens M, Morrison JFB (eds): The Physiology of the Lower Urinary Tract. New York, Springer Verlag, 1987, pp 161–192.

115. Brading AF: Physiology of the urinary tract smooth muscle. *In* Webster G, Kirby R, King L, Goldwasser B (eds): Reconstructive Urology. Cambridge, Blackwell Scientific Publications, 1993, pp 15–26.

116. Bonner TI: The molecular basis of muscarinic receptor diversity. Trends Neurosci 12:148, 1989.

117. Poli E, Monica B, Zappia L et al: Antimuscarinic activity of telemyepine on isolated human urinary bladder: No role for M-1 muscarinic receptors. Gen Pharmacol 23:659, 1992.

118. Levin RM, Ruggieri MR, Wein AJ: Identification of receptor subtypes in the rabbit and human urinary bladder by selective radioligand binding. J Urol 139:844, 1988.

119. Levin RM, Ruggieri MR, Lee W, Wein AJ: Effect of chronic atropine administration on the rat urinary bladder. J Urol 139:1347, 1988.

120. Restorick JM, Mundy AR: The density of cholinergic and alpha and beta adrenergic receptors in the normal and hyperreflexic human detrusor. Br J Urol 63:32, 1989.

121. Lepor H, Gup D, Shapiro E, Baumann M: Muscarinic cholinergic receptors in the normal and neurogenic human bladder. J Urol 142:869, 1989.

122. Brown JH: Atropine, scopolamine and related antimuscarinic drugs. *In* Gilman AG, Rall TW, Nies AS, Taylor P (eds): Goodman and Gilman's The Pharmacological Basis of Therapeutics, 8th ed. New York, Pergamon Press, 1990, pp 150–165.

123. Gibaldi M, Grundhofer B: Biopharmaceutic influences on the anticholinergic effects of propantheline. Clin Pharmacol Ther 18:457, 1975.

124. Levin RM, Staskin D, Wein AJ: The muscarinic cholinergic binding kinetics of the human urinary bladder. Neurourol Urodyn 1:221, 1982.

125. Peterson JS, Patton AJ, Noronha-Blob L: Mini-pig urinary bladder function: Comparisons of in vitro anticholinergic responses and in vivo cystometry with drugs indicated for urinary incontinence. J Auton Pharmacol 10:65, 1990.

126. Zorzitto ML, Jewett MA, Fernie GR, et al: Effectiveness of propantheline bromide in the treatment of geriatric patients with detrusor instability. Neurourol Urodyn 5:133, 1986.

127. Urinary Incontinence Guideline Panel: Urinary Incontinence in Adults: Clinical Practice Guideline. AHCPR Pub. No. 92-0038. Rockville, MD: Agency for Health Care Policy and Research, Public Health Service, U.S. Department of Health and Human Services, March, 1992.

128. Weiner LB, Baum NH, Suarez GM: New method for management of detrusor instability: Transdermal scopolamine. Urology 28:208, 1986.

129. Cornella JL, Bent AE, Ostergard DR, Horbach NS: Prospective study utilizing transdermal scopolamine in detrusor instability. Urology 35:96, 1990.

130. Greenstein A, Chen J, Matzkin H, et al: Transdermal scopolamine in prevention of post open prostatectomy bladder contractions. Urology 39:215, 1992.

131. Lau W, Szilagyi M: A pharmacological profile of glycopyrrolate: Interactions at the muscarinic acetylcholine receptor. Gen Pharmacol 23:1165, 1992.

132. Tonini M, Rizzi CA, Perrucca E, et al: Depressant action of oxybutynin on the contractility of intestinal and urinary tract smooth muscle. J Pharm Pharmacol 39:103, 1986.

133. Kachur JF, Peterson JS, Carter JP, et al: R and S enantiomers of oxybutynin: Pharmacological effects in guinea pig bladder and intestine. J Pharmacol Exp Ther 247:867, 1988.

134. Thompson I, Lauvetz R: Oxybutynin in bladder spasm, neurogenic bladder and enuresis. Urology 8:452, 1976.

135. Moisey C, Stephenson T, Brendler C: The urodynamic and subjective results of treatment of detrusor instability with oxybutynin chloride. Br J Urol 52:472, 1980.

136. Hehir M, Fitzpatrick JM: Oxybutynin and the prevention of urinary incontinence in spina bifida. Eur Urol 11:254, 1985.

137. Gajewski JB, Awad JA: Oxybutynin versus propantheline in patients with multiple sclerosis and detrusor hyperreflexia. J Urol 135:966, 1986.

138. Holmes DM, Monty FJ, Stanton SL: Oxybutynin versus propantheline in the management of detrusor instability. A patient-regulated variable dose trial. Br J Obstet Gynecol 96:607, 1989.

139. Thuroff J, Bunke B, Ebner A, et al: Randomized double-blind multicenter trial on treatment of frequency, urgency and incontinence related to detrusor hyperactivity: Oxybutynin vs. propantheline vs. placebo. J Urol 145:813, 1991.

140. Zeegers A, Kiesswetter H, Kramer A, Jonas U: Conservative therapy of frequency, urgency and urge incontinence: A double-blind clinical trial of flavoxate, oxybutynin, emepronium and placebo. World J Urol 5:57, 1987.

141. Van Doorn ESC, Zweirs W: Ambulant monitoring to assess

the efficacy of oxybutynin chloride in patients with mixed incontinence. Eur Urol 18:49, 1990.

142. Zorzitto ML, Holliday PJ, Jewett MAS, et al: Oxybutynin chloride for geriatric urinary dysfunction: A double-blind placebo controlled study. Age Aging 18:195, 1989.

143. Ouslander JG, Blaustein J, Connor H: Habit training and oxybutynin for incontinence in nursing home patients: A placebo-controlled trial. J Am Geriatr Soc 36:40, 1988.

144. Ouslander JG, Blaustein J, Connor A, et al: Pharmacokinetics and clinical effects of oxybutynin in geriatric patients. J Urol 140:47, 1988.

145. Kato K, Kitada S, Chun A, et al: In vitro intravesical instillation of anticholinergic antispasmodic and calcium blocking agents (rabbit whole bladder model). J Urol 141:1471, 1989.

146. Madersbacher H, Jilg G: Control of detrusor hyperreflexia by the intravesical instillation of oxybutynin hydrochloride. Paraplegia 19:84, 1991.

147. Weese DL, Roskamp DA, Leach GE, Zimmern PE: Intravesical oxybutynin chloride: Experience with 42 patients. Urology 41:527, 1993.

148. Andersson KE, Hedlund H, Mansson W: Pharmacologic treatment of bladder hyperactivity after augmentation and substitution enterocystoplasty. Scand J Urol Nephrol Suppl 142:42–46, 1992.

149. Downie J, Twiddy D, Awad S: Antimuscarinic and non-competitive antagonist properties of dicyclomine hydrochloride in isolated human and rabbit bladder muscle. J Pharmacol Exp Ther 201:662, 1977.

150. Fischer C, Diokno A, Lapides J: The anticholinergic effects of dicyclomine hydrochloride in uninhibited neurogenic bladder dysfunction. J Urol 120:328, 1978.

151. Beck RP, Amausch T, King C: Results in testing 210 patients with detrusor overactivity incontinence of urine. Am J Obstet Gynecol 125:593, 1976.

152. Awad SA, Bryniak S, Downie JW, Bruce AW: The treatment of the uninhibited bladder with dicyclomine. J Urol 117:161, 1977.

153. Ruffman R: A review of flavoxate hydrochloride in the treatment of urge incontinence. J Int Med Res 16:317, 1988.

154. Delaere KP, Michiels HGE, Debruyne FMJ, Moonen WA: Flavoxate hydrochloride in the treatment of detrusor instability. Urol Int 32:377, 1977.

155. Jonas U, Petri E, Kissal J: The effect of flavoxate on hyperactive detrusor muscle. Eur Urol 5:106, 1979.

156. Briggs RS, Castleden CM, Asher MJ: The effect of flavoxate on uninhibited detrusor contractions and urinary incontinence in the elderly. J Urol 123:656, 1980.

157. Benson GS, Sarshik SA, Raezer DM, Wein AJ: Bladder muscle contractility: Comparative effects and mechanisms of action of atropine, propantheline, flavoxate, and imipramine. Urology 9:31, 1977.

158. Forman A, Andersson K, Henriksson L, et al: Effects of nifedipine on the smooth muscle of the human urinary tract in vitro and in vivo. Acta Pharmacol Toxicol 43:111, 1978.

159. Husted S, Andersson KE, Sommer L, et al: Anticholinergic and calcium antagonistic effects of terodiline in rabbit urinary bladder. Acta Pharmacol Toxicol 46:20, 1980.

160. Finkbeiner AE: Effect of extracellular calcium and calcium-blocking agents on detrusor contractility: An in vitro study. Neurourol Urodyn 2:245, 1983.

161. Malkowicz SB, Wein AJ, Brendler K, Levin RM: Effect of diltiazem on in vitro rabbit bladder function. Pharmacology 31:24, 1985.

162. Andersson KE, Fovaeus M, Morgan E, et al: Comparative effects of five different calcium channel blockers on the atropine-resistant contraction in electrically stimulated rabbit urinary bladder. Neurourol Urodyn 5:579, 1986.

163. Abrams P: Terodiline in clinical practice. Urology 36(Suppl):60, 1990.

164. Ekman G, Andersson KE, Rud T, Ulmsten K: A double-blind crossover study of the effects of terodiline in women with unstable bladder. Acta Pharmacol Toxicol 46 (Suppl):39, 1980.

165. Peters D, Multicentre Study Group: Terodiline in the treatment of urinary frequency and motor urge incontinence—a controlled multicentre trial. Scand J Urol Nephrol 87(Suppl):21, 1984.

166. Tapp A, Fall M, Norgaard J, et al: Terodiline: A dose titrated, multicenter study of the treatment of idiopathic detrusor instability in women. J Urol 142:1027, 1989.

167. Levin RM, Scheiner S, Zhao Y, Wein AJ: The effect of terodiline on hyperreflexia (in vitro) and the in vitro response of isolated strips of rabbit bladder to field stimulation, bethanechol and KCl. Pharmacology 46:346, 1993.

168. Veldhuis G, Inman J: Terodiline and torsade de pointes (letter to the editor). Br Med J 303:519, 1991.

169. Connolly MJ, Astridge PS, White EG, et al: Torsade de pointes ventricular tachycardia and terodiline. Lancet 338:344, 1991.

170. Stewart DA, Taylor J, Ghosh S, et al: Terodiline causes polymorphic ventricular tachycardia due to reduced heart rate and prolongation of QT interval. Eur J Clin Pharmacol 42:577, 1992.

171. Palmer J, Worth P, Exton-Smith A: Flunarizine: A once daily therapy for urinary incontinence. Lancet 2:279, 1981.

172. Dykstra D, Sidi A, Anderson L: The effect of nifedipine on cystoscopy-induced autonomic hyperreflexia in patients with high spinal cord injuries. J Urol 138:1155, 1987.

173. Andersson KE: Current concepts in the treatment of disorders of micturition. Drugs 35:477, 1988.

174. Malmgren A, Andersson KE, Fovaeus M, Sjogren C: Effects of cromakalim and pinacidil on normal and hypertrophied rat detrusor in vitro. J Urol 143:828, 1990.

175. Fovaeus M, Andersson KE, Hedlund H: The action of pinacidil in the isolated human bladder. J Urol 141:637, 1989.

176. Hedlund H, Mattiasson A, Andersson KE: Lack of effect of pinacidil on detrusor instability in men with bladder outlet obstruction. J Urol 143:369A, 1990.

177. Nurse D, Restorick J, Mundy A: The effect of cromakalim on the normal and hyperreflexic human detrusor muscle. Br J Urol 68:27, 1991.

178. Longman SD, Hamilton TC: Potassium channel activator drug: Mechanisms of action, pharmacological properties and therapeutic potential. Med Res Rev 12:73, 1992.

179. Levin RM, Hayes L, Zhao Y, Wein AJ: Effect of pinacidil on spontaneous and evoked contractile activity. Pharmacology 45:1, 1992.

180. Downie JW, Karmazyn M: Mechanical trauma to bladder epithelium liberates prostanoids which modulate neurotransmission in rabbit detrusor muscle. J Pharmacol Exp Ther 230:445, 1984.

181. Cardozo L, Stanton S, Robinson H, Hale D: Evaluation of flurbiprofen in detrusor instability. Br Med J 180(1):281, 1980.

182. Cardozo L, Stanton SL: An objective comparison of the effects of parenterally administered drugs in patients suffering from detrusor instability. J Urol 122:58, 1979.

183. Brooks PM, Day RO: Non-steroidal anti-inflammatory drugs—differences and similarities. N Engl J Med 324:1716, 1991.

184. Norlen L, Sundin T, Waagstein F: Beta-adrenoceptor stimulation of the human urinary bladder in vivo. Acta Pharmacol Toxicol 43:5, 1978.

185. Lindholm P, Lose G: Terbutaline (Bricanyl) in the treatment of female urge incontinence. Urol Int 41:158, 1986.

186. Gruneberger A: Treatment of motor urge incontinence with clenbuterol and flavoxate hydrochloride. Br J Obstet Gynecol 91:275, 1984.

187. Castleden CM, Morgan B: The effect of beta adrenoceptor agonists on urinary incontinence in the elderly. Br J Clin Pharmacol 10:619, 1980.

188. Naglo AS, Nergardh A, Boreus LO: Influence of atropine and isoprenaline on detrusor hyperactivity in children with neurogenic bladder. Scand J Urol Nephrol 15:97, 1981.

189. Hollister LE: Current antidepressants. Ann Rev Pharmacol Toxicol 26:23, 1986.

190. Richelson E: Antidepressants and brain neurochemistry. Mayo Clin Proc 65:1227, 1990.

191. Olubadewo J: The effect of imipramine on rat detrusor muscle contractility. Arch Int Pharmacodyn Ther 145:84, 1980.

192. Levin RM, Staskin DR, Wein AJ: Analysis of the anticholinergic and musculotropic effects of desmethylimipramine on the rabbit urinary bladder. Urol Res 11:259, 1983.

193. Levin RM, Wein AJ: Comparative effects of five tricyclic compounds on the rabbit urinary bladder. Neurourol Urodyn 3:127, 1984.

194. Bigger J, Giardino E, Perel J, et al: Cardiac antiarrhythmic effect of imipramine hydrochloride. N Engl J Med 296:206, 1977.

195. Malkowicz SB, Wein AJ, Ruggieri MR, Levin RM: Comparison of calcium antagonist properties of antispasmodic agents. J Urol 138:667, 1987.

196. Akah PA: Tricyclic antidepressant inhibition of the electrical evoked responses of the rat urinary bladder strip-effect of variation in extracellular Ca concentration. Arch Int Pharmacodyn 284:231, 1986.

197. Foreman MM, McNulty AM: Alterations in K(+) evoked release of 3-H-norepinephrine and contractile responses in urethral and bladder tissues induced by norepinephrine reuptake inhibition. Life Sci 53:193, 1993.

198. Cole A, Fried F: Favorable experiences with imipramine in the treatment of neurogenic bladder. J Urol 107:44, 1972.

199. Mahony D, Laferte F, Mahoney J: Observations on sphincter augmenting effect of imipramine in children with urinary incontinence. Urology 2:317, 1973.

200. Raezer DM, Benson GS, Wein AJ, et al: The functional approach to the management of the pediatric neuropathic bladder: A clinical study. J Urol 117:649, 1977.

201. Tulloch AGS, Creed KE: A comparison between propantheline and imipramine on bladder and salivary gland function. Br J Urol 51:359, 1979.

202. Castleden CM, George CF, Renwick AG, Asher MJ: Imipramine—a possible alternative to current therapy for urinary incontinence in the elderly. J Urol 125:218, 1981.

203. Korczyn AD, Kish I: The mechanism of imipramine in enuresis nocturna. Clin Exp Pharmacol Physiol 6:31, 1979.

204. Lose G, Jorgensen L, Thunedborg P: Doxepin in the treatment of female detrusor overactivity: A randomized double-blind crossover study. J Urol 142:1024, 1989.

205. Sant G: Intravesical 50% dimethylsulfoxide in the treatment of interstitial cystitis. Urology 4(Suppl):17, 1987.

206. Kiesswetter H, Schober W: Lioresal in the treatment of neurogenic bladder dysfunction. Urol Int 30:63, 1975.

207. Taylor MC, Bates CP: A double-blind crossover trial of baclofen: A new treatment for the unstable bladder syndrome. Br J Urol 51:505, 1979.

208. James MJ, Birmingham AT, Hill SJ: Partial mediation by NO of the relaxation of human isolated detrusor strips in response to electrical field stimulation. Br J Clin Pharmacol 35:366, 1993.

209. James MJ, Iacovou JW: The case of GTN patches in detrusor instability: A pilot study. Neurourol Urodyn 12:399, 1993.

210. Soulard C, Pascaud X, Roman FJ, et al: Pharmacological evaluation of JO-1870: Relation to the potential treatment of urinary bladder incontinence. J Pharmacol Exp Ther 260:1152, 1992.

211. Haruno A: Inhibitory effects of propiverine hydrochloride on the agonist-induced or spontaneous contractions of various isolated muscle preparations. Drug Res 42:815, 1992.

212. Constantinou CE: Pharmacologic treatment of detrusor incontinence with thiphenamil HCL. Urol Int 48:42, 1992.

213. Constantinou CE: Pharmacologic effect of thiphenamil HCl on lower urinary tract function of healthy asymptomatic volunteers. Urol Int 48:293, 1992.

214. Maggi CA, Barbank G, Santicoli P, et al: Cystometric evidence that capsaicin-sensitive nerves modulate the afferent branch of micturition reflex on humans. J Urol 142:150, 1989.

215. Maggi CA: Capsaicin and primary afferent neurons: From basic science to human therapy? J Auton Nerv Syst 33:1, 1991.

216. Maggi CA: Therapeutic potential of capsaicin-like molecules. Life Sci 51:1777, 1992.

217. Dray A: Mechanism of action of capsaicin-like molecules on sensory neurons. Life Sci 51:1759, 1992.

218. Craft RM, Porreca F: Treatment parameters of desensitization to capsaicin. Life Sci 51:1767, 1992.

219. Fowler CJ, Betts C, Christmas T, et al: Botulinum toxin in the treatment of chronic urinary retention in women. Br J Urol 70:387, 1992.

220. Hoffman BB, Lefkowitz RJ: Catecholamines and sympathomimetic drugs. In Gilman AG, Rall TW, Nies AS, Taylor P (eds): Goodman and Gilman's The Pharmacological Basis of Therapeutics, 8th ed. New York, Pergamon Press, 1990, pp 187–220.

221. Rashbaum M, Mandelbaum CC: Non-operative treatment of urinary incontinence in women. Am J Obstet Gynecol 56:777, 1948.

222. Diokno A, Taub M: Ephedrine in treatment of urinary incontinence. Urology 5:624, 1975.

223. Ek A, Andersson KE, Gullberg B, Ulmsten K: The effects of long-term treatment with norephedrine on stress incontinence and urethral closure pressure profile. Scand J Urol Nephrol 12:105, 1978.

224. Obrink A, Bunne G: The effect of alpha adrenergic stimulation in stress incontinence. Scand J Urol Nephrol 12:205, 1978.

225. Lose G, Lindholm D: Clinical and urodynamic effects of norfenefrine in women with stress incontinence. Urol Int 39:298, 1984.

226. Lose G, Rix P, Diernoes E, Alexander N: Norfenefrine in the treatment of female stress incontinence—a double-blind controlled trial. Urol Int 43:11, 1988.

227. Diernoes E, Rix P, Sorensen T, Alexander N: Norfenefrine in the treatment of female urinary stress incontinence assessed by one hour pad weighing test. Urol Int 44:28, 1989.

228. Lose G, Diernoes E, Rix P: Does medical therapy cure female stress incontinence? Urol Int 44:25, 1989.

229. Awad S, Downie J, Kiruluta H: Alpha adrenergic agents in urinary disorders of the proximal urethra: I. Stress incontinence. Br J Urol 50:332, 1978.

230. Stewart B, Borowsky L, Montague D: Stress incontinence: conservative therapy with sympathomimetic drugs. J Urol 115:558, 1976.

231. Collste L, Lindskog M: Phenylpropanolamine in treatment of female stress urinary incontinence. Urology 30:398, 1987.

232. Mueller S: Neurologic complications of phenylpropanolamine use. Neurology 33:650, 1983.

233. Baggioni I, Onrot J, Stewart CK, Robertson D: The potent pressor effect of phenylpropanolamine in patients with autonomic impairment. JAMA 258:236, 1987.

234. Lasagna L: Phenylpropanolamine and blood pressure. JAMA 253:2491, 1985.

235. Liebson I, Bigelow G, Griffiths RR, Funderbuck M: Phenyl-propanolamine: Effects on subjective and cardiovascular variables at recommended over-the-counter dose levels. J Clin Pharmacol 27:685, 1987.

236. Blackburn GL, Morgan JP, Lavin PT, et al: Determinants of the pressor effect of phenylpropanomaline in healthy subjects. JAMA 261:3267, 1989.

237. Kiesswetter H, Hennrich F, Englisch M: Clinical and pharmacologic therapy of stress incontinence. Urol Int 38:58, 1983.

238. Gilja I, Radej M, Kovacic M, Parazajades J: Conservative treatment of female stress incontinence with imipramine. J Urol 132:909, 1984.

239. Gleason D, Reilly R, Bottaccini M, Pierce MJ: The urethral continence zone and its relation to stress incontinence. J Urol 112:81, 1974.

240. Kaisary AU: Beta adrenoceptor blockade in the treatment of female stress urinary incontinence. J Urol (Paris) 90:351, 1984.

241. Donker P, Van der Sluis C: Action of beta adrenergic blocking agents on the urethral pressure profile. Urol Int 31:6, 1976.

242. Fellenius E, Hedberg R, Holmberg E, et al: Functional and metabolic effects of terbutaline and propranol in fast and slow contracting skeletal muscle in vitro. Acta Physiol Scand 109:89, 1980.

243. Kishimoto T, Morita T, Okamiya Y, et al: Effect of clenbuterol on contractile response in periurethral striated muscle of rabbits. Tohoku J Exp Med 165:243, 1991.

244. Salmon UJ, Walter RI, Geist SH: The use of estrogen in the treatment of dysuria and incontinence in post-menopausal women. Am J Obstet Gynecol 42:845, 1941.
245. Hodgson BT, Dumas S, Bolling DR, Helsch CM: Effect of estrogen on sensitivity of rabbit bladder and urethra to phenylephrine. Invest Urol 16:67, 1978.
246. Levin RM, Shofer FS, Wein AJ: Estrogen induced alterations in the autonomic responses of the rabbit urinary bladder. J Pharmacol Exp Ther 215:614, 1980.
247. Levin RM, Jacobowitz D, Wein AJ: Autonomic innervation of rabbit urinary bladder following estrogen administration. Urology 17:449, 1981.
248. Levin RM, Zderic SA, Ewalt DH, et al: Effects of pregnancy on muscarinic receptor density and function in the rabbit urinary bladder. Pharmacology 43:69, 1991.
249. Tong YC, Wein AJ, Levin RM: Effects of pregnancy on adrenergic function in the rabbit urinary bladder. Neurourol Urodyn 11:525, 1992.
250. Larsson B, Andersson KE, Batra S, et al: Effects of estradiol on norepinephrine-induced contraction, alpha adrenoreceptor number and norepinephrine content in the female rabbit urethra. J Pharmacol Exp Ther 229:557, 1984.
251. Callahan SM, Creed KE: The effects of estrogens on spontaneous activity and responses to phenylephrine of the mammalian urethra. J Physiol 358:35, 1985.
252. Bump RC, Friedman CI: Intraluminal urethral pressure measurements in the female baboon: Effects of hormonal manipulation. J Urol 136:508, 1986.
253. Batra SC, Iosif CS: Female urethra: A target for estrogen action. J Urol 129:418, 1983.
254. Batra S, Byellin L, Sjogren C: Increases in blood flow of the female rabbit urethra following low dose estrogens. J Urol 136:1360, 1986.
255. Rud T: Urethral pressure profile in continent women from childhood to old age. Acta Obstet Gynecol Scand 59:331, 1980.
256. Versi E, Cardozo L, Buncat L, et al: Correlation of urethral physiology and skin collagen in post menopausal women. Br J Obstet Gynaecol 95:147, 1988.
257. Eika B, Salling LN, Christensen LL, et al: Long-term observation of the detrusor smooth muscle in rats—its relationship to ovariectomy and estrogen treatment. Urol Res 18:439, 1990.
258. Raz S, Ziegler M, Caine M: The effect of progesterone on the adrenergic receptors of the urethra. Br J Urol 45:131, 1973.
259. Batra S, Iosif CS: Progesterone receptors in the female lower urinary tract. J Urol 138:1301, 1987.
260. Rud T: The effects of estrogens and gestagens on the urethral pressure profile of urinary continent and stress incontinent women. Acta Obstet Gynecol Scand 59:265, 1980.
261. Raz S, Ziegler M, Caine M: The role of female hormones in stress incontinence. Proceedings of 16th Congress of Societe International d'Urologie, Paris, vol 1, 1973, pp 397–402.
262. Schreiter F, Fuchs P, Stockamp K: Estrogenic sensitivity of alpha receptors in the urethral musculature. Urol Int 31:13, 1976.
263. Beisland HO, Fossberg E, Moer A, et al: Urethral sphincteric insufficiency in postmenopausal females: Treatment with phenylpropanolamine and estriol separately and in combination. Urol Int 39:211, 1984.
264. Bhatia NN, Bergman A, Karram MM: Effects of estrogen on urethral function in women with urinary incontinence. Am J Obstet Gynecol 160:176, 1989.
265. Karram MM, Yeko TR, Sauer MV, Bhatia NN: Urodynamic changes following hormonal replacement therapy in women with premature ovarian failure. Obstet Gynecol 74:208, 1989.
266. Walter S, Wolf H, Barleto H, Jensen HK: Urinary incontinence in post menopausal women treated with estrogens. Urol Int 33:135, 1978.
267. Hilton P, Stanton SL: The use of intravaginal estrogen cream in genuine stress incontinence. Br J Obstet Gynaecol 90:940, 1983.
268. Samsioe G, Jansson I, Mellstrom D, Svanborg A: Occurrence, nature and treatment of urinary incontinence in a 70 year old female population. Maturitas 7:335, 1985.
269. Cardozo L: Role of estrogens in the treatment of female urinary incontinence. J Am Geriatr Soc 38:326, 1990.
270. Kinn AC, Lindskog M: Estrogen and phenylpropanolamine in combination for stress urinary incontinence in post-menopausal women. Urology 32:273, 1988.
271. Walter S, Kjaergaard B, Lose G, et al: Stress urinary incontinence in postmenopausal women treated with oral estrogen (estriol) and an alpha adrenergic stimulating agent (phenylpropanolamine): A randomized double-blind placebo controlled study. Int Urogynecol J 1:74, 1990.
272. Hilton P, Tweddel AL, Mayne C: Oral and intravaginal estrogens alone and in combination with alpha adrenergic stimulation in genuine stress incontinence. Int Urogynecol J 1:80, 1990.
273. Sessions DR, Kelly AC, Jewelewicz R: Current concepts in estrogen replacement therapy in the menopause. Fertil Steril 59:277, 1993.
274. Murray K: Medical and surgical management of female voiding difficulty. In Drife JO, Hilton P, Stanton SL (eds): Micturition. London, Springer-Verlag, 1990, p 179.
275. Norgaard JP, Rillig S, Djurhuus JC: Nocturnal enuresis: An approach to treatment based on pathogenesis. J Pediatr 114:705, 1989.
276. Rew DA, Rundle JSH: Assessment of the safety of regular DDAVP therapy on primary nocturnal enuresis. Br J Urol 63:352, 1989.
277. Asplund R, Oberg H: Desmopressin in elderly subjects with increased nocturnal diuresis: a 2 month treatment study. Scand J Urol Nephrol 27:77, 1993.
278. Kinn AC, Larsson PO: Desmopressin: A new principle for symptomatic treatment of urgency and incontinence in patients with multiple sclerosis. Scand J Urol Nephrol 24:109, 1990.
279. Pedersen PA, Johansen PB: Prophylactic treatment of adult nocturia with bumetanide. Br J Urol 62:145, 1988.

PART V

Surgery for Anatomic Incontinence

CHAPTER 25

Colpocystourethropexy

Emil A. Tanagho, M.D.

Genuine stress urinary incontinence is a specific entity directly related to an anatomic abnormality that results in impaired efficiency of the urethral sphincteric mechanism, allowing loss of urine with any increase in intra-abdominal pressure. Owing to recent advances in urodynamic studies and the appreciation of the pathophysiology of true stress incontinence, the treatment of this problem has become better understood; consequently, the purpose of surgical repair and the means of achieving it can be clearly defined.

Surgical Principles

In pure stress urinary incontinence, the sphincteric mechanism, with its striated somatic component and its smooth sphincteric element, is essentially normal. It is loss of normal anatomic position or normal anatomic support, or both, that weakens the functional efficiency of this sphincteric unit. Accordingly, restoration of normal position and support of the vesicourethral segment usually reestablishes normal sphincteric function.

From this basic principle, it is clear that a suprapubic approach is more effective than an anterior vaginal repair and longer lasting in terms of restoring the position and support of the sphincteric unit. Trying to push the urethrovesical junction into a normal retropubic position from below is obviously less sound than to achieve the same result from above. The latter is the logical approach for placing the urethra and the urethrovesical segment in a secure, well-supported, normal anatomic position.

Preoperative demonstration of the presence of the anatomic abnormality is essential to the evaluation of the patient because in the absence of any anatomic variance there is no reason for a surgical repair primarily intended to restore normal anatomy and support.

A lateral cystogram obtained with a radiopaque, soft red Robinson catheter permits visualization of the vesicourethral segment and its anatomic relationships. Two exposures, first with the patient relaxed and then with maximum straining (Figs. 25–1 and 25–2), will demonstrate the extent of mobility and thus the effectiveness of the support to the vesicourethral segment. The study will permit evaluation of (1) normal resting position and (2) extent of mobility. If the resting position is abnormal (lower than normal), if the mobility of the vesicourethral segment is excessive (Fig. 25–3), or if both conditions are present, the lateral cystogram will confirm the anatomic basis for the existing and clinically established fact of urinary stress incontinence. It must be emphasized that this cystographic study does not permit *diagnosis* of stress incontinence but demonstrates the presence of the basic anatomic abnormality responsible for genuine stress incontinence.

Surgical repair should attempt to restore normal position and support. Urinary stress incontinence is encountered frequently in multiparous women after middle age as a result of weakness of the pelvic floor. As mentioned earlier, the intrinsic sphincteric mechanism is essentially normal. However, owing to the laxity of the pelvic floor and the weakness of the normal mechanism of support to the vesicourethral segment, the latter will tend to lie abnormally low and will exhibit excessive mobility with any increase in intra-abdominal pressure (see Fig. 25–3) or with assumption of the upright position. The intrinsic sphincteric mechanism can be restored to normal function once this anatomic abnormality is corrected without any need to plicate, constrict, or otherwise directly interfere with the sphincteric unit itself.

It is imperative to avoid creation of any obstruction or damage to the delicate intrinsic sphincteric muscular element. If this principle is adhered to, the sphincter will regain and maintain its effectiveness, and the repair will be permanent. In my opinion, the suprapubic approach is the best way to achieve this goal.

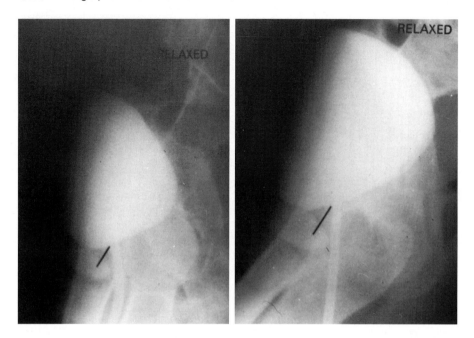

Figure 25-1   Cystogram shows the relationship between the vesicourethral segment and the pubic bone. The perpendicular line from the vesicourethral point over the long axis of the pubic bone will meet the pubic bone opposite its lower third.

Surgical Technique

The patient is supine, with the lower limbs stretched and supported in a slightly abducted position. The footpiece of the operating table is dropped down to permit easy access to the vagina, which is properly prepared and draped into the sterile field. A 22 Fr or 24 Fr 5-ml Foley catheter is passed and kept in the sterile field.

The retropubic space is exposed through a suprapubic transverse or midline incision. In making this incision, one should stay close to the back of the pubic bone, dropping the anterior bladder wall, the urethra (easily palpated with the Foley catheter in place), and the anterior vaginal wall downward. This step is easy in patients who have had no previous surgical intervention in this area but is otherwise extremely difficult, and it is of critical importance. In the latter situation, adhesions are usually dense, and the anterior bladder wall frequently is found displaced downward and adherent to the back of the pubic bone. Unless the anterior bladder wall is freed and pulled upward, one will not be able to expose the urethra and the urethrovesical junction.

VIRGINAL CASES   Once the retropubic space is en-

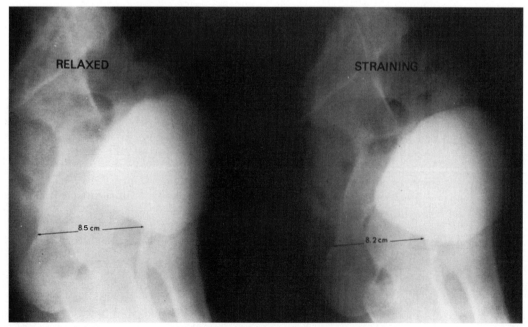

Figure 25-2   Lateral cystogram shows the patient in the relaxed state *(left)*, then straining *(right)*. Note the extent of mobility of the vesicourethral segment in relation to any bony point. Normally it is less than 1.5 cm in any direction.

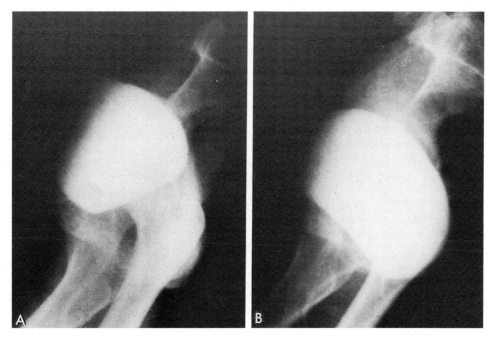

Figure 25-3 Lateral cystourethrogram of a patient with urinary stress incontinence. A, In the relaxed position. B, With straining. Note the excessive drop of the vesicourethral segment and an increase in intraabdominal pressure associated with straining. This is the classic anatomic abnormality of urinary stress incontinence.

tered and the urethra is dropped downward with the anterior vaginal wall, no dissection should be done in the midline over the urethra. Whatever amount of tissue is covering it should be left undisturbed. In this way, the delicate musculature of the urethra is protected from any possibility of surgical trauma. Attention should be directed to the anterior vaginal wall on each side of the urethra—again, easily identified with the catheter in it. Most of the overlying fat should be dissected and cleared away to permit future firm adherence to any tissue brought into contact with it. This area is extremely vascular because it has a rich thin-walled venous plexus that should be avoided as much as possible. As this region is cleared, the vesicourethral junction becomes more apparent. This step can be facilitated by palpating the Foley balloon or, even better, by partially distending the bladder and defining the rounded lower margin of the anterior bladder wall as it meets the anterior vaginal wall. No dissection should be done at the vesicourethral junction itself because at that point all the detrusor muscle fibers are moving downward to encircle the urethra, and every effort should be made to protect them from trauma. More laterally, however, the inferior margin of the bladder is identified and mobilized upward. The extent of this mobilization depends on the extent of downward displacement, but occasionally hardly any is needed at all. Placing fingers in the vagina facilitates this dissection and also is essential to determine the extent of the needed mobilization and freeing of the anterior vaginal wall.

REPEAT CASES The dissection here is most difficult, particularly when three or four previous attempts at repair have failed. Nevertheless, it is in such circumstances that the dissection must be impeccable if good results are to be achieved. Unless the urethrovaginal wall is adequately exposed and all adhesions

are severed, and the lower margin of the bladder, together with the vesicourethral junction, is permitted to slide upward, proper positioning and support will not be obtained. Utmost care must be taken not to lacerate or damage the urethral or vesical musculature. If identification of the lower margin of the bladder is difficult, one should open the bladder and, with a finger inside the cavity, define its limits for easier dissection and mobilization.

SUTURES

Once mobilization is completed and judged adequate (as determined by inserting two fingers in the vagina and lifting the anterior vaginal wall upward and forward, thus revealing adequate mobility and bringing the vesicourethral segment to a normal position), it is time to place the sutures. I prefer absorbable suture material and use No. 1 Dexon on an atraumatic tapered needle. Positioning of sutures is a most important step in the procedure, second only to proper mobilization. The sutures should be placed as far laterally in the anterior vaginal wall as technically possible. I apply two sutures on each side. The distal suture is placed first, opposite the midurethra. The proximal suture is the most essential and is placed just below the reflection of the anterior bladder wall at the level of the vesicourethral junction, yet far laterally from it (Fig. 25–4).

In placing these sutures one should take a good bite in the vaginal wall parallel to the urethra, taking full thickness but sparing the mucosa and being guided by the vaginal finger at the appropriate selected sites. All four sutures are placed in the vagina and left with their needles attached before being placed anteriorly. As noted previously, this area is extremely vascular, and visible vessels should be

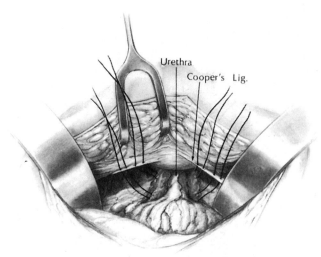

Figure 25-4 Placement of the sutures in the anterior vaginal wall. They are placed lateral to the vesicourethral segment, and there are two on each side. The lower ones are opposite the midurethral segment, and the upper one is exactly at the level of the vesicourethral junction. Sutures are then passed through Cooper's ligament. (From Tanagho EA: Colpocystourethropexy: The way we do it. J Urol 116:751, 1976.)

avoided if at all possible. When excessive bleeding occurs it can be controlled by underrunning with figure-of-eight sutures. Less severe bleeding usually stops once these fixation sutures are finally tied.

The vaginal sutures are then attached to Cooper's ligament. They are not placed in the midline of the symphysis but are pulled straight upward to Cooper's ligament. The distal two sutures are placed first, followed by the two proximal sutures, which are placed in the same ligament but slightly lateral (Fig. 25–5). Once all the sutures are placed, with the operator's fingers in the vagina lifting it upward and forward, the assistant ties the distal sutures and then the proximal ones. In tying the sutures one does not have to be concerned about whether the vaginal wall site of the suture meets Cooper's ligament, and one should not overdo the tension on the vaginal wall. The suture is approximated as close as the supporting fingers in the vagina feel it to be safe. There should be no tension on the sutures beyond that governed by the fingers lifting the vaginal wall. Free suture material between the two points is of no disadvantage (Fig. 25–6). After the two sutures are tied, the vaginal fingers will appreciate immediately how much the vaginal wall is lifted upward and forward, carrying with it the vesicourethral segment. However, the latter is still free in the retropubic space. One should be able to insert two fingers easily between the pubic bone and the urethra. The urethra is in no way compressed against the bone. Its continuing fixation and support are going to be dependent on fibrosis and scarring of opposed tissues rather than on the suture material holding it in place. Absorbable sutures are meant to last only long enough for tissue fixation to take place.

Penrose drains are usually left in the retropubic space lateral to the sutures, and the wound is closed. The catheter is then changed to a 16 Fr 5-ml Foley and left indwelling for 5 days. The patient is restricted to bed for about the same period.

Voiding after removal of the catheter is generally free, without problems of urinary retention or residual urine. If for any unexpected reason the patient has to strain to void, the catheter is replaced for a few more days. This replacement is rarely necessary and has been used only in cases of atonic bladder that did not demonstrate any detrusor activity in preoperative physiologic studies. Postoperative activity is restricted for 3 to 4 months and is then gradually built up to the normal individual level.

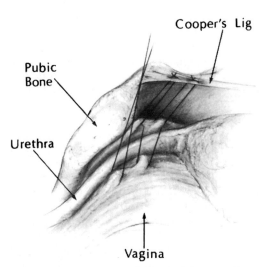

Figure 25-5 Lateral view of the sutures as placed in Figure 25–4 with one side tied. Note that the vaginal wall did not meet Cooper's ligament and that there is a free suture between the two. (From Tanagho EA: Colpocystourethropexy: The way we do it. J Urol 116:751, 1976.)

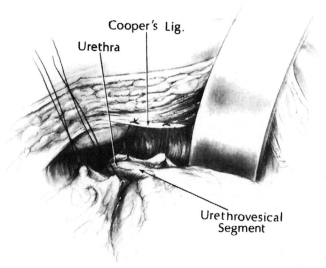

Figure 25-6 Same as Figure 25–5 except at a different projection; this view shows the vesicourethral segment well supported by the vaginal wall behind it. Note that the urethra is free in the retropubic space without being compressed against the pubic bone.

PRECAUTIONS

1. Make every effort to avoid direct dissection of the delicate urethral sphincteric muscular element throughout the entire length of the urethra as well as close to the vesicourethral junction.
2. Avoid by any means creating any compression or obstruction of the urethra while placing the sutures (Fig. 25–7).
3. Keep in mind that healing and permanent support will be achieved by the adherence and fibrosis that will occur and not by the sutures placed at the time of surgery. Accordingly, absorbable suture material is usually advised. Nonabsorbable suture, no matter how far from the bladder, not infrequently finds its way toward the lumen of the urinary tract.

The preexisting funneling of the internal meatus and vesiculation of the proximal urethral segment are a result of the downward and posterior sagging of the vesical neck as well as its poor support. This need not be corrected surgically because the vesical neck will regain tonus and normal configuration once the normal support and position are restored. The posterior urethrovesical angle is not in itself a critical factor in maintaining continence or losing it. It is usually corrected spontaneously with the proper suspension and support of the vesicourethral segment, and thus no special effort should be made to create a posterior angle. At the end of the procedure the retropubic space should be relatively free, and there should be an adequate space for the urethra to move, without being compressed against the pubic bone. There is no need to fix the anterior bladder wall itself because once the entire vesicourethral segment is supported in a normal position, the rest of the bladder will follow suit. Pulling the anterior bladder wall close to the bladder neck (toward the anterior abdominal wall) will probably defeat the free mobility and ability of the muscular tonus to include the internal meatus and keep it open.

Conclusions

The technique described here has been uniformly successful—and highly so in recurrent cases, regardless of the number of previous failures, as long as the urodynamic studies showed an element of active sphincteric musculature. Physiologic studies have confirmed the fact that the only failures were those in which severe intrinsic damage had been inflicted previously on the sphincteric mechanism by surgical repairs that had traumatized and scarred the urethral musculature. The extent of the damage is usually dependent on the techniques used initially. Excessive scarring and fibrosis create a rigid drain pipe that, whatever amount of support or elevation is provided, will never function as an active sphincter unit. There is no remedy possible in these cases except creation of obstruction by compression or slings. What was learned from these cases led to adoption of the technique described, by which one can avoid any close dissection toward the vesicourethral segment, thus sparing its delicate musculature from any surgical damage.

From experience, I believe that adherence to these principles will result in the highest rate of success and the longest lasting repairs.

Urethra Free in Spacious Retropubic Space

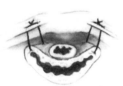

Compressed and Strangulated Urethras

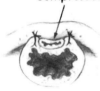 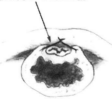

Figure 25-7 Effect of the suspension in the technique described in the text. Top drawing shows urethra free in a widely opened retropubic space; drawings below show other techniques, in which it can be compressed and strangulated between the bone and the vaginal wall. (From Tanagho EA: Colpocystourethropexy: The way we do it. J Urol 116:751, 1976.)

BIBLIOGRAPHY

Bergman A, Koonings PP, Ballard CA: Proposed management of low urethral pressure type of genuine stress urinary incontinence. Gynecol Obstet Invest 27:155, 1989.

Brieger G, Korda A: The effect of obesity on the outcome of successful surgery for genuine stress incontinence. Aust NZ J Obstet Gynecol 32:71, 1992.

Burch JC: Urethrovaginal fixation to Cooper's ligament for correction of stress incontinence, cystocele, and prolapse. Am J Obstet Gynecol 81:281, 1961.

Burch JC: Urethrovaginal fixation to Cooper's ligament in the treatment of cystocele and stress incontinence. Prog Gynecol 4:591, 1963.

Carey MP, Dwyer PL: Position and mobility of the urethrovesical junction in continent and in stress incontinent women before and after successful surgery. Aust NZ J Obstet Gynecol 31:279, 1991.

Durfee RB: The anterior vaginal suspension operation; a report of 110 cases. Am J Obstet Gynecol 92:610, 1965.

Eriksen BC, Hagen B, Eik-Nes SH, et al: Long-term effectiveness of the Burch colposuspension in female urinary stress incontinence. Acta Obstet Gynecol Scand 69:45, 1990.

Fecheco-Mena M, Cedano-Gomez R: Treatment of stress incontinence by vaginopubic urethropexy. Urology 5:536, 1975.

Ferriani RA, Silva de Sa MF, Dias de Moura M, et al: Ureteral blockage as a complication of Burch colposuspension: Report of 6 cases. Gynecol Obstet Invest 29:239, 1990.

Green TH Jr: Development of a plan for the diagnosis and treatment of urinary stress incontinence. Am J Obstet Gynecol 83:632, 1962.

Hilton P, Mayne CJ: The Stamey endoscopic bladder neck suspension: A clinical and urodynamic investigation, including actuarial follow-up over four years. Br J Obstet Gynecol 98:1141, 1991.

Hutch JA: A modification of the Marshall-Marchetti-Krantz operation. J Urol 99:607, 1968.

Imparato E, Aspesi G, Rovetta E, Presti M: Surgical management and prevention of vaginal vault prolapse. Surg Gynecol Obstet 175:233, 1992.

Jeffcoate TNA, Roberts H: Effects of urethrocystopexy for stress incontinence. Surg Gynecol Obstet 98:743, 1954.

Kelly HA: Incontinence of urine in women. Urol Cutan Rev 17:291, 1913.

Kiilholma P, Makinen J, Chancellor MB, et al: Modified Burch colposuspension for stress urinary incontinence in females. Surg Gynecol Obstet 176:111, 1993.

Korda A, Ferry J, Hunter P: Colposuspension for the treatment of female urinary incontinence. Aust NZ J Obstet Gynecol 29:146, 1989.

Kulkarni S: Surgery for post-hysterectomy vaginal prolapse. West Indian Med J 42:65, 1993.

Langer R, Golan A, Arad D, et al: Effects of induced menopause on Burch colposuspension for urinary stress incontinence. J Reprod Med 37:956, 1992.

Langer R, Golan A, Ron-El R, et al: Colposuspension for urinary stress incontinence in premenopausal and postmenopausal women. Surg Gynecol Obstet 171:13, 1990.

Lapides J: Simplified operation for stress incontinence. J Urol 105:262, 1971.

Lapides J: Operative technique for stress urinary incontinence. Urology 3:657, 1974.

Lee RA, Symmonds RE: Repeat Marshall-Marchetti procedure for recurrent stress urinary incontinence. Am J Obstet Gynecol 122:219, 1975.

Lim PH, Brown AD, Chisholm GD: The Burch colposuspension operation for stress urinary incontinence. Singapore Med J 31:242, 1990.

Marchetti AA, Marshall VF, Shultis LD: Simple vesicourethral suspension: A survey. Am J Obstet Gynecol 74:57, 1957.

Marshall VF, Segaul RM: Experience with suprapubic vesicourethral suspension after previous failure to correct stress incontinence in women. J Urol 100:647, 1968.

Miller NF: The surgical treatment of urinary incontinence in the female. JAMA 98:628, 1932.

Murnaghan GF: Colposuspension in the management of stress incontinence. Br J Urol 47:236, 1975.

Penttinen J, Kaar K, Kauppila A: Colposuspension and transvaginal bladder neck suspension in the treatment of stress incontinence. Gynecol Obstet Invest 28:101, 1989.

Pereyra AJ: A simplified surgical procedure for the correction of stress incontinence in women. West J Surg Obstet Gynecol 67:223, 1959.

Pereyra AJ, Lebherz TB: Combined urethrovesical suspension and vaginourethroplasty for correction of urinary stress incontinence. Obstet Gynecol 30:537, 1967.

Read CD: Stress incontinence of urine with special reference to failure of cure following vaginal operative procedure. Am J Obstet Gynecol 59:1260, 1950.

Rosenzweig BA, Bhatia NN, Nelson AL: Dynamic urethral pressure profilometry pressure transmission ratio: What do the numbers really mean? Obstet Gynecol 77:586, 1991.

Stamey TA: Endoscopic suspension of the vesical neck for urinary incontinence. Surg Gynecol Obstet 136:547, 1973.

Symmonds RE: The suprapubic approach to anterior vaginal relaxation and urinary stress incontinence. Clin Obstet Gynecol 15:1107, 1972.

Tanagho EA: Simplified cystography in stress urinary incontinence. Br J Urol 46:295, 1974.

Tanagho EA: Anatomy and physiology of the urethra. In Caldwell KPS (ed): Urinary Incontinence. New York, Grune & Stratton, 1975, p 27.

Tanagho EA: Genuine stress incontinence, the retropubic procedure: A physiologic approach to repair. In Ostergard DR (ed): Gynecologic Urology and Urodynamics. Baltimore, Waverly Press, 1980, p 285.

Tanagho EA: The effect of hysterectomy and periurethral surgery on urethrovesical junction. In Ostergard DR (ed): Gynecologic Urology and Urodynamics. Baltimore, Waverly Press, 1980, p 293.

Tanagho EA: Bladder neck reconstruction for total urinary incontinence: Ten years' experience. J Urol 125:321, 1981.

Tanagho EA: Urinary incontinence management: Neourethra repair. Dialog Pediatr Urol 4:5, 1981.

Tanagho EA: Colpocystourethropexy. AUA Update 12:27, 1993.

Tanagho EA, Miller ER: Functional considerations of urethral sphincteric dynamics. J Urol 109:273, 1973.

Thunedborg P, Fischer-Rasmussen W, Jensen SB: Stress urinary incontinence and posterior bladder suspension defects. Results of vaginal repair versus Burch colposuspension. Acta Obstet Gynecol Scand 69:55, 1990.

Vierhout ME, Mulder AF: De novo detrusor instability after Burch colposuspension. Acta Obstet Gynecol Scand 71:414, 1992.

Wheelahan JB: Long-term results of colposuspension. Br J Urol 65:329, 1990.

Wiskind AK, Creighton SM, Stanton SL: The incidence of genital prolapse after the Burch colposuspension. Am J Obstet Gynecol 167:399, 1992.

CHAPTER 26

Laparoscopic Bladder Neck Suspension

Ashok Chopra, M.D.
Shlomo Raz, M.D.
Lynn Stothers, M.D., M.H.Sc., F.R.C.S.C.

In recent years there has been an explosion in the use of laparoscopic techniques. A variety of urologic procedures have been attempted; this chapter will briefly discuss some of the techniques of laparoscopic bladder neck suspension for stress urinary incontinence (SUI). The reader is referred to other sources for details of the specific techniques, pathophysiology, anatomy, and complications of laparoscopic surgery.

Evaluation and pathogenesis of SUI are outlined in other chapters of this book. In brief, in regard to incontinence, laparoscopic surgery is suitable for patients with no intrinsic sphincteric dysfunction. The goal of laparoscopic surgery in these patients is similar to that of other forms of surgery for type 1 and type 2 SUI—namely, to elevate the bladder neck into a high supported position.

CONTRAINDICATIONS The reader is again referred to other sources for a complete discussion of these issues. In brief, contraindications to laparoscopic surgery include the presence of extensive adhesions, a history of peritonitis or coagulopathy, and patients with a dilated small bowel.[1]

Operative Strategy and Techniques

All patients undergo a bowel preparation that not only provides bowel prophylaxis should inadvertent injury occur but also provides decompression of the bowel. Blood is cross-matched, and intravenous antibiotics are administered preoperatively. A Foley catheter is introduced; a nasogastric tube may be considered. General anesthesia is administered.

One technique of laparoscopic bladder neck suspension is that outlined by Albala and colleagues.[1] The patient is placed in the modified lithotomy position, a small infraumbilical incision is made, and a Veress needle is introduced. Carbon monoxide gas is introduced to insufflate the abdomen at a rate of 1 to 6 liters/minute. Subsequently, four trocars are placed. The initial trocar is placed at the umbilicus with a 10-mm port. The camera is introduced, and the remaining trocar placements are done under direct vision. Three additional ports are placed; the second 10-mm port is inserted midway between the umbilicus and the pubic bone, and a 5-mm trocar is placed on the right side, lateral to the rectus and halfway between the anterior iliac spine and the umbilicus. An identical trocar is placed in a similar position on the left side. Once all trocars are in place, careful inspection of the sites is undertaken to ensure that no injury has occurred. Care is taken with transillumination during trocar placement to avoid injury to the epigastric vessels.

Adhesions are initially lysed as needed. An initial incision is made along the medial border of the left umbilical ligament using the electrocautery scissors. With the peritoneum opened, the posterior aspect of the pubic bone is seen. Using an atraumatic grasper, the surgeon's assistant retracts the bladder while the surgeon develops the retropubic space. Attention to hemostasis is important because blood will accumulate in the space of Retzius. After this dissection has been completed, an Ethibond 2–0 suture is inserted via the suprapubic trocar. This suture is placed just lateral to the urethra. Placement of this suture is facilitated by displacing the vagina away from the pubic bone with the surgeon's hand in the vagina. The needle is next brought through the symphysis of the pubic bone as in the modified Marshall-Marchetti-Kranz (MMK) procedure. If, alternatively, a Burch-type technique is chosen, the sutures may be placed in Cooper's ligament. The bladder neck is elevated under direct vision to the appropriate level by pulling on the suture. The knot is made extracorporally and tied. This maneuver is repeated on the contralateral side. The peritoneal defect may or may not be closed. The trocars are removed, the camera port being the last trocar taken out. All trocar sites are examined prior to removal of the final camera trocar. Wounds are closed with subcuticular sutures.

POSTOPERATIVE COURSE Clear liquids are started when the patient is alert and oriented. Oral antibiotics are given for 5 days, and patients are usually discharged within 18 hours.

RESULTS Vancaille and Schuessler reported on a total of 32 patients with type 1 or 2 incontinence treated as described here.[2] Of these 32, 22 underwent a modified MMK procedure, and 10 underwent a Burch-type suspension. Operative time in their experience was 105 minutes for the Burch and 65 minutes for the MMK. Mean follow-up time was 1 year for the MMK patients and 7 months for the Burch patients. All patients were defined as "cured" (no further data).

COMPLICATIONS No complications occurred in the group undergoing Burch suspension. In the group undergoing the MMK procedure, two patients developed retention that required a cystostomy tube (duration was not specified). Three patients underwent laparotomy; in two patients technical difficulties prevented placement of the periurethral suture. In one patient the bladder was injured during the dissection of the space of Retzius.

Alternative Techniques

Various techniques of laparoscopic-assisted bladder neck suspension have been described in the literature. Chau-Su and coworkers have described a modification using titanium staples and Prolene mesh in place of traditional suture material, allowing them to eliminate the need for laparoscopic suturing.[3] The initial steps in this procedure are similar to those described by Albala. However, in lieu of sutures they use two strips of Prolene mesh measuring 1 × 3 cm. These strips are stapled in place with the EMS disposable endostaple. In this technique the surgeon places one finger in the vagina and exerts pressure anteriorly while the surgeon's assistant places one end of the Prolene strip on the exposed perivaginal fascia and fires the endostapler twice against the surgeon's finger. The other end of the strip is then placed against Cooper's ligament, and two staples are fired to secure this in place. The contralateral side is treated in an identical fashion. Excess mesh is trimmed. When suspension is complete, attention is turned to hemostasis. The endostaples are next used to achieve reperitonealization.

RESULTS Chau-Su reported on 40 patients treated in this fashion with a mean follow-up of 6 months. Mean hospital stay was 1.2 days, and average duration of catheterization was less than 24 hours. In the first 10 cases a cystoscope was placed intraoperatively to measure the urethrovesical angle to ensure proper suspension and to assess for urethral and bladder injury during placement of the staples. In all 10 of these patients no injury was manifest and support was thought to be adequate. The remaining 30 patients were not studied in this fashion. Results were described as follows: "All forty patients reported improved voiding and resolution or improvement of symptoms" (no further specific data were provided in this paper). Complications included one episode of hematuria, urinary retention (outcome not reported) in one patient, urinary tract infection in two patients, and low-grade fever in two patients.

Liu and colleagues reported on their technique of laparoscopic bladder neck suspension using their modification of the Burch-type technique.[4] The patient is placed in the low lithotomy position with the lower extremities supported by Allen stirrups. A 20 Fr Foley catheter with a 30-ml balloon is inserted. Fifty milliliters of indigo carmine are instilled into the bladder to assist in identification of any inadvertent bladder injury. A 10-mm laparoscope is inserted at the umbilicus, and four additional trocars are inserted under direct vision. Two 5-mm ports are introduced on each side; the cephalad port is placed lateral to the rectus at the level of the umbilicus, and the caudal port is placed lateral to the deep inferior epigastric vessels in the suprapubic area. The patient is next placed in a slight Trendelenburg position, and any coexisting pathology is addressed. The cul-de-sac is obliterated by a Moschowitz technique using 3–0 Prolene sutures.

Next, a transverse incision is made in the anterior peritoneum between the two obliterated umbilical ligaments, and the retropubic space is entered and developed. Paravaginal fatty tissue is removed with care to avoid any dissection within 2 to 2.5 cm from the urethra. Two sutures of No. 2 Gore-Tex are placed at the level of the midurethra and urethrovescial junction. These are placed 2.0 cm lateral to the urethra and incorporate the entire vaginal wall (excluding the vaginal cavity). The needle is subsequently passed through Cooper's ligament and the suture tied extracorporeally. During this maneuver the surgical assistant places one hand in the vagina to approximate the tissues and minimize tension on the sutures. Irrigation is performed with lactated Ringer's solution, and a Bonnano suprapubic tube is inserted. The peritoneum is closed with 3–0 polydioxanone. Cystoscopy is performed to check for any violation of the bladder by sutures. Indigo carmine is administered intravenously, and the ureteral orifices are assessed for patency.

RESULTS Fifty-eight patients were treated with this technique with follow-up ranging from 6 to 22 months. Nineteen patients had had previous major abdominal procedures; concomitant major laparoscopic procedures such as hysterectomy or salpingo-oophorectomy were performed in 52 patients. Average operative time was 73.21 minutes excluding time used to perform hysterectomy. Mean hospital stay was 1.22 days, and mean blood loss was 50 ml. At 6 weeks all patients had a negative standing stress test. Patients were otherwise defined as improved if they were subjectively satisfied with their results. Using these definitions, 55 patients were thought to be improved, and 3 were worse; they had symptoms of instability and were treated with oxybutinin and bladder training. Complications included hemorrhage from the suprapubic site in one patient and intraoperative bladder injury in two patients.

Knapp and colleagues described a technique in which extraperitoneal laparoscopic bladder neck mobilization is done through a single port.[5] In this technique the patient is placed in the lithotomy position, and a transverse incision is made in the suprapubic area two fingerbreadths above the symphysis. The subcutaneous tissue is incised and dissected off the rectus fascia. A 2-cm incision is made in the rectus fascia midline. The surgeon's finger next dissects the retropubic space. A 10-mm sheath without the trocar is placed, and a Gaur dissecting balloon introduced. The balloon is positioned behind the symphysis and inflated with 600 to 1000 ml of saline. This maneuver dissects the perivesical space and achieves bladder neck mobilization. Next, the balloon is removed, and the operating laparoscope is introduced into the space. The prevesical space is insufflated with carbon dioxide at 8 mmHg (this pressure allows good visualization and avoids subcutaneous emphysema). Further dissection if necessary may be accomplished using electrocautery scissors. Additional instrument ports are not needed if an offset operating laparoscope is used with scissors through the working port.

A Stamey needle is next placed through the rectus fascia 1 cm above the pubic tubercle on each side. Insertion of the needle is observed through the laparoscope; the needle is placed precisely at the level of the bladder neck taking two or three bites through the full thickness of the vaginal wall in the fashion described by Gittes and Loughlin.[6] The two ends of the Prolene suture are threaded through the eye of the Stamey needle, and the needles on each side are withdrawn into the suprapubic area. Cystoscopy is performed to confirm the integrity of the bladder, and elevation of the bladder neck is assessed cystoscopically and laparoscopically. A single end of each suspension suture is threaded into a No. 5 Mayo needle and passed through the rectus fascia overlying the pubic tubercle on each side. Each suture is tied to itself.

RESULTS Four patients were treated in this fashion. Average follow-up was only 3.8 months; all four patients were dry at that point. Three patients were discharged on postoperative day 1. One patient remained in the hospital (she underwent concurrent rectocele repair). All patients were voiding within 2 weeks. No other complications were reported.

Harewood also presented a modification of laparoscopic bladder neck suspension.[7] With the patient in the low lithotomy position, three lower abdominal ports were inserted. A 10-mm port with camera was inserted at the umbilicus, a 5-mm port was placed in the lower abdominal midline, and a 5-mm port was placed in the left iliac fossa. A 5-cm incision is made at the upper border of the symphysis pubis and deepened to the rectus. The bladder is filled to aid in identification of its margins. Bilateral incisions are made in the peritoneum from the medial umbilical ligament anteromedially to the urachus (the urachus is left intact). The retropubic space is dissected. A Stamey needle is inserted from the suprapubic incision into the retropubic space and subsequently passed into the vagina under vision. No. 1 Ethibond sutures are used to take double bites of the vaginal wall. These sutures are next passed to the suprapubic incision. The suture is tied over a silicon button with no slack and no tension.

RESULTS Seven patients were treated. All patients were described as "cured of their incontinence" at the conclusion of the study. Follow-up was quite short, ranging from 3 to 6 weeks. Mean operative time was 112 minutes. Mean time to discharge was 3.3 days. Six patients voided within 2 days; one patient had a cystotomy at the time of surgery and had the catheter in place for 12 days. The second significant complication was peritoneal irritation with mild fever in one patient, who required readmission for 3 days.

Conclusion

Laparoscopic techniques of bladder neck suspension are somewhat sparsely reported in the literature because they are relatively new. As one would expect, current reports consistently have short follow-up. Additionally, many of the reports in the literature do not provide a specific definition of the terms cure and improved. The complication rate is likely to decrease as familiarity with these techniques increases. The advantages of these techniques over transvaginal techniques are somewhat speculative; clearly, the cost and the incidence of complications are greater with laparoscopy at this time.

REFERENCES

1. Albala DM, Schuessler WW, Vancaillie TG: Laparoscopic bladder suspension for the treatment of stress incontinence. Semin Urol 10(4):222, 1992.
2. Vancaillie TG, Schuessler WW: Laparoscopic bladder neck suspension. J Laparoendoscop Surg 3:169, 1991.
3. Chau-Su O, Presthus J, Beadle E: Laparoscopic bladder neck suspension using hernia mesh and surgical sutures. J Laparoendoscop Surg 3(6):563, 1993.
4. Liu CY: Laparoscopic retropubic colposuspension. J Reprod Med 38(7):526, 1993.
5. Knapp PM, Siegel YI, Lingeman JE: Laparoscopic retroperitoneal needle suspension urethropexy. J Endourol 8(4):279, 1994.
6. Gittes R, Loughlin K: No-incision pubovaginal suspension for stress incontinence. J Urol 138:568, 1987.
7. Harewood LM: Laparoscopic needle suspension for genuine stress incontinence. J Endourol 7(4):319, 1993.

CHAPTER 27

No-Incision Urethropexy

Ruben F. Gittes, M.D.

Rationale

For over 50 years since the popularization of the Marshall-Marchetti procedure,[1] surgeons have cured urinary stress incontinence in women with procedures that accomplish these goals:

1. Keep the bladder neck tethered in place during abdominal straining.
2. Steady the anterior vaginal wall as backing for the proximal urethra, which is compressed during abdominal pressure increases.

It was previously thought that nonabsorbable sutures holding up the anterior vaginal wall and bladder neck must not come through the "outside" vaginal wall to prevent infection and suppuration. But animal research studies[2] demonstrated that heavy monofilament sutures tied down through-and-through the abdominal wall and kept under tension to plicate the skin and muscles longitudinally would cut through the plicated abdominal wall slowly until the abdomen was flat again and there was no more tension. This occurred without suppuration and without infection as long as (1) monofilament suture (nylon or Prolene) was used and (2) the knots were "buried" when first tied. When such animals were subjected later to abdominal distention caused by injection of air (pneumoperitoneum), a waist band appeared at the level of the incorporated sutures, demonstrating their internal "bolster" effect.

Transposing these laboratory studies to the clinic, we modified the existing needle urethropexy techniques (Pereyra, Stamey, Raz) to allow monofilament sutures to pass through-and-through the full thickness of the anterior vaginal wall with the knots tied down and buried in the suprapubic fat just superficial to the rectus fascia (Fig. 27–1). Within days, the loops of monofilament in the vagina cut through the full-thickness wall and disappear from sight. The anterior vaginal wall slowly descends to the neutral position, eliminating the continuous tension but still

"hanging" from the suture loop on each side by a curtain of natural fibrous tissue (Fig. 27–2). The sutures are now internal bolsters that (1) tether the "sling" of anterior vaginal wall and prevent rotational descent with coughing, and (2) provide a "backing" for the pulses of intra-abdominal pressure that flatten out the proximal urethra. Stress incontinence is thus cured.

Of course, in the Marshall-Marchetti procedure or the more recent Burch procedure or in any of the other successful needle urethropexies (Stamey, Raz, and so on), the same internal bolstering and growth of fibrous tissue from the initial insertion site of

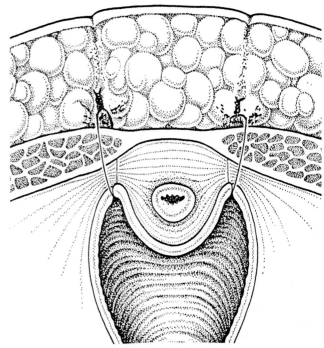

Figure 27-1 Diagrammatic illustration of no-incision urethropexy "just tied," with nonabsorbable monofilament sutures lifting the vaginal wall under tension.

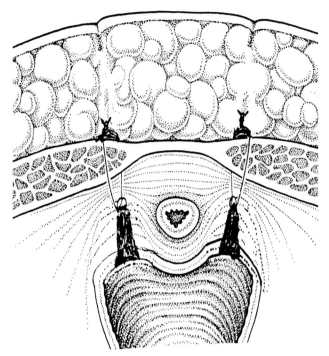

Figure 27-2 Illustration of the position of sutures at about 1 month postoperatively, at which time sutures have been "incorporated." The helical suture slowly cutting through the uplifted vagina and fascia leaves a curtain of scar tissue that protects the bladder neck from rotational descent with abdominal straining.

the sutures occurs. This relocation of the pulled-up tissues occurs universally after an open or closed operation. The angulated, upwardly deformed vaginal wall that is left at the close of those open procedures always settles back slowly to a neutral, nontense position and presumably spins off a similar "curtain" of fibroblasts to bolster it against downward rotation.

Thus, our "no-incision" needle urethropexy is no more and no less than a Marshall-Marchetti or Burch suspension performed from below, tethering the strong full thickness of the vaginal wall "sling" to the rectus muscle fascia above.

TECHNIQUES

Preoperative Evaluation

Preoperative evaluation is common to all the suspension techniques described in this textbook. For straightforward, first-time stress incontinence surgery, our own preference is for merely a careful history and pelvic examination with a Marshall test performed in the office. This need not be defended further here. Patients with previous surgical failures require more circumspection.

ANESTHESIA

A brief general anesthetic is widely used, deep enough to avoid involuntary abdominal strains or

motions during the "blind" advancement of the Stamey needles to the uplifted vaginal wall. However, local anesthesia has been used extensively.[3] Local infiltration of the rectus fascia, prevesical space, and anterior vaginal wall requires a little more time and patience from the physician but eliminates the cost of the anesthetist and overnight observation in some clinics.

INSTRUMENTATION

The following simple instrumentation is required:

1. Cystoscope with lateral and fore oblique lenses
2. Weighted vaginal retractor with a long tongue
3. Foley catheter during the procedure
4. Allis clamps and tooth forceps
5. Needle holder and half-circle free needles (Mayo type)
6. Scalpel blade (pointed No. 11)
7. Stamey (15- and 30-degree) needles
8. Hemostats to be used as suture "tags"
9. Foley-type suprapubic tube (trocar-inserted, with balloon for retention)

PROCEDURE

The patient is placed in the lithotomy position, avoiding exaggerated flexion of the hips onto the abdomen, which deforms the lower abdominal wall. After appropriate preparation, the bladder is emptied with a Foley catheter, and the balloon is palpated to reveal the location of the bladder neck behind the anterior vaginal wall. An Allis clamp is used to grasp that location momentarily on the vaginal wall. To each side of this spot, the vaginal wall is uplifted toward the abdomen, and, in the most mobile part, an Allis clamp is used to grasp the full thickness of the vaginal wall. This will be the location of the helical suspending stitch.

In the procedure modified and improved by Morales and VanCott,[4] the helical bites are taken first, and the Stamey needles are passed down to retrieve the two ends later. We cut off the large needles wedged onto the commercially supplied monofilament retention sutures (No. 1 Prolene or No. 2 nylon) and thread them on a half-circle small and stout Mayo needle. With tooth forceps the full thickness of the mobile anterior vaginal wall is grasped behind or deep to the previously plicating Allis clamp, and the first transverse bite with the suture is placed across it. Then a second bite is taken across it under the Allis clamp. Sometimes a third or rarely even a fourth bite is taken, especially if there is ample redundant vaginal wall (cystourethrocele). The result is a helical suture running parallel to the proximal urethra. The loose ends (front and back) of the just-placed suture are tagged with a small and a large hemostat, respectively. A second helical suture is similarly placed on the other side. It is evident that a vaginal wall sling is formed as soon as these sutures are tethered above.

The suspending sutures are now tied on each side over the rectus muscle fascia close to their pubic bone insertion. To do so we still avoid an "incision" by puncturing the skin with a No. 11 blade 2 inches lateral to each side of the midline and above the mons pubis, just below the suprapubic crease. Some surgeons (see later discussion) prefer a small transverse incision with open exposure of the fascia. The angled, blunt Stamey needle is passed twice on each side through the fascia, medially and laterally, 1 to 2 cm apart. The needle is held with both hands for a controlled "pop" through the fascia; then the tip is levered anteriorly to contact the pubic bone. With one hand the needle tip is "walked" down toward the operator's second hand, which is holding up the vaginal wall. The bladder is avoided by the presence of an open Foley catheter in place and by progressing slowly, making several small lateral to medial waves of the needle tip to "sweep" medially any redundant bladder wall. The recipient hand feels for the tip and guides it against one end of the helical stitch. The needle is then popped through the vagina. The finger lifts and leads out the rounded needle tip. The adjacent loose end of the monofilament suture is passed through the needle's hole, pulled up out of the suprapubic puncture, and tagged. For the second pass on that side, the needle tip is slid alongside the tagged first half of the suture in an attempt to stay within the same needle tract down to the fascia. This is necessary to avoid entrapment of sensory subcutaneous nerves. At the fascia, the needle tip is scraped laterally or medially for 2 cm and popped through as before, using two hands for control, and then passed down to the helical suture to retrieve the remaining loose arm and lift it up through the skin puncture. We usually delay bladder inspection until both sides are done but sometimes prefer an earlier check with the cystoscope, especially if prior surgery has thickened the perivesical tissue. If the cystoscope shows that the bladder was entered, the offending suture arm is visualized and retrieved from below, and the Stamey needle is repassed while the surgeon observes it continuously with a cystoscope in a half-full bladder.

When both suspending sutures are placed and loosely tagged from above, a 70-degree cystoscope is placed in the bladder, and the absence of sutures inside is confirmed. With the bladder full and the cystoscope monitoring the dome, a needle-trocar suprapubic Foley catheter is pushed into the bladder and secured for postoperative drainage.

The bladder suspension is tested by pulling up on each stitch in turn and applying suprapubic Credé pressure. If one stitch is ineffective at preventing leakage it is inspected on the vaginal side to be sure it is not misplaced into the lateral vaginal wall.

The urethral Foley catheter is replaced while the sutures are tied. It helps to prevent excessive lift or kinking of the urethra during typing and also helps to avoid too much tension on the ties. The sutures are tied on each side with five to six square knots, using just enough tension to lift up the vaginal wall when the knot is deep in the subcutaneous fat. It is a common error to crunch the first knot too tight and leave it under so much tension that the suture will cut through too fast and too far as the vaginal wall returns to its normal position, resulting in a curtain of scar tissue of poorer holding quality that may easily be overstretched again in the future. When tied down, each suture is pulled up until the knot shows through the puncture site. The suture is cut above the knot so it pops down into the fat. The procedure is then finished. The suprapubic tube is connected for drainage, and a small gauze dressing covers the suprapubic tube entry site. Small Band-Aids (or nothing) cover the suture puncture sites. No vaginal pack is used (the tension stops any venous oozing there).

POSTOPERATIVE CARE

We usually keep patients overnight because of the following benefits:

1. For pain control hydrocodone plus acetaminophen (Vicodin) is used; it may be supplemented with intramuscular ketorolac.
2. The suprapubic tube can be monitored for bleeding or retention.
3. An opportunity is provided to teach patients how to care for the suprapubic tube and to plug it between voiding after one night of gravity drainage.

Results

Short-term results are excellent and have been confirmed by other groups as providing about 90% cures.[5, 6] Long-term results (over 5 years) are hard to find convincingly demonstrated for any technique. Our own clinical impression is that long-term success with this procedure is equivalent to that of prior techniques. Certainly the underlying cause of long-term failure—slow descent of the bladder neck due to intermittent strains—is the same with all techniques.

Complications

Most complications of this procedure are shared with other needle urethropexy techniques and will not be detailed here. These include prolonged postoperative urinary retention, overlooked or delayed intrusion of suture into the bladder, and, rarely, infection occurring subcutaneously around the knot.

Neurologic complications resulting from entrapment by the blindly placed sutures must be anticipated, prevented if possible, and managed promptly if they occur. These complications are discussed in the following sections.

SENSORY ILIOINGUINAL NEUROPATHY

Avoidance of open exposure of the rectus fascia allows occasional entrapment of branching sensory nerve fibers extending medially from the external inguinal ring. The anatomic factors in this entrapment have been outlined clearly by Ghoniem.[7] Within 2 weeks the patient notices unilateral pubic discomfort, with or without hypesthesia, that is aggravated by walking or abdominal straining. Examination with finger pressure over the buried knot causes sharper pain, which can be contrasted to the usual negative findings on the other side.

Prevention of this superficial entrapment is accomplished by puncturing the fascia at two points that are on a horizontal line to each other. Further, the second puncture is done after the needle tip is slid down *alongside* the just-pulled first half of the monofilament tie; then, at the level of the fascia, the tip is dragged medially on the fascia 1 to 2 cm and "popped" downward to retrieve the second half of the tie. This has reduced the incidence of entrapment in our patients from about 20% to less than 5%. Others prevent it by making a small incision above, as in the original Stamey procedure.[4]

Treatment consists first of reassurance and watchful waiting for the affected sensory nerve to become better spontaneously. Pain and tenderness that persist after 3 to 4 weeks are treated by local injection of a mixture of bupivacaine (Marcaine) and triamcinolone (Kenalog) (9 ml of 0.5% Marcaine and 1 ml/40 mg Kenalog), which can be repeated two to three times if the first injection is only partially effective. Finally, if local "electric" tenderness persists, the offending suture is removed under local anesthesia from above, as described later.

MOTOR OR SENSORY OBTURATOR NEUROPATHY

Rarely but dramatically, a tethering or medical entrapment of the obturator nerve occurs. The patient has from the beginning immediate signs and symptoms of unilateral perineal pain with radiation to the medial thigh and groin. Left leg motion is impaired and exacerbates the complaints. Adductor weakness of the thigh may or may not be demonstrable at first. Electromyographic signs of impairment of the adductors become positive later. We strongly recommend immediate removal of the presumptively offending sutures, even in the recovery room. This is a minor procedure that can prevent a lot of unrewarding, irrelevant testing by neurologic consultants, accompanied by time loss and alienation of the patient.

RETRIEVAL OF THE MONOFILAMENT SUTURE

The surgeon performing any of the needle urethropexies must be quick to recognize the advantage of removing one of the two sutures to solve a complication. We once removed *both* from a patient with pelvic pain complaints. The key point is that the suture is really the only suspected source of any postoperative complaint. In patients with pain it is foolish for the surgeon to dismiss the obvious and hide behind the slim possibility of a coincident "back injury," "positioning trauma," "preexisting radiculopathy," "spinal stenosis," and so on. Investigation of these unlikely possibilities must be done only *after* the stitch is removed if the pain persists.

The usual indications for surgical removal of the offending suture are as follows:

1. Pain syndrome, early or late. See previous discussion of neuropathy.
2. Delayed intrusion of suture into bladder. This may occur months to years after surgery and should be suspected and sought with cystoscopy in follow-up if red cells, inflammatory symptoms, or new bladder irritability appears. If a stone has formed around the suture, it will slip off the monofilament; when the suture is removed, the stone can be withdrawn or passed.
3. Infected or abscessed pubic area around the knot. This infection presumably develops from bacteria (hair?) trapped in the buried knot. We have never heard of it on the vaginal side where there is no knot.

The technique for removal of the sutures is simpler than most practitioners imagine because (1) the knot is always superficial to the rectus fascia, and (2) the suture is always easily pulled out when one leg is cut just below the knot.

To remove the suture in the office, simply

1. Prepare the skin over the usually palpable knot.
2. Infiltrate the area with enough local anesthetic to cover the knot area, but no deeper.
3. Make a 1-cm incision of the skin into the fat overlying the knot.
4. *Feel* through the incision to detect the general location of the knot.
5. Apply an Allis clamp to the fat nodule where the knot is felt.
6. Lift fat into view through the incision and sharply scrape off the fat until the blue or black monofilament is visualized.
7. Grasp the monofilament with a fine hemostat to free the knot and both legs of the stitch.
8. Snip one leg of the suture with fine tip scissors; the stitch in its entirety follows the knot out.
9. Close with a stitch or Steri-Strip.

In my experience, removal of one stitch often leads to early recurrence of some stress incontinence. In that case, replacement has always worked to restore continence.

REFERENCES

1. Marshall VF, Marchetti AA, Krantz KE: The correction of stress incontinence by simple vesicourethral suspension. Surg Gynecol Obstet 88:509, 1949.
2. Gittes RF, Foreman R: Transcutaneous incorporation of nonabsorbable monofilament sutures. Surg Gynecol Obstet 166:545–548, 1988.
3. Gittes RF, Loughlin KR: No-incision urethropexy for stress incontinence under local anesthesia. J Urol 139:270A, 1988.
4. Morales A, VanCott G: The Gittes procedure as an improved simplification of current techniques for vesical neck suspensions. Surg Gynecol Obstet 167:243–254, 1988.
5. Lipshitz S, Burnstein J, Garey-Sage J: Our experience with 135 cases of the no-incision bladder suspension—Gittes procedure. J Urol 143:224A, 1990.
6. Benson JT, Agosta A, McClellan E: Evaluation of a minimal-incision pubovaginal suspension as an adjunct to other pelvic-floor surgery. Obstet Gynecol 75:844–847, 1990.
7. Ghoneim GM: Ilioinguinal nerve entrapment after needle bladder suspension. Surg Gynecol Obstet, in press.

CHAPTER 28

Stamey Needle Suspension for Female Stress Incontinence

Lynn Stothers, M.D., M.H.Sc., F.R.C.S.C.
Shlomo Raz, M.D.
Ashok Chopra, M.D.

The endoscopic needle suspension of Stamey, using a single-pronged needle, was described in 1973.[1] As such, its description preceded that of the Raz bladder neck suspension. Unlike abdominal procedures such as the Burch or the Marshall-Marchetti-Krantz procedure and other vaginal needle suspension operations, the Stamey needle suspension does not require dissection of the bladder or bladder neck. The paraurethral tissues suspending the bladder neck are buttressed with knitted Dacron grafts placed through a vaginal approach and suspended through small suprapubic incisions. The needle used for this procedure is different from the Pereyra or Raz needle. It is single-pronged and is passed a total of four times during the procedure.

Surgical Technique

Excellent descriptions of the technique have been reported by Stamey.[1, 2] To begin, the patient is positioned in the lithotomy position, and the vagina and lower abdomen are prepared with an iodine scrub. A urethral catheter is used to empty the bladder and is left in situ. Two transverse 2-cm incisions are made in the lower abdomen to the left and right of the midline just anterior to the border of the symphysis pubis (Fig. 28–1). The anterior rectus fascia is exposed using blunt dissection with the aid of a clamp. Adequate exposure of the fascia is necessary to aid in tying down the suture material against the rectus fascia and allows for adequate coverage of the sutures when the wounds are closed.

A vaginal incision in the form of a T is made in the anterior vaginal wall. The transverse part of the incision starts near the urethral meatus with the arm of the T in the midline extending to just beyond the bladder neck. Dissection is carried out laterally to expose the glistening periurethral fascia. During this dissection care should be taken not to enter the urethra or bladder, which can result in excess bleeding. The balloon of the Foley catheter may be palpated within the incision, providing a tactile landmark for the region of the bladder neck. Dissection should be carried out until the operator can place a fingertip in the incision so that it rests against the bladder neck on either side of the urethral catheter. Adequate exposure must be allowed for placement of the Dacron pledget so that it may be adequately buried when the vaginal incisions are closed.

The Stamey needle is then inserted into the medial edge of one of the suprapubic wounds through the rectus fascia (Fig. 28–2). The needle is passed adjacent to the periosteum under fingertip control (Fig. 28–3) and advanced into the vaginal incision, passing alongside the bladder neck and through the paraurethral fascia. The Foley catheter is removed, and cystoscopy is carried out with the needle in position to confirm correct placement. Correct positioning of the needle indents the ipsilateral vesical neck when the needle is manipulated suprapubically.[2] A No. 2 nylon suture is threaded through the needle, and the needle is pulled suprapubically. The needle is then passed for a second time, 1 cm laterally on the ipsilateral side, and its position is confirmed once again cystoscopically. The vaginal end of the suture is placed through the 10- by 5-mm Dacron arterial graft and then through the eye of the needle. The Dacron graft is visually guided into the area of the urethrovesical junction while the needle is pulled upward for a second time (Fig. 28–4). A loop of per-

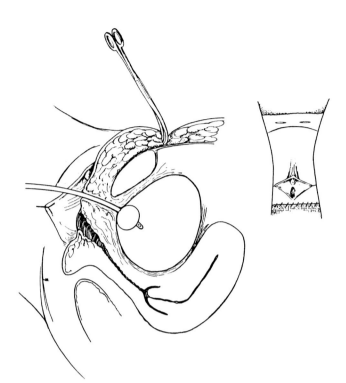

Figure 28-1 With the patient in the lithotomy position, a urethral catheter is placed, and two suprapubic incisions are made into which the single-pronged needle will be passed. (From Shortliffe LMD, Stamey TA: *In* McDougal WS [ed]: Rob & Smith's Operative Surgery. Urology, 4th ed. Andover, Hampshire, England, Chapman & Hall, 1983.)

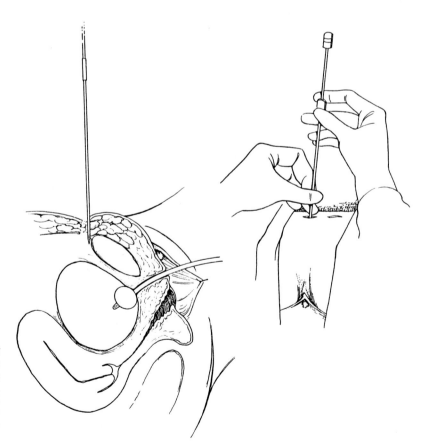

Figure 28-2 Diagrammatic representation of the direction in which the Stamey needle is passed. Two hands are recommended to guide the needle through its perforation of the rectus fascia. (From Shortliffe LMD, Stamey TA: *In* McDougal WS [ed]: Rob & Smith's Operative Surgery. Urology, 4th ed. Andover, Hampshire, England, Chapman & Hall, 1983.)

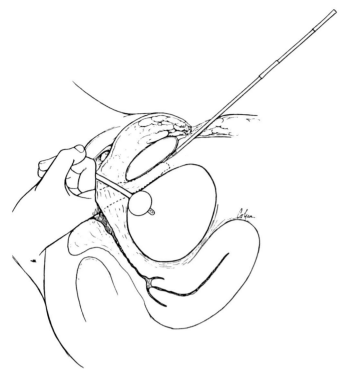

Figure 28-3 As with the Raz bladder neck suspension, the needle is guided under fingertip control to avoid perforation of the bladder. (From Shortliffe LMD, Stamey TA: *In* McDougal WS [ed]: Rob & Smith's Operative Surgery. Urology, 4th ed. Andover, Hampshire, England, Chapman & Hall, 1983.)

manent suture material results that supports the graft material. The procedure is repeated on the contralateral side, resulting in two Dacron grafts on each side of the urethrovesical junction that should be symmetrical in location. Antibiotic solution should be used to irrigate the vaginal wound and graft material prior to closure. The vaginal incision is closed with a running, locking, 2–0 polyglycolic acid suture, and the suspension sutures are tied down without

undue tension following placement of a vaginal pack. A suprapubic catheter is placed, and the suprapubic incisions are closed with 4–0 polyglycolic acid suture following antibiotic irrigation.

On the first postoperative day the urethral Foley catheter is removed along with the vaginal pack. As with other vaginal suspension procedures, the patient checks postvoid residual urines, and the suprapubic tube is removed when adequate bladder emptying is demonstrated. As a general rule, the postvoid residuals should be less than 60 ml.

Important technical points have been outlined by Stamey.[2] Positioning of the Dacron graft well below the suture line to prevent erosion of the graft through the vaginal incisions is critical. Copious irrigation with aminoglycoside solution should be carried out in the vaginal wound prior to closing it to prevent infection of the grafts, which represent foreign bodies. The Stamey needle comes in three forms, each of which has a different angle at the distal end containing the eye of the needle. The straight version of the needle or its 15- or 30-degree angled counterparts can be used in patients in whom the anatomy presents difficult problems. For example, in patients who have previously undergone retropubic suspension, the bladder may be adherent to the symphysis pubis, and careful inspection with the cystoscope is important to ensure that the needle or suture material has not perforated the bladder.

Discussion

RESULTS

Defining cure as the absence of urinary incontinence 6 months postoperatively, Stamey reported a 91% cure rate in 203 consecutive patients.[3] As with the Raz bladder neck suspension, prior hysterectomy was

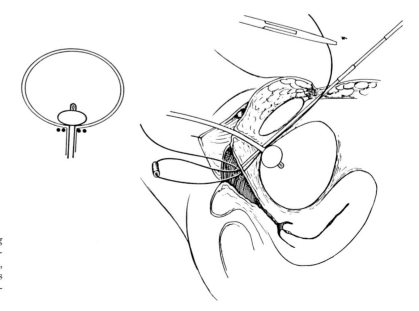

Figure 28-4 Diagrammatic representation showing placement of suture with Dacron graft after the second pass of the Stamey needle. (From Shortliffe LMD, Stamey TA: *In* McDougal WS [ed]: Rob & Smith's Operative Surgery. Urology, 4th ed. Andover, Hampshire, England, Chapman & Hall, 1983.)

not found to affect patient outcome adversely with regard to recurrence of stress incontinence, and the majority of failures occurred in the early postoperative period.

Other authors have reported on the use of the Stamey needle suspension worldwide since its introduction in 1973.[6, 13, 14, 18, 21–23] A summary of contemporary series and their reported results is provided in Table 28–1. All contemporary series in the literature written in the English language or with English language abstracts were of the uncontrolled observational series design. No prospectively randomized trials or case control series were identified using a MEDLINE search of the last 5 years. Comparison of the results of such series is difficult owing to their retrospective, unblinded nature and the authors' varying definitions of "cure." Those reporting follow-up with a mean of 16 months or more report a "cure" rate of 53 to 85%. Several authors report high success rates in elderly patients. Hilton and Mayne reported a higher long-term cure rate in patients aged 65 years or older (76%) than in those aged less than 65 years (53%).[15] Griffith-Jones and Abrams also found a high cure rate of 85% in elderly patients aged 65 to 81 years.[26]

The Stamey needle suspension has been used in combination with vaginal hysterectomy and colpoperineoplasty when uterine prolapse is clinically significant. Ralph and colleagues reported in 1993 on 40 women who underwent vaginal hysterectomy plus colpoperineoplasty for uterine prolapse with a Stamey procedure in 26 patients and without a Stamey procedure in 14.[7] When the Stamey suspension was used as part of the pelvic reconstruction the postoperative continence rate was 83% compared with 43% in the group without bladder neck suspension. The authors correctly emphasized the need to anticipate latent stress incontinence in this group of patients with severe degrees of pelvic and uterine prolapse.

The Stamey needle suspension has been used in surgical reconstruction in some special circumstances.[11, 12] Cardozo and Brindley reported the use of the Stamey needle suspension in two paraplegic patients with anterior nerve root stimulator–driven micturition.[11] Correction of stress urinary incontinence in these patients was possible without interfering with their micturition cycle. A second special use of the Stamey suspension was described by Ganabathi and colleagues, who used a Stamey suspension combined with a Martius flap in the treatment of patients with stress incontinence related to intrinsic sphincter dysfunction (low maximum urethral closing pressure and a scarred, well-supported urethra).[12] The authors reported a 91% cure rate in 13 months mean follow-up.

Questionnaires from 192 patients reporting patient satisfaction as an outcome measure were recently described following the Stamey needle suspension.[10, 28] This figure represented a 72% response rate in a group of 284 questionnaires mailed out. Sixty-five percent of patients reported that they would be willing to have the procedure again, and 82% reported improvement compared with their preoperative status. Obesity, a prior Marshall-Marchetti-Krantz procedure, respiratory disease, and previous abdominal hysterectomy were associated with a lower long-term success rate in this cohort of patients. Concomitant vaginal hysterectomy was reported by the authors not to influence the long-term success rate of the procedure.

POTENTIAL COMPLICATIONS

Suprapubic wound infection should be extremely rare if monofilament nylon sutures are used and the

TABLE 28–1
Contemporary Series Reporting on the Stamey Needle Suspension for Stress Urinary Incontinence

Author	Study Design	Number of Patients	Follow-up	"Cured" According to Authors' Definition (%)	Comments
Hermieu 1994[4]	Uncontrolled observational study	55	21 months (mean)	76	16% of patients had combined SUI and urge incontinence
Valle Gerhold 1993[5]	Uncontrolled observational study	51	35 months (mean)	60	
Ralph 1993[8]	Uncontrolled observational study	24	23 months (mean)	80	Primary procedure for SUI
				52	Second or greater procedure for SUI
Conquy 1993[9]	Uncontrolled observational study	32	29 months (mean)	66	Also reports on Gittes and G-S techniques
Hilton 1991[15]	Uncontrolled observational study	100	27 months	53	Aged <65 years
				76	Aged >65 years Uses actuarial life table analysis
Ralph 1991[16]	Uncontrolled observational study	70	16 months	70	
Kil 1991[17]	Uncontrolled observational study	13	34 months	69	Also reports on Burch and Gittes techniques
Ashken 1990[25]	Uncontrolled observational study	100		80	Pad test for outcome measure

wounds are irrigated with antibiotic solution. Long-term erosion of the suture and bolster material may rarely occur and may cause acute onset of irritative voiding, urinary tract infection, hematuria, or stones in patients 2 to 36 months following the procedure.[24] Cystoscopically, one may see an acute inflammatory reaction of the urethral mucosa, urethral stones, or direct visualization of the foreign body. Bihrle and Tarantino described a successful outcome in such circumstances with endoscopic removal of the eroding sutures or pledgets.[24] One to two percent of patients undergoing the procedure have been reported to require removal of one of the sutures for pain or infection. In this instance, the offending suture may be removed without adversely affecting the outcome of continence. Rarely, the Dacron tubing may erode into the vagina, necessitating its removal. Long-term urinary retention may rarely occur if the sutures are tied too tight, and loosening the nylon loop that forms the suspension under local anesthesia has been reported to result in voiding without recurrence of stress incontinence.[20] When such conservative measures for treating urinary retention fail, the patient may require transvaginal urethrolysis and suture removal. Long-term failures, with recurrent stress incontinence, have been ascribed to suture pull-through and obesity.[19] Osteomyelitis following the Stamey needle suspension is extremely rare but has been reported.[27]

Overall, the Stamey needle suspension continues to be used worldwide for the successful treatment of stress urinary incontinence. Its use of foreign body material requires special care to prevent erosion and infection. Lower success rates have been reported in retrospective case series involving repeat surgery for stress incontinence. Recently, laparoscopic modifications of the Stamey needle suspension have been described, and these are discussed in Chapter 26. When the Stamey suspension is performed as a primary procedure for stress incontinence, high success rates have been reported; the procedure involves a short hospital stay and potentially low morbidity if meticulous technique is utilized.

REFERENCES

1. Stamey TA: Endoscopic suspension of the vesical neck for urinary incontinence. Surg Gynecol Obstet 136:547, 1973.
2. Walsh PC, Retik AB, Stamey TA, Vaughan ED Jr (eds): Campbell's Urology, 6th ed. Philadelphia, WB Saunders, 1992.
3. Stamey TA: Endoscopic suspension of the vesical neck for urinary incontinence in females; report of 203 consecutive patients. Ann Surg 192:465, 1980.
4. Hermieu JF, Van Glabeke E, Patard JJ, et al: Endoscopic retropubic colpopexy for stress urinary incontinence in women (Stamey's operation). 55 cases. Progr Urol, 4(1):63–69, 1994.
5. Valle Gerhold J, Murillo Perez C, Timon Garcia A, et al: Experience with endoscopic urethrocervicopexy: long-term results. Acta Urol Esp 17(9):595–597, 1993.
6. Orozco Farinas R, Osorio Acosta V, Capdevila Viciedo D, et al: The use of vagina and percutaneous surgery in stress urinary incontinence: Description, foundations, and indications. Arch Espanol Urol 46(10): 855–862, 1993.
7. Ralph G, Tamussino K, Michelitsch L: Treatment of stress incontinence with total prolapse of the uterus. Geburtsh Frauenheilk, 53(12):870–872, 1993.
8. Ralph G, Tamussino K, Michelitsch L: Surgical therapy of recurrent stress incontinence. Geburtsh Frauenheilk, 53(4):265–269, 1993.
9. Conquy S, Zerbib M, Younes E, et al: Retrospective comparative study of three surgical procedures in the treatment of urinary stress incontinence in women, apropos of 119 patients treated from 1985 to 1990. J Urol (Paris), 99(1):16–19, 1993.
10. Walker GT, Texter JH Jr: Success and patient satisfaction following the Stamey procedure for stress urinary incontinence. J Urol 147(6):1521–1523, 1992.
11. Cardozo L, Brindley GS: Endoscopically guided bladder neck suspension for continence in paraplegic women with implant driven micturition. Paraplegia 30(5):336–338, 1992.
12. Ganabathi K, Abrams P, Mundy AR, et al: Stamey-Martius procedure for severe genuine stress incontinence. Br J Urol 69(1):34–37, 1992.
13. Yamada T, Mizuo T, Kawakami S, et al: Application of transrectal ultrasonography in modified Stamey procedure for stress urinary incontinence. J Urol 146(6):1555–1558, 1991.
14. Ramon J, Mekras J, Webster GD: Transvaginal needle suspension procedures for recurrent stress incontinence. Urology 38(6):519–522, 1991.
15. Hilton P, Mayne CJ: The Stamey endoscopic bladder neck suspension: A clinical and urodynamic investigation, including actuarial follow-up over four years [see comments]. Br J Obstet Gynaecol 98(11):1141–1149, 1991.
16. Ralph G, Tamussino K: Endoscopic bladder neck suspension—clinical, urodynamic and radiologic results. Geburtsh Frauenheilk 51(10):830–833, 1991.
17. Kil PJ, Hoekstra JW, van der Meijden AP, et al: Transvaginal ultrasonography and urodynamic evaluation after suspension operations: Comparison among the Gittes, Stamey and Burch suspensions. J Urol 146(1):132–136, 1991.
18. Harrison SC, Abrams PH: The endoscopic video camera as an aid to the Stamey procedure. Br J Urol 66(3):329, 1990.
19. Varner RE: Retropubic long-needle suspension procedures for stress urinary incontinence [see comments]. Am J Obstet Gynecol 163(2):551–557, 1990.
20. Araki T, Takamoto H, Hara T, et al: The loop-loosening procedure for urination difficulties after Stamey suspension of the vesical neck [see comments]. J Urol 144(Pt 1):319–322, discussion 322–323, 1990.
21. Navalon P, Llopis B, Picurelli L, et al: Surgical treatment of urinary stress incontinence in women. Acta Urolog Esp 14(4):271–273, 1990.
22. Orozco Farinas R, Perez Poo HR: Modification of Stamey's endoscopic cervicopexy for stress urinary incontinence. Arch Esp Urol 43(2):117–120, 1990.
23. Orozco Farinas R, Oro Ortiz J: Anatomic effects of Stamey's urethrocystopexy as modified by Orozco and Perez Poo. Arch Esp Urol 43(2):121–124, 1990.
24. Bihrle W 3d, Tarantino AF: Complications of retropubic bladder neck suspension. Urology 35(3):213–214, 1990.
25. Ashken MH: Follow-up results with the Stamey operation for stress incontinence of urine. Br J Urol 65(2):168–169, 1990.
26. Griffith-Jones MD, Abrams PH: The Stamey endoscopic bladder neck suspension in the elderly. Br J Urol 65(2):170–172, 1990.
27. Wheeler JS Jr: Osteomyelitis of the pubis: Complication of a Stamey urethropexy. J Urol 151(6):1638–1640, 1994.
28. Stamey TA, Schaeffer AJ, Condy M: Clinical and roentgenographic evaluation of endoscopic suspension of the vesical neck for urinary incontinence. Surg Gynecol Obstet 140:355–361, 1975.

CHAPTER 29

Pathogenesis of Cystoceles— Anterior Colporrhaphy

Ashok Chopra, M.D.
Shlomo Raz, M.D.
Lynn Stothers, M.D., M.H.Sc., F.R.C.S.C.

As described in the chapters on enterocele and vault prolapse repair, cystocele describes a herniation of the bladder base. Cystocele represents an additional aspect of pelvic floor relaxation and prolapse and as such must be seen in the context of the status of the entire pelvic floor. The surgeon must also bear in mind that treatment of cystocele requires evaluation of voiding function. This chapter will discuss the pathogenesis, evaluation, and diagnosis of cystoceles. The techniques of anterior colporrhaphy, Kelly plication, and transabdominal repair will be reviewed. Transvaginal suspension techniques will be reviewed in Chapter 30.

Anatomy

Support of the bladder and anterior vaginal wall is primarily the function of the levator muscle group and its fascia. The specific anatomic features of this area are discussed in detail in Chapter 5; a brief overview is provided here. The levator muscle is composed of two groups of muscles: the pubococcygeus and the iliococcygeus. The pubococcygeus originates from the pubic bone and the anterior portion of the tendinous arch. It extends posteriorly to its insertion at the median raphe between the rectum and the coccyx. The iliococcygeus originates from the tendinous arch of the obturator and inserts into the anococcygeal ligament and the lateral aspect of the coccyx. A central hiatus in this muscle group, the levator hiatus, allows passage of the urethra, vagina, and rectum. Posterior to the rectum the levators form a supportive plate on which lie the rectum, upper vagina, bladder, and uterus.

The levator fascia has the principal responsibility for support of the urethra and bladder. This fascia inserts into the tendinous arch of the obturator laterally and has a vaginal side and an abdominal side. The abdominal leaf has been called the endopelvic fascia; the vaginal leaf is called the urethropelvic fascia at the level of the urethra and the vesicopelvic fascia at the level of the bladder. These layers fuse laterally at the edge of the levator hiatus and insert into the tendinous arch of the obturator internus.

The levator fascia has several significant condensations that provide support. The pubourethral ligaments suspend the midurethra from the undersurface of the pubic bone. The urethropelvic ligament extends to the lateral pelvic wall and suspends the urethra from the external meatus to the bladder neck. The cardinal ligaments extend laterally from the cervix and upper vagina and anchor these structures to the pelvic sidewall. The uterosacral ligaments attach to the posterolateral cervix and extend to the periosteum of the fourth sacral vertebra.

Cystoceles are divided into four groups. Grade 1 cystoceles imply descent toward the introitus. Grade 2 cystoceles are associated with descent to the introitus, and grade 3 with descent outside the introitus on strain. Grade 4 cystoceles exist when the cystocele extends outside the introitus at rest.

Cystoceles are also defined by the location of the primary defect. Isolated central cystoceles are found when the fascia spanning the levator hiatus becomes attenuated without compromising the lateral support (Fig. 29–1). These cystoceles account for 5 to 15% of cystoceles. Lateral cystoceles occur in the presence of weakness or disruption of the lateral attachments of the vesicopelvic or anterior cardinal ligaments to the pelvic sidewall (Fig. 29–2). These cystoceles account

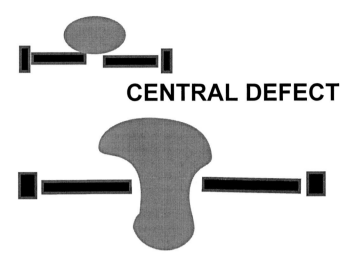

CENTRAL DEFECT

Figure 29-1 Depiction of central defect; area of fascial weakness is located in the midline. Diagram at upper left depicts normal bladder support.

for 70 to 80% of cystoceles.[1] Combinations of lateral and central defects may also occur and are especially common in patients with marked degrees of prolapse. Several authors also discuss the transverse defect (secondary to disruption of the fascial attachments to the pericervical fascia).[1]

Damage to the support of the bladder leads to cystocele formation. The most common cause is obstetric damage. Other causes of prolapse of the bladder are described in the chapter on uterine prolapse (Chapter 43) and underscore the relationships of various manifestations of pelvic relaxation. Indeed, up to 60% of patients with grade 3 cystoceles have other forms of concomitant pelvic prolapse (e.g., rectocele, enterocele, uterine prolapse, vaginal vault prolapse); 95% of patients with grade 4 cystocele have other forms of concomitant pelvic prolapse.[2]

Signs and Symptoms

Because smaller cystoceles tend to be asymptomatic, repair is not generally required. When grade 1 cystoceles are found in association with urethral hypermobility and stress incontinence, therapy should be directed toward treatment of the incontinence alone. Larger cystoceles, however, are frequently quite symptomatic, common complaints being dyspareunia and vaginal bulging. Gardy and colleagues described 33 patients with large cystoceles. In her review she noted that 32 of 33 patients had symptoms or urodynamic evidence of stress incontinence, 18 had significant (at least 80 ml) residual urine, and 24 had urgency incontinence.[3] Stress incontinence may be associated commonly with coexisting rotational descent of the bladder neck and also with large amounts of residual urine.[3, 4] Retention of urine may result from kinking at the bladder neck; this situation is often found when the urethra has been fixed

in place by previous surgery. In these patients incomplete emptying of the bladder may lead to recurrent urinary infection. To minimize the obstructive effect many of these patients manually reduce the cystocele to facilitate emptying. Silent hydronephrosis secondary to ureteral obstruction may occur.

Diagnosis

Physical examination follows many of the caveats outlined in the chapter on vault prolapse. Thorough examination in the sitting and standing positions will provide a great deal of information. Examination of the patient is best performed with the bladder full. Evaluation in the standing position will reveal a mass descending toward the introitus. In the supine position with strain a mass can similarly be seen extending from the anterior wall. If the source of the prolapse is uncertain, examination with a half speculum is often helpful. Determination of the type of cystocele (i.e., lateral or central) can also be made at this point. Examination with the speculum may reveal loss of the lateral supports of the vagina (the H configuration), suggesting a lateral defect. Use of the vaginal defect analyzer is a valuable tool at this point. If the surgeon supports the base of the bladder and no midline descent is found, the patient's defect is central.[5] If the surgeon supports the lateral vaginal attachments with the analyzer and finds prolapse of the bladder between the leaves of the analyzer, a central defect is present. In contrast, if the prolapse resolves with support of the lateral vaginal attachments, a lateral defect is present.[6] Similarly, a tongue blade may be used in place of the defect analyzer.[7] A lateral defect is much more likely to be accompanied by urethral descent, vaginal eversion, and uterine hypermobility.[8] Marked cystoceles (grade 4) present with a combination of these two defects.

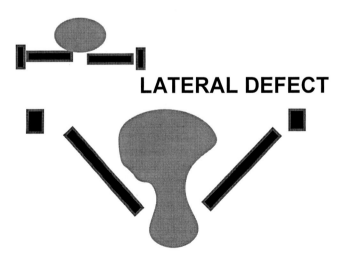

LATERAL DEFECT

Figure 29-2 Depiction of lateral defect; area of weakness is at the lateral attachments to the tendinous arch of the obturator. Diagram at upper left depicts normal bladder support.

Cystography can show the anatomy in the standing position and is useful in analyzing the cystocele. In patients with an isolated central cystocele the urethra maintains a normal relationship with the pubic symphysis and the posterior wall of the bladder. With lateral defects this relationship between the urethra and pubis is lost, and a greater portion of the bladder will prolapse.[8]

Once again, it is important to analyze the cystocele in terms of the entire syndrome of pelvic floor relaxation. Coexisting vault prolapse, urethral hypermobility, and posterior vaginal wall defects must be addressed. The status of the patient's continence must also be noted. Gardy and colleagues stated that "symptoms of stress incontinence are not a reliable indication of the presence or absence of urethral dysfunction in patients with cystoceles."[3] Clearly, if the patient is wet, some type of incontinence procedure is required. However, de novo stress incontinence may appear after repair of a cystocele, partly owing to loss of the obstructive ball-valving effect found with large cystoceles. To avoid this outcome consideration should always be given to providing bladder neck support when a cystocele is repaired in the presence of malposition or hypermobility of the urethra or bladder neck.

Techniques of Surgical Repair

Three primary types of cystocele repair are generally described in the literature: the Kelly plication–anterior colporrhaphy and its modifications, the transabdominal suspension procedures, and the transvaginal suspension procedures. Until Richardson published his landmark paper in 1976 it was thought by most surgeons that midline defects were the cause of most cystoceles.[9] As such, anterior repair and its modifications remained the standard for repair.[7] In 1976 Richardson described the various types and locations of fascial defects involved in the pathogenesis of cystoceles.[7] In his experience, 70 to 80% of all cystoceles resulted from damage to the lateral support. Richardson's technique of transabdominal suspension was aimed specifically at repairing the lateral defect. Other authors followed his lead, using various techniques of transabdominal and transvaginal suspension procedures to repair cystoceles secondary to weakness of the lateral support.

This section addresses only techniques of transabdominal cystocele repair and techniques of anterior colporrhaphy (including the Kelly plication). Transvaginal modifications of operative procedures for cystocele repair are discussed in Chapter 30. The reader is referred to the chapters on vault prolapse and enterocele (Chapters 42 and 44) for modifications in approach in patients with these coexisting pathologies.

ABDOMINAL PROCEDURES FOR CYSTOCELE REPAIR WITH OR WITHOUT STRESS INCONTINENCE

Abdominal approaches allow fixation of the vaginal wall to the lateral pelvic sidewall. As such, they are used in patients with lateral defects; central defects should be repaired transvaginally. Indeed, the plication or reapproximation of the vesicopelvic fascia and cardinal ligaments that is required in a central defect repair cannot be achieved transabdominally. The two primary procedures for transabdominal cystocele repair are the Burch colposuspension and the paravaginal repair described by Richardson and Turner-Warwick. These two techniques differ primarily in the location of the suspension. In the Burch suspension the vaginal wall and fascia are opposed to Cooper's ligaments; in the paravaginal repair the vaginal wall and fascia are approximated to the obturator fascia.

A modification of the Burch procedure is described in the chapter on abdominal suspension procedures (Chapter 25). The paravaginal procedures are performed with the patient in the supine position with access to the vagina. In these repairs entrance into the extraperitoneal retropubic space is achieved in the same fashion as with the Burch procedure. The endopelvic fascia and obturator vessels are initially exposed, and the assistant surgeon's fingers are used to elevate the vagina. The primary surgeon next places a series of interrupted sutures through the lateral vagina and vesicopelvic ligaments along the length of the proximal urethra and bladder. In the Richardson procedure the other ends of the sutures are placed through the obturator fascia; in the Turner-Warwick procedure the lateral vaginal wall is brought through an incision in the endopelvic fascia to reach the obturator fascia.[7]

The basic steps of the Richardson procedure have been outlined by Youngblood.[9] Youngblood suggests the use of permanent 2–0 polyester braided plain (Dacron) suture and small needles. If the uterus is present, total hysterectomy is performed (if indicated). Attention should be given to careful cuff suspension. Uterosacral plication is performed to prevent enterocele formation. The space of Retzius is entered and the bladder reflected medially, exposing the anterior lateral vaginal wall. The left forefinger is inserted into the vagina to direct the needle. At this point a strategic ("key") stitch is placed opposite the vesical neck in the anterolateral vaginal sulcus. This suture should be placed through the vaginal mucosa, being careful to avoid large longitudinal vessels. The needle is passed through the tendinous arch about 1.5 to 2 cm below the obturator foramen, thus completing the key stitch. In a similar fashion two to four sutures are placed distally and one or two sutures proximally. Finally, all the sutures are tied at one time (Fig. 29–3).

Richardson reported continence in approximately 95% of 233 patients. Ten of his patients developed recurrent prolapse. Richardson believed that in four

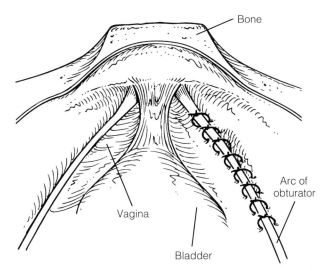

Figure 29-3 Technique of Richardson repair. Sutures approximate the lateral vaginal sulcus and the tendinous arch.

of these the poor results were due to technical errors, one had recurrence of the original defect, four developed central defects after surgery, and one developed a contralateral defect after unilateral repair of the lateral defect.[10]

KELLY PLICATION AND ANTERIOR COLPORRHAPHY (ANTERIOR REPAIR)

The most common operative procedure for repair of a cystocele is the Kelly-type plication with anterior colporrhaphy (anterior repair). These techniques involve midline plication of the fascia and as such are ideally suited for repair of central defects. Kelly initially described his procedure in 1914 as a procedure for the treatment of incontinence (not cystocele).[11] He incised the vaginal wall in the midline and then performed lateral dissection of it for 2 to 2.5 cm at the level of the bladder neck. The "lateral tissues" were reapproximated with silk or linen suture, taking 1.5-cm bites of tissue (Fig. 29–4). Of historical interest, in Kelly's follow-up 80% of his 20 patients reported improved continence. His paper did not comment on anatomic resolution of bladder prolapse.

Nichols points out that the Kelly stitch is in essence a subvesical urethral plication stitch and advocates its use when urethral funneling is present.[12] This suture actually reduces the diameter of the urethra at the site of funneling (in contrast to the pubourethral plication stitch); as such, Nichols recommends placement of a 16 Fr catheter prior to the placement and tying of sutures. He believes that this maneuver prevents stenosis and ensures a urethral diameter of at least 16 Fr.[12]

Similarly, anterior colporrhaphy involves exposure of the pubocervical fascia with reapproximation or plication in the midline with absorbable sutures. In contrast, however, dissection and repair are not limited to the area of the bladder neck but involve the entire anterior vaginal wall. One technique of anterior colporrhaphy is described as follows.[13] The patient is initially placed in the dorsal lithotomy position. If vaginal hysterectomy is to be performed, this is done before the cystocele is repaired. Alternatively, uterine-sparing procedures such as the Manchester procedure may be performed (see Chapter 43). The reader is referred to Chapters 42 and 44 on vault prolapse and enterocele for modifications of this technique when these conditions coexist.

After infiltration of the anterior vaginal wall, the vaginal wall is undermined using scissors in the midline from the underlying vesicopelvic fascia. Subsequently, the anterior vaginal wall is opened from the apex of the vagina to the area of the urethrovesical junction. The cut edges of the vaginal wall are grasped and elevated with Allis clamps, and the vaginal wall is dissected laterally from the underlying fascia. At this point, a Foley catheter is inserted, and the bladder is drained.

Attention is first turned to the area of the bladder neck. At this point, as described previously, Nichols suggests use of the Kelly stitch if funneling of the urethra is present. Next, the fibromuscular tissue of the posteroinferior aspect of the pubic symphysis (the urethropelvic fascia) is grasped with Allis clamps. Plicating sutures are used to approximate this tissue; this maneuver will fix the bladder neck in position. At this point a second plicating stitch may be placed if further support of the bladder neck is thought to be required. Nichols has advocated the use of long-

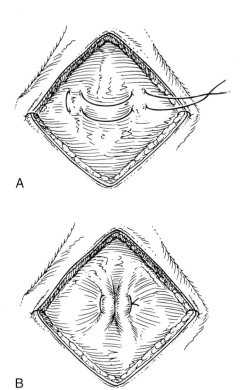

Figure 29-4 Depiction of Kelly plication. (Modified from Kelly HA, et al: Urinary incontinence in women without manifest injury to the bladder. Surg Gynecol Obstet 18:444, 1914.)

lasting synthetic absorbable suture such as polydiaxone (PDS) or polyglyconate (Maxon); Gershenson and colleagues recommend use of 2–0 or 0 polyglycolic acid suture.[13, 14]

After the urethrovesical junction has been supported, attention is turned to the cystocele repair. To reduce the cystocele the attenuated pubovesical (vesicopelvic) fascia is plicated in the midline. It is important to reconstruct the full length of the anterior vaginal wall to the level of the cardinal ligament.[14] If the cystocele is very large, a Gersuny ("tobacco pouch") pursestring suture reinforced by the plicating sutures may be used; additionally, a synthetic mesh may be used to assist with the repair (we prefer Dexon).[14] Finally, the redundant vaginal mucosa is excised, and the edges of the vaginal wall are reapproximated using a continuous 3–0 absorbable suture. Care must be taken to avoid excessive resection of tissue at this point. A vaginal pack is generally left in place for 24 hours postoperatively. Of note, Symmonds and Jordan discuss the importance of avoiding overcorrection of the cystocele because obliteration of the posterior urethrovesical angle may occur with resultant stress incontinence.[14]

Low and Ross and Singleton reported continence rates of 48 to 60% after use of anterior colporrhaphy for treatment of incontinence associated with prolapse.[15, 16] They did not comment on the anatomic resolution of the cystocele.[15, 16] Beck and associates reported a series of 519 patients who were treated with modifications of the anterior colporrhaphy over a 25-year period.[17] In their series some patients had prolapse only, some had incontinence only, and some had a combination of both. Patients with poor tissue (as determined by the primary surgeon) at the time of surgery were treated with alternative techniques. In the first group of 77 patients with stress incontinence a Kelly-Kennedy type of anterior repair was performed using chromic catgut for fascial plication. The results in terms of correction of incontinence were discouraging, with only 75% of the patients becoming dry postoperatively. At this point these authors modified their procedure, treating patients with urethroceles with a vaginal retropubic urethropexy (they also changed the suture material to polyglycolic acid and used suprapubic catheters). Following these changes, continence rates improved to 91% in 122 patients. Overall, in the group of 519 patients (242 of whom were operated on for prolapse only), only 8 patients required repeat surgery for prolapse. Ten percent of 219 patients undergoing anterior colporrhaphy for prolapse without preoperative incontinence were incontinent postoperatively. Of 436 patients, 28 (6%) developed de novo instability. In three patients postoperative onset of spontaneous voiding was delayed for more than 7 days.

Gardy and colleagues reported the results of anterior colporrhaphy (with or without urethral suspension or sling) in 12 patients with grade 1 or 2 cystoceles and in 30 patients with grade 3 or 4 cystoceles (29 of whom underwent bladder neck suspension); mean follow-up time was 24.6 months. Patients with grade 1 or 2 cystoceles had no postoperative stress incontinence and no recurrence of cystocele. Among the patients with grade 3 or 4 cystoceles there were two failures in regard to continence; three patients developed recurrent cystoceles. Of note in this study was the fact that three patients underwent colpocleisis.[3]

In summary, anterior repair and its modifications are successful in the treatment of prolapse in patients in whom the tissues are deemed adequate. Unfortunately, without urethropexy, stress incontinence occurs frequently in as many as 40% of patients.[9] These techniques do not support the urethra in a high retropubic position, a fact that has caused many surgeons to modify their techniques to include some form of bladder neck support, sling, or urethropexy. Finally, anterior colporrhaphy does not address a lateral defect of bladder support (indeed, anterior colporrhaphy may further avulse the lateral attachments from the tendinous arch of the obturator).[9] It is unclear why this type of repair is often successful in treatment of lateral defects. It has been postulated that tightening the fascia underneath the bladder reduces herniation when the lateral attachments are only partially avulsed; late failures of this repair become manifest when the lateral injury is more complete.[10]

Conclusions

Because of the limitations of anterior repair, we tailor our repair to match the type of defect present (i.e., central, lateral, or combined). The operative technique is dictated primarily by this determination. Central defects are repaired by plication or reapproximation of the vesicopelvic ligaments (pubocervical fascia) and the cardinal-uterosacral ligament complex. Lateral defects are repaired by suspending the vesicopelvic ligament, urethropelvic ligament, and cardinal-sacrouterine ligament complex toward the anterior abdominal wall. For combined defects (classically, grade 4 cystocele) we use both central and lateral defect repairs. As emphasized earlier, urethral or bladder neck malposition or hypermobility must be addressed at the time of repair to avoid postoperative incontinence; we use a modified vaginal sling to treat this problem. Specific details of these repairs (six-corner bladder suspension and formal grade 4 cystocele repair) are discussed in Chapter 30.

REFERENCES

1. Macer G: Transabdominal repair of cystocele, a 20-year experience compared with the traditional vaginal approach. Am J Obstet Gynecol 131:203, 1978.
2. Unpublished data, UCLA Medical Center, 1995.
3. Gardy M, Kozminsky M, Delancey J, et al: Stress incontinence and cystoceles. J Urol 145:1211, 1991.

4. Nichols DH: Vaginal Surgery, 3rd ed. Baltimore, Williams & Wilkins, 1989.

5. Shull B: Clinical evaluation of women with pelvic support defects. Clin Obstet Gynecol 36(4):939, 1993.

6. Baden WF, Walker TA: Surgical Repair of Vaginal Defects. Philadelphia, JB Lippincott, 1992.

7. Richardson AC: A new look at pelvic relaxation. Am J Obstet Gynecol 126:568, 1976.

8. Raz S: Operative repair of rectocele, enterocele and cystocele. Adv Urol 5:121, 1992.

9. Youngblood JP: Paravaginal repair for cystourethrocele. Clin Ob-Gyn 36(3):960, 1993.

10. Richardson AC, Edmonds PB, Williams NL, et al: Treatment of stress urinary incontinence due to paravaginal fascial defect. Obstet Gynecol 57(3):357, 1981.

11. Kelly HA, Dumm WM: Urinary incontinence in women without manifest injury to the bladder. Surg Gynecol Obstet 18:444, 1914.

12. Nichols DH: Surgery for pelvic floor disorders. Surg Clin North Am 71:927, 1991.

13. Gershenson DM, DeCherney AH, Curry SL (eds): Operative Gynecology. Philadelphia, WB Saunders, 1993.

14. Symmonds RE, Jordan LT: Iatrogenic stress incontinence of urine. Am J Obstet Gynecol 82:1231, 1961.

15. Low JA: Management of anatomic urinary incontinence by vaginal repair. Am J Obstet Gynecol 97:308, 1967.

16. Ross RA, Shingleton HM: Vaginal prolapse and stress urinary incontinence. West Va Med J 65:77, 1969.

17. Beck RP, McCormick S, Nordstrom L: A 25-year experience with 519 anterior colporrhaphy procedures. Obstet Gynecol 78(6):1011, 1991.

BIBLIOGRAPHY

Bergman A, Ballard CA, Koonings PP: Comparison of three different surgical procedures for genuine stress incontinence: A prospective randomized study. Am J Obstet Gynecol 160:1102, 1989.

Borstad E, Skrede M, Rud T: Failure to predict and attempts to explain urinary stress incontinence following vaginal repair in continent women by using a modified lateral urethrocystography. Acta Obstet Gynecol Scand 70(6):501, 1991.

Chan YT, Ng WD, Yin TF, Kwok TF: Complete prolapse of the urinary bladder. Br J Urol 66(4):436–437, 1990.

Harris TA, Bent AE: Genital prolapse with and without urinary incontinence. J Reprod Med 35(8):792–798, 1990.

Leach GE, Zimmern P, Staskin D, et al: Surgery for pelvic prolapse. Semin Urol 4:43–50, 1986.

Lee RA: Vaginal hysterectomy with repair of enterocele, cystocele, and rectocele. Clin Obstet Gynecol 36(4):967–975, 1993.

Nichols DH: Gynecological and Obstetric Surgery. Chicago, Mosby Year Book, 1987, 334.

Nichols DH: Surgery for pelvic floor disorders. Surg Clin North Am 71(5):927–946, 1991.

Nichols DH: Vaginal prolapse affecting bladder function. Urol Clin North Am 12:329–338, 1985.

Raz S: Modified bladder neck suspension for female stress incontinence. Urology 17:82–85, 1981.

Raz S: Vaginal surgery for stress incontinence. J Am Geriatr Soc 38(3):345–347, 1990.

Raz S, Erickson DR: SEAPI QMM incontinence classification system. Neurourol Urodyn 11:187–199, 1992.

Raz S, Golomb J, Klutke C: Four corner bladder and urethral suspension for moderate cystocele. J Urol 142:712–715, 1989.

Raz S, Little NA, Juma S, Sussman EM: Repair of severe anterior vaginal wall prolapse (grade IV cystourethrocele). J Urol 146(4):988–992, 1991.

Rosenzweig BA, Soffici AR, Thomas S, Bhatia NN: Urodynamic evaluation of voiding in women with cystocele. J Reprod Med 37(2):162–166, 1992.

Sanz L: Gynecological Surgery. New York, Medical Economics Books, 1988.

Thompson J (ed): TeLinde's Operative Gynecology, 7th ed. Philadelphia, JB Lippincott, 1992.

Tovell H: Gynecological Operations. New York, Harper & Row, 1978.

Wahle GR, Young GP, Raz S: Vaginal surgery for stress urinary incontinence [editorial]. Urology 43(4):416, 1994.

Wiskind AK, Creighton SM, Stanton SL: The incidence of genital prolapse after the Burch colposuspension. Am J Obstet Gynecol 167(2):399–404, 1992.

Yang A, Mostwin JL, Rosenshein NB, Zerhouni EA: Pelvic floor descent in women: dynamic evaluation with fast MR imaging and cinematic display. Radiology 179(1):25–33, 1991.

Youngblood JP: Paravaginal repair for cystourethrocele. Clin Obstet Gynecol 36(4):960–966, 1993.

Raz Techniques for Anterior Vaginal Wall Repair

Shlomo Raz, M.D.
Lynn Stothers, M.D., M.H.Sc., F.R.C.S.C.
Ashok Chopra, M.D.

Urinary incontinence in women can result from either detrusor or sphincteric dysfunction. Sphincteric incompetence originates from either anatomic malposition of an intact sphincteric unit (anatomic incontinence) or from intrinsic sphincteric dysfunction (ISD) secondary to multiple surgeries, neurogenic disease, radiation therapy, or direct urethral trauma. With anatomic incontinence there is hypermobility of the midurethral segment and bladder neck. The goal of surgery for anatomic incontinence is to reposition the bladder neck and urethra in a high retropubic position. However, when the sphincter is intrinsically damaged, mere restoration of position may fail to cure the problem. In such a case, the goal of surgery is to provide increased urethral resistance by improving urethral coaptation and compression.

Although this chapter focuses on the treatment of stress urinary incontinence (SUI), it is important for the clinician to understand that stress incontinence is often only one manifestation of pelvic prolapse. The degree of cystocele, rectocele, and uterine prolapse should be considered at the time of patient assessment because this dictates the appropriate surgical option for correction of stress incontinence. One of the advantages of the vaginal approach to the cure of stress incontinence is that it also permits simultaneous correction of all forms of pelvic prolapse.

Many options, both nonsurgical and surgical, exist for the treatment of SUI. We focus this discussion on surgical reconstruction and, more specifically, on vaginal approaches to the correction of stress incontinence and anterior vaginal wall prolapse. The following approach is the surgical method preferred by the authors, but overall, the best procedure for the cure of stress incontinence is the one that works best for the individual surgeon.

ETIOLOGY   The cause of stress incontinence and pelvic prolapse is often multifactorial in any given patient. Mechanical, neurologic, hormonal, and biochemical changes have all been shown in the human to be potential causal factors (Table 30–1).

Trauma to the pelvic floor during vaginal delivery is an important risk factor in the genesis of stress incontinence. Cross-sectional studies have demonstrated that the incidence of stress incontinence in the female population increases during pregnancy and persists in 3% of healthy young women postpartum.[1] The exact mechanism causing stress incontinence in this group is debatable. Some pelvic floor neurophysiologic studies have shown denervation-reinnervation patterns in the urethral striated sphincter musculature. This finding is not consistent, however, and more recent studies have contradicted this theory. Barnick and colleagues performed a prospective observational study to evaluate denervation injury using needle electromyography.[2] They found no differences in the mean motor unit potential duration, the number of changes in polarity, or the amplitude of individual motor unit potentials between stress incontinent women and controls. Deindl and colleagues studied conduction of the pubococcygeus muscles with wire electrodes in nulliparous continent and stress incontinent parous women.[3] Muscle activation patterns in stress incontinent parous women were found to be similar to those of controls with two exceptions. The holding time of a voluntary squeeze was decreased in parous compared with nulliparous continent women. Asymmetrical and uncoordinated levator activation patterns were also seen in parous incontinent women. In addition, conduction of impulses along the pudendal nerves has been studied. Following delivery, intravaginal pressures are de-

TABLE 30–1
**Potential Etiologic Factors for
Stress Incontinence**

1. Anatomic factors following childbirth[3]
2. Thinning of the pelvic floor musculature
3. Stretch Neuropathy[2]
4. Decreased collagen synthesis in the urethra
5. Previous pelvic surgery
6. Smoking[6]
7. Chronic constipation[7]
8. Degeneration of the pelvic floor with aging
9. Estrogen deficiency

creased. Although reduced functional urethral length and urethral closing pressure have been demonstrated in some postpartum urodynamic studies, these findings have not been consistent.

Biochemical collagen composition in incontinent women is different from that in continent controls in several studies. Falconer and colleagues suggested that connective tissue metabolism may result in decreased collagen synthesis in incontinent women compared with controls based on fibroblast cultures.[4] Thirty percent less collagen was found in skin biopsies in these women compared to controls; however, general protein synthesis was similar in the two groups. Other authors have focused on the specific type of collagen that may be affected in stress incontinent patients. Bergman and associates studied type III collagen content of the perineal skin, uterosacral ligaments, and round ligaments.[5] They found that type III collagen was significantly reduced in patients with stress incontinence compared to those

with pelvic prolapse alone or controls with no history of incontinence or prolapse.

Chronic mechanical stressors to the pelvic floor other than childbirth have been identified in epidemiologic studies as potential causal factors for SUI. These include smoking and chronic constipation.[6, 7] When parity was controlled for in both studies, an increased risk of stress incontinence persisted, suggesting an independent effect.

The onset or worsening of stress incontinence with menopause can be recognized clinically in many patients. For example, nulliparous women may develop stress incontinence at the time of menopause without other risk factors. Estrogen therapy may result in clinical improvement in some patients with stress incontinence. Animal studies support this clinical observation. Administration of estrogens to ovariectomized virginal rabbits resulted in increased urethral sensitivity to noradrenaline, increased evoked contractions, and increased urethral responsiveness to nerve stimulation.[8] Administration of estrogen in combination with progesterone did not negate any of these effects.

Classification of Stress Incontinence

Several classifications of stress incontinence used in the modern literature are outlined in Table 30–2. We prefer to use the terms anatomic incontinence and intrinsic sphincter dysfunction. Stress incontinence may be caused by anatomic malposition of an intact sphincter unit (anatomic incontinence, AI) or by in-

TABLE 30–2
Classification of Stress Urinary Incontinence (SUI)

Blaivas	McGuire	Raz
Type O: h/o SUI but no objective SUI. Bladder neck and urethra open during stress.	Type O No true SUI.	Anatomic—due to malposition of intact sphincter unit.
Type I: Bladder neck and urethra open and descend < 2 cm during stress with minimal or no cystocele.	Type I SUI, minimal hypermobility, with/without cystocele, UCP > 20 cm H_2O pressure in supine position at rest.	
Type IIA: Bladder neck and urethra open and descend > 2 cm during stress with cystocele.	Type II SUI, marked hypermobility with rotational descent and horizontal position of the urethra at peak abdominal pressure. UCP > 20 cm, H_2O pressure in supine position at rest.	
Type IIB: Bladder neck and urethra below symphysis at rest. During stress may/may not descend.		
Type III: Bladder neck and urethra are open at rest in the absence of detrusor contraction.	Type III Prior failed bladder neck suspension or UCP < 20 cm H_2O.	Intrinsic sphincter dysfunction—due to malfunction of the sphincter with/without hypermobility.

Abbreviations: h/o history of; UCP, urethral closing pressure.
From Walsh PC, Retik AB, Stamey TA, Vaughan ED Jr (eds): Campbell's Urology, 6th ed. Philadelphia, WB Saunders, 1992.

trinsic sphincteric dysfunction (ISD). ISD may exist with or without associated anatomic abnormalities. A common associated finding in patients with stress incontinence is urgency incontinence, which occurs in approximately 55% of patients.

Anatomic incontinence is the most common type of stress incontinence and is seen in about 90% of all patients with primary stress incontinence. It results from loss of pelvic support of the bladder neck and urethra owing to a number of factors including birth trauma, hysterectomy, lack of estrogen, pelvic denervation, congenital weakness, or aging. A combination of factors frequently exists in a single patient.

In contrast to anatomic incontinence, the cause of ISD is related to damage to the sphincter following prior operations, direct urethral trauma, radiation therapy, or neurogenic disorders. The hallmarks of this form of incontinence are a bladder neck and urethra that are fixed and open, and a low abdominal leak point pressure. This form of incontinence is classified as type III in the McGuire and Blaivas classifications. No pathognomonic test distinguishes this type of incontinence. Rather, the diagnosis is made by a combination of clinical, urodynamic, endoscopic, and radiologic findings. Classically, the therapeutic options for ISD are different from those for anatomic incontinence, and thus the clinical distinction of the two is important. Recent advances have led to a potential to treat both disorders with the use of an anterior vaginal wall sling. This surgical method is discussed in Chapter 35.

Diagnosis of Stress Incontinence

The various ways of diagnosing stress incontinence vary from the simplistic—asking the patient if she leaks urine without warning during activities—to the complex, using multichannel videourodynamic techniques. A detailed discussion of the diagnosis of SUI is found in Chapter 8. Briefly, it is our practice to perform a comprehensive urologic history noting the frequency, type, and severity of urinary incontinence. The presence of any risk factors for stress incontinence as previously outlined in this chapter is determined. Details about any previous surgical procedures for SUI and prolapse are noted. A subjective SEAPI classification score is assigned, and the patient completes a quality of life assessment form.[9] A physical examination including a complete pelvic examination is performed. Following a bimanual examination of the pelvis a single-bladed vaginal speculum is used to assess anterior vaginal wall, posterior vaginal wall, and vault prolapse. Any anatomic distortion due to previous surgical scars in the vagina is noted along with signs of estrogen deficiency. Cystoscopy is performed using 2% lidocaine lubricant for anesthesia. The 0-degree lens is used to inspect the urethra. Urethral support, position, and potential hypermobility are documented. Inspection for any intrinsic urethral lesions and urethral distortion due

to previously placed sutures to correct SUI is carried out. The urethra is palpated manually over the cystoscope to assess for urethral or periurethral masses. The bladder is then inspected with 30- and 70-degree lenses. The size, shape, position, and number of ureteral orifices are noted along with any changes to the mucosa of the bladder. If the patient has undergone previous procedures for correction of stress incontinence the bladder should be inspected carefully for any misplaced sutures. A Marshall test for urinary leakage is then performed.

Videourodynamic examination is performed with the patient in the standing position using a slow-fill rate to instill contrast medium into the bladder. A 7 Fr urethral pressure–monitoring catheter and a rectal pressure balloon are used. The video portion of the study represents the physical examination in the standing position and provides information that complements the physical examination of the patient in the supine position. A cystometrogram, voiding cystourethrogram, and invasive pressure flow studies are included. Following the video study an objective SEAPI score is assigned.[9]

Measuring Outcomes Before and After Treatment of Stress Incontinence

There is currently a voluminous literature on both the surgical and nonsurgical treatment of stress urinary incontinence. A significant problem in the review of this literature becomes evident when one begins to examine the various ways in which the outcome of treatment is measured. For example, a successful outcome of therapy has been defined by various authors as less than one episode of incontinence per week, less than one episode of incontinence per day, use of no pads per day, less than 2 wet pads per day, complete dryness at 3, 6, or 12 months following therapy, and so on. It is evident that it is impossible to make valid comparisons of treatments within and between institutions when such discrepancies in measurement exist. Recent advances in clinical epidemiology have led to sophisticated validation processes for clinical outcome scores. Such outcome scores are particularly relevant to the treatment of stress incontinence because the aim of therapy is based on the ability to improve the patient's quality of life.

The SEAPI incontinence classification system is a scoring system designed for and validated in incontinent individuals. The system is analogous to the TNM system for tumor staging, and each aspect of the score is graded from 0 to 3. Zero indicates no symptom, problem, or abnormality, and 1, 2, and 3 represent correspondingly increased symptoms. When applicable, both a subjective and an objective score can be graded separately for a given patient. Five domains are covered by the SEAPI score as represented by the score name: S represents stress activity-related incontinence; E, emptying ability; A, anatomy; P, protection, and I, inhibition. The score is described in more detail in Tables 30–3 and 30–4.

In addition to a pre- and post-treatment SEAPI score, we use the SEAPI quality of life score (Table 30–5). The quality of life score covers numerous domains including emotional well-being, interpersonal relationships, work, financial factors, physical health, recreation, and overall satisfaction with life as these factors relate to incontinence. The test should be completed by the patients themselves and is not meant to be administered by the practitioner.

Various other methods of measuring the outcomes of stress incontinence therapies are shown in Table 30–6. The pyridium pad test and quantitative weighing of pads to detect urinary leakage has been compared by Wall and colleagues.[10] In this study 23 normal volunteers without SUI were compared with 18 women with urodynamically proven stress incontinence. The accuracy of the qualitative pad test with pyridium staining was compared to the quantitative pad weight to detect the presence of SUI in the two groups. The authors found that in the group with stress incontinence all 18 women had positive pyridium pad tests and positive pad weight gains of over 1.0 g. However, 52% of healthy volunteers had a positive pyridium pad test also. The mean pad weight gain in the volunteer group was 0.1 g. Therefore, the pyridium pad test had a high false-positive rate in continent volunteers and is therefore misleading as an outcome measure if pad weighing tests are not performed in addition.

TABLE 30–3
SEAPI Incontinence Score—Subjective

S	Stress-Related Leakage	0 = No urine loss 1 = Loss with strenuous activity 2 = Loss with moderate activity 3 = Loss with minimal activity or gravitational incontinence
E	Emptying Ability	0 = No obstructive symptoms 1 = Minimal symptoms 2 = Significant symptoms 3 = Voiding only in dribbles or urinary retention
A	Anatomy	0 = No descent during strain 1 = Descent, not to introitus 2 = Descent through introitus with strain 3 = Through introitus without strain
P	Protection	0 = Never used 1 = Used only for certain occasions 2 = Used only for occasional accidents 3 = Used continually for frequent accidents or constant leaking
I	Inhibition	0 = No urgency incontinence 1 = Rare urgency incontinence 2 = Urgency incontinence once a week 3 = Urgency incontinence at least once a day

TABLE 30–4
SEAPI Incontinence Score— Objective Measures

S	Stress-Related Leakage	Observe for leak during Valsalva and cough 0 = No leak 1 = Leak at >80 cm water 2 = Leak at 30–80 cm water 3 = Leak at <30 cm water
E	Emptying Ability	Postvoid residual should be verified by repeat measurement 0 = 0–60 ml 1 = 61–100 ml 2 = 101–200 ml 3 = >200 ml or unable to void
A	Anatomy	Position of bladder neck relative to symphysis during cough or Valsalva seen on lateral cystogram 0 = Above symphysis with strain 1 = <2 cm below symphysis with strain 2 = >2 cm below symphysis with strain 3 = >2 cm below symphysis at rest
P	Protection	0 = Never used 1 = Used only for certain occasions 2 = Used daily for occasional accidents 3 = Used continually for frequent accidents or constant leaking
I	Inhibition	Involuntary rise in pressure during cystometry 0 = No pressure rise 1 = Rise late in filling (>500 ml) 2 = Medium fill rise (150–500 ml) 3 = Early rise (<150 ml)

Surgical Correction

The treatment options for SUI discussed in the literature may be classified as either medical or surgical approaches. A summary of treatment options is provided in Table 30–7. The remainder of this chapter is focused on our personal surgical approach using a transvaginal surgical technique to correct hypermobility-related stress urinary incontinence and anterior vaginal wall prolapse. Other techniques of needle suspension such as the Stamey procedure and the no-incision Gittes suspension as well as other techniques of cystocele repair (such as anterior repair) are described in detail elsewhere in this textbook. Because stress urinary incontinence is one symptom of pelvic dysfunction and prolapse we include a discussion of surgical correction of other anterior vaginal wall prolapse (cystocele).

RAZ BLADDER NECK SUSPENSION

In 1981 and 1985 Raz described two modifications of the Pereyra bladder neck suspension.[11] This procedure is best suited for patients with anatomic incontinence due to urethral and bladder neck hypermobility with minimal or no cystocele. As described in Chapter 35, more common than Raz bladder neck suspension is use of a vaginal wall sling for patients

TABLE 30–5
SEAPI Incontinence Quality of Life Score

1. How much does your incontinence interfere with your ability to perform your usual daily tasks?
   - 0 = No interference; I can do all of the tasks that I need to.
   - 1 = Minimal interference; I can do most of the tasks that I need to.
   - 2 = Moderate interference; there are some tasks that I cannot do.
   - 3 = Severe interference; I cannot do most tasks.

2. How much does your incontinence interfere with your ability to engage in physical recreation (sports, dancing, etc.)?
   - 0 = No interference; I can do all the activities that I want to do.
   - 1 = Minimal interference; I can do most of the activities that I want to do.
   - 2 = Moderate interference; I cannot do some of the activities that I want to do.
   - 3 = Severe interference; I cannot do most of the activities that I want to do.

3. How much does your incontinence interfere with your ability to engage in non-strenuous recreation (movies, dining out, etc.)?
   - 0 = No interference; I can do all the activities that I want to do.
   - 1 = Minimal interference; I can do most of the activities that I want to do.
   - 2 = Moderate interference; I cannot do some of the activities that I want to do.
   - 3 = Severe interference; I cannot do most of the activities that I want to do.

4. How much does your incontinence affect your relationships with your friends?
   - 0 = No problems; my friendships are the same as they would be if I did not leak urine.
   - 1 = Minimal problems; my friendships would be a little better if I did not leak urine.
   - 2 = Moderate problems; my friendships would be somewhat better if I did not leak urine.
   - 3 = Severe problems; my friendships would be much better if I did not leak urine.

5. How much does your incontinence affect your relationship with your spouse/companion?
   - Not applicable; I do not have a spouse/companion.
   - 0 = No problems; the relationship is the same as it would be if I did not leak urine.
   - 1 = Minimal problems; the relationship would be a little better if I did not leak urine.
   - 2 = Moderate problems; the relationship would be somewhat better if I did not leak urine.
   - 3 = Severe problems; the relationship would be much better if I did not leak urine.

6. How much does your incontinence interfere with your sexual activity?
   - Not applicable; I am not sexually active, regardless of incontinence.
   - 0 = No problems; sex is the same as it would be if I did not leak urine.
   - 1 = Minimal problems; sex would be a little better if I did not leak urine.
   - 2 = Moderate problems; sex would be somewhat better if I did not leak urine.
   - 3 = Severe problems; sex would be much better if I did not leak urine.

7. Does your incontinence make it difficult for you to establish new relationships with other people (friends, business associates, etc.)?
   - 0 = My incontinence causes no difficulty when I establish new relationships.
   - 1 = My incontinence makes it slightly more difficult for me to establish new relationships.
   - 2 = My incontinence makes it somewhat more difficult for me to establish new relationships.
   - 3 = My incontinence makes it much more difficult for me to establish new relationships.

8. How does your incontinence affect your financial situation?
   - 0 = No effect; I do not lose any money due to incontinence.
   - 1 = Minimal effect; I have to spend a small amount of extra money for protection, extra clothes, etc.
   - 2 = Moderate effect; I spend a significant amount of money because of incontinence and/or I am losing income because incontinence interferes with my job.
   - 3 = Severe effect; my incontinence costs so much that I cannot afford other necessities and/or I lost my job because of incontinence.

9. How does your incontinence affect your overall health?
   - 0 = No effect; incontinence causes no health problems for me.
   - 1 = Minimal effect; incontinence causes small problems such as a minor skin rash.
   - 2 = Moderate effect; incontinence causes significant problems such as infection or persistent skin rash.
   - 3 = Severe effect; incontinence causes major problems such as skin ulcers, or illness due to infection.

10. Do you feel increased nervousness or anxiety because of your incontinence?
    - 0 = No effect; my incontinence does not increase my feelings of nervousness or anxiety.
    - 1 = Minimal effect; my incontinence makes me feel slightly more nervous or anxious.
    - 2 = Moderate effect; my incontinence makes me feel somewhat more nervous or anxious.
    - 3 = Severe effect; my incontinence makes me feel much more nervous or anxious.

11. How much does your incontinence affect your overall level of energy?
    - 0 = No effect; my energy level is the same as it would be if I did not leak urine.
    - 1 = Minimal effect; I would be a little more energetic if I did not leak urine.
    - 2 = Moderate effect; I would be somewhat more energetic if I did not leak urine.
    - 3 = Severe effect; I would be much more energetic if I did not leak urine.

12. Does your incontinence make you feel less useful?
    - 0 = No effect; I feel just as useful as I would feel if I did not leak urine.
    - 1 = Minimal effect; I would feel slightly more useful if I did not leak urine.
    - 2 = Moderate effect; I would feel somewhat more useful if I did not leak urine.
    - 3 = Severe effect; I would feel much more useful if I did not leak urine.

13. How do you rate the overall quality of your life?
    - 0 = My life is just as good as anyone else's.
    - 1 = Only a few people have a better life than I do.
    - 2 = Several people have a better life than I do.
    - 3 = Most people have a better life than I do.

14. How would you rate the overall quality of your life if you did not leak urine?
    - 0 = My life would be just as good as anyone else's.
    - 1 = Only a few people would have a better life than I would.
    - 2 = Several people would have a better life than I would.
    - 3 = Most people would have a better life than I would.

15. How much does your incontinence affect your overall satisfaction with your life?
    - 0 = No effect; I am just as satisfied with my life as I would be if I did not leak urine.
    - 1 = Minimal effect; my incontinence makes me feel slightly less satisfied with my life.
    - 2 = Moderate effect; my incontinence makes me feel somewhat less satisfied with my life.
    - 3 = Severe effect; my incontinence makes me feel much less satisfied with my life.

From Raz S, Erickson DR: SEAPI QMM incontinence classification system. Neurourol Urodyn 11:187–199, 1992. Copyright © 1992 Wiley-Liss, Inc. Reprinted by permission of Wiley-Liss, Inc., a subsidiary of John Wiley & Sons, Inc.

TABLE 30–6
**Diagnostic Maneuvers Used
to Demonstrate Stress
Urinary Incontinence**

1. International Continence Society pad test
2. Administration of phenazopyridine hydrochloride
3. Voiding diary
4. Valsalva leak point pressure
5. Marshall test
6. Voiding cystourethrogram
7. Multichannel urodynamics

with anatomic incontinence and intrinsic sphincter dysfunction.

SURGICAL TECHNIQUE The patient is placed in the lithotomy position, and the vagina and lower abdomen are prepared with an iodine scrub (Fig. 30–1A–G). A suprapubic tube is placed using the Lowsley retractor. A urethral catheter is connected to suction to empty the bladder and then clamped off. Two oblique incisions are made in the anterior vaginal wall, and the plane between the vagina and the glistening periurethral fascia is dissected. The retropubic space is entered either bluntly or sharply between the pubic bone and the urethropelvic fascia. The urethropelvic fascia is freed from its lateral attachments to the tendinous arch of the obturator. Any adhesions found in the retropubic space are divided using a combination of blunt and sharp dissection. A No. 1 Prolene sture is placed in a helical fashion in the vaginal wall (excluding the epithelium), the pubocervical fascia, and the medial edge of the urethropelvic ligament. Traction on the sutures tests the integrity of

TABLE 30–7
**Classification of Management
Options for Patients with Stress
Urinary Incontinence**

Nonsurgical
  1. Pelvic floor exercise
  2. Estrogen
  3. Biofeedback
  4. Alpha-sympathomimetics
  5. Protective undergarments
  6. Catheter drainage
  7. Pessary
Surgical
  Anatomic incontinence
    Abdominal approach
      1. Burch
      2. Marshal-Marchetti-Krantz
    Vaginal approach
      1. Raz bladder neck suspension
      2. Raz anterior vaginal wall sling
      3. Stamey needle suspension
      4. Gittes needle suspension
      5. Pereyra needle suspension
    Laparoscopic suspension
  Intrinsic sphincter dysfunction
    1. Raz anterior vaginal wall sling
    2. Vaginal wall island sling
    3. Fascial slings—autologous or artificial mesh
    4. Injectable agents (collagen, autologous fat, Teflon)
    5. Artificial urinary sphincter

the anchoring tissue. The contralateral side is approached similarly.

The anterior rectus sheath is exposed through a small suprapubic stab incision just superior to the pubic symphysis in the midline. The double-pronged ligature carrier is guided through the retropubic space by the surgeon's finger and out through the vaginal incision. The sutures are threaded and transferred suprapubically. Indigo carmine is administered intravenously and cystoscopy is carried out. The position of the suprapubic catheter is inspected. Blue efflux should be noted from both ureteral orifices, and the area is inspected to ensure that no suture material has entered the bladder. Finally, with the cystoscope in the urethra, gentle elevation of the Prolene sutures should ensure elevation of the bladder neck. The vaginal incision is closed with a running, locking 2–0 polyglycolic acid suture. A vaginal pack previously covered with sulfa cream is placed, and the Prolene suspension sutures are tied without tension. The suprapubic and urethral Foley catheters are left indwelling.

The urethral catheter and vaginal pack are removed on the first postoperative day, and the suprapubic tube is plugged. The patient is asked to try to void through the urethra, measuring the postvoid residual urine through the suprapubic tube. Patients are maintained on oral antibiotics, a stool softener, and oral analgesics while the suprapubic tube remains in situ. When the postvoid residual urine consistently measures less than 2 ounces, the suprapubic tube is removed. Ninety percent of patients can empty the bladder with less than 2 ounces residual by the end of the first postoperative week.

Several important principles apply to the Raz bladder neck suspension in comparison to other vaginal techniques. The inverted U vaginal epithelial incision was devised to allow dissection to be carried out lateral to the urethra and bladder neck, thus avoiding dissection directly beneath the urethra and bladder neck and facilitating entrance into the retropubic space. The pubocervical and urethropelvic fasciae are conveniently approached from the limbs of the inverted U incision. The medial edge of the urethropelvic ligament, detached from the tendinous arch when the retropubic space is entered, is the most important and reliable structure used in suspension. A potential complication of other suspension procedures, including the Marshall-Marchetti-Krantz, the original Pereyra, and the Stamey procedures, is urethral obstruction secondary to the close proximity of the suspending sutures to the urethra itself, which prevents satisfactory funneling and shortening of the bladder neck during voiding. The principle of the Raz procedure is similar to that of the Burch colposuspension in that the lateral placement of the sutures obviates obstruction. It is important to enter the retropubic space not merely to facilitate fingertip control of the ligature carrier but also to mobilize the urethra and bladder neck sufficiently from adhesions and scars prior to performing the suspension. This is a sine qua non in the patient who has undergone prior procedures, either retropu-

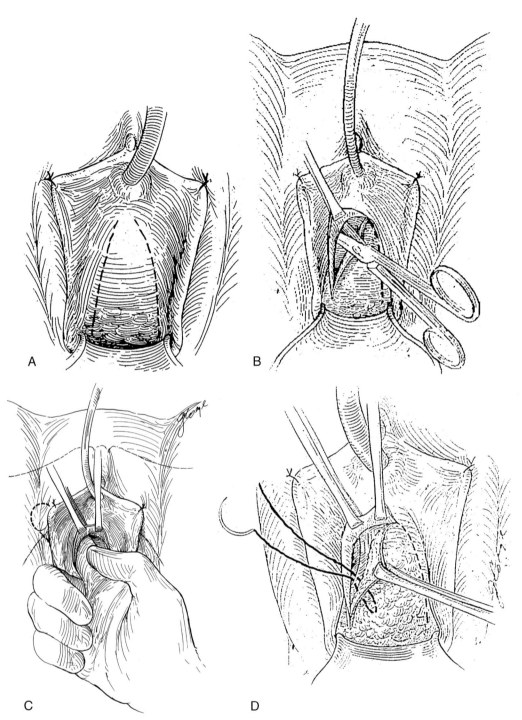

Figure 30-1   *A,* The two parallel incisions for the Raz bladder neck suspension are shown. Exposure is facilitated by the use of silk sutures to retract the labia minora, and a weighted vaginal speculum is placed. Urethral Foley and suprapubic catheters (not shown) are placed prior to making the incisions. *B,* Dissection is carried out over the glistening periurethral fascia. It is important to maintain the dissection superficial to the fascia. Violation of the fascial layer with the scissors may result in increased bleeding. The curved Mayo scissors are used to enter the retropubic space and expose the urethropelvic ligament. *C,* Here a finger is shown in the retropubic space. Adhesions are taken down using a combination of sharp and blunt dissection. Allis clamps are used to retract the anterior vaginal wall and facilitate exposure. (From Raz S: Atlas of Transvaginal Surgery. Philadelphia, WB Saunders, 1992, p 55.) *D,* Prolene sutures are placed to encompass the urethropelvic ligament. Note that these sutures should include the whole depth of the ligament to provide a secure anchor for the suture.

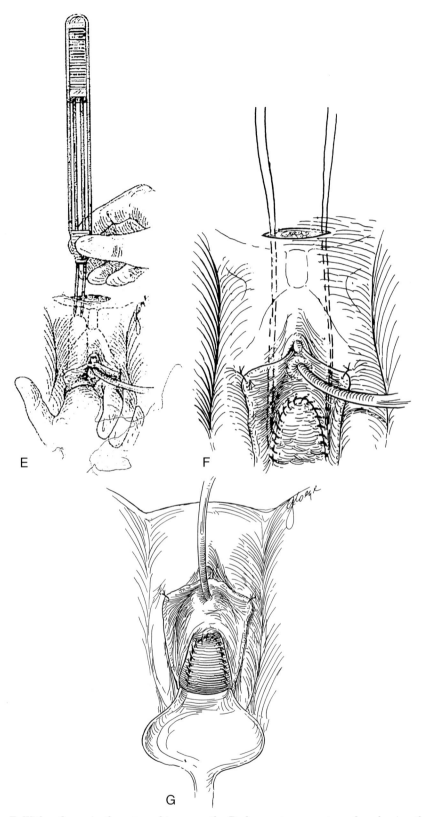

E

F

G

Figure 30-1 *Continued* *E,* With a finger in the retropubic space, the Prolene sutures are transferred using the double-pronged needle carrier. The needle is always passed in the midline in the immobile portion of the insertion of the rectus fascia onto the pubis. The needle should be passed under fingertip control to guide it correctly through the incision in the anterior vaginal wall. *F,* Transfer of the sutures through the midline incision is shown. The anterior vaginal wall is closed with a running, and locking long-lasting absorbable suture. *G,* A vaginal pack is placed prior to tying down the suspension sutures. The sutures should be tied without tension, and the vaginal pack provides support of the anterior vaginal wall. (From Walsh PC, Retik AB, Stamey TA, Vaughan ED Jr [eds]: Campbell's Urology, 6th ed. Philadelphia, WB Saunders, 1992.)

bic or vaginal, to reposition the bladder neck and proximal urethra in a high retropubic position. We routinely use cystoscopy after administration of intravenous indigo carmine to ensure bilateral ureteral efflux, lack of suture penetration of the urethra and bladder, and adequate suspension of the bladder neck when minimal traction is placed on the suspension sutures. Unlike the Stamey procedure, in which the purpose of cystoscopy is to ensure proper placement of the sutures at the level of the bladder neck, the Raz procedure does not rely on cystoscopy for suture placement because the sutures are placed under direct observation.

RESULTS Numerous authors have reported on the success of the Raz bladder neck suspension procedure since its introduction in 1981.[11-19] A prospective cohort of over 400 patients at UCLA based on objective and subjective evaluation revealed a cure rate (S0-1, E0, A0, P0-1, I0) of 85%, with 9% of patients having rare episodes of incontinence. A long-term retrospective review of 225 patients who underwent the Raz bladder neck suspension between 1984 and 1990 was published in 1992.[15] Two hundred and six patients were available for follow-up, the mean follow-up time was 15 months. Eighty-three percent of patients were thought to be cured (S0-1, E0, A0, P0-1, I0). Rare episodes of stress incontinence occurred in 7.3% of patients. Age, number of prior anti-incontinence procedures, hysterectomy, menopause, and the presence of urgency incontinence preoperatively were not found to be significantly predictive of postoperative failures. On the other hand, the preoperative subjective severity of the frequency of stress incontinence (S level, as measured by the SEAPI score) was predictive of postoperative failure. In 23 patients with severe stress incontinence (S3) before surgery, there was a 35% failure rate. The median time to failure was 5 months.[15]

Golomb and colleagues reported in 1994 a comparison of 88 patients undergoing the Raz bladder neck suspension after mean follow-up of 18.2 months.[20] Patients were divided into young (less than 65 years of age) and elderly (over 65 years) groups, and the long-term results were compared between the two groups. Eighty-five percent of young women were completely cured of stress incontinence, and 8.9% were markedly improved. Four percent had recurrence of stress incontinence. Results were similar in the elderly group with 90.4% completely cured, 4.8% improved, and 1 failure.

POTENTIAL COMPLICATIONS Overall, the Raz bladder neck suspension is well tolerated by patients, and over 95% are discharged from the hospital on the first postoperative day. Short-term complications are rare but may include vaginal spotting, urinary tract infection, or urinary irritative symptoms. Potential long-term complications include de novo urgency incontinence (11%), secondary prolapse (6%), prolonged retention (2.5%), and suprapubic pain (3%). Attention to proper patient selection, adequate lysis of adhesions in the retropubic space, and careful technique in passing the double-pronged needle will minimize these complications.

RAZ TRANSVAGINAL TECHNIQUE OF CYSTOCELE REPAIR WITH AND WITHOUT ANATOMIC INCONTINENCE

In the following three sections we discuss the Raz techniques of repair for patients with one of three types of defects—moderate cystocele with a predominantly lateral defect, cystocele with a central defect, and grade 4 cystocele. We also briefly discuss in this section our previous techniques of repair (four-corner bladder suspension and technique of grade 4 cystocele repair with midline incision). The reader is referred to Chapter 29 for a discussion of the significance, location, and implications of the various types of defects. Evaluation and strategy of the management of cystocele are also discussed in Chapter 29.

Our current techniques of repair represent an evolution in our understanding of cystocele development and reflect our concern with the predominance of lateral defects in patients with cystocele (70 to 80%) and our desire to limit the onset of postoperative stress incontinence (which occurs in up to 40% of patients).[21]

Techniques of Repair of Lateral Defect for Moderate Cystocele (Four-Corner and Six-Corner Bladder Suspension)

These repairs are suited for patients with lateral defects and moderate (grade 2 or 3) cystocele. Our previous technique of repair for patients with this type of problem included suspension of the bladder and bladder neck with the use of four Prolene sutures. As discussed later in this section, we have now revised this technique and replaced it with a six-corner technique; for a more detailed description of the four-corner procedure the reader is referred to reference 22.

FOUR-CORNER BLADDER SUSPENSION In the four-corner technique a U-shaped incision is made in the anterior vaginal wall, and the perivaginal tissue is dissected away from the perivesical fascia. At this point two sutures of Prolene are placed on each side; each suture incorporates several passes through the tissues. The more proximal suture is placed at the bladder base and includes the anterior vaginal wall (minus the epithelium), the vesicopelvic fascia, and the cardinal and uterosacral ligaments. The distal suture is placed at the level of the bladder neck. This suture incorporates the vaginal wall (minus the epithelium), the vesicopelvic fascia, and the urethropelvic fascia. Care is taken to ensure that the proximal and distal sutures overlap.

Results Between 1984 and 1988 120 patients with grade 2 or 3 cystocele underwent four-corner bladder and bladder neck suspensions at UCLA. One hundred and seven patients were available for follow-up that ranged from 6 months to 5 years (average, 2 years). Postoperatively, 105 of 107 patients had either complete resolution of cystocele or only grade 1 cystocele. Stress incontinence resolved in 84 of the

89 patients presenting with this complaint. De novo instability occurred in 6 patients; 54 patients with preoperative instability noted clinical improvement. Twelve patients had preoperative retention; of these, 10 patients reported resolution of the obstruction; no other cases of prolonged retention occurred.[23]

As described in Chapter 35 on the vaginal wall sling, one of the major elements in our recent understanding of incontinence has been the role of the midurethral complex. To address the pathology found in this area, we have modified our approach in the last few years and now use what we call the six-corner bladder suspension technique. This technique is now discussed in depth.

SIX-CORNER BLADDER SUSPENSION   The patient is placed in the lithotomy position, care being taken to protect any pressure points. The vagina is prepared, and stay sutures and a posterior weighted speculum are placed. A Lowsley retractor is introduced into the bladder and a suprapubic tube is placed. A Foley catheter is placed next, and the anterior vaginal wall is infiltrated with saline solution. Two oblique incisions are made from the level of the vaginal cuff (paracervical area if the uterus is present) to the level of the bladder neck. The pubocervical and periurethral fasciae are exposed by lateral dissection with Metzenbaum scissors. At the level of the midurethra the retropubic space is entered. In this maneuver, closed, curved Mayo scissors are pointed toward the ipsilateral shoulder and advanced.

At this point three sutures of No. 1 Prolene are placed on each side. Each suture incorporates multiple passes through the tissues. The proximal suture is placed through the vesicopelvic fascia (excluding the vaginal epithelium) and incorporates two additional passes posteriorly to incorporate the cardinal and uterosacral ligaments (Fig. 30–2). This suture should be so strong that the patient can be rocked on the table when tension is applied on the suture. The middle suture is placed at the level of the bladder neck and starts with two passes through the vaginal wall (excluding the vaginal epithelium but including the underlying vesicopelvic ligament). The bladder neck is next held medially, and two additional passes are made through the freed lateral edge of the urethropelvic ligament. The distal suture is placed at the level of the midurethra and incorporates the levator musculature as it inserts in the periurethral tissue, the urethropelvic ligament, and the vaginal wall (minus the epithelium).

At this point a small suprapubic puncture is made, and the double-pronged ligature carrier is inserted. This is passed under direct fingertip control through the retropubic space until it exits from the vaginal incision. The passage is made close to the midline to avoid bleeding or nerve entrapment and scrapes the periosteum of the pubis to minimize postoperative pain. All sutures are transferred.

At this point cystoscopy is undertaken (the patient is given indigo carmine 5 to 10 minutes before passage of the sutures). Cystoscopy is done to confirm the patency of the ureters by visualizing of blue efflux

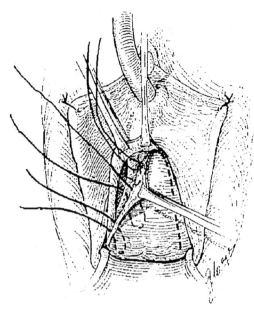

Figure 30–2   The position of the Prolene sutures for a six-corner suspension is shown prior to transfer through a lower abdominal midline stab incision.

from each orifice. Further, the bladder is examined for the presence of any sutures and for the correct location of the suprapubic tube. Finally, anterior tension is placed on the sutures to ensure that good elevation of the bladder will occur.

The vaginal incisions are repaired with a 2–0 Vicryl running interlocking suture. A triple sulfa- or Betadine-impregnated vaginal pack is inserted next. The Prolene suspension sutures are tied sequentially to themselves and their ipsilateral mates. It is important to tie these sutures without tension to avoid postoperative retention of urine. At this point the suprapubic site is irrigated with Betadine solution, and the wound is closed with 4–0 Vicryl. Finally, the suprapubic tube is secured in place. Both urethral and suprapubic catheters are left to gravity drainage.

The Foley catheter and vaginal pack are removed when the patient has fully awakened from anesthesia. The patient is allowed to void immediately postoperatively; postvoid residual urine is measured from the suprapubic tube approximately every 2 hours. When the residual is consistently less than 60 ml, we remove the suprapubic tube. Alternatively, in the unusual case when residuals remain high, we instruct the patient in self-catheterization techniques and remove the suprapubic tube at the end of 4 weeks.

Results   We are currently compiling data on this technique, which represents a relatively new modification of our previous four-corner technique.

Repair of Central Defect

In this repair the lateral support remains adequate, and the defect is caused by laxity of the vesicopelvic ligaments and separation of the cardinal and uterosacral ligaments. This is an unusual situation that occurs in only approximately 5% of patients.[24] Classically, the urethra retains a normal anatomic relationship with the symphysis pubis and the posterior bladder wall.

In this repair a longitudinal midline incision is made from the level of the bladder neck to the level of the vaginal cuff or cervix. The vaginal wall is dissected laterally, exposing the underlying vesicopelvic ligaments and the cardinal-uterosacral ligaments. The initial suture is placed to incorporate the cardinal-uterosacral ligaments. Tension on this suture delineates a rectangle of support, in effect demonstrating the lateral edges of the vesicopelvic fascia. The importance of proper exposure and reapproximation of the cardinal-uterosacral ligaments cannot be understated; technical inadequacy at this point will result in a much greater incidence of surgical failure. At this point Dexon mesh may be used to reduce the bladder and facilitate the remainder of the repair. Mattress sutures of 2–0 Vicryl are subsequently placed, approximating the edges of the vesicopelvic fascia (see Fig. 30–3D). Cystoscopy is undertaken at this time, as in the lateral defect repair. Finally, excess vaginal tissue is excised, and the edges of the vaginal incision are reapproximated using a running interlocking 2–0 Vicryl suture. A vaginal pack is placed at this time. Postoperative care is identical to that described for the lateral defect repair.

Once again, it is important to address any urethral hypermobility; if this is present, a sling or bladder neck suspension should be undertaken.

Repair of Grade 4 Cystocele with Combined Central and Lateral Defects

Grade 4 cystocele implies prolapse of the bladder outside the introitus at rest. Generally, this defect involves three specific problems: urethral hypermobility, lateral defects, and central defects. These three defects are repaired in one operation.

As with the repair for grade 2 and 3 cystocele, our current technique of repair has been in use for only approximately the last 12 months. Again our technique has been modified to account for new interpretations of the mechanisms of continence.

Our previous technique of repair is briefly discussed. In this procedure we made a midline incision and used two suspension Prolene sutures. Each suture incorporated multiple bites through the tissues. The distal suture was placed at the bladder neck and incorporated the anterior vaginal wall (without epithelium) and the freed lateral edge of the urethropelvic ligament. The more proximal suture incorporated the vesicopelvic fascia and the cardinal-uterosacral ligament complex. The central defect was repaired with 2–0 polyglactin mattress sutures. (The reader is referred to reference 22 for a more detailed discussion.)

In 1993, 31 patients underwent grade 4 cystocele repair at UCLA with this technique. Preoperative evaluation included lateral cystography, videourodynamic evaluation, and cystoscopy. Preoperative and postoperative scores of 0 to 3 were assigned using the SEAPI incontinence classification. Follow-up data were available for 29 patients.

Results according to the SEAPI classification are as follows: Subjective stress evaluation showed that 17 patients had SUI preoperatively. Postoperatively four patients had subjective SUI. Only one patient developed de novo stress incontinence (S-1). With regard to emptying ability, 28 of 29 patients emptied the bladder with clinically insignificant residuals (scores of 0 to 1); one patient had preoperative and postoperative retention that required intermittent straight catheterization. In regard to correction of the anatomic defect, 27 of 29 patients had excellent repair of the severe cystocele with scores of 0 to 1, and two patients had recurrence of asymptomatic cystocele. Protection results showed that two patients had a rare need for pads and two patients required daily use of pads for occasional incontinence. Preoperative instability was present in 20 of 29 patients. This instability resolved in 17 patients. Four patients developed de novo instability. In only one patient did the inhibition score progress by more than one point.[24]

Current Technique of Grade 4 Cystocele Repair Using the Goalpost Incision

This technique allows development of an island of vaginal tissue, which is used to create a hammock of support for the urethra. It is our hypothesis that this will assist in the treatment of stress incontinence. A second modification from our previous technique is the placement of sutures at the midurethral complex. A final difference is the use of a Dexon mesh for reduction of the cystocele; this maneuver facilitates the reapproximation of the vesicopelvic fascia and lends support to the repair.

Repair of a grade 4 cystocele begins with placement of a suprapubic tube and a urethral Foley catheter. The anterior vaginal wall is infiltrated with saline, and a goalpost type of incision is then made with the arms distal and the incision extending proximally to the level of the vaginal cuff or paracervical area. This incision creates an island of vaginal wall tissue as seen in Figure 30–3A. Dissection is carried out to expose the perivesical fascia. The extent of this dissection includes the junction of the periurethral fascia with the tendinous arches distally, the junction of the bladder with the peritoneal folds proximally, and the junctions of the vesicopelvic ligaments with the levator muscle laterally. During this dissection careful attention should be paid to the possibility of a coexisting enterocele. The retropubic space is now entered by penetrating the junction of the urethropelvic ligament with the tendinous arches. A proximal set of helical sutures of No. 1

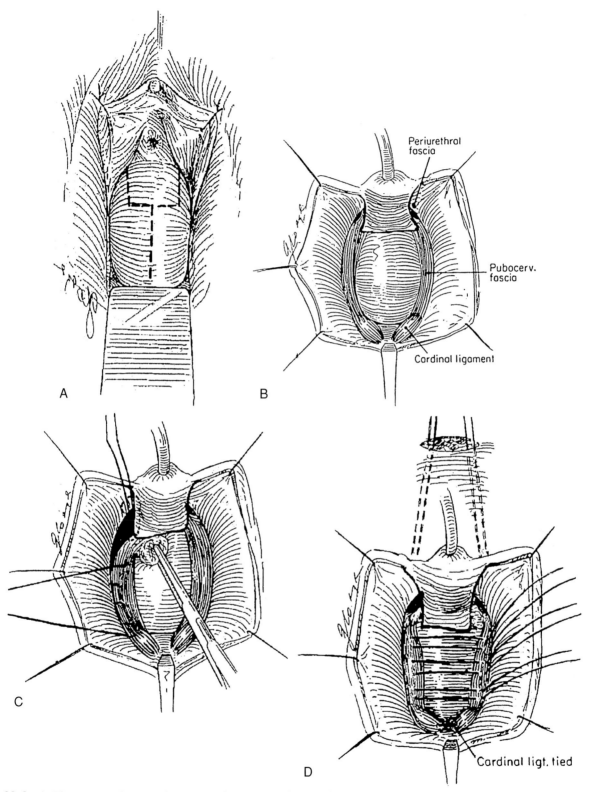

Figure 30-3 *A,* The incision for a grade 4 cystocele repair is shown. The "goal post" incision facilitates central dissection over the cystocele (the midline "post" portion of the incision), and the arms of the goal post provide exposure of the urethropelvic ligament and retropubic space on each side, as in the bladder neck suspension. *B,* Anatomy of the anterior vaginal wall after lateral dissection and creation of an island of vaginal wall anteriorly over the urethra to be used in the sling portion of the repair. *C,* Placement of sutures for the lateral defect repair and vaginal wall sling. *D,* Repair of the central defect with mattress sutures (mesh not depicted). The Prolene sutures for repair of the lateral defect and vaginal wall sling have been transferred to the lower abdominal midline incision.

Prolene is used to incorporate the freed lateral edge of the urethropelvic fascia, the pubocervical (or vesicopelvic fascia), and the cardinal-uterosacral ligaments. A second set of sutures is placed to include the freed lateral edge of the urethropelvic ligament, the levator complex at its insertion into the mid-urethra, and the vaginal wall excluding the epithelium. A suprapubic puncture is made, and these sutures are passed anteriorly to the rectus fascia with a double-pronged ligature carrier. The Prolene sutures are not tied at this time. These maneuvers constitute the repair of the lateral defect and the modified vaginal sling. They provide support for the lateral repair, the bladder neck, and the urethra (see Fig. 30–3*B,C*).

At this point the surgeon's attention is turned to the central defect. The central defect is reduced with a Dexon mesh. Mattress sutures of 2–0 polyglactin are used to reapproximate the cardinal-uterosacral ligament complex. Similar sutures are used to reapproximate the pubocervical fascia (see Fig. 30–3*D*). These two maneuvers constitute the central repair.

Next, indigo carmine is administered, and the ureteral orifices are examined for blue efflux. The bladder is searched for sutures, and the suprapubic tube site is checked. Now the vaginal wall is closed using a running interlocking 2–0 Vicryl suture, and a vaginal pack is placed. Finally, the Prolene suspension sutures are tied down without tension to the level of the rectus fascia.

Postoperative care is similar to that described for repair of the central and lateral defects. The vaginal pack is removed, and the patient is fed and begins ambulation when she has recovered from anesthesia. Intravenous antibiotics are administered for 24 hours postoperatively. Generally, patients are discharged on the first postoperative day with the Foley catheter removed. The guidelines for removal of the suprapubic tube are identical to those used in other cystocele repairs.

RESULTS   As noted earlier, this technique has been in use for only the last few years; at this point data are still being collected.

Complications

Many complications of cystocele repair can be avoided at the time of surgery by careful cystoscopy. Attention should be paid to the presence of blue efflux from both orifices, indicating patency of the ureters. A careful search should be made for sutures to minimize complications of recurrent infection or stone formation. De novo incontinence may occur postoperatively if the urethra is left with poor support. Indeed, it is imperative for the surgeon to assess the adequacy of urethral support prior to operative intervention. De novo bladder instability is found in less than 10 to 15% of patients.[24] Urinary retention with a prolonged or indefinite requirement for intermittent straight catheterization may occur. Inadvertent cystotomy can occur and should be repaired at the time of surgery with drainage of the site and prolonged bladder drainage. Fistula or damage to the rectum is a much less likely complication. Bleeding requiring transfusion is exceedingly rare. Finally, it must be emphasized that proper selection of patients is imperative; use of the appropriate procedure for the appropriate patient minimizes the chance of a recurrent cystocele. A more thorough discussion of complications is found in Chapter 55.

Conclusion

The advent of enhanced pelvic MRI has contributed greatly to our understanding of incontinence. Surgical techniques should be modified to reflect this increased knowledge. The choice of surgical procedure to correct stress incontinence should be based not only on the type and severity of incontinence but

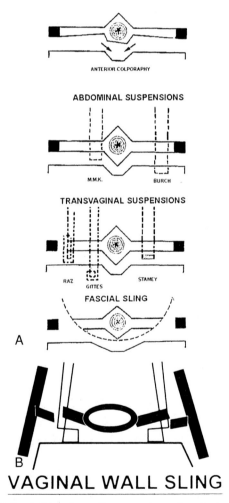

Figure 30–4   *A,* Diagrammatic comparison of vaginal procedures used for the correction of stress urinary incontinence and prolapse. Compare the various procedures noting the depth and distance of suture placement from both the urethra and the insertion of the levator fascia into the tendinous arch (shown as a black square anchoring both ends of the levator fascia). *B,* Compare suture placement of the anterior vaginal wall sling with the procedures shown diagrammatically in *A.*

also on the type and degree of anterior vaginal wall prolapse. A diagrammatic comparison of some of the techniques described for anterior vaginal wall reconstruction is shown in Figure 30–4. This philosophy requires a comprehensive approach to reconstruction of the female pelvis in patients with stress incontinence to provide correction of both incontinence and prolapse.

New methods of quantifying and unifying the results of surgical therapy through validated outcome measures, such as the SEAPI score, will aid clinicians in the scientific study of surgical outcomes. We continue to emphasize the need for such a common language to describe surgical outcomes by reporting the results of surgical therapy in terms of the SEAPI and validated quality of life scores. Although many techniques of surgical therapy for stress incontinence and anterior vaginal prolapse have been described, the best procedure for any individual surgeon is the one that works best in his or her hands.

REFERENCES

1. Meyer S, De Grandi P, Kuntzer T, et al: Birth trauma: Its effect on the urine continence mechanisms. Gynakol Geburtshilf Rundschau 33(4):236–242, 1993.
2. Barnick CG, Cardozo LD: Denervation and re-innervation of the urethral sphincter in the aetiology of genuine stress incontinence: An electromyographic study. Brit J Obstet Gynaecol 100(8):750–753, 1993.
3. Deindl FM, Vodusek DB, Hesse U, Schussler B: Pelvic floor activity patterns: Comparison of nulliparous continent and parous urinary stress incontinent women. A kinesiological EMG study. Br J Urol 73(4):413–417, 1994.
4. Falconer C, Ekman G, Malmstrom A, Ulmsten U: Decreased collagen synthesis in stress-incontinent women. Obstet Gynecol 84(4):583–586, 1994.
5. Bergman A, Elia G, Cheung D, et al: Biochemical composition of collagen in continent and stress urinary incontinent women. Gynecol Obstet Invest 37(1):48–51, 1994.
6. Bump RC, McClish DK: Cigarette smoking and urinary incontinence in women. Am J Obstet Gynecol 167(5):1213–1218, 1992.
7. Spence-Jones C, Kamm MA, Henry MM, Hudson CN: Bowel dysfunction: A pathogenic factor in uterovaginal prolapse and urinary stress incontinence. Br J Obstet Gynaecol 101(2):147–152, 1994.
8. Ekstrom J, Iosif CS, Malmberg L: Effects of long-term treatment with estrogen and progesterone on in vitro muscle responses of the female rabbit urinary bladder and urethra to autonomic drugs and nerve stimulation. J Urol 150(4):1284–1288, 1993.
9. Raz S, Erickson DR: SEAPI QMM incontinence classification system. Neurourol Urodyn 11:187–199, 1992.
10. Wall LL, Wang K, Robson I, Stanton SL: The pyridium pad test for diagnosing urinary incontinence. A comparative study of asymptomatic and incontinent women. J Reprod Med 35(7):682–684, 1990.
11. Raz S: Modified bladder neck suspension for female stress incontinence. Urology 17:82–85, 1981.
12. Nitti VW, Bregg KJ, Sussman EM, Raz S: The Raz bladder neck suspension in patients 65 years old and older. J Urol 149(4):802–807, 1993.
13. Stricker P, Haylen B: Injectable collagen for type 3 female stress incontinence: the first 50 Australian patients. Med J Australia 158(2):89–91, 1993.
14. Hara M, Hiraoka Y, Kimura G, et al: Operation of female stress incontinence—comparison between Raz procedure and Gittes procedure. Hinyokika Kiyo (Acta Urol Jap) 38(10):1117–1121, 1992.
15. Raz S, Sussman EM, Erickson DB, et al: The Raz bladder neck suspension: Results in 206 patients. J Urol 148(3):845–850, 1992.
16. Pastor Sempere F, Cisnal Monsalve JM, Chicote Perez F, et al: Treatment of stress urinary incontinence in women by the Raz technique: Results. Arch Espan Urol 45(1):59–61, 1992.
17. Naudin M, Hauzeur C, Schulman C: S. Raz method of bladder suspension and treatment of cystocele in urinary stress incontinence (short-term results). Acta Urol Belg 60(2):67–75, 1992.
18. Soler Rosello A, Conejero Sugranes J, Abad Gairin C, et al: Modification of the simplified Cobb-Radge and Raz techniques in the treatment of stress urinary incontinence. Description and results. Arch Espan Urol 44(1):15–21, 1991.
19. Zimmern PE, Leach G: Bladder neck suspension using the modified Pereyra-Raz procedure in the treatment of stress urinary incontinence in women. J Urol (Paris) 97(7-8):309–319, 1991.
20. Golomb J, Goldwasser B, Mashiach S: Raz bladder neck suspension in women younger than sixty-five years compared with elderly women: Three years' experience. Urology 43(1):40–43, 1994.
21. Youngblood JP: Paravaginal repair for cystourethrocele. Clin Obstet Gynecol 36(3):960, 1993.
22. Raz S: Operative repair of rectocele, enterocele and cystocele. *In* Advances in Urology, Vol 5. Chicago, Mosby-Year Book, 1992.
23. Raz S, Klutke CG, Golomb J: Four corner bladder and urethral suspension for moderate cystocele. J Urol 142:712–715, 1989.
24. Unpublished data, UCLA Medical Center.
25. Amarenco G, Denys P, Kerdraon J: Neuropathy due to stretching of the internal pudendal nerve and female urinary incontinence. J Urol (Paris) 98(4):196–198, 1992.

BIBLIOGRAPHY

Abarbanel J, Lask D, Benet A, Mukamel E: Pelvic floor training for stress incontinence. Harefuah 126(4):180–182, 240, 1994.
Abos Fanlo P: Colpo-urethral suspension for stress incontinence. Acta Urol Esp 14(5):378–380, 1990.
Abu-Heija AT: Long-term results of colposuspension operation for genuine stress incontinence. Asia-Oceania J Obstet Gynaecol 20(2):179–181, 1994.
Ahlstrom K, Sandahl B, Sjoberg B, et al: Effect of combined treatment with phenylpropanolamine and estriol, compared with estriol treatment alone, in postmenopausal women with stress urinary incontinence. Gynecol Obstet Invest 30(1):37–43, 1990.
Albala DM, Schuessler WW, Vancaillie TG: Laparoscopic bladder suspension for the treatment of stress incontinence. Semin Urol 10(4):222–226, 1992.
Amarenco G, Denys P, Kerdraon J: Active forces of urinary continence and urethral fatiguability. Application to stress urinary incontinence in women. J Gynecol Obstet Biol Reprod 22(4):361–365, 1993.
Amarenco G, Kerdraon J: Decreased urethral pressure after coughing: The concept of urethral fatiguability. Its relationship with active forces of continence. Prog Urol 3(1):21–26, 1993.
Amarenco G, Kerdraon J, Adba MA, Lacroix P: Perineal stretch neuropathy: Its relationship to urinary stress incontinence in women. J Gynecol Obstet Biol Reprod 20(4):501–505, 1991.
Amarenco G, Kerdraon J, Albert T, Denys P: Stretch neuropathy of the internal pudendal nerve. Its relationship to urinary incontinence, anorectal, and genito-sexual disorders in women. Contracep Fertil Sexual 22(4):235–238, 1994.
Amarenco G, Kerdraon J, Lanoe Y: Perineal neuropathy due to stretching and urinary incontinence. Physiopathology, diagnosis and therapeutic implications. Ann Urol 24(6):463–466, 1990.
Appell RA: Urinary incontinence (editorial). J Urol 152(1):103–104, 1994.
Araki T, Takamoto H, Hara T, et al: The loop-loosening procedure for urination difficulties after Stamey suspension of the vesical neck [see comments]. J Urol 144(2 Pt 1):319–322, 1990.
Aran RM, Ortega I: Urinary incontinence. Its prevalence among female health professionals. Rev Enferm 17(188):19–22, 1994.

Ashken MH: Follow-up results with the Stamey operation for stress incontinence of urine. Br J Urol 65(2):168–169, 1990.

Atanasov A, Atanasova Z: The treatment of stress incontinence by Burch's colposuspension. Akusherstvo i Ginekologiia 32(3):1–3, 1993.

Awad SA, Gajewski JB, Katz NO, Acker-Roy K: Final diagnosis and therapeutic implications of mixed symptoms of urinary incontinence in women. Urology 39(4):352–357, 1992.

Bandi G, Larizza U, Rodolico R, et al: Transrectal echography and cystography in the assessment of female stress urinary incontinence. Radiol Med 79(3):228–232, 1990.

Banzhaf E, Hagemeier T, Herrmann K: Sacro-coccygeal meningocele—a case report on differential diagnosis of urinary incontinence in adulthood. Psychiat Neurol Med Psychol 42(11):699–703, 1990.

Barat M, Egon G, Daverat P, et al: Why does continence fail after sacral anterior root stimulator? Neurourol Urodyn 12(5):507–508, 1993.

Barnick CG, Cardozo LD: A comparison of bioelectrical and mechanical activity of the female urethra. Brit J Obstet Gynaecol 100(8):754–757, 1993.

Barrett JA, Oldham JA: Physiotherapy for stress urinary incontinence (letter). Br Med J 302(6786):1208, 1991.

Barrows B, Bavendam T, Leach GE: Ectopically draining dysplastic kidney associated with genuine stress urinary incontinence: Unusual combined cause of incontinence. Urology 40(3):283–285, 1992.

Battcock TM, Castleden CM: Pharmacological treatment of urinary incontinence. Br Med Bull 46(1):147–155, 1990.

Bautrant E, Nadal F, Mollard P, et al: Treatment of urinary stress incontinence by a modified Pereyra procedure: Chrub's operation. Rev Fr Gynecol Obstet 87(2):91–97, 1992.

Beck RP, McCormick S, Nordstrom I: A 25-year experience with 519 anterior colporrhaphy procedures. Obstet Gynecol 78(6):1011–1018, 1991.

Beckingham IJ, Wemyss-Holden G, Lawrence WT: Long-term follow-up of women treated with periurethral Teflon injections for stress incontinence. Br J Urol 69(6):580–583, 1992.

Behr J, Winkler M, Willgeroth F: Functional changes in the lower urinary tract after irradiation of cervix carcinoma. Strahlenther Onkol 166(2):135–139, 1990.

Benderev TV: Anchor fixation and other modifications of endoscopic bladder neck suspension. Urology 40(5):409–418, 1992.

Benjelloun S, Meziane F, el Mrini M, Bennani S: Diagnostic and therapeutic approach to stress urinary incontinence in women. Acta Urol Bel 58(3):53–64, 1990.

Benjelloun S, Meziane F, el Mrini M, Bennani S: Percutaneous fixation of the bladder neck under endoscopic control in the treatment of stress urinary incontinence. J Urol (Paris) 96(6):327–333, 1990.

Benson JT, Agosta A, McClellan E: Evaluation of a minimal-incision pubovaginal suspension as an adjunct to other pelvic-floor surgery. Obstet Gynecol 75(5):844–847, 1990.

Bent AE: Management of recurrent genuine stress incontinence. Clin Obstet Gynecol 33(2):358–366, 1990.

Bercault N, Peneau M, Martin P, et al: Nondilated obstructive anuria complicating urethrocystopexy. J Urol (Paris) 96(8):437–439, 1990.

Bergman A, Bader K: Reliability of the patient's history in the diagnosis of urinary incontinence. Int Gynaecol Obstet 32(3):255–259, 1990.

Bergman A, Karram MM, Bhatia NN: Changes in urethral cytology following estrogen administration. Gynecol Obstet Invest 29(3):211–213, 1990.

Bergman A, Koonings PP, Ballard CA: The Ball-Burch procedure for stress incontinence with low urethral pressure. J Reprod Med 36(2):137–140, 1991.

Bergman A, Ballard CA, Koonings PP, et al: Comparison of three different surgical procedures for genuine stress incontinence: A prospective randomized study. Am J Obstet Gynecol 160:1102, 1989.

Beurton D, Fontaine E, Grall J, Quentel P: Urethro-cervico-cystopexy using aponeurotic colposuspension: an original technic in the treatment of stress urinary incontinence. Apropos of 32 long-term reviewed cases. Progr Urol 3(2):216–227, 1993.

Bihrle W 3d, Tarantino AF: Complications of retropubic bladder neck suspension. Urology 35(3):213–214, 1990.

Blaivas JG: Incontinence (editorial). J Urol 150(5 Pt 1):1455, 1993.

Blaivas JG, Jacobs BZ: Pubovaginal fascial sling for the treatment of complicated stress urinary incontinence. J Urol 145(6):1214–1218, 1991.

Boemers TM, van Gool JD, de Jong TP: Displacement of incontinence device into the bladder. Br J Urol 72(6):985, 1993.

Bolayir K: Suspension of the bladder neck for urinary stress incontinence under local anesthesia. Minerva Urol Nefrol 42(2):95–98, 1990.

Borenstein R, Elchalal U, Goldchmit R, et al: The importance of the endopelvic fascia repair during vaginal hysterectomy. Surg Gynecol Obstet 175(6):551–554, 1992.

Borstad E, Skrede M, Rud T: Failure to predict and attempts to explain urinary stress incontinence following vaginal repair in continent women by using a modified lateral urethrocystography. Acta Obstet Gynecol Scand 70(6):501, 1991.

Bosman G, Vierhout ME, Huikeshoven FJ: A modified Raz bladder neck suspension operation. Results of a one to three years follow-up investigation. Acta Obstetr Gynecol Scand 72(1):47–49, 1993.

Bortel DT: Candida osteomyelitis pubis following a Marshall-Marchetti procedure. Orthopedics 16(12):1353–1355, 1993.

Brieger G, Korda A: The effect of obesity on the outcome of successful surgery for genuine stress incontinence. Austr NZ J Obstet Gynaecol 32(1):71–72, 1992.

Brito CG, Mulcahy JJ, Mitchell ME, Adams MC: Use of a double cuff AMS800 urinary sphincter for severe stress incontinence. J Urol 149(2):283–285, 1993.

Brodak PP, Juma S, Raz S: Levator hernia. J Urol 148(3):872–873, 1992.

Browne DS, Frazer MI: Abdominoperineal urethral suspension: A report of 20 cases. Aust NZ J Obstet Gynaecol 30(4):366–369, 1990.

Brun-Poulsen P: Genital prolapse and urinary incontinence. A clinical assessment of patients with prolapse with particular emphasis on surgical methods and their long-term effects. Ugeskr Laeger 152(46):3460–3463, 1990.

Bump RC, McClish DM: Cigarette smoking and pure genuine stress incontinence of urine: A comparison of risk factors and determinants between smokers and nonsmokers. Am J Obstet Gynecol 170(2):579–582, 1994.

Burgener L: R Lenzi's article, Colpohysteropexy in urinary stress incontinence (letter). Rev Med Suisse Romande, 113(3):256, 1993.

Burns PA, Nochajski TH, Pranikoff K: Factors discriminating between genuine stress and mixed incontinence. J Am Acad Nurse Pract 4(1):15–21, 1992.

Burns PA, Pranikoff K, Nochajski T, et al: Treatment of stress incontinence with pelvic floor exercises and biofeedback. J Am Geriat Soc 38(3):341–344, 1990.

Burns PA, Pranikoff K, Nochajski TH, et al: A comparison of effectiveness of biofeedback and pelvic muscle exercise treatment of stress incontinence in older community-dwelling women. J Gerontol 48(4):M167–174, 1993.

Cabrera JA, Szekely Z, Ospitia JA: Suprapubic or vaginal procedure (letter). Am J Obstet Gynecol 163(6 Pt 1):2025–2026, 1990.

Cammu H, Van Nylen M, Derde MP, et al: Pelvic physiotherapy in genuine stress incontinence. Urology 38(4):332–337, 1991.

Cardozo I, Brindley GS: Endoscopically guided bladder neck suspension for continence in a paraplegic women with implant driven micturition. Paraplegia 30(5):336–338, 1992.

Carey MP, Dwyer PL: Position and mobility of the urethrovesical junction in continent and in stress incontinent women before and after successful surgery. Austr NZ J Obstet Gynaecol 31(3):279–284, 1991.

Casanova JE: Incontinence after use of enalapril (letter). J Urol 143(6):1237–1238, 1990.

Caspi E, Langer R: Colpo-needle suspension for the treatment of urinary stress incontinence—a new surgical technique. Br J Obstet Gynaecol 98(11):1183–1184, 1991.

Cervigni M, Sbiroli C: Transvaginal bladder neck suspension: a safer method. Urology 36(3):219–221, 1990.

Chalouhy E, Dergham R: The artificial sphincter in the treatment of urinary incontinence. J Med Libanais (Lebanese Med J) 40(3):145–148, 1992.

Chan YT, Ng WD, Yin TF, Kwok TF: Complete prolapse of the urinary bladder. Br J Urol 66(4):436–437, 1990.

Chang HC, Chang SC, Kuo HC, Tsai TC: Transrectal sonographic cystourethrography: studies in stress urinary incontinence. Urology 36(6):488–492, 1990.

Conquy S: Treatment of urinary incontinence by feedback in women. J Urol (Paris) 97(7-8):327–331, 1991.

Conquy S, Zerbib M, Younes E, et al: Retrospective comparative study of three surgical procedures in the treatment of urinary stress incontinence in women. Apropos of 119 patients treated from 1985 to 1990. J Urol (Paris) 99(1):16–19, 1993.

Contreras Ortiz O, Lombardo RJ, Pellicari A: Non-invasive diagnosis of bladder instability using the Bladder Instability Discriminant Index (BIDI). Zentralbl Gynakol 115(10):446–449, 1993.

Cornella JL, Ostergard DR: Needle suspension procedures for urinary stress incontinence: a review and historical perspective. Obstet Gynecol Surv 45(12):805–816, 1990.

Couillard DR, Deckard-Janatpour KA, Stone AR: The vaginal wall sling: A compressive suspension procedure for recurrent incontinence in elderly patients. Urology 43(2):203–208, 1994.

Cucchi A: Acceleration of flow rate as a screening test for detrusor instability in women with stress incontinence. Br J Urol 65(1):17–19, 1990.

Cutner A, Cardozo LD, Wise BG: The effects of pregnancy on previous incontinence surgery. Case report. Br J Obstet Gynaecol 98(11):1181–1183, 1991.

Darai F, Benachi A, Meicler P, Colau JC: Transvaginal colposuspension. A series of 49 cases. Rev Fr Gynecol Obstet 89(1):7–10, 1994.

Davila GW, Ostermann KV: The bladder neck support prosthesis: a nonsurgical approach to stress incontinence in adult women. Am J Obstet Gynecol 171(1):206–211, 1994.

Debodinance P, Querleu D: Comparison of the Bologna and Ingelman-Sundberg procedures for stress incontinence associated with genital prolapse: prospective randomized study. Eur J Obstet Gynecol Reprod Biol 52(1):35–40, 1993.

Debus-Thiede G, Kraus K, Klosterhalfen T, Dimpfl T: Success and quality control in prolapse and stress incontinence operations—comparative use of urodynamics and transrectal endosonography. Geburtshilfe Frauenheilk 53(2):115–120, 1993.

Debus-Thiede G, Maassen V, Dimpfl T, et al: Late disorders of bladder function after Wertheim operation—an analysis of urodynamic parameters with reference to surgical radicality. Geburtshilfe Frauenheilkd 53(8):525–531, 1993.

de Gregorio G, Stein B, Kaltenbach FJ, Hillemanns HG: Effect of stress incontinence surgery on urodynamic parameters. 2. Are various surgical methods comparable? Geburtshilfe Frauenheilkd 50(7):548–551, 1990.

De Jong PR, Pontin A, Pillay G: Where is the bladder neck following needle suspension operations? Clin Experi Obstet Gynecol 21(1):10–13, 1994.

DeLancey JO: Structural support of the urethra as it relates to stress urinary incontinence: the hammock hypothesis. Am J Obstet Gynecol 170(6):1713–1720, 1994.

De Muylder X, Claes H, Neven P, De Jaegher K: Usefulness of urodynamic investigations in female incontinence. Eur J Obstet Gynecol Reprod Biol 44(3):205–208, 1992.

Dennis PJ, Rohner TJ Jr, Hu TW, et al: Simple urodynamic evaluation of incontinent elderly female nursing home patients. A descriptive analysis. Urology 37(2):173–179, 1991.

Dewan PA, Byard RW: Re: Long-term follow-up of women treated with periurethral Teflon injections for stress incontinence (letter). Br J Urol 71(1):112, 1993.

Dewan PA, Byard RW: Re: Transurethral Polytef injection for post-prostatectomy urinary incontinence and long-term follow-up of women treated with periurethral Teflon injections for stress incontinence (letter). Br J Urol 71(1):112, 1993.

Dimpfl T, Hesse U, Schussler B: Incidence and cause of postpartum urinary stress incontinence. Eur J Obstet Gynecol Reprod Biol 43(1):29–33, 1992.

Diokno AC, Normolle DP, Brown MB, Herzog AR: Urodynamic tests for female geriatric urinary incontinence. Urology 36(5):431–439, 1990.

Dixon PJ, Christmas TJ, Chapple CR: Stress incontinence due to pelvic floor muscle involvement in limb-girdle muscular dystrophy. Br J Urol 65(6):653–654, 1990.

Donovan JM, Gleason DM: Identifying types of female incontinence with retrograde urethrocystography. Urology 35(5):458–463, 1990.

Dorsey JH, Cundiff G: Laparoscopic procedures for incontinence and prolapse. Curr Opin Obstet Gynecol 6(3):223–230, 1994.

Dougherty M, Bishop K, Mooney R, et al: Graded pelvic muscle exercise. Effect on stress urinary incontinence. J Reprod Med 38(9):684–691, 1993.

Duncan HJ, Nurse DE, Mundy AR: Role of the artificial urinary sphincter in the treatment of stress incontinence in women. Br J Urol 69(2):141–143, 1992.

Dwyer PL, Glenning PP: Anatomy and neurology of the lower urinary tract. Curr Opin Obstet Gynecol 2(4):573–579, 1990.

Dwyer PL, Teele JS: Prazosin: a neglected cause of genuine stress incontinence. Obstet Gynecol 79(1):117–121, 1992.

Eckford SD, Abrams P: Para-urethral collagen implantation for female stress incontinence. Br J Urol 68(6):586–589, 1991.

Elia G, Bergman A: Estrogen effects on the urethra: beneficial effects in women with genuine stress incontinence. Obstet Gynecol Sur 48(7):509–517, 1993.

Elia G, Bergman A: Pelvic muscle exercises: when do they work? Obstet Gynecol 81(2):283–286, 1993.

Elser DM, Fantl JA: Pelvic relaxation of the anterior compartment. Curr Opin Obstet Gynecol 5(4):446–451, 1993.

Enzelsberger H, Helmer H, Seifert M, Kurz C: Results of colposuspension versus lyodura sling operation in therapy of recurrent stress incontinence. Gynakol Geburtshilfliche Rundschau 33 (Suppl 1):241, 1993.

Enzelsberger H, Kurz C, Adler A, Schatten C: Effectiveness of Burch colposuspension in females with recurrent stress incontinence—a urodynamic and ultrasound study. Geburtshilfe Frauenheilkd 51(11):915–919, 1991.

Enzelsberger H, Kurz C, Seifert M, et al: Surgical treatment of recurrent stress incontinence: Burch versus lyodura sling operation—a prospective study. Geburtshilfe Frauenheilkd 53(7):467–471, 1993.

Enzelsberger H, Skodler WD, Wolf G, Reinold E: Comparative study of introital sonography and the urethrocystogram in women before and after surgery for stress incontinence. Ultraschall Med 12(3):149–152, 1991.

Eriksen BC, Hagen B, Eik-Nes SH, et al: Long-term effectiveness of the Burch colposuspension in female urinary stress incontinence. Acta Obstet Gynecol Scand 69(1):45–50, 1990.

Ferguson KL, McKey PI, Bishop KR, et al: Stress urinary incontinence: Effect of pelvic muscle exercise. Obstet Gynecol 75(4):671–675, 1990.

Ferrari A, Frigerio L, Gandini L, et al: Clinical results of the modified Marshall-Marchetti procedure in female urinary incontinence. Ann Obstet Ginecol Med Perinat 111(4):223–227, 1990.

Ferriani RA, Silva de Sa MF, Dias de Moura M, et al: Ureteral blockage as a complication of Burch colposuspension: Report of 6 cases. Gynecol Obstet Invest 29(3):239–240, 1990.

Feyereisl J, Dreher E, Haenggi W, et al: Long-term results after Burch colposuspension. Am J Ob Gynecol 171(3):647–652, 1994.

Feyereisl J, Hanggi W, Dreher E: Terodiline in the treatment of stress incontinence in women. Schweiz Rundschau Med Praxis 79(14):420–422, 1990.

Fischer W: Treatment of stress incontinence. Zentralbl Gynakol 114(4):195–197, 1992.

Fischer W, Pfister C, Tunn R: Histomorphology of pelvic floor muscles in women with urinary incontinence. Zentralbl Gynakol 114(4):189–194, 1992.

Fischer-Rasmussen W: Treatment of stress urinary incontinence. Ann Med 22(6):455–465, 1990.

Fitzpatrick C, Swierzewski SJ 3d, McGuire EJ: Periurethral collagen for urinary incontinence after gender reassignment surgery. Urology 42(4):458–460, 1993.

Foldspang A, Mommsen S: Adult female urinary incontinence and childhood bedwetting. J Urol 152(1):85–88, 1994.

Foldspang A, Mommsen S, Lam GW, Elving L: Parity as a correlate of adult female urinary incontinence prevalence. J Epidemiol Community Health 46(6):595–600, 1992.

Fonda D, Brimage PJ, D'Astoli M: Simple screening for urinary incontinence in the elderly: comparison of simple and multichannel cystometry. Urology 42(5):536–540, 1993.

Fossaluzza V, Di Benedetto P, Zampa A, De Vita S: Misoprostol-induced urinary incontinence. J Int Med 230(5):463–464, 1991.

Foster HE, McGuire EJ: Management of urethral obstruction with transvaginal urethrolysis. J Urol 150(5 Pt 1):1448–1451, 1993.

Fukui J, Hosaka K, Ishizuka O, et al: Results of the conservative treatment of urinary incontinence in women. Nippon Hinyokika Gakkai Zasshi 81(11):1700–1705, 1990.

Ganabathi K, Abrams P, Mundy AR, et al: Stamey-Martius procedure for severe genuine stress incontinence. Br J Urol 69(1):34–37, 1992.

Gardy M, Kozminski M, DeLancey J, et al: Stress incontinence and cystoceles. J Urol 145(6):1211–1213, 1991.

Geirsson G, Fall M, Lindstrom S: The ice-water test—a simple and valuable supplement to routine cystometry. Br J Urol 71(6):681–685, 1993.

Ghoniem GM, Walters F, Lewis V: The value of the vaginal pack test in large cystoceles. J Urol 152(3):931–934, 1994.

Gillon G, Engelstein D, Servadio C: Risk factors and their effect on the results of Burch colposuspension for urinary stress incontinence. Israel J Med Sci 28(6):354–356, 1992.

Golomb J, Lindner A: Surgical treatment of urinary stress incontinence in women. Harefuah 121(3-4):77–79, 1991.

Gonchar MA, Gonchar OM: The pathogenesis and results of the surgical treatment of stress urinary incontinence in women. Urolog Nefrol (3):62–65, 1990.

Gondry J, Gagneur O, Naepels P, et al: Treatment of stress urinary incontinence. Experience at the Gynecology-Obstetrics Center of Amiens. Rev Fr Gynecol Obstet 85(12):684–688, 1990.

Gonnermann D, Pecqeux JC, Huland H: The diagnosis of female stress incontinence—the value of the clinical examination, anamnesis and urodynamics. Urologe [A] 31(2):67–69, 1992.

Gonzalez de Garibay AS, Castillo Jimeno JM, Villanueva Perez I, et al: Treatment of urinary stress incontinence using paraurethral injection of autologous fat. Arch Esp Urol 44(5):595–600, 1991.

Goodno JA Jr, Powers TW: Modified retropubic cystourethropexy. II. Am J Obstet Gynecol 166(6 Pt 1):1678–1681, 1992.

Graham JM, Stresing HA: A modified cystourethropexy in the management of incontinence and dyspareunia. J SC Med Assoc 86(11):578–582, 1990.

Griffith-Jones MD, Abrams PH: The Stamey endoscopic bladder neck suspension in the elderly. Br J Urol 65(2):170–172, 1990.

Griffith-Jones MD, Jarvis GJ, McNamara HM: Adverse urinary symptoms after total abdominal hysterectomy—fact or fiction? Br J Urol 67(3):295–297, 1991.

Griffiths DJ, McCracken PN, Harrison GM, Gormley EA: Relationship of fluid intake to voluntary micturition and urinary incontinence in geriatric patients. Neurour Urodyn 12(1):1–7, 1993.

Grimby A, Milsom I, Molander U, et al: The influence of urinary incontinence on the quality of life of elderly women. Age Ageing 22(2):82–89, 1993.

Grischke EM, Anton H, Stolz W, et al: Urodynamic assessment and lateral urethrocystography. A comparison of two diagnostic procedures for female urinary incontinence. Acta Obstetr Gynecol Scand 70(3):225–229, 1991.

Grischke EM, Stolz W, Anton HW, Bastert G: Urodynamics and the lateral cystogram: value for incontinence diagnosis. Geburtshilfe Frauenheilkd 50(2):145–149, 1990.

Groeneweg JM, Vierhout ME, Mulder AF: Subjective and objective success of Burch's method of colpo-suspension concerning continence, satisfaction and micturition pattern. Ned Tijdsch Geneeskd 138(25):1277–1280, 1994.

Grunberger W, Grunberger V, Wierrani F: Pelvic promontory fixation of the vaginal vault in sixty-two patients with prolapse after hysterectomy. J Am Coll Surg 178(1):69–72, 1994.

Guerinoni L, Treisser A, Klein P, Renaud R: Functional and urodynamic results of Burch's colpopexy. A series of 173 cases. J Gynecol Obstet Biol Reprod 20(2):231–240, 1991.

Guner H, Yildiz A, Erdem A, et al: Surgical treatment of urinary stress incontinence by a suburethral sling procedure using a Mersilene mesh graft. Gynecol Obstet Invest 37(1):52–55, 1994.

Hahn I, Milsom I, Fall M, Ekelund P: Long-term results of pelvic floor training in female stress urinary incontinence. Br J Urol 72(4):421–427, 1993.

Hanzal E, Berger E, Koelbl H: Levator ani muscle morphology and recurrent genuine stress incontinence. Obstet Gynecol 81(3):426–429, 1993.

Hanzal E, Berger E, Koelbl H: Reliability of the urethral closure pressure profile during stress in the diagnosis of genuine stress incontinence. Br J Urol 68(4):369–371, 1991.

Hanzal E, Joura E, Hausler G, Kolbl H: Urethral stress pressure profile in diagnosis of incontinence—a reliable diagnostic parameter? Gynakologisch-Geburtshilfliche Rundschau 33 (Suppl 1):239–240, 1993.

Harewood LM: Laparoscopic needle colposuspension for genuine stress incontinence. J Endourol 7(4):319–322, 1993.

Harris TA, Bent AE: Genital prolapse with and without urinary incontinence. J Reprod Med 35(8):792–798, 1990.

Harrison SC, Abrams PH: The endoscopic video camera as an aid to the Stamey procedure. Br J Urol 66(3):329, 1990.

Harrison SC, Brown C, O'Boyle PJ: Periurethral Teflon for stress urinary incontinence: medium-term results. Br J Urol 71(1):25–27, 1993.

Herbertsson G, Iosif CS: Surgical results and urodynamic studies 10 years after retropubic colpourethrocystopexy. Acta Obstet Gynecol Scand 72(4):298–301, 1993.

Heritier P, Levigne F, Oussoff MP, Gilloz A: Recurrent bladder calculi after colpocystopexy. J Gynecol Obstet Biol Reprod 19(3):307–308, 1990.

Hilton P, Mayne CJ: The Stamey endoscopic bladder neck suspension: A clinical and urodynamic investigation, including actuarial follow-up over four years. Br J Obstet Gynaecol 98(11):1141–1149, 1991.

Hofbauer J, Preisinger F, Nurnberger N: The value of physical therapy in genuine female stress incontinence. Z Urol Nephrol 83(5):249–254, 1990.

Holschneider CH, Solh S, Lebherz TB, Montz FJ: The modified Pereyra procedure in recurrent stress urinary incontinence: A 15-year review. Obstet Gynecol 83(4):573–578, 1994.

Horbach NS: Problems in the clinical diagnosis of stress incontinence. J Reprod Med 35(8):751–757, 1990.

Horbach NS, Ostergard DR: Predicting intrinsic urethral sphincter dysfunction in women with stress urinary incontinence. Obstet Gynecol 84(2):188–192, 1994.

Hosker GL, Mallet VT: Denervation and re-innervation of the urethral sphincter in the aetiology of genuine stress incontinence and a comparison of bioelectrical and mechanical activity of the female urethra (letter). Br J Obstet Gynaecol 101(6):559–560, 1994.

Imachi M, Tsukamoto N, Shigematsu T, et al: Marshall-Marchetti-Krantz operation for urinary stress incontinence. Nippon Sanka Fujinka Gakkai Zasshi 43(7):795–798, 1991.

Iosif CS: Effects of protracted administration of estriol on the lower genitourinary tract in postmenopausal women. Arch Gynecol Obstet 251(3):115–120, 1992.

Irani J, Dore B, Ruscillo MM, et al: Burch's procedure. Value of association with fixation to the promontorium and colpoperineorrhaphy. J Urol 97(3):123–127, 1991.

Jame A, Cabrera F, Szekely S, et al: Reflections on Marshall's operation (letter). Rev Fr Gynecol Obstet 85(12):713, 1990.

Jarvis GJ: Re: Erosion of buttress following bladder neck suspension (letter). Br J Urol 70(6):695, 1992.

Jarvis GJ: Surgery for genuine stress incontinence. Br J Obstet Gynaecol 101(5):371–374, 1994.

Johnson JD, Lamensdorf H, Hollander IN, Thurman AE: Use of transvaginal endosonography in the evaluation of women with stress urinary incontinence. J Urol 147(2):421–425, 1992.

Jonasson A, Larsson B, Pschera H, Nylund L: Short-term maximal electrical stimulation—a conservative treatment of urinary incontinence. Gynecol Obstet Invest 30(2):120–123, 1990.

Jorgensen L, Lose G, Alexander N: Acute effect of norfenefrine on the urethral pressure profile in females with genuine stress incontinence. Urol Int 46(2):176–179, 1991.

Jozwik M: Stress urinary incontinence in women—an overuse syndrome. Med Hypotheses 40(6):381–382, 1993.

Juma S, Little NA, Raz S: Vaginal wall sling: four years later. Urology 39(5):424–428, 1992.

Kadakia SC: Urinary incontinence associated with dysphagia (letter). Gastrointest Endosc 39(6):860–861, 1993.

Karram MM, Angel O, Koonings P, et al: The modified Pereyra procedure: A clinical and urodynamic review. Br J Obst Gynaecol 99(8):655–658, 1992.

Karram MM, Bhatia NN: Patch procedure: Modified transvaginal fascia lata sling for recurrent or severe stress urinary incontinence. Obstet Gynecol 75(3 Pt 1):461–463, 1990.

Karram MM, Rosenzweig BA, Bhatia NN: Artificial urinary sphincter for recurrent/severe stress incontinence in women. Urogynecologic perspective. J Reprod Med 38(10):791–794, 1993.

Kato K, Kondo A, Hasegawa S, et al: Pelvic floor muscle training as treatment of stress incontinence. The effectiveness of vaginal cones. Nippon Hinyokika Gakkai Zasshi 83(4):498–504, 1992.

Kawakami S, Yamada T, Watanabe T, et al: Significance of transrectal ultrasonography in surgery for stress urinary incontinence and cystocele. Assessment of the bladder neck suspension by measuring posterior urethrovesical angle and angle of inclination of the upper urethra. Nippon Hinyokika Gakkai Zasshi J 85(7):1066–1071, 1994.

Keane DP, Eckford SD: Surgical treatment of urinary stress incontinence. Br J Hosp Med 48(6):308–313, 1992.

Keane DP, Eckford SD, Abrams P: Surgical treatment and complications of urinary incontinence. Curr Opin Obstet Gynecol 4(4):559–564, 1992.

Kelly MJ, Knielsen K, Bruskewitz R, et al: Symptom analysis of patients undergoing modified Pereyra bladder neck suspension for stress urinary incontinence. Pre- and postoperative findings. Urology 37(3):213–219, 1991.

Kelly MJ, Zimmern PE, Leach GE: Complications of bladder neck suspension procedures. Urol Clin North Am 18(2):339, 1991.

Kelly MJ: Urinary incontinence in women without manifest injury to the bladder. Surg Gynecol Obstet 18:444, 1914.

Kelvin FM, Maglinte DD, Benson JT, et al: Dynamic cystoproctography: A technique for assessing disorders of the pelvic floor in women. AJR 163(2):368–370, 1994.

Kieswetter H, Fischer M, Wober I, Flamm J: Endoscopic implantation of collagen (GAX) for the treatment of urinary incontinence. Br J Urol 69(1):22–25, 1992.

Kiilholma P, Makinen J: Disappointing effect of endoscopic Teflon injection for female stress incontinence. Eur Urol 20(3):197–199, 1991.

Kiilholma P, Makinen J, Chancellor MB, et al: Modified Burch colposuspension for stress urinary incontinence in females. Surg Gynecol Obstet 176(2):111–115, 1993.

Kiilholma PJ, Makinen JI, Pitkanen YA, Varpula MJ: Perineal ultrasound: An alternative for radiography for evaluating stress urinary incontinence in females. Ann Chir Gynaecol Supple 208:43–45, 1994.

Kil PJ, Hoekstra JW, van der Meijden AP, et al: Transvaginal ultrasonography and urodynamic evaluation after suspension operations: Comparison among the Gittes, Stamey and Burch suspensions. J Urol 146(1):132–136, 1991.

Kirschner-Hermanns R, Wein B, Niehaus S, et al: The contribution of magnetic resonance imaging of the pelvic floor to the understanding of urinary incontinence. Br J Urol 72(5):715–718, 1993.

Klutke C, Golomb J, Barbaric Z, Raz S: The anatomy of stress incontinence: magnetic resonance imaging of the female bladder neck and urethra. J Urol 143(3):563–566, 1990.

Knespl J: The Cobb-Ragde method of a simplified correction of female stress incontinence. Cesk Gynekol 55(4):268–269, 1990.

Koelbl H, Bernaschek G, Deutinger J: Assessment of female urinary incontinence by introital sonography. J Clin Ultrasound 18(4):370–374, 1990.

Kohorn EI: Negative Q-tip test as a risk factor for failed incontinence surgery in women (letter). J Reprod Med 35(1):68, 1990.

Kohorn EI: Surgery for stress urinary incontinence. Curr Opin Obstet Gynecol 3(3):394–397, 1991.

Kolbl H, Bernascheck G: Introital sonography—a new method in the diagnosis of bladder function. Geburtshilfe Frauenheilkd 50(4):295–298, 1990.

Komatsu H: A study on the self-regulation of stress urinary incontinence in middle-aged and elderly women. Seiroka Kango Daigaku Kiyo 20:2–10, 1994.

Koonings PP, Bergman A, Ballard CA: Low urethral pressure and stress urinary incontinence in women: Risk factor for failed retropubic surgical procedure. Urology 36(3):245–248, 1990.

Koonings PP, Bergman A, Ballard CA: Prostaglandins for enhancing detrusor function after surgery for stress incontinence in women. J Reprodu Med 35(1):1–5, 1990.

Korn AP: Does use of permanent suture material affect outcome of the modified Pereyra procedure? Obstet Gynecol 83(1):104–107, 1994.

Krahulec P, Rovny F, Matysek P, et al: Personal experience with colpoureteral suspension using the Burch method. Cesk Gynekol 57(5):197–202, 1992.

Kranzfelder D, Baumann-Muller A, Kristen P: Recurrence following urinary incontinence surgery. Urodynamic and radiologic study. Geburtshilfe Frauenheilkd 50(7):552–559, 1990.

Krasnopol'skii VI, Ioseliani MN, Slobodianiuk AI, Sigua DS: Modification of the Aldrich operation—a method of choice in the surgical treatment of patients with stress-induced urinary incontinence. Akush Ginekol (Mosk) (1):55–58, 1991.

Kursh ED: Factors influencing the outcome of a no-incision endoscopic urethropexy. Surg Gynecol Obstet 175(3):254–258, 1992.

Kursh ED, Angell AH, Resnick MI: Evolution of endoscopic urethropexy: Seven-year experience with various techniques. Urology 37(5):428–431, 1991.

Lagro-Janssen TI, Debruyne FM, Smits AJ, van Weel C: Controlled trial of pelvic floor exercises in the treatment of urinary stress incontinence in general practice. Br J Gen Prac 41(352):445–449, 1991.

Lagro-Janssen AL, Debruyne FM, Van Weel C: Psychological aspects of female urinary incontinence in general practice. Br J Urol 70(5):499–502, 1992.

Largo-Janssen AL, Debruyne FM, van Weel C: Value of the patient's case history in diagnosing urinary incontinence in general practice. Br J Urol 67(6):569–572, 1991.

Lagro-Janssen AI, Smits AJ, van Weel C: Beneficial effect of exercise therapy in urinary incontinence in family practice depends largely on therapy compliance and motivation. Ned Tijdschr Geneeskd 138(25):1273–1276, 1994.

Lahodny J: Anatomic principles of surgical therapy of stress incontinence. Gynakologisch-Geburtshilfliche Rundschau 33(1):44–46, 1993.

Lam TC, Hadley HR: Surgical procedures for uncomplicated ("routine") female stress incontinence. Urol Clin North Am 18(2):327–337, 1991.

Langer R, Golan A, Arad D, et al: Effects of induced menopause on Burch colposuspension for urinary stress incontinence. J Reprod Med 37(12):956–958, 1992.

Langer R, Golan A, Neuman M, et al: The effect of large uterine fibroids on urinary bladder function and symptoms. Am J Obstet Gynecol 163(4 Pt 1):1139–1141, 1990.

Langer R, Golan A, Ron-El R, et al: Colposuspension for urinary stress incontinence in premenopausal and postmenopausal women. Surg Gynecol Obstet 171(1):13–16, 1990.

Leach GE: Urethral resistance after surgery for stress incontinence. Urology 35(4):373–374, 1990.

Leach GE, Zimmern P, Staskin D, et al: Surgery for pelvic prolapse. Semin Urol 4:43–50, 1986.

Lee RA: Vaginal hysterectomy with repair of enterocele, cystocele, and rectocele. Clin Obstet Gynecol 36(4):967–975, 1993.

Lim PH, Brown AD, Chisholm GD: The Burch colposuspension operation for stress urinary incontinence. Singapore Med J 31(3):242–246, 1990.

Llorente C, Linares R, Carnero J, et al: Pubo-vaginal percutaneous suspension by the Gittes technique for stress incontinence. Initial experience. Acta Urol Esp 14(6):418–420, 1990.

Liu CY. Laparoscopic retropubic colposuspension (Burch procedure). A review of 58 cases. J Reprod Med 38(7):526–530, 1993.

Lockhart JL, Ellis GF, Helal M, Pow-Sang JM: Combined cystourethropexy for the treatment of type 3 and complicated female urinary incontinence. J Urol 143(4):722–725, 1990.

Lopez Lopez JA, Valdivia Uria JG, Rosa Arias J, Ucar Terren A: Percutaneous endoscopic urethrocervicopexy. Arch Esp Urol 44(5):591–593, 1991.

Lopez Lopez JA, Valdivia Uria JG, Ucar Terren A: Percutaneous endoscopic urethrocervicopexy. Eur Urol 22(2):167–170, 1992.

Lose G: Urethral pressure and power generation during coughing and voluntary contraction of the pelvic floor in females with genuine stress incontinence. Br J Urol 67(6):580–585, 1991.

Lose G, Colstrup H: Mechanical properties of the urethra in healthy and stress incontinent females: Dynamic measurements in the resting urethra. J Urol 144(5):1258–1262, 1990.

Lotenfoe R, O'Kelly JK, Helal M, Lockhart JL: Periurethral polytetrafluoroethylene paste injection in incontinent female subjects: Surgical indications and improved surgical technique. J Urol 149(2):279–282, 1993.

Lotocki W, Drozdzewicz M, Siekierski A: Results of surgical treatment of stress urinary incontinence in women. Rocz Akad Med Bialymstoku 35–36:89–97, 1990–1991.

Lotocki W, Pieciukiewicz Z, Podziewska I: Results of the evaluation of intracystic and intraurethral pressure in women with stress urinary incontinence. Rocz Akade Med Bialymstoku 35–36:81–87, 1990–1991.

Loughlin KR, Whitmore WF 3d, Gittes RF, Richie JP: Review of an 8-year experience with modifications of endoscopic suspension of the bladder neck for female stress urinary incontinence. J Urol 143(1):44–45, 1990.

Luschin-Ebengreuth G, Ralph G, Tamussino K: Endoscopic bladder neck suspension—clinical, urodynamic and radiologic results. Gynakol Rundschau 31 (Suppl 2):315–317, 1991.

Lycklama a Nijeholt AA: Neuromodulation; a new treatment method for incontinence and micturition disorders. Ned Tijdschr Geneesk 136(2):60–61, 1992.

MacArthur C, Lewis M, Knox EG: Health after childbirth. Br J Obstet Gynaecol 98(12):1193–1195, 1991.

Mantle J, Versi E: Physiotherapy for stress urinary incontinence: A national survey. Br Med J 302(6779):753–755, 1991.

Mark SD, McRae CU, Arnold EP, Gowland SP: Clam cystoplasty for the overactive bladder: A review of 23 cases. Aust NZ J Surg 64(2):88–90, 1994.

Marshall S: Conservative management of stress urinary incontinence (letter). Urology 38(3):294, 1991.

Martan A, Halaska M, Drbohlav P, Voigt R: Ultrasound of the urinary bladder neck: Changes before and after pelvic floor muscle exercise. Cesk Gynekol 59(3):121–124, 1994.

Martan A, Halaska M, Sindlar M, et al: Treatment of stress incontinence using a combination of the parasympatholytics, hexadiphensulphonium and oxyphenonium and the spasmolytic, papaverine. Cesk Gynekol 56(1):27–31, 1991.

Martan A, Halaska M, Voigt R, et al: Kolpexin in the conservative treatment of stress incontinence. Zentralbl Gynakol 113(11):645–648, 1991.

Martan A, Sindlar M, Halaska M, et al: The atropine test in patients with stress incontinence and their treatment with a combination of diltiazem and oxyphenonium. Cesk Gynek 55(6):406–412, 1990.

Martan A, Sindlar M, Halaska M, et al: Treatment of stress incontinence using the tricyclic antidepressive agent imipramine (Melipramin). Cesk Gynekol 55(6):426–430, 1990.

Martan A, Voigt R, Halaska M: Drug therapy of urge incontinence in the female. Zentralbl Gynakol 115(5):205–209, 1993.

Masuda H, Yamada T, Nagamatsu H, et al: Analysis of continence mechanisms by stress urethral pressure profiles. Nippon Hinyokika Gakkai Zasshi 85(3):434–439, 1994.

Masuda H, Yamada T, Nagamatsu H, et al: The correlation of the severity of stress urinary incontinence with static and stress urethral pressure profiles. Hinyokika Kiyo 40(3):209–213, 1994.

McGuire EJ: Identifying and managing stress incontinence in the elderly. Geriatrics 45(6):44–46, 51–52, 1990.

McGuire EJ, Fitzpatrick CC, Wan J, et al: Clinical assessment of urethral sphincter function. J Urol 150(5 Pt 1):1452–1454, 1993.

McIntosh LJ, Mallett VT, Richardson DA: Complications from permanent suture in surgery for stress urinary incontinence. A report of two cases. J Reprod Med 38(10):823–825, 1993.

Meyer S, de Grandi P: Anamnestic, clinical and urodynamic comparative data from a group of patients with urinary stress incontinence. J Gynecol Obstet Biol Reprod 19(6):709–716, 1990.

Meyer S, DeGrandi P, Schmidt N: Effect of occluding the urethra while recording urethral stress profile. Urology 38(2):157–160, 1991.

Meyer S, De Grandi P, Schmidt N, et al: Urodynamic parameters in patients with slight and severe genuine stress incontinence: is the stress profile useful? Neurourol Urodyn 13(1):21–28, 1994.

Meyer S, Dhenin T, Schmidt N, et al: Subjective and objective effects of intravaginal electrical myostimulation and biofeedback in patients with genuine stress urinary incontinence. Br J Urol 69(6):584–588, 1992.

Michelitsch L, Ralph G, Tamussino K: Urodynamic results following incontinence operations. Gynakol Rundschau 30 (Suppl 1):233–234, 1990.

Michelitsch L, Tamussino K, Ralph G: Treatment of stress incontinence in total prolapse of the uterus. Gynakol Geburtshilfliche Rundschau 32 (Suppl 1):140, 1992.

Miyazaki F, Shook G: Ilioinguinal nerve entrapment during needle suspension for stress incontinence. Obstet Gynecol 80(2):246–248, 1992.

Mizuo T, Tanizawa A, Yamada T, et al: Sling operation for male stress incontinence by utilizing modified Stamey technique. Urology 39(3):211–214, 1992.

Mommsen S, Foldspang A, Elving L, Lam GW: Association between urinary incontinence in women and a previous history of surgery. Br J Urol 72(1):30–37, 1993.

Monga M, Ghoniem GM: Ilioinguinal nerve entrapment following needle bladder suspension procedures. Urology 44(3):447–450, 1994.

Mouchel J: Surgical treatment of stress urinary incontinence in women using a suburethral suspension with a polytetrafluoroethylene sling. Apropos of 95 cases. Rev Fr Gynecol Obstet 85(6):399–406, 1990.

Mouritsen L, Frimodt-Moller C, Moller M: Long-term effect of pelvic floor exercises on female urinary incontinence. Br J Urol 68(1):32–37, 1991.

Mouritsen L, Strandberg C: Vaginal ultrasonography versus colpocysto-urethrography in the evaluation of female urinary incontinence. Acta Obstet Gynecol Scand 73(4):338–342, 1994.

Mouritsen L, Strandberg C, Jensen AR, et al: Inter- and intra-observer variation of colpo-cysto-urethrography diagnoses. Acta Obstet Gynecol Scand 72(3):200–204, 1993.

Murphy KP, Kliever EM, Moore MJ: The voiding alert system: a new application in the treatment of incontinence. Arch Phys Med Rehabil 75(8):924–927, 1994.

Navalon P, Llopis B, Picurelli L, et al: Surgical treatment of urinary stress incontinence in women. Acta Urol Esp 14(4):271–273, 1990.

Neikov K, Tachev S: Urethrovesicopexy by the Marshall-Marchetti-Krantz method with urodynamic control in women with stress urinary incontinence. Khirurgiia 46(3):36–38, 1993.

Neri Ruz ES, Azcona Arteaga FJ: Stress urinary incontinence. Its surgical management. Ginecol Obstet Mex 59:302–307, 1991.

Ng RK, Murray A: Can we afford to take short cuts in the management of stress urinary incontinence? Singapore Med J 34(2):121–124, 1993.

Nghiem Toan N: Simplified urethrocystovaginal suspension as treatment for stress urinary incontinence (letter). Am J Obstet Gynecol 168(5):1642, 1993.

Nichols DH: Gynecological and Obstetric Surgery. Chicago, Mosby, 1987, p 334.

Nichols DH: Surgery for pelvic floor disorders. Surg Clin North Am 71(5):927–946, 1991.

Nichols DG: Vaginal prolapse affecting bladder function. Urol Clin North Am 12:329–338, 1985.

Nichols DH: Vaginal Surgery, 3rd ed. Baltimore, Williams & Wilkins, 1989.

Niecestro RM, Wheeler JS Jr, Nanninga J, et al: Use of stresscath for diagnosing stress incontinence. Urology 39(3):266–269, 1992.

Nielsen KK, Kromann-Andersen B, Jakobsen H, et al: The intraurethral plug. A new alternative in the treatment of women with stress incontinence. Ugeskr Laeger 153(51):3608–3610, 1991.

Nielsen KK, Kromann-Andersen B, Jacobsen H, et al: The urethral plug: A new treatment modality for genuine urinary stress incontinence in women. J Urol 144(5):1199–1202, 1990.

Nielsen KK, Walter S, Maegaard E, Kromann-Andersen B: The urethral plug II: An alternative treatment in women with genuine urinary stress incontinence. Br J Urol 72(4):428–432, 1993.

Nito H: Clinical effect of midodrine hydrochloride on the patients with urinary incontinence. Hinyokika Kiyo 40(1):91–94, 1994.

Nitti VW, Raz S: Obstruction following anti-incontinence procedures: Diagnosis and treatment with transvaginal urethrolysis. J Urol 152(1):93–98, 1994.

Nochajski TH, Burns PA, Pranikoff K, Dittmar SS: Dimensions of urine loss among older women with genuine stress incontinence. Neurourol Urodyn 12(3):223–233, 1993.

Norton KR, Bhat AV, Stanton SL: Psychiatric aspects of urinary incontinence in women attending an outpatient urodynamic clinic. Br Med J 301(6746):271–272, 1990.

Nygaard I, DeLancey JO, Arnsdorf L, Murphy E: Exercise and incontinence. Obstet Gynecol 75(5):848–851, 1990.

Nygaard IE, Thompson FL, Svengalis SL, Albright JP: Urinary incontinence in elite nulliparous athletes. Obstet Gynecol 84(2):183–187, 1994.

O'Donnell PD: Combined Raz urethral suspension and McGuire pubovaginal sling for treatment of complicated stress urinary incontinence. J Ark Med Soc 88(8):389–392, 1992.

O'Flynn KJ, Thomas DG: Artificial urinary sphincter insertion in congenital neuropathic bladder. Br J Urol 67(2):155–157, 1991.

Ogundipe A, Rosenzweig BA, Karram MM, et al: Modified suburethral sling procedure for treatment of recurrent or severe stress urinary incontinence. Surg Gynecol Obstet 175(2):173–176, 1992.

Olah KS, Bridges N, Denning J, Farrar DJ: The conservative management of patients with symptoms of stress incontinence: A randomized, prospective study comparing weighted vaginal cones and interferential therapy. Am J Obstet Gynecol 162(1):87–92, 1990.

Orozco Farinas R, Oro Ortiz J: Anatomic effects of Stamey's urethrocystopexy as modified by Orozco and Perez Poo. Arch Esp Urol 43(2):121–124, 1990.

Orozco Farinas R, Osorio Acosta V, Capdevila Viciedo D, et al: The use of vagina and percutaneous surgery in stress urinary incontinence: Description, foundations, and indications. Arch Esp Urol 46(10):855–862, 1993.

Orozco Farinas R, Perez Poo HR: Modification of Stamey's endoscopic cervicopexy for stress urinary incontinence. Arch Esp Urol 43(2):117–120, 1990.

Ou CS, Presthus J, Beadle E: Laparoscopic bladder neck suspension using hernia mesh and surgical staples. J Laparoendosc Surg 3(6):563–566, 1993.

Papa Petros PE, Ulmsten U: An analysis of rapid pad testing and the history for the diagnosis of stress incontinence. Acta Obstet Gynecol Scand 71(7):529–536, 1992.

Parra RO, Shaker L: Experience with a simplified technique for the treatment of female stress urinary incontinence. Br J Urol 66(6):615–617, 1990.

Parys BT, Woolfenden KA, Parsons KF: Bladder dysfunction after simple hysterectomy: Urodynamic and neurological evaluation. Eur Urol 17(2):129–133, 1990.

Penders L, Lombard R, Jehaes C: Reinforced colposuspension (modified Cukier's operation). Immediate results, complications, indications. Acta Urol Belg 58(4):59–70, 1990.

Penders L, Vanstalle-Nelissen G: Bladder instability and kinesitherapy. The concept of deficient bladder instability. Acta Urol Belg 58(2):103–114, 1990.

Petros PE, Ulmsten U: Bladder instability in women: A premature activation of the micturition reflex. Neurourol Urodyna 12(3):235–239, 1993.

Petros PE, Ulmsten UI: Cough transmission ratio: An indicator of suburethral vaginal wall tension rather than urethral closure? Acta Obstet Gynecol Scand Suppl 153:37–39, 1990.

Petros PE, Ulmsten UI: Cure of stress incontinence by repair of external anal sphincter. Two case reports. Acta Obstet Gynecol Scand Suppl 153:75, 1990.

Petros PE, Ulmsten UI: Pregnancy effects on the intravaginal sling operation. Acta Obstet Gynecol Scand Suppl 153:77–78, 1990.

Petros PE, Ulmsten U: Tests for 'detrusor instability' in women. These mainly measure the urethral resistance created by pelvic floor contraction acting against a premature activation of the micturition reflex. Acta Obstet Gynecol Scand 72(8):661–667, 1993.

Petros PE, Ulmsten UI: The role of a lax posterior vaginal fornix in the causation of stress and urgency symptoms: A preliminary report. Acta Obstet Gynecol Scand Suppl 153:71–73, 1990.

Petros PE, Ulmsten UI, Papadimitriou J: The autogenic ligament procedure: A technique for planned formation of an artificial neo-ligament. Acta Obstet Gynecol Scand Suppl 153:43–51, 1990.

Phillips TH, Zeidman EJ, Thompson IM: The fate of buried vaginal epithelium. J Urol 148(6):1941–1943, 1992.

Phua SM, Low JJ, Chew SY: The role of urodynamics in evaluating incontinent females. Singapore Med J 33(2):139–142, 1992.

Pidutti RW, George SW, Morales A: Correction of recurrent stress urinary incontinence by needle urethropexy with a vaginal wall sling. Br J Urol 73(4):418–422, 1994.

Pieber D, Zivkovic F, Tamussino K: Pelvic floor exercises without or with vaginal cones in premenopausal women with mild to moderate stress incontinence. Gynakol Geburtshilfliche Rundschau 34(1):32–33, 1994.

Porjazov K: A ten-year follow-up of postoperative results of the treatment of urinary incontinence. Folia Med 32(2):26–28, 1990.

Poryazov K: The therapeutic effect of treatment of urinary stress incontinence with estriol. Folia Med 32(4):16–19, 1990.

Prat-Pradal D, Costa P, Lopez S, et al: Female urinary stress incontinence and insufficient closing pressures. Results of perineal sphincter electromyography. Prog Urol 1(4):546–553, 1991.

Puchmeltr P, Puchmeltr V Sr, Puchmeltr V Jr: The modified Parent urethrovesicopexy and the results from 1977 to 1988 at the gynecology-obstetrical department in Teplice, Czechoslovakia. Cesk Gynekol 55(3):196–199, 1990.

Raboy A, Hakim LS, Ferzli G, et al: Extraperitoneal endoscopic vesicourethral suspension. J Laparoendosc Surg 3(5):505–508, 1993.

Rachagan SP, Mathews A: Urinary incontinence caused by prazosin. Singapore Med J 33(3):308–309, 1992.

Ralph G: Effect of various operations for incontinence on the dynamics and topography of the bladder and bladder neck. Wien Klini Wochensch Suppl 185:3–14, 1991.

Ralph G: Results of incontinence operations: Comparative study. Gynakol Geburtshilfliche Rundschau 33(1):47–48, 1993.

Ralph G, Tamussino K: Endoscopic bladder neck suspension—clinical, urodynamic and radiologic results. Geburtshilfe Frauenheilkd 51(10):830–833, 1991.

Ralph G, Tamussino K, Michelitsch L: Surgical therapy of recurrent stress incontinence. Geburtshilfe Frauenheilkd 53(4):265–269, 1993.

Ralph G, Tamussino K, Michelitsch L: Treatment of stress incontinence with total prolapse of the uterus. Geburtshilfe Frauenheilkd 53(12):870–874, 1993.

Ramirez CH, Figueroa LA, Hidalgo F: Cystometry in recurrent urinary stress incontinence. Arch Esp Urol Oct, 44(8):985–986, 1991.

Ramirez CH, Figueroa LA, Hidalgo CF: Cystometry in recurrent stress urinary incontinence. Arch Esp Urol 45(10):1009–1010, 1992.

Ramirez JC, Salinas J, Silmi A, et al: Technique of simplified retropubic colpourethrocervicopexy in the treatment of genuine urinary stress incontinence in women. Acta Urol Esp 15(2):149–153, 1991.

Ramirez PH: Therapeutic alternatives in recurrent urinary incontinence. Rev Chil Obstet Ginecol 56(1):48–50, 1991.

Rammer E, Friedrich F, Burger F: Treatment of stress incontinence with Burch colposuspension. Gynakol Geburtshilfliche Rundschau 32 (Suppl 1):136–137, 1992.

Ramon J, Mekras JA, Webster GD: The outcome of transvaginal cystourethropexy in patients with anatomical stress urinary incontinence and outlet weakness. J Urol 144(1):106–108, 1990.

Ramon J, Mekras J, Webster GD: Transvaginal needle suspension procedures for recurrent stress incontinence. Urology 38(6):519–522, 1991.

Ramsay IN, Hilton P, Cox TF: Time-series analysis of urethral electrical conductance measurements in the assessment of unstable urethral pressure: Results in normal patients and in those with genuine stress incontinence. Neurourol Urodyn 12(1):23–31, 1993.

Raz S: Vaginal surgery for stress incontinence. J Am Geriatr Soc 38(3):345–347, 1990.

Raz S, Golomb J, Klutke C: Four-corner bladder and urethral suspension for moderate cystocele. J Urol 142:712–715, 1989.

Raz S, Little NA, Juma S, Sussman EM: Repair of severe anterior vaginal wall prolapse (grade IV cystourethrocele). J Urol 146(4):988–992, 1991.

Raz S, Nitti VW, Bregg KJ: Transvaginal repair of enterocele. J Urology 149(4):724–730, 1993.

Realini JP, Walters MD: Vaginal diaphragm rings in the treatment of stress urinary incontinence. J Am Board Fam Pract 3(2):99–103, 1990.

Rechberger T, Donica H, Baranowski W, Jakowicki J: Female urinary stress incontinence in terms of connective tissue biochemistry. Euro J Obstet Gynecol Reprod Biol 49(3):187–191, 1993.

Resnick NM: Initial evaluation of the incontinent patient. J Am Geriatr Soc 38(3):311–316, 1990.

Resnick NM, Beckett LA, Branch LG, et al: Short-term variability of self report of incontinence in older persons. J Am Geriatr Soc 42(2):202–207, 1994.

Richardson DA, Ramahi A, Chalas E: Surgical management of stress incontinence in patients with low urethral pressure. Gynecol Obstet Invest 31(2):106–109, 1991.

Riss P, Ralph G: Abdominal colposuspension—the gold standard in incontinence therapy? Geburtshilfe Frauenheilkd 54(2):69–74, 1994.

Rockner G: Urinary incontinence after perineal trauma at childbirth. Scand J Caring Sci 4(4):169–172, 1990.

Rosenzweig BA, Bhatia NN: Temporal separation of cough-induced urethral and bladder pressure spikes in women with urinary incontinence. Urology 39(2):165–168, 1992.

Rosenzweig BA, Bhatia NN, Nelson AL: Dynamic urethral pressure profilometry pressure transmission ratio: What do the numbers really mean? Obstet Gynecol 77(4):586–590, 1991.

Rossi D, Nadal F, Serment G, et al: The results of urethro-cervicolysis after surgical over-correction of stress urinary incontinence. Apropos of 10 cases. Ann Urol 24(1):27–31, 1990.

Rosenzweig BA, Pushkin S, Blumenfeld D, Bhatia NN: Prevalence of abnormal urodynamic test results in continent women with severe genitourinary prolapse. Obstet Gynecol 79(4):539–542, 1992.

Rosenzweig BA, Soffici AR, Thomas S, Bhatia NN: Urodynamic evaluation of voiding in women with cystocele. J Reprod Med 37(2):162–166, 1992.

Rychtarech B, Bolgac A, Taufer I, et al: Our results with the Burch method of colposuspension. Cesk Gynekol 56(7-8):411–413, 1991.

Sacco F, Rigon G, Carbone A, Sacchini D: Transvaginal estrogen therapy in urinary stress incontinence. Minerva Ginecol 42(12):539–544, 1990.

Sacco F, Rigon G, Carbone A, et al: Ultrasonographic and urodynamic evaluation in stress incontinence. Minerva Ginecol 45(11):519–525, 1993.

Salinas CJ, Varela E, Prieto CL, et al: Results of perineal electric stimulation in stress urinary incontinence. Arch Esp Urol 44(4):437–440, 1991.

Sampselle CM: Changes in pelvic muscle strength and stress urinary incontinence associated with childbirth. J Obstet Gynecol Neonat Nurs 19(5):371–377, 1990.

Sanchez BE, Diaz RF, Vara TC: Stress incontinence: A new endoscopic approach. Urology 36(5):403–405, 1990.

Sanchez BE, Jimenez GA, Gutierrez CJM, Vara TC: Extraperitoneal laparoscopic urethropexy. Arch Esp Urol 47(4):415–418, 1994.

Sand PK, Bowen LW, Ostergard DR: The prognostic significance of augmentation of urethral closure pressure and functional length. Int J Gynaecol Obstet 33(2):135–139, 1990.

Sand PK, Brubaker LT: Advances in nonoperative treatment of genuine stress incontinence. Curr Opin Obstet Gynecol 2(4):599–604, 1990.

Schar G, Kochli OR, Fink D, Haller U: Surgical strategy in incontinence and prolapse. Gynakol Geburtshilfliche Rundschau 33(2):94–102, 1993.

Schiotz HA: One month maximal electrostimulation for genuine stress incontinence in women. Neurourol Urodyn 13(1):43–50, 1994.

Schmidbauer CP: Vaginal estriol administration in treatment of postmenopausal urinary incontinence. Urologe A 31(6):384–389, 1992.

Schultze H, Wolansky D: Urethral wall pulsation in pregnant patients, continent and stress incontinent females. Zentralbl Gynakol 112(1):19–22, 1990.

Schultze HH, Wolf HD: Spatial urethral rest pressure and stress pressure profile in women with stress incontinence. Doppler microtransducer studies. Zentralbl Gynakol 113(5):245–252, 1991.

Schurmann R, Ralph G: Urodynamic results of Burch colposuspension. Zentralbl Gynakol 112(9):577–581, 1990.

Schussler B: Recommendations of the Urogynecology Study Group on urogynecologic diagnosis and therapy. Gynakolog Geburtshilfliche Rundschau 33(3):193–196, 1993.

Scotti RJ, Myers DL: A comparison of the cough stress test and single-channel cystometry with multichannel urodynamic evaluation in genuine stress incontinence. Obstet Gynecol 81(3):430–433, 1993.

Scotti RJ, Ostergard DR, Guillaume AA, Kohatsu KE: Predictive value of urethroscopy as compared to urodynamics in the diagnosis of genuine stress incontinence. J Reprod Med 35(8):772–776, 1990.

Sethia KK, Webb RJ, Neal DE: Urodynamic study of ileocystoplasty in the treatment of idiopathic detrusor instability. Br J Urol 67(3):286–290, 1991.

Sexton DJ, Heskestad L, Lambeth WR, et al: Postoperative pubic osteomyelitis misdiagnosed as osteitis pubis: Report of four cases and review. Clin Infect Dis 17(4):695–700, 1993.

Shull B: Clinical evaluation of women with pelvic support defects. Clin Obstet Gynecol 36(4):939, 1993.

Shimoura H: A surgical correction of urinary stress incontinence by vaginal route—midline plication of urethral supports. Nippon Sanka Fujinka Gakkai Zasshi 45(7):679–682, 1993.

Smart RF: Polytef paste for urinary incontinence. Aust NZ J Surg 61(9):663–669, 1991.

Snooks SJ, Swash M, Mathers SE, Henry MM: Effect of vaginal delivery on the pelvic floor: A 5-year follow-up. Br J Surg 77(12):1358–1360, 1990.

Sommer P, Bauer T, Nielsen KK, et al: Voiding patterns and prevalence of incontinence in women. A questionnaire survey. Br J Urol 66(1):12–15, 1990.

Srinivasan V, Blackford HN: Genuine stress incontinence induced by prazosin. Br J Urol 72(4):510, 1993.

Stanton SL: Stress urinary incontinence. Ciba Foundation Symposium 151:182–189, 1990.

Stanton SL: Suprapubic approaches for stress incontinence in women. J Am Geriatr Soc 38(3):348–351, 1990.

Steg A, Zerbib M, Conquy S, et al: Stress urinary incontinence in women: Treatment of surgical failures. Prog Urol 1(6):1064–1068, 1991.

Stein M, Weinberg JJ: Polytetrafluoroethylene vs. polypropylene suture for endoscopic bladder neck suspension. Urology 38(2):119–122, 1991.

Suarez GM, Baum NH, Jacobs J: Use of standard contraceptive diaphragm in management of stress urinary incontinence. Urology 37(2):119–122, 1991.

Summitt RL Jr, Bent AE, Ostergard DR, Harris TA: Stress incontinence and low urethral closure pressure. Correlation of preoperative urethral hypermobility with successful suburethral sling procedures. J Reprod Med 35(9):877–880, 1990.

Summitt RL Jr, Sipes DR 2nd, Bent AE, Ostergard DR: Evaluation of pressure transmission ratios in women with genuine stress incontinence and low urethral pressure: A comparative study. Obstet Gynecol 83(6):984–988, 1994.

Susset JG, Galea G, Read L: Biofeedback therapy for female incontinence due to low urethral resistance. J Urol 143(6):1205–1208, 1990.

Swash M: The neurogenic hypothesis of stress incontinence. Ciba Foundation Symposium 151:156–170, 1990.

Swierzewski SJ 3d, McGuire EJ: Pubovaginal sling for treatment of female stress urinary incontinence complicated by urethral diverticulum. J Urol 149(5):1012–1014, 1993.

Swierzewski SJ 3d, McGuire EJ, Podrazik RM, Stanley JC: Aortic occlusion and lower extremity exercise induced stress urinary incontinence. J Urol 149(4):846–847, 1993.

Tamussino K, Ralph G: Late results of surgery for incontinence. Gynakol Geburtshilfliche Rundschau 33 (Suppl 1):242, 1993.

Tamussino K, Ralph G: Surgical therapy of stress incontinence after radical hysterectomy. Gynakol Rundschau 31 (Suppl 2):317–318, 1991.

Taylor JD, Tsokos N: A retroperitoneal approach to surgery for stress incontinence using the laparoscope (letter). Med J Aust 160(1):42, 1994.

Taylor JD, Tsokos N: Retroperitoneal laparoscopic surgery for stress incontinence (letter). Lancet 342(8886-8887):1564–1565, 1993.

Thind P, Colstrup H, Lose G, Kristensen JK: Method for evaluation of the urethral closure mechanism in women during standardised changes of cross-sectional area. Clin Phys Physiol Measurement 12(2):163–170, 1991.

Thind P, Lose G, Colstrup H: Initial urethral pressure increase during stress episodes in genuine stress incontinent women. Br J Urol 69(2):137–140, 1992.

Thind P, Lose G, Colstrup H: Pressure response to rapid dilation of resting urethra in healthy women. Urology 40(1):44–49, 1992.

Thunedborg P, Fischer-Rasmussen W, Jensen SB: Stress urinary incontinence and posterior bladder suspension defects. Results of vaginal repair versus Burch colposuspension. Acta Obstet Gynecol Scand 69(1):55–59, 1990.

Timmons MC, Addison WA: Choice of operation for genuine stress incontinence. Curr Opin Obstet Gynecol 3(4):528–533, 1991.

Tjelum KB, Lose G, Abel I, Pedersen LM: Electrostimulation of the pelvic floor muscles in urinary incontinence. Ugesk Laeger 156(15):2214–2216, 1994.

Tovell H: Gynecological Operations. Philadelphia, Harper & Row, 1978.

Turkington D, Grant J, Tophill P, Johnston J: Psychiatric aspects of urinary incontinence (letter). Br Med J 301(6749):444–445, 1990.

Ulmsten U, Petros P: Surgery for female urinary incontinence. Curr Opin Obstet Gynecol 4(3):456–462, 1992.

Valiquette I, Paquin JM, Perreault JP, et al: Perineal retraining in urinary stress incontinence. Ann Chir 45(9):816–821, 1991.

Valle Gerhold J, Murillo Perez C, Timon Garcia A, et al: Experience with endoscopic urethrocervicopexy: Long-term results. Acta Urol Esp 17(9):595–597, 1993.

Vancaillie TG, Schuessler W: Laparoscopic bladder neck suspension. J Laparoendosc Surg 1(3):169–173, 1991.

van Kerrebroeck PE: Surgical correction of urinary incontinence and (or) prolapse symptoms (letter). Ned Tijdschr Geneesk 137(15):781–782, 1993.

van Waalwijk van Doorn ES, Zwiers W: Ambulant monitoring to assess the efficacy of oxybutynin chloride in patients with mixed incontinence. Eur Urol 18(1):49–51, 1990.

Varner RE: Retropubic long-needle suspension procedures for stress urinary incontinence. Am J Obstet Gynecol 163(2):551–557, 1990.

Varner RE, Sparks JM: Surgery for stress urinary incontinence. Surg Clin North Am 71(5):1111–1134, 1991.

Versi E: Discriminant analysis of urethral pressure profilometry data for the diagnosis of genuine stress incontinence. Br J Obstet Gynaecol 97(3):251–259, 1990.

Versi E: The significance of an open bladder neck in women. Br J Urol 68(1):42–43, 1991.

Versi E, Cardozo I, Anand D, Cooper D: Symptoms analysis for the diagnosis of genuine stress incontinence. Br J Obstet Gynaecol 98(8):815–819, 1991.

Versi E, Cardozo L, Cooper DJ: Urethral pressures: Analysis of transmission pressure ratios. Br J Urol 68(3):266–270, 1991.

Vicente RJ: Critical evaluation of Teflon in urology. Arch Esp Urol 43(4):327–331, 1990.

Vierhout ME, Gianotten WL: Mechanisms of urine loss during sexual activity. Eur J Obstet Gynecol Reprod Biol 52(1):45–47, 1993.

Vierhout ME, Gianotten WL: Unintended urine loss in women during sexual activities: An exploratory study. Ned Tijdschr Geneesk 137(18):913–916, 1993.

Vierhout ME, Mulder AF: De novo detrusor instability after Burch colposuspension. Acta Obstet Gynecol Scand 71(6):414–416, 1992.

Viktrup L, Lose G: Epidural anesthesia during labor and stress incontinence after delivery. Obstet Gynecol 82(6):984–986, 1993.

Viktrup L, Lose G, Rolff M, Barfoed K: The symptom of stress incontinence caused by pregnancy or delivery in primiparas. Obstet Gynecol 79(6):945–949, 1992.

Viktrup L, Lose G, Rolff M, Barfoed KL: Urinary tract symptoms in relation to pregnancy and labor in primiparas. Ugeskr Laeger 155(11):789–793, 1993.

Vinagre M, Pardo H, Roa E, Fuente S: Colposuspension in the treatment of stress urinary incontinence: long-term yield. Rev Chil Obstet Ginecol 56(4):284–290, 1991.

Voigt R, Halaska M: Results of urodynamic studies of patients after the Burch colpopexy operation. Cesk Gynekol 55(4):265–267, 1990.

Wahle GR, Young GP, Raz S: Vaginal surgery for stress urinary incontinence (editorial). Urology 43(4):416–419, 1994.

Walker GT, Texter JH Jr: Success and patient satisfaction following the Stamey procedure for stress urinary incontinence. J Urol 147(6):1521–1523, 1992.

Wall LL: Medical management of pelvic relaxation. Curr Opin Obstet Gynecol 5(4):440–445, 1993.

Wall LL: The muscles of the pelvic floor. Clin Obstet Gynecol 36(4):910–925, 1993.

Wall LL, Addison WA: Prazosin-induced stress incontinence. Obstet Gynecol 75(3 Pt 2):558–560, 1990.

Wall LL, Davidson TG: The role of muscular re-education by physical therapy in the treatment of genuine stress urinary incontinence. Obstet Gynecol Surv 47(5):322–331, 1992.

Wall LL, Hewitt JK: Urodynamic characteristics of women with complete posthysterectomy vaginal vault prolapse. Urology 44(3):336–341, 1994.

Walter JS, Wheeler JS, Morgan C, et al: Measurement of total urethral compliance in females with stress incontinence. Neurourol Urodyn 12(3):273–276, 1993.

Walters MD, Jackson GM: Urethral mobility and its relationship to stress incontinence in women. J Reprod Med 35(8):777–784, 1990.

Walters MD, Realini JP, Dougherty M: Nonsurgical treatment of urinary incontinence. Curr Opin Obstet Gynecol 4(4):554–558, 1992.

Walters MD, Taylor S, Schoenfeld LS: Psychosexual study of women with detrusor instability. Obstet Gynecol 75(1):22–26, 1990.

Warwick DJ, Abrams P: The perineal artificial sphincter for acquired incontinence—a cut and dried solution? Br J Urol 66(5):495–499, 1990.

Webb RJ, Ramsden PD, Neal DE: Ambulatory monitoring and electronic measurement of urinary leakage in the diagnosis of detrusor instability and incontinence. Br J Urol 68(2):148–152, 1991.

Webster GD, Kreder KJ: Voiding dysfunction following cystourethropexy: its evaluation and management. J Urol 144(3):670–673, 1990.

Webster GD, Perez LM, Khoury JM, Timmons SL: Management of type III stress urinary incontinence using artificial urinary sphincter. Urology 39(6):499–503, 1992.

Weil EH, van Waalwijk van Doorn ES, Heesakkers JP, et al: Transvaginal ultrasonography: a study with healthy volunteers and women with genuine stress incontinence. Eur Urol 24(2):226–230, 1993.

Wein AJ: Oral and intravaginal estrogens alone and in combination with alpha-adrenergic stimulation in genuine stress incontinence. J Urol 146(6):1670–1671, 1991.

Weiss RE, Cohen E: Erosion of buttress following bladder neck suspension. Br J Urol 69(6):656–657, 1992.

Wells TJ, Brink CA, Diokno AC, et al: Pelvic muscle exercise for stress urinary incontinence in elderly women. J Am Geriatr Soc 39(8):785–791, 1991.

Wheeler JS Jr: Osteomyelitis of the pubis: Complication of a Stamey urethropexy. J Urol 151(6):1638–1640, 1994.

Whishaw DM, Fonda D: Is there a role for drug therapy in the treatment of urinary incontinence in the elderly? Med J Aust 160(7):430–435, 1994.

Wijma J, Tinga DJ, Visser GH: Perineal ultrasonography in women with stress incontinence and controls: the role of the pelvic floor muscles. Gynecol Obstet Invest 32(3):176–179, 1991.

Will E, Pinaudeau A: Urinary stress incontinence associated with a prolapse. Preoperative rehabilitation. Soins Gynecol Obstet Puericulture Pediatrie 144:15–16, 1993.

Wisard M, Jichlinski P: Long-term results of the Cobb and Badge method of bladder neck suspension in the treatment of urinary stress incontinence in women. Helv Chir Acta 57(3):427–430, 1990.

Wise B, Cardozo L: Urge incontinence and stress incontinence. Curr Opin Obstet Gynecol 3(4):520–527, 1991.

Wiskind AK, Creighton SM, Stanton SL: The incidence of genital prolapse after the Burch colposuspension. Am J Obstet Gynecol 167(2):399–404, 1992.

Winter CC: Re: Review of an 8-year experience with modifications of endoscopic suspension of the bladder neck for female stress urinary incontinence (letter). J Urol 144(6):1481–1482, 1990.

Yamada T, Kura N, Kawakami S, et al: Suburethral sling procedure for urinary stress incontinence. With special reference to determination of tension of suspension from posturethrovesical angle measured by ultrasonography. Nippon Hinyokika Gakkai Zasshi 81(9):1351–1356, 1990.

Yamada T, Masuda H, Nagahama K, et al: Use of ultrasonography in the bladder neck suspension. Nippon Hinyokika Gakkai Zasshi 84(8):1411–1416, 1993.

Yamada T, Mizuo T, Kawakami S, et al: Application of transrectal ultrasonography in modified Stamey procedure for stress urinary incontinence. J Urol 146(6):1555–1558, 1991.

Yamanishi T, Yasuda K, Nagashima K, et al: Clinical effects of clenbuterol-HCL in urge incontinence and stress incontinence. Hinyokika Kiyo 36(2):207–211, 1990.

Yang A, Mostwin JL, Rosenshein NB, Zerhouni EA: Pelvic floor descent in women: dynamic evaluation with fast MR imaging and cinematic display. Radiology 179(1):25–33, 1991.

Yasuda K, Yamanishi T: The pathology and treatment of incontinence. Nippon Ronen Igakkai Zasshi 29(3):161–168, 1992.

Youngblood JP: Paravaginal repair for cystourethrocele. Clin Obstet Gynecol 36(4):960–966, 1993.

Zakhmatov IM, Chepurov AK, Sued AO: The treatment of stress urinary incontinence in women. Urolog Nefrol (4-6):33–35, 1992.

Zivkovic F, Ralph G, Schied G, Auer-Grumbach M: The early effect of anterior colporrhaphy on the innervation of the external sphincter of the urethra. Gynakol Geburtshilfliche Rundschau 33 (Suppl 1):74–75, 1993.

Zivkovic F, Ralph G, Schied G, Tamussino K: Neuro-urodynamic sequelae of vaginal continence surgery. Gynakol Geburtshilfliche Rundschau 34(1):27–28, 1994.

Zerbib M, Younes E, Conquy S, et al: Treatment of urinary stress incontinence in women by percutaneous cervico-cystopexy. Gitte's operation: Contribution of intraoperative ultrasonography. Apropos of 47 patients. J Urol (Paris) 98(2):93–97, 1992.

Zuluaga GA, Nogueras OM, Martinez TJL, et al: Stress urinary incontinence. Our results with the Burch's technique. Arch Esp Urol 45(7):609–612, 1992.

Treatment of Intrinsic Sphincter Dysfunction

Slings

CHAPTER 31

Abdominal Fascial Slings

Edward J. McGuire, M.D.
E. Ann Gormley, M.D.

Historical Perspective

Goebell is credited with performing and describing the first pubovaginal sling in 1910.[1] Initially slings were fashioned from muscle including the pyramidalis, gracilis, levator ani, rectus, and bulbocavernosus muscles.[2] Price described the first fascial sling in 1933.[3] He used a strip of fascia lata, passing the fascia beneath the urethra from a suprapubic approach and fixing the ends of the sling to the rectus muscles. In the 1940s Millen, a urologist, and Aldridge, a gynecologist, described the creation of slings using paired strips of rectus fascia. Millen looped the strips under the urethra and then tied them together over the top of the urethra, whereas Aldridge sutured the strips together underneath the urethra.[2, 4] Aldridge noted that one of the advantages of the procedure the way he did it was automatic compression of the urethra when the rectus muscle contracted during coughing or staining.[2] Now, some 50 years later, the current generation of pubovaginal slings uses this same mechanical advantage to correct urethral dysfunction associated with poor resting closure of the primary proximal sphincter mechanism, a problem that is not adequately addressed by standard suspension operations.

Patient Evaluation

Patients who complain of urinary leakage associated with a change in abdominal pressure such as that associated with coughing, lifting, exercise, and laughing are considered to have a sign of stress urinary incontinence. The diagnosis of stress urinary incontinence rests on the determination that urethral urinary leakage exists in association with an increase in abdominal pressure. How much abdominal pressure is required to cause leakage is also an important part of the assessment of stress incontinence. A normal urethra will not leak at any abdominal pressure, whereas a urethra that moves will leak at a relatively high abdominal pressure, and a poorly closed proximal (intrinsic) urethral sphincter will leak at a low abdominal pressure. The fact that abdominal pressure does not normally cause leakage has been attributed to the function of the external sphincter, but for a number of excellent reasons that cannot be the case. Among these reasons is the observation that individuals in whom function of the external sphincter is absent do not develop stress incontinence.[5]

The diagnosis and quantification of stress incontinence are best done with videourodynamic evaluation. The filling behavior of the bladder is measured, and the ability of the urethra to resist abdominal pressure in the upright position is determined. The minimal pressure required to cause leakage is measured. The technique for determining the amount of abdominal pressure needed to cause leakage is described in another chapter, but the degree of intrinsic sphincteric dysfunction is inversely proportional to the amount of abdominal pressure required to cause leakage. That is, the lower the pressure of leakage, the worse the urethral function. Low-pressure leakage (<60 cm H_2O) is associated with some degree of intrinsic sphincteric dysfunction as opposed to a loss of the normal urethral supporting mechanism. Incontinence associated with intrinsic sphincteric dysfunction has been called type III stress

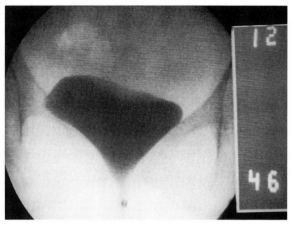

Figure 31–1 A video urodynamic snapshot of a patient with type III incontinence. Note the low abdominal leak point pressure (12 cm H₂O), the open bladder neck, and the dysfunctional proximal urethra.

incontinence (Fig. 31–1). When higher abdominal pressures (>90 cm H_2O) are required to drive urine across the urethral sphincter mechanism, a situation that is typically associated with some degree of urethral hypermobility and displacement, the condition has been called type I or II stress incontinence.[6] If urethral resistance is very low, leakage may occur during filling, and bladder urine storage function may appear to be good when it is in fact poor. When urethral resistance is low and the abdominal pressure needed to cause leakage is also low, a Foley catheter with the balloon inflated and pulled down to occlude the bladder neck may be required to assess accurately the ability of the bladder to store urine at low pressures.[7] Urethral pressure profiles have no role in the evaluation of the patient with stress urinary incontinence. Urethral pressure profiles concentrate on the maximum urethral closing pressure, an area of the urethra that has very little to do with the ability of the urethra to resist abdominal pressure. However, maximum urethral pressure measurement is necessary to fulfill the diagnostic criteria for genuine stress incontinence according to the definition of the International Continence Society (ICS). Genuine stress incontinence is defined by the ICS as "the involuntary loss of urine occurring when, in the absence of a detrusor contraction, the intravesical pressure exceeds the maximum urethral pressure."[8] Simplified, it states that genuine stress incontinence is urine loss that occurs when abdominal pressure (intravesical minus detrusor) exceeds maximum urethral pressure. However, leakage driven by abdominal pressure has no relationship to maximum urethral closing pressure (Fig. 31–2). A poorly closed proximal urethral sphincter can and does leak at abdominal pressures lower than maximum urethral pressure. An additional difficulty with the ICS definition is that subtracted detrusor pressure (intravesical pressure minus abdominal pressure) must be calculated to ensure that a bladder contraction has not occurred. This requires a rectal catheter and a blad-

der catheter. Furthermore, it does not emphasize that abdominal pressure, not bladder pressure, is the most important measurement. We measure abdominal pressure only because it is the expulsive force in stress incontinence. We measure it in the bladder, but it is not detrusor pressure that we are measuring. Bladder activity is monitored fluoroscopically, and a diagnosis of stress urinary incontinence is not made if a bladder contraction is observed.

A pelvic examination is performed in the supine and upright positions to search for a cystocele, rectocele, enterocele, or uterine prolapse. These conditions, when identified, should be repaired when the sling is made.

Patient Selection

Traditionally, slings have been used for patients with intrinsic sphincteric dysfunction. Most patients with low-pressure leakage from the urethra, indicative of intrinsic sphincteric dysfunction, have already failed to respond to one or more operations for stress incontinence.[9, 10] Many of these patients report that the prior procedure not only did not help their incon-

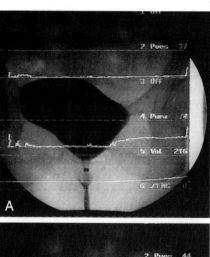
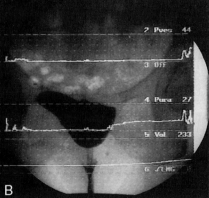

Figure 31–2 Lack of relationship between the abdominal pressure needed to cause leakage and the maximum urethral pressure. *A,* Leakage occurs when abdominal pressure is lower than maximum urethral pressure. *B,* Leakage occurs when abdominal pressure is greater than maximum urethral pressure.

tinence but appeared to make it worse. Intrinsic sphincteric weakness associated with prior operative failure has been attributed to urethral and periurethral scarring and fibrosis, but this has never been documented pathologically. Intrinsic sphincter dysfunction may also be neural in origin, as in individuals with myelodysplasia, sacral agenesis, and T_{12} spinal cord injury. In these conditions usually proximal urethral sphincter closing function is lost, but external sphincter function is preserved. Low abdominal pressure leakage is also seen in 9 to 10% of patients presenting with stress incontinence who have never had an operation for that condition and who do not suffer from neural disease.[11] In addition to patients who have a defect in proximal urethral sphincter function there are some special circumstances that favor the use of a sling because of the strength and durability of that procedure. Among these relative indications are extreme obesity, extreme physical activity such as gymnastics, chronic pulmonary conditions, especially severe asthma or progressive chronic obstructive pulmonary disease. Slings may also be used to effect complete closure of a damaged or nonfunctional urethra in combination with augmentation cystoplasty and construction of an abdominal neourethra or an ileovesicostomy.

A sling is a suitable procedure for patients of any age provided that the patient or caregiver can provide intermittent catheterization should that be required. The procedure has been used in patients ranging in age from 2 to 83 years.

A potential candidate for this procedure must have reasonable bladder storage ability (compliance). Compliance in patients with bladder decentralization or other neurogenic conditions can be adversely affected by the sling. Although that is unusual, it is better to be as certain as possible preoperatively that the bladder stores a reasonable volume at low pressure. A sling is not an effective barrier to bladder pressure as an expulsive force, and leakage driven by bladder pressure will recur at progressively lower bladder volumes after the sling procedure. In patients in whom poor compliance coexists with poor urethral resistance, a sling must be combined with some treatment that either reduces bladder pressure or enlarges bladder capacity.

The relationship between an unstable detrusor, urge incontinence, and stress incontinence is complex. These are not, however, mutually exclusive processes. Indeed, some 30% of patients with videourodynamically identified stress incontinence have both urge incontinence and a demonstrated contraction of the bladder on filling cystometrogram (CMG).[10, 12] Another 20 to 30% of women with stress incontinence diagnosed by a videourodynamic technique also complain of urge incontinence. In this group the filling CMG does not show a contraction. However, if this latter group is subjected to continuous monitoring of bladder pressure, a reflex bladder contraction is very often identified as the cause of the urge incontinence.[13] In addition, some patients evaluated by urodynamic study who have no symptoms of urge incon-

tinence do demonstrate a bladder contraction on a filling CMG. Thus, the CMG is not a method of establishing or confirming the diagnosis of "urge incontinence." A patient with objectively established stress incontinence and a normal CMG is not necessarily a better operative candidate than a patient with stress and urge incontinence with or without a positive CMG.

Seventy percent of patients with both stress and urge incontinence experience relief from both conditions by an operation that cures the stress incontinence.[12] To complicate matters further, about 2 to 6% of all patients undergoing any operation for stress incontinence develop early, usually transient, de novo urge incontinence.[14] In the 20 to 30% of patients with persistent urge incontinence after surgery and in those who develop the problem de novo, treatment with drugs or occasionally operative methods may be required. However, nonoperative treatment of urge incontinence associated with severe stress incontinence is almost never effective and is probably not worthwhile. In other words, women with low abdominal pressure leakage of urine and urge incontinence will not benefit from anticholinergic therapy in lieu of surgery or injection therapy.

Detrusor Function and Stress Incontinence Surgery

Patients with significant residual urine volumes preoperatively, not attributable to a cystocele, are not likely to be able to empty their bladder after a sling procedure. Patients who void habitually by straining will not be able to void in that manner after the procedure because the sling raises the abdominal leak point pressure to infinity (Fig. 31–3). The difficulty here is that some women with severe stress incontinence never void by contracting the bladder.

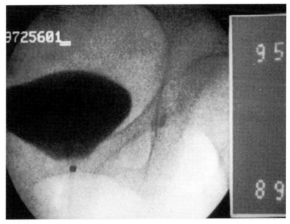

Figure 31–3 A video urodynamic snapshot of a patient following a pubovaginal sling procedure. There is no evidence of leak at an abdominal pressure of 95 cm H_2O, which is the maximum pressure that this patient was able to attain.

After the procedure some of these women may be able to relearn how to void by a contracting the bladder, but it is impossible to predict this on an individual basis.[9] Further complicating the assessment of detrusor function is the fact that many patients who normally do void by a detrusor contraction fail to develop one in the urodynamic testing situation. Thus, even a crude assessment of detrusor power and strength, which requires a bladder contraction, often cannot be done. It is, however, quite reasonable to use a sling for patients with poor or absent detrusor contractile function provided that the patient can perform intermittent catheterization and is willing to do it indefinitely.

Difficult Cases

A patulous urethra surrounded by dense fibrotic tissue may not be completely closed by a sling that provides only a vector force against the back of the urethra. There is a risk that the tension necessary to close such a urethra could result in obstruction or erosion. In some of these cases the sling will prevent stress incontinence. That function of the sling is visible on videourodynamic images, in which the urethra can be seen to be driven into the sling by an increase in abdominal pressure and securely closed. Unfortunately, when the patient is relaxed, even minimal motion, as for example when bending forward, can produce urinary leakage. In these cases, once the urethra is partly closed and immobile as a result of the sling, injection of collagen produces excellent results.

Patients with very wide patulous urethras associated with tissue loss, which may occur following a long period of treatment by an indwelling catheter with a large balloon, may be better served by a formal urethral closure and construction of a continent abdominal stoma or an ileovesicostomy.[10]

Preoperative Care

Patients are told that intermittent catheterization will be required and must be mastered prior to discharge. If there is any question about a patient's ability to perform intermittent catheterization, he or she is taught the technique preoperatively. Patients are told that there is a small risk of permanent urinary retention and a possibility of lifelong catheterization. A clear urinalysis or a sterile urine culture is required prior to surgery. Patients are admitted after the procedure. They receive perioperative parenteral antibiotics 1 hour prior to the procedure.

Procedure

The basic sling procedure has undergone many modifications since the description by Lytton and McGuire

in 1978.[9] At present a combined abdominal and vaginal approach is used. The procedure takes about 40 minutes if two surgical teams are available. Patients are placed in the dorsal lithotomy position with the feet supported by Allen stirrups. An 18 Fr Foley catheter is placed, and the balloon is overfilled with 10 ml of water. A weighted vaginal speculum is placed in the vagina, and an Allis clamp is used to elevate the anterior vaginal wall, which is then infiltrated with normal saline to aid in the dissection (Fig. 31–4). A midline incision about 4 to 5 cm long is made from the area of the midurethra to the bladder neck. The vaginal wall is sharply dissected off the underlying periurethral fascia, which is visible as a glistening white surface. Identification of the periurethral fascia prevents inadvertent entry into a bad plane and bleeding associated with that event as well as inadvertent entry into the bladder during the dissection. The vaginal wall is dissected laterally toward the ischium. The pubocervical fascia is perforated sharply on each side to the urethra, gaining entry into the retropubic space (Fig. 31–5). Perforation of the pubocervical fascia and subsequent blunt dissection frees the attachment of the vagina from the tendinous arch and allows free motion of the urethra and the fascial envelope that contains it. Finger dissection is used to create a tunnel for the sling into the retropubic space toward the rectus muscle bellies.

A transverse suprapubic incision is made and carried down to the rectus fascia, which is opened in the direction of the skin incision (Fig. 31–6). The fascia is lifted off the rectus muscle bellies, and a strip of fascia measuring 1.5 × 4 to 8 cm is taken from either the upper or the lower leaf. The ends of the sling are sutured with several bites of 0 polypropylene suture to trap all of the fibers of the sling. The suture is tied down on the sling, and the needle is removed, leaving the sutures as long as possible. The suprapubic oper-

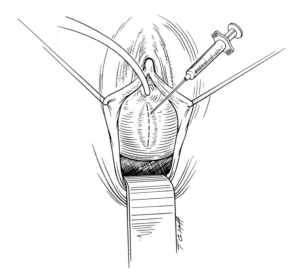

Figure 31–4 The anterior vaginal wall is infiltrated with normal saline to facilitate dissection. (From Hurt WG [ed]: Urogynecologic Surgery. New York, Raven Press, 1992.)

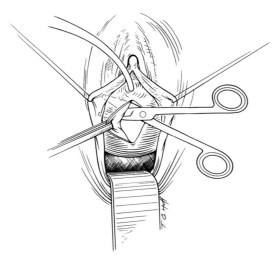

Figure 31-5 The retropubic space is entered from below by perforating the pubocervical fascia. (From Hurt WG [ed]: Urogynecologic Surgery. New York, Raven Press, 1992.)

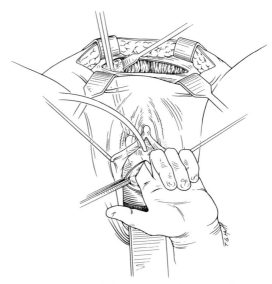

Figure 31-7 A Crawford clamp is passed through the retropubic tunnel. Bimanual palpation is used, and the clamp is kept in contact with the symphysis. (From Hurt WG [ed]: Urogynecologic Surgery. New York, Raven Press, 1992.)

ator then retracts the lateral border of the rectus muscle just above the insertion into the symphysis toward the midline. A triangular area that will permit easy access to the retropubic space is visualized in an area where no previous operative scarring has occurred. Retropubic tunnels are developed in continuity with the previous vaginal dissection. A Crawford clamp is passed from above downward, taking care to keep the nose of the clamp in constant contact with the posterior surface of the symphysis (Fig. 31–7).

If an inadvertent injury to the bladder does occur it will be located at the upper lateral aspect of the anterior bladder wall. Bladder injuries should be suspected if blood is seen when the Foley catheter is irrigated with saline. If this occurs, the interior of the bladder must be inspected with a cystoscope and a new sling tunnel constructed. It is best to irrigate the bladder and perform subsequent cystoscopy if necessary with the Crawford clamp in situ. Visual-

ization of a clamp in the bladder is very dramatic, whereas it is possible to miss seeing a piece of suture peeking through a small hole. If the bladder is entered it is drained for a period of 5 to 7 days rather than the standard 2 days.

The sutures on each end of the sling are grasped in the Crawford clamp, and the sling is gently pulled into the retropubic space bilaterally (Fig. 31–8). This seats the sling at the bladder neck in the correct position. The sling will ultimately arrive at the right position because the entry points into the retropubic space are just at the bladder neck and proximal urethra. The sling can move neither upward toward the trigone nor downward toward the external meatus. At this point, the sling is sutured to the periurethral

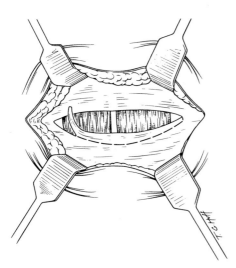

Figure 31-6 A strip of rectus fascia is obtained through a suprapubic incision. (From Hurt WG [ed]: Urogynecologic Surgery. New York, Raven Press, 1992.)

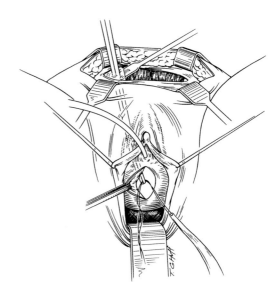

Figure 31-8 The sling suture is grasped and the sling is pulled up into the retropubic tunnel. (From Hurt WG [ed]: Urogynecologic Surgery. New York, Raven Press, 1992.)

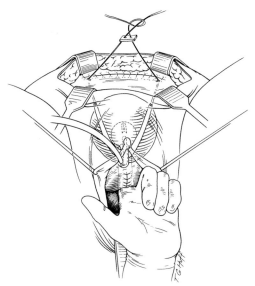

Figure 31-9 The sling tension is assessed by palpation. The sling is then tied over a pledget. (From Hurt WG [ed]: Urogynecologic Surgery. New York, Raven Press, 1992.)

fascia to prevent dislocation and to spread the bearing surface of the fascia on the urethra as widely as possible. This is done with a 3–0 Vicryl or similar suture. The sutures at each end of the sling are brought through two small defects in the inferior leaf of the rectus fascia. The abdominal fascia is closed with 0 polypropylene, and the vaginal wound is closed with 3–0 chromic or similar suture.

The sling tension is adjusted so that gentle traction on the Foley catheter does not result in inferior and posterior urethral mobility (Fig. 31–9). The sling is secured by tying the two sutures over a Teflon pledget. It is better to tie the sling loosely rather than tightly. There is no useful way to measure sling tension intraoperatively that has prognostic value in terms of either achieving continence or preventing long-term use of intermittent catheterization. Previously we applied tension to the sling in an effort to increase urethral pressure beneath the sling by 6 to 10 cm.[9] This method required considerable time and turned out to have no predictive value. Others have described filling the bladder with fluid and then adjusting sling tension so that compression of the full bladder does not result in leakage. This is considerable overkill because a sling does not have to impede the expulsive force of bladder pressure. The purpose of a sling is to oppose abdominal pressure, and that can be achieved by a sling that barely closes the urethra. Coaptation may be assessed endoscopically; however, this ensures neither absence of incontinence nor freedom from retention. The subcutaneous tissues and skin are closed, and the vaginal vault is packed.

Postoperative Care

The vaginal pack is removed on the first postoperative day. Patients are encouraged to walk. As soon as the patient is mobile and reasonably comfortable the Foley catheter is removed, usually on the second postoperative day. When the catheter is removed patients are encouraged to attempt to void frequently. They are told not to strain to void; if they cannot void they are to call the nurse for catheterization. Nurses are asked to catheterize patients at least every 4 hours and more often if requested by the patient. As soon as intermittent catheterization is begun the nurses begin the process of teaching intermittent catheterization to the patient. When patients can perform intermittent catheterization independently they are discharged. In general, this occurs on the third or fourth postoperative day. Intermittent catheterization schedules are determined individually and are adjusted as the patient's voiding ability improves. The patient stops performing catheterization when successive residual urine amounts are 60 ml or less. Intermittent catheterization is performed using a 14 coudé catheter because it avoids trauma to the posterior urethral wall. The shape of the coudé catheter facilitates its passage when the bladder is very full and the sling is tighter than it would be at rest. Every patient is expected to learn (and does learn) intermittent catheterization. Occasionally a patient may develop urinary retention after voiding well and achieving a low residual urine. It is best for the patient to be able to handle this problem herself rather than to rely on a local emergency room for treatment.

Complications

Complications include inadvertent malposition of the sling within the bladder or urethra, wound infection, prolonged retention, pain related to the sling or sling

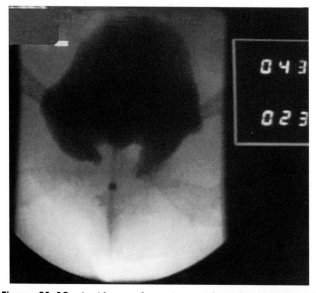

Figure 31-10 A video urodynamic snapshot of a patient with obstruction after a pubovaginal sling procedure. The pressure drop over the obstructed proximal urethra is 20 cm H_2O.

sutures, and potential erosion of the sling into the urethra. Erosion, although fairly common with slings made of synthetic material, has not been reported with autogenous fascial slings to our knowledge. Inadvertent malposition of the sling is associated with bleeding during the operation, which should prompt cystoscopy. Treatment is removal and repositioning of the sling coupled with 7 days of postoperative catheter drainage. In practice, this complication is most likely to occur in patients who are incontinent after pelvic fractures or have failed to respond to retropubic procedures in the past. Wound infections, because they may involve the pledget or the monofilament suture, are a potentially serious complication. Treatment usually requires removal of the foreign material through a small suprapubic incision. Surprisingly, none of the five patients in whom this was done became incontinent.

Patients often complain of a pulling sensation in either inguinal area for 1 to 5 weeks after the procedure. This is usually transient, but if it persists and prevents normal activity, removal of the pledget and the suspension sutures above the rectus fascia will resolve the problem. These patients do not redevelop stress incontinence.

Prolonged urinary retention can be troublesome. It usually occurs because a sling, which prevents leakage, provides too much resistance for a bladder with relatively poor function to overcome. In some instances it is possible to reduce sling tension by having the patient bend forward to void. Attempting to void in the upright position accomplishes the same thing. A full urodynamic investigation is warranted if retention or troublesome urge incontinence or any variety of incontinence develops or persists after a sling procedure. First the ability of the urethra to resist abdominal pressure is determined. If that is satisfactory, the next step is to determine whether the sling is obstructing voiding. Obstruction is assessed by measuring bladder pressure during voiding. When this measurement is made the external sphincter must be demonstrably relaxed and the proximal urethra open. Voiding pressures greater than 30 cm of H_2O are abnormal in a woman and indicate obstruction (Fig. 31–10). Pressures of less than 30 cm H_2O may reflect obstruction in a bladder with poor contractility. Precise identification of obstruction in such a bladder is impossible with the urodynamic equipment that is clinically available. If a bladder contraction cannot be elicited during urodynamic testing, obstruction cannot be assessed. Because management consists of relieving sling tension, it is comforting to have objective evidence of obstruction, although this is not always possible. Take-down of a sling is accomplished using the same steps used in the initial preparation for placement of the sling—namely, transvaginal mobilization of the urethra within its envelope of fascia until urethral mobility has been reobtained.

REFERENCES

1. Goebell R: Zur operativen Besierigung der angeborenen Incontinentia vesical. Z Urol Gynak 2:187, 1910.
2. Aldridge AA: Transplantation of fascia for relief of urinary stress incontinence. Am J Obstet Gynecol 44:398, 1942.
3. Price PB: Incontinence of urine and feces. Arch Surg 26:1043, 1933.
4. Millen T: Stress incontinence in women. *In* Millen TE (ed): Retropubic Urinary Surgery. Baltimore, Williams & Wilkins, 1947, pp 184–193.
5. McGuire EJ, Wagner FC: The effects of sacral denervation on bladder and urethral function. Surg Gynecol Obstet 144:343, 1977.
6. McGuire EJ, Fitzpatrick CC, Wan J, et al: Clinical assessment of urethral sphincter function. J Urol 150:1452, 1993.
7. McGuire EJ, Woodside JR, Borden TA, et al: Prognostic value of urodynamic testing in myelodysplastic patients. J Urol 126:205, 1981.
8. International Continence Society: Standardization of terminology of lower urinary tract function. Neurourol Urodyn 7:403, 1988.
9. McGuire EJ, Lytton B: Pubovaginal sling procedure for stress incontinence. J Urol 119:82, 1978.
10. McGuire EJ, Bennett CJ, Konnak JA, et al: Experience with pubovaginal slings for urinary incontinence at the University of Michigan. J Urol 138:525, 1987.
11. McGuire EJ: Abdominal procedures for stress incontinence. Urol Clin North Am 12:285, 1985.
12. McGuire EJ, Lytton B, Kohorn EI, et al: The value of urodynamic testing in stress urinary incontinence. J Urol 124:256, 1980.
13. Van Waalwijk van Doorn ESL, Remmere A, Janknegt RA: Extramural ambulatory urodynamic monitoring during natural filling and normal daily activities: Evaluation of 100 patients. J Urol 146:124, 1991.
14. McGuire EJ, Savastano JA: Stress incontinence and detrusor instability/urge incontinence. Neurourol Urodyn 4:313, 1985.

CHAPTER 32

Use of Fascia Lata for Pubovaginal Sling

Larry T. Sirls, M.D.
Gary E. Leach, M.D.

Although procedures such as artificial urinary sphincter and periurethral injection are receiving more attention, the pubovaginal sling remains the most commonly used procedure for the management of type III stress urinary incontinence. As discussed in previous chapters, the goal of the pubovaginal sling is to restore sufficient outlet resistance to the intrinsically damaged urethra to prevent urine loss with stress maneuvers while avoiding urethral obstruction and allowing spontaneous voiding. A variety of materials have been used as slings, including muscular and fascial tissues as well as synthetic materials. Goebell first reported the use of transplanted pyramidalis muscle as a sling to provide urethral and bladder neck support for stress urinary incontinence.[1] Frangenheim[2] (by including the overlying pyramidalis fascia) and Stoeckel[3] (by plicating the "muscular structures" around the vesical neck in a vaginal approach) modified the procedure. It was Price, however, in 1933 who first used transplanted fascia lata for a pubovaginal sling in a woman with sacral agenesis and urinary incontinence.[4]

This chapter discusses the rationale for using fascia lata as an alternative fascial source for a pubovaginal sling. The anatomy of fascia lata, the technique of harvesting and the technique of transvaginal placement of the sling, and a review of the literature on the use of fascia lata in the sling procedure are presented.

Two critical points influence the outcome of any sling procedure. First is the proper evaluation of the patient with suspected type III incontinence. As discussed in previous chapters, the history (radiation therapy, previous periurethral surgery, or neurologic injury), severity of incontinence, and objective tests, including videourodynamic evaluation and leak point pressures, are essential to confirm intrinsic urethral dysfunction. Identification of the patient with bladder dysfunction (detrusor overactivity or low compli-

ance) is one of the most important objectives of the preoperative evaluation. Patients with type III incontinence can be difficult to study, and it can be particularly difficult in some cases to demonstrate detrusor instability. When the bladder outlet is so compromised that minimal increases in detrusor pressure cause urine loss across the outlet, the pressure rise indicating a detrusor contraction may not be recorded. In this situation, we find it helpful to use a Foley catheter to fill the bladder during the study.[5] When continuous urine loss is seen across the outlet, particularly at low volumes, gentle traction is applied to the Foley catheter. The inflated balloon occludes the bladder neck and urethra, and any detrusor activity can then be recorded. Should detrusor overactivity be documented in a patient with type III incontinence, two options are available. The clinician can prescribe oral anticholinergic agents and later document whether detrusor overactivity is controlled, or a pubovaginal sling procedure can be performed followed by anticholinergic agents, if needed. However, if a patient has preoperative detrusor overactivity, a response to anticholinergic agents preoperatively does not guarantee a satisfactory response in the postoperative period. Patients with detrusor overactivity, as discussed in the next sections, may be at increased risk of failing to respond to the pubovaginal sling owing to persistent urgency and urge incontinence. It is important for neurologically normal patients to realize that there is a small (5%) risk of permanent urinary retention requiring clean intermittent catheterization after a pubovaginal sling. Similarly, it is important for patients with type III incontinence due to neurologic injury to realize preoperatively that the goal of sling surgery is permanent urinary retention and lifelong performance of clean intermittent catheterization.

The second critical point to be addressed in sling surgery is the amount of tension applied to the fascial sling. Too little tension may result in inadequate outlet resistance and thus recurrent or persistent stress incontinence. Too much tension on the sling can cause prolonged difficulty with bladder emptying or chronic urinary retention. In addition, urethral obstruction resulting from a sling procedure may cause postoperative detrusor instability or exacerbation of preexisting detrusor instability. Symptoms of urgency and urge incontinence after a sling procedure can be debilitating and may require a "take-down" of the sling, anticholinergic therapy, or even augmentation cystoplasty. Unfortunately, no standard parameters exist that identify the appropriate degree of sling tension—it remains more an art than a science. We describe the technique of adjusting sling tension in a later section, Placement of the Fascia Lata Sling.

Fascia Lata: Rationale for Use

We routinely use fascia lata for the pubovaginal sling and prefer it for two reasons. First, fascia lata is uniformly strong regardless of patient age or medical condition. The strength of fascia lata has been studied and compared to that of abdominal rectus fascia.[6] Fascial strips of various widths were harvested and attached to a tensilgraph. Sequential weights were applied, and the weight required to break the strip of fascia was recorded. The results demonstrated that fascia lata had, reproducibly, three to four times more tensile strength than abdominal rectus fascia. Not only is fascia lata stronger than abdominal fascia, the rectus fascia targeted for harvest in patients with type III incontinence is frequently scarred and attenuated.

The second reason we prefer fascia lata for the pubovaginal sling is that less abdominal dissection is required. Instead of the large abdominal incision needed to harvest a 15- to 20-cm segment of abdominal fascia, a small 3-cm abdominal wall incision is sufficient to allow fixation of the fascia lata fascial strip to the pubic tubercle or anterior rectus fascia. Accordingly, there is less chance of anterior abdominal wall nerve injury or entrapment or postoperative hernia. Postoperatively, patients have less abdominal pain and improved ambulation and pulmonary toilet.

Once one is familiar with the technique, harvesting a fascia lata strip is fast and easy. A strip of fascia lata, 20 to 25 cm long, is harvested through two 3-cm transverse incisions in the lateral thigh (the harvest technique will be described in detail later in this chapter). This length provides a strong fascial strip that will support the proximal urethra and bladder neck without an intervening "suture bridge." The additional operating time required for fascia lata harvest is approximately 20 minutes owing to the need to reposition the patient.

Fascia Lata: Anatomy

The fascia lata is the uppermost subdivision of a complete stocking-like fascial investment of the leg (Fig. 32–1). The bony attachments of the fascia lata are located, from medial to posterior, along the pubic crest, the pubic symphysis, and the ischiopubic ramus extending to the ischial tuberosity. From there, further posterior attachments course along the sacrotuberous ligament to the sacrum and coccyx. The lateral attachments travel anteriorly along the posterior superior iliac spine and iliac crest to the anterior superior iliac spine and then medially again along the inguinal ligament and pubic tubercle, completing the circumferential stocking-like investment. Although the fascia lata is a strong membranous fascia, it is particularly strong laterally, where tendinous reinforcements from the tensor fascia lata and the gluteus muscle are incorporated, forming the iliotibial tract (see Fig. 32–1). The iliotibial tract arises from the crest of the ilium and courses distally to insert on the lateral condyle of the tibia, blending with fibers of the vastus lateralis and biceps femoris muscles.

The only relevant anatomic structure to keep in mind when harvesting the fascia lata is the common peroneal nerve. This nerve, originating from L_4–L_5 and S_1–S_2, separates from the sciatic nerve at the popliteal fossa, where it then courses laterally to the back of the head of the fibula. Although normally below the operative field, this nerve could be encoun-

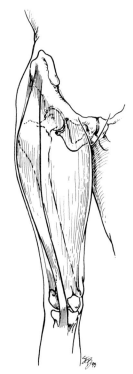

Figure 32-1 Diagrammatic representation of fascia lata. Note the stockinglike investment of the uppermost aspect of the leg. Laterally, the fascia thickens to form the iliotibial tract.

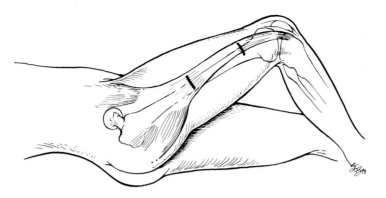

Figure 32–2 Representation of leg positioning for fascia lata harvest. The knee is flexed and the leg internally rotated at the hip. The bony landmarks (greater trochanter of the femur and lateral condyle of the femur) are easily identified. The two incision sites are indicated over the iliotibial tract.

tered with aggressive dissection distally at the insertion of the iliotibial tract onto the lateral tibial condyle. We have never required this much distal dissection because if additional fascial length is required, proximal dissection toward the thigh is easier. However, common peroneal nerve injury, if it occurs, would be manifest as inability to extend the great toe and sensory loss.

Preoperative Preparation

It is very important for the patient to demonstrate the ability to perform clean intermittent catheterization preoperatively. This both reinforces the reality that intermittent catheterization will be necessary and eases the transition to intermittent catheterization postoperatively. Patients are instructed to use a povidone-iodine (Betadine) vaginal douche the night before and the morning of sling surgery. Finally, all patients must understand the potential risks and complications of sling surgery, including prolonged or permanent urinary retention, exacerbated or de novo urgency symptoms, and the 10 to 15% risk of recurrent stress urinary incontinence.

Technique of Fascia Lata Harvest

The patient is placed in the supine position, and anesthesia is administered. The leg from which the fascia is to be harvested is bent at the knee and internally rotated to expose the lateral thigh and allow easy access to the bony landmarks, the lateral condyle of the femur, and the greater trochanter of the femur (Fig. 32–2). Although the lateral condyle and greater trochanter of the femur are not origins or insertions of fascia lata or the iliotibial tract, they are the most useful landmarks for orientation when the leg is flexed. The leg is adequately padded and secured with tape, prepared, and draped. We make two incisions transversely on the lateral thigh (see Fig. 32–2). The first is 5 cm above the lateral condyle of the femur, and the second is 12 to 15 cm proximal to the first along the course of the iliotibial tract. The fascia is identified 2 to 3 cm beneath the skin, and a

combination of blunt and sharp dissection easily cleans off the fatty subcutaneous tissue. A narrow Deaver or other retractor is used, and the subcutaneous tunnel between the two skin incisions is developed. A 2-cm-wide segment is marked in the fascia at the proximal incision site, and the fascia is incised in the direction of its fibers with a knife, being careful not to cut into the underlying muscle. A right-angle clamp is used to elevate the fascia off the muscle, and a small Penrose drain is passed beneath the fascial strip. With the retractor elevating the skin between the two skin incisions, long, straight Metzenbaum scissors are used to extend the fascial incisions (Fig. 32–3). Working from each skin incision, the entire fascial strip is mobilized. It is important not to angle the scissors medially, or the fascial strip will have an hourglass deformity. Additional length is easily obtained, if needed, by continuing mobilization proximally. Care should be taken distally, near the insertion of the fascia at the knee, to avoid potential common peroneal nerve injury. When the fascial harvest is complete, two figure-of-eight absorbable sutures are placed to reapproximate the fascial edges, one suture at each skin incision site. Each incision site is drained and closed, and a pressure dressing is applied.

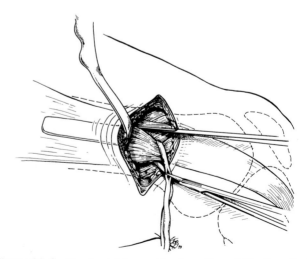

Figure 32–3 The fascial harvest begins with mobilization of a 2-cm-wide segment; a Penrose drain is used to provide upward traction on the fascial strip. A narrow curved retractor is used to elevate the skin bridge between the two incision sites. Long, straight scissors are used to incise the fascia.

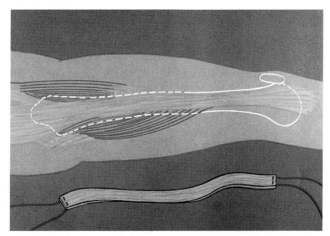

Figure 32–4 A 1–0 nylon suture is secured to each end of the fascial strip. This helps to transfer the fascial strip from the vaginal incision to the suprapubic position and allows fixation of the fascia to the pubic tubercle or abdominal fascia.

Other authors have reported the use of a fascial stripper to harvest the fascia lata.[7-9] This technique may be performed in a fashion similar to that just described. Our technique of making two small thigh incisions and harvesting the strip with long scissors routinely provides a fascial strip 20 to 25 cm in length without the need for special instruments.

Once the fascia has been harvested, it is cleaned of any remaining areolar tissue. A No. 1 nylon suture is secured to each end of the fascia by running the suture back and forth along the end of the fascial strip, distributing suture tension (Fig. 32–4). This suture will assist with the transfer of the fascial strip from the vaginal incision to the suprapubic position. This heavy nylon suture will be the suture anchoring the sling to either the abdominal wall fascia or, as we prefer, the pubic tubercle on each side.

Placement of the Fascia Lata Sling

With the patient in the lithotomy position, a Foley catheter is inserted, the posterior weighted vaginal speculum is placed, and a Scott retractor (Lone Star Medical, Houston, TX) is positioned. After hydrodissection using normal saline, an inverted U incision is made, and an anterior vaginal wall flap is mobilized to expose the proximal urethra and bladder neck. Lateral sharp dissection beneath the vaginal wall, at the level of the bladder neck on each side, exposes the endopelvic fascia at the undersurface of the pubic bone. After the bladder is drained, the endopelvic fascia is penetrated, and the retropubic space is bluntly developed. A 3-cm suprapubic incision is made over the insertion of the rectus fascia and pubic bone, exposing each pubic tubercle. A large blunt curved clamp is passed under finger guidance from the suprapubic incision, adjacent to the pubic tubercle and directed laterally to the empty bladder, through the retropubic space and out through the

ipsilateral vaginal incision (Fig. 32–5). The large curved clamp is used to ensure that the fascial sling can be passed through the anterior fascia without resistance. One end of the sling is transferred to the suprapubic incision, and the nylon suture is secured to the pubic tubercle (Fig. 32–6). With one end of the sling secured, the surgeon can place the sling in position over the proximal urethra and bladder neck using gentle traction and fasten the fascial strip in place to the periurethral fascia using two interrupted 4-0 Vicryl sutures. This step is particularly important to maintain an even distribution of tension and to prevent the sling from curling or rolling proximally toward the bladder neck. The large clamp is then used to transfer the free end of the sling from the vagina to the suprapubic incision adjacent to the pubic tubercle. At this point, intravenous indigo carmine is given, and cystoscopy is performed to confirm bilateral ureteral efflux and exclude inadvertent bladder injury from the large clamp. With the 20 Fr female cystourethroscope in the midurethra (using the 0-degree lens), the surgeon applies gentle traction to the free end of the sling to ensure that the sling position (under the proximal urethra and bladder neck) is correct. Sling tension is then adjusted under cystoscopic control by elevating the free end of

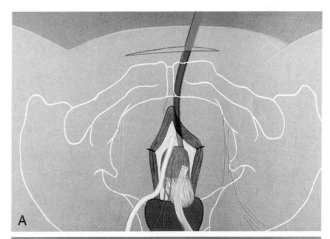

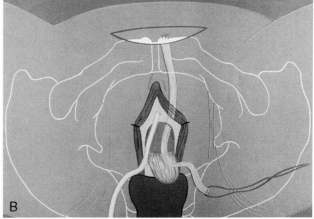

Figure 32–5 *A,* A large curved clamp is used to transfer the fascia to the suprapubic position. *B,* One end of the sling is secured to the pubic tubercle.

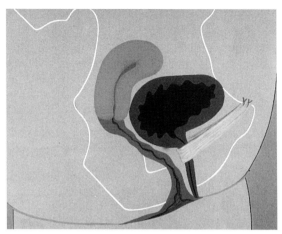

Figure 32–6 Using fascia lata, adequate outlet resistance is restored to the proximal urethra and bladder neck without an intervening suture bridge.

the sling just enough to see a minimal indentation on the floor of the proximal urethra. When there is excess sling length, a new No. 1 nylon suture is used to secure the fascial strip to the pubic tubercle adjacent to the sling at the appropriate level to maintain the desired tension. Any excess fascia is then "tacked" to the abdominal fascia. The anterior vaginal wall is closed with 2–0 Vicryl in a running locking fashion. The Foley catheter is left to allow gravity drainage, and an antibiotic-soaked vaginal pack is placed.

Postoperative Care

The Foley catheter and vaginal pack are removed on the first postoperative morning. A trial of voiding is instituted, and the patient is placed on a 1500 ml/day fluid restriction. All patients are reinstructed in the technique of clean intermittent catheterization (which they learned preoperatively) to monitor residual urine volumes. The lateral thigh pressure dressing and the Penrose drain are removed on the second postoperative morning. Patients are routinely discharged from the hospital after 48 hours.

Results

A review of the literature reporting the efficacy of the pubovaginal sling using fascia lata illustrates two important points.[7, 8, 10–12] First, the efficacy of the fascia lata sling for the treatment of genuine stress incontinence has remained high over the years (Table 32–1). Second, the major cause of failure, resulting in recurrent or persistent incontinence, is detrusor overactivity.

As mentioned, the majority of patients who fail to respond to the pubovaginal sling are found to have detrusor overactivity. Of 35 reported failures, 23

(66%) were attributed to detrusor overactivity. We have evaluated the results of the pubovaginal sling using fascia lata compared to the pubovaginal sling using abdominal fascia. Long-term efficacy in curing stress urinary incontinence and patient satisfaction with outcome were similar. However, the reported incidence of postoperative urgency and urge incontinence had a negative impact on overall patient satisfaction.

Two studies have compared the pubovaginal sling using fascia lata to a sling using foreign material (Mersilene and Gore-Tex).[7, 13] Both fascia lata and the foreign materials were equally effective in curing stress incontinence; however, both series reported an increased risk of complications with the synthetic material. In one series of 17 patients who underwent a pubovaginal sling using synthetic material, three subsequently required removal of the sling, two for erosion into the bladder or urethra.[7]

Complications

Although urethral erosion is a theoretical concern, only one case of urethral erosion in the 365 cases of fascia lata pubovaginal slings reported in the literature has been recorded.[9] There are three technical points that help minimize the risk of urethral erosion by a fascial sling. First, a wide fascial strip secured in place to ensure an even distribution of tension over the bladder neck and proximal urethra is used. Second, it is important to avoid excessive tension on the sling. Third, synthetic materials should be used with caution. As previously stated, it has been demonstrated that the use of synthetic materials increases the risk of urethral erosion.

No data exist to assess the risk of fascial harvest from the lateral thigh. Beck and colleagues reported eight wound infections in 170 patients but did not indicate whether these were suprapubic or thigh infections.[12] Smith[11] reported two women with lateral thigh "muscle herniation," although this has not been seen by us or mentioned by other authors. In our series, 3 of 18 patients undergoing fascia lata slings have had postoperative cellulitis of one thigh incision, and all responded to outpatient oral antibiotic therapy. Pain from the fascia lata harvest is usually described as an aching, lateral thigh pain. However, all patients are ambulatory on the first postoperative day. Duration of the thigh pain is usually 2 to 4 weeks, but it may last as long as 6 weeks.

Conclusion

The most important factors in ensuring success in sling surgery are patient selection and proper sling tension. There are definite advantages to the use of fascia lata. Harvesting fascia lata is fast and easy and is associated with minimal morbidity. Sufficient

TABLE 32–1
Fascia Lata Experience with Pubovaginal Sling

Investigator	No. Patients	No. Cured (%)	Reason for Failure (No. Failed from SUI or DI)	Follow-up
Ridley (1966)	36	31 (84)	Not stated	Not stated
Low (1969)	43	37 (86)	2 SUI, 4 DI	6 months–7 years (no mean)
Parker (1979)	50 (38 fascia lata)	42 (82)	3 SUI, 2 DI	1–21 years (no mean)
Smith (1982)	66	53 (80)	Not stated	Not stated
Beck (1988)	170	157 (92)	3 SUI, 10 DI	6 weeks–2 years (no mean, only 17 patients with more than 2 years follow-up)

Abbreviations: SUI, stress urinary incontinence; DI, detrusor instability.

fascial length is routinely obtained, allowing a strong fascial support without an intervening suture bridge. Finally, fascia lata is inherently stronger than rectus fascia and is not subject to the same factors that compromise abdominal fascial integrity such as previous surgical procedures and radiation, which are prevalent in the patient population with type III urinary incontinence.

REFERENCES

1. Goebell R: Zur operativen Behandlung der Incontinenz mannlichen Harnrohre. Verb Dtsch Gee Chir 2:187, 1910.
2. Frangenheim P: Zur operativen Behandlung der Incontinenz mannlichen Harnrohre. Verb Dtsch Gee Chir 43:149, 1914.
3. Stoeckel W: Über die Verwendung der Musculi pyrimidales bei der operativen Behandlung der Incontinentia urinae. Zentralbl Gynakol 41:11, 1917.
4. Price PB: Plastic operations for incontinence of urine and feces. Arch Surg 26:1043, 1933.
5. Woodside JR, McGuire EJ: Technique for detection of detrusor hypertonia in the presence of urethral sphincteric incompetence. J Urol 127:740, 1982.
6. Crawford JS: Nature of fascia lata and its fate after implantation. Am J Ophthmol 67:900, 1969.
7. Ridley JH: Appraisal of the Goebell-Frangenheim-Stoeckel sling procedure. Am J Obstet Gynecol 95:714–721, 1966.
8. Parker RT, Addison WA, Christopher JW: Fascia lata urethrovesical suspension for recurrent stress urinary incontinence. Am J Obstet Gynecol 135:843–852, 1979.
9. Beck RP, Grove D, Arnusch D, Harvey J: Recurrent stress urinary incontinence treated by the fascia lata sling procedure. Am J Obstet Gynecol 120:613, 1974.
10. Low JA: Management of severe anatomic deficiencies of urethral sphincter function by a combined procedure with fasica lata. J Obstet Gynecol 90:934–939, 1969.
11. Smith JL: Fascia lata paraurethrovesical suspension for the correction of stress urinary incontinence. Am J Surg 143:542, 1982.
12. Beck RP, McCormick S, Nordstrom L: The fascia lata sling procedure for treating recurrent genuine stress incontinence of urine. Obstet Gynecol 72:699, 1988.
13. Ogundipe A, Rosenzweig BA, Karram MM, et al: Modified suburethral sling procedure for treatment of recurrent or severe stress urinary incontinence. Surg Gynecol Obstet 175:173, 1992.

CHAPTER 33

The Use of Artificial Material for Sling Surgery in the Treatment of Female Stress Urinary Incontinence

Lindsey A. Kerr, M.D.
David R. Staskin, M.D.

The choice of a sling procedure for the correction of genuine stress urinary incontinence (GSI) in the female patient involves placement of autologous or artificial material beneath the bladder neck or proximal urethra. In theory, this graft restores continence not only by suspending the bladder neck and increasing transmission of intra-abdominal pressure to the proximal urethra but also by facilitating coaptation of the urethra and increasing intrinsic urethral closure pressure. There are many materials and techniques available to meet this goal. The evaluation of incontinence leading to the decision to pursue surgery is described elsewhere in this text. Here we will briefly review the findings and indications for sling surgery as well as the choices available and the approaches used when synthetic materials have been selected for sling surgery. Finally, we will describe in detail our choice of sling material, preferred approach, and expected results.

Indications for Sling Surgery

The most commonly accepted application of sling surgery has been for the treatment of type III stress urinary incontinence. Type III GSI signifies decreased intrinsic urethral closure pressure without altered support of the bladder neck, base, and urethra.[1, 2] It is most commonly associated with decreased urethral integrity affecting the ability of the submucosal and muscular layers to coapt and compress the urethral lumen. This deficiency in closure pressure often is the result of devascularization, denervation, or trauma. The underlying cause is vari-

able but can be due to scarring from previous surgery, radiation therapy, catheter trauma, myelodysplasia, or radical pelvic surgery.

Patients with type III GSI classically present with a well-supported pipestem urethra, although type III GSI can occur in patients who have concomitant loss of bladder neck and urethral support (type II GSI). A properly performed sling procedure will also correct the coexisting bladder neck and urethral motion. Another situation in which a sling procedure might be of benefit is type II GSI in a patient in whom poor periurethral tissue makes suture anchoring problematic. These patients often have a history of prior vaginal surgery or vaginal atrophy secondary to hormonal deprivation. Patients with severe obstructive lung disease or obesity who challenge classic type I or II repairs with frequent high-pressure "stress" maneuvers should be considered candidates for sling procedures also. Artificial graft material increases the strength of the repair and prevents erosion of suspension sutures from deficient periurethral or paraurethral tissues. A sling, by creating a stronger "backboard" for the absorption of transmitted intra-abdominal pressure by the urethra, restores continence without allowing the same degree of bladder neck motion. The sling repair prevents "sagging" between the suspension sutures, which is occasionally observed in a classic type II repair.

The last category of patients who may benefit from a sling are those with neurogenic disease and indwelling Foley catheters with leakage around the catheter.[3] These patients are at risk for total urethral erosion because repeated propulsion of the Foley balloon, secondary to detrusor hyperreflexia, leads to loss of urethral integrity. We have found that relocation of the catheter to the bladder dome through a suprapubic tube, along with anticholinergic therapy and sling placement, decreases both the detrusor hyperreflexia and urinary leakage. We prefer this to bladder neck closure with suprapubic tube placement because bladder neck closure has a high incidence of fistula and leakage.[4]

Patient Evaluation and Selection

Patients with type III GSI classically present with more severe symptoms of stress incontinence, often with urinary loss at rest. However, many patients with type III GSI may have more typical symptoms of moderate stress incontinence. These patients typically void frequently in an attempt to keep the bladder empty, so their condition can be mistakenly diagnosed as detrusor instability with urgency and frequency. Conversely, in patients with type III GSI and coexisting detrusor instability, detrusor instability may be underdiagnosed because the patients never allow their bladders to fill to a volume that elicits an unstable contraction. This is especially true if GSI is severe and the bladder remains relatively empty. Severe urethral incompetence also permits urine loss during low-pressure bladder contractions—so low, in fact, that the patient may be unaware of the contraction and not report the sensation at the time of urinary leakage. Preoperative instability, if it persists in the postoperative period, will be unmasked as urethral resistance is increased. In these cases, high intravesical pressures may be reached during uninhibited contractions before actual urinary loss occurs. The diagnosis of detrusor instability or hyperreflexia should be established preoperatively so that it can be managed appropriately if it remains postoperatively (see later discussion).

A history of prior failed incontinence surgery should raise a suspicion of intrinsic urethral dysfunction. Previous suspension procedures or cystocele repairs may attenuate or destroy the periurethral tissue planes and limit the surgeon's ability to elevate the anterior wall during subsequent repair without undue tension. Tension predisposes to suture erosion through the periurethral tissue and subsequent failure of the suspension procedure. Prior radiation therapy to the pelvis affects tissue integrity and healing, increasing the incidence of suture erosion and failure. Spinal surgery or radical pelvic surgery predisposes to denervation and subsequent urethral dysfunction. Even events considered less traumatic, such as a simple hysterectomy, vaginal delivery, or postmenopausal urethral atrophy, can lead to type III GSI.

The physical examination should focus on both the relevant anatomy and any neurologic abnormalities. A neurologic examination of the lower spinal segments should be part of any evaluation for stress incontinence. In the genitourinary examination the physician should specifically assess the mobility of the urethra and anterior vaginal wall as well as any intravaginal pathology, including the presence of a cystocele, rectocele, enterocele, or uterine prolapse. Suspension of the bladder neck without concomitant cystocele repair may lead to postoperative urethral kinking and urinary obstruction. Any contemplated anterior vaginal wall repair should include evaluation for posterior vault defects because anterior repair only will lead to accentuation of these defects.

In the urodynamic assessment the bladder and outlet must be evaluated during both urine storage and emptying. The tests we perform are the urine flow rate, postvoid residual urine (PVR), cystometry (CMG), and voiding cystourethrography (VCUG). A poor flow rate and increased PVR indicate poor bladder emptying and the possibility of prolonged postoperative urinary retention. The preoperative CMG serves several functions. It is essential to confirm adequate bladder capacity. Actual obstruction of the bladder neck may be required to obtain this measurement, and this is easily performed if a Foley catheter, placed on mild tension, is used during the study rather than a straight urodynamic catheter. If urethral resistance is low, decreased bladder compliance and bladder instability may be missed if fluid is unknowingly allowed to leak around the urodynamic catheter.

Some degree of decreased bladder compliance may be expected in type III GSI patients for a variety of reasons. Severe incontinence that has prevented bladder distention, recurrent infections with bladder fibrosis, or a chronic indwelling Foley catheter or bladder denervation may result in decreased compliance. Conversely, fast-fill cystometry (100 to 150 ml/minute) may artifactually produce low compliance. If low compliance is observed, the study should be repeated at a slower filling rate (20 to 40 ml/minute). Accurate assessment of bladder filling pressures is essential in these patients. Elevated intravesical filling pressures put the upper tracts at risk, especially if the pressures maintained are chronically above 35 to 40 cm H_2O. Anticholinergic medication will not help the compliance of a fibrotic bladder. These patients may need a bladder augmentation in addition to sling surgery. Demonstrable detrusor instability or hyperreflexia, on the other hand, can be managed with anticholinergics. One of the proposed causes of detrusor instability is the entrance of urine into the proximal urethra, which is presumed to stimulate a bladder contraction. Demonstration of normal detrusor contractility suggests that adequate postoperative bladder emptying can be obtained. However, the inability to elicit a voluntary bladder contraction is common during cystometric evaluation of women patients. It should not be cause for alarm if the history and physical examination are otherwise unremarkable. Patients with a prior history of peripheral neurologic disease often present with a noncontractile bladder, and long-term intermittent catheterization should be anticipated in these patients after surgical intervention.

The major postoperative complications are persistent urgency, frequency, and possibly urge incontinence. Postoperative instability may be classified as persistent or de novo. McGuire and colleagues noted improvement in the symptoms of bladder instability in 20 of 29 patients who underwent sling procedures.[5] The development of de novo instability has been reported in 10 to 40% of patients and may be secondary to bladder outlet obstruction, although it is possible that a diagnosis of detrusor instability was missed on preoperative cystometric assessment. Preoperative detrusor hyperreflexia should not be expected to resolve, because its neurogenic origin will be unaffected by the surgery. The decision to place a sling in a patient with detrusor instability or hyperreflexia is based on the expectation that the uninhibited contractions will resolve postoperatively or that they can be controlled with anticholinergic medication.

Selection of a Surgical Procedure

A variety of techniques have been described for the performance of sling surgery. The placement of autologous, heterologous, or artificial material beneath the urethra is presumed to provide an increase in urethral compression and a sturdier "backboard" than classic suspension procedures. This backboard functions to transmit abdominal pressure efficiently to the bladder neck and proximal urethra, thereby increasing urethral closure pressure during stress maneuvers.

Differences in sling techniques can be classified by the surgical approach and by the sling material employed. We concentrate on artificial materials in this chapter. The selection of surgical approach should be made with several considerations in mind. The first is the need to minimize morbidity and ensure the optimal rate of success. The surgeon should therefore use an anatomically familiar approach to ensure meeting both these criteria. Technically, accurate placement of the sling beneath the bladder neck and proximal urethra with a broad base of compression, and the simple and safe passage of the supporting arms of the sling through the retropubic space for attachment to the rectus fascia, pubic bone, or various other ligaments are required. The optimal approach minimizes the risk of damage to the bladder, bladder neck, urethra, and vagina. Abdominal, abdominovaginal, and vaginal approaches have been described.

The pure abdominal approach involves entrance into the retropubic space and placement of the sling beneath the proximal urethra and bladder neck without making a vaginal incision. The abdominovaginal approach combines dissection into the retropubic space through the abdomen with a vaginal incision that aids in accurate perforation of the arms of the sling and in placement of the body of the sling beneath the urethra. The vaginal approach requires a vaginal incision for placement of the body of the sling, and blind instrument passage of the arms of the sling through the retropubic space to a location above the rectus fascia without opening the rectus muscles. The approach to placement of the sling should be determined prior to performance of the procedure to place the patient in the optimal position (supine, relaxed lithotomy, full lithotomy) for surgical exposure.

THE ABDOMINAL APPROACH

Use of the pure abdominal approach should be limited to patients in whom the lithotomy position is contraindicated (e.g., decreased mobility of the hip or severe spinal problems), the rare circumstance when a sling is elected intraoperatively (e.g., inability to obtain sufficient periurethral or paraurethral tissue mobilization to perform a classic suspension), or when positioning of the legs in the lithotomy position limits the exposure needed for concomitant abdominal procedures (e.g., bladder augmentation, abdominal hysterectomy). If the lithotomy position is contraindicated, a frog-legged position is preferred because it affords vaginal access for intraoperative palpation of the bladder neck during sling passage.

The tissue superficial to the mid and distal urethra consists of periurethral fascia and overlying anterior vaginal wall. There is limited fibroareolar tissue space for dissection in this plane. Anatomically, this space is too distal to be used for sling placement because postoperative obstruction is the all-too-common result. The proper plane for dissection is at the level of the proximal urethra or vesical neck in the vesicovaginal plane. If prior incontinence surgery or cystocele repair has been performed, dissection within this plane beneath the bladder neck may be more difficult because of scar tissue. In a pure abdominal approach, the bladder should be opened prior to dissection of the tunnel for the sling. Transvesical exposure of the bladder neck allows palpation during the dissection beneath the bladder neck and visualization of the bladder neck area to ensure that the sling has not been placed within the bladder or urethra. Early postoperative sling erosion into the urethra is too often a misnomer for a sling that was placed through the urethral wall at the time of surgery. To avoid damage to the urethra or bladder neck, the plane for dissection of the sling tunnel should begin proximal to the level of the bladder neck where the vesical fascia can be separated more easily from the anterior vaginal wall. Distal dissection beneath the urethra is facilitated once this plane has been developed more proximally.

When the plane beneath the bladder neck and proximal urethra is difficult to develop, it may be best to enter the vagina. The vaginal wall will subsequently have to be mobilized to cover the artificial sling because the vagina will not granulate over the foreign material, but this choice avoids the more ominous urethral injury.

THE ABDOMINOVAGINAL APPROACH

The addition of a vaginal counterincision for sling placement is highly recommended when the abdominal approach is used because it provides improved exposure. The abdominovaginal approach (Fig. 33–1) combines an abdominal incision, which is used for dissection within the retropubic space, with an anterior vaginal wall vertical flap incision, which allows direct exposure beneath the bladder neck. This approach permits formation of the paraurethral tunnels by combined abdominal and vaginal routes. A relaxed lithotomy position provides adequate exposure for the abdominal and vaginal portions of the surgery. The ability to pass the sling below the urethra and bladder neck without fear of unintentionally perforating the anterior vaginal wall significantly decreases the amount of retropubic space dissection required for exposure of the bladder neck. A vertical or Pfannenstiel skin incision can be performed, the size of the incision being determined solely by the

need for retropubic space exposure. However, the need for an abdominal incision to allow entrance into the retropubic space is obviated by the pure vaginal approaches.

THE VAGINAL APPROACH

Like the abdominovaginal approach, the vaginal approach uses a vertical or flap incision in the vaginal wall for placement of the sling at the level of the bladder neck under direct vision. Using this strategy, the supporting arms of the sling are passed with a clamp, a pilot suture, or a suspension needle through tunnels or canals formed by instrument or finger dissection within the retropubic space. The tunnels can be formed from above (abdominally to vaginally) or below. The tunneling maneuver eliminates the need for splitting the rectus musculature and opening the retropubic space. A more acute lithotomy position can be employed for improved vaginal exposure. A small abdominal skin incision to the level of the rectus fascia is required for securing the arms of the sling.

The advantage of the vaginal approach is the decreased exposure of the retropubic space compared with that in the previously discussed approaches. The primary disadvantage of the vaginal approach is the increased chance of bladder, bladder neck, or urethral injury during blind passage of the arms of the sling. The vaginal approach is reviewed in detail later in this chapter.

Choice of Sling Material

Artificial slings have been fashioned as continuous pieces of material that comprise both the body and the arms of the sling or, alternatively, as patches or grafts placed beneath the urethra with the supporting arms provided by nonabsorbable suture. One obvious advantage over autologous material is the availability of the material and lack of dependence on factors such as previous surgery, body habitus, or experience in harvesting the chosen graft. The use of artificial material increases the risk of infection and possibly subsequent erosion into the urethra or vagina, but the biocompatibility of Marlex, Silastic, Gore-Tex, and Mersiline has been demonstrated. Broad-spectrum intravenous and oral antibiotics that provide gram-positive, gram-negative, and anaerobic coverage and thorough preoperative vaginal preparation can significantly decrease the incidence of infection. Risk of infection is also decreased by employing the least amount of foreign material necessary to correct the incontinence. We typically use a patch of sling material suspended beneath the urethra by nonabsorbable suture. If infection occurs it is easier to remove a patch (leaving the sutures in place) than to try to remove a full-length sling. In our experience, patients who have had the patch removed because of

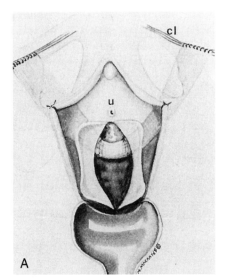

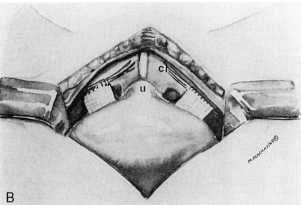

Figure 33-1 Abdominovaginal approach using a Marlex polypropylene mesh sling. Marlex is attached to Cooper's ligament after extensive dissection of the bladder neck. *A,* Vaginal incision. u, urethra; cl, Cooper's ligament. *B,* Abdominal incision. See text for discussion. (From Morgan JE: A sling operation using Marlex polypropylene mesh for the treatment of recurrent stress incontinence. Am J Obstet Gynecol 106[3]:369, 1970.)

infection have remained dry. Presumably their continence is due to continued support from scar tissue that has formed. We have not removed any patches until after a waiting period of 3 months from the original date of surgery, so that scarification is maximal. Urethrovaginal erosion caused by artificial material is often related to uneven compresson of the urethra (a thin strip beneath the urethra placed on excessive tension) or to technical errors in sling placement (entrance into the urethra or bladder neck during sling placement). The durability of the sling material and the contribution of scarring around the sling to the long-term surgical result have not been established. Vaginal erosion may be caused by infection of the graft material, necessitating its removal. Scarring is probably significant and may account for success in cases in which the sling has had to be removed, yet the patient remains continent.

Synthetic Slings Placed Using an Abdominal or Abdominovaginal Approach

Mersilene was the first artificial material used as a sling to support the vesicourethral junction for continence (Fig. 33–2).[6, 7] Unfortunately, Mersilene gauze was reported to erode and cause obstruction when used with these techniques.[7, 8] The use of Silastic, Gore-Tex, and Marlex in surgery has been demonstrated in a variety of capacities with some of the same problems. Morgan and coworkers reported on their experience with a Marlex sling procedure.[9, 10]

The procedure was based on a two-team, abdominovaginal operative technique, unchanged since its description 15 years before, wherein the bladder neck is extensively dissected and replaced in a midretropubic position on a hammock of Marlex mesh attached to Cooper's ligament (see Fig. 33–1). The success rate was 81% in the 208 patients followed for more than 5 years. Success was defined as lack of need for pads and the ability to resume normal activity without stress incontinence. Two slings eroded into the urethra, requiring revision in these patients. Treatment of persistent outlet obstruction in 12 patients was noteworthy in that anterior transurethral resection of the bladder neck was the procedure of choice.

Stanton and colleagues described the use of a Silastic sling.[11, 12] A 19- × 1-cm sling was fashioned from a medical-grade Silastic sheet with a double thickness of sheeting used for the central portion and a triple thickness used for the arms. Through a Pfannensteil incision the sling was anchored to the pectineal ligament bilaterally. Objective and subjective cures were achieved in 81% of patients at 3 years. Of concern was the high frequency of de novo instability occurring postoperatively. Eleven percent of patients complained of severe voiding difficulty postoperatively and required release or removal of the sling. Complications included vaginal entry or bladder and urethral injury and in some cases development of urethrovaginal fistula that required removal of slings in 8 of 125 cases. In all, 20% of slings had to be removed.

Horbach and associates and Bent and colleagues reviewed their experience with a Gore-Tex suburethral sling in 115 patients (Fig. 33–3).[13, 14] The

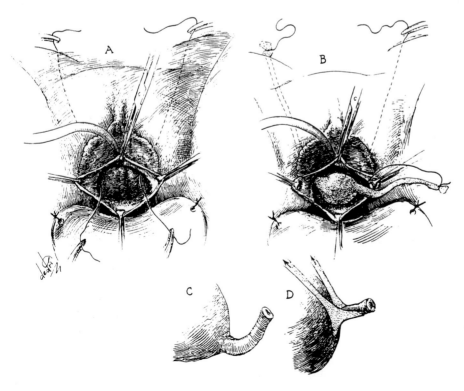

Figure 33-2 Abdominally placed Mersilene gauze mesh hammock. *A,* Two inguinal incisions have been made and the rectus aponeuroses incised bilaterally. The anterior vaginal wall is opened, and two silk sutures now traverse the retropubic space from vagina to abdomen. *B,* The Mersilene gauze is tacked in the periurethral fascia in the midline and the ends are sewn to the rectus aponeurosis. *C* and *D,* Correction of vesicourethral support by the hammock. (Reprinted with permission from the American College of Obstetricians and Gynecologists [Obstet Gynecol 1973, 41:88.])

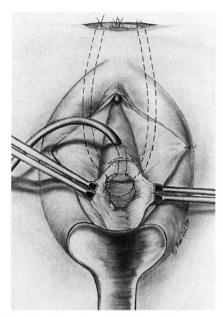

Figure 33-3 Gore-Tex suburethral sling. Placement at the level of the urethrovesical junction after plication of the suburethral fascia in the midline at this point. See text for more detail. (Reprinted with permission from the American College of Obstetricians and Gynecologists [Obstet Gynecol 1988, 71:648.])

vagina was incised longitudinally from near the vaginal apex to 1.5 cm proximal to the urethral meatus. The vaginal epithelium was dissected laterally off the underlying fascia to the descending pubic rami. After plication of the periurethral fascia over the proximal urethra, the Gore-Tex graft was fixed in place at the level of the urethrovesical junction. The endopelvic fascia was perforated, and counterincisions were made through the rectus fascia so that the arms of the sling could be secured to this fascia after they had been passed through the retropubic space. A cure rate of 82.4% was obtained, but a number of rejections occurred. Twenty-four patients experienced vaginal or abdominal reaction to the sling material, and 23 required removal of the sling. It may be postulated that reaction to the sling material is related to the large amount of sling surface area exposed to the body (66 cm^2). Two other patients had pain or urinary retention necessitating sling removal. Seventy-four percent of these patients remained continent. Histologic examination revealed gram-positive cocci in all Gore-Tex slings that were examined after removal.

Gore-Tex Patch Placement Using the Vaginal Approach

Our preferred approach to patients with type II and type III stress incontinence is vaginal dissection and placement of a suburethral patch fashioned from Gore-Tex and suspended by two nonabsorbable Gore-Tex sutures (Fig. 33–4). Rather than the large strip

of Gore-Tex used by Bent and colleagues, a small patch suspended by bilateral sutures is fashioned (7 cm^2 exposed surface area). This vaginal approach is a modification of the Pereyra operation as described by Raz and incorporates many of the principles that have been described for the transvaginal needle bladder neck suspension.[15]

PREOPERATIVE PREPARATION

The patient is instructed to have a clear liquid dinner, use a limited enema, and perform a Betadine douche the night before surgery. Preoperative intravenous antibiotics are administered 1 hour prior to surgery and include a third-generation cephalosporin or gentamicin and ampicillin.

POSITIONING AND EXPOSURE

The patient is positioned in a full lithotomy position. After a weighted vaginal speculum is inserted, a 16 Fr Foley catheter is placed for drainage. The bladder neck is identified by palpating the Foley balloon, taking care not to place any tension on the catheter (see Fig. 33–4B). Ten to twenty-five ml of sterile saline is injected into the vesicovaginal space at the level of the bladder neck and laterally to facilitate dissection. An Allis clamp is placed 1.5 cm distal to the bladder neck, and a 5- to 6-cm longitudinal incision is made. Antibiotic solution is used to irrigate all incisions during the surgery. Dissection is undertaken laterally in the vesicovaginal plane, parallel to the periurethral fascia, as far as the inferior aspect of the pubic rami. Care should be taken not to dissect superficially, or troublesome bleeding may be encountered as one mistakenly dissects into the medial aspect of the labia minora. If this occurs, a figure-of-eight suture may be placed through the superior and inferior portions of the labia, to be removed at the end of the surgery.

ENTRANCE INTO THE RETROPUBIC SPACE AND DISSECTION THEREIN

The retropubic space is entered by sharp perforation at the 2 o'clock and 10 o'clock positions by cupping the Metzenbaum scissors with the left hand, points curved outward, and guiding them with the left index finger along the internal aspect of the inferior pubic ramus (see Fig. 33–4C). The points of the scissors are used to perforate the attachment of the periurethral fascia on the inferior pubic ramus, allowing entrance into the retropubic space. The scissors are opened and then withdrawn in the open position, and the left index finger is placed in the defect. Blunt perforation is not used because it creates a defect through the weakest portion of the periurethral tissue, resulting in poor tissue for anchoring sutures. The index finger is advanced laterally through the perfora-

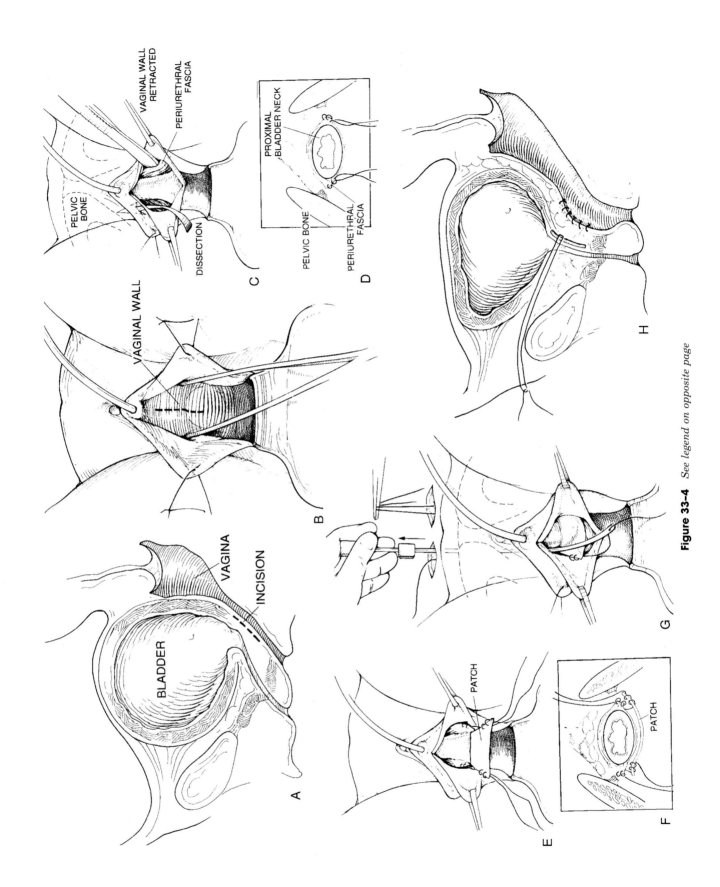

Figure 33-4 *See legend on opposite page*

tion lateral to the pubourethral attachments and then immediately superiorly along the surface of the pubic bone within the retropubic space. The bladder neck is further mobilized by sweeping the periurethral attachments from the inferior surface of the pubic rami.

The pubourethral ligaments may be palpated medial to the dissecting finger, and dissection of these structures or dissection across the midline above these structures is not required. The same maneuver is now performed on the patient's right side. The now-completed mobilization of the bladder neck and anterior vaginal wall is a distinct advantage that is provided only with entrance into the retropubic space. Mobilization of the anterior vaginal wall and bladder neck allows elevation with decreased tension on the suspending sutures.

Bleeding during these maneuvers is usually encountered at the edge of the periurethral fascia, which has been mobilized from the pubic bone. Attempts to obtain hemostasis by clamping or cauterizing should be reserved until after the bladder neck suspension sutures have been placed because they often incorporate the area responsible for the majority of the bleeding. Frequently passage and elevation of suspension sutures may be necessary to appreciate the full hemostatic effect of the placement of suspension sutures.

SUTURE AND PATCH PLACEMENT

A 2–0 Gore-Tex suture on a curved needle (THX-26) is used to secure the medial edge of the periurethral fascia at the level of the bladder neck (see Fig. 33–4C, D). The needle is left intact for incorporation of the patch. A trapezoid (4- × 3- × 1.5-cm) Gore-Tex soft tissue patch (1 mm thick) is placed suburethrally in the vesicovaginal plane beneath the periurethral fascia, and the base edges are incorporated into the suspension sutures (see Fig. 33–4E). If periurethral tissue is found to be severely deficient, a free Gore-Tex stitch is incorporated into the posterior surface of the anterior vaginal wall at the bladder neck level and then attached to the patch for suspension. The advantage of incorporating periurethral fascia is that it fixes the patch and prevents it from sliding into

the retropubic space during suture elevation. The patch is then advanced into a suburethral position. An antibiotic-soaked sponge is placed in the vaginal incision, and attention is turned to the abdomen.

THE ABDOMINAL INCISION AND PASSAGE OF THE SUTURES

Two 2-cm horizontal abdominal incisions are made down to the rectus fascia one fingerbreadth above the pubic bone, each 1 cm from the midline. A suspension needle is then placed through the medial aspect of one of the skin incisions and through the rectus fascia near the midline. Using finger guidance from below, the needle is guided out of the ipsilateral vaginal incision, taking care not to enter the bladder (see Fig. 33–4F, G). The suture is threaded through the eye of the needle and transferred out of the abdominal incision with withdrawal of the needle. The second ipsilateral transfer is begun 2.5 to 3 cm laterally to the first. The same procedure is carried out on the opposite side. Cystoscopy confirms the absence of sutures within the bladder and accurate placement of a 12 Fr cystocath tube for suprapubic urinary drainage. Evidence of intravenously administered indigo carmine in the urine excreted from both ureteral orifices and elevation and compression of the bladder neck by the patch is sought at this time as well.

Following anterior vaginal wall closure with absorbable suture, the patch is secured by tying the ipsilateral sutures under minimal tension and then by tying the suture strands to the contralateral sutures under the midline skin bridge (see Fig. 33–4H). The lack of appreciable tension cannot be overemphasized because minimal elevation and compression are needed, and too much tension will result in obstruction. The abdominal incisions are closed with absorbable suture, and a vaginal pack may be inserted.

OTHER DIFFICULTIES ENCOUNTERED

Dense scarring from prior surgery may be encountered near the area of the bladder neck or pubovesical attachments, especially in the area of prior suture

---

Figure 33-4 Gore-Tex patch suspension. *A,* Sagittal view of bladder and vaginal incision. *B,* The labia are sutured laterally (optional). A Foley catheter is placed in the bladder. The location of the bladder neck can be determined by palpating the Foley balloon, using extreme care not to pull the catheter during this maneuver. Forceps measure the distance between the vaginal fornices at the level of the bladder neck. This measurement is used to determine the width of the patch. The vaginal incision (5 to 6 cm) begins just proximal to the bladder neck. *C,* Lateral dissection is performed in the vesicovaginal plane. The periurethral fascia is dissected from the internal surface of the pubic bone using a combination of sharp and blunt dissection. *D,* Transverse view at the level of the bladder neck after suture placement. *E* and *F,* Following placement of the suspension suture in the periurethral fascia, the sutures are incorporated into the patch in a helical fashion (three bites). *G,* The patch is advanced along the suspension sutures, and at the level of the bladder neck it is placed loosely beneath the periurethral fascia. Two stab incisions are made one fingerbreadth above the pubic bone; dissection is taken down to the rectus fascia. The Gore-Tex sutures are transferred suprapubically, using the suspension needle via the stab incisions. *H,* Completed repair with Gore-Tex patch in place.

placement. We have found that a renal pedicle clamp cupped within the right hand and with the points slightly extended provides a controlled way to mobilize this scar tissue off the bone as one proceeds superiorly. If the scarring is extremely dense, mobilization can be stopped just superior to the bladder neck area without proceeding to the inferior surface of the rectus muscles. The suspension needle can be relied on to traverse this scarred area aided by cystoscopic guidance. The advantage of complete bladder neck mobilization is that it facilitates bladder neck repositioning and allows finger guidance of the needle through the entire retropubic space, thus avoiding entrance into the bladder. In the presence of dense scarring, this mobilization may have to be less aggressive to avoid bladder neck perforation.

If the bladder neck or urethra is entered during dissection, use of the Gore-Tex patch may be contraindicated because of the increased risk of graft infection. It is our routine practice to switch to a vaginal wall or fascial graft in these circumstances.

POSTOPERATIVE CARE

A vaginal pack is not used routinely, but if one is placed it is removed on the first postoperative day. The suprapubic tube is clamped the day after surgery, and voiding trials begin. The patient is taught how to open the suprapubic tube and check the postvoid residual urine every 2 to 4 hours. When the postvoid residual urine remains less than 100 ml, the suprapubic tube is removed. If this period of time lasts longer than 2 weeks, self-intermittent catheterization is begun.

OPERATIVE RESULTS

We have used a Gore-Tex patch suspension procedure for correction of primary (42 first operations) and recurrent (39 second and 19 third operations) type II genuine stress incontinence in 100 patients.[16] The age of the patients (6 patients aged 30 to 39, 26 aged 40 to 49, 24 aged 50 to 59, 25 aged 60 to 69, 14 aged 70 to 79, and 5 aged 80 to 89) did not affect the decision about use of the graft material. All patients underwent preoperative videourodynamic evaluation (uroflow, PVR, provocative CO_2-CMG, urethral pressure profile [UPP], VCUG) as described earlier; those with persistent symptoms had postoperative videourodynamic evaluation. The initial 32 patients had a history of unsuccessful prior surgery, chronic obstructive pulmonary disease, obesity, or corticosteroid use, making them excellent candidates for sling repair. Of the next 62 patients, 39 were undergoing their first repair for stress urinary incontinence. These patients had either poor anterior vaginal wall mobility or deficient periurethral tissue (or both), which limited the ability to elevate and fix the bladder neck. We followed the technique described earlier without modification.

Follow-up was more than 2 years for 11 of 14 patients, more than 1 year for 53 of 60 patients, more than 9 months for 72 of 81 patients, and more than 6 months for 91 of 100 patients. Either phone contact or office visits were undertaken as well as repeat urodynamic evaluation if patients were symptomatic postoperatively. In three patients the Gore-Tex patches (but not the sutures) were removed owing to patch infection. All three reported significant vaginal discharge within 8 weeks of surgery. Two remain continent. Four patients had persistent symptoms of obstructive voiding (confirmed by pressure-flow studies), and their patches were vertically incised (6, 8, 12, and 14 weeks postoperatively) but not removed. All four remain continent without obstruction (three patients are continent more than 1 year after the incision). Presumably, continence in these patients is due to continued support from scar tissue formation. Six patients experienced onset of symptoms of urinary urgency and frequency, and two of these had urge incontinence demonstrable on postoperative CMG. These patients were managed by anticholinergic therapy. One patient has persistent incontinence, which is type III by urodynamic evaluation.

In summary, 89 of 91 patients available for follow-up were cured of stress urinary incontinence with the use of the Gore-Tex patch sling. This procedure eliminates the major cause of surgical failure for type II GSI, namely, suture failure. The procedure is well tolerated, with a second procedure being required in 7 of 91 patients. In only 2 patients of 91 was de novo detrusor instability seen.

Conclusion

We have reviewed the indications for sling surgery and the evaluation of patients thought to be surgical candidates for this procedure. We have discussed the options available for surgical approach, namely, the abdominal, abdominovaginal, or vaginal routes. We have presented our choice of the Gore-Tex patch sling as an evolution of prior techniques and materials that provides the best results in properly selected patients.

REFERENCES

1. Staskin DR, Zimmern PE, Hadley HR, Raz S: The pathophysiology of stress incontinence. Urol Clin North Am 12(2):271, 1985.
2. Blavis J, Olsson C: Stress incontinence: Classification and surgical approach. J Urol 139:727, 1988.
3. Kerr LA, Witt M, Staskin DR: Transvaginal bladder neck closure versus a transvaginal obstructive sling as an adjunct to the treatment of total urethral incontinence managed with suprapubic tube drainage. In press, 1995.
4. McGuire EJ, Woodside JR, Borden TA, Weiss RM: Prognostic value of urodynamic testing in myelodysplastic patients. J Urol 126:205, 1981.
5. McGuire EJ, Bennet C, Konnak J, et al: Experience with pubovaginal slings for urinary incontinence at the University of Michigan. J Urol 138:525, 1987.

6. Moir JC: The gauze-hammock operation. J Obstet Gynaecol Br Commonwlth 75:1, 1968.

7. Nichols DH: The Mersilene mesh gauze hammock for severe urinary stress incontinence. Obstet Gynecol 41:88, 1973.

8. Melnick I, Lee RE: Delayed transection of urethra by Mersilene tape. Urology 8(6):580, 1976.

9. Morgan JE: A sling operation using Marlex polypropylene mesh, for treatment of recurrent stress incontinence. Am J Obstet Gynecol 106(3):369, 1970.

10. Morgan JE, Farrow GA, Stewart FE: The Marlex sling operation for the treatment of recurrent stress urinary incontinence: A 16-year review. Am J Obstet Gynecol 151(2):224, 1985.

11. Stanton SL, Brindley GS, Holmes DM: Silastic sling for urethral sphincter incompetence in women. Br J Obstet Gynecol 92:747, 1985.

12. Stanton SL: Suprapubic approaches for stress incontinence in women. J Am Geriatr Soc 38:348, 1990.

13. Horbach NS, Blanco JS, Ostergard DR: A suburethral sling procedure with PTFE for the treatment of genuine stress incontinence in patients with low urethral closure pressure. Obstet Gynecol 71:648, 1988.

14. Bent AE, Ostergard DR, Zwick-Zaffuto M: Tissue reaction to expanded polytetrafluoroethylene suburethral sling for urinary incontinence: Clinical and histologic study. Am J Obstet Gynecol 169(5):1198–1201, 1993.

15. Raz S: Modified bladder neck suspension for female stress incontinence. Urology 17:82, 1981.

16. Staskin DR, Kerr LA: The Gore-Tex patch transvaginal needle suspension: Indications, technique, results and followup of 100 consecutive patients. J Urol 149:291A, 1993.

CHAPTER 34

Technique of Rectangular Fascial Sling

Ashok Chopra, M.D.
Shlomo Raz, M.D.
Lynn Stothers, M.D.

The use of fascial slings has a distinct role in the treatment of incontinence, as described in Chapters 31 to 33. This chapter will not repeat the points these authors have raised but rather will present a simplified technique of performing an abdominal rectus fascial sling.

Considerations

Different surgeons use formal fascial slings with various degrees of emphasis. Some authors use this procedure for all patients with stress urinary incontinence (SUI); others restrict its use to patients with type III incontinence. Since techniques of vaginal wall sling were developed, we have limited the use of formal fascial strip slings in our practice. At UCLA we use these slings primarily for patients with poor vaginal tissues, for some patients who have had radiation to the pelvis, for those undergoing creation of a neourethra, and for those who have failed to respond to previous vaginal sling surgery.

Our technique of fascial sling suspension is quite similar to that described in Chapter 31. Three primary differences exist: (1) A smaller segment of fascia is used with Prolene sutures attached to allow suspension; (2) the technique of transfer and fixation of the suspension sutures makes use of the Raz suture carrier in a fashion identical to that used for bladder neck suspension and modified vaginal sling; and (3) the fascial strip is fastened at the level of the bladder neck by creating a tunnel in the anterior vaginal wall and using additional fixation sutures to avoid migration of the strip.

SURGICAL TECHNIQUE

The patient is placed in the dorsal lithotomy position and prepared from the abdomen to the perineum (including the vagina). The labia are retracted laterally with stay sutures, and a suprapubic catheter is placed (as described in the section on anterior vaginal wall slings). A urethral Foley catheter is inserted, the bladder is drained, and a weighted speculum is placed. The anterior vaginal wall is infiltrated with saline solution, and two parallel oblique incisions are made. Lateral dissection is carried out over the urethropelvic fascia. The retropubic space is entered bilaterally by advancing curved Mayo scissors toward the ipsilateral shoulder. The retropubic space is freed from adhesions, and the surgeon's fingertip is advanced toward the suprapubic area. At this point a right-angle clamp is used to connect the two vaginal incisions at the level of the bladder neck; this maneuver creates a tunnel (Fig. 34–1). Later in the procedure the harvested fascial strip will be placed within this tunnel, ensuring its fixation and correct location. Of note, if an anterior vaginal flap has been devel-

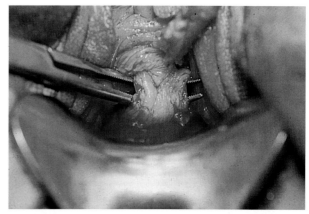

Figure 34–1 The anterior vaginal wall "tunnel." This is used as the site of placement of the fascial sling.

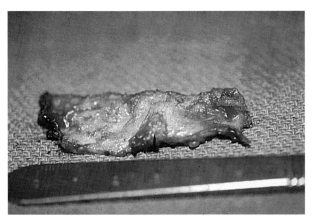

Figure 34–2 The rectus fascial strip.

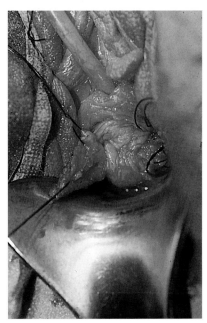

Figure 34–4 Insertion of the fascial strip into the anterior vaginal wall tunnel.

oped as the "bed" for the strip, absorbable sutures will be needed to fix the fascia in the correct location.

A vaginal pack is now introduced to tamponade any bleeding, and attention is turned to the harvesting of the fascial strip. A number of different donor sites may be used; we prefer to use the rectus fascia. A 5-cm incision is made in the suprapubic area, and dissection is carried down to the level of the rectus fascia. A 2- × 5-cm rectangle of fascia is harvested and the rectus is subsequently repaired with sutures of polyglycolic acid (Fig. 34–2). The suprapubic incision is next closed. At this point four sutures of No. 1 Prolene are placed in the harvested fascial strip; one suture is placed in each corner of the graft (Fig. 34–3). The fascial strip is placed in the anterior vaginal tunnel and adjusted to ensure correct orientation (Fig. 34–4). A suprapubic puncture is made, and the Raz suture carrier is passed under fingertip control to the vaginal incision. Next, the sutures are passed anteriorly (Figs. 34–5 and 34–6). During this portion of the procedure it is important that the surgeon be aware of the location and orientation of the fascial segment within its tunnel.

Cystoscopy is performed after administration of indigo carmine. The examination should ensure patency of the ureters (blue efflux from both orifices);

also, coaptation of bladder neck with traction on the untied sutures should be appreciated. Finally, the examination should ensure that the Prolene sutures do not violate the bladder wall and that the suprapubic catheter is in a good position.

The wounds are irrigated with dilute Betadine, and the vaginal incisions are closed with a running interlocking 2–0 Vicryl suture. During this portion of the closure the rectus fascial strip should be incorporated in the running suture to prevent its migration and ensure proper positioning. A sulfa- or Betadine-impregnated vaginal pack is next introduced. The untied Prolene sutures exiting the suprapubic incision are now tied sequentially to themselves and to their ipsilateral mates. It is important to tie these sutures without tension. At this point the suprapubic puncture is closed. A schematic diagram of the final repair is shown in Figure 34–7.

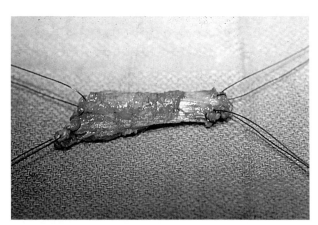

Figure 34–3 The rectus fascial strip with one No. 1 Prolene suture in each corner.

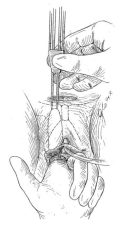

Figure 34–5 Drawing of passage of the Raz suture carrier.

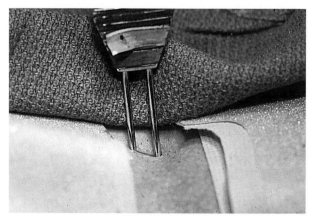

Figure 34–6 Intraoperative photo of passage of the Raz suture carrier.

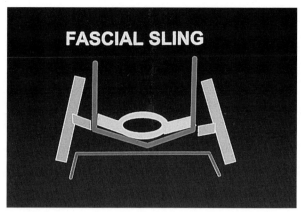

Figure 34–7 Schematic diagram of the fascial sling.

Postoperatively, the Foley catheter and vaginal pack are removed when the patient awakens from anesthesia. The patient is allowed to eat and ambulate when alert and oriented. Discharge usually occurs on the first postoperative day. The patient uses the suprapubic tube for postvoid residual urine checks until the residual is less than 2 ounces; if residual urine remains large for more than 2 to 4 weeks, the patient is instructed in the technique of intermittent straight catheterization. Patients are generally discharged on an oral antibiotic and a mild analgesic.

Karram and Bhatia described a similar technique in their paper on patch procedure using fascia lata.[1] In their procedure a midline vaginal incision was made, and the fascia lata was secured to the suburethra and bladder base using Dexon sutures. An additional difference was their use of only one No. 1 Prolene suture at each side of the strip. This suture was applied to the fascia lata by taking at least four bites in a helical fashion. They described 10 patients treated with this technique; 9 were continent at follow up 1 to 2 years later.

As stated in the introduction to this chapter, this procedure is presented as an optional technique when a fascial sling is thought to be indicated. Because of its basic conformity to other techniques of fascial sling, we would expect results similar to those reported by McGuire[4] and by Blaivas and colleagues (i.e., 90% or greater success).[2]

Postoperative complications are described elsewhere in this book. The surgeon should be aware of the 5% risk of permanent urinary retention associated with fascial sling procedures.[3] Postoperative incontinence may be secondary to inadequate urethral coaptation or detrusor instability.

REFERENCES

1. Karram MM, Bhatia NN: Patch procedure: Modified transvaginal fascia lata sling for recurrent or severe stress urinary incontinence. OB Gynecol 75(3):461, 1906.
2. Blaivas JG, Jacobs BZ: Pubovaginal sling; Long-term results and prognostic indicators. J Urol 149:313, 1993.
3. Raz S, Siegel AL, Short J: Vaginal wall sling. J Urol 139:727, 1989.
4. McGuire EJ Lytton B: Pubovaginal sling procedure for stress incontinence. J Urol 119:82, 1978.

BIBLIOGRAPHY

Blaivas JG, Olsson CA: Stress incontinence: Classification and surgical approach. J Urol 139:727, 1988.
Juma S, Little N, Raz S: Vaginal wall sling; four years later. Urology 36:424, 1992.
Leach GE: Vaginal surgery for the urologist. Urol Clin North Am 2(1):61, 1994.
Raz S: Atlas of Transvaginal Surgery. Philadelphia, WB Saunders, 1992.
Smith JL: Fascia lata paraurethral suspension for the correction of stress urinary incontinence. Am J Obstet Gynecol 95:714–721, 1966.

CHAPTER 35

Anterior Vaginal Wall Sling

Lynn Stothers, M.D., M.H.Sc., F.R.C.S.C.
Shlomo Raz, M.D.
Ashok Chopra, M.D.

The diagnosis of intrinsic sphincter dysfunction (ISD) is based on a combination of factors including history, physical examination, voiding cystourethrogram, and urodynamic parameters. Unlike anatomic incontinence, ISD exists when the bladder neck and proximal urethra are open at rest in the absence of detrusor contractions. This has been called type III incontinence by Blaivas and McGuire.[1] However, the urethra may be radiologically closed in some patients who present clinically with ISD. Whether the urethra is open or closed at rest, the abdominal leak-point pressure is typically low in patients with ISD. The cause of ISD may be multifactorial; possible etiologic factors are damage to the sphincter mechanism from multiple prior surgeries, radiation, direct trauma, or neurologic dysfunction. The diagnosis is made by a combination of historical, physical, and urodynamic parameters because no pathognomonic test currently exists.

Management options for patients with ISD include injection agents (collagen, autologous fat), various sling techniques, or insertion of an artificial urinary sphincter. As a basic principle, a sling can be created by the use of autologous fascial strips (rectus fascia, fascia lata, and so on) or synthetic materials (Marlex), by burying the vaginal mucosa, or by using permanent sutures placed in the periurethral supporting structures. The last technique, known as the anterior vaginal wall sling, is a relatively new technique developed since 1992. It creates a sling without burying the vaginal epithelium or using autologous fascial strips. The techniques for inserting an artificial urinary sphincter and periurethral injectable agents are described elsewhere in this text. This chapter focuses on the surgical technique of making an anterior vaginal wall sling using permanent suture material to create a hammock of support from the anatomic structures adjacent to the bladder neck and urethra.

The factors that led to the development of the anterior vaginal wall sling included (1) the need to correct a defect of midurethral support, (2) a better understanding of the anatomy of the levator musculature as it envelops the urethra just distal to the pubourethral ligaments, and (3) evidence suggesting that the bladder neck is not the only mechanism controlling urinary continence. Examples supporting this latter principle include the observations that 30 to 50% of postmenopausal women have an open bladder neck on a straining cystourethrogram with no incontinence and the observation that Y-V plasty does not produce stress incontinence. Most bladder neck suspension procedures elevate the bladder neck, creating a valvular effect, but do not affect the most important area of continence, the midurethral area. The Raz anterior vaginal wall sling involves construction of a sling from the anterior vaginal wall and underlying fascia that provides both compression and support for the urethra.

Surgical Technique

The surgical goals of the anterior vaginal wall sling are (1) to provide elastic support to the urethra and (2) to create a strong hammock of vaginal wall and underlying tissues that provide a backboard to increase coaptation and support to the midurethra and bladder neck.

TECHNIQUE The patient is placed in the lithotomy position, with the heels padded in protective boots and suspended from the supporting stirrups. The vagina and lower abdomen are prepared with an iodine scrub, which extends inferiorly from the level of the umbilicus and includes the entire perineum. The vagina should be scrubbed with iodine-based soap and painted with an iodine-prep solution. A weighted vaginal speculum and silk labial retraction sutures are used for exposure as in the bladder neck suspension procedure. A suprapubic tube is placed using the curved Lowsley retractor. A 16 Fr Foley catheter is typically used for the suprapubic tube, which should be placed approximately 2 cm above the symphysis pubis in the midline. The incision for the suprapubic tube should be just the width of the catheter and is made using a stab with a knife blade over the tip of the curved Lowsley retractor held by the assistant. Once the suprapubic tube is in position, it is placed on slight traction and the bladder is emptied. A second Foley catheter is placed in the urethra.

Following saline infiltration of the anterior vaginal wall tissues to facilitate dissection, two longitudinal incisions are made in the anterior vaginal wall (Fig. 35–1). These incisions extend from the level of the midurethra to beyond the level of the bladder neck and are 1 cm medial to the folded margin of the anterior vaginal wall throughout their entire length. If the incisions are made too lateral it will be difficult to close them owing to the natural folding of the anterior vaginal wall. Incisions made too medially result in difficult dissection and a greater potential for entering the bladder during dissection.

After the incisions have been made the dissection is carried out over the glistening surface of the periurethral fascia using the Metzenbaum scissors. The attachment of the urethropelvic fascia to the tendinous arch of the obturator is identified. Using the curved Mayo scissors, the retropubic space is entered at the level of the tendinous arch, and the urethropelvic ligament is exposed (Fig. 35–2). Any adhesions encountered in the retropubic space are divided using

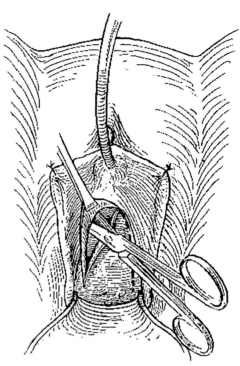

Figure 35-2 Dissection is carried out over the glistening periurethral fascia. The curved Mayo scissors are shown entering the retropubic space. The scissors are pointed toward the shoulder of the patient. Misdirecting the scissors too far medially could result in perforation of the bladder.

a combination of blunt and sharp dissection. Sutures found in the retropubic space from previous suspension procedures are divided. Adequate urethrolysis should permit a finger entering the retropubic space from either incision to palpate the pubic bone.

Two pairs of No. 1 Prolene sutures are placed during creation of the anterior vaginal wall sling. The first pair of Prolene sutures is placed at the level of the bladder neck. Each suture includes helical bites of the vesicopelvic fascia, the urethropelvic ligament, and the anterior vaginal wall without epithelium (Fig. 35–3). The arc of the needle should include a large area of tissue in both the vesicopelvic fascia and the urethropelvic ligament. When passing the needle to encompass the vesicopelvic fascia, the direction of the needle should be kept parallel to the vaginal wall. Failure to keep the needle parallel to the vaginal wall may result in suture material's entering the bladder.

To pass the second pair of Prolene sutures, the forceps are opened in the retropubic space. Gentle downward traction with the open forceps aids in exposure of the levator musculature. The second pair of Prolene sutures includes the levator ani musculature as it inserts onto the midurethral segment, the medial edge of the urethropelvic ligament, and the anterior vaginal wall without epithelium (Fig. 35–4). To obtain an adequate amount of levator tissue the needle must be placed deep into the retropubic space. The levator should be visualized on the arc of the needle. When the anterior vaginal wall without epithelium is taken, the arc of the needle should not

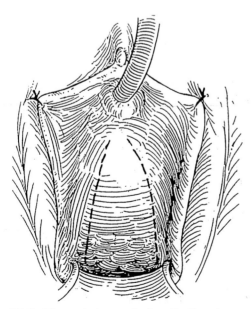

Figure 35-1 The anterior vaginal wall sling is approached through two lateral incisions in the anterior vaginal wall. A urethral Foley catheter and a suprapubic catheter are placed before these incisions are made. Allis clamps are used on the anterior vaginal wall to aid in exposure.

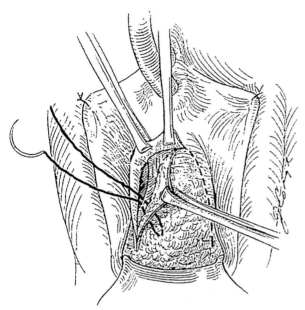

Figure 35-3 The first pair of Prolene sutures placed at the level of the bladder neck is shown. These sutures include the vesicopelvic fascia, the urethropelvic ligament, and the anterior vaginal wall without epithelium.

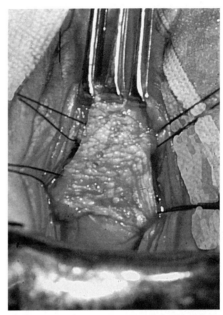

Figure 35-5 Intraoperative photograph after placement of the four Prolene sutures before they are transferred through the lower abdominal stab incision. They demonstrate the complete rectangle of vaginal wall, which will provide a backboard of support for the urethra and bladder neck during increases in abdominal pressure.

cross the midline but should include a generous amount of tissue. As with the vesicopelvic fascia, when the needle is passed to include the anterior vaginal wall without epithelium, the arc of the needle should stay parallel to the anterior vaginal wall to avoid entering the spongy tissue of the urethra itself.

After the four Prolene sutures are in place, a rectangle of support for the bladder neck and urethra can be visualized (Fig. 35–5). To transfer the Prolene sutures, a stab incision in the lower abdomen is made just anterior to the symphysis pubis in the midline.

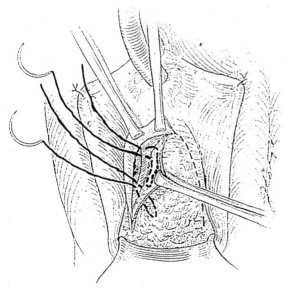

Figure 35-4 The second pair of Prolene sutures is placed at the level of the midurethra. These sutures include the levator musculature, the edge of the urethropelvic ligament, and the anterior vaginal wall without epithelium.

Blunt dissection with a clamp facilitates exposure of the rectus fascia. A double-pronged needle is passed, scratching the symphysis into the retropubic space and onto the operator's finger, which is placed in the retropubic space through the vaginal incision. Under fingertip control, the needle is advanced through the ipsilateral vaginal incision, and the ends of the Prolene suture are passed through the eyes of the needle. The suture is then transferred to the lower abdomen by pulling up on the needle. After all four Prolene sutures have been transferred through the single lower abdominal stab incision, the urethral catheter is temporarily removed to allow cystoscopy.

Just prior to cystoscopy, indigo carmine is administered, and blue efflux should be noted from both ureteral orifices. The location of the suprapubic catheter is noted, and the side walls of the bladder and trigone are inspected to ensure that no suture has passed within the bladder. The urethral Foley catheter is then replaced, and the anterior vaginal wall incisions are closed using a running locking 2–0 polyglycolic acid suture. A vaginal pack covered with sulfa cream is placed, and the suspension sutures are tied down without undue tension following placement of the vaginal pack. Each suture is tied to itself and its neighbor for security. The skin edges are loosened with a clamp to prevent dimpling of the skin over the Prolene sutures. The suprapubic stab wound is closed with a subcuticular 4–0 absorbable suture, and Steri-Strips are applied. Both the suprapubic tube and the urethral catheter are placed to straight drainage.

POSTOPERATIVE CARE This procedure is currently performed as outpatient surgery. Within 6 to 20 hours postoperatively the patient is prepared for discharge. The vaginal pack and urethral catheter are removed, and the suprapubic tube is plugged. The patient should maintain the suprapubic tube taped on slight traction to prevent leakage around the tube. The patient is asked to try to void through the urethra and to check her own postvoid residual urine after each voiding. Oral antibiotics, stool softeners, and oral analgesics are given to the patient for use after discharge. Antibiotics are continued while the suprapubic tube is in place. The urethral catheter is removed once the postvoid residual urine is consistently less than 2 ounces.

Results

One hundred and thirty-seven women underwent the sling procedure between June of 1992 and June of 1994.[2] Preoperative evaluation included history, physical examination, urinalysis, lateral cystography, videourodynamics, cystoscopy, quality of life measures, and SEAPI incontinence classification (S, activity-related incontinence; E, emptying ability; A, degree of anatomic defect; P, use of protection, and I, instability). Postoperative outcome measures were prospectively assigned on a 6-month basis by a third party and included SEAPI score, quality of life scores, and assessment of any complications.[3] Statistics were applied using SPSS* computer software to create regression models for outcome variables of interest.

The median follow-up has been 11 months (range, 3 to 24 months) in the 137 patients. Age ranged from 32 to 81 years. Three patients were lost to follow-up. Of the 134 patients who could be evaluated, 91 had ISD, and 42 had anatomic incontinence (AI). Overall, 54% of patients had undergone an average of 2.5 prior procedures for stress incontinence. Associated urge incontinence was common preoperatively and was seen clinically in 47% of these patients. One hundred and twenty-nine patients were considered

---

*SPSS is a registered trademark of SPSS Inc., 444 North Michigan Avenue, Chicago, IL

cured at last follow-up; they had clinical SEAPI scores of S0-1, E0, A0, P0-1. Five of 134 patients were considered failures; they had recurrent incontinence on follow-up that was unrelated to instability and required further therapy. Time to failure in ISD and AI patients was modeled using Kaplan Meier survival curves, and the logrank test showed no significant difference between these two groups ($p >$ .05). Conditional logistic regression covariates revealed no significant predictive factors for postoperative failure. Seven percent of patients developed de novo instability and were treated with anticholinergics orally. Three percent had SEAPI inhibition scores $\geq I_2$ prior to anticholinergic therapy. Preoperative patient age was the only predictive factor of de novo instability identified by the logistic regression model ($p <$ .05). Preoperative and postoperative within-patient changes of quality of life scores were statistically and significantly different for patients with AI and ISD.

CONCLUSION   These initial results indicate that excellent continence was achieved in patients with both ISD and AI using the anterior vaginal wall sling. Advantages of this surgical technique include the absence of vaginal flaps and the lack of a transverse incision over the urethra as used in other techniques. No vaginal tissue is buried. Other advantages of this technique are its simplicity, avoidance of laparotomy, short hospital stay, lateral placement of permanent nonreactive sutures, and the ability to correct mild cystocele. The technique relies on healthy well-vascularized supporting tissues.

Further follow-up is required to establish the longevity of these results; however, the procedure has been shown to be safe and effective in short-term follow-up and allows outpatient surgical management of both ISD and AI.

REFERENCES

1. Blaivas JG, Olsson CA: Stress incontinence: Classification and surgical approach. J Urol 139:727, 1988.
2. Stothers L, Chopra A, Raz S: Vaginal wall sling for anatomic incontinence and intrinsic sphincter damage—efficacy and outcome analysis. J Urol 153:525A, 1995.
3. Raz S, Erickson DR: SEAPI QMM Incontinence Classification System. Neurourol Urodynam 11:187, 1992.

Injections

CHAPTER 36

Collagen Injections

Rodney A. Appell, M.D.

Definition of Problem

The approach to correcting the problem of failure to store urine may be simplified by considering the location of the cause. Treatment modalities can then be directed at the dysfunctional location in the lower urinary tract, either the bladder itself or its outlet. When the problem originates in the outlet, the difficulty is often related to the competency of the urethral sphincteric mechanism at the neck of the bladder. Although this incompetence may be the result of some defect in anatomic support (so-called genuine stress urinary incontinence secondary to hypermobility of the urethra with resultant inadequate transmission of intra-abdominal pressure to the urethra), it may also be related to a problem in the intrinsic urethral closure mechanism itself due to sympathetic neurologic injury, surgical trauma, or myelodysplasia. Urodynamically, in these cases of intrinsic sphincteric deficiency (ISD) or type III stress urinary incontinence, the bladder neck and the proximal segment of the urethra are open at rest without a detrusor contraction. However, it must be recognized that ISD may exist concomitantly with an anatomic abnormality of the position of the bladder neck and urethra.

The treatment of urinary incontinence due to an incompetent outlet has been a challenging problem. When ISD has been identified as the cause of a woman's urinary incontinence, treatment has been aimed at increasing outflow resistance based on the premise that the incontinence occurs because resistance to the flow of urine has decreased below that of normal detrusor tonus or any increases in intra-abdominal pressure. Various surgical procedures and devices have been developed that have been used with varying degrees of success in augmenting intraurethral pressures. The primary procedures currently employed include various types of suburethral slings and, to a lessor degree, implantation of an artificial urinary sphincter. Another technique used to treat this type of female urinary incontinence is the injection of bulk-enhancing agents into the periurethral tissues to compress the urethral lumen, resulting in an increase in resistance to the outflow of urine. This is accomplished by promoting reapposition of the urethral mucosa, thus enhancing the mucosal seal effect and protecting against increases in intravesical pressure. Because the type of incontinence described as ISD is nonresistant urinary leakage, the goal in treatment should be only to coapt the urethra by passive occlusion, and this can be accomplished by the injection of collagen. The procedure outlined later in this chapter is done under direct vision and is considered a minimally invasive procedure that can be performed using local anesthesia alone. This form of therapy is potentially less costly than major surgery if patients are selected properly, and it offers a genuine alternative to surgery in the elderly and those who are poor surgical risks without jeopardizing the ability to perform surgery later if it is required.

Pertinent Anatomic and Physiologic Aspects

The precise anatomic and physiologic mechanisms of urinary continence are still poorly understood. Nevertheless, it has been well documented that urinary continence is achieved because maximum urethral pressure remains greater than intravesical pressure during bladder filling and that increases in intraabdominal pressure are transmitted approximately equally to the bladder and proximal urethra.[1] The vesical neck and proximal urethra lie above a well-supporting pelvic diaphragm and are positioned to promote equal distribution of forces to the bladder and urethra during increases in intra-abdominal pressure. In restoring continence one tries to accomplish precisely this same goal of protecting against increases in intra-abdominal pressure. It follows that stress-type urinary incontinence can occur by two mechanisms. In the first (and by far the most common) condition, the vesical neck and proximal urethra retain their basic sphincteric function; however, transmission of intra-abdominal pressure becomes unequal owing to descent of the proximal urethra below the pelvic diaphragm, and intravesical pressure exceeds urethral pressure, resulting in urinary leakage. In the second condition, ISD, the urethra no longer functions as a sphincter. Recognition of this difference and of the fact that both conditions can occur in the same patient is the only way to be successful in choosing the correct modality of treatment for the patient's problem.

Patient Selection

As discussed previously, the choice of the correct approach for treating urinary incontinence depends on determining the underlying cause of the problem. Therefore, before initiating therapy, it is important to take a thorough history, conduct a complete physical examination, and subject the patient to a careful urodynamic evaluation.

DIAGNOSTIC EVALUATION

Fluoroscopy or urethral pressures (or both) are accurate ways of diagnosing proximal urethral sphincter failure. Put more simply, the purpose of urodynamics evaluation is to classify the disproportion between the bladder and urethral pressures. This volume tolerance equals the leak point, and the pressure within the bladder when urine leaks through the continence mechanism is the urethral opening pressure, which can be recorded as the leak point pressure; simple methods for making this determination have been discussed earlier in Chapter 10 and elsewhere.[2] When ISD is demonstrated on evaluation, treatment must be directed toward correcting this specific problem; resuspending the vesicourethral junction by standard procedures (e.g., Marshall-Marchetti-Krantz, Burch colposuspension, Stamey, Pereyra, and Gittes procedures) will not accomplish this end. Patient evaluation and selection for bladder outlet incompetence is no different for patients being considered for injectable procedures than for patients considered for slings or artificial sphincters except that these latter two modalities may also be used when there is concomitant hypermobility of the urethra. Injectables are not as successful as slings or artificial sphincters when this concomitant hypermobility is present.

Endoscopic evaluation to determine whether viable tissue is present at the prospective injection site is mandatory and helpful in determining the proximity of the ureteral orifices to the bladder neck and posterior urethra.

CONTRAINDICATIONS

Injectable agents are not a panacea for all types of incontinence. Strict criteria for their consideration as a treatment modality have been ascertained.[3] Candidates for injections to augment bladder outlet pressure are patients with a primary incompetent urethra or a loss of sphincteric function secondary to either surgery or trauma. Injectables are most suitable for patients with sphincter incompetency and normal detrusor muscle function. However, patients with decreased detrusor muscle contractility may still be candidates if they accept and can perform self-intermittent catheterization. Success in achieving continence is influenced by the status of bladder function. A normal bladder or poor detrusor contractility, with unaltered compliance, is associated with a high degree of success. Detrusor hyperreflexia or instability must be controlled prior to injection to prevent treatment failure. Adequate bladder capacity (greater than 125 ml) is essential, but residual urine is not a factor in those patients capable of self-catheterization. The only total contraindication to the use of any specific injectable is hypersensitivity to the chosen agent. Any urinary tract infection must be adequately treated prior to an injection session.

Preoperative Preparation

One of the major advantages of treatment with injectables is that the use of local anesthesia alone is sufficient to accomplish the procedure in an outpatient setting. Preoperative antimicrobials have not been used routinely. The procedure is performed with the patient in the dorsal lithotomy position using a routine povidone-iodine preparation as for any routine cystourethroscopy.

Surgical Technique

The minimally invasive endoscopic methodology is not difficult but requires precision to ensure an optimal therapeutic response. Regardless of the material chosen, the injection can be performed suburothelially through a needle placed directly through a cystoscope (transurethral injection), transvaginally with the needle placed through the biopsy port of the ultrasound probe, or periurethrally with a spinal needle inserted percutaneously and positioned in the

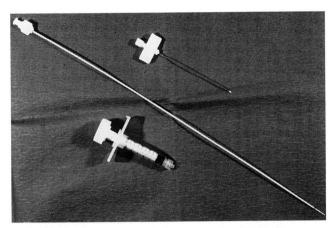

Figure 36-1 Injection delivery systems for Contigen.

tissues adjacent to the urethra while the manipulation is observed cystoscopically (Fig. 36–1). The cause of the incontinence, the tissue at the injection site, and the plane of delivery of the injectable collagen will affect the treatment results. Nearly every patient can be injected under local anesthesia, which has the added advantage of allowing the patient to stand and perform a few provocative maneuvers immediately after the injection in an attempt to cause urinary leakage, which can then be addressed before the patient is released from that particular treatment session.

COLLAGEN

Attempts to treat urinary incontinence with a variety of injectables have been made for decades since the first report by Murless using a sclerosing agent.[4] Most investigators have concluded that the basic approach is effective, but problems with the bulking agents themselves have limited the use of the procedure up to this time. A multicenter study of the efficacy and safety of glutaraldehyde cross-linked bovine collagen (Contigen) has now been completed.

THE SUBSTANCE Contigen is a biocompatible and biodegradable substance consisting of a sterilized, nonpyrogenic, purified bovine dermal collagen that has been cross-linked with glutaraldehyde and dispersed in phosphate-buffered physiologic saline. This cross-linking process increases the length of time before degradation takes place and reduces the immunogenic potential. Glutaraldehyde binds adjacent collagen fibrils to improve the integrity of the implant after injection. This cross-linked form of bovine collagen has 90 to 100% net weight persistence as a stable implant suburothelially compared to less than 50% for the noncross-linked bovine collagen,[5] and there has been no correlation between this degree of histologic change with time.[6] In addition, there appears to be a significantly lower potential for local immune-type reactions after collagen has been cross-linked with glutaraldehyde.[7, 8] As a substance for injection into humans, this material has the additional positive attribute of not eliciting a foreign body reaction. Although a minimal inflammatory response results from this noncytotoxic material, there has been no evidence of particle migration.

ADVANTAGES OF CONTIGEN IMPLANT The low viscosity of the suspension allows Contigen to be easily injected through a relatively small-gauge needle. The entire procedure can be performed using local anesthesia alone. The delivery system (see Fig. 36–1) consists of two types of needles and a 3-ml Luer-Lok syringe containing 2.5 ml of Contigen. The needle used for transurethral injection or transvaginal ultrasound-guided injection is a beveled 20-gauge, 1.5-cm long needle attached to a 5 Fr thermoplastic catheter that looks like a ureteral catheter with a needle on the end. Periurethral injections are performed using a simple 22-gauge spinal needle. The syringe of Contigen easily attaches to either needle.

The material has been demonstrated in the multicenter trials to be efficacious and safe as well as simple to use and durable for a biodegradable substance. The material is biocompatible, and the minimal inflammatory response elicited by Contigen allows eventual successful replacement of the bovine collagen with the patient's own collagen[5, 9] as the injected Contigen is transformed into living connective tissue.[10]

If therapy with Contigen is unsuccessful, its presence in the patient does not preclude the use of follow-up surgical procedures as any such surgery is made no more difficult by the presence of previously injected Contigen.

DISADVANTAGES OF CONTIGEN IMPLANT As stated previously, the use of Contigen is contraindicated in patients with an active, untreated cystitis or urethritis, uncontrolled detrusor instability, or known hypersensitivity to bovine collagen. All patients are skin-tested 30 days prior to treatment to eliminate those with preexisting hypersensitivity. In the multicenter trial, only 11 of 427 patients who were tested demonstrated this preexisting hypersensitivity and were excluded from treatment on this basis alone.

The fact that Contigen is biodegradable is both an advantage and a disadvantage. As stated earlier, the biodegradability of the substance eliminates any concerns about migration and granuloma formation. However, the biodegradation of the material raises questions about the potential need for repeated injections when the material degrades in patients who have been rendered continent. It is thought that replacement of Contigen by the individual's own collagen explains the durability of the results obtained in the multicenter study because the injected Contigen is transformed into living connective tissue.[10]

TRANSURETHRAL INJECTIONS

The patient is placed in a semilithotomy position, and the surgical field is prepared in the usual sterile fashion used for the standard cystoscopic procedure. Local anesthesia consists of 2% plain lidocaine jelly

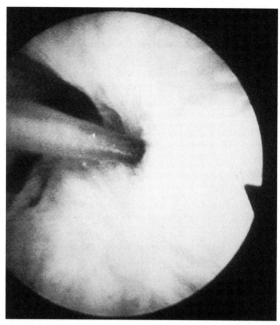

Figure 36-2 Endoscopic view of the bladder neck during transurethral injection of Contigen. (From Appell RA: Use of collagen injections for treatment of incontinence and reflux. Adv Urol 5:145, 1992.)

placed over the introitus and intraurethrally and left in place at least 10 minutes prior to instrumentation. This may be augmented by the use of 2 ml of 1% plain lidocaine injected periurethrally at the 3 and 9 o'clock positions. Cystourethroscopy with a 21 Fr sheath and a 30- or 0-degree lens can be used comfortably. The thermoplastic catheter with the needle described earlier is placed through the panendoscope, and the Contigen is delivered suburothelially under direct vision on either side until the urethral mucosa nearly coapts in the midline. This requires several placements of the needle (Fig. 36-2). Each time the needle is advanced under the mucosa with the beveled portion facing the urethral lumen. Extrusion of Contigen into the urethral lumen from the needle hole as the needle is withdrawn may occur; however, the loss of injected Contigen is minimal and inconsequential and may be minimized by not traversing the injected area with the distal end of the cystoscope once the Contigen has been injected. If Contigen extravasation is visible in all quadrants in any given patient, the procedure should be terminated and another injection session scheduled in 2 weeks or more.

PERIURETHRAL INJECTIONS

The possible complications of bleeding and extrusion of Contigen during transurethral injection are eliminated by injecting the material through a periurethral approach. In this periurethral injection technique a smaller 17 Fr panendoscopic sheath may be used with the spinal needle positioned periurethrally at approximately the 4 o'clock position, again with the bevel of the needle directed toward the lumen.

The needle is advanced into the urethral muscle but remains suburothelially in the lamina propria, where it advances with very little force. The needle may also be introduced between the urethral fascia and the vaginal epithelium at 6 o'clock and advanced toward the bladder neck—again, fully observed endoscopically (Fig. 36-3). During advancement of the needle, bulging of the tip of the needle against the lining of the urethra can be observed to ensure proper position prior to injection of the Contigen. When the needle tip is properly positioned 0.5 cm below the vesical neck, the Contigen syringe is attached to the spinal needle, and the material is injected until swelling is visible in the urethra on each side (Fig. 36-4). It is quite easy to inject the substance with one hand while stabilizing the cystoscope with the other hand. Endoscopically, the Contigen layering outside the lining of the urethra will be observed to occlude the urethral lumen gradually. When the urethra appears to be approximately 50% occluded, the needle is removed and reinserted on the opposite side, and additional Contigen is injected until the urethral mucosa coapts in the midline and has the endoscopic appearance of two lateral prostatic lobes (Fig. 36-5A and B). Again, the cystoscope should not be introduced proximal to the injection site to avoid disturbance of the injected material and prevent flattening or molding of the urethra.

TRANSVAGINAL ULTRASOUND-GUIDED INJECTIONS

Using a multiplanar probe with a biopsy port (the standard transrectal ultrasound probe for prostate

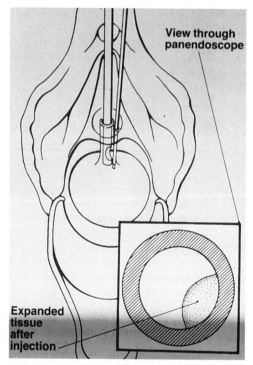

Figure 36-3 Periurethral injection. (From McGuire EJ, Appell RA: Collagen injection for the dysfunctional urethra. Contemp Urol 3[9]:11, 1991, copyright Medical Economics.)

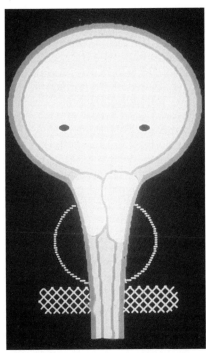

Figure 36-4 Schematic representation of cushions of Contigen just below the bladder neck. (From Appell RA: Use of collagen injections for treatment of incontinence and reflux. Adv Urol 5:145, 1992.)

examination and biopsy) passed vaginally, the open bladder neck can be identified (Fig. 36–6A), the transurethral needle placed accurately through the biopsy port, and the injection followed through closure of the bladder neck (Fig. 36–6B) by longitudinal (sagittal) scanning. This technique avoids the need for instrumentation of the urinary tract, thus reducing the likelihood of disturbing the position of the injected material.

Postoperative Management

One of the beneficial aspects of performing the procedure under local anesthesia is the fact that there is very little concern about causing permanent urinary retention because it is recognized that Contigen will lose some of its bulking owing to resorption of water and local anesthetic. Therefore, there is the added advantage of having the patient stand immediately after the injection and perform provocative maneuvers to induce urinary loss; if any should occur, she can immediately be repositioned and more Contigen can be injected. Additionally, after injection most patients void with little difficulty and indwelling catheters are usually unnecessary and should be avoided to prevent molding of the Contigen-filled urethra around the catheter. If the patient cannot void, then transient self-catheterization with a small (10–14 Fr) catheter or a trocar cystotomy should be considered. This temporary self-catheterization has been required infrequently in the multi-center trial and no

patients had a trocar cystotomy. Prophylactic antimicrobials are administered for 2 days post-procedure. In the event where reinjection is necessary this can be effectively performed between 7 and 30 days following the initial injection session.

Results

The purpose of the procedure is to render the patient completely continent. Most women (and, therefore, most investigators) will accept a certain amount of urinary leakage. This "social continence" allows for

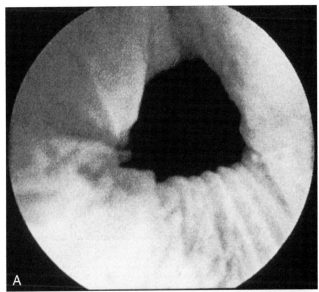

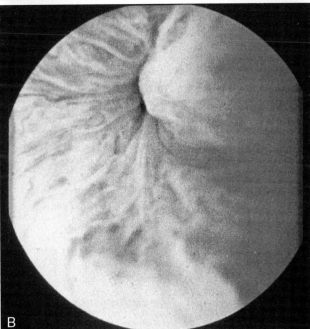

Figure 36-5 *A,* Bladder neck before injection with Contigen. *B,* Bladder neck after injection with Contigen. (From Appell RA: Periurethral collagen injection for female incontinence. Probl Urol 5[1]:134, 1991.)

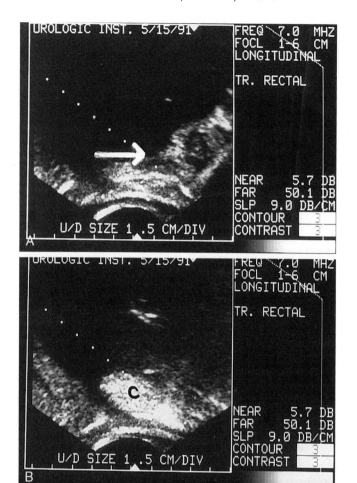

Figure 36-6 *A,* Transvaginal identification of bladder neck *(white arrow). B,* Ultrasound evaluation of bladder neck after injection of Contigen; note hyperechoic appearance of Contigen (C).

urinary loss handled by tissues or a minipad at most and is included in reports of treatments for urinary incontinence as success. Because the results of slings, artificial sphincters, and injectables are comparable, the question arises as to why injectables, which are easier for both the patient and the surgeon, have not been universally accepted and performed. The answer involves two objections to injectables: (1) the inability to quantify the amount of material needed in any individual patient, and (2) concerns about the safety of the injectable substance.

EFFICACY

With respect to the first problem regarding the quantity of material needed for each patient, I have no answers, and, sadly, one does not get better at judging the quantity with experience. With Contigen continence was achieved in 55% of women with a single treatment.[11] Additional Contigen injections may be necessary to establish complete urinary continence. The need for more Contigen may be related to several issues, not the least of which is the surgeon's inability to determine in advance the quantity of

Contigen required in any given patient. In some cases the severity of urethral dysfunction may cause detrusor abnormalities to be unrecognized, but these are then unmasked with the marked improvement in urethral closure. However, less than 20% of patients injected have evidence of short-term detrusor muscle instability on follow-up cystometric examination after 1 to 3 months.[12] Some of these patients are symptomatic and require treatment with anticholinergic drugs for a short period. Whether this is due to an underlying detrusor functional abnormality or to a certain degree of obstruction has yet to be determined. Some of the need for more Contigen may be explained by the loss of some of the initial bulking owing to resorption of the water content of Contigen. Just as important in patient evaluation after the injection is the fact that she may have increased her activity level, and this may result in even greater intra-abdominal forces that must be opposed, thus requiring more bulk. Attesting to this is the fact that only 5 of 155 women withdrew from the study owing to lack of improvement.[12] Of the 155 women (aged 7 to 87) injected with Contigen between October 1987 and September 1991, 34 required less than 10 ml of Contigen whereas 30 required more than 30 ml.[12] Again, the cause of the defect, the state of the tissue at the injection site, and the plane of placement of the Contigen are all significant factors affecting the degree of correction of incontinence and the volume of material required to effect the correction. Women require an average of 1.8 injections and 18.4 ml of Contigen to attain continence.[13] The simplicity of the procedure performed with local anesthesia on an outpatient basis should offset this inconvenience as long as the patient is aware of the probable need for additional injections preoperatively. The 24-month duration of treatment efficacy is 77% in patients with ISD and 57% in women with hypermobility, which is to be expected because 96.4% of patients with ISD are dry or socially continent compared to 82.3% of those with detrusor hypermobility.[13] It is expected that those with a fixed, open bladder neck will have better short- and long-term results with Contigen (or any other injectable) than those with anatomic hypermobility.

SAFETY

In analyzing the safety of Contigen, two types of events were considered: (1) local hypersensitivity responses and (2) the occurrence of other adverse events and their relationship to the use of the injectable. Prior to treating any patient hypersensitivity to bovine collagen was assessed by skin testing. Of 427 total patients 11 were excluded from the study because they demonstrated hypersensitivity to bovine collagen on the skin test. In addition, all patients were evaluated with enzyme-linked immunosorbent assay (ELISA) for humoral antibodies before and after exposure to Contigen. No significant anticollagen antibody responses were found, which was as expected owing to the cross-linking with glutaraldehyde.[7, 8] The primary safety concern with Contigen is related to its immunogenicity. Some patients who have had bovine collagen injections for soft tissue augmentation have complained of signs and symptoms of collagen vascular disorders such as dermatomyositis and have made claims that have led to litigation. Despite these claims, there has been no evidence linking injections of bovine collagen with any disorder. The patient population receiving bovine collagen has actually had a lower incidence of such disorders than would be expected in the general population.[14] None of the patients in the multicenter trial (many of whom have been followed for more than 5 years) have had an adverse event related to immunogenicity.

The only adverse events have been transient and treatable. These include urinary retention and urinary tract infection. Urodynamic changes following successful injection for restoring continence showed a mean rise in leak point pressure of 37 cm of water, demonstrating that Contigen permits closure of the internal sphincter at the lowest effective pressure and protects the upper urinary tract. In other words, when Contigen is properly injected between the bladder neck and the external sphincter, passive continence against increased intra-abdominal pressure will be maintained with no risk to upper tract function.

Conclusions

The goal of treatment in women with outflow incompetence is to allow coaptation of the urethral mucosa without causing urethral obstruction. Urodynamically, this means that the pressure necessary to open the urethra (leak point pressure) increases while no appreciable change occurs in the closure pressure of the urethra. Periurethral injections have the potential to accomplish this goal. The technical aspects of the actual injection process are easily learned, and no special equipment is needed. More important than technique is patient selection. The best results are attained in patients who do not have detrusor problems, have an adequate bladder capacity, and have minimal anatomic abnormality (urethral hypermobility). Because therapy with Contigen is less invasive than surgery, a significant number of patients can benefit from this modality of therapy, especially if the patient is an unsuitable surgical candidate. Injectables are still in the developmental stage, and their role in the management of incontinence remains to be defined more precisely. With respect to the materials currently studied, the injection procedure with Contigen has been easy to perform with local anesthesia, is efficacious, and appears to be durable while free of significant complications. It is anticipated that Contigen will become a valuable adjunct in the management of both adult and pediatric incontinence problems.

REFERENCES

1. McGuire EJ, Herlihy E: The influence of urethral position on urinary continence. Invest Urol 15:205, 1977.
2. Badlani GH, Ravalli R, Moskowitz MO: A tool for the objective assessment of passive incontinence. Contempo Urol 5(7):29, 1993.
3. Appell RA: Injectables for urethral incompetence. World J Urol 8:208, 1990.
4. Murless BC: The injection treatment of stress incontinence. J Obstet Gynaecol Br Empire 45:67, 1938.
5. Canning D, Peters C, Gearhart J, et al: Local tissue response to glutaraldehyde cross-linked collagen in the rabbit bladder. J Urol 139:258, 1988.
6. Gearhart JP: Endoscopic management of veisoureteral reflux. Probl Urol 4:639, 1990.
7. Griffiths R, Shakespeare P: Human dermal collagen allografts: A three year histological study. Br J Plast Surg 35:519, 1982.
8. McPhearson JM, Wallace DG, Piez KA: Review: Development and biochemical characterization of injectable collagen. J Dermatol Surg Oncol 14:13, 1988.
9. Ford CN, Martin DW, Warner TF: Injectable collagen in laryngeal rehabilitation. Laryngoscope 95:513, 1984.
10. Remacle M, Marbaix E: Collagen implants in the human larynx. Arch Otorhinolaryngol 245:203, 1988.
11. Appell RA: New developments: Injectables for urethral incompetence in women. Int Urogynecol J 1:117, 1990.
12. Appell RA: Use of collagen injections for treatment of incontinence and reflux. Adv Urol 5:145, 1992.
13. Bard CR: Updated PMAA amendment to submission to US Food and Drug Administration for IDE G850010, Bethesda, Maryland. 1992.
14. Lyon MG, Bloch DA, Hollak B, et al: Predisposing factors in polymyositis-dermatomyositis: Results of a nationwide survey. J Rheumatol 16:1218, 1989.

CHAPTER 37

Periurethral Injections of Autologous Fat for the Treatment of Incontinence

Jerry G. Blaivas, M.D., F.A.C.S.
Dianne M. Heritz, M.D., F.R.C.S.C.

Submucosal urethral injection is an evolving technique for the treatment of urinary incontinence due to sphincteric abnormalities. Although it has been used successfully to treat both types of sphincteric incontinence, urethral hypermobility and intrinsic sphincteric deficiency (ISD) in women, and postprostatectomy incontinence in men, its role in the therapeutic armamentarium has not been clearly defined. The ideal substance used for injection should be (1) biocompatible, (2) nonbiodegradable, (3) easily administered, and (4) cost-effective.

Historical Perspective

Periurethral injection for the treatment of urinary incontinence is not a new concept. During the last 100 years a variety of substances, including fat, wax, cartilage, bone dust, cod liver oil, metal, Teflon, inflatable spheres, and protein, have been tried.

Paraffin was used as a periurethral injection for stress incontinence almost a century ago.[1] A 39-year-old woman developed sloughing of the urethral mucosa following silver nitrate treatment. Subsequently, she underwent multiple procedures for urinary incontinence and also developed a 2- by 3-cm vesical ulcer. Howard Kelly, the pioneering gynecologist, excised the ulcer and injected paraffin under the urethra to control the incontinence. At the time of discharge from the hospital 1 month later she remained continent.

Prior to Kelly's report Gersuny had reported a successful fistula repair with paraffin.[2] Quackels injected paraffin into the periurethral tissues of two men following prostatectomy and reported its success in 1955.[3] In 1938 Murless presented a series of 20

women with urinary incontinence who were treated with the sclerosing agent morrhuate sodium.[4] Morrhuate sodium is the sodium salt of the fatty acids in cod liver oil. It had previously been used for the treatment of varicose veins. An intentional fibrosis was created by injecting the agent into the anterior vaginal wall, causing compression of the urethra by secondary scarring. As expected, many of these patients had painless sloughing of the anterior vaginal wall. Subsequent periurethral injections were delayed until the ulcer healed. Murless believed that this sloughing was a favorable prognostic sign! He used a urethral sound to guide the periurethral injections. None of these patients developed urethral stricture or direct sloughing of the urethra. Patients were followed at 2-week intervals to determine the need for further injections. The number of injections per patient varied from one to seven. Murless cited a 60% success rate; however, the methods of treatment and duration of follow-up were not documented.

Another sclerosing agent, Dondren, was used by Sachse for the treatment of incontinence in both men and women.[5] Four patients developed clinical and radiographic findings of pulmonary emboli. Signs of emboli were apparent 3 days after injection and continued to progress up to 30 days later. The nature of the pulmonary emboli was identified in animal experiments as lipoid pneumonia.

In the 1950s Arnold initiated a series of experiments to determine the best material for intracordal injection for the treatment of vocal cord paralysis.[6] He sought a substance that could be suspended in liquid to facilitate passage through a long needle. He initially harvested cartilage from the patient's nasal septum, crushed it, and suspended it in gelatin. The use of heterologous bone dust, also suspended in gelatin, spared the patient the harvesting procedure.

The processing of cartilage and bone dust proved to be too tedious, and exogenous substances were sought. Tantalum powder and glycerin were tried next. Patients who underwent intracordal injection with these substances experienced transient fevers associated with an acute illness. They did have vocal improvement, but the acute reaction was too great to continue using tantalum.

Teflon powder was found to be the most inert of all plastic materials. Arnold prepared the Teflon by adding glycerin and sterilizing the mixture.[7] Teflon had been described as a lubricant that was injected into joints for the treatment of arthritis. It was also used in vascular grafts and prostheses. In 1973, both Berg[8] and Politano and associates[9] described the use of polytef paste (polytetrafluoroethylene micropolymer particles and polysorbate) for the purpose of increasing urethral resistance. Berg treated three female patients with polytef and reported his series in 1973. He injected glycerin through an 18-gauge needle submucosally at two separate urethral sites in four quadrants. The injection was completed when the urethral walls apposed each other and there was no demonstration of stress incontinence. If the patient remained dry for 24 hours after the glycerin injection, she was injected with polytef paste. Berg reported three patients who were treated on an outpatient basis. All three required more than one injection. They remained dry, one patient at 6-month follow-up and two at follow-up 18 months later. Berg theorized that the initial treatment episode was limited by the inflammatory response and potential migration of polytef particles. The subsequent injections were placed in a scarred area that prevented migration.

In 1974 Politano and associates reported a larger series of 17 men and 15 women.[10] Women were injected periurethrally at the bladder neck with 10 to 14 ml of polytef, and men were injected through the perineum. These procedures were carried out under panendoscopic guidance. Of the 17 men, 15 were incontinent after prostatectomy, 11 after transurethral resection, 4 after open prostatectomy, and 1 after radical prostatectomy. One man was incontinent following fracture of the pelvis. Most of the women had recurrent stress incontinence. Three women had large cystourethroceles, and they all had failed previous incontinence surgery. Overall, 18 of 32 patients were cured of their urinary incontinence. The actual number of cured men and women was not stated. In this first series, the complications reported were urethritis, periurethral abscess, and temporary urinary retention lasting less than 2 days. In a follow-up report of 165 patients, 111 men and 54 women, Politano used, on average, a larger amount of paste and thought that this improved the cure rate.[11] Patients who received only one injection had a higher failure rate. He advised an interval of 4 to 6 months between reinjections because some patients had restoration of continence following transient episodes of incontinence after injection. The methods of follow-up in this series are not stated. Complications

reported were urinary retention in "a large number of patients" lasting a few days, and dysuria and perineal discomfort in approximately one-fourth of patients. A "substantial" number of patients had transient fevers lasting up to 24 hours.

Experience with Teflon during the last 20 years has revealed other potential complications. Granulomas can form both locally and distantly.[12] Experimentally, migration of Teflon particles has been documented in the pelvic nodes, lungs, brain, kidney, and spleen of animals.[13] There has been a case report of a woman who developed pulmonary migration after her third injection.[14] A 76-year-old man who underwent radical prostatectomy 4 years prior to his death (he committed suicide) had a total of three Teflon injections.[15] At autopsy granulomas were found at the injection site, and areas of interstitial granulomatous inflammation were dispersed throughout the lungs. The largest granuloma measured 2.0×0.5 mm.[15]

From a technical standpoint, the Teflon paste itself is difficult to inject. It is very thick and viscous and must be injected under high pressure to pass through the needle. A special ratchet-gun has been devised and is the most practical delivery system.

Another approach at developing an injectable substance was the use of small inflatable spheres that were placed percutaneously in the periurethral tissues under fluoroscopic guidance.[16] Once positioned next to the vesical neck, the spheres were inflated with a radiographic contrast agent and left in place. One sphere was placed on each side of the vesical neck. The spheres proved difficult to place accurately and had a tendency to migrate out of position. Some extruded into the urethra or bladder. The initial multicenter study reported in an abstract that 77% of 39 women were either dry or moderately improved.[17] The dependence on fluoroscopy, the potential for extrusion, and the disappointing long-term results were sufficient reasons for the manufacturer to halt production and discontinue clinical trials.

Collagen was first used as a biomaterial in the midnineteenth century in the form of catgut sutures.[18] Other collagen devices include heart valves and hemostatic agents. A form of collagen called Zyderm had been used for the treatment of facial defects and deformities. Zyderm is not cross-linked with glutaraldehyde and can be more rapidly resorbed by collagenase.[19] Collagen has many advantages over polytef for the treatment of incontinence. It is easy to inject, and it is treated to reduce immunogenicity.

Shortliffe and colleagues[20] described the use of highly purified bovine collagen or glutaraldehyde cross-linked collagen for periurethral injections in 1989. Her initial series consisted of 16 men with postprostatectomy sphincteric incontinence and one woman with grade 3 incontinence. A suprapubic tube was placed during the procedure. Collagen was injected into the area of sphincteric deficit or at the bladder neck in patients without an apparent sphincter. The suprapubic tube drained the bladder for 2 to 4 days following the procedure. Seven patients had one injection, and 10 had two injections. The average total amount injected per patient was 28.40 ml. Follow-up ranged from 9 to 23 months. The frequency of follow-up visits was not stated. Nine of the seventeen patients were cured or improved. There was no change in bladder or urethral function based on urodynamic studies of 14 patients at 3 months or 9 patients at 3 to 6 months after collagen injection.

There are a few studies in the current literature with short-term follow-up. McGuire and colleagues reported a multicenter series of 30 men and 35 women who were followed for 1 year.[21] The abstract cited an 83.3% and 94.3% cure or improvement in men and women, respectively. Eckford and Abrams cited an 80% success rate at 3 months in 25 women with stress incontinence treated with periurethral collagen injection.[22] Kieswetter and associates reported a series of 18 patients (16 women and 2 men), 16 of whom received only one 8-ml injection.[23] Seven of eighteen patients remained cured at 9 months, and eight remained improved. One of the "improved" patients had received a second injection. Herschorn and colleagues reported the early results of collagen injection in 41 patients (10 men and 31 women).[19] Women had, on average, two treatments, and the total mean amount of collagen used was 12.7 ml. Thirteen women had not had prior surgery for incontinence. Male patients in this study had an average of six treatments with a total mean of 51.8 ml of collagen. Twenty-eight, or 90.3% of the women, and 70% of the men were cured or improved. Follow-up ranged from 2 to 15 months. The use of collagen shows promise, but many more definitive studies need to be done to document its efficacy and define the indications for its use. The very high cost of collagen casts doubt on its cost-effectiveness.

Other products such as silicone microparticles (vulcanized methyl siloxane, Uroplastique)[24] and silicone macroparticles (polydimethyl siloxane, Macroplastique)[25] are injected submucosally and heal within a fibrin capsule, thereby preventing migration. They are claimed to be effective in some patients for the treatment of postprostatectomy and female urinary incontinence. This product is easily injected, nonmigratory, and permanent. Clinical trials are under way, but no long-term results are yet available.

One hundred years ago Neuber first transplanted fat from a patient's upper arm to fill out a depressed facial scar and reported this in the German literature.[26] Ellenbogen, in his extensive review, eloquently describes the multiple uses of human autologous fat during the last century.[26] Fat has been used to correct facial defects and deformities, to treat dural scars secondary to epilepsy, to cover severed nerves, to reconstruct breasts, to replace testicles, to perform procedures to buttress open renal wounds, and to provide material for omental or labial fat flaps for fistula repairs.[26] The use of fat for periurethral and transurethral injection for incontinence has been described only recently.[27–37]

Periurethral Fat Injections

Periurethral injection of autologous fat was first described by Gonzalez-de-Garibay and colleagues for the treatment of urinary stress incontinence in 1989.[27, 28] The advantages of autologous fat include its ready availability at virtually no cost, its lack of antigenicity, and its ease of use. Additionally, all women treated to date have been enthusiatic donors, and most have expressed a willingness to donate their fat to other, less fortunate patients.

The injected fat either remains in situ or stimulates an inflammatory response that leads to subsequent reabsorption of the fat and eventual fibrosis. The final result is a decrease in the lumen of the urethra with either fat or fibrosis remaining under the mucosa. Optimally, more fat than scar will remain. The ideal method of fat preservation at the injection site has not been determined.

Numerous authors have studied this problem and have showed that no more than 30% of the fat survives after injection. Most studies show a 10 to 20% survival.[30] Bartynski and associates used a rabbit ear model to look at fat injection grafts.[30] A predictable progressive series of histologic events following free fat graft injections was outlined. Graft fibrosis followed a progressive course, with capsule formation initially followed by fibrous septation and extensive fibrosis of the entire graft. The fibrous reaction peaked at 40 days after transplant of the graft and remained constant afterward with only slight progression noted at 100 days. Viability of the fat itself also diminished over time from 80 to 100% initially to 40% after 20 days. Final viability appeared to be 20 to 30% in this study.[30] Neovascularization began along the graft periphery but was never adequately achieved at the center to maintain long-term viability. Progressive fibrosis does occur in these autografts and probably accounts for the final volumes obtained.

Some surgeons who use fat for filling soft tissue defects routinely transplant 50% more fat than they believe necessary for the desired result in anticipation of a variable amount of reabsorption.[31] Several techniques aimed at improving graft survival have been devised. These include mixing the harvested fat with Ringer's solution and insulin prior to injection,[32] cutting harvested fat into "pearls,"[26] or simply minimizing trauma to aspirated fat.[31, 33] No method has been shown to improve graft survival consistently or minimize resorption, nor has there been any explanation for the wide variations in graft survival seen from patient to patient. Factors that may account for this variability include the type of soft tissue bed the graft is injected into, the degree of recipient site scarring, and the amount of fat used. No studies controlled for these factors have shown consistent results to date. A study by Nguyen and colleagues, however, demonstrated the potential importance of a well-vascularized recipient site in promoting fat graft survival.[32]

Horl and associates noted that despite the addition

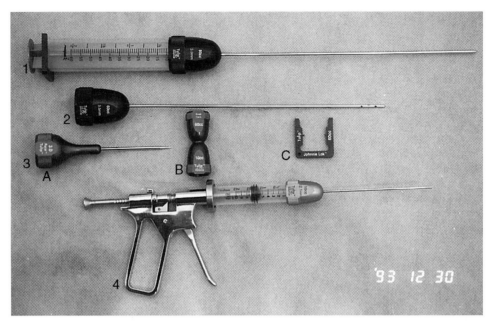

Figure 37-1 The Tulip Company instruments designed specifically for abdominal wall liposuction, fat processing, and injection. (1) Liposuction cannula (attached to 35-ml syringe); (2) needle for injection of local anesthesia; (3A) "punch" for making a small opening in skin to pass a cannula, (3B) 10- to 60-ml anaerobic transfer (for transferring aspirated fat to a periurethral or transurethral needle), (3C) Johnnie Loks (to keep traction on the syringe during aspiration); and (4) 10-ml reinjection gun (for periurethral injection).

of hyaluronidase and the use of an atraumatic technique, microscopic examination revealed defective membranes in 40% of aspirated cells.[34] Follow-up showed that a 49% volume loss was seen at 3 months, a 55% volume loss at 6 months, and then no further volume loss at 9 and 12 months. Chajchir and Benzaquen reported on a 4-year follow-up of pathology specimens in patients who had fat injection for soft tissue augmentation.[35] Specimens obtained 3 months after surgery showed zones of cystosteatonecrosis, lipophagic granulomas (a granuloma attended by the loss of subcutaneous lipid), lymphocytes, adipocytes, giant cells, and new vessel formation. Biopsies taken 1 year later showed large amounts of connective tissue and a fibrotic reaction as the final result. The tissue that followed the cystosteatonecrotic process showed a cicatricial reaction that maintained the desired volume of the area for a considerable time. To our knowledge, no reports of fat migration have been reported.

Indications

Definitive indications for periurethral fat injections have not been formulated. As our experience continues to evolve, we believe that the most important consideration is to characterize the nature of sphincteric incontinence as accurately as possible. The best results have been attained in patients with sphincteric incontinence without appreciable urethral hypermobility; this encompasses both type I and type III stress incontinence.[36] In type I stress incontinence, urinary leakage occurs during an increase in abdominal pressure unaccompanied by urethral hypermobility. Type III stress incontinence is also known as intrinsic sphincter deficiency (ISD). It occurs when there is functional damage to the urethra

and is characterized by a low leak point pressure and an open vesical neck at rest. The urethra retains its gross anatomic integrity but no longer maintains adequate sphincteric capability. ISD may coexist with urethral hypermobility. The efficacy of autologous fat injection in women with stress incontinence due to urethral hypermobility is less favorable.[37]

Operative Technique

The procedure is performed with the patient in the dorsal lithotomy position under local anesthesia. The abdomen and perineum are prepared and draped. The liposuction technique is greatly facilitated by the use of special instruments designed specifically for this purpose (Fig. 37–1). A site on the lower lateral abdominal wall is chosen for the liposuction, and a skin wheal is raised with 1% lidocaine. A 2-mm skin incision is made, and the subcutaneous tissue is stabilized by grasping it with the index finger and forefinger of the left hand (Fig. 37–2). A long Tulip local anesthesia needle is inserted through the incision and advanced subcutaneously as approximately 10

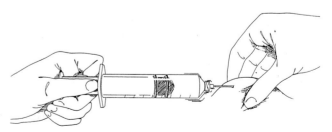

Figure 37-2 Fat aspiration is performed by pinching the skin of the anterior abdominal wall between the index finger and the thumb. (From Santorosa RP, Blaivas JG: Building continence with periurethral fat injections. Contemp Urol 5 [4]: 96–102, 1993, copyright Medical Economics.)

to 15 ml of 1% lidocaine is injected. The liposuction needle is attached to a 35-ml catheter tip syringe and rinsed with saline. Approximately 5 ml of saline is left in the syringe, and the needle is advanced through the skin incision into the subcutaneous tissue between the index finger and the thumb. The plunger of the syringe is pulled back, applying negative pressure, and is locked into place with a special adapter. The needle is moved rapidly back and forth in a radial direction. Approximately 20 ml of fat is aspirated in a few minutes. The fat may also be harvested with a 60-ml syringe and 16-gauge needle while manual traction is placed on the plunger of the syringe. However, this may require two or three insertions with the needle in different sites.

The fat is mixed with saline in the syringe and placed in a vertical position (Fig. 37–3). Fat floats to the top, and after several minutes the excess saline is squirted off. The procedure is repeated a number of times until the fat is reasonably pure. The fat is then injected into a 10-ml syringe through a special adapter that accommodates the two different sized syringes.

Two percent lidocaine (Xylocaine) jelly is introduced into the urethra, and the periurethral area is anesthetized with 2% Xylocaine. Approximately 5 ml of Xylocaine is injected at the 3 and 9 o'clock positions at each side of the urethra, staying as far lateral as possible. Under cystoscopic guidance, the fat is injected submucosally at the bladder neck and proximal urethra. This is accomplished by inserting the needle into the periurethral tissue at about the 3 and 9 o'clock positions. The needle tip advances

obliquely toward the bladder neck with the bevel facing the urethral lumen. The position of the needle can be seen cystoscopically. This part of the operation is technically difficult, and great care must be taken not to perforate the urethra lest the fat be extruded. The procedure is repeated on the opposite side. The goal is to cause complete coaptation of the urethra, giving an appearance similar to an "obstructing prostate." This usually requires 5 to 15 ml of fat.

The first injection is the most difficult from a technical standpoint because the target submucosal area is small, probably no more than a few millimeters in breadth. Nevertheless, it is almost always possible to inject at least some of the fat in the submucosa during the first injection; subsequent injections are that much easier because the target is larger. Our intention is to perform sequential injections at 1- to 3-month intervals until enough fatty bulk is retained to effect a more permanent cure. Subsequent injections are directed to build up symmetrical tissue bulk around the proximal urethra.

Results

To date, there have been very few clinical studies, and follow-up has been short. During the past 3 years we have prospectively followed 51 women. Patients have been evaluated at 4-week intervals. If incontinence persists after the first injection, reinjections are performed as often as every 4 weeks, or whenever there is recurrent stress incontinence that requires treatment. Results were assessed by subjective patient score (percent improvement), diaries, pad tests, and clinical evaluation. Follow-up ranged from 3 months to $3\frac{1}{2}$ years with a mean of 12 months. Preoperatively, 6 women had incontinence due to urethral hypermobility, 42 had intrinsic sphincter deficiency or type III stress incontinence, and 3 had both urethral hypermobility and intrinsic sphincter deficiency.

Overall, 70% of the women were dry or improved after an average of 2.7 fat injections. Twenty-eight percent of those with ISD, and 10% of those with urethral hypermobility were cured. Improvement occurred in 51% of those with ISD and 30% of those with urethral hypermobility. "Dry" was defined as totally continent; "improved" was defined as a subjective patient score of more than 50% improvement and a decrease in pad score of 50%. Four of the six women with urethral hypermobility did not achieve these improvement goals and were considered failures. Minimal complications included temporary urinary retention in two patients, cystitis in two patients, and transient irritative bladder symptoms in one patient.

The results presented here do not necessarily represent end points in therapy because many patients may elect continued reinjection as long as progressive improvement is noted.

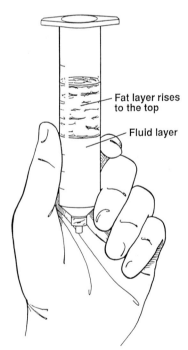

Fat layer rises to the top

Fluid layer

Figure 37-3 The fat is processed by rinsing it with saline and then standing a 60-ml syringe upright to allow the fat to float to the top. (From Santarosa RP, Blaivas JG: Periurethral injection of autologous fat for the treatment of sphincteric incontinence. J Urol 151:607–611, 1994.)

Summary

Autologous fat is a biocompatible, easily administered, cost-effective agent. It fulfills many of the criteria for an ideal injectable agent for the control of incontinence. Further research is required to develop the best technique to prevent resorption. There are many advantages for the use of autologous fat as a periurethral injectable. The fat is readily available, usually in surplus amounts, and is easily harvested with special instruments designed for this purpose. Injections are carried out under local anesthesia on an outpatient basis. There is minimal risk, and the cost of the procedure is negligible. The highest success rate is seen in women with intrinsic sphincter deficiency. Its effectiveness in patients with urethral hypermobility is not as encouraging. We believe that the most important determinant of a successful outcome is accurate placement of fat submucosally in sufficient quantity to effect coaptation of the urethra in a woman without urethral hypermobility.

REFERENCES

1. Kelly HA: Medical Gynecology. Appleton and Company, 1908.
2. Gersuny R: Paraffine Inspritzung bei Incontinentia urinae. Zentralb Gynakol 24:1281, 1900.
3. Quackels R: Deux cas d'incontinence après adénomectomie guéries par injection de paraffine dans le périnée. Acta Urol Belg 23:259, 1955.
4. Murless BC: The injection treatment of stress incontinence. J Obstet Gynaecol Br Commonwlth 45:67, 1938.
5. Sachse H: Sclerosing therapy in urinary incontinence: Indications, results, complications. Urol Int 15:255, 1963.
6. Arnold R: Vocal rehabilitation of paralytic dysphonia v.i. Further studies of intracordal injection materials. Arch Oto., 73:290, 1961.
7. Arnold R: Vocal rehabilitation of paralytic dysphonia i.x. Technique of intracordal injection. Arch Otolaryngol 76:358, 1962.
8. Berg S: Polytef augmentation urethroplasty. Arch Surg 107:379, 1973.
9. Politano VA, Small MP, Harper JM, et al: Periurethral Teflon injection for urinary incontinence. Trans Am Assoc Genitourin Surg 65:54, 1973.
10. Politano VA, Small MP, Harper JM, Lynn CM: Periuretheral Teflon injection for urinary incontinence. J Urol 111:180, 1974.
11. Politano VA: Periurethral polytetrafluoroethylene injection for urinary incontinence. J Urol 127:439, 1982.
12. Ferro MA, Smith PHF, Smith PJB: Periurethral granuloma: Unusual complication of Teflon periurethral injection. Urology 21:422, 1988.
13. Malizia AA, Reinman HM, Myers RP, et al: Migration and granulomatous reaction after periurethral injection of polytef (Teflon). JAMA 251:3277, 1984.
14. Claes H, Stroobants D, Van Meerbeek J, et al: Pulmonary migration following periurethral polytetrafluoroethylene injection for urinary incontinence. J Urol 142:821, 1989.
15. Mittelman RE, Marraccini JV: Pulmonary Teflon granulomas following periurethral Teflon injection for urinary incontinence. Arch Pathol Lab Med 107:611, 1983.
16. Barrett DM, Parulkar BG, Malizia AA: The genitourinary spheroidal membrane: An experimental study of a new percutaneously inserted prosthetic device for the control of urinary incontinence. J Urol 142:1615, 1989.
17. Barrett DM, Ghoniem G, Bruskewitz R, et al: The genisphere: A new percutaneously placed anti-incontinence device. J Urol 143:141A, 1990.
18. Cooperman L, Michaeli D: The immunogenicity of injectable collagen. 1. A 1-year prospective study. J Am Acad Dermatol 10:4, 638, 1984.
19. Herschorn S, Radomski SB, Steele DJ: Early experience with intraurethral collagen injections for urinary incontinence. J Urol 148:1797, 1992.
20. Shortliffe LM, Freiha FS, Kessler R, et al: Treatment of urinary incontinence by the periurethral implantation of glutaraldehyde cross-linked collagen. J Urol 141:538, 1989.
21. McGuire E, Wang SC, Appel R, et al: Treatment of urethral incontinence by collagen injection—one year follow up. J Urol (pt 2) 143:224A, 1990.
22. Eckford SD, Abrams P: Para-urethral collagen implantation for female stress incontinence. Br J Urol 68(6):586–589, 1991.
23. Kieswetter H, Fischer M, Wober L, Flamm J: Endoscopic implantation of collagen (GAX) for the treatment of urinary incontinence. Br J Urol 69(1):22–25, 1992.
24. Buckley JF, Scott R, Lingham V, et al: Injectable silicone microparticles: A new treatment for female stress incontinence. J Urol 147:280A, 1992.
25. Buckley JF, Lingam K, Lloyd SN, et al: Injectable silicone macroparticles for female urinary incontinence. J Urol 149:402A, 1993.
26. Ellenbogen R: Free autogenous pearl fat grafts in the face—a preliminary report of a rediscovered technique. Ann Plast Surg 16:179, 1986.
27. Gonzalez-de-Garibay AS, Jimenco C, York M, et al: Endoscopic autotransplantation of fat tissue in the treatment of urinary incontinence in the female. J Urol (Paris) 95:363, 1989.
28. Santiago-Gonzalez-de-Garibay AM, Castro-Morrando I, Castillo-Jimenco JM, et al: Endoscopic injection of autologous adipose tissue in the treatment of female incontinence. Arch Esp Urol 42:143, 1989.
29. Gonzalez-de-Garibay AS, Castillo-Jimenco JM, Villanueva-Perez I, et al: Treatment of urinary stress incontinence using paraurethral injection of autologous fat. Arch Esp Urol 44:595, 1991.
30. Bartynski J, Marion MS, Wang TD: Histopathologic evaluation of adipose autografts in a rabbit ear model. Otolaryngol Head Neck Surg 102:314, 1990.
31. Ersek RA: Transplantation of purified autologous fat: A 3-year follow-up is disappointing. Plast Reconstr Surg 87:219, 1991.
32. Nguyen A, Pasyk KA, Bouvier TM, et al: Comparative study of survival of autologous adipose tissue taken and transplanted by different techniques. Plast Reconstr Surg 85: 378, 1990.
33. Gasperoni C, Salgarello M, Emiliozzi P, Gorgani G: Subdermal liposuction. Aesth Plast Surg 14:137, 1990.
34. Horl HW, Feller AM, Biemer E: Technique for liposuction fat reimplantation and long-term volume evaluation by magnetic resonance imaging. Ann Plast Surg 26:248, 1991.
35. Chajchir A, Benzaquen I: Fat-graft injection for soft tissue augmentation. Plast Reconstr Surg 84:921, 1989.
36. Blaivas JG, Olsson CA: Stress incontinence: Classification and surgical approach. J Urol 139:727, 1988.
37. Santarosa R, Blaivas JG: Periurethral injection of autologous fat for the treatment of sphincteric incontinence. J Urol 151:607, 1994.

CHAPTER 38

The Use of Silicon Particles for the Treatment of Urinary Incontinence

David R. Henly, M.D.
David M. Barrett, M.D.

Urinary incontinence is a distressing medical, social, and economic problem. The true prevalence figures for urinary incontinence are difficult to assess because of the social embarrassment associated with the condition. A large population-based study in Great Britain by Thomas and associates surveyed 22,430 persons.[1] Recognized incontinence occurred in 0.2% of women and 0.1% of men aged 15 to 64 and in 2.5% of women and 1.3% of men aged 65 and over. However, "unrecognized" incontinence (existing socially unacceptable urinary incontinence that had previously been unreported to a physician) had a prevalence of 8.5% in women and 1.6% in men aged 15 to 64 years and 11.6% in women and 6.9% in men aged 65 and over. These figures have been confirmed by other large population-based studies.[2, 3]

The magnitude of the problem of urinary incontinence should not be underestimated. Urinary incontinence in the elderly is not only common but morbid, costly, and neglected. Its prevalence increases strikingly in older people who are functionally impaired. Approximately half of the 1.6 million nursing home residents in the United States are incontinent.[4] Counting only direct costs, the expense of urinary incontinence overall was recently estimated to be a staggering $10.5 billion.[4]

Urinary incontinence restricts social and physical activity and can be a significant handicap. It demands the wearing of pads or diapers and may require the use of a condom catheter or permanently indwelling urinary catheter. Continuous perineal wetness can lead to a persistent rash, skin excoriation or ulceration, and intractable infection. It contributes to falls, pressure sores, social isolation, and the increased risk of institutionalization, especially among the elderly.

Consequently, a cost-effective, safe, and efficacious method of alleviating stress urinary incontinence in women has been sought. Techniques that are noninvasive and require a minimum of cost and inconvenience to the patient have been developed. At the forefront of these procedures are periurethral injections. Numerous materials have been used to coapt the urethral tissues in women, thereby relieving stress urinary incontinence. The most widely used injectable material is polytetrafluoroethylene. This material has been used extensively in the management of incontinence.[5] Institutions that favor the use of this material have not reported clinical complications related to its use.[6] However, in animals migration of the material has been reported,[7] as have pulmonary granulomas found at autopsy[8] and clinically significant pulmonary migration.[9] These reports, however isolated, have prompted the search for a material with fewer migratory and inflammatory tendencies.

Many injectable products are currently being used by urologists in treating urinary incontinence. Since relatively inert materials became available, periurethral injections have been used to provide bladder neck support, a periurethral mass effect, and thus continence. Paraffin wax was used by Quackels in 1955,[10] and in 1963 Sachse used sclerosing agents.[11] Currently, the most widely used material is polytetrafluoroethylene, or polytef. First described by Berg[12] and popularized by Politano, this compound was formulated in a 50:50 mixture with glycerol to form a paste that was injected periurethrally adjacent to the bladder neck. Its effectiveness in treating stress incontinence in women[13] and postprostatectomized men[14] has been reported.

Polytef is effective but has two major drawbacks as an injected agent for incontinence. First, marked chronic inflammatory reaction and fibrosis contribute to the mass effect of the injection. Thus, further surgical procedures may become more difficult.[15] Second, polytef particles migrate from the site of injection to adjacent lymph nodes and distant solid organs such as the spleen, lung, and choroid plexus. The clinical significance of this migration is unclear, but the possibilities of lymphatic obstruction and fibrotic lung disease exist.[8]

In an effort to overcome these shortcomings, other materials have been injected in a similar fashion. Collagen[16] enjoys popularity, but due to its rapid resorptive properties repeated injections are often required to maintain any long-term effect.[17] Autologous fat[18] injections have met with similar difficulties. Recently, saline-filled silicon spheres have been described as a treatment for female incontinence.[19] These have shown promise but require intraoperative fluoroscopic equipment for insertion.

The purpose of our study is to examine several properties of particulate silicon (Uroplastique), a new injectable material. We aimed to (1) analyze the actual particle size of the injected silicon; (2) determine (in animals) whether the particles remain at the periurethral site of injection; and (3) observe the presence and extent of any tissue reaction, both locally (in the pelvis) and in distant organs. The study evaluates both short-term (4-month) and long-term (9-month) findings.

Materials and Methods

SILICON PARTICLES

The material is a 60:40 mixture of povidone gel (polyvinyl pyrrolidinone, or PVP) and silicon particles. A thick yellow paste, it becomes tacky on exposure to air. Povidone is a gel used as a carrier for the silicon particles. It has a molecular weight of 24,000 daltons and is produced by GAF (United Kingdom). Presently, its most widespread use is as a vehicle for

iodine in the surgical solution Betadine. Silicon particle size was measured by electron microscopy. The paste was spread on aluminum stubs and allowed to dry. A sputter coating of gold palladium dust was applied and several samples of particles were examined with the Jeol 6400 scanning electron microscope. Multiple electron microscipic photographs were taken, and particle size was measured by obtaining computer-assisted outlines of individual silicon particles and quantifying each particle's greatest dimension (Fig. 38–1).

Two batches of silicon particles (one small, one large) were injected periurethrally in female mongrel dogs using the same delivery device that would be used in human patients. Waiting periods of 4 and 9 months were used to determine short- and long-term histologic effects. The silicon particles were then examined at the periurethral site, areas of migration were identified, and observation of any associated tissue reaction was documented.

To aid in the search for silicon particles undergoing distant migration, radiolabeled cobalt-57 microspheres that corresponded in size to the mean silicon particle size of the two batches were added to each injection. (Two control batches without radiolabeling were also injected.) A total activity of 1.4 millicuries (mCi) of cobalt-57 was used in the preparation of the beads, and each batch was subdivided into 14 lots of approximately 100 microcuries (μCi) per lot. Cobalt (^{57}Co) has a half-life of 240 days and emits only gamma radiation, which is safely, easily, and sensitively detected by a scintillation counter. Direct radiolabeling of the silicon particles was not possible owing to the inert character of the material. Microspheres were used to accurately guide the search for distant migration by specifically targeting anatomic regions of radioactivity. All animals were imaged at 1 week, at monthly intervals, and immediately prior to sacrifice. Imaging was performed using the Searle pho-gamma camera with a low-energy diverging collimator. The energy analyzer was set to detect the 122-keV emissions from cobalt-57. Images were ac-

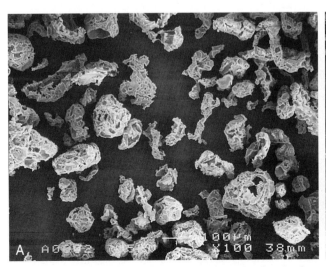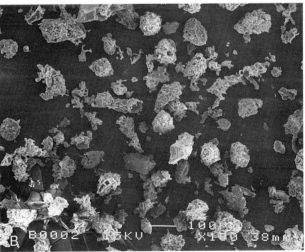

Figure 38-1 Electron micrographs showing large-particle silicon *(A)* and small-particle silicon *(B)*.

quired on the Medasys computer system, and all data were acquired on a 256 × 256 pixel matrix at approximately 10 minutes per image.

INJECTIONS

Female mongrel dogs, 20 to 25 kg in weight, were used. This animal model has been successfully used in other periurethral studies.[7] The amount of silicon paste injected into each animal mimicked the amount used for human injection (5 ml). One hour prior to anesthesia the dog received an intramuscular injection of 60 mg of gentamicin and 600,000 units of benzyl penicillin. Anesthesia was induced with 2 mg/kg of intravenous thiopentone, an endotracheal tube was placed, and anesthesia was maintained with 1.5% halothane and oxygen using a controlled ventilation volume of 350 ml with a respiratory rate of 18 to 20 breaths/minute. The animal was placed in the lithotomy position, and the perineal area and vagina were prepared with povidone-iodine (Betadine) solution. Cystourethroscopy was carried out with an 18 Fr Storz cystoscope available in the urology department.

The injections were accomplished in the manner described by Politano and colleagues using an 18-gauge, 9-cm needle and a syringe loaded with silicon paste.[20] The needle was inserted 2 to 3 cm lateral to the urethral meatus and advanced parallel to the urethra 1 cm toward the bladder neck. Aspiration ensured extravascular placement. The paste was injected along the length of the urethra as the needle was withdrawn. A similar injection was carried out on the opposite side of the urethra. A total of 2.5 ml of paste was injected on each side of the urethra. Cystoscopic inspection after each injection ensured a lack of bladder perforation or particle extravasation and adequate formation of periurethral silicon bleb.

IDENTIFICATION OF SILICON PARTICLES

The dogs were sacrificed with an intravenous injection of 10 ml of 20% pentobarbital (Sleepaway).

Five animals were sacrificed at 4 months and the others at 9 months. (One animal died from an anesthetic-related complication.) Immediately after death, the pelvic organs were removed en bloc and fixed in a 40% formaldehyde solution. The lymph nodes, liver, lungs, spleen, kidneys, and brain were placed in separate containers of a similar composition. After fixation, the pelvic block was dissected and the silicon injection site identified. The surrounding tissues of the injection site, adjacent lymph nodes, lungs, spleen, kidneys, and brain were prepared for histologic examination. To avoid a "needle-in-the-haystack" approach to histologic sectioning, the search for migratory particles was aided by the scintillation counter. The separate organ blocks to be studied were placed on top of the Searle pho-gamma camera to determine the presence of activity in each organ. To increase the sensitivity of the gamma camera, the collimator was removed, thereby increasing sensitivity by a factor of 10,000. A protective covering was placed over the gamma camera, and the total counts were recorded over a 5-minute period for each organ. Specific areas of organs showing uptake of cobalt-57 as well as multiple random samples from each organ were examined histologically.

Light microscopy was performed with routinely stained hematoxylin-eosin sections to determine the presence of silicon and the extent of histologic reaction. Silicon particles were most easily recognized using phase contrast microscopy.

X-ray energy dispersive spectroscopy was performed on unstained sections mounted on titanium grids. The Kevex Micro-X 7000 x-ray spectrometer interfaced with a Philips 400 transmission electron microscope was used. Spectra of the emitted energy from particles in selected biopsy specimens were collected at an accelerating voltage of 60 kv, specimen tilt of 25 degrees, and an electron beam spot of 50 nm in diameter.

Results

PARTICLE SIZE Electron microscopy determined the size of the particles injected in both the small and

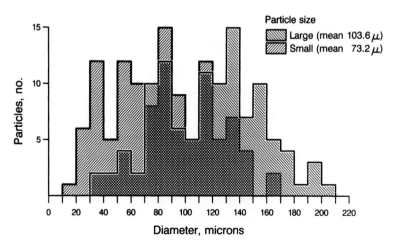

Figure 38-2 Silicon particle size distribution (in microns). (By permission of Mayo Foundation.)

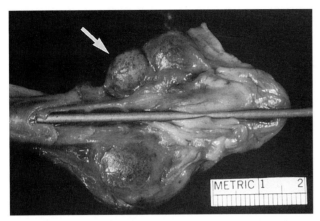

Figure 38-3 Large-particle injection site at 4 months. The peri-urethral bleb is intact *(arrow).*

large batches (see Fig. 38–1). The large-particle batch had a median diameter of 110 microns (μ) with a range of 32 to 270 μ. The small-particle batch had a median size of 73 μ (range, 11 to 160 μ) (Fig. 38–2).

LOCATION OF INJECTED PARTICLES Initial gamma camera images of all animals 1 week after injection revealed focused activity only in the pelvis. Prior to sacrifice, images were obtained that confirmed the presence of primary activity in the pelvis for the animals labeled with the larger microspheres. There was no increased uptake on images of the thorax or head in any of these large-particle animals. Increased radioactivity was apparent over the thorax of the animals with the smaller microspheres, and there was decreased uptake in the pelvis of these animals.

LOCAL EFFECTS Large-particle injection sites were palpable as two distinct periurethral blebs during dissection of the pelvic block in all six animals at the 4- and 9-month intervals (including one long-term nonradiolabeled control animal). Figure 38–3 demonstrates the palpable silicon blebs typically seen in the large-particle animals. Subsequent sectioning after fixation confirmed the persistent aggregation of the

material in the animals with large particles. The animals injected with small particles showed some loss of material at 4 months and significant dissipation at the 9-month period (Fig. 38–4). This was also true of the small-particle control animal sacrificed at 9 months.

At the large-particle aggregation site a well-encapsulated fibrous sheath surrounding the injected area was visualized without local migration in all animals at both time intervals. There was a typical histiocytic–giant cell reaction within the injection site but no granuloma formation (Fig. 38–5). The small-particle injection site was smaller and showed evidence of leaching out of the material into the surrounding tissues in four of the seven pelvic blocks (Fig. 38–6).

DISTANT MIGRATION Areas of interest for histologic sectioning were determined by gamma camera images of individual organs. Silicon particles were demonstrated in many sites in all dogs with the small-particle injections—lung (in seven animals), lymph nodes (five), kidney (three), and brain (two). All observed areas of migration simply revealed the presence of the silicon particles (Fig. 38–7). No inflammatory reaction was noted. No migratory particles were found in the spleen, liver, ovaries, or heart.

Discussion

This study demonstrates that periurethral injection of small silicon particles (<70 μ) is followed by local and distant tissue migration in the female dog. The tissue response to injection of larger silicon particles (>100 μ) differs markedly. Local encapsulation without distant migration was almost complete in the animals injected with the larger particles. The periurethral mass effect at the injection site maintained its integrity for up to 9 months. When seen at distant migratory sites the silicon particles produced a noninflammatory nongranulomatous response.

Numerous investigators have chronicled case re-

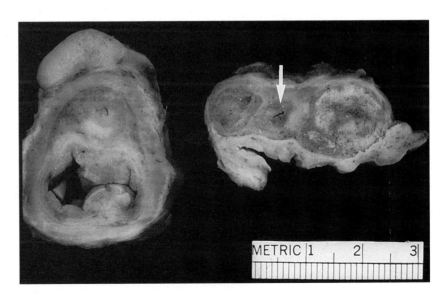

Figure 38-4 Cross-section of periurethral injection sites. Small particles *(left)* and large particles *(right)* *(arrow* points to urethra).

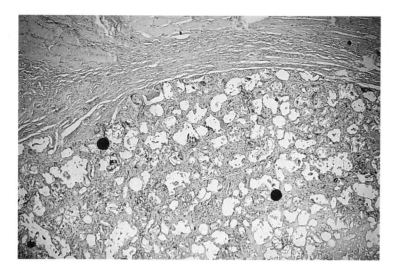

Figure 38-5 Large-particle injection site at 4 months. Circumferential fibrous sheath surrounds silicon particles and microspheres (magnification 40×).

ports of the adverse effects of silicon in human tissues.[21, 22] The majority of postulated associations of rheumatologic disorders and silicon have been related to the inflammatory response of leaking silicon gel in breast implants.[23, 24] Few of these publications have documented the actual particle size of the migratory or inflammation-producing silicon. Our data point to particle size as a determining factor in the migratory activity of silicon within the canine body. Histologically, the apparent inability of phagocytic macrophages to surround or encompass these larger silicon particles and thereby transport them into the reticuloendothelial system may account for the relative stability of the large particles in the periurethral injection site.

It has been shown that particles less than 80 μ have a tendency to migrate.[7] This investigation substantiated the presence of local migration in all animals with small-particle injections, but no such local migration in dogs with large-particle injections was

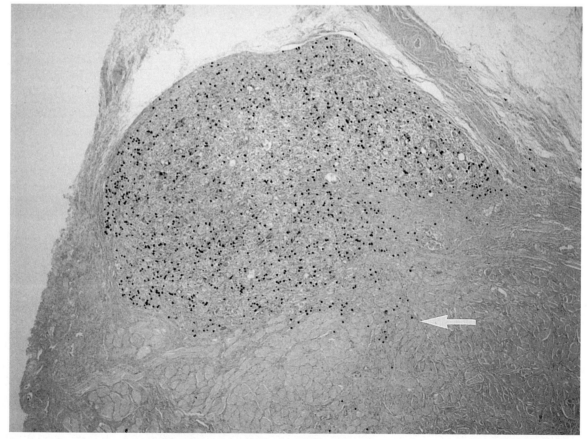

Figure 38-6 Small-particle injection site at 4 months. Lack of fibrous capsule and area of migration are present *(arrow)*.

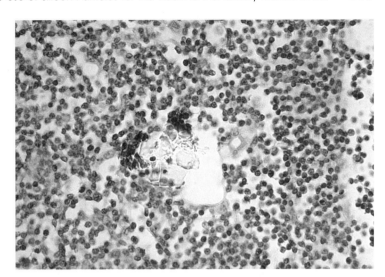

Figure 38–7   Silicon particle (35 μ in diameter) in para-aortic lymph node in a dog injected with small particles at 9 months after injection (magnification 200×).

discovered. To the contrary, a well-encapsulated silicon bleb with a thick circumferential fibrous sheath was observed. In these animals lymphadenopathy was not seen, and multiple sequential lymph node sectioning revealed no silicon particles.

To suggest that these large-particle periurethral injection sites are permanently immutable or that they would maintain their integrity in human tissues would be premature. However, their observed inertness bodes well for the potential use of this material in incontinent patients.

CLINICAL TRIALS

Injectable silicon has not been approved in this country for clinical use. However, the material is being used in incontinent patients in Europe.[25] Buckley and associates used particles with an average size of 150 μ (range, 100 to 600 μ).[26] Injections of 2.0 to 4.5 ml of silicon paste were placed periurethrally at the 3, 6, and 9 o'clock positions in 50 women with stress urinary incontinence. Seventeen patients had type II (prolapsing urethra) incontinence and 33 had type III (stable nonprolapsing urethra.) Five patients had had previous procedures to correct incontinence. Follow-up on these patients is short, ranging from 1 week to 6 months. The results are encouraging. Forty patients (80%) were dry after the initial injection. Five patients (10%) were "improved," and five patients (10%) "failed" to respond; an additional treatment is planned for all of these women. Side effects included mild dysuria, frequency, and hematuria in all patients for a maximum of 2 days. Two patients were unable to void following injection. One required a single "in and out" catheterization, and the second required three "in and out" catheterizations prior to normalization of the voiding pattern. Both patients subsequently became dry and voided efficiently.

In addition to incontinent women, a group of children with vesicoureteral reflux were treated by Buckley and associates with subureteric injection of silicon paste.[26] To date, 22 refluxing ureters in 16

patients (six bilateral) have been treated with the cystoscopically guided injection of between 0.2 and 2.0 ml (average, 1.0 ml) of silicon paste per ureter. The grade of the reflux was grade III in 3 ureters, grade IV in 15 ureters, and grade V in 4 ureters. Follow-up was available on the first 18 ureters. Reflux was cured in 17 ureters (95%) as evaluated by voiding cystourethrogram. In one patient reflux was reduced from grade V to grade I. Transient side effects of urinary frequency and hematuria were noted in all patients for the first 2 days after the procedure but resolved. There was no evidence of upper tract obstruction. No repeat procedures have been required.

These early results from the Scottish group are encouraging. Long-term follow-up will be required to determine the retreatment rate and and other untoward sequelae of these silicon injections.

REFERENCES

1. Thomas TM, Plymat KR, Blannen J: Prevalence of urinary incontinence. Br Med J 281:1243, 1980.
2. Feneley RCL, Shepherd AM, Powell PH: Urinary incontinence: Prevalence and needs. Br J Urol 51:493, 1979.
3. Yarnell JWG, Voyle GJ, Richards CJ: The prevalence and severity of urinary incontinence in women. J Epidemiol Community Health 35:71, 1981.
4. Consensus Panel: Urinary incontinence in adults. JAMA 261:2685, 1989.
5. Politano VA: Periurethral polytetrafluoroethylene injection for urinary incontinence. J Urol 127:439, 1982.
6. Lockhart JL, Walker RD, Vorstman B, Politano VA: Periurethral polytetrafluoroethylene injection following urethral reconstruction in female patients with urinary incontinence. J Urol 140:51, 1988.
7. Malizia AA, Reiman HM, Myers RP, et al: Migration and granulomatous reaction after periurethral injection of polytef (Teflon). JAMA 251:3277, 1984.
8. Mittleman RE, Marraccini JV: Pulmonary Teflon granulomas following periurethral Teflon injection for urinary incontinence. Arch Pathol Lab Med 107:611, 1983.
9. Claes H, Stroobants D, Van Meerbeek J, et al: Pulmonary migration following periurethral polytetrafluoroethylene injection for urinary incontinence. J Urol 142:821, 1989.
10. Quackels R: Deux cas d'incontinence après adénomectomie gué-

ries par injection de paraffine dan la périnée. Acta Urol Belg 23:259, 1955.

11. Sachse H: Die Behandlung der Harninkontinenz mit der Sklerotherapie: Indikations stellulung—Ergebnisse—Komplikationem. Urol Int 15:225–244, 1963.

12. Berg S: Polytef augmentation urethroplasty: Correction of surgically incurable urinary incontinence by injection technique. Arch Surg 107:379, 1973.

13. Lim KB, Ball AJ, Fenerley RCL: Periurethral Teflon injection: A simple treatment for urinary incontinence. Br J Urol 55:208, 1983.

14. Kaufman M, Lockhart SL, Silverstein J, Politano VA: Transurethral polytetrafluoroethylene injection for post-prostatectomy incontinence. J Urol 132:403, 1984.

15. Boykin H, Rodriguez FR, Brizzolura J, et al: Complete urinary obstruction following periurethral polytetrafluoroethylene injection for urinary incontinence. J Urol 141:1199, 1989.

16. Shortliffe LM, Freiha FS, Kessler R, et al: Treatment of urinary incontinence by the periurethral implantation of glutaraldehyde cross-linked collagen. J Urol 141:538, 1989.

17. Herschorn S, Radomski DB, Steele DJ: Early experience with intraurethral collagen injections for urinary incontinence. J Urol 148:1797, 1992.

18. Gonzalez de Garibay AM: Endoscopic injection of autologous adipose tissue in the treatment of female incontinence. Arch Esp Urol 42:143, 1989.

19. Barrett DM, Parulkar BG, Malizia AA Jr: The genitourinary spheroidal membrane: An experimental study of a new percutaneously inserted prosthetic device for the control of urinary incontinence. J Urol 142:1615, 1989.

20. Politano VA, Small MP, Herper JM: Periurethral Teflon injection for urinary incontinence. J Urol 111:180, 1974.

21. Endo LP, Edwards NL, Longley S, et al: Silicone and rheumatic diseases. Semin Arthritis Rheum 17(2):112, 1987.

22. Spiera H: Scleroderma after silicone augmentation mammoplasty. JAMA 260:236, 1988.

23. Varga J, Schumacher HR, Jimenez SA: Systemic sclerosis after augmentation mammoplasty with silicone implants. Ann Intern Med 111:377, 1989.

24. Sergott TJ, Limoli JP, Baldwin CM Jr, Laub DR: Human adjuvant disease, possible autoimmune disease after silicone implantation; a review of the literature, case studies, and spectulation for the future. Plast Reconstr Surg 78:104, 1986.

25. Buckley JF, Scott R, Meddings R, et al: Injectable silicone microparticles: A new treatment for female stress incontinence [abstract]. J Urol 147:280A, 1992.

26. Buckley JF, Azmy A, Fyfe A, et al: Endoscopic correction of vesicoureteric reflux with injectable microparticle silicone [abstract]. J Urol 147:356A, 1992.

Artificial Sphincters

CHAPTER 39

Artificial Sphincter: Abdominal Approach

Robert L. Long, M.D.
David M. Barrett, M.D.

The artificial genitourinary sphincter (AGUS) has now been in use since 1972, when it was first introduced by Scott and colleagues.[1] According to data provided by American Medical Systems (AMS, the manufacturer of the AGUS), over 15,000 artificial urinary sphincters have been implanted in men and women. The primary indication in female patients has been type III sphincteric incompetence. Although relatively uncommon compared to other types of female incontinence, its treatment requires a thorough understanding of the mechanism of incontinence, very careful patient preparation, evaluation, and selection, in-depth knowledge of the treatment options available, and technical knowledge of the AGUS. The AGUS provides the clinical urologist with a unique treatment option for the female patient with type III incontinence.

History

The history of the AGUS shows a constant evolution from the first AS-721 to the current AS-800 manufactured by AMS. The AS-800 has been in production since 1982. Recent modifications to the device include a delayed activation device, a dip coating, a cuff that has been modified to decrease the chance of urethral erosion, color-coded kink-resistant tubing, and various connectors. Several texts provide an excellent review of the chronologic development of the AGUS since 1972.[2-4]

Patient Selection

The AS-800 has been implanted in children and adults. Very careful patient selection, knowledge of alternative options, technical expertise with the device and implantation technique, and education of the patient are essential requirements for a satisfactory surgical outcome. The typical patient is one who complains of both daytime and nighttime incontinence and is socially disabled by the incontinence. Female candidates for AGUS fall into three basic categories of sphincter incontinence: (1) type III stress incontinence, (2) neurogenic incontinence, and (3) posttraumatic incontinence. Multiple previous pelvic operations or pelvic radiation therapy increase the difficulty and risk of artificial sphincter placement.

Type III stress urinary incontinence is a direct result of intrinsic urethral dysfunction from failed anti-incontinence procedures resulting in injuries to the intrinsic urethral mechanism, extensive pelvic surgery, or pelvic irradiation.[5-7] The continence mechanism in women is complex and is the net result of a neurologically functional bladder neck and proximal urethra and a stable competent detrusor.[8, 9] Anatomic changes in the urethra such as scarring and fixation further compromise the continence mechanism.

The work-up for suspected type III incontinence includes a detailed history and physical examination, pelvic examination, urinalysis, urine culture and sensitivity results, cystoscopic examination paying careful attention to the bladder neck, which is usually open or gaping in appearance, and video imaging studies such as a lateral voiding cystourethrogram and urodynamic evaluation, which will document a nonfunctioning urethra. Studies evaluating detrusor contractility and compliance are also recommended.

The ideal patient has sphincter incontinence with normal detrusor function.[10] Among those presenting with urinary incontinence, only 10% have problems related to intrinsic sphincter deficiency.[7] See Table

39–1 for patient selection criteria. Preoperative evaluation should determine which patients are at risk for developing detrusor hyperreflexia in the postoperative period, which could result in excessive intravesical pressure and deterioration of the upper urinary tract secondary to reflux. Women with myleodysplasia are at increased risk for development of unsuspected detrusor hyperreflexia.[6, 11, 12, 13] Management of sphincter incompetence is illustrated in Figure 39–1.[14]

For patients with type III incontinence who are candidates for an AGUS but have noncompliant, small-capacity bladders or are at risk for development of detrusor hyperreflexia, a concurrent or staged augmentative cystoplasty is indicated. In selected cases an antireflux procedure for patients with grade II or higher reflux should be performed.[14]

Treatment Options

Treatment options depend on the surgeon's experience and the patient's preference. Steroid dependency, previous irradiation, and lack of manual dexterity are relative contraindications to the use of

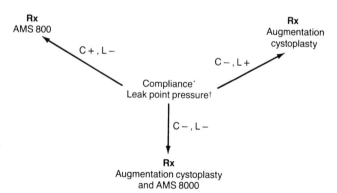

Figure 39–1 Management of sphincteric incompetence (C, compliance; L, leak point pressure; +, high; −, low; *, normal = 15 cm H₂O; high = 40 cm H₂O or above leak point pressure). (From Barrett DM, Parulkar BG: The artificial sphincter [AS-800]. Experience in children and young adults. Urol Clin North Am 16:119, 1989.)

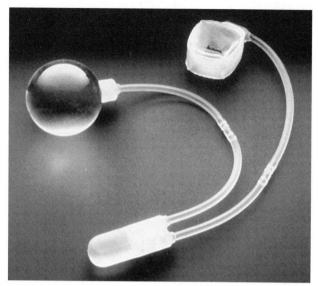

Figure 39-2 AS-800 sphincter. (From Barrett DM, Parulkar BG: The artificial sphincter [AS-800]. Experience in children and young adults. Urol Clin North Am 16:119, 1989.)

the AGUS. Other options include vesicourethral sling procedures, bladder neck and urethral tubularization, and periurethral injection techniques.[6, 12, 15, 16]

Advantages of each technique vary, but according to the Clinical Practice Guideline prepared by the U.S. Department of Health and Human Services in March, 1992, the continence results and complications of the sling procedures and the AGUS are comparable, both having approximately a 90% continence rate and a 30% complication rate. With periurethral injections approximately 75% of patients are either cured or improved with a 6% complications rate, and with collagen upward of 90% report good to excellent continence for up to 18 months.[17]

All procedures result in continence by increasing outlet resistance, whereas with the AGUS resistance can be temporarily eliminated for voiding or intermittent catheterization.

The AS-800

The AS-800 sphincter (Fig. 39–2) is manufactured by AMS in Minnetonka, Minnesota. The current price per unit is $3990, and the CPT Manual code is 53445. The prosthesis is composed of silicone elastomer, has an internal Dacron cuff, and should be filled with a combination of sterile water and contrast medium unless the patient has an allergy to contrast media. The manufacturer will provide personnel support, an operating room manual, and an instructional video to assist the operative surgeon in the use, preparation, and placement of the AGUS.

The AGUS has three components including the pressure regulatory dip-coated balloon, the pump with the deactivation button, and the occlusive Dacron-reinforced cuff and the tubing connectors. The system should be filled with saline or iso-osmotic contrast medium.

Continence or cuff inflation is maintained by continuous pressure in the cuff, which is modulated by the pressure balloon, which in turn is usually positioned in the prevesical space. The cuff is positioned around the bladder neck in women, and the pump is placed subcutaneously in the labia.

To release pressure on the cuff, the pump is squeezed several times, emptying the cuff and pumping fluid into the pressure regulatory balloon. Pressure slowly refills the cuff in 3 to 5 minutes through a resistor valve in the pump. With a transient increase in intra-abdominal pressure (e.g., with cough or Valsalva maneuver), additional pressure is transmitted through the balloon into the cuff, thereby temporarily increasing outflow resistance. Five pressure-regulating balloons are available in 10-cm H_2O gradients ranging from 41 to 90 cm H_2O. There are 10 cuff sizes, from 4.5 to 10 cm, in 0.5-cm increments. Cuff sizers and tubing connectors are included in the prepackaged kits.[19] Selection of cuff size is determined by the measurement obtained around the bladder neck. Although various pressure-regulating balloons are available, the 61 to 70 cm H_2O size is the one most commonly selected.

AGUS Implantation

PATIENT PREPARATION

After patient selection, patient preparation is the most important factor in achieving an acceptable surgical outcome. The patient should be prepared both mentally and physically for AGUS placement. Mental preparation includes instruction in the use of the valve and deactivation button, the technique of clean intermittent catheterization, infection precautions, and counseling about the mechanical limitations of the AGUS and the potential for corrective surgical procedures in the future.

Patients are admitted on the day of surgery and placed on broad-spectrum preoperative parenteral antibiotics such as ampicillin and gentamicin.[20] The urine should be sterile. A bowel preparation with an osmotic agent (e.g., GoLYTELY) and a clear liquid diet the day prior to surgery have proved to be adequate if a concurrent cystoplasty is planned. Antibiotic coverage is designed to cover gram-negative, gram-positive, and anaerobic organisms. One recommended regimen by Appell and associates is vancomycin for gram-positive coverage, gentamicin for gram-negative coverage, and metronidazole for anaerobes.[21] Although practically any bacterium can cause a wound or genitourinary prosthetic infection, *Staphylococcus epidermidis* is the most common organism isolated from infected prostheses.[20–22] Other organisms isolated include *Proteus* species, *Pseudomonas* species, *Escherichia coli*, *Serratia* species, *Corynebacterium* species, and *Enterobacter* species.[22]

Most implanting surgeons recommend a skin preparation the night before surgery with a surgical scrub solution such as iodoform or hexachlorophene soap. Shaving the skin is done in the operating room to decrease the likelihood of bacterial colonization of skin knicks. Surgical hoods are used, and attempts to keep operating room traffic to a minimum are strongly recommended.

During the procedure liberal use of an antibiotic spray or irrigant is recommended (e.g., 50 mg of neomycin, 100,000 units of polymixin B, and 80 mg of gentamicin per 100 ml of 0.9% sodium chloride solution[22] or a solution of neomycin 0.1% and 50,000 units of bacitracin in 1 liter of 0.9% sodium chloride solution).[20] Note: The ends of the connector tubing should not be sprayed with antibiotic solution because this causes an increased risk of intraluminal crystal formation resulting in prosthetic malfunction at a later date.

OPERATIVE PROCEDURE

Two operative approaches are currently used in placing the AGUS. The most commonly employed is a retropubic extraperitoneal approach. Recently, a combined suprapubic transvaginal technique has been recommended by Appell and colleagues.[3, 15] Abbassian has suggested a new retropubic approach through a periurethral inverted U incision going through the anterior vaginal vestibule.[23]

Abdominal Approach

The patient is placed in a low lithotomy position that provides access to the abdomen and perineal area. Vaginal preparation is performed with povidone-iodine solution. A vaginal pack soaked in the same solution is left in the vaginal vault during the procedure. The operating surgeon should pay careful attention to the AMS AS-800 Operating Room Manual for device preparation.

A 16 Fr, 5-ml balloon Foley catheter is introduced preoperatively in the urethra. The lithotomy position is adjusted to place the knees at the level of the abdomen. Access to the retropubic space is gained with a Pfannenstiel or midline incision, which is then deepened to the bladder neck region. The place of entry of the cuff is below the insertion of the ureters into the native bladder. The vesicovaginal plane is next dissected at a point superior to the endopelvic fascia (Fig. 39–3). Fingers placed in the vagina may aid in this step of the dissection. Extreme care is taken to identify this plane, especially in prepubertal or postmenopausal women and in patients with a history of bladder neck tubularization and sling procedures. The bladder is next filled with antibiotic solution containing methylene blue to detect points of leak, if any. If the vesicovaginal plane is not readily identified, the bladder is opened by a high midline incision to visualize carefully the bladder neck re-

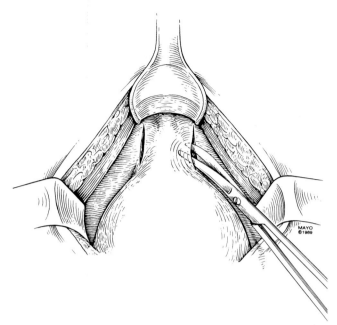

Figure 39-3 Sharp dissection of the vesicovaginal plane. (By permission of Mayo Foundation.)

gion. The cutter clamp may also be used for the dissection of this plane.

An accidentally opened bladder neck or vagina is sutured in two continuous layers with 3–0 chromic catgut sutures to achieve a watertight closure. The cuff sizer is used to measure the circumference of the bladder neck so that the cuff is neither too loose nor too tight (Fig. 39–4). The snap-on cuff is drawn around the bladder neck (Fig. 39–5). The inner surface of the cuff (bladder contact surface) is kept away from sharp instruments. The pump is placed in a subcutaneous position within the labia majora, and the pressure-regulating balloon reservoir (PRBR) is placed in the preperitoneal retrorectus muscle space (Fig. 39–6). The PRBR is first filled with properly

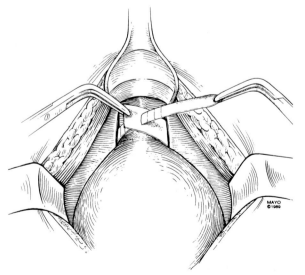

Figure 39-4 Cuff sizer. (By permission of Mayo Foundation.)

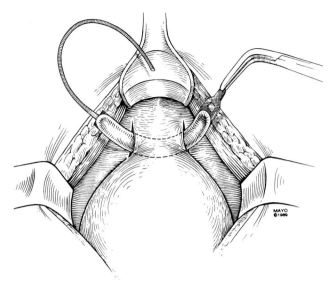

Figure 39-5 Cuff placement (inflatable surface facing inward). (By permission of Mayo Foundation.)

constituted ionic contrast medium to a volume of 20 ml, which is temporarily used to prime the cuff. It is then refilled to a total volume of $20\frac{1}{2}$ ml. The system is deactivated and the cuff left in an open position. Appropriate tie-on connectors are used with 2–0 Prolene (polypropylene) fixation. The 16 Fr silicone Foley catheter is left indwelling without tension overnight. A Jackson-Pratt drain (3.2-mm diameter) may be placed in the retropubic space for 48 to 72 hours or until drainage stops. Ice packs applied locally help to decrease local edema and pain.

The patient usually voids without undue difficulty after removal of the Foley catheter. A careful check is made of the residual urine after each void. If residual urine volume is equal to or more than 100 ml persists, self-administered or assisted intermittent catheterization with a 12 Fr soft rubber catheter is recommended to the patient.

The sphincter is activated about 4 to 6 weeks postoperatively. A roentgenogram verifies the normal function of the sphincter in the cuff-inflated position (Fig. 39–7).[7] Parenteral antibiotics are continued postoperatively for at least 4 days before the patient is switched to oral antibiotics. If the patient undergoes a concurrent cystoplasty, systemic antibiotics are continued for 2 weeks.

Transvaginal Approach

Because of concern about urethral or vaginal injury during creation of the urethral vaginal plane, an alternate approach has recently been popularized using a combined suprapubic and transvaginal approach[3, 15, 21] employing a similar preparation and position and an inverted U incision made in the anterior vaginal wall. The urethra and bladder neck are mobilized to the ischial tuberosity, and the retropubic space is entered in a fashion similar to a modified

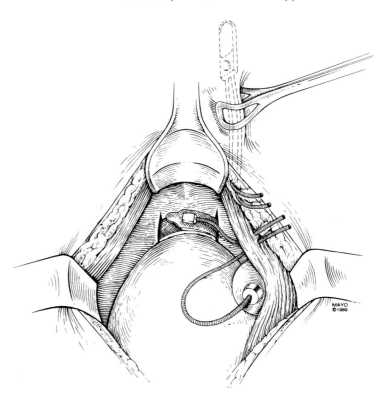

Figure 39-6 Final anatomic position of cuff, pressure-regulating balloon reservoir, and pump assembly. (By permission of Mayo Foundation.)

Pereyra or Raz procedure.[3, 8, 24] Measurement of anatomy and device preparation are similar. The balloon and pump are implanted through the suprapubic incision as they are in the standard abdominal approach.

In performing either operation the surgeon should be aware of conditions that will render cuff placement either very difficult or impossible. Any previous procedures involving the urethra or anterior vaginal wall such as external beam radiation therapy, pelvic trauma, fistula repair, multiple stress urinary incontinence (SUI) procedures, bladder neck tubularization, or sling procedures may result in extremely poor tissue integrity, which increases the risk of operative injury or postoperative cuff erosion. In certain circumstances a urinary diversion may be the only option.

The AGUS and Complex Reconstructive Procedures

Until recently, small-capacity, noncompliant neurogenic bladders or detrusor hyperreflexia with uninhibited contractions were relative contraindications to the use of the AGUS. In some cases, particularly in children and young adults with neurogenic bladders, the AGUS was implanted but the patient subsequently developed reflux and upper urinary tract deterioration secondary to unacceptably high intravesical pressure.

To prevent upper urinary tract deterioration and leakage from overcoming the cuff pressure, augmentative cystoplasties have been employed to increase vesical storage capacity and to decrease in-travesical pressures. Selection of the shape of the cystoplasty is important to prevent unacceptable intravesical pressure.[25] Barrett and colleagues advocate consideration of four technical considerations to decrease the risk of unacceptably high intravesical pressure after cystoplasty:[20]

1. Detubularization of the bowel segment
2. Large-diameter cystoplasty
3. Large-capacity cystoplasty
4. Direct peristaltic wave away from trigone.

A prime consideration in a patient who is a candidate for an AGUS is that the neurogenic bladder should have a capacity of at least 400 ml and still maintain an intravesical pressure of less than 40 cm H_2O pressure.[10] If these parameters cannot be met, augmentative cystoplasty is indicated to decrease the risk of reflux and upper urinary tract deterioration (Fig. 39–8).

Two groups of patients who may benefit from an AGUS are those who are candidates for neobladder reconstruction and those with a small-capacity neurogenic bladder and low leak pressures. In women who require cystectomy the continence mechanism may be damaged, and either concurrent or delayed placement of the AGUS around the neourethra or bladder neck can be considered. After constructing the neobladder, it is essential to use a healthy unharvested efferent limb of small bowel.[26] The AGUS should fit snugly around the surgeon's finger, and either a 51 to 60 or 61 to 70 cm H_2O pressure cuff should be used. Avoid placing the AGUS over the suture line to decrease the risk of erosion and fissure formation. Infection precautions are essential to minimize the risk of prosthetic infection. The remainder of the prosthesis is placed in a routine fashion, taking care to place the tubing anteriorly to allow greater ease of accessibility in case of possible later revision. Atrophy and erosion of the neobladder neck is a genuine concern because bowel and not bladder neck is used. At the end of the procedure the pump is deactivated with the cuff left open, and a suprapubic cystotomy is placed away from the bladder neck. With adequate attention to detail and infection precautions, there is no increased risk of infection when the AGUS is placed at the same time the bladder reconstruction is performed. The infection rate remains constant at around 2 to 5%, but the risk of erosion doubles to approximately 10 to 20%.[26]

Artificial urinary sphincters have also been implanted in patients with neurogenic bladders with low leak pressures and low compliance. The work-up includes radiographic evaluation of both the upper and lower urinary tracts and urodynamic evaluation. Despite the preoperative work-up, progressive changes in bladder function can occur, and close long-term follow-up is mandatory with particular attention paid to the upper tracts.[28] In occasional patients with borderline sphincteric competence, placement of the cuff alone provides continence with an option to place the remaining prostheses at a later date.[29]

Patients with reflux of grade II or greater usually undergo an antireflux procedure at the same time as augmentative cystoplasty and AGUS placement.[20] Although the numbers are small, Strawbridge and

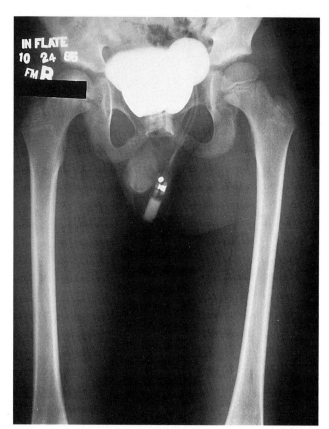

Figure 39-8 Voiding cystourethrogram shows no vesicoureteral reflux or urinary leakage. (From Barrett DM, Parulkar BG: The artificial sphincter [AS-800]. Experience in children and young adults. Urol Clin North Am 16:119, 1989.)

colleagues in a Mayo Clinic study reported on seven female patients undergoing placement of the AGUS and augmentative cystoplasty.[29] Five patients underwent simultaneous cystoplasty and AGUS placement with no deaths, 88% reporting fair to good continence with 0.6% revision procedures per patient.[14] Five patients had myelodysplasia, and two had a neurogenic bladder. Modifying procedures were necessary for mechanical failure, surgical or technical failure, erosion and infection, and total reimplantation of the prosthesis.[14, 29]

Results and Complications

The results of placement of the AGUS for female urinary incontinence are encouraging. Numerous researchers have reported either good or excellent continence in approximately 90% of their patients. Revisions are common, varying between 0.3 and 0.6 per patient.[6, 9, 21, 30, 31] Reasons for revision include infection, cuff erosion, mechanical malfunction, and technical revision. In the event of infection, usually heralded by induration, erythema, or tenderness at the pump site, the entire prosthesis should be removed, and at least 3 months should transpire before reimplantation is considered.[22, 32] Nurse and Mundy rec-

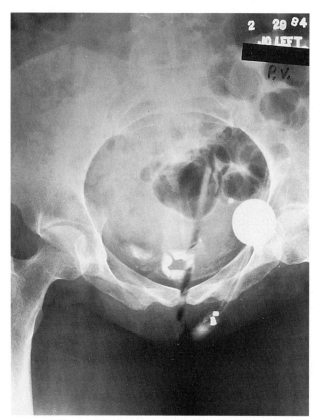

Figure 39-7 Roentgenogram with activated sphincter in cuff inflate position.

ommend placing omentum around the cuff site after removal to facilitate future dissection and subsequent cuff placement.[32]

Considering that there is no easily created surgical plane between the vagina and urethra and that some neurogenic bladders and most SUI candidates have had previous bladder, pelvic, and urethral surgery, it is not surprising that intraoperative injuries to the urethra, bladder, and vagina can occur owing to altered anatomy and fibrosis. Salisz and Diokno reported six intraoperative injuries among 57 female patients, with four vaginal perforations, one anterior bladder perforation, and one urethral injury. All six were repaired at the time of the injury with absorbable suture and subsequent AGUS placement. By using pre- and postoperative antibiotics, vaginal antiseptic packs, and delayed sphincter activation, they reported no infections, and five of six patients were dry after initial sphincter placement.[33]

Continued or persistent incontinence after placement of the AGUS is a relatively common occurrence.[34-36] Diagnosis and treatment require a logical and systematic approach. The algorithm developed by Kreder and Webster provides an approach to the diagnosis and treatment of incontinence after AGUS placement (Fig. 39–9).[6]

Medicolegal Implications

Medicolegal implications are a serious consideration when dealing with all genitourinary prosthetic de-

vices, including artificial urinary sphincters. Factors contributing to the surgeon's risk of litigation include (1) complexity of the procedure, (2) risk of mechanical (device) failure, (3) the patient's clinical status necessitating use of the AGUS, (4) the possibility of delayed problems (e.g., infection, tissue atrophy), (5) the prevailing public attitude toward medical malpractice, and (6) current controversy about and federal government investigations into the use of implantable silicone products.

Informed consent is necessary before proceeding with any surgical procedure. It is briefly defined as a patient's agreement to a procedure after adequate disclosure. Patients about to receive an AGUS should be made particularly aware of alternative procedures including Teflon and collagen injections, sling procedures, indwelling catheters, urinary diversion, the risk of AGUS infections (both immediate and delayed), the possibility and likelihood of mechanical failure, AGUS erosion, and general information about the likelihood of future replacement of the AGUS.

General controversy about implantable silicone devices should be taken into consideration when implanting an AGUS regardless of whether the prosthesis is a solid silicone elastomer or is composed of silicone gel or oils. The AS-800 AGUS has been available since 1982 and comprises a solid silicone elastomer that has been dip coated. Although silicone-based prostheses have been used for more than 20 years and have been viewed as relatively inert, recent controversy about the possible immunologic as-

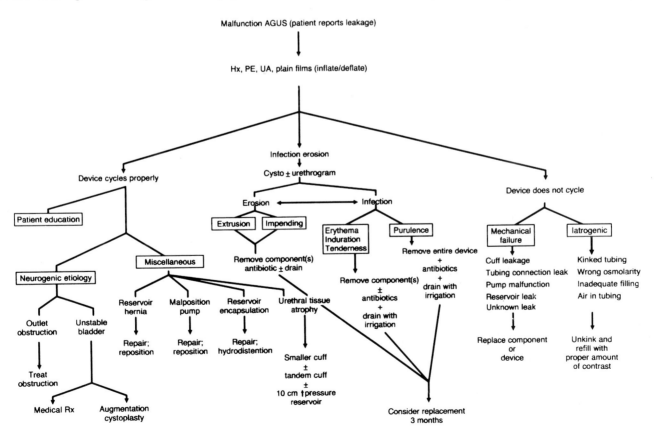

Figure 39-9 Algorithms for evaluation of the malfunctioning artificial urinary sphincter. (By permission of Mayo Foundation.)

pects of implanted breast prostheses has raised questions about the safety of these prostheses and the use of silicone gel.

Barrett and colleagues' study of 26 patients who underwent revision or repair of a genitourinary prosthetic device showed silicon particle shedding in 18 of 25 patients (72%) in the periprosthetic sheath and silicon particles in regional lymph nodes in 4 patients. The particles were detected under electron microscopy. They concluded that the implications of particle shedding were unclear, but to date the benefits of the prosthesis appear to outweigh the potential risks.[39]

Summary

The AGUS offers an alternative treatment for female incontinence secondary to sphincter incompetence. The implanting surgeon should be familiar with female pelvic and vaginal anatomy. Alternative treatment methods such as pubovaginal slings and injection therapy should be understood. Patient selection and preparation are essential to success, and particular attention should be paid to the work-up. Halstedian surgical technical procedures and meticulous attention to detail are essential to decrease the risk of prosthetic infection, cuff erosion, and iatrogenic mechanical malfunction. Although complex reconstructive procedures can be performed in association with AGUS placement, the complications increase as the complexity increases. All things considered, in the hands of an experienced surgeon, the AGUS offers the closest option to a natural sphincter and can be a solution to the distressing and debilitating condition of sphincteric urinary incontinence.

REFERENCES

1. Scott FB: The use of the artificial sphincter in the treatment of urinary incontinence in the female patient. Urol Clin North Am 12:305, 1985.
2. Barrett DM, Furlow WL: Artificial urinary sphincter in the management of female incontinence. In Raz S (ed): Female Urology, Philadelphia, WB Saunders, 1983, pp 284–292.
3. Furlow W: Two decades of experience: AMS sphincter 800 now accessible to all urologists. Colleagues Urol 9:4, 1992.
4. Siegel SW: History of the prosthetic treatment of urinary incontinence. Urol Clin North Am 16:99, 1989.
5. Leach GE, Zimmern P: Surgical treatment of female incontinence. In Leach GE (chair): Management of urinary incontinence in the female. Presented at the 86th Annual Meeting of the American Urological Association, Toronto, June, 1991.
6. Kreder KJ, Webster GD: Evaluation and management of incontinence after implantation of the artificial urinary sphincter. Urol Clin North Am 18:375, 1991.
7. Parulkar BG, Barrett DM: Application of the AS-800 artificial sphincter for intractable urinary incontinence in females. Surg Gynecol Obstet 171:131, 1990.
8. Staskin DR, Zimmern PE, Hadley HR, et al: The pathophysiology of stress incontinence. Urol Clin North Am 12:271, 1985.
9. Massey A, Abrams P: Urodynamics of the female lower urinary tract. Urol Clin North Am 12:231, 1985.
10. Petrou SP, Barrett DM: The expanded role for the artificial

11. sphincter. In Barrett DM (chair): Artificial urinary sphincters. Presented at the Annual Meeting of the American Urological Association, Washington, DC, May, 1992.
11. McGuire EJ, Woodside JR, Borden TA, et al: Prognostic value of urodynamic testing in myelodysplastic patients. J Urol 126:205, 1981.
12. Mitchell ME, Rink RC, Adams MC: Augmentation cystoplasty implantation of artificial urinary sphincter in men and women and reconstruction of the dysfunctional urinary tract. In Walsh PC, Retik AB, Stamey TA, Vaughan ED (eds): Campbell's Urology, 6th ed. Philadelphia, WB Saunders, 1992, pp 2630–2653.
13. McGuire EJ, Woodside JR, Borden TA, et al: Upper urinary tract deterioration in patients with myelodysplasia and detrusor hypertonia: A follow-up study. J Urol 129:823, 1983.
14. Barrett DM, Parulkar BG: The artificial sphincter (AS-800): Experience in children and young adults. Urol Clin North Am 16:119, 1989.
15. Appell RA: The artificial urinary sphincter and periurethral injections: Role in treatment of female incontinence. Ob/Gyn Report 2:334, 1990.
16. Appell RA: Implantation of artificial urinary sphincters. In Hurt WG (ed): Urogynecologic Surgery. Gaithersburg, MD, Aspen Publishers, 1992, pp 147–155.
17. Urinary Incontinence Guideline Panel: Urinary Incontinence in Adults: Clinical Practice Guideline. AHCPR Pub. No. 92-0038. Rockville, MD: Agency for Health Care Policy and Research, Public Health Service, U.S. Department of Health and Human Services, March 1992.
18. AMS Sphincter 800 Urinary Prosthesis: U.S. price list (Order No. 0580). Minnetonka, MN, American Medical Systems, February 1993.
19. AMS Sphincter 800 Urinary Prosthesis: Operating Room Manual (Publication 90630), 4th ed. Minnetonka, MN, American Medical Systems, 1989, pp 1–17.
20. Barrett DM, Furlow WL, Goldwasser B: Artificial urinary sphincters. In Rous SN (ed): Urology Annual. Norwalk, CT, Appleton and Lange, 1988, pp 117–141.
21. Appell RA: Techniques and results in the implantation of the artificial sphincter in women and type III stress urinary incontinence by a vaginal approach. Neurourol Urodyn 7:613, 1988.
22. Carson CC: Infections in genitourinary prostheses. Urol Clin North Am 16:165, 1989.
23. Abbassian A: A new surgical approach for the correction of female stress urinary incontinence. J Urol 139:554, 1988.
24. Pereyra AJ, Raz S: Vaginal needle suspension. In Hinman F (ed): Atlas of Urologic Surgery. Philadelphia, WB Saunders, 1989, pp 445–448.
25. Goldwasser B, Webster GD: Augmentation and substitution enterocystoplasty. J Urol 135:215, 1986.
26. O'Sullivan DC, Barrett DM: Artificial bladder and the use of the artificial sphincter. Urol Clin North Am 18:677, 1991.
27. Light JK, Reynolds JC: Impact of the new cuff design on reliability of the AS-800 artificial urinary sphincter. J Urol 147:609, 1992.
28. Roth DR, Vyas PR, Kroovand RL, et al: Urinary tract deterioration associated with the artificial urinary sphincter. J Urol 135:528, 1986.
29. Strawbridge LR, Kramer SA, Castillo OA, et al: Augmentation cystoplasty and the artificial genitourinary sphincter. J Urol 142:297, 1989.
30. Webster GD, Perez LM, Khoury JM, et al: Management of type III stress urinary incontinence using artificial urinary sphincter. Urology 39:499, 1992.
31. Goldwasser B, Furlow WL, Barrett DM: The model AS-800 artificial urinary sphincter: Mayo Clinic experience. J Urol 137:668, 1987.
32. Nurse DE, Mundy AR: One hundred artificial sphincters. Br J Urol 61:318, 1988.
33. Salisz JA, Diokno AC: The management of injuries to the urethra, bladder or vagina encountered during difficult placement of the artificial urinary sphincter in the female patient. J Urol 148:1528, 1992.
34. Diokno AC, Hollander JB, Alderson TP: Artificial urinary

sphincter for recurrent female urinary incontinence: indications and results. J Urol 138:778, 1987.

35. Fishman IJ, Shabsigh R, Scott FB: Experience with the artificial urinary sphincter model AS-800 in 148 patients. J Urol 141:307, 1989.
36. Wang Y, Hadley HR: Management of persistent or recurrent urinary incontinence after placement of artificial urinary sphincter. J Urol 146:1005, 1991.
37. Irwin JR: Legal aspects of urologic prosthetic devices. Urol Clin North Am 16:165, 1989.
38. Nora PF (ed): Professional Liability / Risk Management: A Manual for Surgeons. Chicago, American College of Surgeons, 1991, p 115.
39. Barrett DM, O'Sullivan DC, Malizia AA, et al: Particle shedding and migration from silicone genitourinary prosthetic devices. J Urol 146:319, 1991.

BIBLIOGRAPHY

Anderson RU: Neurogenic bladder. Monogr Urol 13:111, 1992.
Barrett DM: Female incontinence and the artificial urinary sphincter. *In* Kaufman JJ (ed): Current Urologic Therapy, 2nd ed. Philadelphia, WB Saunders, 1986, pp 273–275.
Bauer SB, Reda EF, Colodny AH, et al: Detrusor instability: A delayed complication in association with the artificial sphincter. J Urol 135:1212, 1986.
Bent AF: Evaluation of the urinary incontinence. *In* Hurt WG (ed): Urogynecologic Surgery, Gaithersburg, MD, Aspen Publishers, 1992, pp 35–46.
de Badiola FI, Castro-Diaz D, Hart-Austin, et al: Influence of preoperative bladder capacity and compliance on the outcome of artificial sphincter implantation in patients with neurogenic sphincter incompetence. J Urol 148:1493, 1992.
Karram MM: Transvaginal needle suspension. *In* Hurt WG (ed): Urogynecologic Surgery. Gaithersburg, MD, Aspen Publishers, 1992, pp 61–72.
Light JK, Pietro T: Alteration in detrusor behavior and the effect on renal function following insertion of the artificial urinary sphincter. J Urol 136:632, 1986.
McGuire EJ, Wan J: Pubovaginal slings. *In* Hurt WG (ed): Urogynecologic Surgery. Gaithersburg, MD, Aspen Publishers, 1992, pp 97–105.
Perez LM, Webster GD: Successful outcome of artificial urinary sphincters in men with post-prostatectomy urinary incontinence despite adverse implantation features. J Urol 148:1166, 1992.
Perry MD, Husmann DA: Urethral injuries in female subjects following pelvic fractures. J Urol 147:139, 1992.
Roth DR, Vyas PR, Kroovand RL, et al: Re: urinary tract deterioration associated with the artificial urinary sphincter (Letter to the editor). J Urol 137:1011, 1987.
Scott FB: The artificial urinary sphincter: Experience in adults. Urol Clin North Am 16:105, 1989.
Wang Y, Hadley HR: Experiences with the artificial urinary sphincter in the irradiated patient. J Urol 147:612, 1992.
Wein AJ: Neuromuscular dysfunction of the lower urinary tract. *In* Walsh PC, Retik AB, Stamey TA, Vaughan ED (eds): Campbell's Urology, 6th ed. Philadelphia, WB Saunders, 1992, pp 625–626.

CHAPTER 40

Artificial Sphincter: Transvaginal Approach

Yu Wang, M.D.
H. Roger Hadley, M.D.

The artificial urinary sphincter is an effective alternative to the urethral sling or periurethral injection therapy for the treatment of urinary incontinence in women due to primary urethral sphincter insufficiency (type III stress urinary incontinence).[1, 2] The artificial urinary sphincter should not be used in patients with anatomic stress urinary incontinence (type I or II) resulting from poor bladder neck or proximal urethral support because this is typically managed by a bladder neck suspension procedure performed through either a transvaginal or a transabdominal approach.

Primary urethral sphincter dysfunction in women may be associated with scarring following multiple prior anti-incontinence operations, neurologic causes (myelomeningocele, sacral cord tumor, or peripheral neuropathy), radical pelvic operations (abdominoperineal resection or radical hysterectomy), pelvic radiation therapy, and possibly estrogen deficiency or senile changes. Because the problem is inadequate urethral closure, a standard bladder neck suspension will not alleviate the incontinence.

The artificial urinary sphincter is a synthetic device that includes a cuff designed to provide a uniform circumferential compression on the urethra and bladder neck. The patient manipulates a labially placed pump to open the cuff prior to voiding. The American Medical System AS-800 is the currently used model; it can be implanted using either a transvaginal or transabdominal approach.

This chapter describes the technique of transvaginal implantation of the artificial urinary sphincter in the treatment of type III stress urinary incontinence. The results achieved are compared with those reported with the urethral sling and periurethral injection therapy.

Evaluation of the Patient

Preoperative evaluation of the patient should include a history, physical examination, radiographic evaluation, and urodynamic studies. The patient with genuine stress urinary incontinence due to primary urethral insufficiency will report loss of urine with abdominal straining that may or may not be associated with urgency. Previous anti-incontinence procedures, radical pelvic operations, and orthopedic or neurologic disorders are important historical information.

The physical examination includes measurement of postvoid residual urine and demonstration of objective stress urinary incontinence with the bladder full in the supine or upright position or both. The Q-tip deflection test is used to assess urethral mobility. Neurologic examination of the lower extremities and perineum is performed to evaluate the lower lumbar and sacral cord segments. Cysto-urethroscopy is done to assess urethral coaptation, bladder trabeculation, and the unlikely presence of a fistula.

Radiographic evaluations should include a standing voiding cystourethrogram with resting and straining views. A well-supported urethra with an open bladder neck not associated with a bladder contraction is consistent with primary urethral insufficiency.

Urodynamic studies include a filling cystometrogram and measurement of urethral leak point pressure. Leakage of urine associated with a leak point pressure of less than 30 to 40 cm H_2O in the absence of a detrusor contraction supports the diagnosis of intrinsic sphincter insufficiency.

The patient best suited for implantation of an artificial urinary sphincter is one who has genuine stress urinary incontinence despite a well-supported bladder neck and no significant bladder instability. If the incontinent patient has concomitant vesical instability, simultaneous pharmacologic or operative management may be required to achieve urinary continence.

In the patient with urinary incontinence due to primary urethral insufficiency, conservative measures should be tried before operative intervention. These nonoperative measures include timed voiding, fluid restriction, pelvic floor exercises, systemic or topical estrogens, alpha-receptor agonists, and anticholinergic medications. If the patient continues to be incontinent despite conservative treatment, placement of the artificial urinary sphincter may be considered.

Technique

The artificial urinary sphincter is composed of three parts: the inflatable cuff, the pressure-regulating balloon, and the pump (Fig. 40–1). The cuff is placed circumferentially around the bladder neck, the pressure-regulating balloon is positioned in the prevesical space, and the pump is put in the labia majora. When the pump is squeezed, fluid moves from the cuff to the balloon reservoir. This decompression of the cuff opens the bladder neck and allows the patient to void. After 1 to 2 minutes the pressure-regulating balloon automatically reinflates the cuff, which then reestablishes urethral coaptation and continence.

Three different techniques have been described for the transvaginal placement of the artificial urinary sphincter.[1, 3, 4] The inherent advantage of the transvaginal approach is the possibility of dissection of the urethrovaginal plane, which is often obliterated after previous anti-incontinence procedures. The transvaginal technique allows dissection of the urethrovaginal plane under direct vision.

The patient is admitted to the hospital on the same day as the operation. Preoperative parenteral antibiotics (cefazolin, gentamicin, and metronidazole) are given 1 hour prior to the operation. After a regional or general anesthetic has been given, the patient is placed in the modified dorsal lithotomy position. The lower abdomen and vagina are shaved and prepared with povidine-iodine in the usual manner. The labial minora are sutured with silk to the skin laterally, and a posterior-weighted vaginal retractor is placed for exposure of the anterior vaginal wall. After insertion of a Foley catheter to drain the bladder, saline is injected into the subepithelial tissue of the anterior vaginal wall near the bladder neck to facilitate dissection of the vaginal flap.

A vertical incision is made in the anterior vaginal wall (Fig. 40–2). The incision extends from a point midway between the bladder neck and the external meatus to the proximal bladder neck. A plane under the vaginal wall is created on each side of the incision with sharp dissection. The dissecting scissors are first pointed laterally to the pubis ramus and then upward toward the ipsilateral shoulder of the patient (Fig. 40–3). Sufficiently thick vaginal flaps are created in anticipation of closure of the vagina over the soon-to-be-placed cuff of the artificial urinary sphincter. If the patient has not had a previous bladder neck operation, blunt finger dissection may be per-

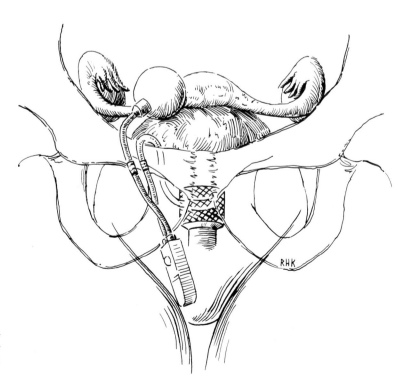

Figure 40-1 The AS-800 artificial urinary sphincter in a woman. The cuff is placed around the bladder neck, the pressure-regulating balloon in the prevesical space, and the pump in the labia majora.

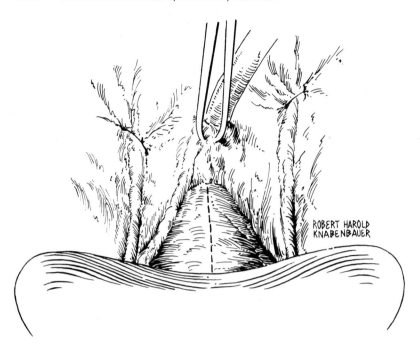

Figure 40-2 With the patient in the modified dorsolithotomy position, a vertical incision is made in the anterior vaginal wall.

formed to separate the endopelvic fascia from its lateral attachments to the pubic rim. The finger should sweep from lateral to medial, creating a window into the retropubic space. In the patient who has dense scar tissue, sharp dissection will be required to enter the retropubic space. The urethra and bladder neck can then be separated posteriorly and laterally from the vagina and the pelvic side wall with sharp and blunt dissection. A similar procedure is followed on the opposite side.

Attention is next directed to the anterior aspect of the proximal urethra or bladder neck to free its attachments from the overlying symphysis pubis. If

possible, blunt finger dissection should be used to perform this part of the procedure. However, in the patient who has had a previous retropubic operation, dense scarring may be encountered in the anterior portion of the urethra. Overly aggressive dissection may lead to unintentional bladder opening or urethral tear. The dissection on the anterior side of the urethra may be particularly difficult because of its relative inaccessibility through the transvaginal approach. To facilitate exposure of the top side of the urethra a separate suprameatal incision may be used. The Foley catheter is retracted downward, and a small (1 to 2 cm) crescent-shaped incision is made

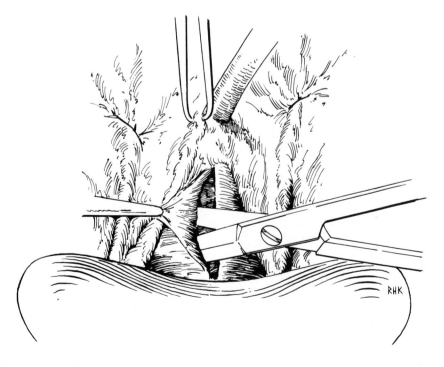

Figure 40-3 Using a combination of sharp and blunt dissection, the retropubic space is entered lateral to the bladder neck.

above the external meatus (Fig. 40–4A). Sharp dissection is then done in the midline below the symphysis pubis (Fig. 40–4B). After the bladder is allowed to drop away from its attachments to the symphysis, lateral blunt dissection can easily be performed to complete the dissection to the retropubic space previously opened through the vaginal incision. Thus, a circumferential dissection is completed around the bladder neck. However, if one is readily able to free the urethra from its anterior attachments through the vaginal incision alone, this suprameatal dissection is not necessary.

After the proximal urethra has been freed circumferentially, a broken-back small vascular clamp (Dale femoral-popliteal anastomosis clamp, Pilling 35-3543) is passed around the urethra from left to right. The cuff-measuring tape is grasped and passed around the urethra (Fig. 40–5), and the circumference of the urethra is measured. If the circumference is equivocal, it is best to err in favor of a slightly larger cuff size. Using a curved clamp, the appropriate size cuff of the artificial urinary sphincter is placed around the proximal urethra (Fig. 40–6). If the pump of the artificial urinary sphincter is to be inserted into the right labium majus, the cuff is withdrawn from right to left. If, however, the pump is to be placed in the left labia majora, the cuff should be withdrawn from left to right. The cuff is then

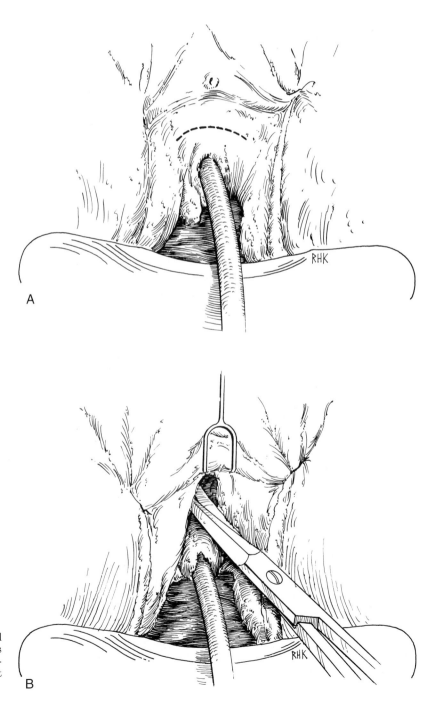

Figure 40-4 *A,* If dense scarring is encountered anterior to the urethra, a separate incision is made above the urethral meatus. *B,* The suprameatal dissection is done in the midline just below the symphysis pubis.

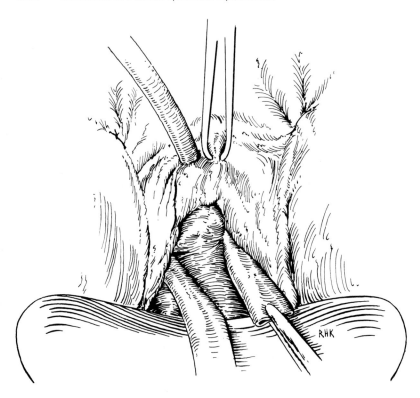

Figure 40-5 A Penrose drain is placed around the bladder neck to demonstrate the completed circumferential dissection.

locked in place (see Fig. 40–6) and rotated 180 degrees so that the hard-locking button lies on the anterior aspect of the urethra, away from the anterior vaginal wall (Fig. 40–7).

On the side on which the pressure-regulating balloon and pump mechanism will be implanted, a 4-cm transverse suprapubic incision is made. The tubing passer is passed antegrade under fingertip guidance from the suprapubic incision lateral to the midline down to the vaginal incision on the ipsilateral side of the bladder neck. (This operative step is similar to passing a needle carrier under fingertip guidance during a Pereyra-type bladder neck suspension.) The cuff tubing is attached to the tubing passer and then withdrawn up to the suprapubic incision. The anterior rectus sheath is incised transversely, and the

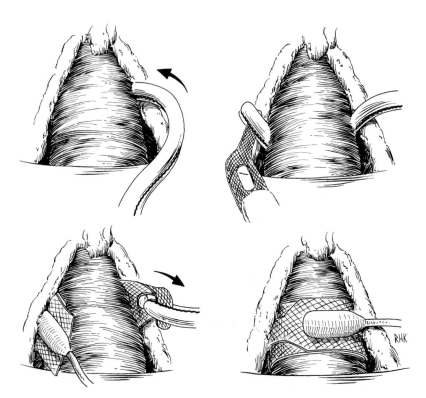

Figure 40-6 The cuff of the artificial urinary sphincter is passed around the bladder neck and then locked in place.

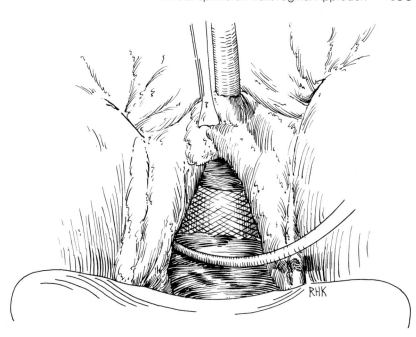

Figure 40-7 The cuff is rotated 180 degrees clockwise so that the hard-locking button lies anterior to the urethra, away from the anterior vaginal wall.

prevesical space is developed adjacent to the bladder. The pressure-regulating balloon is then inserted in the prevesical space. In women, the 51 to 60 cm H_2O pressure balloon reservoir is routinely used.

From the suprapubic incision a subcutaneous tunnel is created through which the pump will be inserted into the labia majora. The pump is passed into the labia majora to the level of the urethra with the deactivation button facing anteriorly. A Babcock clamp is used to secure the pump in position.

The tubings are trimmed to the appropriate lengths and then irrigated to remove any air or debris from the system. Filling of the cuff and reservoir are performed according to the instructions specified by the manufacturer. A straight connector is placed between the pump and the balloon reservoir. A right-angle connector attaches the pump to the cuff. Several 3–0 monofilament suture ties or Quick Connectors are used to secure these attachments.

The suprapubic and vaginal wounds are irrigated with copious amount of antibiotic solution. The wounds are then closed in multiple layers with absorbable sutures to ensure good coverage of the prosthesis with healthy overlying tissue. If the integrity of the vaginal wall appears to be compromised, an interposition of a vascularized flap (e.g., Martius flap) should be considered. The pump is left in the deactivated mode for 6 weeks.

A vaginal gauze pack is placed and removed on the first postoperative day. The Foley catheter is removed on the third postoperative day. The principles and technical steps of the transvaginal placement of the artificial urinary sphincter are outlined in Table 40–1.

Discussion

The few published reports of the artificial urinary sphincter implanted through the transvaginal approach reported favorable outcomes. Appell reported a series of 34 patients in whom the artificial urinary sphincter was placed through simultaneous vaginal and abdominal incisions.[1] Nineteen patients underwent follow-up of 3 years. The overall continence rate was 100%. Three patients, however, required revisionary operations for inadequate cuff compression and connector leak. Abbassian described the implantation of the artificial urinary sphincter in four patients utilizing the vaginal incision alone.[4] At mean follow-up of 14 months all patients were dry.

The potential advantage of the artificial urinary sphincter over the urethral sling is the capability to place a known circumferential compressive force around the entire urethra rather than only on the posterior surface of the urethra. Also a decreased likelihood of urinary retention and bladder instability is associated with the artificial urinary sphincter. The incidence of prolonged postoperative urinary retention after the urethral sling operation has been

TABLE 40–1
Principles and Technical Steps for the Placement of the Artificial Urinary Sphincter

1. Vertical incision in the anterior vaginal wall.
2. Entrance into the retropubic space lateral to the bladder neck.
3. If dense scar tissue is encountered, the circumferential bladder neck dissection is completed with a suprameatal incision to facilitate direct vision of the anterior surface of the urethra and bladder neck.
4. Placement of the cuff around the bladder neck with rotation of the hard-locking button of the cuff 180 degrees away from the vaginal wall incision.
5. Placement of the low-pressure balloon reservoir (51- to 60-cm water pressure) and the labial pump through a small suprapubic incision.
6. Interposition of Martius flap if necessary.
7. Delayed cuff activation for 6 weeks.
8. Patients with prior pelvic radiotherapy are excluded.

reported to be up to 10%, especially in patients with preoperative hypotonic bladder.[5] Persistent postoperative frequency and urgency due to bladder instability has been demonstrated in 6 to 18% of patients after placement of the pubovaginal sling in the treatment of type III stress urinary incontinence.[6, 7] In our experience of 25 patients who underwent transvaginal placement of the AS-800 artificial urinary sphincter for primary urethral insufficiency, seven patients had preoperative hypotonic bladder documented on urodynamic studies. Follow-up lasted from 3 to 16 months (mean, 7.3 months). None of the patients developed clinically significant postoperative frequency or urgency. All seven patients were dry and able to void spontaneously with or without abdominal straining. Prolonged (i.e., more than 1 month) urinary retention requiring intermittent catheterization was not demonstrated by any of the patients who had hypocontractile bladders preoperatively.[8]

One major disadvantage of the artificial urinary sphincter is the risk of erosion of the device. This complication can occur if the pump erodes through the skin of the labium or the cuff erodes into the urethra or the vagina. Device erosion has been attributed to poor circulation, low-grade infection, technical difficulties, and shifting of the cuff.[4] Cuff erosion commonly occurs in patients who have undergone prior pelvic irradiation.[9] Our earlier experience included two patients who had been previously irradiated for cervical carcinoma. Both patients developed repeated cuff erosion into the vagina despite multiple revisionary operations. With the use of a low-pressure–regulating balloon (51 to 60 cm H_2O pressure), delayed primary activation of the cuff, and exclusion of the patient with prior pelvic radiotherapy, the incidence of device erosion may be much reduced.[1, 9] In the past, mechanical malfunction of the artificial urinary sphincter has been common, revision occurring in 31 to 43% of women with the device.[10, 11] However, since the introduction of the newly improved cuff design and the in situ activation-deactivation control assembly of the AS-800 model in 1983, the incidence of mechanical malfunction has dramatically decreased.[2]

Summary

The management of women with stress urinary incontinence associated with a nonmobile well-supported urethra and bladder neck is certainly a challenge to the surgeon. Many of these patients have undergone previous unsuccessful anti-incontinence operations. The artificial urinary sphincter is a viable alternative treatment modality to the urethral sling or periurethral injection therapy for these difficult patients.

The advantage of the transvaginal approach in the placement of the artificial urinary sphincter is that it offers the surgeon the ability to dissect through the difficult urethrovaginal plane under direct vision. In the patient with abundant scar tissue, the addition of a suprameatal incision reduces the likelihood of an inadvertent cystotomy or urethral injury during the anterior dissection of the urethra. With familiarization of implantation technique, the use of a low-pressure–regulating balloon reservoir (51 to 60 cm H_2O pressure), delayed primary activation of the cuff, and selective patient criteria (e.g., exclusion of patients with prior pelvic irradiation), the artificial urinary sphincter can result in reasonable long-term social continence in patients with urinary incontinence due to intrinsic urethral insufficiency. In the subgroup of patients with a combination of hypotonic bladder and intrinsic sphincteric incompetence, the artificial urinary sphincter may be the initial treatment of choice over the urethral sling because of its lower incidence of prolonged postoperative urinary retention and vesical instability.

REFERENCES

1. Appell RA: Techniques and results in the implantation of the artificial urinary sphincter in women with type III stress urinary incontinence by a vaginal approach. Neurourol Urodyn 7:613, 1988.
2. Webster GD, Perez LM, Khoury JM, et al: Management of type III stress urinary incontinence using artificial urinary sphincter. Urology 39(6):499, 1992.
3. Hadley R: Transvaginal placement of the artificial urinary sphincter in women. Neurourol Urodyn 7:292, 1988.
4. Abbassian A: A new operation for insertion of the artificial urinary sphincter. J Urol 140:512, 1988.
5. Blaivas JG, Jacobs BZ: Pubovaginal fascial sling for the treatment of complicated stress urinary incontinence. J Urol 145:1214, 1991.
6. Blaivas JG, Olsson CA: Stress incontinence: Classification and surgical approach. J Urol 139:727, 1988.
7. McGuire EJ, Bennett CJ, Konnak JA, et al: Experience with pubovaginal slings for urinary incontinence at the University of Michigan. J Urol 138:525, 1987.
8. Wang Y, Hadley HR: Artificial urinary sphincter in the female: Is it procedure of choice for the patient with type III urinary incontinence associated with an acontractile bladder? J Urol 147(4):377A, 1992.
9. Duncan HJ, Nurse DE, Mundy AR: Role of the artificial urinary sphincter in the treatment of stress incontinence in women. Br J Urol 69:141, 1992.
10. Donovan MG, Barrett DM, Furlow WL: Use of the artificial urinary sphincter in the management of severe incontinence in females. Surg Gynecol Obstet 161:17, 1985.
11. Light JK, Scott FB: Management of urinary incontinence in women with the artificial urinary sphincter. J Urol 134:476, 1985.

CHAPTER 41

Why Anti-incontinence Surgery Succeeds or Fails

David F. Penson, M.D.
Shlomo Raz, M.D.

The overall goal of any surgery for stress urinary incontinence (SUI) is to correct the anatomic and functional abnormalities of the bladder neck or urethra and to re-create conditions conducive to an effective continence mechanism. To this end, more than 100 different procedures designed to treat SUI have been described in the literature.[1] Since the first description of the Kelly plication in 1918,[2] our surgical techniques have evolved and improved as our understanding of the female anatomy and the continence mechanism has grown. There is still, however, a 5 to 15% failure rate, defined as persistent SUI, recurrent SUI, de novo detrusor instability (DI), obstructive or irritative voiding symptoms, urinary retention, or persistent postoperative pain, associated with these operations.[3-5] In this chapter, we examine the facets of a successful anti-incontinence operation and discuss how and why these procedures fail.

Mechanisms of Continence

In women, an effective urinary continence mechanism depends on a complex interaction among four factors: effective urethral closing pressure, functional urethral length, anatomic support of the bladder outlet (urethrotrigonal anatomy), and urethral and pelvic floor compensation for increased intra-abdominal pressure.

The first factor, effective urethral closing pressure, is defined as a urethral pressure that exceeds intravesical pressure, thereby preventing the flow of urine into and through the urethra. This pressure depends on a number of components, including complete urethral coaptation and tensile forces provided by the urethropelvic ligaments and levator musculature. The healthy, infolding urethral mucosa and rich submucosal vascular plexus create an effective mucosal sphincter similar to the washer of a faucet. In addition, mucous secretions contribute to the development of surface tension that further promotes complete urethral coaptation.[6] Effective urethral closing pressure is increased further by tensile forces provided by a two-layered condensation of the levator ani fascia that we call the urethropelvic ligaments. These ligaments enclose the urethra and provide compression for the proximal and midurethra (Fig. 41–1). These structures are essential in providing support for the mechanism of passive continence and also during periods of increased intra-abdominal stress. Furthermore, voluntary or reflex contractions of the levator ani or obturator musculature increase the tensile forces exerted by these ligaments and increase bladder outlet resistance.

The second factor, functional urethral length, is

URETHRAL SUPPORT

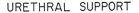

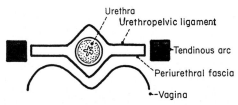

Figure 41-1 The periurethral fascia and levator ani fascia form an envelope around the urethra and are collectively termed the urethropelvic ligaments. These structures provide elastic support for the passive mechanism of continence. Furthermore, they contract during periods of increased intra-abdominal pressure and increase coaptation of the urethral wall. (Adapted from Raz S, Little NA, Juma S: Female urology. *In* Walsh PC, Retik AB, Stamey TA, Vaughan ED Jr [eds]: Campbell's Urology, 6th ed. Philadelphia, WB Saunders, 1992, pp 2782–2827.)

defined as the total length of urethra in which urethral pressure exceeds bladder pressure as measured by the urethral pressure profile. This definition is critically different from that for anatomic urethral length, which is the length of urethra from the internal to the external urethral meatus. The anatomic length of the urethra is approximately 3 to 4 cm, but the functional length is only 2.8 cm.[7] Although the importance of adequate urethral length may seem obvious, the overall contribution of functional urethral length to the mechanism of continence may be less than expected. This statement is based on the following evidence. First, many patients with shortened urethral lengths are continent.[8] Second, isolated resection of the distal third of the urethra for treatment of malignancy does not necessarily result in incontinence.[9] This implies that the distal third of the urethra serves only as a conduit for urine. Third, Y-V plasty or incision of the bladder neck does not result in incontinence in otherwise well-supported bladders.[6] Removal of the bladder neck and midurethral area together, however, will result in incontinence.[10] Although the bladder neck does provide continence, its removal or destruction does not result in incontinence because the middle third of the urethra acts as a secondary continence zone. This suggests that a certain minimal length in the midurethra is critical to the continence mechanism. Henriksson and Ulmsten showed that most patients with SUI showed little change in functional urethral length or maximal closure pressure following successful bladder neck suspension.[11] On a urethral stress profile, however, improvements in maximal closure pressure and functional urethral length were noted.[11] This indicates that the role of functional urethral length

may be to provide continence in the presence of increased intra-abdominal stress.

The third factor, anatomic support of the bladder outlet, has been well described elsewhere in this book and in the literature.[5, 6, 12, 13] In the standing position, the bladder base is maintained in the horizontal position above the level of the inferior ramus of the symphysis. When hypermobility and descent of the bladder neck are present, SUI is often noted. The internal urethral orifice is normally supported in a fixed retropubic "nondependent" position with regard to the bladder base (Fig. 41–2). This creates a valvar effect in the bladder neck.[5] This valvar effect is of particular importance in the presence of increased intra-abdominal pressure because it allows "through transmission" of this pressure to the bladder base and prevents leakage of urine through the urethra. In addition, on coughing or straining, continence is improved by further posterior rotation of the bladder, which can also lead to urethral closure.

Recent reports have indicated the importance of proper support of the midurethral complex in maintaining both passive continence and continence in the presence of increased intra-abdominal pressures.[14] We believe that the midurethral complex may play a greater role in the continence mechanism than was previously thought and that anti-incontinence surgery should be performed with this in mind.

The fourth factor, pelvic floor muscular activity in response to stress, also plays an important role in maintaining continence. When faced with a sudden increase in intra-abdominal pressure, a reflex contraction of the muscle fibers of the levator ani and obturator groups and of the urogenital diaphragm occurs in neurologically intact women that results in

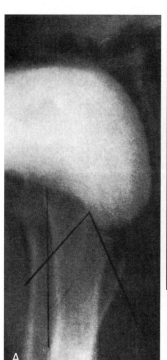
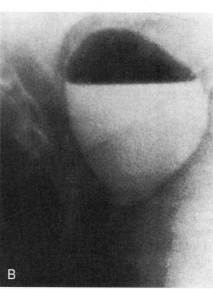

Figure 41–2 Straining cystourethrograms in normal and incontinent patients. In the normal patient *(A)*, note that the internal urethral orifice is fixed in a retropubic "nondependent" position. This allows pressure to be directed at the bladder base and creates a valvar effect. In the incontinent patient *(B)*, the internal urethral orifice is in a dependent position. This creates funneling at the bladder neck and leads to leakage of urine with straining. (From Smith RB, Ehrlich RM: Complications of Urologic Surgery, 2nd ed. Philadelphia, WB Saunders, 1990.)

closure at the level of the midurethra and increased elastic tension on the urethropelvic ligaments. This in turn leads to stabilization of the bladder neck and increased closure of the proximal urethra. In a properly supported bladder, the contracted pelvic floor acts as a "backboard," providing a stable surface for urethral compression.[6] The pelvic floor muscles also contribute to the continence mechanism through voluntary contraction, which allows the woman to voluntarily stop the urinary stream or to prevent urinary escape. Finally, the pelvic floor muscles contribute to the mechanism of continence through their basic underlying tone, like any other skeletal muscle. These muscles provide support mainly to the middle third of the urethra and are probably responsible for 30 to 50% of the closing pressure in this area.[15] This point is demonstrated when the effect of spinal anesthesia on the muscles of the pelvic floor is examined. In men, if one performs transurethral resection of the prostate (TURP) under spinal anesthesia and fills the bladder, the application of pressure to the suprapubic area leads to the leakage of urine. In the awake patient or the patient under general anesthesia without muscle relaxation, pressure on the suprapubic area does not lead to incontinence. This is true in males and females. This example illustrates the contribution of the pelvic floor musculature to the continence mechanism. The contribution of proper pelvic floor repair to the long-term outcome of antistress incontinence interventions cannot be overstated. If the patient is left with a weak pelvic floor, proper transmission of increased intravesical pressures will not occur, and less efficient urethral closure and recurrent stress urinary incontinence will ensue.

Characteristics of a Successful Anti-incontinence Operation

As mentioned earlier, most procedures designed to treat SUI attempt to restore the anatomy of the bladder neck and urethra to a position that is conducive to continence. This in turn affects the urethral function of the patient and allows transmission of increased intra-abdominal stress to areas away from the urethrovesical junction.[1] Most anti-incontinence procedures, including the Marshall-Marchetti-Krantz (MMK) procedure, the Burch colposuspension, the anterior repair procedure, and transvaginal procedures such as needle suspensions (Raz, Stamey, Gittes), attempt to elevate the bladder neck above the lowest level of the bladder base. These procedures direct any increased pressure away from the previously dependent bladder neck to the lowest point at the bladder base, creating a valvar effect at the bladder neck and preventing the leakage of urine. It is important to note that this is a dynamic effect and is active only during periods of increased intra-abdominal and intra-pelvic pressures. We can see this valvar effect in action from the fact that stress

urinary incontinence can be reproduced in more than 50% of patients following successful surgery to realign the urethrovesical junction.[4] Following a successful bladder neck suspension, elevation of the bladder base in the patient with a full bladder can lead to recurrent SUI. This occurs because the bladder neck becomes the most dependent position, and the valvar effect is therefore negated. This result confirms the fact that the major mechanism of continence in surgical procedures that elevate the bladder neck is a valvar effect. It is also important to note that the valvar effect is not obstructive in nature. In general, anti-incontinence operations do not work by causing obstruction.

The MMK procedure, the Burch colposuspension, the Raz four-corner bladder neck suspension, and most sling procedures, including the vaginal wall sling procedure that we have described elsewhere,[14] move the dependent bladder neck, trigone, and proximal urethra to a position behind the symphysis. Sling procedures, such as the vaginal wall and fascia sling, not only change the anatomic position but also create a "backboard" for the urethra. Thus, any increased intra-abdominal forces cause increased compression of the proximal urethra. This backboard effect ensures that intraurethral pressure is higher than intravesical pressures and therefore provides continence in the presence of increased intra-abdominal pressure. In effect, these operations provide a stable and strong "hammock" of urethral support (Fig. 41–3). Any changes in intra-abdominal pressure compress the urethra against this support and ensure continence.

Although the importance of the anatomic effects of these operations is without question, our experience with these procedures has led us to believe that restoration of normal anatomy is not always sufficient to produce continence. It is our belief that all patients who suffer from SUI have some degree of intrinsic sphincter dysfunction (ISD). It has been our experience using fluoroscopy that 30 to 50% of continent women have open bladder necks while straining and in the standing position. This fact implies that there are many women with anatomic abnormalities who do not suffer from SUI. There must, therefore, be a

SLING PROCEDURES

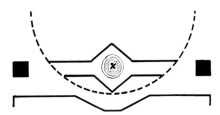

Figure 41–3   Schematic diagram of the effect of sling procedures. These operations provide stable elastic support for the urethra and create a "hammock" to improve coaptation. (From Raz S, Little NA, Juma S: Female urology. *In* Walsh PC, Retik AB, Stamey TA, Vaughn ED Jr [eds]: Campbell's Urology, 6th ed. Philadelphia, WB Saunders, 1992, pp 2782–2827.)

component of ISD in every patient with anatomic incontinence. It is important that the clinician bear in mind that SUI cannot be explained on the basis of anatomic changes alone. There are many patients, particularly among the elderly population, who suffer from incontinence but still have normal anatomy, including a well-supported urethra.

Anatomic changes are related to several factors including hysterectomy, childbirth, hormonal changes, and aging. The anatomic changes associated with SUI are often a result of childbirth. It is widely accepted that multiparous women are more likely to suffer SUI than nulliparous women.[5] If this is the case, why do most women who suffer from SUI first become symptomatic in their fifties and sixties, many years after childbirth and usually after the onset of menopause? Estrogen deficiency associated with menopause has been shown to affect urethral function by causing atrophy of the urethral seal, leading to a compromise in the coaptability of the urethra.[6, 16–19] In addition, the lack of estrogen affects anatomic support by worsening an already poor situation, causing weakness and loss of elasticity in the urethropelvic and pubourethral ligaments. All of this information again implies that some element of ISD must be present in this patient population; otherwise, they would all be incontinent immediately after childbirth when the anatomic changes described elsewhere in this book occur.

Our belief that all women who suffer from SUI have some degree of ISD has led us to support the use of the vaginal wall sling procedure for most cases of SUI. We have based this conclusion on several facts: (1) The most important segment of urethra needed for compensation against an increase in abdominal pressure is not the bladder neck. We know this from the fact that the bladder neck is often found to be open in continent women, as mentioned earlier. (2) During bladder neck suspension procedures we reposition the bladder neck in a more superior position. In so doing, we increase the valvar effect without truly affecting urethral function, thereby recreating continence in an indirect way. (3) Most discussions about the causes of SUI seem to center on bladder neck hypermobility, yet most patients suffer from a second anatomic defect, the separation of the urethra from the inferior ramus of the symphysis pubis. The increased distance between these two structures is due to a weakness of the midurethral complex (levator muscle and pubourethral ligaments). Very few surgical procedures affect this segment of the urethra. Our vaginal wall sling procedure is an attempt to modify midurethral function. In our sling we not only elevate the bladder neck but also provide support, elevation, and increased resistance in the midurethral area, which, in our view, is the most important compensatory or secondary area of continence. It is this attention to the midurethral complex that clearly distinguishes our vaginal wall sling from other sling procedures, in-

cluding those that use rectus fascia, fascia lata, and synthetic materials such as Marlex or Gore-Tex.

Why Do Anti-incontinence Operations Fail?

The goal of surgery for anatomic SUI is to reposition and support the bladder base. The goal of surgery for ISD is to provide compression and coaptation to the failed sphincteric unit. Failure of anti-incontinence surgery of either type is defined as persistent SUI, recurrent SUI, de novo detrusor instability, obstructive or irritative voiding symptoms, urinary retention, or persistent postoperative pain. These failures can occur regardless of whether the goal of the operation is achieved. The causes of failure to correct stress incontinence can be categorized into four groups: anatomic failures in general due to technical reasons (e.g., the bladder neck was not properly supported); functional failures (the bladder was properly supported but nevertheless incontinence exists); inappropriate patient selection; and failures due to postoperative complications.

ANATOMIC FAILURES DUE TO TECHNICAL REASONS

In technical failures resulting in poor anatomic support (recurrent anatomic defect), the defect was never corrected or it recurred after a period of good support. Misplacement of the suspension sutures (not at the bladder neck) can lead to symptomatic failure secondary to recurrent anatomic defect. Placement of the sutures too far distal to the bladder neck (well below the level of the urethrovesical junction or the midurethra) may result in obstructive symptoms secondary to urethral kinking. Even if the patient does not complain of obstructive symptoms, placement of the suspension sutures in this position may result in inadequate elevation of the proximal urethra and bladder neck. Although the patient may report some relief, any remaining SUI is a result of insufficient elevation of the bladder neck due to improper distal placement of the supporting sutures (Fig. 41–4). There is a similar danger in placing the suspension sutures too far laterally, away from the important periurethral tissue. By placing the sutures far away from the urethra, too much lax tissue may be left between the suture and the proximal urethra and bladder neck. This will create a situation similar to the one described previously, in which the patient may report some relief, but SUI will persist despite moderate elevation of the affected anatomy.

Another cause of technical failure is the use of poor vaginal anchoring tissue. In these cases, the sutures are placed in the right place but break from the anchor in the vaginal site. This is the most common

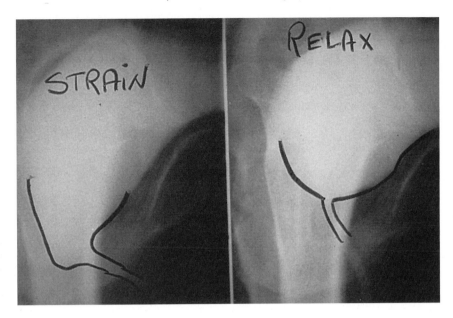

Figure 41-4 A relaxed and straining cystourethrogram in a patient following a failed bladder neck suspension. Note that there is insufficient elevation of the bladder neck on straining, leading to recurrent incontinence. (From Raz S: Atlas of Transvaginal Surgery. Philadelphia, WB Saunders, 1992.)

cause of failure. This occurs not only because of failure or breakage of the suture material but also because the intact suture pulls through the vaginal anchoring site.[20] This situation is almost always due to the inclusion of poor-quality tissue in constructing the vaginal anchor and leads to recurrence of anatomic abnormalities.

Technical failures can also result from failure of the pubic bone anchor tissue. In the case of the Burch procedure or MMK procedure, a weakened Cooper's ligament or pubic periosteum can lead to the sutures' pulling through and recurrence of anatomic abnormalities. In needle suspension procedures the sutures can pull through the abdominal wall fascia if an inadequate amount of this tissue is used. Finally, in sling procedures, the anchoring tissue used in securing the flap may be inadequate, leading to technical failure. Our experience has proved that use of the periosteum of the symphysis pubis, as in the MMK procedure, is often unreliable to maintain support of the bladder neck and proximal urethra. For this reason, it is preferable to use Cooper's ligament, as described in the Burch colposuspension, when using a suprapubic approach (Fig. 41-5). Bavendam and Leach have described using the pubic tubercle in place of the periosteum in needle suspension procedures.[21]

Another technical reason for surgical failure secondary to recurrent anatomic abnormalities is inappropriate selection of suture material. Numerous authors have supported the use of absorbable suture material, such as Dexon or Maxon, when performing anti-incontinence surgery, such as colpocystourethropexy.[22] We routinely use nonabsorbable suture material when performing these procedures. The use of absorbable suture material introduces the risk that the supporting sutures may dissolve prior to the formation of adequate scar tissue. The bladder neck and proximal urethra may then return to their previous dependent positions, resulting in recurrent SUI. We

believe that the use of cystoscopy effectively eliminates the possibility that the sutures could be intravesical and makes nonabsorbable suture material safe. Breakage of the suture material can also lead to recurrence of anatomic abnormalities. This is often caused by early mobilization and overexertion by the patient, leading to increased intra-abdominal stress and breakdown of the repair. Some patients can report the exact instant of failure, when they felt something rip or pop and then suffered recurrent SUI.[23] As a general rule, sutures should not be tied too tightly because this will lead to pain or urethral obstruction and can damage the suture material. At the same time the surgeon must not tie the suture too loosely or the knot might come undone. When

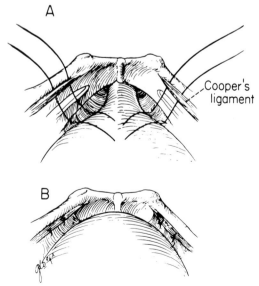

Figure 41-5 Burch colposuspension. (From Raz S, Little NA, Juma S: Female urology. In Walsh PC, Retik AB, Stamey TA, Vaughn ED Jr [eds]: Campbell's Urology, 6th ed. Philadelphia, WB Saunders, 1992, pp 2782–2827.)

placing the knot, the surgeon should bear in mind that the goal of surgery is to gently reposition the bladder neck and to provide stabilization and prevent the urethra from dropping down during periods of increased stress. There is nothing to be gained by placing unnecessary tension on the sutures.

FUNCTIONAL FAILURES

In functional failures in the presence of restored anatomy, the bladder neck is properly supported but recurrent incontinence occurs nonetheless. There are many reasons for functional failures. One cause of a functional failure is misplacement of the suspension sutures. The importance of proper placement of these sutures in all types of anti-incontinence surgery cannot be overemphasized. We always use intraoperative cystoscopic evaluation of the bladder neck to ensure proper placement of the sutures. Placement of sutures too proximally (above the level of the urethrovesical junction) will fix the bladder neck in the open position and result in worsened or continuous SUI postoperatively. Placement of the sutures too medially (close to the urethra wall itself) can result in an intense scarring reaction and can lead to the formation of a fibrotic "pipestem" urethra (Fig. 41–6). This is the most common form of failure following the MMK procedure. If the surgeon places the sutures too close to the urethral wall, the normal anatomy may be restored, but periurethral fibrosis may occur, resulting in incomplete coaptation of the urethra with subsequent ISD and continued SUI. The urethra must be able to contract properly for the continence mechanism to function correctly. Placement of suture material too close to the urethra can also lead to obstructive voiding symptoms, resulting in failure in this way as well. The urethra must shorten, funnel, and open during voiding. Periurethral fixation as described earlier will impair this function and lead to the symptoms we have just described. The use of intraoperative cystoscopy, after placement of the sutures but prior to tying them down, allows the surgeon to assess their position and ensure that they have not been placed intravesically. In addition, cystoscopy is of great importance when using nonabsorbable suture material because intravesical placement can lead to stone formation, irritative voiding symptoms, and surgical failure. If the surgeon thinks that the sutures have been placed improperly, they should be removed and replaced to ensure a successful outcome.

Failure to lyse adhesions from previous failed procedures is another reason for functional failure in the presence of restored anatomy. In patients who have undergone previous surgery, an intense periurethral fibrosis can occur, particularly if the suspension sutures have been placed immediately adjacent to the urethra, as described previously. If these adhesions are not lysed, the urethra will remain fixed in a dependent position, resulting in continued SUI. We think that it is important for the surgeon to lyse all retropubic adhesions and detach the urethropelvic ligament from its pubic attachments. Failure to do this may prevent optimal restoration of the bladder neck and proximal urethra to a more superior position. With lysing the inferolateral fixation applied by this structure secondary to its insertion on the tendinous arch of the obturator fascia is removed, and the suspension sutures are able to draw the urethra more superiorly, resulting in better postoperative continence.

The presence of persistent SUI in the presence of a well-supported urethra postoperatively is usually indicative of some degree of ISD. This is often secondary to postoperative atrophy of the urethral mucosa and the spongy tissue of the submucosa. ISD leads to inadequate coaptation of the urethra despite good apposition of the muscular layer and is the most common cause of functional failure. One could compare this situation to that of a new faucet with a bad washer. You can apply unlimited pressure, but the faucet will still leak if the washer is faulty and does not create a good seal. If one changes the washer, however, only minimal pressure is required to stop the leak. ISD is the main indication for the use of injectables. They increase the bulk of the inner urethral layer (mucosal sphincter), thereby improving continence.

When a patient presents with persistent incontinence despite restoration of normal anatomy, the surgeon should also consider the possibility of iatrogenic vesicovaginal or urethrovaginal fistula. A voiding cystourethrogram is helpful in confirming this diagnosis.

INAPPROPRIATE PATIENT SELECTION

The proper selection of patients cannot be stressed enough. A complete history and physical examination, cystography, and cystoscopy can provide the surgeon with invaluable information about the type of SUI that is present and help guide the choice of surgical procedure. The main diagnostic task is to separate stress incontinence due to sphincter incompetence from bladder instability. Often the difference is not clear despite a good history, physical examination, and urodynamic evaluation. A full videourodynamic work-up is particularly helpful in more complicated cases when the initial evaluation is not adequate. The surgeon must determine if the cause of the patient's incontinence stems from anatomic incontinence, ISD, or a combination of these causes. Patients with stress incontinence due to hypermobility of the bladder neck and proximal urethra (anatomic incontinence) can expect an 80 to 90% rate of cure from surgery that restores the bladder neck to a high anatomic position.[5, 20] In a patient who suffers from ISD, however, an operation designed to restore normal anatomy alone is of minimal value.[24] Patients with ISD often have a history of multiple operations, both abdominal and vaginal, resulting in periurethral fibrosis and a pipestem urethra.[3] This patient

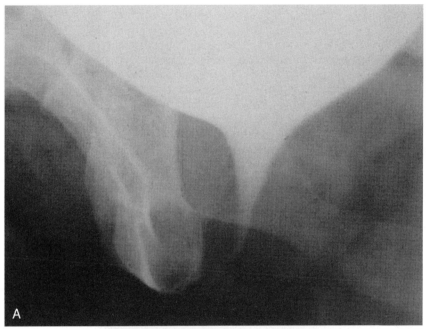

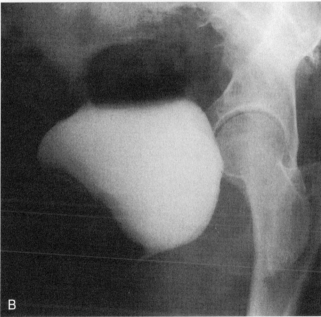

Figure 41-6 *A* and *B*, Standing cystourethrograms in two patients following multiple failed anti-incontinence procedures. Note that both patients have adequate anatomic support. In both cases, however, the urethra is in a fixed and open position, leading to recurrent severe type III stress incontinence. (*A* from Raz S: Atlas of Transvaginal Surgery. Philadelphia, WB Saunders, 1992; *B* from Smith RB, Ehrlich RM: Complications of Urologic Surgery, 2nd ed. Philadelphia, WB Saunders, 1990.)

population can expect a similar cure rate (95%) with the use of injectables such as collagen or a sling procedure (fascial, Gore-Tex, or vaginal wall).[14] It is therefore inappropriate to perform bladder neck suspension in a patient with isolated ISD.

Patients often present with a combination of symptoms, including frequency and urgency, in addition to genuine stress incontinence. Further evaluation often reveals a wide-open posterior urethra when the patient is in the standing position. This dilatation of the urethra leads to a constant sensation of impending micturition. A complete history usually reveals that the patient's symptoms of urgency and frequency are positional in nature and improve when the patient is supine. Vesicourethral suspension not only cures the patient's SUI but also relieves the

patient's symptoms of urgency, frequency, and urge incontinence in at least 50% of cases.[25, 26] In contrast to this is the patient who presents with stress-induced detrusor instability. In these cases, a sudden increase in intra-abdominal pressure will trigger a detrusor contraction, simulating SUI. Urodynamic evaluation allows the surgeon to differentiate between bladder hyperreflexia and anatomic incontinence with associated urgency and frequency. Patients suffering from bladder hyperreflexia predominantly are usually not surgical candidates and will benefit from medical therapy.

There are many other conditions that cause or may be confused with SUI that may lead to improper selection of patients for anti-incontinence surgery. These include urethral diverticula, ureteral ectopia, and bladder calculi. Furthermore, overflow incontinence secondary to a neurologic deficit can easily be mistaken for SUI, leading to inappropriate intervention and surgical failure. A complete preoperative evaluation, including a thorough history, physical examination, and videourodynamics and cystoscopy, when indicated, will identify these entities and is absolutely essential to determine the true nature of the patient's stress incontinence and to guide the choice of surgical technique.

POSTOPERATIVE COMPLICATIONS

Finally, anti-incontinence surgery can fail because of postoperative complications resulting in new symptoms such as obstruction or de novo instability. Although these topics are discussed at greater length elsewhere in this book, a few words are indicated here. Postoperative urinary retention is most commonly due to placement of the suspension sutures too far distally or too close to the urethra, resulting in scarring. If the sutures are inadvertently placed intraurethrally, they can result in stone formation and obstruction as well. Obstructive symptoms can also be caused by pelvic hematoma. Most cases are temporary and can be managed by self-intermittent catheterization if a suprapubic catheter is not present. If the problem persists for an extended period of time, reoperation and urethrolysis are indicated and have been shown to produce good results in 71% of cases.[27]

De novo bladder instability is a well-known complication of anti-incontinence surgery. Most often, symptoms were present preoperatively and became more pronounced in the postoperative period. These are often temporary and resolve over time. There are patients who develop new-onset bladder instability causing them to be classed as surgical failures. The cause of this is unclear, and the treatment is medical in nature. In isolated cases, augmentation cystoplasty can be considered.

REFERENCES

1. Stanton SL: Stress incontinence: Why and how operations work. Clin Obstet Gynecol 12(2):369, 1985.
2. Kelly HA: Incontinence of urine in women. Urol Cutan Rev 17:291, 1918.
3. Raz S, Maggio AL, Kaufman JJ: Why Marshall-Marchetti operation works . . . or does not. Urology 14(2):154, 1979.
4. Stanton SL, Tanagho EA (eds): Surgery of Female Incontinence, 2nd ed. New York, Springer-Verlag, 1986, chaps. 3, 5.
5. Raz S, Little NA, Juma S: Female urology. In Walsh PC, Retik AB, Stamey TA, Vaughan ED Jr. (eds): Campbell's Urology, 6th ed, vol 3. Philadelphia, WB Saunders, 1992, pp 2782–2827.
6. Staskin DR, Zimmeren PE, Hadley HR, Raz S: The pathophysiology of stress incontinence. Urol Clin North Am 12(2):271, 1985.
7. Siegel AL, Raz S: Surgical treatment of anatomical stress incontinence. Neurourol Urodyn 7:569, 1988.
8. Kjolhede P, Ryden G: Prognostic factors and long-term results of the Burch colposuspension. A retrospective study. Acta Obstet Gynecol Scand 73(8):642, 1994.
9. Reid GC, DeLancey JO, Hopkins MP, et al: Urinary incontinence following radical vulvectomy. Obstet Gynecol 75(5):852, 1990.
10. Myers RP: Practical pelvic anatomy pertinent to radical retropubic prostatectomy. AUA Update Series, 13(4):25, 1994.
11. Henriksson L, Ulmsten U: A urodynamic evaluation of the effects of abdominal urethrocystopexy and vaginal sling urethroplasty in women with stress incontinence. Am J Obstet Gynecol 113:78, 1978.
12. Delancey JL: Anatomy and embryology of the lower urinary tract. Obstet Gynecol Clin North Am 16:717, 1989.
13. Raz S: Atlas of Transvaginal Surgery. Philadelphia, WB Saunders, 1992, pp 1–23.
14. Young GPH, Wahle GR, Raz S: Modified vaginal wall sling. Presented at the Eighty-Ninth Annual Meeting of the American Urological Association, San Francisco, California, 1994.
15. Klutke C, Golomb J, Barbaric Z, Raz S: The anatomy of stress incontinence: Magnetic resonance imaging of the female bladder neck and urethra. J Urol 143(3):607, 1990.
16. Caine M, Raz S: The role of female hormones in stress incontinence. Communication to the 16th Congress of the International Society of Urology, Amsterdam, 1973.
17. Faber P, Heidenreich J: Treatment of stress incontinence with estrogen in postmenopausal women. Urol Int 32:221, 1977.
18. Smith PCM: Age changes in the female urethra. Br J Urol 44:667, 1972.
19. Tulloch AGS: The vascular contribution to intraurethral pressure. Br J Urol 46:659, 1974.
20. Wahle GR, Young GPH, Raz S: Vaginal surgery for stress urinary incontinence. Urology 43(4):416, 1994.
21. Bavendam TG, Leach GE: Urogynecologic reconstruction. Probl Urol 1(2):295, 1987.
22. Tanagho EA: Colpocystourethropexy. AUA Update Series, 12(27):210, 1993.
23. Wall LL, Norton PA, Delancey JOL: Practical Urogynecology. Baltimore, Williams & Wilkins, 1993.
24. McGuire EJ, Appell RA: Transurethral collagen injection for urinary incontinence. Urology 43(40):416, 1994.
25. Stamey TA, Schaeffer AJ, Condy M: Clinical and roentgenographic evaluation of endoscopic suspension of the vesical neck for urinary incontinence. Surg Gynecol Obstet 140:355, 1975.
26. McGuire EJ, Lytton B, Kollorn EI, Pepe V: The value of urodynamic testing in stress urinary incontinence. J Urol 124:256, 1980.
27. Nitti VW, Raz S: Obstruction following anti-incontinence procedures: Diagnosis and treatment with transvaginal urethrolysis. J Urol 152:93, 1994.

Pelvic Prolapse

CHAPTER 42

Pelvic Floor Relaxation

Joseph W. Babiarz, M.D.
Shlomo Raz, M.D.

Patients presenting with urinary incontinence frequently have complaints or findings of coincidental pelvic prolapse. The combination of rectocele, weakness of the levator ani, loss of the normal near-horizontal vaginal axis, and damage to the perineal body is termed pelvic floor relaxation. A clear understanding of the anatomy, pathophysiology, and repair of pelvic floor weakness will assist the surgeon performing anti-incontinence surgery because attention to anterior prolapse without attention to the pelvic floor predisposes to an increased occurrence of postoperative enterocele, uterine prolapse, and rectocele. Secondarily, coincidental repair of pelvic floor weakness may improve pressure transmission to the proximal urethra, thereby improving results of anti-incontinence surgery. Complete restoration of the normal anatomic relationships of the vagina and pelvic organs by simultaneous repair of anterior and posterior vaginal wall weakness should be the goal of all vaginal reconstructive surgery. Genitourinary surgeons who do not feel comfortable in performing these repairs should invite their gynecologic colleagues to assist them in obtaining this goal.

Anatomy

Female pelvic anatomy has previously been described but will be reviewed here because an understanding of the pelvic floor support system and its fascial relationships is paramount for an understanding of the pathophysiology and treatment of pelvic floor relaxation. Bonney[1] was the first to describe the importance of both the suspensory apparatus and the lower support system in preventing pelvic organ prolapse. Attenuation of the suspensory apparatus is manifest as uterine prolapse and is considered separately. Weakness of the lower support system or pelvic floor is manifest as rectocele and perineal weakness, and its occurrence may facilitate prolapse of the vagina or small bowel. The pelvic floor consists of two separate layers, the pelvic diaphragm and the urogenital (UG) diaphragm and the investing fascia of the rectum and posterior wall of the vagina.

PELVIC DIAPHRAGM

The pelvic diaphragm is the superior shelf of the lower support system and can be divided into the levator ani and the coccygeus muscles and their fasciae. The levator ani with its component parts, the pubococcygeus, iliococcygeus, and ischiococcygeus, forms a broad plate beneath the urethra, bladder, vagina, and rectum. These muscles take origin from the posterior pubis, the tendinous arch of the obturator, and the ischial spine and sweep posteriorly behind the rectum to unite with their mates on the opposite side, forming a broad horizontal plate on which the rectum and subsequently the vagina lie. In the central portion of this muscular plate there is a central hiatus through which pass the urethra, vagina, and rectum. This rectal-genital hiatus represents the weak point of the pelvic diaphragm through which the pelvic organs may herniate. Some muscle fibers of the levator ani and the investing fascia unite anterior to the rectum between the rectum and the vagina and are called the prerectal fibers of the levator ani[2, 3] (Fig. 42–1). They are important in maintaining a narrow levator hiatus. Bustami has noted the attachment of the anterior portion of the levator ani to the central tendon of the UG diaphragm, which serves as the central insertion point of the entire pelvic support system.[4] This connection also serves to maintain a narrow hiatus.

UROGENITAL DIAPHRAGM

The urogenital diaphragm forms the second layer of pelvic floor support and consists of the bulbocaverno-

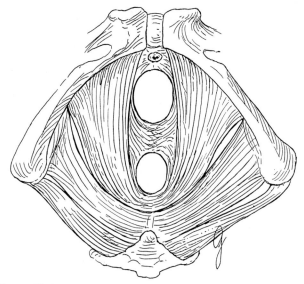

Figure 42-1 The pelvic diaphragm consisting of the levator ani and the coccygeus muscles and their investing fascia. In the central portion is the levator hiatus, an area of relative weakness. Between the rectum and the vagina are the important prerectal fibers of the levator ani, which help to maintain a narrow hiatus that resists prolapse of pelvic organs. (From Raz S, Little NA, Juma S: Female urology. *In* Walsh PC, Retik AB, Stamey TA, Vaughan ED Jr [eds]: Campbell's Urology, 6th ed. Philadelphia, WB Saunders, 1992, pp 2782–2828.)

sus, superficial and deep transverse perinei, and external anal sphincter muscles. These muscles join together with the anterior fibers of the levator ani to form the pyramidal central tendon of the perineum (Fig. 42–2). This structure has a posteriorly oriented base, supports the distal portion of the vagina, and is of great importance in repair of the pelvic floor because it forms the central fixation point for the entire pelvic support system. The UG diaphragm, reinforced by the superior and inferior perineal fas-

cia, fills the space between the pubic rami and reinforces the pelvic diaphragm at its weakest point. In the erect position the UG diaphragm is horizontal and aids in support of the urethra, which rests on it.[5]

FASCIA

The vagina is separated from the rectum by a fibromuscular extension of the peritoneum extending from the pouch of Douglas to the central tendon.[6] This structure, called the rectovaginal septum or prerectal fascia, prevents protrusion of the rectum into the vagina. The anterior surface of the prerectal fascia fuses with the posterior vaginal wall, while posterior to the prerectal fascia is a potential space, the rectovaginal space, which offers a convenient plane of dissection in repair of the rectocele component of pelvic floor weakness.

A second layer of fascia of the posterior pelvic compartment consists of the pararectal fascia, rectal pillars, or lateral rectal ligament, which represents the fibromuscular tissue accompanying the blood vessels, nerves, and lymphatics that supply the rectum. This fascia takes origin from the lateral pelvic sidewall and sweeps posteromedially to the rectum, where it splits into the anterior and posterior sheets forming a fibrous capsule for the rectum. The pararectal fascia and the fibrous capsule surrounding the rectum together form the perirectal fascia.[7, 8] Use of these layers further strengthens repair of a rectocele. Anteromedial to the pararectal fascia is the rectovaginal space, and posterior to it is the pararectal space (Fig. 42–3).

VAGINAL AXIS

In the well-supported erect woman two vaginal angles can be described. The distal vagina forms an

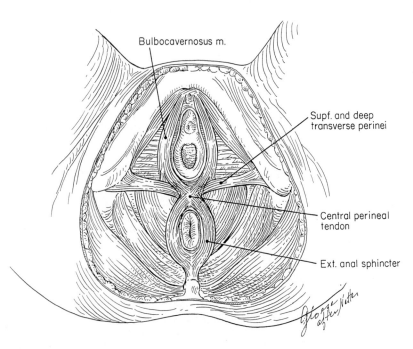

Bulbocavernosus m.

Supf. and deep transverse perinei

Central perineal tendon

Ext. anal sphincter

Figure 42-2 The urogenital diaphragm, consisting of the bulbocavernosus, superficial and deep transverse perinei, and external anal sphincter muscles and their investing fasciae, provides the second layer of pelvic support and is anchored in the middle by the central perineal tendon. (From Raz S, Little NA, Juma S: Female urology. *In* Walsh PC, Retik AB, Stamey TA, Vaughan ED Jr [eds]: Campbell's Urology, 6th ed. Philadelphia, WB Saunders, 1992, pp 2782–2828.)

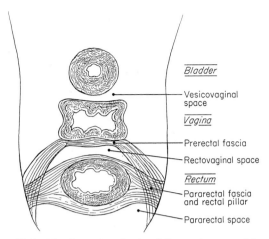

Figure 42-3 The investing fascia of the rectum consists of the prerectal fascia, which runs anterior to the rectum from the cul-de-sac to the central tendon and forms the anterior border of the rectovaginal space. The pararectal fascia or rectal pillars sweep medially from the pelvic side wall to surround the rectum in a fibromuscular envelope, called the perirectal fascia. Posterior and lateral to the pararectal fascia is the pararectal space.

angle of 45 degrees from the vertical. More proximally, the vagina lies in a near-horizontal position on top of the rectum and horizontal levator plate (Fig. 42–4), forming a midvaginal angle of 110 to 130 degrees.[9–12] The upper vagina is held over the levator plate by the cardinal and uterosacral ligaments, while the angle is maintained by a strong horizontal levator plate and the anterior pull of the levator sling including the prerectal fibers. This horizontal proximal vaginal position is of paramount importance in preventing pelvic prolapse, and its restoration is critical during repair of the pelvic floor.

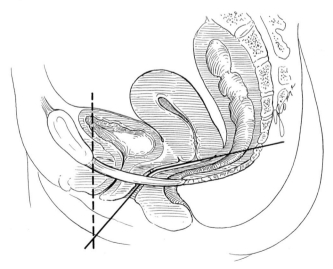

Figure 42-4 Lateral view of the pelvis. The distal vagina forms an angle of 45 degrees from the vertical. The proximal half of the vagina lies on top of the nearly horizontal levator plate and rectum, forming an angle of 110 degrees from the distal vagina. (From Raz S, Little NA, Juma S: Female urology. *In* Walsh PC, Retik AB, Stamey TA, Vaughan ED Jr [eds]: Campbell's Urology, 6th ed. Philadelphia, WB Saunders, 1992, pp 2782–2828.)

Normal Physiology and the Pathophysiology of Pelvic Floor Weakness

In the well-supported upright position, bulging of the rectum into the posterior vaginal wall is prevented by strong prerectal and perirectal fasciae. The levator plate has not been weakened and maintains a broad horizontal plate on which rest the rectum and consequently the proximal vagina. With increases in intra-abdominal pressure, two important compensation mechanisms occur. First, the levator muscle contracts reflexly, pulling the midvagina forward while forcing the proximal vagina more posteriorly, both of which actions increase the midvaginal angle and resist pelvic organ prolapse. Second, the reflex contraction of the levator ani and muscles of the UG diaphragm narrow the anogenital hiatus in the levator muscle and vaginal introitus, closing the opening through which prolapse may occur.[13, 14]

With childbirth, several events weaken the pelvic floor support system. Changes wrought by childbirth are further enhanced by aging, loss of estrogen stimulation, strenuous work, and chronic abdominal straining. First, with passage of the child's head through the birth canal there is stretching of the prerectal and perirectal fasciae as well as detachment of the prerectal fascia from the perineal body, leading to the formation of a rectocele.[15] Midvaginal and high rectoceles tend to push the vagina forward, altering the normal near-horizontal vaginal axis. Second, childbirth damages and weakens the levator musculature and its fascia, especially the decussating prerectal levator fibers and the attachment of the levator ani to the central tendon, which allows the levator hiatus to widen (Fig. 42–5). This combination causes sagging of the levator plate (Fig. 42–6) and loss of the normal horizontal vaginal axis[14] (Fig. 42–7). The result is a tendency for the pelvic organs to slide downward along the new vaginal axis.[11] Furthermore, the loss of the horizontal vaginal axis exposes the pouch of Douglas to the forces of increased intra-abdominal pressure, facilitating enterocele formation. Third, with widening of the anogenital hiatus and damage to the UG diaphragm and central tendon, the normal compensatory narrowing of the vaginal opening is rendered ineffective, further facilitating prolapse.

Correction of anterior prolapse and bladder neck hypermobility by suspension of the bladder neck without paying attention to pelvic floor weakness may further alter the vaginal axis as the vagina is pulled forward by the anterior repair. This predisposes the patient to a high incidence of subsequent uterine prolapse, enterocele, and rectocele formation. Indeed, this result has been recognized by several authors, who have reported an incidence of pelvic prolapse after anti-incontinence surgery alone of 12 to 26%.[16–18] Therefore, the degree of posterior pelvic floor weakness must be assessed in all patients being

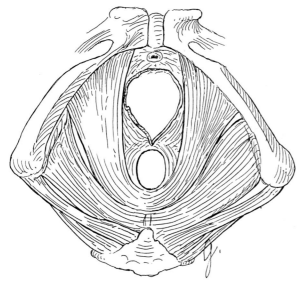

Figure 42–5 Attenuation of the prerectal fibers of the levator by trauma during childbirth leads to widening of the levator hiatus. (From Raz S, Little NA, Juma S: Female urology. *In* Walsh PC, Retik AB, Stamey TA, Vaughan ED Jr [eds]: Campbell's Urology, 6th ed. Philadelphia, WB Saunders, 1992, pp 2782–2828.)

considered for anti-incontinence surgery or repair of anterior prolapse.

In summary, then, the critical changes that occur with pelvic floor weakness are formation of a recto-

cele, loss of normal horizontal axis of the levator plate and vagina, and weakness of the UG and pelvic diaphrams. Each of these must therefore be addressed in repair of the pelvic floor, which is more than a simple rectocele repair.

Classification and Prevalence

Classification of pelvic floor weakness relies on a physical assessment of the degree of rectocele and perineal tear. A saccular protrusion of the posterior rectal wall at the level of the hymenal ring with depression of the perineum is termed grade I. Protrusion at the level of the hiatus is termed grade II, and protrusion beyond the introitus is termed grade III.[19] Perineal tears are graded on a basis of I to IV as follows: I, a tear in the hymenal ring; II, a tear involving the perineal body but not the anal sphincter; III, a tear involving the anal sphincter; IV, a tear extending into the anal mucosa.[20]

Rectoceles may also be classified according to their position in the vagina as low, medium, or high. Low rectoceles generally result from obstetric forces that disrupt the attachment of the prerectal fascia and levator musculature from the central tendon and also from damage to the central tendon. Midvaginal rectoceles arise from attenuation and stretching of the perirectal and prerectal fasciae and are most common. High rectoceles are often associated with enteroceles because the enterocele weakens the upper portion of the rectovaginal septum or prerectal fascia, which is a continuation of the peritoneum from the Pouch of Douglas. When one of these is present, the other must always be sought and corrected if found.

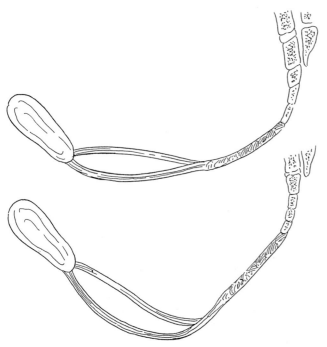

Figure 42–6 The normal levator plate lies in a near-horizontal plane with a narrow hiatus that provides a shelf for support of the pelvic organs. Trauma to the levator plate causes laxity and widening of the levator hiatus, leading to a downward sloping plate. The pelvic organs tend to slide downward through the widened hiatus. (From Raz S, Little NA, Juma S: Female urology. *In* Walsh PC, Retik AB, Stamey TA, Vaughan ED Jr [eds]: Campbell's Urology, 6th ed. Philadelphia, WB Saunders, 1992, pp 2782–2828.)

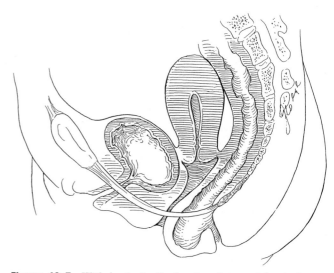

Figure 42–7 With laxity in the levator plate and forward pressure of the rectocele, the vaginal axis assumes a near-vertical position that facilitates the downward prolapse of the pelvic organs. Failure to correct the vaginal axis and rectocele at the time of anti-incontinence surgery leads to a predisposition to symptomatic postoperative prolapse.

The prevalence of rectocele is variable depending on the population studied. Clearly, there is a high incidence of rectocele in asymptomatic patients. However, the true incidence is unknown. In patients complaining of urinary incontinence Wells and colleagues found an incidence of rectocele of 12% on physical examination.[21] In patients found to have stress urinary incontinence Raz and colleagues found that a higher percentage of patients had a rectocele and also that the incidence increased with the degree of associated prolapse.[22, 23] For example, the authors repaired rectoceles or enteroceles in 35% of patients undergoing a Raz bladder neck suspension with no cystocele or a grade I cystocele, but they repaired a rectocele in 65% of patients who were undergoing repair of a grade IV cystocele.[22, 23]

Evaluation

HISTORY

Many symptoms are attributed to rectoceles, but few studies have correlated surgical correction with symptomatic relief. For example, constipation is often attributed to rectoceles, although defecation is a complex process in which any number of abnormalities can contribute to the symptom of constipation. Arnold and colleagues recently reviewed the results of 64 rectocele repairs for the primary complaint of constipation; 54% of patients reported persistent constipation postoperatively.[24] Complaints that do seem to correlate with rectocele include sufficient difficulty in evacuating stool to require digitalization of the vagina to facilitate stool passage, a feeling of blockage at the outlet or a sensation of stool pocketing,[25] and symptoms attributable to prolapse including the feeling of a "bulge" or "sitting on a ball." Although in general these symptoms tend to occur primarily in patients with moderate or large rectoceles,[26] size does not always correlate with symptoms. Caps reported that of 51 patients with a symptomatic rectocele, 8% had a mild rectocele.[27] Additionally, vaginal outlet laxity may contribute to coital dissatisfaction, but one must keep in mind the complexity of this problem and realize that most problems are secondary to psychosocial causes and not pelvic floor weakness.

PHYSICAL EXAMINATION

In any patient being examined for correction of incontinence or pelvic prolapse, an assessment of the posterior compartment must be included. Assessment of the posterior compartment includes evaluation for enterocele, rectocele, and perineal weakness, which is best accomplished using half of the vaginal speculum to displace the anterior vaginal wall anteriorly to allow visualization of the posterior vaginal wall. Rectocele and perineal weakness are graded as pre-

viously described. The vaginal axis is assessed by digital examination of the vagina. In a nulliparous patient with a well-supported pelvic floor, the examiner will note a definite posterior curvature of the proximal vagina, whereas in a patient with pelvic floor weakness the vagina will appear straight when the patient is examined in the lithotomy position. Bimanual examination with a finger in the vagina and rectum is necessary to rule out coincidental enterocele, which should always be suspected in a patient with a high rectocele. Finally, it is important to perform any evaluation for rectocele and pelvic floor weakness prior to anesthetizing the patient because virtually all patients manifest weakness under anesthesia.

RADIOGRAPHIC EVALUATION

Evaluation of a plain upright pelvic radiograph such as that obtained at the start of a voiding cystourethrogram (VCUG) frequently demonstrates gas more than 3 to 4 cm below the pubococcygeal line. This suggests the presence of a rectocele, an enterocele, or both and should be searched for in all patients undergoing VCUG.

Proctography is a second means of assessing a patient for rectocele but when used alone has not proved superior to physical examination in diagnosing rectocele.[26] However, the addition of colpography to proctography may prove valuable in assessing the degree of alteration in the vaginal axis, thereby assisting in the assessment of pelvic floor weakness (Fig. 42–8B). Colpography can be accomplished by injecting a low-pH vaginal gel (Aci-Jel, Ortho Pharmaceutical Canada, Don Mills, Ontario, Canada) and a high-density, water-soluble contrast medium (Hypaque 75 or Omnipaque 350, Winthrop Diagnostic Imaging, Aurora, Ontario, Canada) in a 50:50 mixture.[28] This technique can easily be combined with voiding cystourethrography during a videourodynamic evaluation to yield a complete assessment of the anterior, middle, and posterior compartments.

Evacuation proctography, or defecography, is being used more frequently to assess patients with abnormalities of defecation. It is hoped that this technique will help to select patients with defecation difficulties who will benefit from rectocele repair. Results to date have been less than optimal. For example, Kelvin and colleagues found no correlation between the degree of barium trapping and the need for vaginal digitalization with defecation.[26] Furthermore, Freimanis and associates found that 67% of asymptomatic patients had an abnormal evacuation proctogram and that there was no difference in the frequency of rectocele in patients with more than 40% barium trapping and those with less than 40% barium trapping.[29] Additionally, Yoshioka and colleagues also measured resting anal pressures, rectal pressures, and rectal compliance and found no difference between controls and patients with rectoceles,

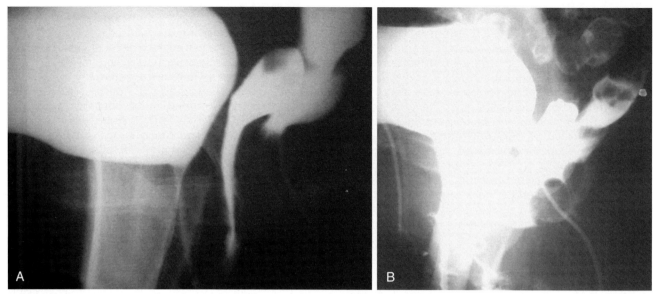

Figure 42-8 *A,* Normal vaginal axis on colpography showing the proximal vaginal axis in the near-horizontal plane. The rectum is poorly filled. *B,* With a moderate rectocele and weakness in the levator plate, the vaginal axis is now nearly vertical.

either symptomatic or asymptomatic.[30] Thus it would appear that further studies of evacuation proctography are needed to define the physiologic correlates of a symptomatic rectocele.

Recently, a group of patients with pelvic prolapse were studied using fast dynamic magnetic resonance imaging (MRI) with graded abdominal straining.[31] The authors studied a group of controls to define the limits of normal descent in the anterior, middle, and posterior compartments and then used these normal values for comparison with patients with pelvic prolapse. This technique appeared to be most helpful in delineating enteroceles that were not noted on physical examination. It is likely that these enteroceles would have been discovered at the time of vaginal reconstruction on opening the vaginal vault or posterior vaginal wall, and it is unclear how much beneficial information is obtained compared with standard evaluations. This technique, however, is noninvasive and allows simultaneous assessment of all three compartments. Unfortunately, it assesses patients in a supine position, whereas prolapse is a disease of the upright position and at this time does not allow simultaneous urodynamic evaluation. Further studies will help to define the role of this technique in assessing pelvic floor weakness, and it will certainly be important in helping us understand the pathophysiology of pelvic floor weakness and changes that occur after repair.

Indications for Repair

Clearly, patients with symptomatic pelvic floor weakness manifested by difficult evacuation or bothersome prolapse should undergo surgical correction. More controversial is the indication for repair of asymptomatic pelvic floor weakness coincident with anti-incontinence surgery, correction of anterior prolapse, or vaginal hysterectomy. Opponents argue that patients risk a high incidence of postoperative dyspareunia or complete loss of coital function. Indeed, Jeffcoate has described a 30% rate of discontinued coitus or dyspareunia in patients undergoing simultaneous anterior and posterior repair.[32] Coital difficulties resulted from overnarrowing of the vaginal introitus and senile contracture of the vagina. However, Jeffcoate's survey of patients was done during a period when posterior repair relied on nonanatomic suturing together of the entire levator plate between the vagina and the rectum, resulting in overnarrowing of the vagina and a painful vaginal ridge.[33] More recent surveys have found dyspareunia in 0 to 9% of patients undergoing anterior and posterior repairs.[33-35] In Haase and Skibsted's review there was a 9% incidence of dyspareunia, but an equal number of patients experienced improvement in sex life. Modern series, then, tend to lessen the strength of this argument, especially if patients are counseled to resume coitus early at 3 to 6 weeks postoperatively. Although rectal injury is a concern, we have found none in our recent review.[36]

On the other hand, proponents argue that leaving a lax pelvic floor unrepaired when repairing anterior prolapse or incontinence or performing a vaginal hysterectomy leaves a portion of the vaginal hernia unrepaired, exposing it to increased forces and resulting in even faster enlargement.[37] In addition, repair of the pelvic floor deficit will restore the normal near-horizontal axis and therefore decrease the likelihood of postoperative prolapse, especially after anti-incontinence surgery, which further orients the vagina in a vertical axis. In correcting even asymptomatic grade II and III rectoceles we have found an incidence of postoperative rectocele, enterocele, or uterine prolapse of 7.4% in patients undergoing Raz bladder neck suspension in combination with repair of grade I to IV cystoceles with a mean follow-up of 18 months,[38] substantially less than other series not including coincidental correction of pelvic floor weakness.[16–18]

Finally, because the urethra and bladder neck are secondarily supported by the pelvic floor it can be argued that repair of the lax pelvic floor will improve the results of anti-incontinence surgery by providing a backboard against which the urethra and bladder neck can be compressed. Because no randomized study comparing the results of anti-incontinence surgery with and without coincidental pelvic floor repair has been undertaken, this will remain a theoretical advantage only.

We strongly favor simultaneous repair of even asymptomatic moderate or severe pelvic floor weakness with anti-incontinence surgery because it restores the normal anatomic vaginal axis, resists postoperative occurrence of pelvic prolapse, and may improve the results of anti-incontinence surgery without introducing significant complications such as dyspareunia, rectal injury, or rectovaginal fistula.

Technique of Repair

The essential goals of pelvic floor reconstruction include reduction of the rectocele by plication of the prerectal and perirectal fasciae, narrowing of the levator hiatus by reapproximation of the prerectal levator fibers, and repair of the urogenital diaphragm (Fig. 42–9). Reduction of the rectocele and reconstruction of the prerectal levator fibers in the distal vagina restore the normal horizontal levator plate and vaginal axis. Three nights and two nights prior to surgery the patient takes a laxative such as bisacodyl. The patient begins a clear liquid diet 48 hours prior to surgery and receives cleansing tap water enemas on admission along with broad-spectrum intravenous antibiotics to cover anaerobes, gram-negative bacilli, and group D enterococcus.

The patient is placed in a lithotomy position, and vaginal and perineal preparation are accomplished. A Betadine-soaked rectal packing is placed to aid in identification of the rectum and to avoid rectal injury. The patient is then draped, the labia are retracted laterally with stay sutures, and a Foley catheter is placed. Anti-incontinence surgery, repair of cystocele, vaginal hysterectomy, and enterocele repair are accomplished first. Attention is then turned to repair of the posterior pelvic floor weakness.

The procedure is simplified by use of a Scott retractor. Upward retraction of the anterior vaginal wall will improve visualization and help prevent overnarrowing of the vagina. The repair begins with the placement of two Allis clamps on the posterior margin of the introitus such that when the clamps are brought together the introitus will easily admit two fingers. A triangular segment of the mucocutaneous junction is then excised between the Allis clamps, exposing the attenuated perineal body (Fig. 42–10). The Allis clamps are used to grasp the rectocele at its midpoint and elevate it. Saline is injected in the posterior vaginal wall. A triangular incision in the posterior vaginal wall is made with the base of the triangle at the site of the previous incision and the apex at the apex of the rectocele (Fig. 42–11).

Sharp dissection from the lateral margin of the triangle exposes the prerectal fibers of the levator in the distal third of the vagina. Proximally, the dissection enters the rectovaginal space (Fig. 42–12) to expose the perirectal fascia and prerectal fascia, which are attenuated or absent medially but present laterally. It is imperative that the dissection go beyond the apex of the rectocele to ensure an adequate

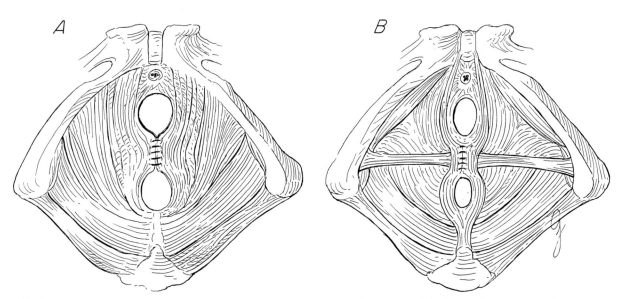

Figure 42-9 The goals of pelvic floor repair are reduction of the rectocele, narrowing of the levator hiatus *(A),* and reconstruction of the urogenital diaphragm *(B).* (From Raz S, Little NA, Juma S: Female urology. *In* Walsh PC, Retik AB, Stamey TA, Vaughan ED Jr [eds]: Campbell's Urology, 6th ed. Philadelphia, WB Saunders, 1992, pp 2782–2828.)

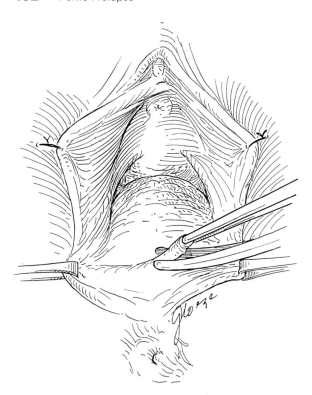

Figure 42–10 Pelvic floor repair begins with the excision of a triangle of skin at the junction of the posterior vaginal wall and perineal skin. With reconstruction, the introitus should easily admit two to three fingers. (From Raz S, Little NA, Juma S: Female urology. *In* Walsh PC, Retik AB, Stamey TA, Vaughan ED Jr [eds]: Campbell's Urology, 6th ed. Philadelphia, WB Saunders, 1992, pp 2782–2828.)

repair. As previously mentioned, one must always actively search for an enterocele that can be repaired at the same time. At this point, the remaining triangular island of posterior vaginal wall is sharply dissected off the prerectal levator fascia and fibers and is discarded (Fig. 42–13).

Repair of the rectocele is then accomplished. The rectum is protected by downward and contralateral retraction while the sutures are placed. The first suture, generally placed at the apex of the vagina, commonly incorporates the uterosacral ligaments and the prerectal and perirectal fasciae. The repair is carried out to the distal third of the vagina using a running locking 2–0 polyglycolic acid suture that incorporates the vaginal wall and prerectal and perirectal fasciae in a single bite (Fig. 42–14). This suture is tied at the level of the levator hiatus. A second short running locking or figure-of-eight suture of 2–0 polyglycolic acid is used to close the distal third of the posterior vaginal wall to the level of the perineal incision; it incorporates the same layers described earlier and reapproximates the prerectal fibers of the levator, which usually represent fascia at this level. This suture narrows the levator hiatus. During repair of the rectocele and narrowing of the levator hiatus it important that these sutures create a smooth posterior vaginal wall without creating painful ridges.

The final step is repair of the perineal weakness by reapproximating the central tendon. Appropriate repair will lengthen the posterior vaginal wall, recreate the connection of the anterior portion of the levator ani to the central tendon, help to narrow the vaginal introitus, and bring together the muscles of the UG diaphragm. This repair is accomplished by two to three vertical mattress sutures of 2–0 polyglycolic acid (Fig. 42–15). The skin of the perineum is then closed with a running suture (Fig. 42–16). If the repair is found to be too tight, relaxing incisions through the full thickness of the vaginal wall in the 3 and 9 o'clock positions can be made. An antibiotic-impregnated vaginal packing is then placed to aid in hemostasis.

Alternatively, the repair can be approached through a single midline incision entering the rectovaginal space directly and eliminating the triangular posterior vaginal wall incision, although this approach fails to preserve the prerectal fibers of the levator in the midline of the distal vagina. Another alternative is to dissect the vaginal wall off the prerectal fascia, staying out of the rectovaginal space. Repair is then accomplished in two layers, the first plicating the attenuated prerectal fascia in the midline and the second reapproximating the narrowed posterior vaginal wall.

Postoperative Considerations

On the first postoperative day the Foley catheter and vaginal packing are removed, and the patient resumes a normal diet. Intravenous antibiotics are continued for 48 hours followed by oral antibiotics for several days. Stool softeners are prescribed for 1 month postoperatively. One may consider the use of estrogen cream to facilitate wound healing and improve viscoelasticity. Finally, the patient is encouraged to resume early postoperative coitus if there are

Text continued on page 456

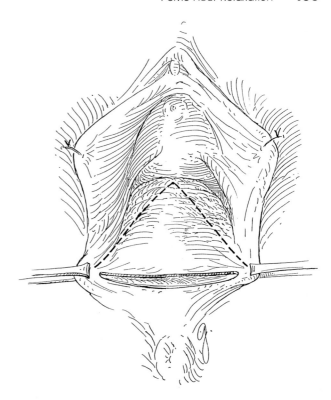

Figure 42-11 A triangle of posterior vaginal wall is incised with its base at the perineum and its apex at the apex of the vagina.

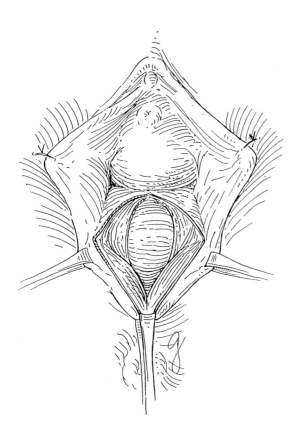

Figure 42-12 Lateral dissection from this incision exposes the underlying pararectal and prerectal fasciae, which will be used in the rectocele repair.

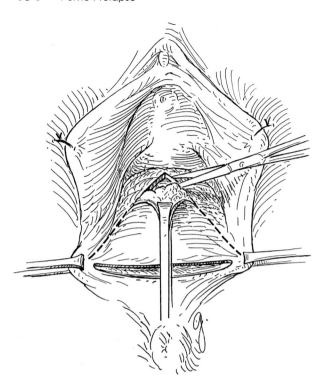

Figure 42-13 The triangle of excess posterior vaginal wall is then excised and discarded. (From Raz S, Little NA, Juma S: Female urology. *In* Walsh PC, Retik AB, Stamey TA, Vaughan ED Jr [eds]: Campbell's Urology, 6th ed. Philadelphia, WB Saunders, 1992, pp 2782–2828.)

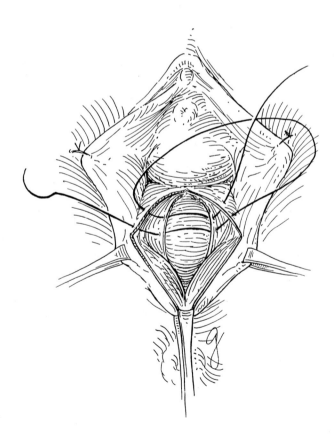

Figure 42-14 A running locking absorbable suture is used to plicate the pararectal fascia across the midline to reduce the rectocele. At the level of the levator hiatus a lateral bite of prerectal fascia is taken in a figure-of-eight fashion to narrow the levator hiatus to two to three fingerbreadths. (From Raz S, Little NA, Juma S: Female urology. *In* Walsh PC, Retik AB, Stamey TA, Vaughan ED Jr [eds]: Campbell's Urology, 6th ed. Philadelphia, WB Saunders, 1992, pp 2782–2828.)

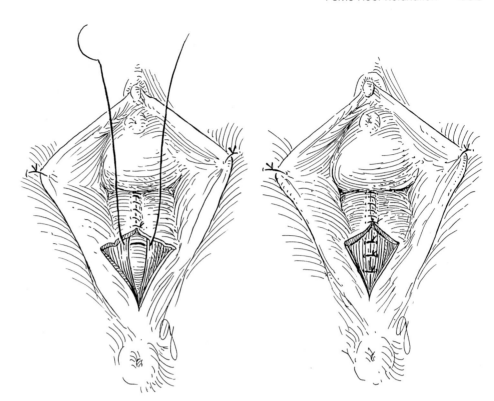

Figure 42-15 Vertical mattress sutures are used to reconstruct the urogenital diaphragm. (From Raz S, Little NA, Juma S: Female urology. *In* Walsh PC, Retik AB, Stamey TA, Vaughan ED Jr [eds]: Campbell's Urology, 6th ed. Philadelphia, WB Saunders, 1992, pp 2782–2828.)

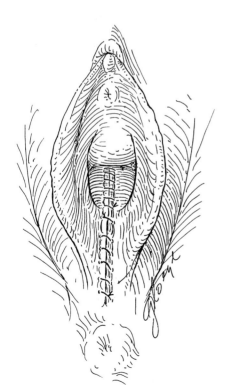

Figure 42-16 The completed repair recreates the near-horizontal vaginal axis, reduces the rectocele, and reconstructs the urogenital diaphragm, leaving adequate vaginal width for normal postoperative sexual function. (From Raz S, Little NA, Juma S: Female urology. *In* Walsh PC, Retik AB, Stamey TA, Vaughan ED Jr [eds]: Campbell's Urology, 6th ed. Philadelphia, WB Saunders, 1992, pp 2782–2828.)

no complications in the early postoperative period to ensure normal resumption of sexual function.

Complications

Recurrent rectocele is very uncommon, occurring in none of the 95 patients we recently reviewed.[38] The most frequent complication of rectocele repair alone is urinary retention, which occurred in 12.5% of patients.[24] Vaginal narrowing and dyspareunia generally can be avoided by adhering to meticulous technique, by not overnarrowing the vagina, by not leaving painful ridges, and by not placing sutures directly into the levator musculature. Rectovaginal fistula did not occur in our series but has been reported in up to 5% of patients undergoing pelvic floor repair.[34] Despite aggressive repair of even asymptomatic pelvic floor weakness, recurrent pelvic prolapse can still be expected in as many as 7.5% of patients.

REFERENCES

1. Bonney V: The sustentacular apparatus of the female genital canal, the displacements from the yielding of its several components and their appropriate treatment. J Obstet Gynaecol Br Emp 45:328, 1914.
2. Halban J, Tandler J: Anatomie und Atiologie der Genitalprolapse beim Weibe. Vienna, Wilhelm Braumuller, 1907; translated by Porges RF, Porges JC: Obstet Gynecol 15:790, 1960.
3. Tindall VR: Anatomy. In Tindall VR: Jeffcoate's Principles of Gynaecology, 5th ed. London, Butterworth & Co, 1987, pp 16–52.
4. Bustami FM: A reappraisal of the anatomy of the levator ani muscle in man. Acta Morphol Neerl-Scand 26:255, 1988-89.
5. Nichols DH, Randall CL: Vaginal Surgery, 3rd ed. Baltimore, Williams & Wilkins, 1989, pp 1–45.
6. Milley PS, Nichols DH: A correlative investigation of the human rectovaginal septum. Anat Rec 163:443, 1969.
7. Uhlenhuth E, Day EC, Smith RD, et al: The visceral endopelvic fascia and the hypogastric sheath. Surg Gynecol Obstet 86:9, 1948.
8. Uhlenhuth D, Wolfe WM, Smith EM, et al: The rectovaginal septum. Surg Gynecol Obstet 86:148, 1948.
9. Dickinson RL: Studies of the levator ani muscle. Am J Obstet Dis Wom 22:897, 1889.
10. Morgan KF Jr: Casts of the vagina as a means of evaluation of structural changes and treatment. Calif Med 94:30, 1961.
11. Nichols DH, Milley PS, Randall CL: Significance of restoration of normal vaginal depth and axis. Obstet Gynecol 36:251, 1970.
12. Funt MI, Thompson JD, Birch H: Normal vaginal axis. South Med J 71:1534, 1978.
13. Sturmdorf A: Gynoplastic Technology. Philadelphia, FA Davis, 1919, pp 109–114.
14. Berglas B, Rubin IC: Study of the supportive structures of the uterus by levator myography. Surg Gynecol Obstet 97:677, 1953.
15. Kuhn RJ, Hollycock VE: Observations on the anatomy of the rectovaginal pouch and septum. Obstet Gynecol 59:445, 1982.
16. Kiilholma P, Makinen J, Chancellor MB, et al: Modified Burch colposuspension for stress urinary incontinence in females. Surg Gynecol Obstet 176:111, 1993.
17. Gillon G, Stanton SL: Long-term follow-up of surgery for urinary incontinence in elderly women. Br J Urol 56:478, 1984.
18. Wiskind AK, Creighton SM, Stanton SL: The incidence of genital prolapse after the Burch colposuspension. Am J Obstet Gynecol 167:399, 1992.
19. Beecham CT: Classification of vaginal relaxation. Am J Obstet Gynecol 136:957, 1980.
20. Baden WF, Walker TA, Lindsey JH: The vaginal profile. Tex Med 64:56, 1968.
21. Wells TJ, Brink CA, Diokno AC: Urinary incontinence in elderly women: Clinical findings. J Am Geriatr Soc 35:933, 1987.
22. Raz S, Sussman EM, Erickson DB, et al: The Raz bladder neck suspension: Results in 206 patients. J Urol 148:845, 1992.
23. Raz S, Little NA, Juma S, Sussman EM: Repair of severe anterior vaginal wall prolapse (grade IV cystourethrocele). J Urol 146:988, 1991.
24. Arnold MW, Stewart WR, Aguilar PS: Rectocele repair: Four years experience. Dis Col Rect 33:684, 1990.
25. Siproudhis L, Lucas RJ, Raoul JL, et al: Defecatory disorders, anorectal disorders and pelvic floor dysfunction: A polygamy? Int J Colorectal Dis 7:102, 1992.
26. Kelvin FM, Maglinte DD, Hornback JA, et al: Pelvic prolapse: Assessment with evacuation proctography (defecography). Radiology 184:547, 1992.
27. Caps WR Jr: Rectoplasty and perineoplasty for the symptomatic rectocele: A report of fifty cases. Dis Colon Rectum 18:237, 1975.
28. Archer BD, Somers S, Stevenson GW: Contrast medium gel for marking vaginal position during defecography. Radiology 182:278, 1992.
29. Freimanis MG, Wald A, Caruna B, et al: Evacuation proctography in normal volunteers. Invest Radiol 26:581, 1991.
30. Yashioka D, Mausie Y, Yamada O, et al: Physiologic and anatomic assessment of patients with rectocele. Dis Colon Rectum 34:704, 1991.
31. Yang A, Mostwin JL, Rosen NB, et al: Pelvic floor descent in women: Dynamic evaluation with fast MR imaging and cinematic display. Radiology 179:25, 1991.
32. Jeffcoate TN: Posterior colpoperineorhaphy. Am J Obstet Gynecol 77:490, 1958.
33. Nichols DH: Posterior colporrhaphy and perineorhaphy: Separate and distinct operations. Am J Obstet Gynecol 164:714, 1991.
34. Pratt JH: Surgical repair of rectocele and perineal lacerations. Clin Obstet Gynecol 15:1160, 1972.
35. Haase P, Skibsted L: Influence of operations for stress incontinence and/or genital descensus on sexual life. Acta Obstet Gynecol Scand 67:659, 1988.
36. Babiarz JW, Payne CK, Raz S: The importance of posterior vaginal repair in correction of stress urinary incontinence. J Urol 149:403a, 1993.
37. Nichols DH, Randall CL: Vaginal Surgery, 3rd ed. Baltimore, Williams & Wilkins, 1989, pp 82–97.
38. Unpublished data.

CHAPTER 43

Uterine Prolapse

Ashok Chopra, M.D.
Lynn Stothers, M.D., M.H.Sc., F.R.C.S.C.
Shlomo Raz, M.D.

Hysterectomy is one of the most common operative procedures in the United States. In 1975 approximately 750,000 of these procedures were performed. In a review of data from the National Center for Health Statistics for the years 1970 to 1984, the most common indications for hysterectomy were as follows: leiomyomas, 26.8%; prolapse, 20.8%; endometriosis, 14.7%; carcinoma, 10.7%; endometrial hyperplasia, 6.2%. Most surgeons have some familiarity with the techniques of abdominal hysterectomy, specifically those involved in anterior exenterative surgery. Vaginal prolapse, however, is particularly suited to transvaginal hysterectomy. This chapter addresses specifically the various issues of prolapse and the technique of vaginal hysterectomy. This chapter does not take into account such confounding factors as bleeding or dysplasia.

Pathogenesis of Prolapse

Many factors influence the development and progression of prolapse. Racial and social differences are highlighted by the lower incidence of prolapse in blacks and Asians as opposed to whites. Differences in pelvic architecture, inherent quality of the pelvic musculature, and character of tissue response to injury are also significant. Social patterns of behavior may lessen or exacerbate stress and trauma to the perineum. Neurogenic or congenital factors play a role, as demonstrated by the incidence of prolapse in nulliparous patients with multiple sclerosis and spina bifida.[4] Conditions affecting physical status such as chronic constipation, lung disease, and other conditions that increase abdominal pressure all tend to increase prolapse.

Trauma from childbirth is the most obvious factor contributing to prolapse. Modern obstetric care has lessened this trauma by techniques designed to avoid prolonged labor, cesarean section for women with cephalopelvic disproportion, and treatment for malposition of the fetus. The patient with a significant history of pelvic inflammatory disease may have a decreased incidence of prolapse by virtue of both lower parity and scar tissue due to inflammation and infection of the paracervical and parametrial tissues.

Despite the multiplicity of etiologic factors, the primary one is parity. Stretching of the various paravaginal, parauterine, and paracervical tissues during parturition causes significant trauma. In the majority of women the tissues recover. However, as time passes the original trauma may become manifest. A deficiency of estrogen in the postmenopausal woman contributes to the delay between pelvic trauma and the onset of clinical prolapse.

Anatomic Considerations

The normal uterine position in a standing woman is anteverted with the corpus posterior and superior to the bladder. The cervix points posteroinferiorly, and the uterine corpus lies horizontally.

The muscles comprising the floor of the pelvis are commonly referred to as the levator group, and among their functions is assistance in the prevention of prolapse. These muscles form the levator plate on which rest the uterus and upper vagina. These muscles form the boundaries for the levator hiatus and displace the lower rectum and vagina anteriorly to deflect intra-abdominal pressure away from the hiatus.

The primary supporting ligaments are the uterosacral and cardinal ligaments. The cardinal, or

Mackenrodt's, ligament extends from each side of the cervix and upper vagina to the sides of the pelvis. This tissue is found within the lower part of the broad ligament and is designed to hold the cervix and upper vagina at that level. The uterosacral ligaments are found beneath the peritoneal folds on each side of the pouch of Douglas. These ligaments are attached to the posterolateral surface of the cervix and extend backward to each side of the rectum. Here they insert into the periosteum of the sacrum, thus holding the cervix back. In this fashion the corpus lies anteriorly so that intra-abdominal pressure falls on the posterior surface of the corpus, maintaining its anteverted position. The round ligaments provide little support in terms of uterine descent. They do, however, contribute to holding the uterus in anteversion. The lateral vaginal fornices are supported in their position by the fibers of Luschka, which are fixed to the tendinous arch of the levators.

It is important to note that other anatomic structures support the uterus and vagina as well. These include the bony pelvis, the urogenital diaphragm including the pubourethral ligaments, and the perineal body and perineum.[1] Certain aspects of the role of the supporting ligaments in the pathogenesis of prolapse can be more easily interpreted when this understanding of ligament function is kept in mind. With weakness of the uterosacral ligaments the cervix moves anteriorly, thereby compromising the position of the uterus over the levator plate. The axis of the uterus changes, with the corpus swinging backward on a relatively fixed transverse axis. When this occurs the intra-abdominal pressure falls on the anterior surface of the uterus, thus further exacerbating the retroversion and leading to the development of prolapse. Stress on the cardinal ligaments encourages prolapse by causing loss of support over the levator plate. It is vital to note that despite the distinct identities of the uterosacral and cardinal ligaments, their tissues are to a large measure enmeshed, making separation essentially impossible and creating a single complex useful for surgical therapy.[1]

Diagnosis

The patient with uterine prolapse often presents with a history of a mass in the vagina. Further questioning may elucidate a history of pain, dyspareunia, urinary retention, or incontinence. Discomfort in the lower back is common. Symptoms are classically aggravated by standing and may decrease when the patient assumes a recumbent position. The diagnosis is established by physical examination by the finding of significant uterine descent. Pelvic examination under anesthesia should immediately precede hysterectomy. This examination will confirm earlier impressions of the size of the uterus, mobility, position of the posterior cul-de-sac, and the length and strength of the cardinal and uterosacral ligaments.[4] The clinician will at this time appreciate the marked increase in relaxation of the ligamentous support during anesthesia. Minimal traction often reveals descent that is not clinically apparent in the awake patient. Attentive bimanual examination often reveals other pathology germane to the planned operation (i.e., enterocele, rectocele, cystocele, urethral hypermobility, perineal body laxity). The bony structure of the pelvis should be assessed to obtain some estimation of the degree of technical difficulty of transvaginal delivery of the uterus. Rarely, imaging modalities such as ultrasound may be required to fully evaluate the pelvis. Progressive hydronephrosis is associated with procidentia. Rates of this complication in the literature vary from 2% to 92%.[2] In general, this dilation is associated with low-grade obstruction and is insidious in onset and symptoms. Repeated renal infections may draw attention to this problem.

CLASSIFICATION

Prolapse is classically divided into four stages. First-degree prolapse occurs when the cervix descends toward the orifice of the vagina. Second-degree prolapse is present when the cervix descends to the level of the outlet of the vagina. Third-degree prolapse exists when the cervix is actually outside the vagina. Fourth-degree prolapse or procidentia is present when the uterus extends outside the introitus.[3]

INDICATIONS

Many patients with prolapse are seen by the physician for complaints of urinary incontinence, instability, or retention. Most have a variety of anatomic defects including cystocele, urethrocele, rectocele, and enterocele. These patients require a comprehensive plan of reconstruction. Individualized repair of a cystocele or suspension of the bladder neck may create significant problems in such patients.

Treatment of the prolapsed uterus varies according to the patient's symptomatology, degree of prolapse, and desire to maintain fertility. Minimal degrees of prolapse may respond to hormonal treatment or Kegel exercises. Mildly symptomatic patients may require no therapy at all. Patients with severe prolapse, moderate prolapse and associated enterocele, moderate prolapse and large cystocele, and significant discomfort constitute the ideal population for hysterectomy.

CONTRAINDICATIONS TO VAGINAL HYSTERECTOMY

Specific contraindications to transvaginal hysterectomy include size disproportions (i.e., enlarged uterus, stenotic vagina), obliteration of the cul-de-sac, adnexal tumor, pelvic inflammatory disease, and malignancy of the uterus or ovaries (extrafascial vaginal hysterectomy may be done in selected patients with low-grade tumor of the uterus).[1] Fixation of the uterus by infection or inflammation may make hysterectomy difficult. A history of endometriosis of unknown extent may be considered an absolute contraindication.[4] To these contraindications one must add the patient who has a strong desire to maintain fertility (in these patients uterine fixation to the sacrum may be considered).

Nonsurgical Options

The primary nonsurgical treatment for prolapse of the uterus involves use of a pessary. This may be an attractive option in the high-risk patient. Unfortunately, success is dependent on the adequacy of perineal outlet support, and this is often lacking in this patient population. Complications of pessary use include mechanical irritation or ulceration of the vaginal mucosa. A pessary may also be used as a diagnostic tool. Use for a few weeks often assists in determining whether a patient's symptoms of discomfort are secondary to prolapse or some other source. It should be noted that the pessary may become imbedded in the vaginal wall, requiring operative intervention to remove.

Surgical Treatment of Prolapse

The underlying principle guiding surgical repair of uterine prolapse is that the problem is not with the uterus but with the pelvic support. As such, repair should be directed toward these structures. Nichols characterizes these themes as follows:[1]

1. Damage to the upper support group (the round and broad ligaments) interferes with the anteversion of the uterus. This type of damage is commonly associated with retroversion and hypermobility of the uterus in this plane. This type of injury is usually nonprogressive and requires no therapy.
2. Damage to the middle support group (uterosacral and cardinal ligaments) results in progressive eversion of the upper vagina with elongation of the cervix and descent of the uterus. Of note, the pelvic diaphragm is usually intact with such an injury, and as such rectocele is not a characteristic finding in these situations.
3. Damage to the lower support group (pelvic and urogenital diaphragms) usually results in eversion of the vagina with development of a cystocele or rectocele.

As one would expect, injury can occur to any combination or group of these supports, resulting in various clinical pictures. Prolapse of the cervix can occur without prolapse of the fundus of the uterus.

Surgical Options

Various operative procedures have been described to treat prolapse. For our purposes they will be divided into uterus-sparing procedures and those that involve hysterectomy.

UTERUS-SPARING PROCEDURES

Uterus-sparing procedures may be performed through a number of techniques. In recent years techniques of vaginal vault support such as sacrospinous fixation or abdominal sacral colpopexy have become more common.[2] Various operations require repair of the ligamentous uterine support and entail round ligament suspension with shortening of the uterosacral ligaments. These procedures may be performed either transvaginally or transabdominally. The Manchester-Fothergill operation may be used in the patient with cervical elongation and strong uterosacral ligaments. This procedure includes amputation of the cervix, repair of the freed cervical supporting ligaments anterior to the cervix, and finally, appropriate colporrhaphy. Of concern in this procedure is the potential for postoperative incompetence of the os; repair of an associated enterocele is difficult. If the cervix is not elongated, transabdominal sacrocervical colpopexy is useful.[1] Other operations include the LeFort procedure in which a portion of the vaginal mucosa is excised and the denuded anterior and posterior walls are sewn together. This procedure, although quick and effective, has several disadvantages, including loss of coital function and difficulty in accessing the uterus should bleeding or other uterine pathology develop. Obviously, this procedure is suitable for only a very small number of patients. Techniques that have fallen into disfavor include the Watkins operation. This procedure was described as an interposition technique that used the uterine corpus as an obturator for the pelvic diaphragm.[2] In this procedure the corpus of the uterus was placed beneath the bladder (invariably requiring amputation of the cervix).[3] Ventral fixation techniques were also used in the past but were found to be ineffective.[2]

HYSTERECTOMY

Many techniques of hysterectomy exist. This chapter does not attempt to describe all techniques of treatment for prolapse. Instead, we focus on one technique of vaginal hysterectomy that we have used with success.

Evaluation and Preparation

Issues of size disproportion, mobility of the uterus, and status of the pelvic floor and ligamentous support should be addressed preoperatively. The bimanual examination should be repeated intraoperatively to confirm earlier assessments. Elongation of the cervix and the depth and angle of the vagina should be noted prior to the initial incision.

Selection of the ideal procedure depends on the pathology coexisting with prolapse of the uterus. In patients with coexisting grade 1 cystocele we perform vaginal hysterectomy with simple bladder neck suspension. For those with moderate cystocele with a primarily lateral defect we perform vaginal hysterectomy with a six-corner bladder suspension and bladder neck suspension. For grade 4 cystocele we incise vertically in the anterior vaginal wall. We then dissect laterally over the pubocervical fascia, thus freeing the bladder from the cervix. This technique allows us to elevate the bladder base, thus facilitating the hysterectomy and subsequent closure of the cul-de-sac. The grade 4 cystocele is then repaired in our standard fashion with repair of both lateral and central defects.

Technique

Initially the labia are retracted, and a weighted speculum is inserted. A ring retractor is used for exposure. A tenaculum is used to grasp the cervix, and the mobility of the uterus is checked. If bladder neck suspension or cystocele repair is planned, a suprapubic tube is inserted at this point. A urethral catheter

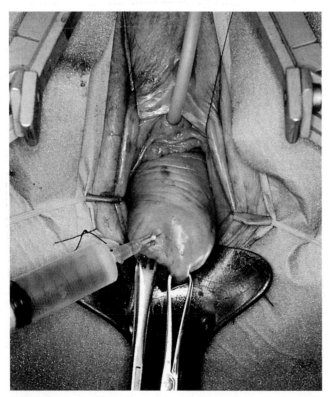

Figure 43-1 Infiltration around the cervix with normal saline. The cervix has been grasped with a tenaculum. (From Raz S: Atlas of Transvaginal Surgery. Philadelphia, WB Saunders, 1992.)

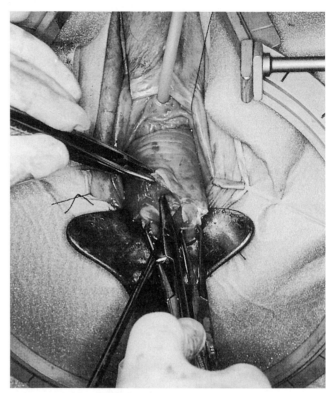

Figure 43-2 Anterior dissection. (From Raz S: Atlas of Transvaginal Surgery. Philadelphia, WB Saunders, 1992.)

is also inserted. Normal saline is injected around the cervix to help create cleavage planes (Fig. 43–1). Next, a circumferential incision is made at the cervix, and anterior dissection is begun (Fig. 43–2). Sharp dissection of the cervix from the bladder is safer than blunt stripping. This dissection may be aided by exerting anterior traction on the bladder and performing dissection with the scissors pointing toward the uterus. As the vesicoperitoneal fold is approached, the peritoneum usually becomes apparent (Fig. 43–3). Occasionally, the operator enters the wrong plane in an attempt to stay as far away from the bladder as possible. This error is particularly likely if the initial incision is too close to the cervical os. In these instances the surgeon may inadvertently mistake the peritoneum for the undersurface of the bladder.

At this point the surgeon turns his or her attention to the posterior dissection. In a similar fashion the posterior peritoneal fold is exposed (Fig. 43–4). The posterior peritoneum is now opened sharply, and the cul-de-sac is explored through a small peritoneotomy for unsuspected adhesions, carcinoma, or other pathology. Sometimes the operator may have difficulty in identifying the posterior cul-de-sac. In these instances it is often advisable to begin the hysterectomy in an extraperitoneal fashion, initially severing the uterosacral and caudal portions of the cardinal ligaments close to the cervix. This maneuver allows the uterus to descend, providing better visualization. Once the posterior peritoneum is opened, a retractor

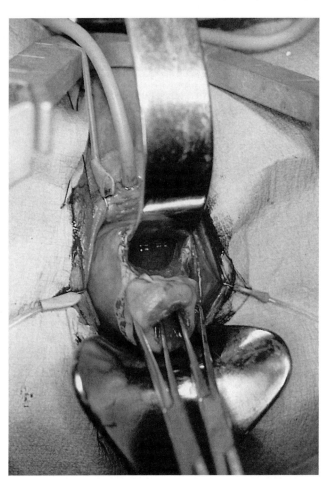

Figure 43-3 Exposure of the vesicouterine fold. (From Raz S: Atlas of Transvaginal Surgery. Philadelphia, WB Saunders, 1992.)

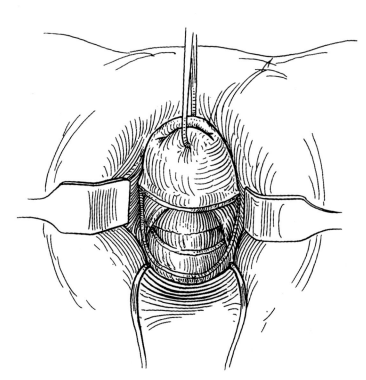

Figure 43-4 Posterior dissection toward the pouch of Douglas. (From Raz S: Atlas of Transvaginal Surgery. Philadelphia, WB Saunders, 1992.)

is placed. Tagging the peritoneum at this point may make later closure simpler.

Next, attention is turned to the division of the ligamentous attachments. With the cervix under slight retraction, the cardinal and sacrouterine ligaments are identified. The tip of a right-angle retractor is introduced into the cul-de-sac at the level of the cervix. Pointing anteriorly, the ligaments are isolated at their point of attachment to the cervix. The ligaments are individually clamped, divided, and ligated 1 cm lateral to the cervix using a figure-of-eight suture ligature (Fig. 43–5). The uterine vessels should be ligated separately. The sutures on the ligaments are left long and anchored to the grooves in the retractor ring. Any traction on the cardinal ligaments implies traction on the uterine vessels. This maneuver brings the ureters closer to the operator's field.

At this point the uterus should be markedly mobile because the round ligaments provide little resistance to movement. If free descent of the uterus does not occur, the surgeon should consider confounding factors such as ventral fixation, endometriosis, adhesions, carcinoma, size disproportion, and fibrosis.

The surgeon should next evert the uterus, bringing it outside the introitus (Fig. 43–6). Attention is now turned to entry to the anterior peritoneum. This portion of the procedure entails the risk of inadvertent entry into the bladder. It is advantageous to insert the finger anteriorly over the fundus of the uterus to tent the peritoneum. An incision can then be made over the finger, allowing safe entry into the anterior peritoneum.

Further parametral ligation is then undertaken to the level of the peritoneal folds. With the anterior retractor elevating the bladder and mild posterior

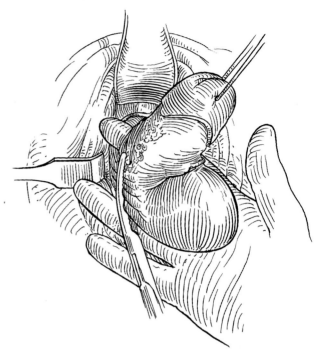

Figure 43–6 Eversion of the uterus. (From Raz S: Atlas of Transvaginal Surgery. Philadelphia, WB Saunders, 1992.)

traction placed on the uterus, the thin attaching folds of peritoneum can be seen. These are divided, leaving the broad ligaments as the only attachments. The broad ligaments are next divided close to the uterine body. If the adnexa are to be left behind, their attachments are now divided. The utero-ovarian ligament, the fallopian tube, and the round ligament are visible from anterior to posterior and are divided and ligated sequentially.

At this point the uterus is removed. Three pedicles are identified on each side—the broad ligaments, the cardinal ligaments, and the uterosacral ligaments (Fig. 43–7). The vaginal vault is secured in place by reapproximating the ligaments and performing a culdoplasty. Closure of the cul-de-sac is essential to prevent formation of an enterocele and to provide support for the vaginal vault. A number of techniques exist. We use a modified McCall culdoplasty, placing matching sutures through the vaginal wall at the lateral fornices. These sutures incorporate both sacrouterine-cardinal complexes and the prerectal fascia. The sutures exit approximately 1 cm from the site of entry (Fig. 43–8). Two pursestring sutures are placed cephalad to this area to close the pouch of Douglas. These sutures incorporate the prerectal and prevesical fasciae and the broad and sacrouterine-cardinal ligaments. If simultaneous vaginal surgery is planned, it is performed now. The vaginal mucosa is finally closed with a running 2–0 Vicryl suture, and vaginal packing with antibiotic cream is used.

Complications

Complications of vaginal hysterectomy are known to the urologist, who may be consulted about their re-

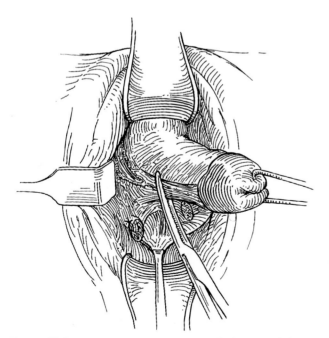

Figure 43–5 Retraction on the cervix with division of the cardinal and sacrouterine ligaments. (From Raz S: Atlas of Transvaginal Surgery. Philadelphia, WB Saunders, 1992.)

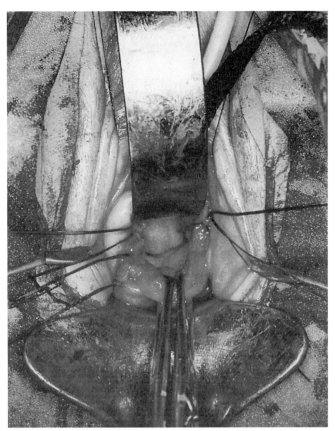

Figure 43-7 Demonstration of pedicles after hysterectomy; anterior (broad ligament), middle (uterine artery), and posterior (cardinal and sacrouterine ligaments). (From Raz S: Atlas of Transvaginal Surgery. Philadelphia, WB Saunders, 1992.)

pair. It is important to note that as long as the uterus is freely movable the difficulty of hysterectomy increases with increasing degrees of prolapse. The primary reason for this difficulty is the lack of consistent anatomy.[1]

One of the interesting points about the transvaginal hysterectomy concerns the lower incidence of ureteral injury associated with this technique as opposed to transabdominal hysterectomy. Hofmeister and Wolfgram studied this phenomenon and determined that traction applied to the cervix, combined with adequate retraction of the anterior vesicouterine peritoneal folds, provides a superior degree of displacement of the ureters.[5]

Bladder injury may occur during development of the anterior planes; it occurs in approximately 0.5% of patients undergoing vaginal hysterectomy. Bladder injury occurs approximately six times as frequently with transabdominal hysterectomy.[2]

Vaginal prolapse is quite frequent following vaginal hysterectomy. Usually this prolapse is asymptomatic and involves only the upper third of the vagina. More significant prolapse is much more unusual and occurs in less than 0.5% of cases.[2] Often the finding of prolapse after hysterectomy indicates that an enterocele was missed at the time of surgery. Ureteral fistulas occur with a frequency of .09 to 0.5%, and bladder fistulas are seen in between .05 and 0.6% of cases. As one would expect, the most common site of a ureteral fistula is at the distal portion just preceding entrance into the intramural tunnel. Bladder fistulas occur at the trigone or along the bladder base.

REFERENCES

1. Nichols D, Randall CL: Vaginal Surgery, 3rd ed. Baltimore, Williams & Wilkins, 1989.
2. Thompson J (ed): TeLinde's Operative Gynecology, 7th ed. Philadelphia, JB Lippincott, 1992.
3. Gray LA: Vaginal Hysterectomy, 3rd ed. Springfield, Charles C Thomas, 1989.
4. Kursh ED, McGuire E: Female Urology. Philadelphia, JB Lippincott, 1994.
5. Hofmeister FJ, Wolfgram RL: Methods of demonstrating measurement relationships between vaginal hysterectomy ligatures and the ureters. Am J Obstet Gynecol 83:938–948, 1962.

BIBLIOGRAPHY

Baden WE, Walker J: Surgical Repair of Vaginal Defects. Philadelphia, JB Lippincott, 1992.
Brett KM, Madans JH: Hysterectomy use: The correspondence between self-reports and hospital records. Am J Publ Health 84(10):1653–1655, 1994.
Feldman GB, Birnbaum SJ: Sacral colpopexy for vaginal vault prolapse. Obstet Gynecol 53:399, 1979.
Hendee AE, Berry CM: Abdominal sacropexy for vaginal vault prolapse. Clin Obstet Gynecol 24:1217–1226, 1981.
Jeffcoate TNA: Posterior colporrhaphy. Am J Obstet Gynecol 77:490, 1959.
Kuhn RJP, Hollyock VE: Observations of the anatomy of the rectovaginal pouch and septum. Obstet Gynecol 59:445, 1982.
Leach GE, Zimmern P, Staskin D, et al: Surgery for pelvic prolapse. Semin Urol 4:43–50, 1986.
McCall ML: Posterior culdeplasty. Obstet Gynecol 10:595, 1957.
Nezhat C, Bess O, Admon D, et al: Hospital cost comparison between abdominal, vaginal, and laparoscopy-assisted vaginal hysterectomies. Obstet Gynecol 83(Pt 1):713–716, 1994.
Randall CL, Nichols DH: Surgical treatment of vaginal inversion. Obstet Gynecol 38:502, 1971.

Bladder

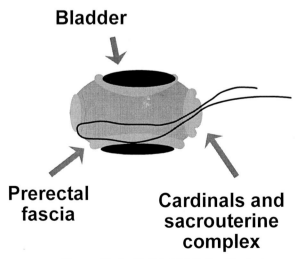

Prerectal fascia

Cardinals and sacrouterine complex

Figure 43-8 Modified McCall culdoplasty.

Raz S: Operative repair of rectocele, enterocele and cystocele. Adv Urol 5:121–144, 1992.

Richardson AC, Lyon JB, Williams NL: A new look at pelvic relaxation. Am J Obstet Gynecol 126:12, 1976.

Smith HO, Thompson JD: Indications and technique for vaginal hysterectomy. *In* Sanz LE (ed): Gynecological Surgery. Oradell, NJ, Medical Economics Books, 1988, pp 227–290.

Smout CFV, Jacoby F, Lillie EW: Gynaecological and Obstetrical anatomy. London, Lewis Publishers, 1969.

Staskin DR, Hadley HR, Zimmern P, et al: Anatomy for vaginal surgery. Semin Urol 4:2, 1986.

TeLinde RW: Prolapse of the uterus and allied conditions. Am J Obstet Gynecol 94:444–463, 1966.

Tovell H: Gynecological Operations. Philadelphia, Harper & Row, 1978.

Uhlenhuth E, Wolfe WM, Smith EM, et al: The rectogenital septum. Surg Gynecol Obstet 76:148, 1948.

Wall LL: A technique for modified McCall culdeplasty at the time of abdominal hysterectomy. J Am Coll Surg 178(5):507–509, 1994.

Zacharin RF: Pulsion enterocele: Review of functional anatomy of the pelvic floor. Obstet Gynecol 55:135, 1980.

CHAPTER 44

Enterocele and Vault Prolapse

Ashok Chopra, M.D.
Shlomo Raz, M.D.
Lynn Stothers, M.D., M.H.Sc., F.R.C.S.C.

An enterocele is defined as a herniation of the peritoneum and its contents at the level of the vaginal apex. To understand the development and treatment of enterocele it is vital to be familiar with the normal anatomy of the cul-de-sac and the upper vagina.

Anatomy

In the normal woman the vagina lies cephalad to the rectum with the potential space of the pouch of Douglas lying sandwiched between them. Increases in intra-abdominal pressure compress the vagina against the rectum, effectively obliterating this potential space. The vaginal orientation is posterior and cephalad and is maintained by traction of the cardinal and uterosacral ligaments. The horizontal orientation of the rectum is maintained by the integrity of the levator plate.

Alterations in anatomy lead to the formation of enterocele. Anterior displacement of the vagina with widening of the hiatus between the uterosacral ligaments opens the cul-de-sac as does weakness of the levator plate. Prolapse of the uterus in a similar fashion opens the cul-de-sac and widens the uterosacral hiatus.

Classification

Enteroceles are classically divided into four types.[11] (1) *Congenital enteroceles* result from failure of fusion of the layers of peritoneum at the level of the rectovaginal septum. In this situation there is no cystocele or rectocele. (2) *Traction enteroceles* occur when prolapse of the vaginal vault or uterus pulls the peritoneum caudally. (3) *Pulsion enteroceles* exist when chronic pressure is exerted on the vault of the vagina. This pressure creates a hernial sac and often pushes the vaginal vault caudally. This herniation represents a sliding-type hernia with the vaginal vault and anterior vaginal wall sliding downward on the anterior surface of the rectum.[1] This type of enterocele is unusual in the patient with a uterus; as such, prolapse of the uterus is rarely associated. (4) *Iatrogenic enteroceles* follow a surgically induced change in vaginal axis, thus leaving the cul-de-sac unprotected.

We prefer to classify enteroceles according to anatomic findings. These findings eventually determine the course of treatment. The majority of enteroceles occur in posthysterectomy patients; accordingly, we divide our patients into categories based on the presence or absence of vault prolapse. (1) *Simple enteroceles* exist when there is no vault prolapse and the cuff is well supported. No cystocele or rectocele is found. (2) *Complex enteroceles* are associated with vault or uterine prolapse. The cuff is poorly supported, and prolapse may include either the anterior wall (cystocele) or posterior wall (rectocele) of the vagina (Table 44–1).

Pathogenesis

Congenital enteroceles arise from defects of fusion of the rectovaginal peritoneum. Iatrogenic enteroceles are usually caused by anterior displacement of the vagina as occurs in the Burch procedure. Indeed, the incidence of enterocele after the Burch suspension may be as high as 15%. To avoid this complication it is important to enter the peritoneum at the time of colposuspension and close the cul-de-sac. Traction

TABLE 44-1
Classification of Posthysterectomy Enterocele

Simple Enterocele
No vault prolapse
Cuff well-supported
No rectocele or cystocele

Complex Enterocele
Vault prolapsed
Cuff poorly supported
Associations:
1. Anterior wall prolapse—cystocele
2. Posterior wall prolapse—rectocele
3. Both walls

enteroceles reflect weaknesses in the supporting tissues of the pelvis. These issues have been described elsewhere in the section on vaginal prolapse.

Chronic increases in intra-abdominal pressure contribute to the development of pulsion enteroceles. These enteroceles are also commonly found after hysterectomy if closure of the peritoneum is inadequate. Pulsion enteroceles are also found after prolapse repair when excision or treatment of the peritoneum is inadequate. Caveats of vaginal surgery should include restoration of the proper vaginal axis and proper evaluation of the overall status of pelvic floor relaxation.

Symptoms

Symptoms of prolapse are minimal until descent reaches the grade 2 hymenal level.[7] At this point the patient may begin to complain of a sensation of fullness in the perineal area. Dyspareunia and vaginal discomfort are common. Low back discomfort, accentuated in the standing position, is also common. Rarely, complications of bowel obstruction may be found. If rectocele and cystocele are present, constipation and urinary complaints may be present.

Diagnosis

Diagnosis of an enterocele is made on the basis of physical examination. Observation of the introitus may reveal a bulging mass. Bimanual examination reveals a herniating sac at the apex of the vagina. During the rectovaginal examination straining often reveals an impulse of the enterocele sac against the fingertip. This mass is classically found posterior to the cervix (in patients who have undergone hysterectomy this sac is found at the apex of the vagina). Bimanual examination also often reveals thickness of the high rectal-vaginal septum.

Examination in the standing or sitting position may be valuable in some cases. A kidney-ureter-bladder (KUB) film may reveal bowel gas in the prolapsing mass. A rectogram may provide data about prolapse of the rectum. Finally, a cystogram will rule out the bladder as a source of the mass.

Difficulty may be encountered in differentiating enterocele from high rectocele; indeed, these conditions are often found together. It is helpful to have, therefore, some familiarity with the anatomy of the posterior vaginal wall. The posterior vaginal wall is approximately 8 to 9 cm in length from apex to hymen. With some degree of accuracy the wall can be divided into segments of 3 cm each. The proximal 3 cm is the cul-de-sac floor, the middle 3 cm is the rectum, and the distal 3 cm is the perineal body.[2] Classically, if both enterocele and rectocele are present, a small furrow divides the two. Use of a Sims speculum may be helpful in making this distinction. In this examination the patient is asked to bear down as the speculum is slowly withdrawn. This maneuver usually reveals the site of the bulge. Alternatively, the vaginal defect analyzer may be used to help localize the site of the herniation.

Nonoperative Therapy

Nonoperative therapy is often indicated in patients who have minimal symptoms. This therapy may involve changes in activities, treatment of constipation (and other circumstances that increase intra-abdominal pressure), Kegel exercises, and hormonal replacement. Pessaries may be used; if vaginal support is inadequate, a perineorrhaphy may be performed.

Operative Strategy

Prior to surgery a thorough understanding of the patient's functional and anatomic status must be achieved. The presence of incontinence or constipation and the patient's desire to have vaginal intercourse must be addressed. Anatomic defects must be recognized and repair considered (i.e., rectocele, cystocele, vault or uterine prolapse, perineal body abnormalities). The degree of prolapse must also be considered.

Nichols presents four principles of enterocele repair: (1) Identify the lesion and its probable cause. Careful preoperative evaluation is required with emphasis on examination with strain or in the standing position. (2) Mobilize and excise or obliterate the entire sac. (3) Occlude the sac by ligation as high as possible. (4) Provide adequate support from below and restore the normal axis of the vagina.[3]

We prefer the vaginal approach because it allows broader treatment of the many manifestations of vaginal prolapse (e.g., repair of cystocele, rectocele, bladder neck suspension). The abdominal approach, however, may be more appropriate if coexisting pathology mandates it. In patients with no vaginal vault prolapse, simple correction of the enterocele is the indicated procedure. In patients with uterine prolapse we perform vaginal hysterectomy. In patients with vault prolapse we perform sacrospinous fixation (sacral colpopexy may be used alternatively). If anterior vaginal prolapse is found concurrently we perform a six-corner suspension (formal repair for a grade 4 cystocele).

Simple Repair of Enterocele Without Vault Prolapse

After general or spinal anesthesia has been induced, the patient is placed in the dorsal lithotomy position. The lower abdomen and vagina are prepared and draped in sterile fashion. The rectum is packed with Betadine-impregnated lubricated gauze and then isolated from the surgical field. A weighted posterior vaginal retractor is placed in the vagina, and the labia are retracted laterally with stay sutures. A ring retractor is positioned and secured with hooks. A Foley catheter is inserted to empty the bladder.

The enterocele bulge is grasped with two Allis clamps, and normal saline is injected to facilitate dissection. A vertical incision is performed in the vaginal wall over the bulge (Fig. 44–1). When there is significant descent of the uterus or when the cervix alone is present, the enterocele repair is performed in conjunction with hysterectomy.

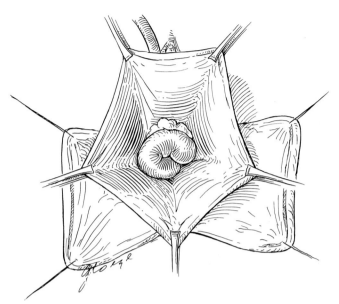

Figure 44-2   The sac has been dissected and opened. (From Raz S, Little NA, Juma S: Female urology. *In* Walsh PC, Retik AB, Stamey TA, Vaughan ED Jr [eds]: Campbell's Urology, 6th ed. Philadelphia, WB Saunders, 1992, pp 2782–2828.)

After the vaginal wall has been incised and dissected laterally, the peritoneal hernia sac is defined and separated from the vaginal wall, bladder, and rectum using blunt and sharp dissection. The sac is opened and its contents are reduced to facilitate definition of the peritoneal sac and neck of the sac (Fig. 44–2). A small, moist laparotomy pad is inserted into the peritoneal cavity to protect the bowel during obliteration of the enterocele.

The uterosacral ligaments and cardinal ligament complex are identified laterally and posteriorly. Two sets of interrupted No. 1 Vicryl sutures are placed to include these structures and the prerectal fascia. The sutures are initially transferred from the vaginal lumen and extended through the vaginal wall into the peritoneal sac and sacrouterine ligaments and back outside to the vaginal lumen, in a fashion similar to that used in the McCall procedure (Fig. 44–3). The sutures are secured with a clamp to be tied later. They are intended to provide depth and support to the vaginal cuff by relying on the strength of the sacrouterine ligaments.

Two pursestring sutures of No. 1 Vicryl are placed from the open enterocele sac, incorporating prerectal fascia posteriorly, uterosacral ligaments and the cardinal ligament complex laterally on each side, and the superficial bladder wall and the peritoneum underlying the bladder base anteriorly. With proper retraction of the trigone, care is taken to avoid injury to the ureters (Fig. 44–4).

After all sutures have been carefully placed, the pursestring sutures are tied in a proximal to distal direction, thus obliterating the pouch of Douglas. The preplaced sutures that include the sacrouterine complex, prerectal fascia, and rectal wall are tied last. The remainder of the peritoneal sac is suture-ligated at its base and excised. A running suture of the

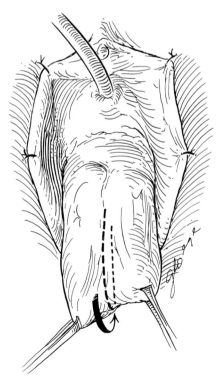

Figure 44-1   The enterocele is grasped with Allis clamps and the vaginal wall infiltrated with saline solution. An incision is made in the vaginal wall, and dissection of the peritoneal sac is begun. (From Raz S, Little NA, Juma S: Female urology. *In* Walsh PC, Retik AB, Stamey TA, Vaughan ED Jr [eds]: Campbell's Urology, 6th ed. Philadelphia, WB Saunders, 1992, pp 2782–2828.)

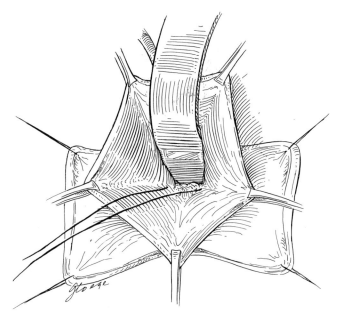

Figure 44-3 A pursestring suture is applied to close the peritoneal sac. (From Raz S, Little NA, Juma S: Female urology. *In* Walsh PC, Retik AB, Stamey TA, Vaughan ED Jr [eds]: Campbell's Urology, 6th ed. Philadelphia, WB Saunders, 1992, pp 2782–2828.)

prerectal fascia will include the peritoneal stump; if a rectocele is present it is repaired at this time.

The redundant vaginal epithelium is trimmed. The vaginal wall is closed with a running 2–0 Vicryl suture, incorporating the area of underlying repair to eliminate any dead space. Vaginal packing is placed for 24 hours.

Repair of Enterocele with Concurrent Cystocele

An enterocele may be found with concurrent cystocele and requires modification of the operative procedure. The type and degree of cystocele also affect the planned operation.

Bladder

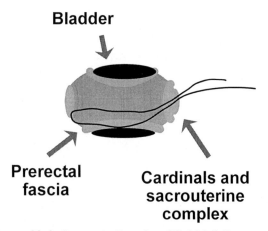

Prerectal fascia

Cardinals and sacrouterine complex

Figure 44-4 Demonstration of modified McCall suture for suspension of the vaginal vault.

ENTEROCELE AND MODERATE CYSTOCELE WITH MAINLY LATERAL DEFECT

The first steps of the operation are similar to those used for simple enterocele repair. After completion of the enterocele repair, the vaginal wall is not closed. The anchoring sutures of the sacrouterine and cardinal complex are left tagged on a clamp after being tied. At this point, the procedure becomes identical to that used for repair of cystocele with lateral defect. Two oblique incisions are made in the anterior vaginal wall, the periurethral fascia is dissected, and the retropubic space is entered. A first pair of No. 1 Prolene suspending sutures is placed at the level of the midurethra to incorporate the levator complex, the urethropelvic ligament, and the vaginal wall excluding the epithelium. A second pair of Prolene sutures is applied to the vaginal wall at the level of the bladder neck (minus the epithelium) and the urethropelvic ligaments. A third pair of sutures is applied to the bladder base including the pubocervical fascia and the area of the cardinal and sacrouterine ligaments (previously tagged by a clamp). A small suprapubic puncture is made, and, using a double-pronged ligature carrier, the sutures are transferred from the vaginal to the suprapubic area. The ligature carrier is passed very close to the symphysis of the pubis in the midline to avoid postoperative pain. Cystoscopy is performed to ensure bladder integrity, normal ureteral efflux, and good support of the bladder neck and bladder. After closing the vaginal wall, the sutures are tied independently in the suprapubic area using multiple knots. After repair of pelvic floor relaxation and rectocele, the vault of the vagina should be well supported and should preserve a normal 110-degree vaginal axis. During this procedure, as in all vaginal surgery, care must be taken to avoid shortening the vagina or performing excessive resection of vaginal wall tissue.

ENTEROCELE WITH SIGNIFICANT GRADE 4 CYSTOCELE

If the cystocele is severe (grade 4), a goalpost incision is made in the anterior vaginal wall, and the bladder is dissected laterally and posteriorly (Fig. 44–5). The retropubic space is entered on each side at the level of the bladder neck, exposing the medial edge of the urethropelvic ligaments. The enterocele sac is dissected from the posterior aspect of the bladder. The sac is opened, and the intra-abdominal contents are reduced. Two pursestring sutures close the peritoneum by incorporating the prerectal fascia, sacrouterine and cardinal ligament complex, and pubocervical fascia over the bladder wall. Another pair of No. 1 delayed absorption sutures includes the cardinal and uterosacral ligaments and prerectal fascia as in the modified McCall technique. These sutures are applied from the epithelial side of the vaginal lumen to the inside of the sac. After including the sacrouterine and cardinal ligament complex, they

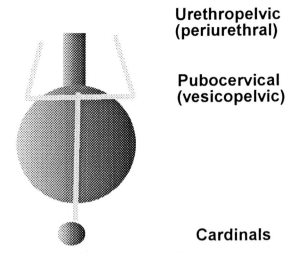

Urethropelvic (periurethral)

Pubocervical (vesicopelvic)

Cardinals

Figure 44-5   Goalpost incision as used in repair of grade 4 cystocele.

are brought back from inside the sac to the vaginal lumen so both threads emerge at the epithelial side separated by a healthy bridge of 1 to 2 cm of vaginal wall. The sutures are tied in a sequential fashion, thus closing the cul-de-sac. The sacrouterine and cardinal ligament sutures are tagged with a clamp. The excess peritoneal sac is excised.

Attention is now turned to repair of the cystocele. The lateral defect is repaired by applying two pairs of Prolene sutures as described earlier in the section on repair of grade 4 cystocele. A small suprapubic puncture is made, and the Prolene sutures are transferred from the vaginal to the suprapubic area using a double-pronged ligature carrier. The central defect is corrected by approximation of the cardinal ligaments and pubocervical fascia to the midline with absorbable sutures (refer to section on repair of grade 4 cystocele). After injection of indigo carmine intravenously, cystoscopy is performed to ensure ureteral and bladder integrity and good support and coaptation of the bladder and urethra. The central defect sutures are tied, the vaginal tissue is trimmed, and the vaginal wall is closed with a running suture of 2–0 absorbable material. The Prolene sutures are tied individually over the fascia without tension, and the suprapubic wound is closed with intradermal sutures.

Sacrospinous Fixation of the Vagina

INDICATIONS

In patients with massive vaginal vault prolapse in whom there is limited cardinal and uterosacral ligament strength, the transvaginal sacrospinalis vaginal suspension is a suitable procedure for restoring a functional vagina. We restrict the use of this procedure to patients with vault prolapse without concom-

itant cystocele (no surgery required to the anterior vaginal wall). Because of the potential for bowel injury, patients who undergo this repair must have proper bowel preparation and perioperative intravenous antibiotics.

SURGICAL TECHNIQUE

The patient is placed in a dorsal lithotomy position. The lower abdomen and vagina are prepared and draped in a sterile fashion. The rectum is packed with Betadine-impregnated lubricated gauze and then isolated from the operative field. The bladder is drained with a suprapubic cystostomy or a urethral catheter. A ring retractor is positioned, and the hooks are applied to the vaginal introitus. A longitudinal incision is made over the enterocele sac extending to the posterior vaginal wall. The enterocele sac is exposed and dissected free from the vaginal wall, bladder, and rectal wall. The sac is opened and the small bowel is packed cephalad. Two Vicryl pursestring sutures are placed close to the pouch of Douglas (but not tied). Then the posterior wall dissection is carried out laterally over the prerectal fascia (Fig. 44–6). The rectal pillars are penetrated, and the pararectal space is entered (the pararectal space is beneath the peritoneum, above the levator floor and lateral to the rectum). The opening in the rectal pillar is widened posteriorly, exposing the superior surface of the pelvic diaphragm, including the coccygeus muscle, which covers the sacrospinous ligament. Deep retractors such as the Breisky-Navratil retractor are required to retract the rectum medially and displace the bladder and peritoneum anteriorly (Fig. 44–7). Loose areolar tissue is pushed to one side, and the pelvic surface of the coccygeus muscle is identified running posterolaterally from the ischial spine toward the sacrum (Fig. 44–8). Buried within this muscle is the sacrospinous ligament. It is unnecessary, difficult, and potentially dangerous to dissect the muscle from the sacrospinous ligament. The sacrospinous ligaments run between the ischial spine and the lateral side of the sacrum in close proximity to a number of vital vessels and nerves (Fig. 44–9). The pudendal nerve and vessels are located just under the ischial spine (any suture applied to the sacrospinous ligament should be placed 1 to 2 cm medial to the ischial spine to avoid injury to these structures). Sutures applied higher than the level of the ischial spine run the risk of injuring the sciatic nerve as it courses beneath the piriformis muscle.

Using a long needle holder, Deschamps ligature carrier, or Mayo hook with No. 1 absorbable sutures, two threads are passed through the substance of the coccygeus muscle and into the sacrospinous ligament, keeping a distance of 1 cm between the two sutures. Gentle traction on the free ends of the suture will test the strength of the anchor. Superficial application of the suture to the coccygeus muscle or more proximal application into the levator musculature will not provide a strong anchor, and the suture will pull out. An

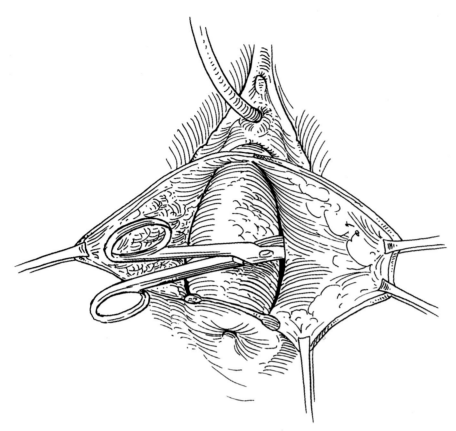

Figure 44-6 The posterior vaginal wall is opened, exposing the prerectal fascia. The pararectal space is entered by opening the rectal pillar. (From Raz S: Atlas of Transvaginal Surgery. Philadelphia, WB Saunders, 1992.)

appropriate anchor into the sacrospinous ligament will essentially allow rocking of the patient over the operating table when the sutures are tested. The two free ends of the sutures are left on a clamp for use at the end of the operation.

Attention is now turned to the enterocele purse-string sutures. These are tied sequentially after removal of the laparotomy pad (as in the standard fashion for enterocele repair). The vaginal wall, however, is not excised at this point. The two free ends of each suture on the sacrospinous ligaments are individually passed through the full thickness of the vaginal wall at the dome with the threads emerging at the epithelial side. The two sutures are placed in healthy vaginal tissue that is not traversed by an incision or suture line with a distance of 1 to 2 cm between the two sutures. The sutures are temporarily left untied and secured with a clamp. The posterior vaginal wall and vaginal vault area are closed. The previously placed sutures in the sacrospinous ligament are tied individually, the vaginal vault be-

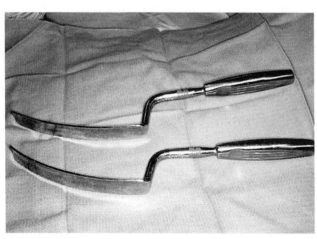

Figure 44-7 Breisky-Navratil retractor. (From Raz S: Atlas of Transvaginal Surgery. Philadelphia, WB Saunders, 1992.)

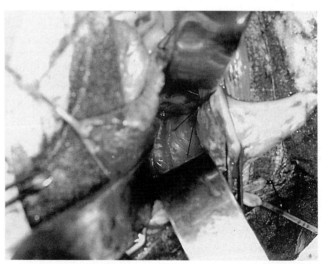

Figure 44-8 The coccygeus muscle is demonstrated within the pararectal space. The bladder and peritoneum are displaced anteriorly and the rectum medially. (From Raz S: Atlas of Transvaginal Surgery. Philadelphia, WB Saunders, 1992.)

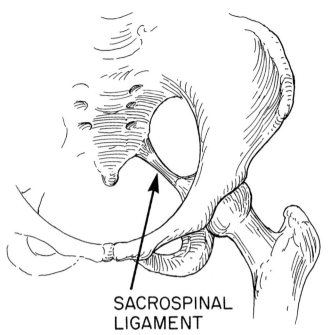

Figure 44-9 Course of the sacrospinal ligament. (From Raz S: Atlas of Transvaginal Surgery. Philadelphia, WB Saunders, 1992.)

ing directed under finger guidance to the uppermost position, where a square knot of the suspension sutures affixes it to the sacrospinous ligament on one side (Fig. 44–10).

Clinical note: If bladder neck surgery is required, it is done before the sacrospinous fixation is performed.

POSTOPERATIVE CARE

The vagina is packed with a vaginal packing coated with an antibiotic cream. The urethral and suprapu-

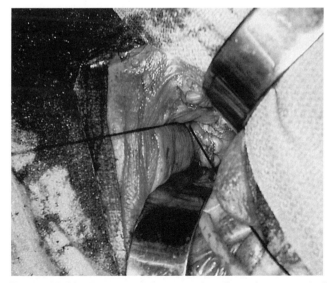

Figure 44-10 Fixation of the vaginal wall to the sacrospinal ligament. (From Raz S: Atlas of Transvaginal Surgery. Philadelphia, WB Saunders, 1992.)

bic catheters are connected to closed bag drainage. The suprapubic tube is secured in place with a 2–0 nylon suture. The Foley catheter and vaginal packing are removed the next morning following surgery. Intravenous antibiotics are given for 24 hours, followed by oral antibiotics for several days. Normal activities like walking and driving are allowed immediately after discharge from the hospital.

INTRAOPERATIVE COMPLICATIONS

A potential complication is bleeding, which can be significant if the levator is damaged or if the pudendal vessels are penetrated. A branch of the internal iliac venous system can be injured as well. Damage to the pudendal nerve may occur if the sutures are placed too far laterally; the sciatic nerve may be injured if sutures are placed too far cephalically (in the area of the piriformis). The pudendal artery may follow a variable course; in order to avoid injury to this structure, sutures should be placed through the sacrospinous ligament, as opposed to posterior to it. Another potential complication is rectal injury during the dissection or retraction of the pararectal space (this surgery should be performed only with complete lower bowel preparation and parenteral antibiotics). Ureteral injury may occur because of the severe distortion of pelvic anatomy associated with significant prolapse.

POSTOPERATIVE COMPLICATIONS

Some patients may complain of low back pain radiating to the back of the thigh following the procedure. This is a self-limiting phenomenon that should respond to analgesics and time. Recurrent prolapse of the vaginal dome may occur owing to laxity of the tissues. Another reason for failure is incomplete or poor anchoring of the vaginal dome into the sacrospinous ligament area. A transabdominal approach may be necessary in patients with recurrent problems. Vaginal shortening and stenosis are potential complications.

Abdominal Repair of Enterocele and Vault Suspension

Abdominal repair of an enterocele may be performed when other intra-abdominal procedures are required; vault suspension may likewise be performed transabdominally. The Moschcowitz procedure involves closure of the cul-de-sac. This procedure was designed initially to treat rectal prolapse by securing the rectum to the relatively fixed vagina. The same logic has been used to fix the vagina in place by securing it to the rectum. Unfortunately, the rectum is not as well secured in place.

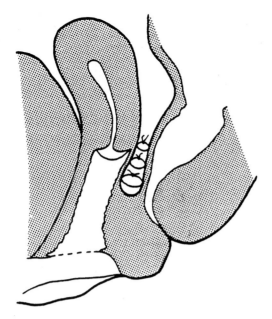

Figure 44–11 Moschcowitz procedure. Sagittal section of the pelvis showing three successive sutures inserted in the pouch of Douglas peritoneum for correction of an enterocele. (From Stanton SL: Vaginal prolapse. *In* Raz S [ed]: Female Urology. Philadelphia, WB Saunders, 1983.)

The basis of this operation involves closure of the cul-de-sac. The patient is placed in the frog leg or abdominoperineal position, and laparotomy is performed. If the uterus is present, it is grasped and pulled forward. If the uterus is absent, the posterior wall of the vagina is grasped with Allis clamps and held anteriorly under traction. Starting at the base of the sac, pursestring sutures of 2–0 Vicryl are placed to close the pouch of Douglas. Included in the suture are any remnants of the uterosacral ligaments, the serosa of the vagina, the lateral peritoneum, and the serosal surface of the rectum. Special care is taken to avoid ureteral injury. The sutures are then tied successively without placing excessive tension on them (Fig. 44–11).

Vault suspension techniques include sacral colpopexy in which the vault or uterus is fixed or directed to the sacrum at the S3–S4 level. This technique may be performed using a bridge of fascia or synthetic material if there is inadequate length to directly appose the two structures. If concurrent repair of cystocele or rectocele is planned this should be performed first transvaginally. Repair of these lesions after colpopexy increases the level of technical difficulty. Finally, it is vital for the surgeon to assess the presence or absence of perineal or rectal abnormalities accurately because failure to repair these may compromise the long-term results of the repair.

One technique of repair is described by Nichols.[3] The patient is put in the lithotomy position, and a pelvic examination is performed to reassess earlier impressions of anatomy. Preparation should allow easy access to the vagina. A Foley catheter is inserted. Either a midline or a transverse incision may be used. The peritoneal cavity is entered, and the bowel is packed out of the field. The vaginal apex is grasped with Allis clamps and the overlying peritoneum incised. The bladder and rectum are dissected away from the vaginal apex to expose at least a 3 × 4 cm area of vaginal wall. Four sutures of figure-of-eight Tevdek material are placed in the thickness of the vaginal wall. At this point the surgeon may wish to place his hand in the vagina to assist with placement of these sutures.

If a graft is to be used, these sutures are next inserted into the graft. At this point a second row of 2–0 Vicryl sutures is placed through the graft into the posterior vaginal wall. Closure of the cul-de-sac is performed next using the Moschcowitz technique. This technique may be modified to a hemi-Moschcowitz technique on one side of the sigmoid to avoid constriction of the sigmoid. The parietal peritoneum over the sacrum is next opened longitudinally in the midline from the promontory to a point caudal to S3. The sacral fascia is exposed by careful dissection, taking care to avoid the presacral vessels. If a graft is used, this is next secured to the presacral fascia and tied without tension. The sigmoid colon should be assessed at this point for compression. The peritoneum is sutured over the repair. Finally, after closure of the anterior peritoneum, attention is turned to a suprapubic colpopexy. This procedure is performed in the standard Burch fashion to minimize the potential for postoperative stress incontinence following a change in the posterior urethropelvic angle.

COMPLICATIONS

Complications may result from inadequate preoperative assessment and include postoperative incontinence or exacerbation or development of rectocele or cystocele. Vault suspension results are generally good if wide approximation of the vaginal apex is achieved using a durable suture such as Tevdek. Other complications may include excessive bleeding during presacral dissection or bowel injury during the initial exposure.

REFERENCES

1. Sanz L: Gynecological Surgery. Oradell, NJ, Medical Economics Books, 1988.
2. Baden WE, Walker J: Surgical Repair of Vaginal Defects. Philadelphia, JB Lippincott, 1992.
3. Nichols DH: Vaginal Surgery, 3rd ed. Baltimore, Williams & Wilkins, 1989.

BIBLIOGRAPHY

Farrell SA, Scotti RJ, Ostergard DR, Bent AE: Massive evisceration: A complication following sacrospinous vaginal vault fixation. Obstet Gynecol 78(Pt 2):560–562, 1991.
Hiller RI: Repair of enterocele with preservation of the vagina. Am J Obstet Gynecol 64:409, 1952.

Hofmeister FJ: Prolapsed vagina. Obstet Gynecol 42:773, 1973.

Jeffcoate TNA: Posterior colporrhaphy. Am J Obstet Gynecol 77:490, 1959.

Leach GE, Zimmern P, Staskin D, et al: Surgery for pelvic prolapse. Semin Urol 4:43–50, 1986.

Lee RA: Vaginal hysterectomy with repair of enterocele, cystocele, and rectocele.

McCall ML: Posterior culdeplasty. Obstet Gynecol 10:595, 1957.

Moschcowitz AV: The cure of prolapse of the rectum. Surg Gynecol Obstet 15:7–21, 1912.

Nichols DH: Types of enterocele and principles underlying choice of operation for repair. Obstet Gynecol 40:257, 1972.

Ranney B: Enterocele, vaginal prolapse, pelvic hernia: Recognition and treatment. Am J Obstet Gynecol 140:53, 1981.

Raz S: Operative repair of rectocele, enterocele and cystocele. Adv Urol 5:121–144, 1992.

Richardson AC: The rectovaginal septum revisited: Its relationship to rectocele and its importance in rectocele repair. Clin Obstet Gynecol 36(4):976–983, 1993.

Richardson AC, Lyon JB, Williams NL: A new look at pelvic relaxation. Am J Obstet Gynecol 126:12, 1976.

Staskin DR, Hadley HR, Zimmern P, et al: Anatomy for vaginal surgery. Semin Urol 4:2, 1986.

Staskin DR, Hadley HR, Zimmern P, et al: Preoperative intraoperative and postoperative management of vaginal surgery. Semin Urol 4:7–12, 1986.

Thompson J (ed): TeLinde's Operative Gynecology, 7th ed. Philadelphia, JB Lippincott, 1992.

Tovell H: Gynecological Operations. New York, Harper & Row, 1978.

Valaitis SR, Stanton SL: Sacrocolpopexy: A retrospective study of a clinician's experience. Br J Obstet Gynaecol 101(6):518–522, 1994.

Wiskind AK, Creighton SM, Stanton SL: The incidence of genital prolapse after the Burch colposuspension. Am J Obstet Gynecol 167(2):399–404, 1992.

Zacharin RF: Pelvic Floor Anatomy and the Surgery of Pulsion Enterocele. New York, Springer-Verlag, 1985.

Zacharin RF: Pulsion enterocele: Review of functional anatomy of the pelvic floor. Obstet Gynecol 55:135, 1980.

PART VIII

Other Conditions

CHAPTER 45

Female Urethral Diverticulum

George P. H. Young, M.D.
Gregory R. Wahle, M.D.
Shlomo Raz, M.D.

The occurrence of female urethral diverticulum was first described by Hey in 1805 but was a rarely recognized entity until the 1930s. A handful of cases were reported in the literature before 1935. Prior to 1950, just over 100 cases total had been noted in the historical records of three major medical centers: Johns Hopkins, Mayo Clinic, and Cleveland Clinic.[1] Since 1950, with the advent of positive pressure urethrography, the general awareness and recognition of this disorder have heightened. Davis and TeLinde reported in 1958 as many cases as had been recognized in the previous 60 years.[2]

Incidence

Female urethral diverticulum is estimated to occur in between 1 and 6% of all adult women. It generally occurs between the ages of 20 and 60, the average age being approximately 40 years. A definite racial predilection of blacks to whites in a ratio of 3.5 to 6:1 has been noted.[3]

This condition probably occurs more frequently than it is diagnosed. In 1964, Adams obtained positive pressure urethrograms in 129 consecutive female patients without active urinary tract symptoms and found the incidence of diverticula to be 4.7%.[4] Andersen noted an incidence of 3% in a group of 300 women undergoing treatment for cervical carcinoma.[5]

Etiology and Pathophysiology

Even though urethral diverticula are found in the usual location of the periurethral glands, the cause and pathogenesis of this entity have been vigorously debated throughout this century. The theories of origin of urethral diverticula are chiefly related to whether they are congenital or acquired and, if acquired, whether they are secondary to infection or parturition or are iatrogenic.

The arguments for a congenital origin have been weakened by the fact that urethral diverticula are rarely found in children.[2, 6] In the study of 121 female patients with urethral diverticula performed by Davis and TeLinde, no diagnoses were made prior to the age of 20 years.[2] Only 6.5% of these patients dated the onset of symptoms prior to the age of 20 years. Some reported cases, however, point to a congenital origin in certain instances. A urethral diverticulum has been reported at the site where an ectopic ureter emptied into the urethra.[1] Urethral diverticula have been located in areas containing remnants of Gartner's ducts.[7] These have been noticed when Gartner's duct carcinomas have been discovered within the diverticula. Several patients have also been treated for diverticula containing cloagenic rests.[3] In a case cited by Silk and Lebowitz, an anterior diverticulum was postulated to represent an aborted attempt at urethral duplication.[8]

Various theories explaining the development of female urethral diverticula have been advanced. Although female urethral diverticula have been described in young infants, presumably occurring as congenital diverticula, the majority certainly appear to be acquired.

Earlier in this century the origin was usually attributed to the trauma of childbirth.[9] It was postulated that pressure from the fetal head or delivery forceps ruptured the intrinsic musculature of the urethra, leading to consequent herniation of the mucosa and diverticular formation. However, studies since then have shown that urethral diverticula are

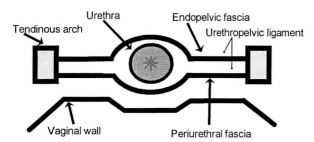

Figure 45–1 Schematic representation of normal urethral support as seen in a coronal plane. Note the support of the urethra by the endopelvic fascia from above and the periurethral fascia from below with the urethropelvic ligament in between.

just as likely to arise in nulliparous patients, and this earlier hypothesis has generally been rejected. More readily accepted now is the explanation offered by Routh, who in 1890 postulated that repeated infection and obstruction of the periurethral glands resulted in the formation of suburethral cysts.[10] These cysts eventually ruptured and drained back into the urethral lumen. Continued irritation of pooled urine retained during each voiding in these abscess cavities would then lead to eventual epithelialization and formation of a permanent diverticulum. Acceptance of this explanation now causes most investigators to consider urethral diverticula an acquired lesion of infectious etiology.

Two of the most probable causes are gonococcal infection and infection of the periurethral glands from normal vaginal flora.[11] The most commonly cultured organisms are *Escherichia coli* and other gram-negative bacilli as well as *Staphylococcus aureus* and *Streptococcus fecalis*. In a study by Peters and Vaughan of 32 patients, patients had either proven gonorrhea or a history suggestive of gonorrhea.[12] Other studies have not been so persuasive, and it is generally concluded now that any urethral infection involving the periurethral glands can lead to eventual diverticula formation, although gonorrhea may often be the etiologic factor.

Many other possible causes of urethral diverticula have been suggested, including trauma from childbirth, high intravesical pressures on voiding against a closed or spastic external sphincter in neurogenic cases, instrumentation, urethral calculus, urethral stricture, and any urethral or anterior vaginal surgery complicated by inadequate wound closure or infection. Congenital factors, including Gartner's duct, faulty union of the primal folds, cell nests, and wolffian ducts or vaginal cysts that rupture into the urethra, may be involved.

Huffman constructed wax models of an infected urethra and found periurethral openings.[13] His experiments support the concept of a suburethral infection's developing into an abscess that becomes lined with epithelium. The periurethral glands become infected and obstructed and rupture into the urethra, forming a communication site between the diverticulum and the urethra itself. Microscopic studies have shown that periurethral glands can be found along much of the length of the urethra.[13] These glands are

located primarily posterolaterally, and the majority open into the distal third of the urethra. They constitute a complex system of tubuloalveolar structures that may number more than 30. Skene's glands, the largest of the periurethral glands, empty at the external meatus and are often considered separately.

Diverticula develop beneath the well-defined periurethral fascia. The periurethral glands are tubuloalveolar structures found predominantly throughout the distal two-thirds of the urethra that open mainly into the distal one-third of the urethra. Up to 90% of diverticula open into the mid or distal urethra.[14] Morphologically, the periurethral glands range from simple saccular structures to complex branching sinus tracts. When they become infected, the associated obstruction of drainage of the gland into the urethra may cause a urethral diverticulum in the distal two-thirds of the urethra. Occasionally, female urethral diverticula may be extremely proximal and may extend beneath the bladder neck and trigonal area as well as anteriorly.[8, 15]

In the last 10 years we have developed a better understanding of the pathophysiology and surgical anatomy of urethral diverticula. Our observations are based mostly on our experience during careful surgical dissection in patients requiring urethral reconstruction, repair of urethral diverticula, and magnetic resonance imaging of the pelvis. To clarify our concept of the pathogenesis of female urethral diverticula, we will briefly summarize our understanding of the surgical anatomy of the female urethra. The urethra consists largely of a rich vascular sponge surrounded by an envelope consisting of smooth and skeletal muscle and fibroelastic tissue. It is supported to the lateral pelvic wall by a urethropelvic ligament that has two components: an abdominal side, the endopelvic fascia, and a vaginal side, the periurethral fascia (Fig. 45–1). Acquired urethral diverticula result from infected and obstructed periurethral glands, normally found in the submucosal layer of the spongy tissue of the distal two-thirds of the urethra. Cystic and abscess formation from repeated infection and obstruction of periurethral glands slowly expands in size. Initially, the expansion occurs by displacing the vascular sponge tissue and urethral musculature; further enlargement of the diverticulum weakens the urethral envelope, causing

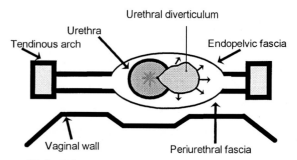

Figure 45–2 Schematic representation of urethral diverticulum and its location between the fascial layers of the urethropelvic ligament.

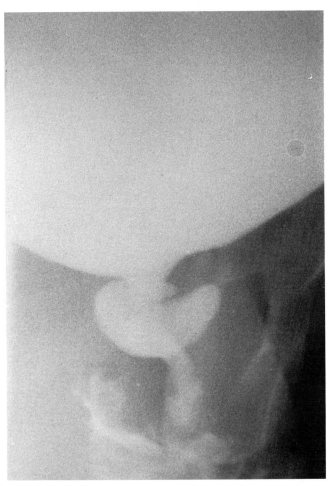

Figure 45-3 Radiograph of a urethral diverticulum with a horseshoe appearance.

herniation and dissection between these two fascial layers of the urethropelvic ligament (Fig. 45–2). The most common expansion of the diverticular sac occurs posteriorly to the urethra, creating the typical finding of a cystic tender mass in the anterior vaginal wall. Also common is the lateral expansion, which can create less of a mass effect but more dissection and separation between the vaginal and abdominal layers of the urethropelvic ligaments. Rarely, expansion occurs anteriorly to the urethra or, even less frequently, encloses completely the urethra like a horseshoe (Fig. 45–3). Eventually, rupture of the diverticulum content into the urethral lumen will occur, establishing the communication between the diverticulum and the urethra. In some cases, rupture may occur into the vagina, leading to a urethrovaginal fistula. These concepts are particularly important for an understanding of the surgical technique used in the excision of urethral diverticula.

Clinical Presentation

The woman with a urethral diverticulum sometimes presents with a tender, cystic suburethral swelling from which retained urine or purulent material can be milked through the meatus by digital pressure. Patients often more typically present with a myriad of symptoms associated with most common lower urinary tract disorders.[2, 6, 12, 16]

The patient frequently notes signs of lower urinary tract irritation. Dysuria, frequency, urgency, and hematuria occur in the majority of cases. The complaint most characteristic of urethral diverticulum, however, appears to be postmicturition dribbling. Dribbling accompanied by dyspareunia and dysuria seems to constitute a classic triad for urethral diverticula. A history of recurrent urinary tract infections refractory to antibiotic therapy may be a clue. Other symptoms include dyspareunia, swelling in the vagina, and urethral discharge and pain with ambulation. Pyuria and cystitis may also occur, depending on the location of the diverticular orifice. Frequently, patients may present with associated symptoms of urinary incontinence (stress or urgency incontinence), and occasionally these may be the only presenting symptoms.

The rare finding of urinary retention usually results from large proximal diverticula that impinge on and obstruct the bladder neck or is subsequent to stricture formation secondary to repeated infections. Hematuria is also usually secondary to active infection; however, Palagiri reported a diverticulum in which the sac after excision was found to contain endometrial stroma and blood clots.[17]

None of the symptoms routinely appear to be proportional to the size of the diverticulum. A large diverticulum is often unnoticed by the patient, whereas a small sac, when actively infected, may be extremely symptomatic. The chronicity of the complaint is not uniform. Prolonged periods of spontaneous remission are not uncommon.

More than 30 cases of carcinoma have been associated with urethral diverticula in women. The patient may be totally asymptomatic, and the diverticulum itself may be detected only on physical examination.

Diagnosis

The diagnosis of urethral diverticulum can be made by a combination of history, physical examination, cystourethroscopy, and urethrography. However, the diagnosis depends on a high index of suspicion because this entity has an incidence that is not insignificant.[1, 18] The history may be quite suggestive, although the patient may be asymptomatic.

Routine urologic evaluation, including urologic history, physical examination, urinalysis, cystourethroscopy, and excretory urogram showing the upper tracts and bladder, often is not diagnostic for urethral diverticulum. The presentation of this disorder is rarely typical, and these tests are not sufficiently specific. The history of irritative symptoms is common for most lower urinary tract disorders.

On physical examination it is extremely important

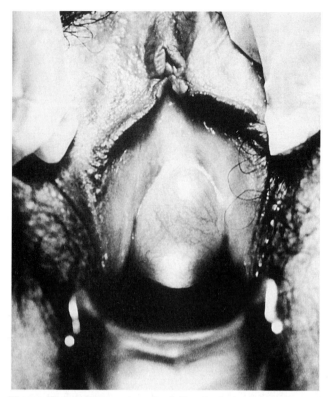

Figure 45-4 Midline suburethral diverticulum on vaginal examination.

to examine specifically the suburethral area in women. The urethra is generally tender, and a suburethral mass may be palpated (Fig. 45–4). Manual compression may lead to the expression of purulent material from the external meatus. The diverticulum may also appear as a stony hard mass, especially if the sac contains a calculus[19] or, infrequently, a malignancy.

While examining the urethra it is also important to determine the position of the proximal urethra and bladder base to assess hypermobility. A preoperative diagnosis of anatomic stress incontinence may warrant a combined operation to correct both the diverticulum and the stress incontinence. When a diagnosis of female urethral diverticulum is suggested on the basis of the history and physical examination, further studies are helpful to delineate the size and location of the diverticulum.

Urethroscopy should be performed using a zero-degree lens and a sheath with a very short beak, allowing the entire urethra to be distended for adequate visualization of the entire urethral lumen. Constant water flow and bladder neck compression at the time of urethroscopy may force the contents of the diverticulum into the urethra, allowing visualization of the orifice (Fig. 45–5). Inflammatory edema may prevent visualization of the orifice. At the time of endoscopy, the urethra is compressed to determine the presence of any active drainage of pus from the mouth of the diverticulum. On rare occasions when the standard radiologic and endoscopic work-up is not confirmatory, a small amount of a mixture of methylene blue and contrast solution can be injected through the anterior vaginal wall directly into the suspected urethral diverticulum. This can help to identify the diverticulum by fluoroscopy and urethroscopy.

The postvoid film of an intravenous pyelogram often reveals a collection of contrast material in the subvesical area (Fig. 45–6). The voiding cystogram under fluoroscopic control in the standing oblique position is the most reliable diagnostic tool and best defines the location, size, and number of diverticula. Frequently, any irregularity of the urethra is demonstrated during the voiding phase of the vesicourethrogram (VCUG) (Fig. 45–7). When the study is monitored fluoroscopically, the exact positioning of the patient can be controlled to obtain an ideal oblique view, so that the diverticulum can be rotated away from the urethra to avoid superimposing both

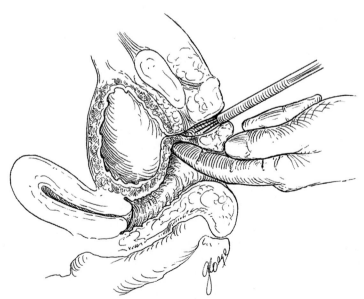

Figure 45-5 Diagram of urethroscopy with a zero-degree lens, showing the occlusion of the bladder neck when constant perfusion of fluid distends the urethra. This maneuver can enhance the chances of detecting urethral diverticula. (From Raz S: Atlas of Transvaginal Surgery. Philadelphia, WB Saunders, 1992.)

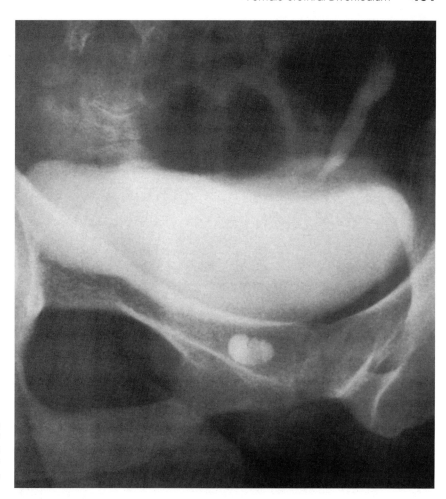

Figure 45-6 Postvoid film after intravenous pyelogram in a patient with recurrent urinary tract infection. A diverticulum is seen in the midurethral area. (From Raz S: Atlas of Transvaginal Surgery. Philadelphia, WB Saunders, 1992.)

on the x-ray film. Should the VCUG not show a suburethral mass that is clinically suggestive of a urethral diverticulum, other radiographic studies may be helpful.

If a postvoid film from a voiding cystourethrogram does not demonstrate the diverticulum, positive pressure urethrography should be performed. In 1959, Lang and Davis introduced their method of positive pressure urethrography.[14] Today, this study coupled with voiding cystourethrography constitutes the optimal method of detection of urethral diverticula in women. Positive pressure urethrography is accomplished using a double-balloon catheter. Today in the United States, a single-unit model, usually either the Davis-TeLinde or the Trattner catheter, is used.[20] A double-balloon catheter blocks the urethra proximally and distally. The proximal and distal balloons have separate inflation conduits, and a third conduit opens to a slit between the balloons to allow positioning in the urethra (Figs. 45–8 and 45–9).

Following a scout film, the catheter is inserted into the bladder. The proximal balloon is inflated with 20 ml of saline or dilute contrast medium. The distal balloon is then inflated with approximately 30 ml to ensure a snug fit at the meatus and to seal the proximal balloon against the bladder neck. The urethra is filled with 4 to 8 ml of contrast medium. Fluoroscopy is used during injection, and anteropos-

terior and oblique radiographs are obtained. The proximal balloon is deflated, and the catheter is removed. Next, a voiding cystourethrogram is performed. A Robinson catheter is inserted in the urethra, and the bladder is filled. With the catheter in place, upright anteroposterior and lateral films are obtained during rest and straining maneuvers. After this catheter has been removed, the important voiding films are taken in the oblique position. The postvoid film is obtained in the anteroposterior projection.

During radiographic examinations it was noted that the double-balloon catheter study could maximally outline the sac of a diverticulum. The diverticulum would appear as a large, rounded, or lobulated collection of contrast material. However, the relationship of the diverticulum to the urethra and the presence of multiple diverticula were often obscured by the catheter. This problem was overcome by obtaining the voiding cystourethrograms after the double-balloon catheter was removed. The collections of contrast material in the diverticulum were usually retained on postvoid films. Voiding studies also allow evaluation of other genitourinary pathology, such as cystourethroceles and fistulas.

An alternative diagnostic scheme has been devised by Borski and Stutzman.[21] The patient is instructed to empty the bladder. The anterior vaginal wall is

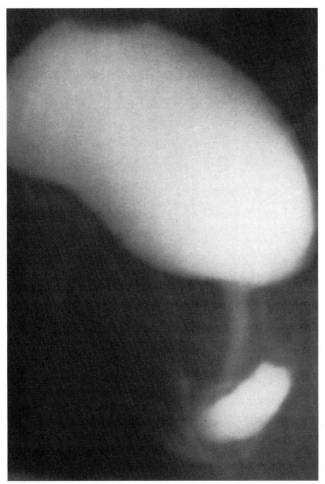

Figure 45–7   Voiding cystogram in a patient with recurrent urinary infection and pain during intercourse. A distal diverticulum is present. (From Raz S: Atlas of Transvaginal Surgery. Philadelphia, WB Saunders, 1992.)

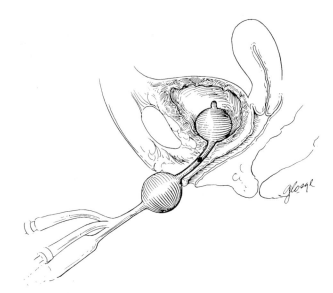

Figure 45–8   Diagram of the double-balloon urethrography. Good occlusion of the bladder neck and urethra must be obtained to avoid leak of the contrast agent around the balloons.

third of the urethra beneath the bladder.[23] Urethral pressure profilometry has also been recommended. A characteristic biphasic shape of the urethral pressure profile has been noted in women with urethral diverticula.[24] The central depression of this biphasic profile is thought to correspond to the weakened ure-

compressed and milked to empty any diverticula. A Foley catheter is inserted, and a solution containing 5 ml of indigo carmine, 60 ml of radiopaque contrast medium, and 100 ml of water is instilled into the bladder. The catheter is removed, and the patient is instructed to void while occluding the urethral meatus with one finger. Radiographs are obtained in the anteroposterior and oblique projections. Urethroscopy with urethral compression is performed to identify any diverticular orifices from which the blue dye is ejected.

Coupling positive pressure urethrography with cystourethroscopy thus provides the basis for diagnostic evaluation of this disorder. Lately, we have also employed endovaginal and transperineal ultrasonography in patients with a suburethral mass not clearly diagnosed by routine radiologic studies.[22] We find it quite helpful in demonstrating a fluid collection in the diverticulum, its size, and whether it is single or multiple. Excretory urography is useful in ruling out upper tract duplication or ectopic ureteral insertion. The appearance of bladder base elevation on an excretory urogram may represent a large fluid collection in a diverticulum located in the proximal

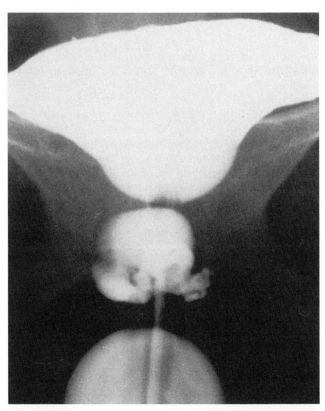

Figure 45–9   Double-balloon urethrogram in a patient with terminal dribbling and urinary tract infection. A large midurethral diverticulum is well seen. (From Raz S: Atlas of Transvaginal Surgery. Philadelphia, WB Saunders, 1992.)

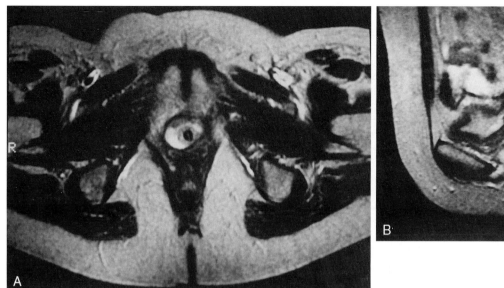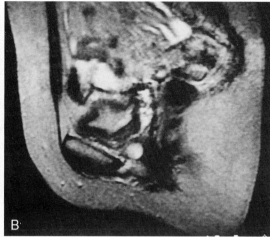

Figure 45-10 Magnetic resonance image of urethral diverticulum. *A,* Transaxial view. *B,* Midsagittal view.

thral wall at the site of communication with the diverticulum. Other radiologic modalities such as MRI[25, 26] have helped us develop a better understanding of the surgical anatomy of urethral diverticula but do not offer any significant clinical diagnostic value (Fig. 45–10).

Differential Diagnosis

Although the history and physical examination may strongly suggest a suburethral diverticulum, other clinical entities may mimic this condition. Simple bacterial cystitis should be considered, as should the lower urinary tract irritative symptoms that usually accompany interstitial cystitis. Other intravaginal and suburethral masses that may mimic female urethral diverticulum include Skene's gland abscesses, which are located in the distal urethra without diverticulum formation. These are usually lateral to the midline. An ectopic ureter may extend to the suburethral area. Occasionally, a urethral neoplasm may appear as a suburethral palpable mass.[12, 27] Gartner's duct cysts of the anterior vaginal wall may be confused with urethral diverticulum, although these cysts usually arise more laterally in the anterior vaginal wall.[28] A hyperreflexic neurogenic bladder, bladder calculus, or bladder neoplasm may also occur with irritative urinary symptoms.

Thorough urologic evaluation with urinalysis, cystourethroscopy, urography, and biopsy may be required to differentiate among them.[29] The differential diagnosis must also include any lesion manifesting as a suburethral mass. Cystourethroceles are best evaluated with voiding cystourethrograms. An ectopic ureter that opens with a cystic dilation into the urethra can be excluded by excretory urograms, voiding cystourethrograms, and cystourethroscopy.

Gartner's duct cysts are usually found lateral to the urethra and do not communicate with it. Periurethral cysts likewise have no demonstrable urethral communication but are very likely remnants of diverticula with closed orifices.

Indications for Surgery

Surgery is indicated in a patient with significant symptoms related to the presence of a urethral diverticulum. They include recurrent urinary tract infections, severe pain, dyspareunia, frequency, urgency, and postvoid dribbling.

Preoperative Care

Once the diagnosis of urethral diverticulum is confirmed, various preoperative factors are worthy of consideration. Should the patient have significant documented genuine stress urinary incontinence (SUI) and a low, poorly supported, hypermobile urethra and bladder neck, it is advisable to consider the option of initial transvaginal needle suspension of the bladder neck and proximal urethra followed by urethral diverticulectomy during the same procedure. Simultaneous performance of both procedures provides the optimal chance of obtaining adequate postoperative continence.

If both procedures are indicated, it is important to perform the needle suspension first to avoid the risk of contaminating the retropubic space after the diverticulum is manipulated. The technique of transvaginal needle suspension of the bladder neck and proximal urethra has been described in detail in Chapter 30. We have performed simultaneous transvaginal needle suspension of the proximal urethra and bladder neck and urethral diverticulectomy in numerous women with excellent results.

The surgeon should be especially alert when a preoperative history of severe urinary urgency and frequency is present. In patients with a significant component of detrusor instability on preoperative cystometric evaluation that is not treated appropriately during the postoperative period, high intravesical pressures certainly increase the risk of postoperative breakdown at the urethral reconstruction site with subsequent formation of a urethral-vaginal fistula or recurrent urethral diverticulum. When significant detrusor instability is documented, we consider anticholinergic therapy to help decrease the risk of postoperative failure. After the diagnosis of female urethral diverticulum has been confirmed and the various preoperative surgical considerations have been thoroughly examined, surgical intervention may then be undertaken.

Prior to surgery, proper antibiotic therapy is mandatory. Reconstructive surgery in a patient with active urinary and diverticular infection may lead to fistula formation and recurrent diverticula. A suprapubic catheter should be inserted at the time of surgery to ensure safe and uninterrupted bladder drainage. This suprapubic catheter functions as a safety valve during the postoperative period should the urethral catheter become occluded, and it facilitates performance of a voiding cystourethrogram by allowing filling of the bladder through the suprapubic catheter. Povidone-iodine (Betadine) douches are administered the night before surgery.

Basically, except for the small, noninfected, benign diverticulum, optimal therapy consists of obliteration or surgical extirpation of the intact sac. Very small diverticula can probably be handled by transurethral incision (widening the orifice intraluminally). In the patient whose surgery must be delayed, the urethra can be stripped intravaginally after each urination (keeping the diverticulum empty), and antibiotics are provided prophylactically. Otherwise, surgical excision is the goal.

Treatment

HISTORICAL PERSPECTIVE

The reported surgical treatments have taken several different approaches to diverticula in the past. Furniss incised the diverticulum transvaginally and packed its sac with gauze.[30] Later, a second operation was performed to excise the resultant urethrovaginal fistula and the granulated sac. Both Hunner and Young passed a sound into the urethra that was kept in place while the diverticulum was excised transvaginally.[31, 32] Hunner then created a vaginal flap to cover the incision line so that the suture lines were not superimposed. Hyams and Hyams packed the diverticulum transurethrally with gauze to facili-

tate transvaginal excision.[33] Cook and Pool suggested passing a urethral catheter transurethrally into the diverticulum and allowing it to coil up as an aid to transvaginal excision.[34] Moore exposed the diverticulum transvaginally, incised it, and inserted a Foley catheter with its tip removed into the sac.[1] He inflated the Foley catheter balloon to fill the diverticulum and secured it with a pursestring suture before excision. Moore thought that this better outlined the sac and permitted traction on it to ease the dissection.[1]

Edwards and Beebe incised the urethra and vaginal wall up to and including the diverticulum.[35] A urethroplasty was then performed to repair the incision. Ellik devised a technique for incising diverticula near the bladder neck.[36] He incised the sac transvaginally, packed the cavity with Oxycel, and oversewed the incision. Subsequently, the surrounding tissues healed by fibrosis. Hirschhorn injected a liquid Silastic material into the diverticulum prior to its excision.[37] O'Connor and Kropp used firm fibrin that was formed from human fibrinogen clotted with thrombin to fill the diverticular sac.[38]

Spence and Duckett saucerized the diverticulum and the distal urethra to the external meatus and sutured the edges to the surrounding incised vaginal mucosa.[29] This maneuver created, in effect, a generous meatotomy. They reported no problem with incontinence if the diverticulum was in the distal two-thirds of the urethra, stating that sphincteric control

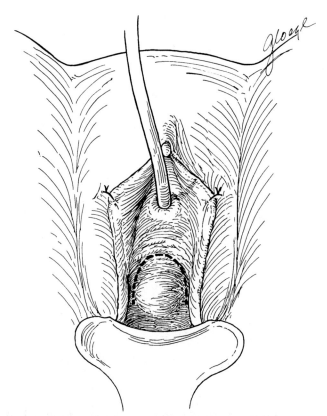

Figure 45-11 Inverted U-shaped incision in anterior vaginal wall with the apex distal to the urethral diverticulum and proximal to the meatus.

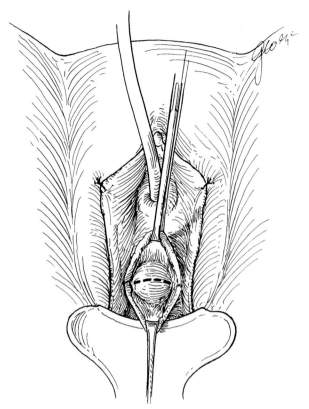

Figure 45-12 Anterior vaginal wall flap is reflected posteriorly, exposing the periurethral fascia.

resided in the region bounded by the bladder neck and the proximal third of the urethra. Flocks and Culp emphasized that in a transvaginal excision a multilayer closure with no overlapping suture lines was required.[39] Sasnett and coworkers advocated the jackknife position instead of the lithotomy position to maximize exposure and to permit a downward perspective on the operative field.[40]

EXCISION

At UCLA, the technique most commonly used is similar to that described by Busch and Carter[41] and illustrated by Benjamin and coworkers[3] but with important modifications. It is based on optimizing the exposure, totally excising the diverticulum, and obtaining a watertight supported closure.

Technique

The procedure preferred by us for the treatment of female urethral diverticulum is that of transvaginal excision using a vaginal flap technique.[42] The patient is placed in the dorsal lithotomy position and draped, paying careful attention to isolation of the rectum from the operative field.

After insertion of a posterior weighted vaginal retractor and urethral and suprapubic catheters, an inverted U incision is made with the apex distal to

the diverticulum and proximal to the urethral meatus (Fig. 45–11). An anterior vaginal wall flap is reflected posteriorly from the urethral meatus to the bladder neck, exposing the periurethral fascia (Fig. 45–12). Care is taken to avoid any perforation or entry into this fascia or the diverticulum by performing dissection directly on the vaginal wall flap itself. This flap is raised as proximally as necessary to allow complete exposure of the diverticulum and to avoid any overlapping suture lines after the urethral reconstruction is completed.

The periurethral fascia is a distinct layer that surrounds the urethral diverticulum and should be preserved to keep a second layer available for reconstruction after completion of the diverticulectomy. The periurethral fascia is incised transversely, and dissection is performed between the periurethral fascia and the diverticulum itself (Fig. 45–13). This fascia may be very attenuated in patients with large diverticula.

Two flaps are created by dissection of the periurethral fascia proximal and distal to the incision. Thus, the periurethral fascia is opened in an anterior and posterior direction, like opening the leaves of a book, to completely expose the urethral diverticulum. With sharp dissection, the wall of the diverticular sac is freed from the surrounding structures (Fig. 45–14). The wall of the diverticulum should be left intact until dissection has reached the neck of the sac. Should there be a significant degree of scarring

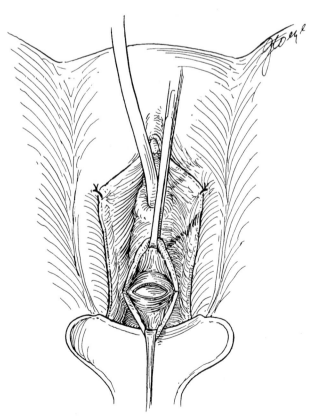

Figure 45-13 Periurethral fascia is opened transversely, exposing the spongy tissue of the submucosal layer of the urethral wall and the diverticular sac.

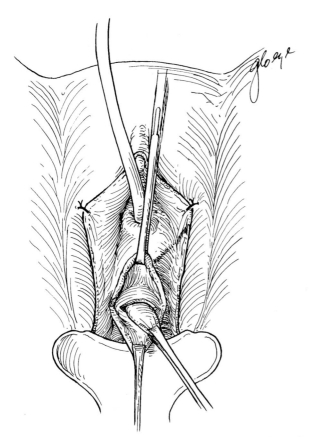

Figure 45-14 After the periurethral fascia is opened, the wall of the diverticular sac is freed from the surrounding structures.

and fibrosis in this area due to chronic inflammation, the diverticulum itself can be opened to define more clearly the extent of the diverticulum and the location of the communication between the diverticulum and the urethra. It is possible that the diverticulum may extend in a circumferential fashion around the urethra, and complete excision of all diverticular tissue is extremely important to minimize the risk of any recurrent diverticulum formation. The communication to the urethral lumen is isolated and excised flush with the urethral wall (Fig. 45–15). All abnormal tissue at this junction is totally excised to decrease the risk of any recurrent diverticulum formation. The lumen of the urethra and the indwelling catheter must be seen.

The mucosal and submucosal layers of the urethra are closed longitudinally with a running 3–0 absorbable suture over a 12 Fr catheter (Fig. 45–16). No patient has developed urethral stenosis when the urethra has been closed over a catheter of this size. The closure should be watertight and tension-free. This step minimizes the risk of postoperative extravasation and urethral-vaginal fistula formation. The periurethral fascia is trimmed and closed horizontally, using a 3–0 absorbable suture (Fig. 45–17). This second layer of closure runs perpendicularly to the first and provides a strong second layer of tissue to aid in the reconstruction of the urethra. Also during closure of this layer the space between the fascial

layers of the urethropelvic ligaments left from excision of the diverticulum must be closed to restore urethral support and prevent formation of a dead space that could facilitate common complications such as recurrence, fistula, and incontinence (Fig. 45–18). The anterior vaginal wall flap is advanced well distally over the suture line of the periurethral fascia and trimmed if necessary. This layer is closed with a running locking 2–0 absorbable suture (Fig. 45–19). The flap advancement brings fresh tissue to cover the reconstruction in a third layer and prevents overlapping lines of sutures. After the procedure is completed, an antibiotic-soaked vaginal pack is placed. Both the suprapubic and urethral catheters are left for gravity drainage.

Identification of the diverticulum at the time of surgical removal has not presented any particular difficulty. Various techniques have been suggested to aid in the identification of the diverticulum, including injection of a coagulum into the diverticulum intraoperatively and coiling a catheter within the diverticulum.[43] In general, we have found that once the periurethral fascia has been opened, the site of the diverticulum is quite obvious, and these further maneuvers are usually not necessary. Should it be difficult to identify the communication site between the diverticulum and the urethra, intraoperative ure-

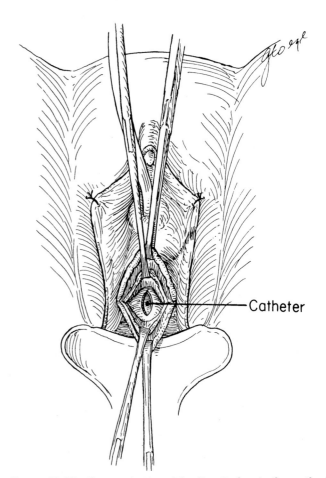

Catheter

Figure 45-15 Communication of the diverticulum to the urethral lumen is excised flush with the urethral wall.

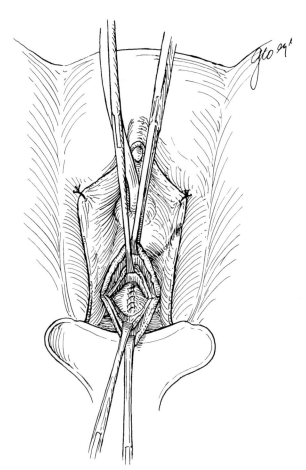

Figure 45-16 Urethra is closed longitudinally with a running 3–0 absorbable suture.

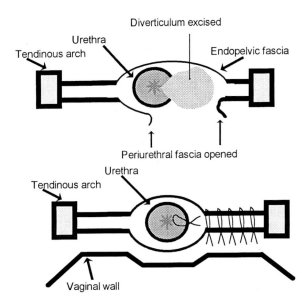

Figure 45-18 Schematic representation of urethral diverticulum. *Top,* After the diverticular sac is excised, a dead space is left between the fascial layers of the urethropelvic ligament. *Bottom,* The space between the fascial layers of the urethropelvic ligament must be closed.

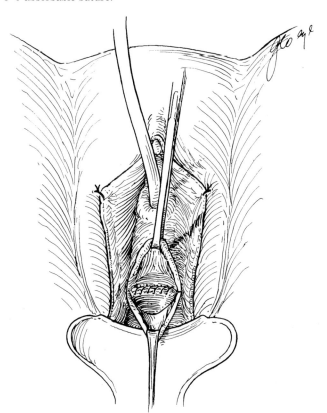

Figure 45-17 Periurethral fascia is closed horizontally with a running 3–0 absorbable suture.

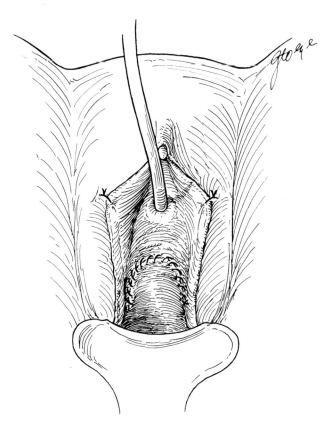

Figure 45-19 Anterior vaginal wall flap is advanced over the suture line in the periurethral fascia.

throscopy can be performed. A pediatric sound can be passed through the communication site into the diverticulum to help facilitate its identification, although this has rarely been necessary.

ENDOSCOPIC TREATMENT

Urethrotomy is performed by splitting the floor of the urethra from the meatus proximally to the diverticular orifice.[44, 45] This maneuver allows better visibility of the diverticular sac during dissection. This technique requires closure and healing of the floor of the urethra along its entire length, which may be tenuous with an infected diverticulum.

SPENCE MARSUPIALIZATION

In 1970, Spence and Duckett suggested marsupialization of the diverticulum to prevent recurrence, minimize operating time, and reduce blood loss.[29, 46] This procedure is useful for diverticula in the distal third of the urethra, away from the intrinsic and external sphincters.

Postoperative Care

After the procedure is completed, a vaginal pack is placed, and the suprapubic and urethral catheters are connected to a drainage bag. Intravenous antibiotics are administered as indicated. The patient may be discharged from the hospital 1 to 2 days after surgery. Patients are routinely placed on anticholinergic therapy after the operative procedure to decrease the risk of any bladder spasms related to catheter drainage. It is hoped in this way to protect the urethral reconstruction site from high intravesical pressures. Anticholinergic medication is discontinued 24 hours before a postoperative voiding cystourethrogram is obtained. About 10 to 14 days after surgery the urethral catheter is removed, and a voiding cystourethrogram is performed through the suprapubic catheter. This radiographic examination is performed in the standing position. When the patient experiences the first urge to urinate, voiding is allowed while the urethra is monitored fluoroscopically, and spot radiographs are obtained as indicated.

Three potential results are possible at the time of voiding cystourethrography. First, the patient may void to completion with no extravasation at the urethral reconstruction site. In this situation, all catheters are removed. Second, the patient may void without extravasation but without complete bladder emptying. The suprapubic catheter is left in place and opened three times daily to monitor postvoid residual urine. When residuals are consistently less than 100 ml, the suprapubic catheter is removed. Third, the patient may have a small degree of extravasation at the urethral reconstruction site. In these patients the urethral catheter is not reinserted, but the suprapubic catheter is placed for drainage. The radiographic study is then repeated 1 week later. No patient in our series has had persistent extravasation when the voiding cystourethrogram has been repeated.

Complications

INTRAOPERATIVE

Bleeding in the form of profuse oozing is not uncommon, particularly in patients with active infection and abscess formation. Vaginal packing should control this oozing well.

If it is difficult to close the urethral mucosa because of the large defect created during excision of the diverticulum, it may be necessary to further expose the urethral wall and close the urethral mucosa over a 5 to 8 Fr feeding tube. We have not encountered urethral strictures following this procedure.

In cases of difficult closure due to severely inflamed or poor quality tissue, a fibrofatty labial (Martius) flap can be used between the periurethral fascia and the vaginal wall. A watertight closure is critical to avoid postoperative extravasation and fistula formation. Precise anatomic dissection and closure of the urethral layers that avoids overlapping suture lines are crucial.

The finding of a large periurethral abscess may require a staged procedure in which the abscess is drained and excision of the diverticulum is performed as a secondary procedure.

Large proximal urethral diverticula may extend into the trigone. Should dissection proceed in an improper plane when the diverticulum extends beneath the trigonal area, bladder or ureteral injury could occur. Instillation of indigo carmine into the bladder in such cases will demonstrate bladder and ureteral integrity, and cystoscopy may then be performed in selected cases.

POSTOPERATIVE

The usual complications of postoperative pain, bleeding, infection, and bladder spasm related to catheters are noteworthy. We believe that appropriate preoperative preparation and perioperative antibiotic therapy as well as postoperative anticholinergics are essential.

New onset of incontinence after diverticulectomy, as well as potential exacerbation of preexisting incontinence, is a complication worthy of consideration. Adequate evaluation of the position of the urethra, bladder neck, and bladder base as well as evaluation of the possibility of SUI prior to diverticulectomy is of utmost importance if this complication is to be avoided.

Urethral stricture may result if too much urethral

wall is removed in dissection of a large diverticulum. Urethrovaginal fistula formation is the most important complication of this surgery, and it should be treated after a period of healing. Anterior vaginal wall infection is rare and responds well to antibiotic therapy. Infection may cause the urethral mucosa to become friable. If an abscess is formed, surgical drainage is required despite the potential damage to the repair.

Recurrent urethral diverticula may occur particularly in a patient with active urethral infection, difficult dissection, and suture line tension and in those in whom postoperative difficulties with catheter drainage are encountered. Secondary surgery should be performed after a prudent period of observation.

Stress incontinence prior to surgery should be well documented and may be corrected in selected cases at the time of excision of the diverticulum. Secondary SUI not present prior to surgery is rare but may develop in a patient with anatomic defects due to dissection of the urethral support. Severe incontinence due to intrinsic sphincteric dysfunction may result from the extensive dissection of the urethral support. Surgery for this condition may require a sling procedure or periurethral injection.

REFERENCES

1. Moore TD: Diverticulum of female urethra: An improved technique of surgical excision. J Urol 68:611, 1952.
2. Davis HJ, TeLinde RW: Urethral diverticula: An assay of 121 cases. J Urol 80:4, 1958.
3. Benjamin J, Elliot L, Cooper JF, Bjornson L: Urethral diverticulum in adult female. Clinical aspects, operative procedures, and pathology. Urology 3:1, 1974.
4. Adams WE: Urethrography. Bull Tulane Med Fac 23:107, 1964.
5. Andersen MJF: The incidence of diverticula in the female urethra. J Urol 98:96, 1967.
6. Davis BL, Robinson DG: Diverticula of the female urethra: Assay of 120 cases. J Urol 104:850, 1970.
7. Hinman F Jr, Cohlan WR: Gartner's duct carcinoma in a urethral diverticulum. J Urol 83:414, 1960.
8. Silk MR, Lebowitz JM: Anterior urethral diverticulum. J Urol 101:66, 1969.
9. McNally A: Diverticula of the female urethra. Am J Surg 28:177, 1935.
10. Routh A: Urethral diverticulum. Br Med J 1:361, 1890.
11. TeLinde RW: Operative Gynecology. Philadelphia, JB Lippincott, 1953, p 777.
12. Peters WH, Vaughan ED Jr: Urethral diverticulum in the female. Obstet Gynecol 47:549, 1976.
13. Huffman JW: The detailed anatomy of the paraurethral ducts in the adult human female. Am J Obstet Gynecol 55:86, 1948.
14. Lang EK, Davis HJ: Positive pressure urethrography: A roentgenographic diagnostic method for urethral diverticula in the female. Radiology 72:401, 1959.
15. Dretler SP, Vermillion CD, McCullough DL: The roentgenographic diagnosis of female urethral diverticula. J Urol 107:72, 1972.
16. Leach GE, Bavendam TG: Female urethral diverticula. Urology 30:110, 1987.
17. Palagiri A: Urethral diverticulum with endometriosis. Urology 11:271, 1978.
18. Bretland PM: A device and technique for urethrography in the female. Br J Radiol 46:311, 1973.
19. Presman D, Rolnick D, Zumerchek J: Calculus formation within a diverticulum of the female urethra. J Urol 91:376, 1964.
20. Greenberg M, Stone D, Cochran ST, et al: Female urethral diverticula: Double-balloon catheter study. Am J Radiol 136:259, 1981.
21. Borski AA, Stutzman RE: Diverticulum of female urethra: A simplified diagnostic aid. J Urol 93:60, 1965.
22. Keefe B, Warshauer DM, Tucker MS, Mittelstaedt CA: Diverticula of the female urethra: Diagnosis by endovaginal and transperineal sonography. Am J Radiol 156:1195, 1991.
23. Lee TG, Keller FS: Urethral diverticulum: Diagnosis by ultrasound. Am J Roentgenol 128:690, 1977.
24. Bhatia NN, McCarthy TA, Ostergard DR: U.P.P.'s in women with urethral diverticula. Proceedings International Continence Society, Los Angeles, 1980, pp 25–28.
25. Klutke C, Golomb J, Barbaric Z, Raz S: The anatomy of stress incontinence: Magnetic resonance imaging of the female bladder neck and urethra. J Urol 143:563, 1990.
26. Hrick H, Secaf E, Buckley DW, et al: Female urethra: MR imaging. Radiology 178:527, 1991.
27. Marshall S, Hirsch K: Carcinoma within urethral diverticula. Urology 10:161, 1977.
28. Drieger JS, Poutasse EF: Diverticulum of the female urethra. Am J Obstet Gynecol 68:706, 1954.
29. Spence HM, Duckett JW: Diverticulum of the female urethra: Clinical aspects and presentation of a simple operative technique for cure. J Urol 104:432, 1970.
30. Furniss HD: Suburethral abscesses and diverticula in female urethra. J Urol 33:498, 1935.
31. Hunner GL: Calculus formation in a urethral diverticulum in women. Report of three cases. Urol Cutan Rev 42:336, 1938.
32. Young HH: Treatment of urethral diverticulum. South Med J 31:1043, 1938.
33. Hyams JA, Hyams MN: New operative procedures for treatment of diverticulum of female urethra. Urol Cutan Rev 43:573, 1939.
34. Cook EN, Pool TL: Urethral diverticulum in the female. J Urol 62:495, 1949.
35. Edwards EA, Beebe RA: Diverticula of the female urethra. Obstet Gynecol 5:729, 1955.
36. Ellik M: Diverticulum of the female urethra: A new method of ablation. J Urol 77:234, 1957.
37. Hirschhorn RC: A new surgical technique for removal of urethral diverticula in the female patient. J Urol 92:206, 1964.
38. O'Connor VJ Jr, Kropp KA: Surgery of the female urethra. In Glenn JF, Boyce WH (eds): Urologic Surgery. New York, Harper & Row, 1969, p 572.
39. Flocks RH, Culp DA: Surgical Urology, 4th ed. Chicago, Year Book, 1975, p 428.
40. Sasnett RB, Mins WW, Witherington R: Jackknife prone position for urethral diverticulectomy in women. Urology 11:183, 1978.
41. Busch FM, Carter FH: Vaginal flap incision for urethral diverticula. Western Section Meeting, American Urological Association, Honolulu, June 29, 1973.
42. Leach GE, Schmidbauer H, Hadley HR, et al: Surgical treatment of female urethral diverticulum. Semin Urol 4:33, 1986.
43. Mueller EJ, Drake GL: A new surgical procedure for the removal of the wide-mouthed urethral diverticulum in females. Surg Gynecol Obstet 168:269, 1989.
44. Miskowiak J, Honnens de Lichtenberg M: Transurethral incision of urethral diverticulum in the female. Scand J Urol Nephrol 23:235, 1989.
45. Spencer WF, Streem SB: Diverticulum of the female urethral roof managed endoscopically. J Urol 138:147, 1987.

CHAPTER 46

Vesicovaginal Fistula

Lynn Stothers, M.D., M.H.Sc., F.R.C.S.C.
Ashok Chopra, M.D.
Shlomo Raz, M.D.

Etiology

A vesicovaginal fistula is an abnormal communication between the bladder and the vagina (Fig. 46–1). Numerous conditions resulting in formation of a vesicovaginal fistula have been reported (Table 46–1). The etiology predominating in any given country is related to the quality of obstetrical care given to its female population. Prior to 1900 the most common cause of vesicovaginal fistula in North America was obstructed labor. The original descriptions of surgical repair for this condition were reported by Sims in 1849.[1] Since that time, sophisticated obstetrical care has resulted in a shift in the predominant etiologies. Currently 70% of vesicovaginal fistulas occur following total abdominal hysterectomy for benign disease. Unfortunately, recent World Health Organization estimates still reveal obstructed labor as a significant cause of both maternal and fetal mortality worldwide, with over 5 million women affected each year.[2] Such obstetrical vesicovaginal fistulas occur in a different population from that in the developed world and differ with regard to mechanism of injury, associated injuries, and method of surgical reconstruction. Because obstetrical fistulas are rare in developed countries and represent a different pathophysiologic process (pressure necrosis), we will not include them in this discussion. Rather, we will focus on the diagnosis and surgical options for treating vesicovaginal fistulas unrelated to prolonged labor.

Surgical trauma following gynecologic procedures currently causes approximately 90% of vesicovaginal fistulas in North America. Recent case reports of bladder injury with secondary fistula formation have been rising as laparoscopic surgery in the pelvis becomes more common.[3, 4] The remaining 10% of causes include a mixture of radiation-induced or local pelvic disease such as infections, foreign bodies,[5, 6] and pelvic carcinoma. The three most common locally advanced carcinomas leading to vesicovaginal fistula include cervical, vaginal, and endometrial carcinoma. A congenital vesicovaginal fistula in a 5-year-old girl has been reported.[7]

Prevention

Prior to discussing diagnosis and treatment of vesicovaginal fistulas, it is worthwhile to discuss the principles of prevention. Risk factors for fistula formation include prior uterine surgery (cesarean section), endometriosis, previous cervical conization, and prior radiation therapy.[18] The bladder is most commonly injured during total abdominal hysterectomy at the level of the cuff of the vagina. Sharp dissection to isolate the bladder, use of an indwelling catheter during dissection, and filling the bladder when injury is suspected to check for leakage may all be useful in individual circumstances. Indigo carmine or methylene blue may be given intravenously during the operation to aid in the location of a potential fistula. If a bladder injury is identified, adequate mobilization of the tissues prior to intraoperative repair is imperative. The first operation to repair a vesicovaginal fistula has the best chance of success.

Diagnosis

SYMPTOMS

The differential diagnosis of fluid draining from the vagina includes both urine and lymph. Other fluids

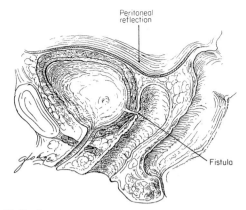

Figure 46-1 Diagram demonstrating a vesicovaginal fistula following hysterectomy.

that can drain and confuse the clinician including serosanguineous drainage in the postoperative period, secretions from the fallopian tube, or profuse vaginal discharge.[8]

Leakage of urine can be confirmed if there is sufficient leakage to send a sample to the laboratory for creatinine measurement. Urine has a creatinine content many times that of serum, whereas other sources of vaginal secretions such as lymph have a creatinine content equal to or less than that of serum. Physical examination with the aid of a speculum assists in isolating the point source of leakage into the vaginal vault. A Foley catheter may be placed into the bladder through the urethra. Palpation or visualization of the balloon may be possible. Methylene blue–tinted sterile saline may be introduced through the Foley catheter and the vagina visually inspected for leakage. If blue-tinged leakage is not immediately apparent, vaginal packing may be placed and the patient asked to ambulate for a short time. The packing may then be inspected for the blue dye. If this maneuver fails to diagnose a bladder source of leakage, a ureterovaginal fistula must be ruled out. The vagina is packed with clean white gauze, and the patient is given 5 ml of indigo carmine

TABLE 46–1
Classification of the Causes of Vesicovaginal Fistula

Congenital
Acquired
  Postoperative
    Total abdominal hysterectomy
    Vaginal hysterectomy
    Bladder neck suspension
    Anterior colpography
    Radical hysterectomy
    Pelvic laparoscopy
    Cone biopsy of the cervix
  Radiation-induced
  Advanced carcinoma
  Obstructed labor
  Infectious—tuberculous
  Vaginal or bladder foreign body
  Subtrigonal injection therapy (phenol)

intravenously. (Pyridium may be given orally as a substitute, but several hours must be allowed for it to become visible in the urine, as noted by its orange color.) The blue color of the indigo carmine should be present in the urine 15 minutes after it is injected intravenously.

In contrast to ureterovaginal fistulas, which tend to become clinically apparent later, vesicovaginal fistulas are clinically evident in two-thirds of cases within 10 days following the time of the injury. Ten percent are associated with a ureterovaginal fistula or ureteral obstruction.

Cystoscopy and upper tract evaluation should be completed in every patient with a urinary fistula. At the time of cystoscopy the location of the ureteral orifices in relation to the fistula should be noted. The size of the fistula and the bladder capacity are assessed. The presence of an unsuspected foreign body in the bladder or vagina that may lead to a vesicoureterovaginal fistula should be ruled out.

SIGNS

The classic presentation of a vesicovaginal fistula in North America is continuous, day and night incontinence following a recent pelvic operation. An unaccounted-for increase in drainage or the occurrence of bloody urine may be suggestive of fistula formation. In the case of a small fistula, a watery vaginal discharge accompanied by normal voiding may be the only sign.

Fistulas related to radiation therapy or obstetrical injury may present years following the insult. Radiation fistulas have been reported to occur as late as 20 years following therapy. Perineal dermatitis may result from long term exposure to urine.

DIAGNOSIS AND TREATMENT OPTIONS

The dye test should be performed following a complete history and physical examination. Cystoscopy and vaginoscopy should be carried out in all patients, and particular attention should be paid to the quality and quantity of vaginal tissue as well as the bladder capacity and location of the ureteral orifices. Attention should be paid to the potential for multiple fistulas, particularly when the cause is related to obstetrical injury, radiation therapy, or anterior repair. An intravenous pyelogram or computed tomographic (CT) urogram must be performed to rule out concomitant ureteral injury and/or obstruction. A biopsy of the fistula site is mandatory in any patient with a history of pelvic neoplasm. A voiding cystourethrogram may demonstrate not only the extent of the fistula but also associated vesical prolapse, vesicoureteral reflux, or stress incontinence that may require simultaneous repair (Fig. 46–2).

Proper and undisturbed bladder drainage may result in closure of the small post-hysterectomy fistula in up to 10% of patients. Such cases require pro-

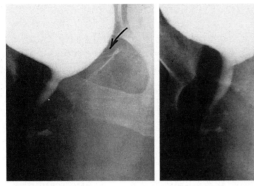

Figure 46-2 Voiding cystourethrogram demonstrating a vesicovaginal fistula in a 45-year-old woman 10 days following hysterectomy. Note the leakage of contrast medium *(arrow)* into the vaginal vault.

longed antibiotic coverage.[9, 10] Bladder drainage may be prolonged (for up to 54 days), and most of these fistulas require surgical correction. If a fistulous tract remains open after 3 weeks of adequate drainage, prolonged catheterization is unlikely to resolve the problem and may lead to persistent irritation, urinary tract infection or severe perineal dermatitis. At this point, the catheter may be removed and definitive repair planned. Another conservative measure includes fulguration of the fistulous tract. Fulguration is an option in a selected group of patients with uncomplicated fistulas in which the tract is solitary and small. This technique has been rarely successful according to reports in the world literature.[11]

Preoperative Considerations

Numerous patient factors must be assessed before performing repair of a vesicovaginal fistula (Table 46–2). Consideration of all of these factors as they relate to any given patient allows an individual approach that will maximize success of the repair.

TIMING OF THE REPAIR

The timing of repair has been debated in the literature for years. The classic strategy is to wait for 3 to

TABLE 46–2
Preoperative Considerations

1. Timing of repair
2. Abdominal versus vaginal approach
3. Estrogen and antibiotics
4. Excision versus no excision of fistula tract
5. Use of grafts or flaps for interposition
6. Sexual function
7. Presence or absence of stress incontinence
8. Postoperative drainage
9. Presence of radiated tissues
10. Need for concomitant procedures (augmentation cystoplasty, etc.)

6 months following the injury to allow maximum healing of the surgically induced inflammatory reaction. This waiting period is particularly important if an abdominal approach is contemplated and the injury is the result of an abdominal hysterectomy. The status of the vaginal cuff is important in this instance. Fistula repair in the presence of cuff infection may lead to an increased failure rate. The disadvantage of a long waiting period is the continued distress and constant wetting experienced by the patient.

In contrast to the delayed repair is the "short wait" approach, in which the repair is done 2 to 3 weeks following the time of injury. Early repair of vesicovaginal fistula is primarily indicated in postabdominal hysterectomy patients in whom a vaginal approach is used. Retrospective series have compared early transvaginal repair with delayed abdominal and vaginal repairs. The success rates of fistula closure appear to be comparable in the two groups. Raz and colleagues have reported their results with early transvaginal repair of postoperative fistulas and found no additional risks attributable to the short waiting period.[12] The major advantage of the early repair is the avoidance of continued psychological grief of the patient. Early vaginal repair is not indicated in the patient with infection of the vaginal cuff or pelvic infection after abdominal hysterectomy. This pathology requires prolonged antibiotic therapy before any attempt at reconstruction can be made.

ABDOMINAL VERSUS VAGINAL APPROACH

It is worth emphasizing that the best chance of success of repair of a vesicovaginal fistula is achieved not only with the first repair but also with the approach that is most familiar to the surgeon. The choice between a vaginal and an abdominal approach depends on the surgeon's training and experience. The advantages of the vaginal technique include avoidance of a laparotomy incision and bivalving of the bladder as well as a quicker recovery with less morbidity. The abdominal approach is best suited to patients in whom intra-abdominal pathology requires simultaneous care—for example, a patient with postradiation cystitis and fistula with a small contracted bladder that requires concomitant augmentation cystoplasty with fistula closure. We use the abdominal approach in patients with associated ureteral fistula or obstruction or with associated bowel fistula when there is a need for concomitant augmentation cystoplasty or when other intra-abdominal pathology requires simultaneous exploration. Although simple fistulas (small, nonrecurrent, well vascularized, nonradiation, or nonischemic) may be treated equally well with either the vaginal or the abdominal approach without adjuvant tissue interposition, complex fistulas require adjuvant techniques of tissue interposition that are described later in this chapter.

ESTROGENS AND ANTIBIOTICS

Preoperative preparation includes estrogen replacement in the postmenopausal or posthysterectomy patient. Broad-spectrum antibiotics such as an aminoglycoside combined with a cephalosporin should be instituted 24 hours prior to surgical repair. An iodine scrub and douche the night before and in the operating room are performed because the vagina is usually contaminated and infected secondary to continuous urinary drainage. If cuff infection is present an additional antibiotic directed against anaerobes (such as metronidazole) is indicated. Culture of the urine should be performed routinely prior to surgery to document sensitivity to any urinary infection, particularly when the patient has been on prolonged oral antibiotic therapy and resistance is possible.

EXCISION OF THE FISTULOUS TRACT

The classic approach to repair of a vesicovaginal fistula includes excision of the fistulous tract to provide fresh edges to aid in the success of the repair. Excision of the fistulous tract is not always necessary for a successful repair, however. Raz and associates have reported 65 cases of early transvaginal repair of vesicovaginal fistulas in which the fistulous tract was not excised with no apparent adverse effect on outcome.[12–14] Disadvantages of excising the tract include conversion of a small fistulous opening into a larger one following excision as well as an increased need for coagulation if bleeding of the freshly exposed areas occurs, which may impede healing. If the fistulous tract is close to the ureteral orifices, excision of the tract may require reimplantation of the ureter, which might have been avoided if the tract had been left in situ. If the fistulous tract is not excised the ureteral orifice can be catheterized with a ureteral stent and transvaginal closure of the fistula can be accomplished, thereby avoiding reimplantation. The fibrous ring of a long-standing fistula may help to improve the strength of the repair.

POSTOPERATIVE DRAINAGE

Use of a urethral Foley catheter as well as a suprapubic catheter is recommended whether one uses an abdominal or a vaginal approach. In selected cases involving difficult technical repair or postradiation fistulas the surgeon may wish to provide additional postoperative drainage. In such cases, single J stents may be inserted; these permit prolonged dryness of the surgical site for several days following the repair.

INTERPOSITION OF TISSUE

Before beginning surgery for repair of a vesicovaginal fistula the surgeon should be aware of several techniques that allow for interposition of tissue. It may not always be possible to predict ahead of time which fistulas require additional coverage to close the defect. Tissue interposition is most commonly used in large, postradiation, obstetrical, and previously failed repairs. Technical descriptions of several interposition techniques are provided in the last section of this chapter.

SEXUAL FUNCTION

The age of the patient and her desire to engage in sexual relations are important preoperative considerations. Preservation of vaginal depth is required in patients who will be sexually active. This may require the use of rotational flaps in patients with large fistulas or who have vaginal stenosis secondary to radiation therapy. In patients who are not sexually active a partial colpocleisis may be performed to maximize tissue coverage in the area of the fistula when the tract is large.

PRESENCE OF STRESS INCONTINENCE

Simultaneous correction of anatomic abnormalities giving rise to stress urinary incontinence may be performed with fistula repair. This avoids the need for a second surgical procedure and reportedly does not increase fistula recurrence rates.[15]

Operative Techniques

A review of the literature on the technical aspects of vesicovaginal fistula repair highlights the ingenuity of surgeons faced with this complex problem (Table 46–3). We will describe our basic technique for repair of a single uncomplicated vesicovaginal fistula following abdominal hysterectomy using a vaginal approach. Following this, a modification of the technique using an abdominal approach will be described, as will numerous techniques for interposing tissue and flaps that can be incorporated into the repair.

VAGINAL APPROACH (RAZ TECHNIQUE)

The Raz technique involves a six-step process for vaginal closure of a simple, uncomplicated vesicovaginal fistula. This repair results in a three-layer fistula closure.

STEP 1 The patient is placed in the lithotomy position following skin preparation with an iodine-based wash and vaginal douche. Cystoscopy and ureteral catheterization are carried out if the fistulous tract is close to the ureteral orifices. A suprapubic catheter is placed using the curved Lowsley retractor through a puncture wound in the suprapubic area. Prior to placement of a posterior vaginal weighted speculum, the posterior vault is assessed. If the vault is nar-

TABLE 46–3
Classification of Management Options for Vesicovaginal Fistula

Nonoperative
    Catheter drainage
Operative
    Closed techniques
        Fulguration of the fistula tract
        Endoscopic fibrin glue insertion
    Open techniques
        Vaginal
            Raz vaginal approach
            Latzko approach
        Abdominal approach
            Extraperitoneal transvesical
            Intraperitoneal transvesical
            Laparoscopic repair
            Urinary diversion
    Interposition of tissue
        Martius flap
        Peritoneal flap
        Gracilis flap
        Seromuscular intestinal patch graft
        Gastric and omental segments
        Dura patch

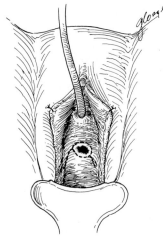

Figure 46–4 Diagram showing the incision for vesicovaginal fistula repair. The incision is made to circumscribe the fistulous tract and extends in an inverted J shape toward the vaginal cuff. (From Raz S, Little NA, Juma S. Female urology. *In* Walsh PC, Retik AB, Stamey TA, Vaughan ED Jr [eds]: Campbell's Urology, 6th ed. Philadelphia, WB Saunders, 1992, pp 2782–2828.)

rowed a relaxing incision (posterolateral episiotomy) may be fashioned to aid in exposure. The labia are sutured apart, and a ring retractor is placed to aid in further exposure.

STEP 2 Saline is injected into the anterior vaginal wall surrounding the fistulous tract. The fistulous tract is dilated using metal sounds, and a small catheter is inserted into the tract, which aids in retraction during dissection (Fig. 46–3). An inverted J inci-

sion that circumscribes the fistulous tract is made (Fig. 46–4). The long end of the J should extend to the apex of the vagina. The asymmetrical nature of the incision allows later advancement and rotation of the posterior flap over the fistula repair. (For fistulas high in the vaginal cuff the incision may be inverted with the base of the flap facing the urethral meatus.)

STEP 3 Two flaps are dissected in an anterior and posterior direction on each side of the fistulous tract (Fig. 46–5). The ring of vaginal tissue at the fistula opening is left intact. Creation of the flaps is begun in healthy tissue away from the opening of the fistulous tract. This technique allows dissection of proper tis-

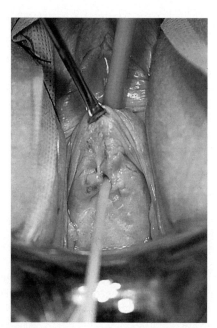

Figure 46–3 Vesicovaginal fistula repair begins with exposure of the anterior vaginal wall and location of the fistula tract. Following insertion of a urethral Foley catheter, an Allis clamp is used to elevate the anterior vaginal wall, and a weighted vaginal speculum is placed. The fistulous tract is dilated using metal sounds to allow insertion of a small Foley catheter into the tract to aid in dissection.

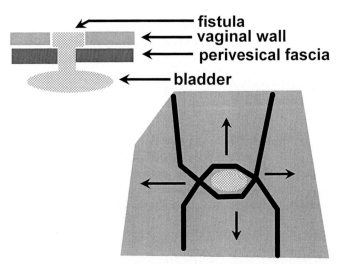

Figure 46–5 Schematic diagram showing incision in the anterior vaginal wall and dissection in an anterior and posterior direction on each side of the fistulous tract. The ring of the fistula is left intact. The vaginal flap should be generous in size and should be mobilized 2 to 4 cm from the fistulous tract, exposing the underlying perivesical fascia.

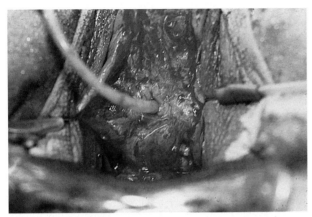

Figure 46-6 Intraoperative photograph showing the extent of dissection around the catheter inserted into the fistulous tract. The fibrous ring of the tract can be seen and is left intact. Excellent hemostasis should be maintained to avoid hematoma formation.

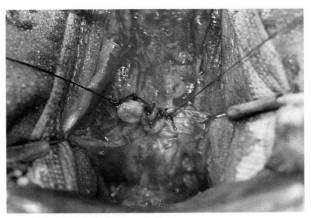

Figure 46-8 Intraoperative photograph of the first layer of closure of a vesicovaginal fistula using a tension-free interrupted absorbable suture.

sue planes and avoids potential bladder perforation or expansion of the fistulous tract. Each flap is dissected 2 to 4 cm from the fistulous tract, exposing the perivesical fascia (Fig. 46–6).

STEP 4 The first layer of the repair is closed (Fig. 46–7). The scarred edges of the fistulous tract are closed with interrupted 2–0 absorbable sutures (Vicryl or Dexon) in a transverse fashion. A strong bite of tissue 2 to 3 mm away from the margin of the fistula is included in this layer, which results in closure of the tract after the intrafistula catheter is removed (Fig. 46–8). These sutures incorporate the bladder wall and the fistulous tract itself. The second layer of the repair (Fig. 46–9) is then accomplished using interrupted absorbable sutures, which are placed to invert the prior layer. These sutures include the perivesical fascia and the deep musculature of the bladder. The sutures are applied at least 1 cm from the prior suture line and should be free of ten-

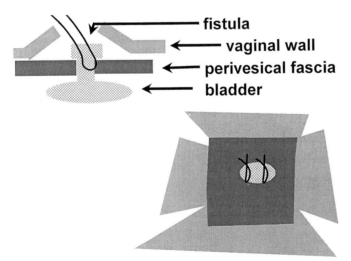

Figure 46-7 Schematic diagram showing the first layer of the fistula closure done with interrupted 2–0 absorbable sutures in a transverse fashion. This layer includes the fistulous tract itself and the bladder wall.

sion; they are placed in a line 90 degrees from the first incision line to minimize the overlapping components. The integrity of the repair is then tested by filling the bladder with indigo carmine.

STEP 5 The posterior flap is rotated to extend beyond the closure of the fistula, covering the site with fresh vaginal tissue and avoiding the overlapping suture lines (Fig. 46–10). The vaginal wall should be advanced at least 3 cm beyond the fistula closure (Fig. 46–11).

STEP 6 A running locking absorbable 2–0 suture (Dexon or Vicryl) is used to close the vaginal wall if no further adjuvant tissue interpositon is to be used. The vagina is packed with triple sulfa–soaked gauze for 24 hours postoperatively. A urethral Foley catheter and the suprapubic catheter are left to straight drainage for 10 days (Fig. 46–12).

INTRAOPERATIVE COMPLICATIONS Potential intraoperative complications include bleeding and injury to the ureters. It is important to control bleeding and attain perfect hemostasis. Hematoma formation may result in disruption of the suture line and recurrent fistula formation. Bleeding encountered during dissection of the vaginal flaps should be controlled with fine absorbable sutures, and the use of cautery should be avoided. If there is doubt about injury to the ureters, 5 ml of indigo carmine should be injected and cystoscopy or ureteral catheterization carried out. The strength of the first two layers of closure is crucial to the success of the procedure.

POSTOPERATIVE CARE Postoperative care includes placement of a vaginal pack and urethral and suprapubic catheters left to straight drainage. Continuous bladder drainage is essential to the success of any fistula repair. Anticholinergics are given to decrease bladder spasm, and oral antibiotics are continued until the catheters are removed 10 to 14 days after the reconstruction. A cystogram is performed prior to catheter removal to document vesical integrity. Sexual intercourse is avoided for 3 months postoperatively.

POSTOPERATIVE COMPLICATIONS Postoperative complications may be classified as early or late. Early com-

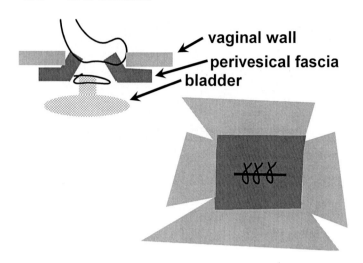

vaginal wall
perivesical fascia
bladder

Figure 46-9 Schematic diagram showing the second layer of closure with interrupted absorbable 2–0 suture (Vicryl or Dexon) created using well-vascularized tissue 1 cm away from the margin of the fistula. These sutures should be tension-free and should invert the first layer of closure.

plications such as vaginal infection, bladder spasms, or bleeding should be treated aggressively to avoid recurrence of the fistula. Bladder spasms should be treated with anticholinergics and local anesthetics if required. Vaginal bleeding is treated with bed rest and vaginal packing. Delayed complications include vaginal shortening and stenosis, unrecognized ureteral injury, or leak and recurrence of the fistula. Vaginal stenosis and shortening result from excessive resection of the vaginal wall and are treated with vaginoplasty. Initially unrecognized ureteral obstruction or leak should be treated with percutaneous nephrostomy drainage to allow a prolonged healing period. Retrograde procedures such as retrograde pyelograms and ureteroscopy in the immediate postoperative period should be avoided because they may result in disruption of the repair. Recurrence of the fistula is the most important postoperative complication. The fistula may be repaired again through a vaginal approach using adjuvant measures such as placement of a Martius or peritoneal flap (see later section, Operative Techniques for Interposition of Tissue).

ABDOMINAL APPROACH

An abdominal approach to repair of a vesicovaginal fistula is indicated when (1) the abdomen requires opening for other concomitant procedures (such as associated augmentation cystoplasty for a contracted postradiation bladder); (2) when ureteral reimplantation is anticipated; (3) in complex or multiple fistulas involving both the ureter and the bladder; or (4) when the surgeon feels most comfortable with this technique. An abdominal approach is not always necessary when a previous vaginal approach has failed. Successful secondary vaginal procedures have been reported.[12] The issues of timing and preoperative preparation apply as much to the abdominal approach as to the vaginal approach. Bowel preparation is required when augmentation cystoplasty is anticipated. The position of the patient should be a modified lithotomy position that allows access to the vagina. Both the vagina and the lower abdomen should be prepared with an iodine-based solution. The intraoperative principles of repair of a vesicovaginal fistula are the same as those described for the vaginal approach.

STEP 1 The patient is positioned in the supine position with the legs slightly separated and the knees abducted to allow intraoperative access to the vagina (modified lithotomy position). The vagina and lower abdomen are draped into the field, and a suprapubic catheter is placed using a Lowsley retractor. A ure-

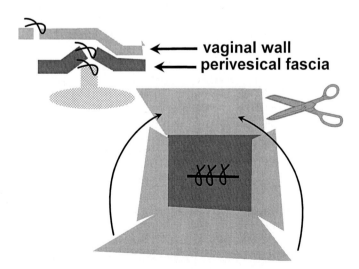

vaginal wall
perivesical fascia

Figure 46-10 Schematic diagram demonstrating the first two layers of closure of a vesicovaginal fistula. The outermost layer consisting of the vaginal flap has not yet been closed.

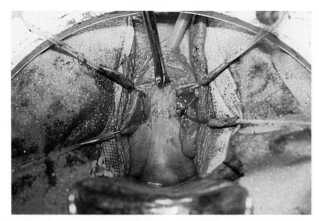

Figure 46-11 Intraoperative photograph demonstrating the vaginal flap created by the inverted J incision, which is advanced over the first two layers of closure.

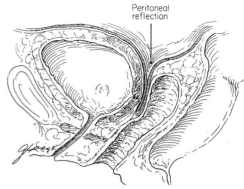

Figure 46-13 Diagram demonstrating closure of a vesicovaginal fistula following an abdominal approach. Suprapubic and Foley catheters are left for drainage following the repair.

thral Foley catheter is also inserted. The vagina is then packed and the bladder filled. A lower abdominal midline or Pfannenstiel incision is made, and the retropubic space is entered. In general, an extraperitoneal approach can be used; however, the peritoneum may be opened to facilitate exposure or to gain access to the omentum if necessary.

STEP 2 The bladder dome is elevated with Allis clamps, and dissection is carried out in the plane between the bladder base and the vagina toward the site of the fistulous tract. Dissection should be started in the lateral aspect of the vagina in normal tissue and move toward the site of the fistula.

STEP 3 When the fistulous tract is identified a small opening in the tract is made, and the bladder wall is dissected free from the tract. A catheter may then be placed in the fistula opening into the vagina to facilitate dissection toward the bladder base. At this time one is left with an opening in the bladder and a opening in the vagina. These two openings are closed in two layers with interrupted Vicryl suture (Fig. 46–13). An omental flap is placed between the bladder and the vagina to add another layer to the closure. The abdominal wound is then closed in the

usual fashion, and the patient is left with suprapubic and urethral catheter drainage as in the vaginal approach.

A modification of the transperitoneal transvesical approach to fistula closure has been reported by Gil-Vernet and colleagues.[16] In this technique the bladder is opened and the fistulous tract identified and excised. An interposing bladder "auto" flap is used to provide additional coverage to the fistula and avoids overlapping suture lines between the bladder and vaginal layers in the closure. One hundred percent success has been reported using this technique in a series of 42 patients with complex, large, or postirradiation fistulas.[16]

Many authors have reported on the success rates of the abdominal approach for vesicovaginal fistula repair. Success rates for primary closure range from 86%, reported by Udeh and colleagues,[17] to 100%.[18] These high success rates are generally reported in patient series that involved no prior radiation. Hedlund and Lindstedt[19] reported that multiple repairs were required in 2 of 14 patients with prior radiation, and 3 were complete failures. Thus, lower success rates for primary closure in postradiation patients of about 60 to 70% can be expected.

RADIATION FISTULAS

Radiation-induced vesicovaginal fistulas are reported to occur in 1 to 5% of patients who have undergone radiation therapy for carcinoma of the cervix or uterus. In patients who subsequently undergo a pelvic procedure such as Wertheim's hysterectomy, fistula formation is even more likely. The site of fistula formation is typically the trigonal area because this area is a fixed area in the bladder, making radiation effects more likely. Radiation fistulas may present in a very delayed fashion and have been reported to occur 15 years or more following radiation exposure.[12]

The pathology leading to fistula formation involves obliterative endarteritis, which makes the area poorly vascularized, and this in turn makes spontaneous healing of the defect less likely. Repair of the

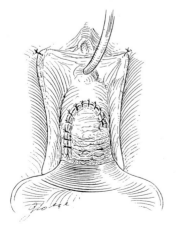

Figure 46-12 The use of an inverted J incision with advancement of the flap over the first two layers of fistula closure avoids overlapping suture lines.

fistula with surrounding tissue is difficult because the surrounding tissue also has been affected by the arteritis. More sloughing and an even larger fistula may result.[20]

Modifications for correction of these fistulas should include the use of interposed tissues (such as omentum or a Martius graft) and a longer period of postoperative catheterization before testing the integrity of the fistula with a cystogram. Augmentation cystoplasty in addition to fistula closure may be required if bladder contraction has occurred following radiotherapy. Virtually all segments of the bowel have been used by various authors to augment the bladder in this fashion. Most importantly, a nonirradiated segment should be used for the augmentation to minimize any compromise to the blood supply of the segment, which can result in suture line breakdown and failure of the reconstruction.

Operative Techniques for Interposition of Tissue

Special techniques are required for complex fistulas. Use of one of the following techniques is advised in fistulas that are recurrent; located high in the vaginal vault; associated with postradiation therapy; ischemic (obstetrical fistulas); large; or associated with poor tissue quality due to lack of estrogens, severe atrophy, or a difficult or doubtful closure. Any one of these techniques (Table 46–4) may enhance the quality of the repair by providing another layer of closure for the reconstruction.

MARTIUS GRAFT

The Martius graft, or fibrofatty labial flap, was first described by Heinrich Martius in 1928.[21] Since then it has become a versatile technique used by many practitioners to repair defects and aid in the reconstruction of many areas of the perineum. Examples of its versatility include its use in rectovaginal fistulas, reconstruction of a destroyed urethra, rectal strictures, vaginal stenosis, urethrovaginal fistulas, and radiation fistulas of the bladder and rectum. Margolis and colleagues described its use in the reconstruction of 10 complex fistulas.[22] The overall success rate was 100% in this group of patients. Adequate

TABLE 46–4
Operative Techniques for Interposition of Tissue In Vesicovaginal Fistula Repair

Martius graft
Omental interposition
Gluteal skin flap
Myocutaneous gracilis muscle flap
Peritoneal flap

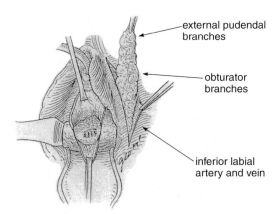

Figure 46–14 The blood supply to the fibrofatty labial (Martius) graft is supplied by the inferior labial artery and vein inferiorly, branches of the external pudendal artery superiorly, and branches of the obturator artery and vein laterally. (By permission of Gwynne Goege.)

vaginal depth was thought to be maintained in all patients.[22]

Anatomically, the Martius graft is a long, broad band of adipose tissue. The strength of the graft is provided by its contents, which include the terminal fibers of the round ligament of the uterus. There are three main sources of blood supply as shown in Figure 46–14. Posteroinferiorly, the internal pudenal artery and vein give rise to the posterior labial vessels. Branches of the external pudendal artery enter the graft superiorly and anteriorly. Branches of the obturator artery and vein enter the lateral border of the graft adjacent to the ischiopubic ramus. This lateral blood supply is sacrificed during mobilization of the graft. The clinical importance of the blood supply lies in the fact that the graft may be divided at either its most superior or its inferior margin, depending on whether the graft will be transferred to the superior or the inferior perineal area.

After the initial longitudinal incision over the labia majora has been made, three borders of dissection are defined. The lateral border of dissection is the labiocrural fold. At this point are located attachments of the fascia lata with the superficial fascia from the skin of the labial fold. Medially the border of dissection is the labia minora and the bulbocavernosus muscle. The posterior border is just superficial to Colles fascia, which covers the urogenital diaphragm.

STEP 1 The first three steps are carried out to close the fistula opening, as described earlier. At this point the fistula has a two-layer closure, and the vaginal flaps are developed. The sutures previously placed in one of the labia for retraction are removed, and the ring retractor is repositioned to remove tension from the labium that will provide the flap.

STEP 2 A vertical incision is made over the labia majora, and the subcutaneous tissues are dissected laterally. The base of the labia majora is the location of the main vascular supply to the graft. The entire thickness of the fibrofatty flap is included in a small Penrose drain. The dissection is continued, and gentle downward traction is applied on the graft as more and more subcutaneous tissue is removed from the most superior portion of the graft. The anterior segment is clamped and transected anterior to the pubic symphysis. The free segment of the flap is dissected from the underlying structures (Fig. 46–15).

STEP 3 Dissection is carried out between the vaginal wall and the perivaginal tissues, creating a tunnel to the area of the fistula. A hemostat is used to pass the graft through the tunnel, transferring the fibrofatty pad from the labial area to the vaginal area (Fig. 46–16). The graft is placed over the fistula site and secured with interrupted absorbable sutures in a tension-free manner.

STEP 4 The vaginal flap is advanced over the Martius graft and closed as in the simple transvaginal repair. Good hemostasis is important, and a small Penrose or Jackson-Pratt drain is left in the labial incision during the early postoperative period. A light pressure dressing may be applied to the labial skin incision for 12 to 24 hours postoperatively.

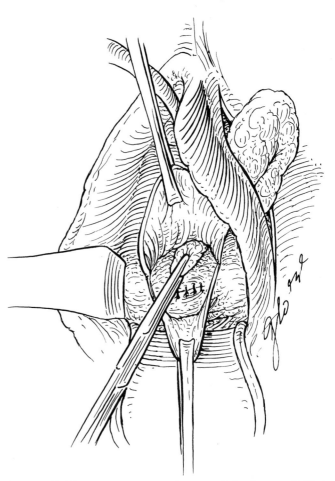

Figure 46-16 The superior attachments of the flap are divided and allow for transfer of the flap to the fistula site using a clamp. Blood supply to the flap is maintained through its inferior and lateral arterial branches. (From Raz S: Atlas of Transvaginal Surgery. Philadelphia, WB Saunders, 1992.)

OMENTAL INTERPOSITION

Omental interposition is a particularly useful technique in the repair of complex fistulas. The omentum is particularly well suited as a material for interposition because of its ability to establish neovascularity and aid in the healing of intra-abdominal infections. Animal experiments have demonstrated that the bladder mucosa may regenerate over the omentum when a bladder defect is created and plugged with an omental graft. Mesenchymal cells from the omentum are thought to contribute to the new mucosa in addition to cells from the bladder mucosa itself.

The omentum can be used in the abdominal approach for fistula repair or in the vaginal approach if it was brought down into the pelvis in a prior procedure. The key to its success lies in familiarity with its unique blood supply, which allows easy mobilization when used carefully.

The blood supply to the omentum comes from the right gastroepiploic artery (a branch of the gastroduodenal artery) and the left gastroepiploic artery (a branch of the splenic artery). The corresponding right and left omental arteries take origin from the gastroepiploics and extend inferiorly to meet at the most

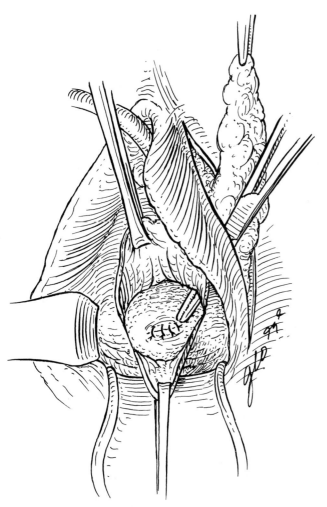

Figure 46-15 Diagram demonstrating the vertical incision used to expose the fibrofatty tissue to be mobilized in the creation of a Martius flap. Note the site of the fistula in the bladder base (shown in black and visible through the vaginal introitus). (From Raz S: Atlas of Transvaginal Surgery. Philadelphia, WB Saunders, 1992.)

inferior extent of the omentum, forming a U-shaped border. The middle omental artery is variable and extends centrally to divide the U into two sections (Fig. 46–17). A small right accessory omental artery that lies lateral to the right omental artery may or may not be present. The right gastroepiploic artery is usually dominant, and therefore most flaps are based on it, although in practice either artery may be used.

In some individuals the omentum is extremely redundant and may reach down into the pelvis without much mobilization. If the omentum is of medium length and only a small amount of mobilization is required, the technique used to obtain a flap comprises an L-shaped incision fashioned below the transverse colon and based on the right omental artery (Fig. 46–18). Further length can be obtained by dissecting the omentum off its attachments to the transverse colon. If the omentum is very short, the left short gastrics may be taken down, the attachments to the transverse colon dissected off, and an incision extended down the center of the omentum to unfold it into a long flap.

GLUTEAL SKIN FLAPS

Gluteal skin flaps are used in patients with postradiation fistulas or when there is severe vaginal atrophy and no other viable skin source is available. The first two steps of fistula closure are accomplished as described earlier (see Vaginal Approach, Raz Techniques). At this point the vaginal flaps have been raised, and the fistulous tract has a two-layer closure. A longitudinal incision is then made in the vaginal wall toward the midportion of the labia majora. The labia are divided into two parts and separated with self-retaining retractors. A semicircular skin incision is made in the gluteal skin in continuity with the labial incision. After proper dissection and undermining of the skin, a flap is rotated and advanced into the vaginal canal. The area of the fistula is covered with the gluteal skin and underlying subcutaneous tissue, and the edges of the vaginal incison are sutured to the edges of the flap (Fig. 46–19).

MYOCUTANEOUS GRACILIS MUSCLE FLAP

Use of the gracilis flap has been most frequently described in association with repair of postradiation fistulas or in the presence of vaginal atrophy or absence secondary to injury or estrogen deficiency. The principle involves rotation of a bulky, well-vascu-

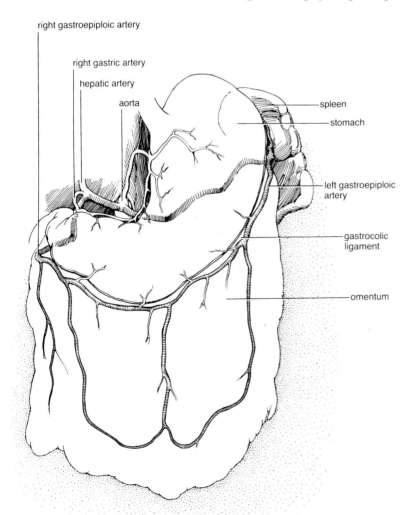

right gastroepiploic artery
right gastric artery
hepatic artery
aorta
spleen
stomach
left gastroepiploic artery
gastrocolic ligament
omentum

Figure 46–17 Diagram of the blood supply of the omentum through the right and left gastroepiploic arteries. The corresponding right and left omental arteries take origin from their gastroepiploic counterparts and extend inferiorly into a U shape. The middle omental artery, which is variable, divides the U-shaped omentum into two sections. (From Hinman F: Atlas of Urologic Surgery. Philadelphia, WB Saunders, 1989.)

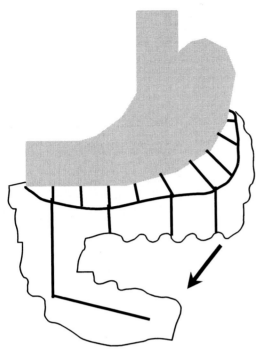

Figure 46-18 Schematic diagram showing mobilization of the omentum to facilitate its use in the deepest parts of the pelvis. An L-shaped flap based on the right gastroepiploic artery is most commonly used, although the left side may be used if it appears dominant. Arrow shows the direction of rotation for the omental flap.

larized flap of skin along with the underlying gracilis muscle, which is transferred to the vaginal area. The gracilis flap has two advantages. Not only does it provide coverage of the fistula site, but also it reconstructs a functional vagina. Bilateral flaps may be used. The anatomy and blood supply to the gracilis muscle are depicted in Figure 46–20. The gracilis is a long slender muscle that extends from the medial condyle of the femur to the inferior border of the symphysis pubis. It lies between the adductor longus laterally and the adductor magnus posteromedially.

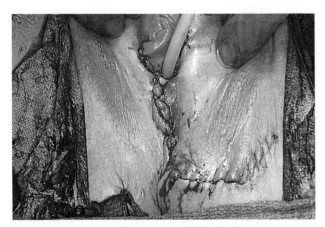

Figure 46-19 Intraoperative photograph showing the gluteal area after completion of a gluteal flap for the closure of a large vesicovaginal fistula. The urethral catheter is in situ, and the gluteal area is elevated superiorly by the operator's hands to fully demonstrate the shape of the incision.

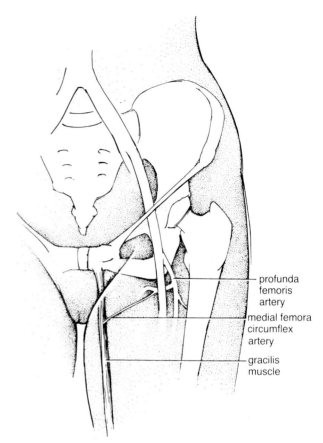

- profunda femoris artery
- medial femora circumflex artery
- gracilis muscle

Figure 46-20 The gracilis muscle lies superiorly in the most medial aspect of the thigh and medial to the adductor longus. Its origin is the inferior ramus of the pubis, and it extends to insert on the medial tibial shaft, inferior to the medial condyle. Blood supply to the gracilis is through the medial femoral circumflex artery, which arises from the deep femoral artery. (From Hinman F: Atlas of Urologic Surgery. Philadelphia, WB Saunders, 1989.)

The blood supply, which is preserved during the dissection, lies along the lateral border. The most distal portion of the muscle, which assumes a tendinous insertion, is the site of transection.

A tennis racquet incision is made on the medial aspect of the thigh over the gracilis muscle (Fig. 46–21). Dissection is carried out to preserve the blood supply while mobilizing the muscle. The gracilis is detached at its distal tendinous insertion point. A tunnel is fashioned underneath the skin to transfer the graft to the vaginal area (Fig. 46–22). The gracilis flap provides cover for the fistulous tract and is used to reconstruct the vaginal canal (Fig. 46–23).

PERITONEAL FLAP FOR HIGH FISTULAS

The technique for use of a peritoneal flap begins with preparation of the fistula site as described in the first two steps of the transvaginal technique. At this point the fistula has been circumscribed, and the two vaginal flaps have been developed. A catheter should be placed through the fistula to aid in the dissection of the peritoneal flap. Gentle traction is placed on the fistula catheter to aid in dissection of the vaginal

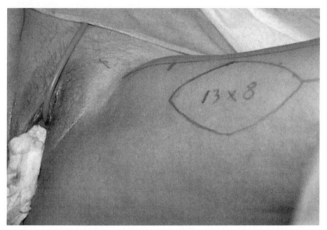

Figure 46-21 The patient is placed in the modified lithotomy position. Palpable landmarks prior to the incision include the pubic tubercle and the medial condyle of the femur. The incision is oval; it begins 10 cm below the pubic tubercle and extends for 20 cm toward the knee as depicted. (From Raz S: Atlas of Transvaginal Surgery. Philadelphia, WB Saunders, 1992.)

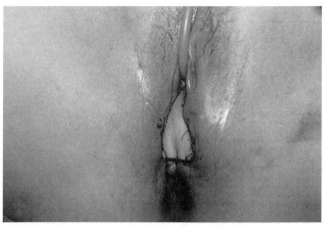

Figure 46-23 Following creation of a tunnel into the area of the vagina, the flap is rotated into position. (From Raz S: Atlas of Transvaginal Surgery. Philadelphia, WB Saunders, 1992.)

dome. The peritoneum including the preperitoneal fat is isolated using sharp dissection (Fig. 46–24A). The fistulous tract is then closed in two layers as previously described, the second layer inverting the fistulous tract (Fig. 46–24B). The peritoneum including the preperitoneal fat is advanced to cover the fistula repair. Interrupted sutures are used to anchor the peritoneum to the perivesical fascia. The sutures should be tension-free. The vaginal flap is then advanced and anchored as previously described, providing a fourth layer of coverage (Fig. 46–24C).

The use of a peritoneal flap using a vaginal approach for correction of vesicovaginal fistula was reported to be successful in 9 of 11 patients with complex recurrent fistulas.[23] The major advantage of this technique lies in its simplicity and the lack of an extravaginal harvesting incision such as is needed for a Martius flap. It is particularly well suited for high-lying vesicovaginal fistulas.

Conclusion

Vesicovaginal fistula represents a significant cause of morbidity in the female population worldwide. The majority of vesicovaginal fistulas seen in developed countries are secondary to surgical intervention and radiation injury. Regardless of the mechanism of injury, urinary fistulas lead to significant physician and patient distress. Techniques of tissue interposition may increase the success rates of closure of complex and postradiation fistulas. Closure of vesicovaginal fistulas is highly successful when the principles of fistula repair are maintained (Table 46–5).

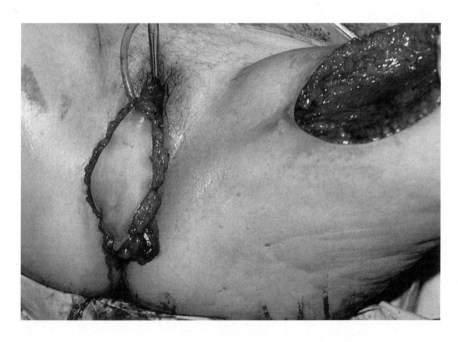

Figure 46-22 Detachment of a gracilis flap from its point of insertion. (From Raz S: Atlas of Transvaginal Surgery. Philadelphia, WB Saunders, 1992.)

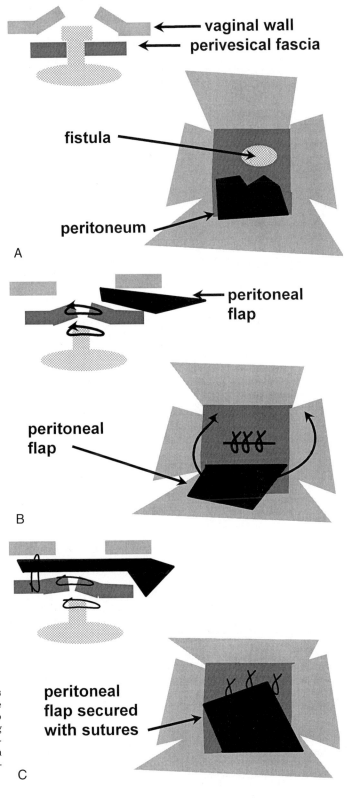

Figure 46-24 To perform a peritoneal flap, one first prepares the fistulous tract, illustrated schematically and described in the first two steps of a vaginal approach to fistula repair *(A)*. Sharp dissection is used to expose the peritoneum and its overlying peritoneal fat *(B)*. The first two layers of closure are accomplished using interrupted absorbable suture, and the peritoneum provides a third layer of coverage. It is held in place by absorbable suture and covered with the vaginal wall *(C)*.

TABLE 46–5
Principles of Vesicovaginal Fistula Repair

1. Adequate exposure of the fistula tract
2. Watertight closure
3. Well-vascularized tissue used for the repair
4. Multiple layer closure
5. Tension-free, nonoverlapping suture lines
6. Adequate urinary drainage early after repair
7. Lack of infection

REFERENCES

1. Ojanuga D: The medical ethics of the "father of gynaecology," Dr J Marion Sims. J Med Ethics 19(1):28–31, 1993.
2. Kelly J: Fistulae of obstetric origin. Midwifery 7(2):71–73, 1991.
3. Wood C, Maher P, Hill D, Lolatgis N: Laparovaginal hysterectomy. Aust NZ J Obstet Gynaecol 34(1):81–84, 1994.
4. Kadar N, Lemmerling L: Urinary tract injuries during laparoscopically assisted hysterectomy: Causes and prevention. Am J Obstet Gynecol 170(Pt 1):47–48, 1994.
5. Binstock MA, Semrad N, Dubow L, Watring W: Combined vesicovaginal-ureterovaginal fistulas associated with a vaginal foreign body. Obstet Gynecol 76(5):918–921, 1990.
6. Goldstein I, Wise GJ, Tancer ML: A vesicovaginal fistula and intravesical foreign body. A rare case of the neglected pessary. Am J Obstet Gynecol 163(2):589–591, 1990.
7. Lefort G, Bouche-Pillon MA, Lefebvre F, et al: Congenital vesicovaginal fistula. Commentary and review of the literature apropos of a case. Chirurg Pediatr 31(2):96–99, 1990.
8. Muntz HG, Goff BA, Thor AD, Tarraza HM: Post-hysterectomy carcinoma of the fallopian tube mimicking a vesicovaginal fistula. Obstet Gynecol 79(5):853–856, 1992.
9. Kliment J, Berats T: Treatment of vesicovaginal fistulas. Cesk Gynekol 57(6):267–271, 1992.
10. Davits RJ, Miranda SI: Conservative treatment of vesicovaginal fistulas by bladder drainage alone. Br J Urol 68(2):155–156, 1991.
11. Geertsen UA, Nielsen HV: Vesicovaginal fistulas with special reference to therapeutic possibilities and time. Ugeskr Laeger 155(26):2046–2049, 1993.
12. Zimmern PE, Hadley HR, Staskin DR, Raz S: Genitourinary fistulae: Vaginal approach for repair of vesicovaginal fistulae. Urol Clin North Am 12(2):361–367, 1985.
13. Leach GE, Raz S: Vaginal flap technique: A method of transvaginal vesicovaginal fistula repair. In Raz S (ed): Female Urology. Philadelphia, WB Saunders, 1992, pp 372–377.
14. Hadley HR, Zimmern PE, Raz S: Transvaginal repair of vesicovaginal fistulae [abstract 101]. Proceedings of the Western Section, American Urological Association, Reno, Nevada, 1984.
15. Arrowsmith SD: Genitourinary reconstruction in obstetric fistulas. J Urol 152(Pt 1):403–406, 1994.
16. Gil-Vernet JM, Gil-Vernet A, Campos JA: New surgical approach for treatment of complex vesicovaginal fistula. J Urol 141:513, 1989.
17. Udeh FN: Simple management of difficult vesicovaginal fistulae by the anterior transvesical approach. Int Urol Nephrol 17(2):159–163, 1985.
18. Kursh ED, Morse RM, Resnick MI, Persky L: Prevention of the development of a vesicovaginal fistula. Surg Gynecol Obstet 166(5):409–412, 1988.
19. Hedlund H, Lindstedt E: Urovaginal fistulas: 20 years of experience with 45 cases. J Urol 137(5):926–928, 1987.
20. Twombly, Surg Gynecol Obstet 83:348, 1946.
21. Martius H: Die operative Wiedeherstellung der volkommen fehlenden Harnrohre und des Schiessmuskels derselben. Zentralbl Gynakol 52:480, 1928.
22. Margolis T, Elkins TE, Seffah J, et al: Full-thickness Martius grafts to preserve vaginal depth as an adjunct in the repair of large obstetric fistulas. Obstet Gynecol 84(1):148–152, 1994.
23. Raz S, Bregg KJ, Nitti VW, Sussman E: Transvaginal repair of vesicovaginal fistula using a peritoneal flap. J Urol 150(1):56–59, 1993.

BIBLIOGRAPHY

Ampofo EK, Omotara BA, Otu T, Uchebo G: Risk factors of vesicovaginal fistulae in Maiduguri, Nigeria: A case-control study. Trop Doct 20(3):138–139, 1990.

Ampofo K, Otu T, Uchebo G: Epidemiology of vesico-vaginal fistulae in northern Nigeria. West Afr J Med 9(2):98–102, 1990.

Attah CA, Ozumba BC: Management of unrepairable urinary vaginal fistulae in a developing country. Aust NZ J Sur 63(3):217–220, 1993.

Ba-Thike K, Than-Aye, Nan-Oo: Tuberculous vesico-vaginal fistula. Int J Gynaecol Obstet 37(2):127–130, 1992.

Benchekroun A: Hydraulic valve for continence and antireflux. A 17-year experience of 210 cases. Scand J Urol Nephrol Suppl 142:66–70, 1992.

Benchekroun A, Faik M, Marzouk M, et al: Continent urinary diversions. J Urol (Paris) 97(4–5):167–177, 1991.

Bergsjo P: Acta fifty years ago. Fistulas, pelvic hyperalgesia, uterine rupture and giant babies. Acta Obstet Gynecol Scand 70(6):423–424, 1991.

Bergsjo P: Acta sixty years ago. On abortions in Oslo, fistulas in Helsinki, elderly primiparas in Stockholm, and more. Acta Obstet Gynecol Scand 70(2):101–102, 1991.

Bhandari M, Dalela D: Complexities of a vesico-vaginal fistula editorial. Arch Esp Urol 47(3):303–306, 1994.

Bissada SA, Bissada NK: Repair of active radiation-induced vesicovaginal fistula using combined gastric and omental segments based on the gastroepiploic vessels. J Urol 147(5):1368–1370, 1992.

Blandy JP, Badenoch DF, Fowler CG, et al: Early repair of iatrogenic injury to the ureter or bladder after gynecological surgery. J Urol 146(3):761–765, 1991.

Carrington BM, Johnson RJ: Vesicovaginal fistula: Ultrasound delineation and pathological correlation. J Clin Ultrasound 18(8):674–677, 1990.

Chapple CR, Hampson SJ, Turner-Warwick RT, Worth PH: Subtrigonal phenol injection. How safe and effective is it? Br J Urol 68(5):483–486, 1991.

Cowie AG: Ureterosigmoidostomy? Trop Doct 24(1):46, 1994.

Demirel A, Polat O, Bayraktar Y, et al: Transvesical and transvaginal reparation in urinary vaginal fistulas. Int Urol Nephrol 25(5):439–444, 1993.

Diako P, Van Langen J, Bonkoungou B, Gazin P: Malaria following surgery in an endemic region. Sante 4(2):115–117, 1994.

Dovlatian AA: Intestinal plastic repair in vesicovaginal fistula. Urol Nefrol Mosk 3:24–27, 1994.

Elkins TE: Surgery for the obstetric vesicovaginal fistula: A review of 100 operations in 82 patients. Am J Obstet Gynecol 170(4):1108–1120, 1994.

Elkins TE, DeLancey JO, McGuire EJ: The use of modified Martius graft as an adjunctive technique in vesicovaginal and rectovaginal fistula repair. Obstet Gynecol 75(4):727–733, 1990.

Elkins TE, Ghosh TS, Tagoe GA, Stocker R: Transvaginal mobilization and utilization of the anterior bladder wall to repair vesicovaginal fistulas involving the urethra. Obstet Gynecol 79(3):455–460, 1992.

Emembolu J: The obstetric fistula: Factors associated with improved pregnancy outcome after a successful repair. Int J Gynaecol Obstet 39(3):205–212, 1992.

Enzelsberger H, Gitsch E: Repair of vesico-vaginal fistulas using the Chassar Moir method. Geburtshilfe Frauenheilkd 50(9):722–725, 1990.

Enzelsberger H, Gitsch E: Surgical correction of vesicovaginal fistulas with the Chassar Moir method. Urologe [A] 30(3):204–206, 1991.

Enzelsberger H, Gitsch E: Surgical management of vesicovaginal fistulas according to Chassar Moir's method. Surg Gynecol Obstet 173(3):183–186, 1991.

Falandry L: Double autoplasty of the labium majus in the surgical repair of vesico-recto-vaginal fistula of obstetric origin. Apropos of 17 cases. J Chir (Paris) 127(2):107–112, 1990.

Falandry L: Repair of large urogenital necrosis of obstetrical origin by pedicled myocutaneous plasty of the greater lip. Technique and results. J Chir (Paris) 128(3):120–126, 1991.

Falandry L: Treatment of post-partum urogenital fistulas in Africa. 261 cases observed in 10 years. Prog Urol 2(5):861–873, 1992.

Falandry L: Uretero-vaginal fistulas: Diagnosis and operative tactics. Apropos of 19 personal cases. (Paris) 129(6–7):309–316, 1992.

Falandry L: Vesicovaginal fistula in Africa. 230 cases. Presse Med 21(6):241–245, 1992.

Falandry L, Lahaye F, Marara C: A pedicled musclefat flap of the major labia in the treatment of complex vesicovaginal fistula. Apropos of 11 cases. J Urol (Paris) 96(2):97–102, 1990.

Fan WN, Zou SZ: Raising the cervix by finger for closure of vesicovaginal fistulae. Br J Urol 68(6):662, 1991.

Fichtner J, Voges G, Steinbach F, Hohenfellner R: Ureterovesicovaginal fistulas. Surg Gynecol Obstet 176(6):571–574, 1993.

Fischer W: Long-term analysis of causes, sites and results of treatment of urogenital fistulas at the Charite Gynecologic Clinic. Zentralbl Gynakol 112(12):747–755, 1990.

Gerber GS, Schoenberg HW: Female urinary tract fistulas. J Urol 149(2):229–236, 1993.

Ghosh TS, Kwawukume EY: A new method of achieving total continence in vesico-urethro-vaginal fistula (circumferential fistula) with total urethral destruction—surgical technique. West Afri J Med 12(3):141–143, 1993.

Girotra S, Kumar S, Rajendran KM: Postoperative analgesia in children who have genito-urinary surgery. A comparison between caudal buprenorphine and bupivacaine. Anaesthesia 45(5):406–408, 1990.

Goldstein AM: Re: Female urinary tract fistulas [letter]. J Urol 150(4):1255, 1993.

Grigovich IN, Otvagina GA, Berezhanskaia TI: Complete duplication of the urethra and bladder. Urol Nefrol (Mosk) (4):62–64, 1990.

Grogan JL, Wells PR: A nursing intervention for intractable incontinence [letter]. J et Nursing, 20(5):228, 1993.

Gueye SM, Ba M, Syllac C, et al: Vesicovaginal fistulas: Etiopathogenic and therapeutic aspects in Senegal. Med Trop 52(3):257–261, 1992.

Gueye SM, Ba M, Syllae C, et al: Vesicovaginal fistulas. Etiopathogenic and therapeutic aspects in Senegal. J Urol (Paris) 98(3):148–151, 1992.

Hubner W, Knoll M, Porpaczy P: Percutaneous transrenal ureteral occlusion: Indication and technique. Urol Radiol 13(3):177–180, 1992.

Iloabachie GC: 260 cases of juxta cervical fistula. East Afri Med J 69(4):188–190, 1992.

Islam AI, Begum A: A psycho-social study on genito-urinary fistula. Bangladesh Med Res Council Bull 18(2):82–94, 1992.

Kelly J: Vesico-vaginal and recto-vaginal fistulae. J R Soc Med 85(5):257–258, 1992.

Kerr-Wilson R: Terminal care of gynaecological malignancy. Br J Hosp Med 51(3):113–118, 1994.

Khanna S: Posterior bladder flap plasty for repair of vesicourethrovaginal fistula. J Urol 147(3):656–657, 1992.

Kiilholma PJ, Haarala M, Soilu-Hanninen M, et al: Urinary tract fistulas following abdominal hysterectomy. Ann Chir Gynaecol Suppl 208:40–42, 1994.

Kliment J, Berats T: Urovaginal fistulas: Experience with the management of 41 cases. Int Urol Nephrol 24(2):119–124, 1992.

Kucera H, Vavra N, Weghaupt K: Benefit of external irradiation in pathologic stage I endometrial carcinoma: A prospective clinical trial of 605 patients who received postoperative vaginal irradiation and additional pelvic irradiation in the presence of unfavorable prognostic factors. Gynecol Oncol 38(1):99–104, 1990.

Kuhlman JE, Fishman EK: CT evaluation of enterovaginal and vesicovaginal fistulas. J Comp Assist Tomogr 14(3):390–394, 1990.

Langenscheidt P, Mast GJ, Becht E, Ziegler M: Complexity-oriented surgical strategies in vesicovaginal fistulas. Urologe A 30(2):94–98, 1991.

Lawson J: Vaginal fistulae [editorial]. J R Soc Med 85(5):254–256, 1992.

Loran OB, Briskin BS, Zaitsev AV, Bunin VA: The surgical treatment of patients with complex intestinal-urogenital fistulae. Urol Nefrol [Mosk] 1:41–45, 1994.

Loran OB, Gazimagomedov GA: Uretero-vesicovaginal fistula. Akush Ginekol [Mosk] (5):51–53, 1991.

Loran OB, Pushkar DO: Treatment of vesicovaginal fistula, simple or complicated by urethral destruction. Experience apropos of 903 cases. J Urol (Paris) 97(6):253–259, 1991.

Mannel RS, Braly PS, Buller RE: Indiana pouch continent urinary reservoir in patients with previous pelvic irradiation. Obstet Gynecol 75(5):891–893, 1990.

Masuda F, Yoshida M, Yamazaki H, et al: Partial colpocleisis for vesicovaginal fistulas. Hinyokika Kiyo. Acta Urol Japon 39(7):611–614, 1993.

Menchaca A, Akhyat M, Gleicher N, et al: The rectus abdominis muscle flap in a combined abdominovaginal repair of difficult vesicovaginal fistulae. A report of three cases. J Reprod Med 35(5):565–568, 1990.

Methfessel HD, Retzke U, Methfessel G: Urinary fistula after radical hysterectomy with lymph node excision. Geburtshilfe Frauenheilkd 52(2):88–91, 1992.

Methfessel HD, Retzke U; Schwarz R, Methfessel G: Occlusion of a vesicovaginal fistula with Latzko-repair. Geburtshilfe Frauenheilkd, 52(10):606–610, 1992.

Meziane F, Diouri M, Larabi K: A new technic of continent urinary diversion: Preliminary results. Progr Urol 4(3):384–390, 1994.

Mhiri MN, Rekik S, Trifa M, Bouzid F: Urogenital lesions and fistulas. What's going on in Tunisia? J Gynecol Obstet Biol Reprod 22(2):157–161, 1993.

Miao YZ: Bladder flap urethroplasty for vesicovaginal fistula with urethral loss. Chung-Hua Wai Ko Tsa Chih 29(2):135–136, 144, 1991.

Moriel EZ, Meirow D, Zilberman M, Farkas A: Experience with the immediate treatment of iatrogenic bladder injuries and the repair of complex vesico-vaginal fistulae by the transvesical approach. Arch Gynecol Obstet 253(3):127–30, 1993.

Motiwala HG, Amlani JC, Desai KD, et al: Transvesical vesicovaginal fistula repair: A revival. Eur Urol 19(1):24–28, 1991.

Mraz JP, Sutory M: An alternative in surgical treatment of postirradiation vesicovaginal and rectovaginal fistulas: The seromuscular intestinal graft (patch). J Urol 151(2):357–359, 1994.

Ndirangu K: Bladder calculus causing vesicovaginal fistula in pregnancy. Br J Urol 68(4):433–434, 1991.

Nezhat CH, Nezhat F, Nezhat C, Rottenberg H: Laparoscopic repair of a vesicovaginal fistula: A case report. Obstet Gynecol 83(Pt 2):899–901, 1994.

Nwabineli NJ, Davis JA: Fistula injury to the bladder at repeat cone biopsy by laser. Eur J Obstet Gynecol Reprod Biol 43(3):245–246, 1992.

Ojanuga DN: Education: The key to preventing vesicovaginal fistula in Nigeria letter. World Health Forum 13(1):54–56, 1992.

Ojanuga D: Preventing birth injury among women in Africa: Case studies in northern Nigeria. Am J Orthopsychiat 61(4):533–539, 1991.

Ojanuga D: Social work practice with childbirth-injured women in Nigeria. Health Social Work 19(2):120–124, 1994.

Onuora VC, al-Mohalhal S, Youssef AM, Patil M: Iatrogenic urogenital fistulae. Br J Urol 71(2):176–178, 1993.

Outwater E, Schiebler ML: Pelvic fistulas: Findings on MR images. AJR 160(2):327–330, 1993.

Pantaleo-Gandais M, Osorio D: Reconstruction of the urinary tract after radiation fistulae. Progr Clin Biol Res 370:151–155, 1991.

Perry EP, Smart JG: Hydrops tubae profluens—not a genitourinary fistula but a diagnosis to be missed. Br J Urol 66(5):547–548, 1990.

Peters J, Lorcher U: Computerized tomography of a vesico-vaginal fistula caused by a foreign body. Zentralbl Gynakol 113(13):789–793, 1991.

Ramos C, de la Rosa F, Castro M, et al: Vesicovaginal fistulas: Correction using lyophilized dura mater. Acta Urol Esp 15(2):143–147, 1991.

Raut V, Bhattacharya M: Vesical fistulae—an experience from a developing country. J Postgrad Med 39(1):20–21, 1993.

Ravi R, Dewan AK, Pandey KK: Transverse colon conduit urinary diversion in patients treated with very high dose pelvic irradiation. Br J Urol 73(1):51–54, 1994.

Redman JF: Female urologic diagnostic techniques. Urol Clin North Am 17(1):5–8, 1990.

Richardson DA: Ethics in gynecologic surgical innovation. Am J Obstet Gynecol 170(Pt 1):1–6, 1994.

Sabnis RB: Re: Conservative treatment of vesicovaginal fistulas by bladder drainage alone [letter]. Br J Urol 70(3):339, 1992.

Sale JM, Claude R, Rigondet G: Simple vesico-vaginal fistulas. Repair technique. Discussion on case reports. Prog Urol 1(6):1069–1072, 1991.

Salup RR, Julian TB, Liang MD, et al: Closure of large postradiation vesicovaginal fistula with rectus abdominis myofascial flap. Urology 44(1):130–131, 1994.

Schneider JA, Patel VJ, Hertel E: Closure of vesicovaginal fistulas from the urologic viewpoint with reference to endoscopic fibrin glue technique. Zentralbl Gynakol 114(2):70–73, 1992.

Schurawitzki H, Hobarth K, Gebauer A, Kratzik C: Therapeutic transrenal occlusion of the ureter: Solution of plug migration problem. Urol Radiol 12(4):181–183, 1991.

Scott R, Gorham SD, Aitcheson M, et al: First clinical report of a new biodegradable membrane for use in urological surgery. Br J Urol 68(4):421–424, 1991.

Shull BL: Urologic surgical techniques. Curr Opin Obstet Gynecol 3(4):534–540, 1991.

Stelmachow J, Borkowski A, Zawada E, Wypych K: Late vesicovaginal fistula after colporrhaphy for urinary incontinence. Ginekologia Polska 63(4):204–206, 1992.

Tancer ML: Observations on prevention and management of vesicovaginal fistula after total hysterectomy. Surg Gynecol Obstet 175(6):501–506, 1992.

Tsiv'ian AL: One-stage bilateral plastic repair of the pelvic ureters and vesicovaginal fistuloplasty. Urol Nefrol Mosk 5:42–43, 1993.

Thorvinger B, Horvath G, Samuelsson L: CT demonstration of fistulae in patients with gynecologic neoplasms. Acta Radiol 31(4):357–360, 1990.

Vinee P, Hauenstein KH, Noldge G, et al: Uretero-arterial fistula. A rare cause of massive hematuria. J Urol (Paris) 98(3):165–166, 1992.

Waaldijk K: The immediate surgical management of fresh obstetric fistulas with catheter and/or early closure. Int J Gynaecol Obstet 45(1):11–16, 1994.

Wang Y, Hadley HR: Nondelayed transvaginal repair of high lying vesicovaginal fistula. J Urol 144(1):34–36, 1990.

Wang Y, Hadley HR: The use of rotated vascularized pedicle flaps for complex transvaginal procedures. J Urol 149(3):590–592, 1993.

Warwick RT: Functional restoration and reconstruction of the incontinent female urethra. Rev Med Suisse Romande 112(9):775–785, 1992.

Westendorp AK: Always damp (letter). Ned Tijdschr Geneeskd 136(2):98–99, 1992.

Yang JM, Su TH, Wang KG: Transvaginal sonographic findings in vesicovaginal fistula. J Clin Ultrasound 22(3):201–203, 1994.

Zimmern P: Urology in women: News and developments in 1992. J Urol (Paris) 99(2):94–97, 1993.

Zoung-Kanyi J, Sow M: Focus on vesicovaginal fistulas at the Yaounde Central Hospital. Apropos of 111 cases seen in 10 years. Ann Urol 24(6):457–461, 1990.

Ureteral Injuries in the Female: Fistulas and Obstruction

Christopher K. Payne, M.D.

Ureteral injury is among the most feared complications of pelvic surgery in women. When a seemingly routine operation results in ureteral obstruction, fistula, or urinary sepsis the patient loses confidence in her surgeon and the doctor-patient relationship is threatened. Because of the common embryologic origin of the lower urinary tract and the female genital tract, the ureter is intimately related to all of the female reproductive organs and is at risk during all gynecologic surgery. Ureteral injuries can also occur during general surgical and vascular procedures. Although modern techniques have all but eliminated obstetrical ureteral injuries, there are now new causes of injuries including surgical laparoscopy and urologic endoscopy. This chapter summarizes the etiology, pathophysiology, prevention, and management of ureteral injuries in women. The information was originally gathered for another source[1] and has been condensed here; interested readers should refer to the original for more detail.

Anatomy

Knowledge of ureteral anatomy is the key to preventing injury. The ureter is a muscular tube approximately 25 cm long that propels urine from the renal pelvis to the bladder by active peristalsis. Pathology outside the ureter (inflammation and fibrosis) may affect its function by interfering with normal peristalsis. It is a retroperitoneal structure and is adherent to the peritoneum through most of its length. The ureter is commonly divided into two segments—the abdominal portion, which runs from the renal hilum to the pelvic brim, and the pelvic portion, which extends from the pelvic brim to the bladder. The unique blood supply of the ureter is diagrammed in Figures 47–1 and 47–2. Arterial inflow comes from a

number of arteries that approach the ureter medially in the abdomen and laterally in the pelvis. The vessels ramify, running longitudinally up and down the ureter, anastomosing freely. The vessels are typically intimate with the peritoneum, and thus, whenever possible, the peritoneum should be preserved with the ureter.

The abdominal ureter generally lies within abun-

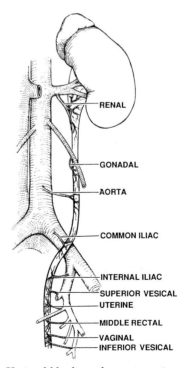

Figure 47-1 Ureteral blood supply, gross anatomy. Feeding vessels enter medially in the abdominal ureter, laterally in the pelvic ureter. (From Kabalin JN: Surgical anatomy of the genitourinary tract. *In* Walsh PC, Retik AB, Stamey TA, Vaughan ED Jr [eds]: Campbell's Urology, 6th ed. Philadelphia, WB Saunders, 1992.)

507

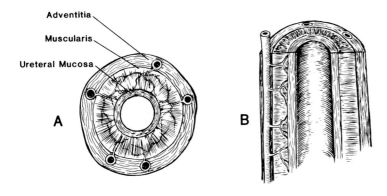

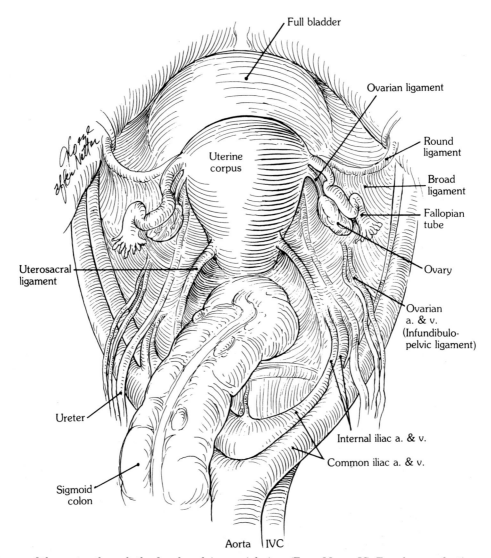

Figure 47-2 Ureteral blood supply, cross sectional *(A)* and sagittal *(B)* views of the longitudinal arteries in the ureteral adventitia and their perforating branches. Through free interanastomoses of these vessels the ureter obtains good collateral circulation. (From Thompson JD: Operative injuries to the ureter. *In* Mattingly RF, Thompson JD [eds]: TeLinde's Operative Gynecology, 7th ed. Philadelphia, JB Lippincott, 1992.)

Figure 47-3 Course of the ureter through the female pelvis, cranial view. (From Moore JG: Female reproductive anatomy. *In* Hacker NF, Moore JG [eds]: Essentials of Obstetrics and Gynecology. Philadelphia, WB Saunders, 1986.)

dant areolar fatty tissue and is not closely adherent to other major structures. The major causes of ureteral injury at this level are sigmoid colectomy, retroperitoneal lymph node dissection, excision of retroperitoneal tumors, and, most importantly, operations on the great vessels. Para-aortic lymphadenectomy for gynecologic malignancies is a new cause of ureteral injury. The pelvic ureter usually begins almost directly over (or a bit laterally on the left) the bifurcation of the common iliac artery. The obliterated umbilical artery, the first branch of the hypogastric artery, provides a convenient and reliable path for the surgeon trying to locate the pelvic ureter. In the female pelvis the ureter is intimately related to the genital tract (Fig. 47–3). Cranially, it is found in the posterior peritoneal layer of the broad ligament, parallel and medial to the infundibulopelvic ligament and the ovarian vessels. Moving caudally, it is at the lateral edge of the uterosacral ligament and crosses the uterine artery ventrally. The ureter continues caudally, just lateral to the cervix and fornix of the vagina. In this area, the uterine artery crosses back over the ureter (ventrally), and the ureter is often enveloped closely by the veins of the vesical and vaginal plexuses.[2] Thus, for a distance of about 2 cm, the ureter and the uterine artery lie adjacent to one another. The ureters then turn ventrally and medially to enter the trigone of the bladder, lying in a thin plane between the vagina and bladder. The vast majority of ureteral injuries occur in the pelvic ureter, primarily during gynecologic surgery. The full course of the ureters and the common sites of injury are displayed in Figure 47–4.

Etiology and Pathophysiology

The most common types of injuries, roughly in descending order of frequency, are ligation, angulation or kinking by suture, division, partial laceration, crushing, and devascularization leading to delayed necrosis (cautery injuries are included here)[3, 4] (Fig. 47–5). In general, the initial manifestation of ureteral injury is obstruction due to edema and tissue trauma. This may result in chronic obstruction, resolve as the edema decreases, or progress to fistula formation. A clean laceration, on the other hand, results in immediate urinary extravasation. Any injury that exposes the ureteral lumen in either an immediate (laceration) or delayed (ischemic necrosis) fashion may lead to a fistula. The usual stages of fistula formation are (1) extravasation and urinoma formation, (2) dissection of the tissue planes, and (3) drainage through the incision. The presence of local infection or prior local irradiation probably predisposes to fistula formation because these factors may prevent a partial injury from healing appropriately.

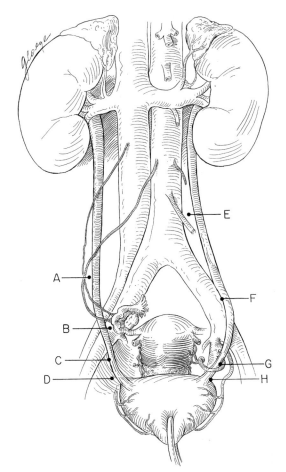

Figure 47–4 Common sites of ureteral injury. *A,* Division of the gonadal vessels and infundibulopelvic ligament. *B,* Resection of adnexal masses adherent to the ureter within the broad ligament, *C,* At the apex of the obturator fossa in pelvic lymphadenectomy, *D,* Division of the lateral ligaments of the rectum in abdominoperineal resection, *E,* Division of inferior mesenteric vessels in sigmoid resection, *F,* At pelvic brim during vascular bypass procedures, *G,* Division of the uterine artery during hysterectomy. *H,* At the lateral vaginal fornix, entry into trigone of the bladder during hysterectomy and vaginal procedures. (From Payne CK, Raz S: Ureterovaginal and related fistulae. *In* McAninch JW [ed]: Traumatic and Reconstructive Urology. Philadelphia, WB Saunders, in press, 1996.)

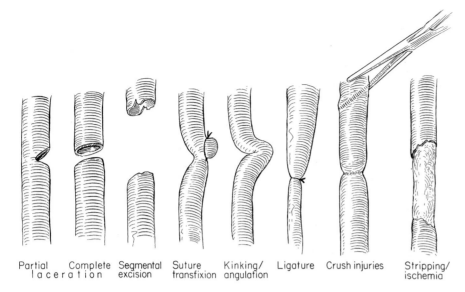

Partial laceration | Complete laceration | Segmental excision | Suture transfixion | Kinking/angulation | Ligature | Crush injuries | Stripping/ischemia

Figure 47-5 Types of ureteral injuries. All injuries must be evaluated for extent of direct mechanical wound and any effect on the blood supply that may lead to delayed icshemia and necrosis. With lacerations and excisions there is generally little ischemic injury. When the ureter is kinked, transfixed, or ligated, the injury is assessed after the suture has been removed; often no other treatment is necessary. Crush injuries caused by sutures, clamps, or other instruments often involve some ischemic insult. When the adventitia of the ureter is stripped during dissection there is a high likelihood of ischemia. (From Payne CK, Raz S: Ureterovaginal and related fistulae. *In* McAninch JW [ed]: Traumatic and Reconstructive Urology. Philadelphia, WB Saunders, in press, 1996.)

Thus, ureteral fistulas may drain cutaneously through abdominal, flank, perineal, or vaginal incisions. Fistulas may form between the ureter and the uterus by the same mechanism. Urinary extravasation may be detected as a large collection in the peritoneum or retroperitoneum, still contained by the skin. In all these cases, however, the pathophysiology is essentially the same.

CAUSES OF IATROGENIC URETERAL INJURY IN THE FEMALE

The causes of iatrogenic ureteral injury are summarized in Table 47-1.[1] Gynecologic surgery accounts for approximately two-thirds of all ureteral injuries. Most occur during surgery for benign disease (Table 47-2).[1] The estimated frequency of ureteral injury during major gynecologic surgery is 0.5 to 2.5%.[5-7]

Ureteral injuries also occur during general surgical operations for colorectal cancer, pelvic abscess and other inflammatory conditions, and retroperitoneal tumors. Vascular reconstruction, especially repair of aortic aneurysms and aortoiliac bypass, also endangers the ureters. General surgical and vascular patients are significantly more likely to be male, however. Reports of ureteral injuries slightly understate the actual incidence of the problem because some injuries produce obstruction, hydronephrosis, and renal atrophy without symptoms. Review of the studies in which series of patients were prospectively screened for such injuries reveals that the incidence of silent injury is approximately 1 in 200 cases.[1]

Abdominal hysterectomy is far and away the most common cause of surgical ureteral injuries, accounting for over half of the total. The rate of ureteral injury during abdominal hysterectomy for benign disease is about 1 in 200 cases.[1] In early radical hyster-

TABLE 47-1
Ureteral Injuries: Etiology (Bilateral Injuries Counted Separately if Possible)

Author	Year	Practice	GYN	Rectal Surg	Other Gen Surg	Vascular	GU Endoscopy	Other	Total
Prentiss and Mullenix	1951	GU	17	4	2	0	0	1	24
Newman	1957	GU	22	4	0	0	0	0	26
Spence	1959	GU	30	0	1	0	0	0	31
Higgins	1967	GU	60	11	1	8	3	4	87
Hoch	1975	GU	17	2	3	2	0	0	24
Bright	1977	GU	12	2	5	1	3	0	23
Brown	1977	GU	18	9	1	2	7	1	38
Zinman (pelvic)	1978	GU	30	8	0	0	0	0	38
(abdominal)			0	0	7	9	5	8	29
Sieben	1978	GU	29	2	1	0	0	0	32
Fry	1983	Gen Surg	18	8	1	0	0	0	27
Total			253	50	22	22	18	14	379
Percentage			67	13	6	6	5	4	100

Approximately two-thirds of iatrogenic ureteral injuries occur during gynecologic surgery (injuries during bladder suspensions are included in this category). The majority of such injuries in men are due to surgery for rectal cancer and for various vascular procedures. From Payne CK, Raz S: Ureterovaginal and related fistulae. *In* McAninch JW (ed): Traumatic and Reconstructive Urology. Philadelphia, WB Saunders, 1996.

TABLE 47-2
Gynecologic Ureteral Injuries: Etiology (Bilateral Injuries Counted Separately)

Author	Year	Disease Process Cancer	Disease Process Benign	Total
Conger	1954	7	10	17
Benson and Hinman	1955	20	16	36
Everett	1956	8	32	40
Newman	1957	5	17	22
Spence	1961	11	19	30
Charles	1967	7	18	25
Lee and Symmonds	1971	18	50	68
Bright	1977	1	9	10
Brown	1977	5	13	18
Seiben	1978	7	22	29
Zinman	1978	9	21	30
Fry	1983	2	16	18
Badendoch	1987	7	33	40
Mann	1988	9	8	17
Total		116	284	400

Note: Some deliberate resections of the ureter during cancer surgery are included here.
From Payne CK, Raz S: Ureterovaginal and related fistulae. *In* McAninch JW (ed): Traumatic and Reconstructive Urology. Philadelphia, WB Saunders, 1996.

ectomy series an incidence of significant ureteral injury of 10% was standard. In a radical hysterectomy, "stripping" of the distal ureter resulting in delayed necrosis is the major risk. Now, however, with refinements in surgical technique, ureteral injury rates of about 2 to 3% are typical, and fistulas occur in less than 1 in 100 cases. Some of these reported "injuries" are actually deliberate resections performed to effect cure of the cancer. The ureter is at risk in the excision of adnexal masses. Ovarian cysts and tumors can displace the ureter anteriorly; it may thus be obscured as it is draped over the mass. The ureter may be densely adherent to an inflammatory mass or to the remaining adnexae after a simple hysterectomy. The ureter may be injured in retropubic bladder neck suspensions of all types including Marshall-Marchetti-Krantz, Burch, and paravaginal repairs. Finally, the ureter can be injured in any vaginal operation on the anterior vaginal wall in which dissection extends proximal to the bladder neck. This includes vaginal hysterectomy, needle bladder neck suspensions, anterior colporrhaphy or cystocele repair, enterocele repair, and vault prolapse. Patients with high-grade prolapse may have severe hydroureteronephrosis; this should be expected when planning the surgical procedure. The incidence of ureteral injury in vaginal hysterectomy is about 1 in 300 cases.[1]

SURGICAL URETERAL INJURIES—RISK FACTORS

Many factors have been postulated to increase the risk of ureteral injury during surgery. These can be divided into five categories—type of operation required, disease factors, complicating factors, surgical

technique, and patient factors[5] (Table 47-3). There is, however, a paucity of data with which to evaluate these purported risk factors and no conclusive evidence that any of them actually present extraordinary risk. It appears that most patients suffering from iatrogenic injuries have no risk factors.[8] In one study of fistulas occurring after radical hysterectomy, obesity and age were not significantly associated with fistula formation, and in half of the patients with ureteral complications no risk factor was identified.[9] Patients with endometriosis (10.9% fistula) and pelvic radiation (13% fistula, 7.6% stricture) demonstrated a slightly increased risk of ureteral complications. Symmonds notes that generally the patient with ureteral injury has had a technically easy hysterectomy for minimal disease.[6] Except for those oncologic cases in which a segment of ureter is deliberately excised, most ureteral injuries represent errors in technique.

Prevention of Ureteral Injury in Pelvic Surgery

Prevention of ureteral injuries begins prior to surgery with a proper urologic history and careful physical examination. When the patient reports a history of urinary tract disease or has symptoms referable to the urinary tract, a urologic evaluation is warranted. All palpable masses must be adequately defined with appropriate radiographic studies. Routine preoperative urologic investigation—cystoscopy, intravenous urogram (IVU), vesicoureterogram (VCUG), and so on—is of dubious value in the vast majority of patients undergoing gynecologic and other pelvic procedures

TABLE 47-3
Risk Factors for Iatrogenic Ureteral Injury

Disease factors
  Inflammatory—severe endometriosis, pelvic inflammatory
    disease, inflammatory bowel disease
  Advanced malignancy—tumor adherent to adjacent structures
  Pelvic prolapse—ureteral anatomy distorted
Type of operation
  Radical surgery—must achieve adequate margin of resection
Complicating factors
  Prior local therapy
    Redo surgery, tissue planes and landmarks destroyed
    Therapeutic radiation
  Adhesions
  Pregnancy—distorts anatomy, limits exposure
  Mass lesion—distorts anatomy
Patient factors
  Obesity
  Age
  Congenital urologic or gynecologic abnormalities
Technical factors
  The most important cause

Although surgical difficulty is influenced by many factors, most ureteral injuries occur during routine operations and are due to errors in technique.
Adapted from Williams TJ: Urologic injuries. *In* Wynn RM (ed): Obstetrics and Gynecology Annual. New York, Appleton-Century-Crofts, 1975, pp 347–368.

dures. Although some surgeons advocate routine placement of ureteral stents prior to pelvic surgery, there are clear morbidity and cost associated with this procedure, and no definite benefit has ever been demonstrated. Likewise, routine postoperative urologic imaging has never been shown to be helpful.

SURGICAL TECHNIQUE

If the incidence of iatrogenic ureteral injury is to be reduced, surgeons must take care to positively identify the ureter throughout its course during all pelvic surgery, even "routine" operations. "It is an axiom of surgical dissection that important contiguous structures subject to inadvertent injury must be dissected and exposed."[6] Adequate exposure is mandatory. Although cosmesis is a legitimate concern, the incision must always be adequate to assess and treat the pathology properly. When difficulties are encountered unexpectedly, small incisions must be promptly extended to gain control of the operation. Many ureteral injuries stem from trying to stop bleeding when the exposure is inadequate to define the source. In most cases, the ureters need only be identified, not completely dissected. In thin patients with little retroperitoneal fat, the ureter is easily visible through the peritoneum and peristalsis can be seen when it is touched by forceps. In the routine case, the easiest point at which to identify the ureter is at the pelvic brim. However, depending on the operation and the pathology involved, it may be necessary to start higher in the abdominal portion of the ureter and trace its course down to the pelvis, where it may be involved with the disease process. When the retroperitoneum must be opened to expose the ureter, the surgeon should remember that the ureteral blood supply is intimate with the peritoneum, and every effort should be made to keep the peritoneum with the ureter. Superior to the bifurcation of the common iliac artery, the blood supply to the ureter comes in medially; thus, the peritoneum should be incised laterally. Below this point the blood supply enters laterally, and the peritoneum is incised medially. The preserved edge of peritoneum provides a handle for traction and prevents crush injury from forceps. Great care should be taken to avoid handling the ureter directly; the "no touch" technique is always best.

In vaginal surgery the ureters may be injured during any operation on the anterior vaginal wall. The greatest risk occurs in high-grade prolapse with *Providencia*, grade 4 cystocele, and vault prolapse. Careful dissection, anterior retraction of the bladder, and accurate placement of clamps and sutures minimize the risk of ligating or kinking the ureters. As in abdominal surgery, injuries are often caused by blind attempts to control bleeding or by clamping large chunks of tissue to prevent bleeding. Hemorrhage should be controlled with pressure until bleeding points are identified and can be handled with precision. Symmonds has argued that direct palpation of the ureter is valuable,[6] but we and others have not had such success with palpation and in fact have noted difficulty in palpating ureteral stents vaginally.[10] We strongly recommend the routine use of intravenous indigo carmine and cystoscopy to assess ureteral integrity in all operations on the anterior vaginal wall.

In summary, excellence in surgical technique is the best safeguard against ureteral injury. Generous exposure, positive identification of the ureters, atraumatic ureteral manipulation, accurate hemostasis, and active intraoperative thinking are far more valuable than preoperative radiographs or stents. At the conclusion of surgery, extraperitoneal drainage, antibiotics, and reperitonealization of ureters securely against the pelvic sidewall help to create optimal conditions for ureteral healing.[9]

Presentation

The early signs and symptoms of ureteral injury are, for the most part, nonspecific. This is because obstruction may be incomplete, and injuries that ultimately lead to fistula formation usually go through sequential stages of obstruction, local extravasation, urinoma formation, and dissection through the tissue planes before sudden drainage of urine from the incision appears. Two exceptions are total bilateral obstruction presenting with anuria in the recovery room and early drainage of urine (within the first 48 hours) from a major ureteral laceration. The general early signs, which may be associated with all types of ureteral injuries, include flank and abdominal pain, fever, nausea, ileus, and localized fluctuance and tenderness.

Unfortunately, these symptoms are often masked in the immediate postoperative period by analgesics. When any postoperative problems emerge, the patient must be evaluated for flank tenderness, which may indicate renal obstruction. Unexplained fever mandates radiographic examination of the urinary tract. An early rise in the creatinine level may be a sensitive indicator of ureteral obstruction and should prompt investigation. In a Mayo Clinic series of 13 patients with unilateral ureteral suture entrapment, a mean rise of 0.8 mg/dl in serum creatinine was observed in the immediate postoperative period.[11] Similar data are not available for patients with injuries other than total obstruction. Although these points make useful guidelines, a high index of suspicion remains the surgeon's most valuable tool.

Diagnosis and Evaluation of Ureteral Injuries

All women with urinary tract injuries should undergo a complete evaluation to establish the integrity of the entire urinary system. Approximately 10% of ureteral injuries are bilateral,[1] and the incidence of concomitant bladder injuries is probably about the same. The same factors predispose to all types of urinary tract injuries, and thus complex injuries should always be suspected.

When a ureteral injury is suspected the best initial study is an intravenous urogram (IVU). Abnormalities on the IVU range from delay to nonfunction to frank extravasation of contrast. The level of the injury can usually be determined, and the anatomic detail is important in planning treatment. Unfortunately, there can be false-positive and false-negative urograms. Thus, whenever the study is suboptimal or clinical suspicion is high, further investigation with retrograde pyelography is indicated. Ultrasonography is useful for diagnosing established obstruction but is not sensitive when a fistula is present because there may not be hydronephrosis. It also does not provide the anatomic detail needed to plan treatment. Thus, ultrasound is preferred as an initial test only when the patient has a contrast allergy or a marked elevation of serum creatinine. Cystoscopy and retrograde pyelography are mandatory whenever the initial study is indeterminate or does not completely define an injury. The retrograde pyelogram is the single best test for diagnosing a ureteral injury and should be almost 100% sensitive and specific when it is technically adequate; it also provides the anatomic detail required to plan treatment. On some occasions, direct injection of contrast into a vaginal fistula tract may be helpful. Cystoscopy is useful, primarily because of its value in excluding a bladder injury and in evaluating the bladder for use in repair. Nuclear medicine renography is very sensitive for urinary extravasation and provides functional information but lacks anatomic precision. Another consideration is that any patient with a ureteral injury may have an undrained collection of urine or pus. Patients with persistent fever or pain should undergo computed tomography to search for an abscess or urinoma. Ultrasound and magnetic resonance imaging (MRI) may also be used in selected patients but should not usually be the initial study.

The prime directives in evaluating a patient with a urinary fistula are to determine the number, type, and location of injuries, ascertain the status of each kidney, and assess the overall condition of the patient. "Any study that neglects a full survey risks failure on the basis of an unrecognized second or third defect."[12] The patient's health, life expectancy, and overall renal function become important factors when a difficult repair is anticipated. At times a trial of a percutaneous nephrostomy will clarify the status of what appears to be a borderline functioning kidney. Although percutaneous drainage and antegrade stenting are indicated for many ureteral fistulas, these procedures are indicated from a therapeutic standpoint, not as part of the evaluation. When a decision is made to proceed with immediate surgical repair, there is no need to place a nephrostomy if the IVU and retrograde studies have adequately defined the extent of the injury.

Management of Ureteral Injuries

OBSERVATION

For many years the only common methods of managing ureteral fistulas were observation and nephrectomy. In some cases spontaneous closure can be predicted. When ureteral continuity is preserved and no significant obstruction or infection is present, the fistula often closes. Radical surgery, which predisposes to devascularization of the ureter, and prior radiation make spontaneous closure less likely. Although approximately 20% of ureterovesical fistulas close spontaneously,[1] closure does not necessarily imply a good result for the patient. After a fistula closes there may be stricture formation, hydronephrosis, and silent renal atrophy. With modern endourologic techniques there is virtually no reason to observe a fistula. The patient should undergo either early surgical repair or nephrostomy placement and ureteral stenting, as discussed subsequently.

Similarly, observation alone is rarely a prudent course for managing the kidney with ureteral obstruction. Fistulas will form in almost half the cases[1] (based on series with deliberate ureteral ligation for lacerations), and infection of the obstructed unit can be fatal. Percutaneous nephrostomy protects renal function and provides access for later endourologic management of the obstruction if necessary. In some cases, obstruction may than resolve as absorbable sutures dissolve.

NONSURGICAL METHODS

Dramatic advances in endourologic and percutaneous techniques make these minimally invasive procedures the treatment of choice for most ureteral fistulas. We recommend an endourologic approach for the majority of patients with unilateral injuries when the continuity of the ureter is maintained. When there is complete disruption of the ureter with separation of the two ends, a satisfactory result is less likely, and surgery is preferred in the healthy patient. Endourologic techniques are also unlikely to be successful in treatment of established fistulas. Once the fistula tract is epithelialized it is not likely to close with conservative measures.

Endourologic management of ureteral injury is discussed in detail in Chapter 48.

Surgical Treatment of Ureteral Injury

IMMEDIATE RECOGNITION

It has been said that "the venial sin is injury to the ureter, but the mortal sin is failure of recognition."[13] Intraoperative recognition of injury may not guarantee a good outcome but does present the best possible opportunity for success. Unless there has been gross contamination of the field, inflammation and scarring are minimal and the tissues will never be in better condition. When an injury is detected and successfully repaired, there is little additional morbidity for the patient. On the other hand, delayed recognition, with fistula formation, obstruction, and sepsis, represents an enormous burden. Despite this, the majority of ureteral injuries continue to go unrecognized. Only one-third of such injuries are detected in the operating room; optimistically, our review shows a trend toward improved recognition over the past 10 years.[1]

The intraoperative approach to an injured ureter depends on the level, mechanism, and severity of injury and is significantly different from that taken when an identical injury is discovered in the postoperative period. When the surgeon encounters such an injury it is often best to simply remove any offending agent (clamp, ligature, and so on), complete the planned operation, and then return to assess the damage. This allows better evaluation of ischemic tissue and prevents undue traction on the ureteral repair. The types of ureteral injuries mentioned earlier (see Fig. 47–5) can be divided into four basic groups—sutures and ligatures, crush injuries, laceration and excision, devascularization—which are discussed next.

Sutures and Ligatures

When the ureter is ligated or transfixed by a suture, the first step in management is always to remove the offending suture and assess the integrity of the ureter. Deligation alone is usually sufficient therapy. When penetration by a suture has occurred, it may be helpful to give indigo carmine intravenously to look for extravasation. Whenever the integrity of the ureter is in question, a stent should be placed. A double-J stent or feeding tube can be placed through a ureterotomy or by opening the bladder to provide internal or external drainage. A Penrose drain placed a few centimeters away from the ureter will prevent the fibrosis that can result if urine extravasates. It is rare for an injury caused by either ligation or suture transfixion not to completely resolve with stenting.

Crush Injuries from Clamps

The severity of a clamp injury depends on the size of the clamp, the length of time it was applied, and the amount of tissue enclosed by the clamp. Although an occasional good result can be obtained by simply removing a small clamp, almost all of these injuries should be stented and drained. When the viability of the ureter is in question, the injured segment should be resected and the case handled in the same manner as a laceration or segmental excision.

Laceration and Excision

Because sharp division of the ureter results in little or no ischemic injury, management depends only on the level and extent of the injury. Partial injuries are repaired directly with fine absorbable suture at all levels except the very distal ureter where reimplantation is often easier. With the larger partial injuries it is best to completely divide and spatulate the ureter to prevent wound contracture and stricture. Complete transection of the distal ureter is treated by ureteroneocystotomy; mid and upper ureteral transections are repaired by direct anastomosis. Repairs should always be drained; stenting is a matter of the surgeon's preference.

Deliberate or accidental excision of a segment of the ureter may result in a significant defect. When the two ends are separated by more than a few centimeters, ureteroureterostomy is inadvisable. All ureteral repairs must be spatulated and tension-free; this cannot be accomplished with such a gap. In these cases the psoas hitch and reimplantation procedure detailed in the next section will bridge almost any defect. In rare cases a Boari bladder flap, transureteroureterostomy, ileal ureter, or nephrectomy may be the procedure of choice.

Devascularization

When surgical dissection compromises the longitudinal blood supply of the ureter running in the adventitia, delayed necrosis and fistula formation may result. When the segment is obviously nonviable, it is excised and a repair performed at the level of healthy tissue using the criteria outlined earlier. In borderline cases the ureter should be stented and covered with omentum or peritoneum. Healthy well-vascularized tissue supports and speeds proper healing and contains urinary extravasation.

Injuries During Vaginal Surgery

Injuries to the ureter detected during vaginal surgery (usually because no indigo carmine is seen during cystoscopy) present a special problem. If the operation was a needle bladder neck suspension, one need only remove and replace the offending suture or sutures. In other cases the situation is evaluated with retrograde pyelography or stent placement. When there is complete obstruction the repair may be redone if the procedure has been a cystocele or enterocele repair. One should not, however, take down the vaginal cuff after a difficult hysterectomy or extensive reconstruction of the vault because significant bleeding can ensue. When these injuries cannot be stented, reimplantation is necessary. When a ureteral catheter cannot be passed through a partial obstruction, ureteroscopy may allow stent placement under direct vision. In selected cases, percutaneous nephrostomy placement alleviates the immediate problem and allows delayed repair in a preferable setting.

In summary, the key principles in the repair of acute ureteral injury are as follows:

1. Debride questionably viable tissue and stent if still in doubt.
2. Strive for a tension-free and watertight anastomosis.
3. Isolate the repair from infection, retroperitoneal fibrosis, and cancer (use omentum as needed).
4. No cancer or radiated tissue should be present at the anastomosis
5. Minimize ureteral mobilization.
6. If simple repair is not possible and a specialist is not available, then divert temporarily.[8]

By adhering strictly to these principles the surgeon should be able to save almost all kidneys in patients with ureteral trauma, and fistula formation should be a rare complication.

DELAYED RECOGNITION

Timing

Although there was considerable controversy in the past about the optimum time to repair ureteral injuries, especially fistulas, the debate has all but ended. As discussed earlier, endourologic and percutaneous techniques allow a trial of nonoperative management and provide a good chance for ultimate success. Renal function is preserved by drainage. The social problem of urine leakage is relieved by nephrostomy or stent placement. In patients in whom nonoperative management fails, the patient is in the delayed repair group by default. When these techniques are technically impossible or surgery is chosen as the most suitable therapy, immediate reconstruction is appropriate for the majority of patients. Surgery should be delayed until local infection has been adequately treated. Injuries in a radiated field and after radical hysterectomy are relative indications for a delay of at least 3 months, and a concerted effort should be made to treat these patients nonoperatively. In the majority of patients who have injuries after gynecologic surgery for benign disease, there is no need to postpone repair.

Planning the Operation

In planning surgical treatment of ureteral injuries, the following factors must be assessed: status of the ipsilateral and contralateral kidneys, length of injured segment and type of injury, level of injury, and status of the bladder for possible use in repair. Mitigating factors such as retroperitoneal fibrosis, infection, and radiation exposure also influence the surgical decision-making process. Even in light of these factors, however, 80 to 90% of ureteral injuries can be successfully reconstructed using two standard

techniques—ureteral reimplantation and the vesicopsoas hitch. Almost all the other lesions are amenable to a modification of the psoas hitch to form a Boari-Ockerblad bladder flap. These three procedures are outlined later and can be mastered by any accomplished pelvic surgeon. Only when the bladder cannot be used in the reconstruction are more elaborate techniques required.

Ureteroneocystostomy

When the ureter can easily be reimplanted into the bladder without tension, ureteroneocystostomy is the preferred procedure. I limit use of the simple reimplant to cases in which the ureter can be implanted into a fixed posterior portion of the bladder so that there will be no kinking and obstruction with filling. Still, injuries in the area of the uterine artery or vaginal fornix and at the beginning of the intramural ureter within about 6 cm of the ureterovesical junction are amenable to this technique. There has been extensive debate in the literature about the optimal type of reimplantation. As a rule, gynecologists favor refluxing methods, and urologists prefer nonrefluxing techniques. Because cystitis is such a common problem in this patient population, the extra effort required to prevent reflux may prevent the long-term morbidity of pyelonephritis, but obstruction is more common with nonrefluxing repairs. The LeDuc reimplant is illustrated and annotated in Figure 47–6. It is a simple nonrefluxing technique that is easy to learn and teach; because it employs a very short tunnel, obstruction is rare. Several points deserve emphasis. Dissection of the proximal ureter should be kept to a minimum. The distal ureter is ligated to prevent reflux and extravasation. It is always safer to move the bladder to the ureter than vice versa. This repair should not be used if there is evidence of infection or significant inflammation; the anastomosis should always be done in a clean field. In the LeDuc procedure the tunnel is short. Normal bladders have low storage pressures; a short tunnel will reliably prevent reflux when pressures are low. Other techniques may be required in patients with an abnormal bladder. The area of the anastomosis must be drained. We stent the anastomosis with a catheter brought out alongside a suprapubic tube, but excellent results are reported with unstented anastomoses. The advantages of stenting include ease of follow-up studies, minimal extravasation and resultant fibrosis, and maintenance of a straight ureter to prevent adhesions and kinking.[14]

Vesicopsoas Hitch

A normal bladder can be easily mobilized above the iliac vessels for use in reconstruction, a technique popularized by Turner-Warwick and Worth.[15] The vesicopsoas hitch has since become the procedure of choice for nearly all injuries to the pelvic ureter

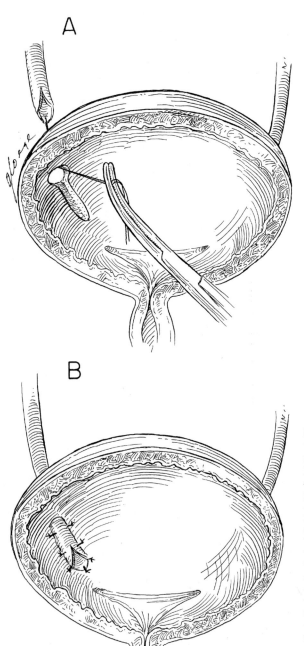

Figure 47-6 LeDuc ureteroneocystostomy. In preparation for reimplantation the ureter is spatulated anteriorly, and a holding stitch is placed in the apex of the posterior wall. The bladder is opened anteriorly and a psoas hitch performed if necessary. The distal end of the ureter is ligated. *A,* At a comfortable site in the posterior wall of the bladder a neohiatus is created, and the only mucosa of the bladder is incised distal to the hiatus for a distance of about 3 cm. The mucosa is then elevated off the muscle of the bladder for several millimeters on each side, creating a small trough. The ureter is passed into the bladder. *B,* The reimplantation is secured using three sutures of 3–0 polyglycolic acid that include the full thickness of the ureter and generous bites of the bladder muscle. The free edges of the bladder mucosa are then secured to the adventitia of the ureter using fine absorbable suture. No effort is made to completely cover the ureter with the mucosa; rather, the ureter is splayed laterally to flatten it against the strong backing of bladder muscle. The bladder is closed in routine fashion, and extraperitoneal drainage is always employed. This has been our preferred method of ureteral reimplantation for several years. It is adaptable to a wide variety of situations, provides a secure antireflux mechanism, and is associated with very rare complications. (From Payne CK, Raz S: Ureterovaginal and related fistulae. *In* McAninch JW [ed]: Traumatic and Reconstructive Urology. Philadelphia, WB Saunders, in press, 1996.)

(combined with ureteroneocystostomy). A tension-free reimplantation can be ensured in essentially all of these cases. A variation of the standard technique is illustrated in Figure 47–7. The following points are emphasized. The contralateral side of the bladder is dissected down to the level of the endopelvic fascia until adequate mobility is achieved. The contralateral superior vesical artery is sacrificed, but the inferior vesical artery is generally preserved. The bladder is opened with a curvilinear incision as if to create a small Boari flap. With the hand inside the bladder, the site for the anastomosis of the ureter and bladder is chosen to allow an adequate length of ureter. Only then are the interrupted Vicryl sutures placed between the bladder and the psoas tendon, taking care not to injure the ilioinguinal nerve.

Ureteroneocystostomy, with psoas hitch whenever necessary, is the most reliable method of reconstructing the lower urinary tract. In patients with unilateral ureteral fistula, success has been achieved in 94% of cases on the first attempt.[1]

Boari-Ockerblad Bladder Tube Flap

Whereas the bladder flap had once been a chief method of repairing ureteral injuries before wide-

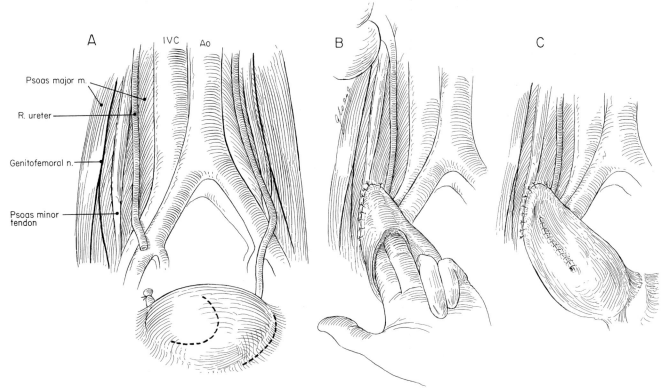

Figure 47-7 Psoas hitch. *A,* In preparation for mobilization of the bladder, all of the lateral attachments on the contralateral side are divided down to the endopelvic fascia. We do not sacrifice the inferior vesical pedicle, although the superior pedicle is divided. A curved incision is then made in the anterior wall of the bladder, which creates a wide-based bladder flap. *B,* With two or three fingers inside the bladder, the posterior-superior portion of the bladder wall is guided across the iliac vessels to the psoas muscle. Multiple interrupted absorbable sutures are then taken to secure the back wall of the bladder to the psoas tendon. To prevent postoperative neuralgia, the genitofemoral nerve must be identified and avoided. Here, the small bladder flap can be "rolled over" to almost any spot below the pelvic brim, giving a great deal of flexibility in reconstruction. *C,* After completing the repair by reimplantation or other procedure, the bladder incision is closed transversely by the standard technique. Extravesical drains are placed alongside the reconstruction. (From Payne CK, Raz S: Ureterovaginal and related fistulae. *In* McAninch JW [ed]: Traumatic and Reconstructive Urology. Philadelphia, WB Saunders, in press, 1996.)

spread use of the psoas hitch, it is now reserved for cases in which the healthy proximal ureter is above the pelvis. When the bladder is normal, a bladder flap with the aid of a psoas hitch can reach at least the lower pole of the kidney, and in some cases the renal pelvis. As such, it remains an exceedingly valuable tool in the surgeon's armamentarium. The technique is illustrated in Figure 47–8. The procedure always begins with creation of a psoas hitch. At that point the remaining defect is assessed and the flap outlined, always making the base of the flap twice as wide as the apex. Again, a nonrefluxing LeDuc-type reimplantation is preferred, but a simple end-to-end anastomosis may be all that is possible.

Results with the Boari flap are consistently good, if not quite so good as those with a psoas hitch and reimplant. Reflux and voiding dysfunction are somewhat more common, as is prolonged urine leakage. Nonetheless, superior results have been achieved by authors who use the procedure frequently, and success rates of close to 90% should be expected.[16–18] Gross infection in the pelvis is a strong indication for creation of a flap to "ensure a tension-free anastomosis far away from the infective focus.[18]

Other Procedures

When the bladder is not normal, other methods of reconstruction must be employed. Radiation therapy and scarring from multiple prior pelvic operations are the two most common factors that prevent adequate bladder mobilization. Transitional cell carcinoma has been considered by some a relative contraindication to a bladder flap, and a variety of inflammatory diseases can preclude its use in reconstruction. In these cases only the most distal lesions can be managed with a reimplant, and other injuries require a variety of other techniques. Direct reanastomosis is almost never possible more than 2 to 3 days from the initial operation, and it has a high complication rate. Transureteroureterostomy may be employed for midureteral lesions with excellent results.[19, 20] The ileal ureter is the most versatile technique; it can be adapted to almost any clinical situation including high bilateral injuries and has excellent reliability in experienced hands. Ileum is almost always available, but an appendix interposition can be used similarly on the right side, avoiding a bowel anastomosis. Disadvantages include the mor-

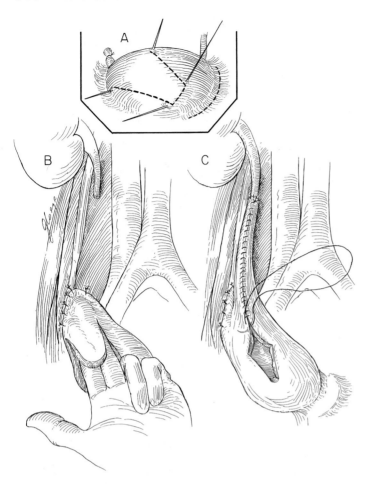

Figure 47-8 Boari flap. *A,* As in a psoas hitch, the contralateral side of the bladder is mobilized from its lateral attachments. Holding sutures are placed in the anterior bladder wall to mark the flap. The flap encompasses nearly the entire breadth of the anterior wall and may be extended somewhat superiorly. The base of the flap should be roughly twice as wide as the apex to ensure good blood supply. *B,* The flap is incised using cautery, and a standard psoas hitch is performed. *C,* The flap is "turned over" and is also secured to the psoas muscle to keep tension off the anastomosis. The proximal ureter is reimplanted into the back wall of the flap using the LeDuc technique when possible. In many cases only a simple end-to-end anastomosis can be achieved. The flap is then rolled into a tube and closed side to side with a single-layer running suture. Ideally, the repair is covered with omentum or peritoneum. The bladder and extravesical spaces must be well drained. (From Payne CK, Raz S: Ureterovaginal and related fistulae. *In* McAninch JW [ed]: Traumatic and Reconstructive Urology. Philadelphia, WB Saunders, in press, 1996.)

bidity of opening the gastrointestinal tract, mucus obstruction, and reflux in about 70% of cases.[21] The potential for electrolyte abnormalities and absorption difficulties limits use of the procedure in patients with renal failure. Reflux is rarely a clinical problem as long as the bladder empties efficiently because the ileal ureter maintains its peristalsis. Because of mucus production the bladder should be drained with both a Foley and a suprapubic tube and the ileum stented with a red rubber catheter. Urinary diversion is indicated only when the bladder cannot be rehabilitated.[22] The primary indication for nephrectomy is palliation in the patient with recurrent or unresectable cancer. We agree with Mandal that "neither poor visualization on IVU nor severe ureteropyelocaliectasis" is to be regarded as an absolute indication for nephrectomy in the patient with a fistula.[18] The presence of a fistula indicates at least partial relief of pressure on the nephrons and thus the potential for good recovery of function. A patient who has had total obstruction for more than a month or so should have a trial of percutaneous drainage prior to reconstruction because ultimate renal function may be marginal. Nephrectomy should be seriously considered in a frail or elderly patient with a compromised ipsilateral kidney or a severe ureteral deficit providing the contralateral kidney is normal.[22] In such patients, however, renal artery embolization should be

considered; this has been reported to cure two patients with a ureteral fistula.[23]

Bilateral Ureteral Injuries

Bilateral ureteral injuries present a special management problem. Regardless of whether the patient has anuria, bilateral fistulas, or a combination of obstruction and extravasation, there is an impetus toward quick and definitive management to preserve renal function and prevent septic complications. Although conservative management is still an option, particularly as a temporizing maneuver, it is somewhat less attractive in these patients. The ultimate likelihood of avoiding open surgery is significantly reduced in a patient with a bilateral injury; at the same time, the morbidity of bilateral stents is significantly greater than in those with a unilateral injury.

When confronted with an anuric patient in the recovery room or a bilateral injury diagnosed during convalescence, I prefer immediate surgical intervention in a stable patient. Nephrostomy drainage is indicated when the patient is septic, uremic, or otherwise unstable. Early surgical intervention was thought earlier to be risky, primarily because of a report by Aschner.[24] His literature review of cases of bilateral ligation showed 83% mortality for patients undergoing immediate deligation compared to 23% for nephrostomy placement and 100% for those with no treatment. Aschner thought that nephrostomy was far preferable to deligation because of the risk of hemorrhage and fistula formation with the latter. However, the safety of immediate therapy was demonstrated in a subsequent report of five consecutive cases of anuric obstruction managed by primary reimplantation without nephrostomy, all of which were successful and free of serious complications.[25] Significant ureteral dilation occurs in the first 24 hours, which facilitates reconstruction.

Bilateral injuries usually occur in the distal third of the ureter. They should always be approached via a midline transperitoneal incision. In many cases repair can be effected with a unilateral psoas hitch to the side of the shorter ureter and reimplantation of both ureters into the bladder at a convenient site. When both ureters are injured at or above the iliac vessels, considerable ingenuity and flexibility are required. The surgeon must be familiar with all possibilities for reconstruction. There are numerous reports of creative procedures combining intestinal segment interposition, transureteroureterostomy, bladder flap, and psoas hitch.[18, 22, 26–28]

Postradiation and Other Complex Fistulas

Repair of a fistula in a radiated field or repair of a complex fistula involving both the urinary and gastrointestinal tracts is among the most challenging cases faced by the pelvic reconstructive surgeon. Although no randomized trials have been conducted, there is considerable evidence that radiation decreases the success of fistula repair. In the Mayo Clinic series initial cure of all nonradiated urinary vaginal fistulas ranged from 93 to 100%, whereas only 67 to 69% of irradiated fistulas were closed on the first attempt.[12]

Several issues are critical to successful management of these cases. Recurrent malignancy must always be considered in the irradiated patient and ruled out by appropriate biopsies. Gross infection must be treated before reconstruction. This may require a temporary diverting colostomy. Adequate drainage is paramount because healing may be delayed in irradiated tissue. We stent all anastomoses and leave the stents until we are sure that the repair is intact. The repair should be done in a well-vascularized field, and whenever necessary, vascularized tissue flaps are interposed to support healing. Omentum, peritoneum, rectus muscle, and mesentery of a bowel segment may be used. Again, imagination and flexibility are the keys to success.

Results and Follow-up

With current techniques, more than 90% of ureteral injuries are successfully repaired with one opera-

tion. Most failures are apparent within the first 6 months[18, 29] and can be salvaged with a second operation if the patient is willing to undergo further surgery.

Little has been written about the follow-up of patients after fistula repair. Careful surveillance is imperative for the first 6 months. An IVU is obtained 1 month after all stents and tubes have been removed. If that study is normal, an ultrasound examination is obtained between 3 and 6 months postoperatively. An abnormal IVU is repeated every 4 to 6 weeks until there is clear evidence of progression, resolution, or stabilization. The urine is examined at each visit. After 1 year asymptomatic patients are seen annually or if there is a clinical problem. An annual pyelogram has been recommended[30] but is probably not necessary in a patient who is doing well. As mentioned earlier, any upper tract infection signals the need for a full work-up.

Progressive hydronephrosis signals stenosis of the anastomosis, usually due to a technical problem. Yeates estimated that half of follow-up urograms demonstrate normal upper tracts, and half show no more than moderate dilation of the ureter.[22] It should be noted that in many of these cases mild to moderate dilation actually represents an improvement over the preoperative morphology. True progressive dilation is very uncommon. Pyelonephritis should make the surgeon suspect stenosis and obstruction. The percentage of patients with reflux depends on the type of reconstruction employed, but reflux in and of itself is not a complication. Patients with reflux and sterile urine typically have no or minor symptoms. Any complications occurring more than 6 to 12 months postoperatively should alert the surgeon to the possibility of tumor recurrence in the cancer patient.

When progressive hydronephrosis is detected, endourologic methods offer an excellent option for treatment. Balloon dilation and stenting or endoscopic incision usually obviates the need for further surgery.

Summary

The close anatomic and embryologic relationship of the ureter to the female genital tract places the ureter at risk during most pelvic operations in women. Improvements in surgical technique have decreased the incidence of ureteral injury during this generation, and rapid progress in percutaneous and endoscopic surgery is currently minimizing morbidity in patients suffering such injuries. Our challenge as pelvic surgeons is to carry this trend forward with excellence in surgical technique and imagination in developing new therapy.

REFERENCES

1. Payne CK, Raz S: Ureterovaginal and related fistulae. *In* McAninch JW (ed): Traumatic and Reconstructive Urology. Philadelphia, WB Saunders, in press, 1996.

2. McVay CB: Abdominal cavity and contents. *In* Anson BJ, McVay CB (eds): Surgical Anatomy, 6th ed. Philadelphia, WB Saunders, 1984, p 760.

3. Van Nagel JR Jr, Roddick JW Jr: Vaginal hysterectomy, the ureter and excretory urography. Obstet Gynecol 39(5):784, 1972.

4. Higgins CC: Ureteral injuries during surgery: A review of 87 cases. JAMA 199(2):118, 1967.

5. Williams TJ: Urologic injuries. *In* Wynn RM (ed): Obstetrics and Gynecology Annual. New York, Appleton-Century-Crofts, 1975, pp 347–368.

6. Symmonds RE: Ureteral injuries associated with gynecologic surgery: Prevention and management. Clin Obstet Gynecol 19(3):623, 1976.

7. Mattingly RF, Borkowf HI: Acute operative injury to the lower urinary tract. Clin Obstet Gynecol 5(1):123–149, 1978.

8. St. Lezin MA, Stoller ML: Surgical ureteral injuries. Urology 38(6):497, 1991.

9. Green TH, Meigs JV, Ulfelder H, Curtin RR: Urologic complications of radical Wertheim hysterectomy: Incidence, etiology, management, and prevention. Obstet Gynecol 20(3):293, 1962.

10. Hofmeister FJ: Pelvic anatomy of the ureter in relation to surgery performed through the vagina. Clin Obstet Gynecol 25(4):821, 1982.

11. Stanhope CR, Wilson TO, Utz WJ, et al: Suture entrapment and secondary ureteral obstruction. Am J Obstet Gynecol 164(6):1513, 1991.

12. Massee JS, Welch JS, Pratt JH, Symmonds RE: Management of urinary-vaginal fistula—ten-year survey. JAMA 190(10):124, 1964.

13. Higgins CC: Ureteral injuries: Etiopathogenesis, prophylaxis, diagnosis, and treatment. JAMA 182(3):225, 1962.

14. Sieben DM, Howerton L, Amin M, et al: The role of ureteral stenting in the management of surgical injury of the ureter. J Urol 119:330, 1978.

15. Turner-Warwick R, Worth PHL: The psoas bladder hitch procedure for the replacement of the lower third of the ureter. Br J Urol 41:701, 1969.

16. Badenoch DF, Tiptaft RC, Thakar DR, et al: Early repair of accidental injury to the ureter or bladder following gynecological surgery. Br J Urol 59:516, 1987.

17. Wallace DM: Uretero-vaginal fistula. Br J Urol 44:617, 1972.

18. Mandal AK, Sharma SK, Vaidyanathan S, Goswami AK: Ureterovaginal fistula: Summary of 18 year's experience. Br J Urol 65:453, 1990.

19. Hendren WH, Hensle TW: Transureteroureterostomy: Experience with 75 cases. J Urol 123:826, 1980.

20. Hodges CV, Barry JM, Fuchs EF, et al: Transureteroureterostomy: 25-year experience with 100 patients. J Urol 123:834, 1980.

21. Boxer RJ, Fritzsche P, Skinner DG, et al: Replacement of the ureter by small intestine: Clinical application and results of the ileal ureter in 89 patients. J Urol 121:728, 1979.

22. Yeates WK: Ureterovaginal fistulae. *In* Stanton SL, Tanagho EA (eds): Surgery of Female Incontinence, 2nd ed. Berlin, Springer-Verlag, 1986, pp 212–227.

23. Long MA, McIvor J: Renal artery embolization with ethanol and Gelfoam for the treatment of ureteric fistulae with one year follow-up. Clin Radiol 46:270, 1992.

24. Aschner PW: Accidental injury to ureters and bladder in pelvic surgery. J Urol 69(6):774, 1953.

25. Harrow BR: Management of ureteral injuries causing anuria. J Urol 101:694, 1969.

26. Goodwin WE, Scardino PT: Vesicovaginal and ureterovaginal fistulas: A summary of 25 years of experience. J Urol 123:370, 1980.

27. Weems WL: Combined use of bladder flap and transureteroureterostomy: Report of a case. J Urol 103:50, 1970.

28. Yokoyama M, Iio S, Hidenobu I, Takeuchi M: Bilateral ureterovaginal fistula treated by psoas hitch and uretero-appendico-cystostomy. J Urol 147:1102, 1992.

29. Lee RA, Symmonds RE: Ureterovaginal fistula. Am J Obstet Gynec 109(7):1032, 1971.

30. Smith AM: Injuries of the pelvic ureter. Surg Gynecol Obstet 140:761, 1975.

CHAPTER 48

Endoscopic and Percutaneous Management of Ureteral Injuries, Fistulas, Obstruction, and Strictures

Anup Patel, M.S., F.R.C.S. (Urol.)
Philip E. Werthman, M.D.
Gerhard J. Fuchs, M.D.
Zoran L. Barbaric, M.D.

Endourologic expertise is often required for the management of ureteral lesions that may be the cause of crippling disability and silent loss of renal function. These may be related either to the primary disease process itself or to operative or nonoperative therapeutic interventions.

Iatrogenic ureteral injury is a well-established potential complication of surgery for benign and malignant diseases of the female pelvic organs. It may be associated with sequelae such as obstruction and fistula formation. The incidence of iatrogenic ureteral injury has varied from 0.4 to 30% in historical series[1-6] and continues to remain in this range despite heightened awareness of possible urologic complications from pelvic surgery in women.

How then, in an era characterized by advanced surgical techniques combined with a better understanding of pelvic anatomy, can this perplexing conundrum be explained? Abdominoperineal and low anterior resections, primary debulking procedures for ovarian cancer and salvage surgery for residual or recurrent disease after primary radiation therapy for locally advanced gynecologic malignancy (such as cervical cancer), are technically demanding operations and leave little margin for error. If meticulous care is not employed in defining the course of the pelvic ureters without devitalizing the tissues, the risk of iatrogenic ureteral injury is significantly increased. The surgical complexity in some patients is compounded by the greater incidence of late radiation toxicity after older external beam and brachytherapy regimens that have resulted in a frozen pel-

vis or a tenuous blood supply to the lower ureter. Nevertheless, in the current decade, ablative surgery in combination with procedures such as continent urinary diversion has been used with greater frequency in such situations, as surgeons seek to attain the twin goals of surgical cure and improved quality of life in younger patients with locally advanced pelvic cancer. More recently, orthotopic neobladder reconstruction has also been possible in selected female patients as knowledge of urethral continence mechanisms has improved and operative techniques have been refined with regard to dissection around the bladder neck and urethra at the pelvic floor. With the contributions of improved anesthesia and pain control, these surgical developments have led to an increase in the number and magnitude of complex radical pelvic and retroperitoneal procedures, either with curative intent or with a neoadjuvant goal in sicker patients. Together, these facts may partly help to explain the paradox of a relatively undiminished incidence of iatrogenic ureteral damage in the modern era.

The types of iatrogenic ureteral injuries most frequently encountered include ureteral laceration, avulsion, complete division, crush, mural or transmural incorporation in suture ligation of vascular pedicles at the pelvic side walls, and obstruction secondary to excessive angulation coupled with secondary fibrosis from misplaced sutures. Benign ureteral strictures are usually the sequela of local ischemic injury resulting either from direct surgical devitalization of periureteral and axial arterial branches or from radiation effect leading to endarteritis and fibrosis.

Most iatrogenic injuries to the ureter are occult and are diagnosed only in the convalescent period. Only one-third are recognized intraoperatively so that immediate appropriate repair or reconstruction can be undertaken by a urologist or an experienced pelvic surgeon. Complete ureteral transection invariably leads to distraction of the cut ends. This injury is rarely amenable solely to endourologic management in the postoperative period. If immediate or early open repair is not undertaken or desirable, it may be necessary to perform external urinary diversion for a time. Partial damage to the ureters may be undetected for weeks or months because acute postoperative symptoms are often absent in such cases. The frequently silent course of such an injury may ultimately result in a ureteral stricture, which may be followed by an irreversible loss of functioning nephrons if complete and unrelieved obstruction continues unabated for 4 or more weeks. Delayed urinary fistula formation, on the other hand, may lead to regular nocturnal fever, persistent unexplained flank pain with renal angle tenderness, pelvic pain associated with a boggy pelvic mass on digital rectal examination, or copious unremitting urinary discharge from dependent parts of the wound, drain sites, or the vaginal vault. These signs are often coupled with abdominal distention and ileus[7] and are early indicators of ureteral injury. Renal salvage is likely to be better in these symptomatic patients as a result of earlier intervention.

Many factors may ultimately influence lasting success in the management of ureteral injury. These include the site of injury, the length of the ureteral wall involved, the status of the contralateral kidney or ureter, the age and comorbidity of the patient, the existence of previous pelvic and abdominal radiation, the presence of a fresh vascular prosthesis or other prosthetic material in the surgical field, the presence of retroperitoneal or pelvic fibrosis or pelvic abscess, and the presence of a concomitantly produced vesicovaginal fistula.[8]

As soon as a ureteral injury is suspected postoperatively, urine should be sent for culture and systemic antibiotic prophylaxis started. The diagnosis must be confirmed without further delay and its site and severity elucidated. These functional and anatomic objectives can be attained most easily by obtaining a high-dose, contrast-enhanced intravenous pyelogram (IVP) or computerized tomographic urogram (CTU), which allows more detailed imaging of the lesion for a lower total radiation dose. The cardinal features of ureteral mishap with urinary extravasation in the IVP are delayed contrast excretion and dilatation of the upper tract above the injury site (Fig. 48–1). Extravasation of contrast medium may be seen in patients with larger ureteral defects. The severity of obstruction can often be judged by the degree to which the upper tract drains the contrast agent when the bladder is decompressed by a Foley catheter. If intravenous contrast administration is contraindi-

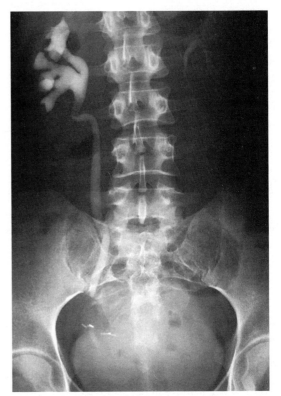

Figure 48-1 Intravenous urogram showing a dilated right ureter above the site of the ureteral fistula at the level of the infundibulopelvic ligament.

cated (e.g., in patients with an elevated serum creatinine level) or is inconclusive, cystoscopy with retrograde pyelography should be performed to delineate the severity of injury and extravasation (Fig. 48–2) so that definitive therapeutic intervention may be carefully planned.

Ureteral damage that is recognized intraoperatively should be repaired primarily without further delay.[9–12] The available open surgical options in this

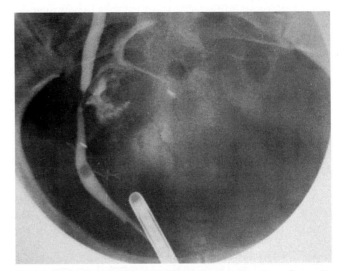

Figure 48-2 Retrograde pyelogram showing the site and severity of the ureteral injury.

context are addressed elsewhere. Unfortunately, the majority of injuries are not recognized immediately. Litigation may be involved in these instances, and it is essential for the treatment options and potential outcomes to be clearly outlined to the satisfaction of the patient through frank discussion before intervention is undertaken. In this chapter we discuss the role of contemporary minimally invasive urologic techniques (endourologic, percutaneous, and laparoscopic) in the diagnosis and management of ureteral injuries, fistulas, and obstruction.

Urinary Fistulas

In a woman, a fistulous communication between the urinary tract and an adjacent pelvic viscus or the skin is usually the end result of transmural iatrogenic injury that fails to heal and is perpetuated by distal obstruction. The cause of noniatrogenic primary ureteroenteric or vesicoenteric fistulas is related to an acute inflammatory phlegmon arising from an adherent colonic diverticulum (including the vermiform appendix), to chronic inflammatory processes of the gastrointestinal tract such as Crohn's disease, or to contiguous local malignant invasion (e.g., from colon cancer).[13, 14] Ureterovaginal and vesicovaginal fistulas develop most often after radical pelvic surgery or primary brachytherapy radiation treatment for locally advanced pelvic malignancy.[3, 15] The resulting constant total urinary incontinence is both disabling and socially unacceptable.

In contrast, ureterocutaneous fistulas usually occur after sharp penetrating trauma, invariably iatrogenic.[14] In these patients, it is often impossible to maintain hygiene or cutaneous adherence of external collecting appliances. When no curative surgical remedy can be rendered, ureteral occlusion coupled with urinary diversion may be the best means of preventing lasting social disability.

In very select circumstances, ureterovaginal fistulas can be managed expectantly.[16] This course should be attempted only when there is unilateral injury with minimal obstruction, mild urinary extravasation that does not affect the patient's quality of life, and an ability to maintain adequate control of urinary tract infection. Regular and frequent microbiologic evaluation of the urine in conjunction with sonographic imaging of the pelvis and upper urinary tract every 2 weeks is essential, however, if such a conservative strategy is undertaken. The cost of such management to both the patient (in terms of the burden of compliance) and the health care provider (in terms of the uncertainty of outcome) is undoubtedly high.

Malignant and chronic inflammatory ureteral fistulas, on the other hand, are most unlikely to heal spontaneously after internal or external urinary diversion alone. Successful open surgical repair or reconstruction may break down as a result of the poor healing properties of irradiated tissue, ischemia, untreated sepsis from prior surgical procedures, or tumor recurrence. Endoscopic management alone rarely delivers a lasting cure under these circumstances, but staged drainage procedures may be indicated frequently. Because many of these patients are poorly nourished, cachectic, or poor surgical candidates, the treatment of fistulas in this particular population can be very difficult or frustrating and requires a multidisciplinary team approach to optimize the outcome. Palliation of symptoms may be all that is possible, but this is often a worthwhile end point for a debilitated but grateful patient.

The primary goals of therapy for urinary fistulas are preservation of renal function, prevention or drainage of localized urinary sepsis, maintenance of hygiene, and eradication of symptoms. After diagnosis of a fistula, it is important to rule out obstruction in the ureter distal to the fistula site, as previously mentioned. This requires treatment in its own right because it discourages spontaneous resolution of the fistula in most instances.[12]

If no significant distal obstruction is present, internalized urinary drainage by means of an indwelling ureteral stent inserted in a retrograde fashion over a safety guidewire may be all that is necessary to allow a benign iatrogenic fistula to heal. This should be attempted as first-line treatment. The stent may also provide a template for healing and reepithelialization at the site of a partial ureteral injury when the defect is small (on the principle of a Davis intubated ureterostomy), provided that local or general patient factors for healing are unimpaired.

If a retrograde stent cannot be placed owing to ureteral distortion, or if sufficient fulcrum cannot be obtained from the ureteral orifice to bypass any element of obstruction that may be present, there are two possible additional methods of achieving successful stent placement. In one technique, rigid ureteroscopy using low-flow rates of irrigant and passage of a second floppy-tipped 0.035-inch guidewire (or Glide wire) across the defect may be attempted under direct vision to obtain better stability across the fistula and enable safe passage of a retrograde stent. Edema at the fistula site makes this a rather difficult procedure that should be attempted only by a skilled endourologist. If undue resistance is encountered, however, the procedure should be curtailed because excessive force or angulation may easily extend a tear in an inflamed edematous ureter. Both wires should be retained, and a 5 Fr angiographic or single-J catheter should be passed over the working guidewire before both wires are secured in place by "piggy-backing" them into a small puncture at the hub of the Foley bladder catheter. This ureteral intubation maneuver may allow sufficient passive dilatation of the ureter to occur over the next 10 to 14 days to allow successful delayed retrograde stent placement. Bladder drainage by Foley catheter is essential for a minimum of 5 days after retrograde stenting to prevent refluxing urinary extravasation from the fistula site. A voiding cystourethrogram thereafter will indicate whether the fistula site has sealed and whether it is safe to dispense with further bladder drainage.

As a second strategy when primary retrograde stenting fails, antegrade percutaneous nephrostomy drainage under local anesthesia allows temporization of an acute problem. This mode of urinary diversion may in itself allow spontaneous healing of a small fistula. It is particularly useful in the sick patient who is unable to tolerate further general anesthesia, or when special endourologic expertise (in terms of both personnel and equipment) is not immediately available. Ideally, once temporary drainage has been achieved, the need for prolonged external drainage is undesirable for the majority of patients, and elective antegrade stenting may be attempted by an experienced uroradiologist.[14, 17–19]

In difficult cases, when even antegrade stent placement is not feasible after nephrostomy drainage, it may be necessary to combine uroradiologic expertise in the placement of antegrade safety and working wires that can be retrieved by the urologist from the native bladder or neobladder (Fig. 48–3). Tension at either end of the working wire can then provide sufficient fulcrum to allow successful passage of a ureteral stent across the fistula site in retrograde fashion. This form of internal drainage has proved to

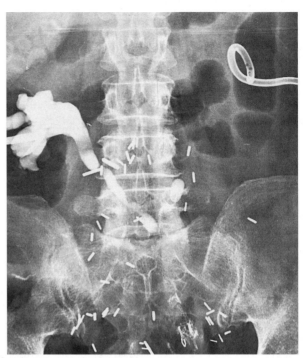

Figure 48–4 Radiograph showing bilateral placement of detachable ureteral occlusion balloons and an antegrade nephrostogram to check the adequacy of occlusion. (From Barbaric ZL: Principles of Genitourinary Radiology. New York, Thieme Medical Publishers Inc., 1991.)

be an excellent alternative to open surgical repair, achieving success in approximately 70% of our patients. Others[20] have used a combined retrograde-antegrade approach to salvage a ureteral leak.

New advances in endourology and invasive uroradiology have provided a variety of options for complete diversion of the flow of urine in patients in whom the fistula fails to heal with conservative methods. These techniques comprise a combination of total occlusion of the ureter proximal to the fistula with creation of a proximal percutaneous urinary diversion. Because ureteral access to the fistula site is obtained through a percutaneous approach, these procedures may be performed under local anesthesia or intravenous sedation. Their usefulness is greatest in unstable or end-stage cancer patients who are at high operative risk and in whom rapid palliation of symptoms is desired, or in patients in whom planned adjuvant local treatment or the management of other complications may interfere with early open surgical repair.

OCCLUSIVE TECHNIQUES

Occlusive techniques have the advantage of being reversible and therefore are useful when only temporary ureteral occlusion is warranted. Transparenchymal ureteral occlusion can be achieved using detachable or nondetachable balloons. Detachable balloons are usually inserted through a 14 Fr nephrostomy tract (Fig. 48–4). An inflatable latex rubber balloon is attached to a 3 Fr, 60-cm-long Teflon catheter by a

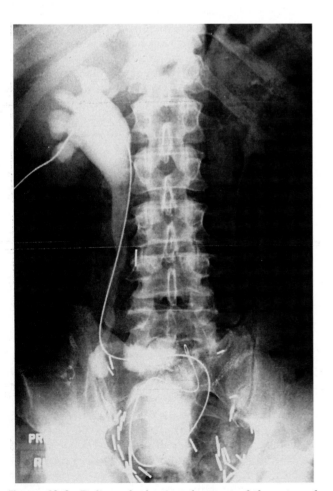

Figure 48–3 Radiograph showing placement of the antegrade safety wire prior to retrieval from the orthotopic neobladder.

fine latex rubber string. An outer coaxial 5 Fr Teflon catheter is used to detach the balloon and stabilize the inner catheter. Fluoroscopic control is used to position the balloon in the distal ureter before it is slowly filled with a mixture of silicone elastomer and silicone fluid 360 (Dow Corning Corp). This is activated with 2 drops/ml of catalyst M and rendered radiopaque by the addition of tantalum powder (1 g/ml). The resulting mixture polymerizes within 15 minutes, and the balloon can then be detached in situ. A nephrostomy tube is retained in the renal pelvis for external urinary diversion. Short-term follow-up in seven patients in whom this technique was used showed good ureteral occlusion with cessation of the urinary leak. The only reported complication in this report was that of balloon rupture during placement in one patient.[21] Others have reported problems with balloon migration.[22]

Temporary balloon occlusion of the ureter can also be easily achieved by improvising with a nondetachable balloon.[23] The size of the balloon should be chosen individually according to ureteral size. A 7 Fr Swan-Ganz catheter or a 4 Fr Fogarty balloon catheter can be positioned over a guidewire placed in the ureter through a percutaneous nephrostomy tract. Because there are no drainage holes in these catheters proximal to the occluding balloon, a nephrostomy tube is placed in the renal pelvis over a second guidewire. Contrast medium should be injected at the end of the procedure to ensure that complete ureteral occlusion has been attained. Both catheters are then secured to the skin with sutures. The occluding balloon should be inflated enough to tamponade flow but not enough to overdistend the ureter. Prolonged placement and overinflation of these devices can lead to local ischemic pressure necrosis of the ureteral wall and extravasation, compounding the problem. Provided appropriate precautions are taken and the efficacy of the occlusion is evaluated from time to time by contrast studies performed with antibiotic prophylaxis (Fig. 48–5), this technique offers the advantage of allowing constant access and easy readjustment or repositioning of the balloon.

Permanent antegrade closure of the ureter was first attempted by Gunther and associates[24] using the tissue adhesive butyl-2-cyanoacrylate. Palliation was attempted in three patients with inoperable vesicovaginal and vesicosacral fistulas secondary to advanced pelvic malignancy. The technique they described began with the placement of an 8 Fr percutaneous nephrostomy tube to decompress the collecting system. This tube was exchanged for a 9 Fr Teflon sleeve, 25 cm long, that allowed access to the renal pelvis. Next, a 5 Fr Swan-Ganz catheter was inserted through the access sheath into the ureter under fluoroscopic control. The balloon was inflated in the distal ureter using 0.2 to 0.3 ml of saline to minimize proximal reflux of the occlusive material. A mixture of butyl-2-cyanoacrylate, lipiodol, and tantalum powder was injected through the sleeve into the distal ureter, again under fluoroscopic guidance. After 1 minute the temporary occlusive balloon was

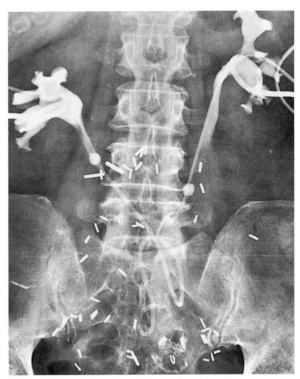

Figure 48–5 Antegrade pyelogram of bilateral ureteral occlusion using nondetachable balloon occlusion catheters.

deflated and removed. These investigators found that two or three injections of sclerosant over the course of 2 days may be necessary to achieve complete ureteral occlusion. As soon as successful occlusion had been achieved, the Teflon access sleeve was replaced by a 10 to 12 Fr nephrostomy tube that provided permanent antegrade drainage. The short-term results of this technique were reportedly favorable, but with constant exposure to urine the occlusive plug may soften and migrate with ureteral peristalsis. This event would jeopardize a successful outcome in the longer term.[25]

Another innovative and minimally invasive technique developed to achieve permanent ureteral occlusion by Kinn and associates was the antegrade insertion of hydrogel-nylon plugs, which had previously been used with success to plug oviducts for the purpose of sterilization.[26] This procedure was combined with injection of a sclerosant above and below the plug to prevent migration. The nephrostomy tract was dilated to 24 to 26 Fr, and after placement of a Lunderqvist wire, a tapered polyethylene catheter 4.0 mm in diameter was introduced into the ureter. A flexible injection needle was then inserted through the catheter and advanced into the distal ureter. Multiple sclerosant (polidocanol) injections in aliquots of 0.5 to 1.5 ml were made intramurally in a circumferential manner. A 6.9-mm outer diameter catheter was then inserted coaxially over the thinner catheter, which was then removed. A 1-cm-long plug of hydrogel mixed with liquid nylon 6 was pushed through the catheter with the aid of the finer catheter and extruded above the injection site. Additional plugs may be introduced into the ureter above the iliac vessels. More sclerosant was then injected into the ureteral wall above the most proximal nylon plug above the level of the iliac vessels. At the end of the procedure, the "working" catheters were removed, and a nephrostomy tube was left in place. Contact with urine allowed the dry plug to swell within 2 to 4 hours, and the original transverse diameter increased from 4.8 mm to 11 mm. Nine failures resulted from recurrence of fistula or plug migration in a series of 15 reported cases treated with this method. One plug had migrated into the calyceal system, causing obstruction. Percutaneous extraction was required in this case.

Complete and permanent ureteral occlusion proximal to a fistula was most simply performed by Reddy and coworkers,[22] who fulgurated the ureter using a percutaneous transparenchymal approach. The nephrostomy tract was created in the upper or mid-pole calyces with the patient sedated by intravenous narcotics supplemented with local anesthesia; the tract was sequentially dilated to allow placement of a 20 Fr Amplatz sheath. A flexible endoscope was passed through this access sheath into the dilated proximal ureter, and a 5 Fr Bugbee electrode was advanced through the work channel. A 2-cm portion of the proximal ureter was then fulgurated under direct vision using coagulation current set on an incident power of 4 on a Valleylab machine. The average time needed for adequate fulguration as determined by mucosal whitening was reported to be 15 minutes. The proximal ureter was chosen for fulguration to avoid possible complications from a static column of urine between the distal ureter and the renal pelvis. A completion nephrostogram was then performed to detect extravasation from both the track site and the ureteral fulguration site. After reinsertion of a secured nephrostomy tube, and confirmation of its position within the renal pelvis by a final contrast study, the Amplatz sheath was removed. Functional occlusion was reliably produced by this method in all three patients.

Percutaneous manipulation of the ureter was first described by Gumpinger and colleagues, who performed percutaneous ureterolithotomy for an otherwise inaccessible calculus.[27] This was followed by a similar report in the American literature.[28] Based on this approach, Smith and associates performed percutaneous ureterolysis and creation of a cutaneous ureterostomy.[29] With the patient in the prone position, a pigtail catheter was inserted into the renal pelvis through a nephrostomy tract. Contrast agent was infused into the kidney to delineate the course of the ureter. Under fluoroscopic guidance, a translumbar aortography needle was passed into the flank, the ureter was punctured, and a guidewire was placed. The needle track was then enlarged with serial Amplatz dilators to 34 Fr. The upper third of the ureter was mobilized for 10 to 15 cm through this sheath and grasped with a Babcock clamp to exteriorize it to the skin. It was then transected, and the distal portion was oversewn and dropped back into the retroperitoneum. The proximal portion was formed into a cutaneous ureterostomy stoma. A ring nephrostomy was finally inserted to ensure proximal drainage until healing had occurred. This procedure was performed bilaterally in two patients with beneficial results. The two caveats to this procedure are that the patients must be of thin body habitus and the ureters must be tortuous in order to create a tension-free stoma. The high risk of vascular injury with this procedure requires readiness by the surgeon to convert the procedure to open surgery. In hindsight, the complexity and technically demanding nature of this surgical method has firmly placed it in the realm of a surgical curio.

As a variation on the theme, a definitive therapeutic method of complete extrinsic ureteral occlusion was developed by Darcy and colleagues in 1987.[30] Here, a clip consisting of two stainless steel springs attached at the base and connected to a screw-off insertion rod was placed around the ureter. Placement of this clip was achieved as follows. Percutaneous access to the kidney was obtained, and a guidewire was advanced into the bladder. A 5 Fr catheter was inserted into the renal pelvis, and contrast medium was injected. An 18-gauge needle was then inserted into the flank and advanced toward the ureter 6 to 7 cm below the ureteropelvic junction. A guidewire was passed through the needle into the retroperitoneal space surrounding the ureter. This track was dilated up to 30 Fr to permit placement of an Amplatz sheath. The ureter was mobilized, grasped, and invaginated into the sheath using laparoscopic grasping forceps. The ureteral clip was then applied, and the applicator handle was unscrewed. Both guidewires and sheath were then removed. A completion nephrostogram was obtained to confirm the presence of total ureteral occlusion. This procedure was performed in one patient with a ureteral fistula, and at 6 months the ureter remained occluded.

Aside from issues of cost, the success of a minimally invasive measure saves the patient from the threat of yet more major open surgery and its attendant physical and psychological morbidity. Furthermore, in the event of significant and persistent fistula, the outcome of complex major open surgical reconstruction in a sick patient may be maximized by the judicious use of temporizing and minimally invasive methods of external or extraperitoneal urinary diversion that minimize pelvic sepsis and relieve azotemia. Valuable time gained in this way can be used to improve the patient's general health and nutritional status so that a major surgical insult subsequently can be better withstood. Most minimally invasive procedures described here can be performed under local or regional anesthesia in combination with sedative-analgesics. This feature increases the attractiveness of these procedures as curative or palliative steps in the management of ureteral fistulas, particularly in critically ill patients with short life expectancies, those who do not wish to undergo repeated major open surgery within short succession, and those who desire expeditious discharge from inpatient hospital stay to spend their remaining time in the comfort of their own home or in hospice care.

Ureteral Obstruction

Obstruction of the ureter is a common source of urologic morbidity and tertiary referral. A careful history should include thorough documentation of all previous surgical procedures and close scrutiny of medical records to provide clues to etiology and any complications from past treatment. After abdominal and gentle pelvic examination, evaluation of urine by microscopy, culture and sensitivity, and appropriate serologic tests, the diagnosis is usually confirmed first by office ultrasonograms that demonstrate dilatation of the calyces and renal pelvis and any thinning of the renal parenchyma due to long-standing pressure atrophy. Because dilatation does not always indicate obstruction and pressure-flow studies are often impractical as first-line studies, additional contrast imaging with or without diuretic challenge is often necessary. Knowledge of the level, length, and severity of the ureteral stricture may be obtained by intravenous urography in patients with a normal or mildly elevated serum creatinine. CTU may provide additional information about the cause and duration of the obstruction, any coexisting pelvic or retroperitoneal pathology, and the functional integrity of the contralateral upper urinary tract and bladder. This information is of paramount importance in planning the definitive management strategy. In patients with abnormal renal function, computed tomography (CT) may be combined with invasive contrast studies (retrograde or antegrade pyelograms). Isotope scans with labeled DMSA (^{99m}Tc-dimercaptosuccinic acid) give an estimation of differential renal function, whereas ^{99m}Tc-mercaptoacetyltriglycine (MAG3) allows accurate estimation of both uptake and excretion to characterize the severity of obstruction. These, together with an estimation of glomerular filtration rate (GFR) in patients with long-standing obstruction, are useful baseline studies. In equivocal cases of idiopathic obstruction, diuretic renography and pressure-flow studies may provide additional diagnostic clues. Obstruction may be categorized as acute or chronic, unilateral or bilateral, and intrinsic or extrinsic (Table 48–1). In this chapter we discuss the definitive minimally invasive options for ureteral obstruction caused by factors that are exclusive to female patients or are secondary to iatrogenic injury.

Intraoperative Ureteral Injury

Iatrogenic ureteral strictures are invariably the end result of any direct ureteral or periureteral injury that leads to ischemic tissue damage. Both open and laparoscopic surgical trauma are common underlying causes. There is a 0.5 to 1% stricture rate following common pelvic operations, but this increases dramatically to 10% for radical pelvic surgery[31] or surgery in patients with previous pelvic fibrosis due to peritonitis, pelvic inflammatory disease, or endometriosis. In comparison, the overall risk of ureteral stricture formation after elective endoscopic surgery is between 0.5 and 3.0%. Attention to detail and gentle but meticulous technique during endoscopy of the upper urinary tract are of paramount importance if ureteral tears or perforation caused by rough instrumentation, inappropriate use of energy sources and accessories for stone treatment, or overzealous balloon dilation of the ureteral orifice are to be avoided. Meretyk and coworkers reported that trauma from open urologic surgery was the most common cause of ureteral stricture, whereas ureteroscopy accounted for 23% of the strictures treated at their institution.[32] We are skeptical of the theory put forward in this paper that a reduction in the size of rigid ureteroscopes in itself will reduce this incidence because this result is unlikely unless proctored expertise in ureteroscopy is first acquired.

The mechanism of stricture formation after local trauma is healing by intrinsic fibrosis extending to the vascular layer of the ureteral wall or extrinsic fibrosis secondary to urinary extravasation from a full-thickness injury. High-velocity gunshot wounds are the leading cause (95%) of external penetrating injury to the ureter. Because of its retroperitoneal location, stab wounds and blunt abdominal trauma rarely affect the ureter unless there is a concurrent severe bony injury to the spine or pelvis.

Intraoperative ureteral injury can be prevented in the majority of instances by routine performance of preoperative baseline intravenous urograms in all women who are candidates for major surgery of the pelvic organs. Scrutiny of these images and the availability of hard copies in the operating room should inform the surgical team about the presence and level of preexisting ureteral obstruction and delineate the course of the ureters. If ureteral dilatation is present or if difficulty is anticipated from fibrosis due to previous surgery or radiation or large tumor bulk, prudence dictates that a urologist should intubate each ureter. Retrograde catheters or indwelling stents can be placed before laparotomy is undertaken to minimize the risk of inadvertent injury. Lighted stents have also been useful in indicating the location and course of the pelvic ureters in this situation.[33] Careful dissection and mobilization of the ureters as they course over or just proximal to the iliac vessel bifurcation at the pelvic brim and the placement of slings to allow gentle traction facilitate the atraumatic distal dissection of these structures. During this dissection the surgeon must take care to preserve the segmental major feeding vessels that course in the periureteral adventitial envelope because damage to these may lead to a late ischemic stricture of the pelvic ureter. When these surgical

TABLE 48–1
Etiology of Ureteral Obstruction in Women

Intrinsic Ureteral Obstruction

Calculi
Primary ureteropelvic junction (UPJ) stenosis
Benign strictures
Ureterocele
Urothelial tumor (benign vs. malignant)
Endometriosis

Extrinsic Ureteral Obstruction

Vascular lesion
    Abdominal aortoiliac aneurysms
    Aberrant segmental renal vessels (UPJ) stenosis
    Ovarian vein syndrome
    Postpartum ovarian vein thrombophlebitis
    Retrocaval ureter
    Angiosarcoma or hemangiopericytoma of iliac veins
Benign conditions of the female reproductive organs
    Endometriosis
    Gartner's duct cyst
    Mass lesions of the uterus (fibroids)
    Ovarian cysts (Meigs' syndrome)
    Ovarian remnants
    Ovarian dermoid tumors
    Pregnancy (extrauterine and intrauterine)
    Periureteral inflammation associated with contraception
    Tubo-ovarian abscess
    Pelvic inflammatory disease
    Uterine prolapse
Diseases of the gastrointestinal tract
    Diverticulitis
    Inflammatory bowel disease
    Inflammatory disease of the appendix
    Pancreatic tail lesions (left kidney)
Diseases of the retroperitoneum
    Lymphocele
    Pelvic lipomatosis
    Retroperitoneal fibrosis
    Radiation-induced fibrosis
    Retroperitoneal infections or abscess
    Retroperitoneal hematoma
    Retroperitoneal tumors (benign or malignant)
        Primary
        Secondary

Malignant pelvic tumors
    Carcinoma of the cervix
    Carcinoma of the uterus
    Carcinoma of the ovary (primary)
    Ovarian metastases (Krukenberg's tumors)
    Carcinoma of the urinary bladder
    Carcinoma of the colon or rectum (Dukes' B stage)
    Sarcoma
    Other rare pelvic tumors
    Secondary pelvic or retroperitoneal nodal tumor metastases

Iatrogenic Ureteral Injury

Routine abdominal or vaginal hysterectomy
Wertheim hysterectomy
Excision of cervical stump
Oophorectomy
Tubal sterilization
Cesarean section
Uterine suspension
Anterior colporrhaphy
Therapeutic abortion
Ureterolithotomy or pyelolithotomy
Ureteral reimplantation
Traumatic ureteroscopy
Balloon dilation of the ureter
Resection of enterovaginal fistula
Abdominoperineal resection of the colon
Low anterior resection of the colon
Hartmann procedure for the colon
Resection of the left colon
Duodenal resection
Aortic or vena caval surgery
Surgery for retroperitoneal fibrosis
Spinal fusion
Excision of herniated intervertebral disc
Lumbar sympathectomy
Laparoscopic pelvic or retroperitoneal lymphadenectomy
Transurethral resection of invasive bladder tumor

---

principles are circumvented by undue or inappropriately directed haste, the risk of iatrogenic ureteral injury rises.

From a historical perspective, some authors have suggested that if absorbable suture material has been used to transfix inadvertently or cause excessive ureteral angulation intraoperatively, a careful "wait and see" approach may be employed after deligation provided that no deterioration of renal function is present.[34] Suture material should be absorbed completely by 8 weeks.[35] If obstruction persists as a result of fibrous scar tissue, either delayed open surgical repair or definitive endourologic treatment should be undertaken. In the current era, the consequences of a failed expectant policy are hard to defend, particularly in light of the low morbidity and high success rate associated with immediate endourologic treatment. In our view, if intraoperative obstruction by a poorly placed suture or ligature is recognized, immediate release of the suture followed by retrograde transvesical ureteral stent placement is mandatory if the ureters have not been previously intubated.

In patients in whom retrograde catheters have been placed preoperatively, these can be cannulated with a 0.035-inch Bentson guidewire before exchanging them for an indwelling stent under fluoroscopic control. A bladder catheter retained for 5 days will serve additionally to minimize leakage of refluxing bladder urine from the site of ureteral injury. The stent should not be removed for at least 6 weeks (benign disease) or until any adjuvant therapy (radiotherapy or chemotherapy) has been completed for malignant disease. Thereafter, the upper urinary tract should be reexamined by an intravenous urogram within 2 weeks of stent removal, followed by renal ultrasound examination every 3 months for 1 year to rule out late-onset hydronephrosis due to delayed stricture formation. This policy has replaced the need for deligation and ureteroneocystostomy.

When ureteral obstruction is suspected early in the postoperative course, the diagnosis should be confirmed by intravenous urography. Retrograde pyelography may better delineate the ureteral injury and at the same time permit placement of a therapeutic stent. Although older series have advocated immediate open exploration and repair,[9–12] the optimal strategy has not been tested in the context of a randomized study to date.

Open surgical repair is unquestionably a hazardous undertaking when ureteral obstruction is discovered 1 to 3 weeks after surgery. Access to the site of injury and subsequent repair is hampered by sticky adhesions and other acute inflammatory changes associated with the natural healing process. Furthermore, difficulty in distinguishing healthy from nonviable tissue and edema around the injury site may prevent secure retention of sutures. Thus, retrograde ureteral stent placement or antegrade percutaneous nephrostomy drainage of the renal pelvis is the treatment of choice in these patients. Delayed open surgical repair, if necessary, can then be safely undertaken at 6 to 8 weeks.

Pelvic and Retroperitoneal Tumors

Retroperitoneal or pelvic masses may cause ureteral obstruction at the pelvic brim or below by means of distortion or external compression. Obstruction after contiguous direct invasion of the ureteral wall by adjacent tumor is rare. Invasive cervical, uterine, or colon cancers are the most common causes of extrinsic ureteral obstruction in women. Para-aortic lymph node metastases from a variety of pelvic or lower limb malignancies may also cause obstruction of the retroperitoneal ureter. The insidious nature of this process is such that renal impairment may already be established by the time of diagnosis. An elevated serum creatinine will occur either if bilateral obstruction is present or if the remaining functioning kidney is obstructed after previous silent unilateral loss of renal function.

Many of these patients have developed an advanced stage of disease and are poor candidates for definitive surgery. Before irreversible interventional decisions for palliation, such as placement of bilateral nephrostomy drainage tubes, are made, the lead clinician should seek the advice of a urologist and determine which kidney has the best functional reserve by isotope scans (using DMSA or MAG3). Consultation with the patient and the family about the consequences of external urinary diversion is often wise. Many such patients are ill-equipped to cope with external drainage in the home environment or terminal care facility, and occasionally these patients may be condemned to a slow and painful demise from locally advanced pelvic cancer that has a poor prognosis. Minimally invasive palliative drainage procedures may also fail to deliver improved quality of life or may remove the possibility of a faster but relatively painless death from uremia.

In patients with bilateral ureteral obstruction who are keenly in favor of active intervention and who may be candidates for either palliative radiation or experimental chemotherapy, often with nephrotoxic drugs, retrograde stent placement may be tried. If this fails, a unilateral nephrostomy tube should be inserted in the kidney with the best function, the thickest parenchyma, or the shortest duration of obstruction (if this is known from serial imaging studies) in the first instance. Tube placement is very effective in the short term provided that urinary sepsis is prevented and high-output salt-wasting diuresis is corrected. Patient weight, fluid balance charts, serum creatinine level, and electrolytes should be monitored on a daily basis so that drug therapy can begin as soon as improvement in creatinine clearance allows. Bilateral nephrostomies (which are more difficult for the patient to manage) are seldom required if this management strategy is followed. Once the patient's condition has been stabilized with a nephrostomy tube, an attempt to internalize drainage by placing antegrade or retrograde stent can be done safely. In patients in whom retrograde stent placement for malignant ureteral obstruction has failed, antegrade insertion has a 95% success rate (compared to a 69% success rate for benign strictures).[36] Failure of antegrade stent placement can usually be attributed to poor angulation of the percutaneous track (success is lower with lower pole access than with midpole access), a tortuous dilated redundant ureter, or high tissue resistance resulting in kinking or angulation of the guidewire and wedging of the stent or pusher.

Early stent failure with recurrent obstruction (within the first 30 days) is rare but has been documented.[37] This unusual complication is more commonly encountered when smaller-caliber or polyurethane stents are used; these may require frequent stent changes. The placement of metallic meshed stents for the purpose of relieving malignant ureteral obstruction and maintaining ureteral patency secondary to extrinsic tumor compression is a recent innovation.[38] The appeal of these devices ultimately rests with the prospects for coverage of the smooth inert stent material (woven surgical steel) by a process of reepithelialization. Contact with the flow of urine and the associated problems of surface encrustation and urinary sepsis are therefore avoided. Short-term results have demonstrated a high patency rate after a 27-week follow-up, but long-term outcomes are unknown. The insertion technique is uncomplicated. After delineating the site and length of the obstruction by antegrade or retrograde pyelography, the stenosis is dilated using an Olbert balloon of sufficient length, positioned across the stricture over a guidewire and inflated to 12 atmospheres (atm). The Wallstent, which is self-expandable to a diameter of 7 mm, is slowly extruded in stages and implanted at the site of dilatation under fluoroscopic control. It is important to choose a stent length greater than the length of the stricture because expansion after release leads to stent shortening. Although a single stent is often sufficient (Fig. 48–6), several stents can be successively telescoped to allow the treatment of longer strictures. At the end of the procedure, a soft single-J or double-J stent or a covering nephrostomy tube is temporarily left in place to prevent blood clot or hyperplastic regenerating epithelium from obstructing the upper tract. The Wallstent is fully incorporated into the ureteral wall by 8 weeks by means of regression of the hyperplastic epithelium to smoother transitional cell epithelium, and stent migration is unlikely thereafter.

This new application of expandable permanent meshed metallic stents may be a better remedy than temporary stents, which require changing every 3 to 6 months, provided that the early promise of minimal morbidity is borne out by long-term results. Problems may arise from mismatch between the stent diameter and that of the native ureter. Once such a stent is placed in the ureter, however, the antegrade flow of urine depends on the hydrostatic forces and intact pacemaker activity of the renal pelvis and calyces. Inappropriate use of these ureteral endoprostheses for benign ureteral obstruction can invite disaster later. In our experience, the major drawback of this technique is the need for major open excisional or reconstructive surgery to remove the stent in the presence of persistent urosepsis. This makes it unsuitable as a first-line treatment for patients with a solitary upper tract or a reasonably long life expectancy.

Palliative external urinary diversion through an anterior cutaneous nephrostomy as a replacement for percutaneous nephrostomy has also been reported[39] and has achieved some success in a small series of eight patients. In this procedure, an autostatic silicone-coated, coiled, expanded polytetrafluoroethylene tube (Impra) is inserted percutaneously into the renal pelvis and tunneled subcutaneously to an anterior exit site where a stoma appliance can be applied. Preliminary results showed no failure of insertion or secondary displacement and no abdominal wall complications, kinking, or encrustation, but one case of intrarenal obstruction occurred at 3 months. The advantage of this method is the ease of access to the urinary stoma gained by the patient and the ability to lie supine comfortably. This same group[40] has also reported the initial clinical experience with palliative subcutaneous nephrovesical bypass in 14 patients. This procedure is possible only in patients in whom bladder function has not been compromised by pelvic tumor. The prosthesis consists of two glued coaxial tubes (an external Impra tube and an internal silicone tube). One end is inserted into the renal pelvis through a percutaneous tract dilated to 30 Fr, and the other end, after subcutaneous tunneling, is inserted into the bladder through a short cystotomy. Vesicorenal reflux in this first group of patients was invariably present but had no clinical significance in the short term compared to the quality of palliation achieved. The long-term risks of encrustation with this procedure may not have a significant impact in patients with a short life expectancy. No experience with changing the prosthesis is available at the present time.

Pregnancy and Ureteral Obstruction

Maternal ureteral dilatation is commonly encountered in the second and third trimesters of pregnancy as an incidental finding in women with flank pain. It is maximal at 28 weeks' gestation and is maintained up to 36 weeks. Urine microscopy and culture are essential to rule out bacteriuria requiring appropriate antibiotic therapy to prevent pyelonephritis. It is important to distinguish gravid hydronephrosis (which is a physiologic phenomenon resulting from a combination of hormonal and mechanical factors in up to 90% of pregnant women) from stone or other causes of obstruction. Dilatation is more common on the right side because of the midterm dextrorotation of the uterus and the exposed position of the right ureter in front of the iliac vessels. The left ureter is cushioned by the sigmoid colon. If an obstruction cannot be excluded by renal ultrasound it may be necessary to resort to more sophisticated studies such as diuretic serial nephrosonography (which should show progressive upper tract dilatation and

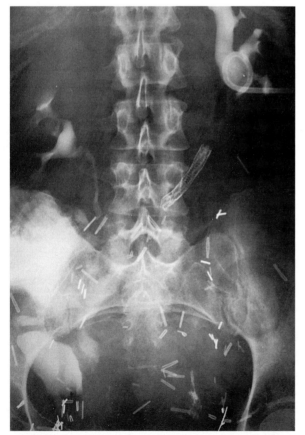

Figure 48-6 Wallstent in the ureter for management of ureteral stricture after pelvic exenteration and continent urinary diversion.

calyceal clubbing in the presence of a significant ureteral obstruction). The sensitivity and specificity of this investigation is unknown, and if findings are equivocal, other imaging is required. Transvaginal sonography may be able to detect whether there is dilatation of the pelvic ureter, which should be absent in patients with gravid hydronephrosis. If all else fails, a one-shot retrograde pyelogram with fetal shielding can be performed with relative safety after the first trimester. It must be noted that a few centers have reported a slightly increased risk of childhood cancers after fetal radiographic exposure.[41] The alternative is empirical cystoscopic stent placement under sonographic guidance.[42] In this circumstance, the upper tract should be reevaluated by a contrast study 4 to 6 weeks after delivery, after the stent has been removed. Percutaneous nephrostomy may be necessary if all else fails, but once again, the cause of the obstruction must be determined by an antegrade nephrostogram after delivery.

Ureteral injury during cesarean section has a reported incidence of 0.09%[43] and occurs when the uterine incision is extended into the broad ligament or during attempts at hemostatic suture ligation. When a short bilateral ureteral injury has occurred after obstetrical surgery, early stent placement or open reconstruction is the treatment of choice. Open surgical diversion should be avoided if at all possible[44] because it is associated with a poor at outcome in 50% of patients.

Other Causes of Ureteral Strictures

Obstructive congenital anomalies such as ureterocele in adult women are rare and may be treated by endoscopic incision at the risk of subsequent reflux. Ovarian vein syndrome was initially associated with pregnancy but has also been described in girls before the onset of menses and in older women after the administration of progestins.[45] It may be caused by hormonally induced chronic venous engorgement of the right ovarian vein after closely spaced pregnancies, use of oral contraceptives, or increased vascularity from gynecologic disease. Both this entity and that of a retrocaval ureter are not direct causes of ureteral strictures in the truest sense. They cause ureteral obstruction through compromise of the ureteral lumen, primarily by external compression, excessive angulation, and chronic periureteral fibrosis from irritation.

Ureteral strictures that are insidious in onset cause slow "silent" hydronephrosis that causes irreversible destruction of the renal parenchyma by the time of diagnosis. Inflammatory processes (e.g., retroperitoneal fibrosis and radiation-induced endarteritis), in contrast, usually induce symptomatic ureteral strictures. Common features of inflammatory strictures are flank pain, which may become worse during periods of diuresis, mimicking stone colic; obstructive pyonephrosis; and urosepsis causing unexplained persistent fever. Infection combined with obstruction of the urinary tract can be lethal and represents a urologic emergency, particularly in patients who are constitutionally or therapeutically immunocompromised (renal transplant recipients).

Diagnostic investigations are used to determine the cause of the stricture, the presence of salvageable ipsilateral renal function, and, in the case of malignant disease, the presence of recurrent or residual disease. The guiding principles of ureteral stricture management are immediate antegrade relief of the obstruction and treatment of any potential systemic consequences of urosepsis with concomitant parenteral antibiotics that attain high urinary concentrations. Before definitive repair of the stricture is undertaken with endoscopic surgery, the urine must be sterile and any associated calculi that may have formed secondary to long-standing obstruction must be addressed and removed to minimize the risk of subsequent septic complications. If successful surgical correction is not possible or prudent (as in patients with end-stage cancer disease) the patient may occasionally be managed with external urinary drainage alone, as previously discussed.

In general, short strictures less than 1.5 cm long are ideally suited to endoscopic management, whereas longer strictures do not respond as well to incisional treatment alone and may require dismembered repair or complex reconstruction by substitution or internal or external urinary diversion. In a retrospective analysis of 137 ureteral injuries, Cormio and associates found that the length of the injury was the single most important prognosticator, whereas previous radiotherapy or delayed treatment contributed to an adverse outcome.

The short length of the female urethra permits safe access to ureteropelvic junction strictures and strictures of the upper or middle third of the ureter with rigid instruments. Retrograde lateral endopyelotomy can be performed under direct visual control with a 12.5 Fr operating ureteroscope and an angled "hot knife" electrode (Fig. 48–7). In this way bleeding can be minimized,[46] and the depth of the incision can be precisely controlled in a stepwise fashion through the entire thickness of the stricture until periureteral fat is visible, which is an advantage over the "cold" knife. Electrocoagulation should be used very sparingly to avoid deep coagulative thermal injury to the local ureteral blood supply. The procedure is completed with balloon dilatation, which ensures complete separation of the cut edges. Prior placement of an indwelling ureteral stent for 2 weeks helps the drainage of infected urine and the restoration of residual renal function, and passive ureteral dilatation facilitates the passage of instruments.

The outcome after retrograde ureteroscopic endopyelotomy in most contemporary series is equivalent to the results achieved with antegrade endopyelotomy and open surgery, both of which yield an 80 to 100% success rate.[47, 48] In the series from Meretyk and colleagues,[47] however, failure of prestenting was associated with a 16% incidence of intraoperative

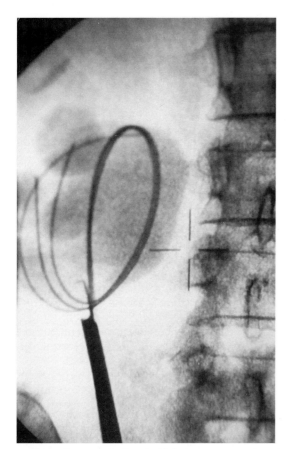

Figure 48-7 Retrograde "hot-knife" electrocautery incision of stricture at the ureteropelvic junction.

during subsequent manipulations, this safety wire allows placement of an antegrade single-J stent to minimize urinary extravasation and limit bleeding. Ideally, the placement of a second working wire alongside the safety wire facilitates entry of a 10.4 Fr flexible ureteroscope into the ureter to visualize the stricture. This instrument may be passed either alongside the wires or backloaded over the working wire until the proximal limit of the stricture has been reached. Contrast can then be injected through the instrument to define the length of the stricture. The stricture can then be incised anteriorly with electrocautery under direct vision (12.5 Fr rigid ureteroscope with hook knife, 10.4 Fr flexible ureteroscope with 2.0 Fr Bugbee electrode or 3 Fr Holmium

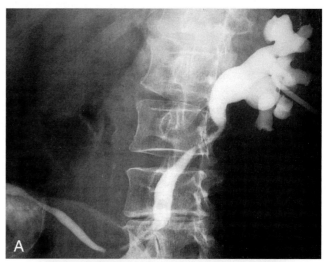

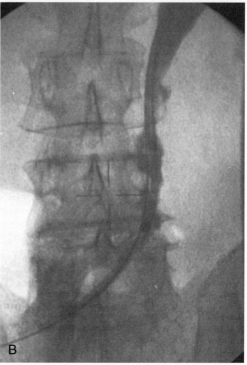

Figure 48-8 Antegrade contrast study showing preaortic left ureteral stricture after cystectomy and continent urinary diversion to skin (*A*) and contrast extravasation after antegrade incision (*B*).

hemorrhage and a 20% incidence of distal ureteral strictures. Others have reported 82 to 92% success using a cold-knife ureteroscopic approach.[49, 50]

If endopyelotomy fails or is not possible in a retrograde manner (in patients with neobladders or urinary diversions), alternatives such as percutaneous antegrade endopyelotomy, laparoscopic, or open dismembered pyeloplasty may ultimately be necessary in 10 to 15% of patients.

In patients with neobladders, ureteral strictures invariably have an ischemic cause and are more common in the left ureter. At this site the stricture has been routed under the base of the sigmoid mesentery and in front of the aorta or common iliac vessels (Fig. 48–8). The other common site of stricturing is at the distal point of anastomosis into the new urinary reservoir, and this may depend partly on the length of the antireflux tunnel. Recurrence of cancer is usually excluded prior to endoscopic treatment by CT or magnetic resonance imaging (MRI) scans. Retrograde treatment of strictures is rarely possible in patients with tumor recurrence.

Antegrade stricturotomy is usually performed after percutaneous placement of a safety wire into the ureter under fluoroscopic guidance. The wire is advanced into the reservoir so that it can be retrieved and secured by retrograde flexible endoscopy. If unexpected ureteral or renal bleeding injury is incurred laser fiber) or under fluoroscopic control using the Acucise device.

After the cut edges have been successfully separated (with a balloon, rigid dilators, or ureteroscope), two single-J stents (8 Fr and 5 Fr) are passed antegradely over the working and safety wires, respectively, into the neobladder under fluoroscopic guidance. Finally the procedure is completed with maximal urinary diversion by placing a proximal draining nephrostomy tube and a catheter distally in the neobladder, which serve to minimize urinary extravasation. The latter can be removed after 5 days. Patency of the ureter is checked by an antegrade nephrostogram at 6 weeks. This is performed after ensuring that the neobladder reservoir is empty of urine and mucus and that the larger single-J stent has been cannulated with a guidewire before both stents are removed if the treatment has failed. In this eventuality, a stent can be easily replaced before other treatment is undertaken. Because it is likely that the stents have been covered by bacterial biofilm, broad-spectrum parenteral antibiotic administration is prudent before any manipulations are undertaken.

Recent developments in imaging technology and probe design have led to the introduction of endoluminal ultrasound (ELUS) for the evaluation of ureteral stricture disease. The Sonicath (Boston Scientific) is a 6.2 Fr diameter, 12- to 20-MHz probe (Fig. 48–9) that can be introduced into the ureter over a guidewire (0.025 inch). It may allow determination of the true length of a ureteral stricture as well as visualization of the site and orientation of the point of maximal thickness of the scar tissue and any crossing vessels that may be intimately related and there-

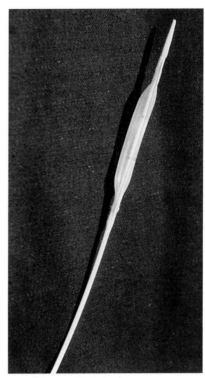

Figure 48-10 Acucise catheter.

fore at risk of injury. Furthermore, imaging immediately after stricturotomy has allowed us to assess the depth and effectiveness of the incision without having to visualize it directly, and it may provide a better end point for endoscopic treatment. Unfortunately, at present the therapeutic applications are limited because it is not possible to target the incision accurately in real-time away from large vessels by endoluminal ultrasound.

Alternative devices can also be used to treat such strictures in an antegrade or retrograde fashion. These include balloon disruption of the stricture using a 30 Fr balloon (ENDOBRST) and other similar devices of 18 to 30 Fr size. Although this technique was originally described by Kadir and colleagues in 1982 in a patient with secondary ureteropelvic junction obstruction,[51] significant testing did not take place until 1989.[52, 53] Short-term follow-up revealed success in 68 to 73%, poorer results occurring in secondary ureteropelvic junction strictures. This concept has more recently been extended in the Acucise device to incorporate a hot electrical cutting wire that rests above the surface of a low-pressure balloon (Fig. 48–10) and is activated at low power for a short period of 3 seconds to incise the stricture at the time of maximal dilatation. Nadler and coworkers reported a 76% objective success rate at 2 years with this device.[54] In this series of 16 patients, 100% success was achieved in patients with secondary ureteropelvic junction strictures, and all failures occurred in the first year.

Our own experience with balloon disruption alone has been disappointing. We reserve the use of the

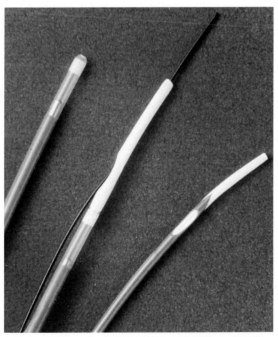

Figure 48-9 Sonicath mounted in "side-saddle" fashion over 0.025-inch guidewire.

Acucise device for difficult ureteral strictures that cannot be reached endoscopically either antegradely or retrogradely with rigid instruments such as ureteroenteric anastomotic strictures in patients with urinary diversions or orthotopic or cutaneous continent neobladders.

Because both balloon dilatation and balloon incision are performed entirely under fluoroscopic control, the end point is arbitrary and must be related to the disappearance of "waisting" (Fig. 48–11) or visible contrast extravasation on antegrade or retrograde pyelography. The Acucise device makes a precise incision rather than a ragged-edged tear with a larger surface area that may be more liable to restenosis. It is our current practice to evaluate the depth of the Acucise incision visually with rigid or flexible ureteroscopy, so that an inadequate stricturotomy can be repeated at the same sitting if necessary or the cut can be completed under direct vision. Long-term prospective comparisons of the relative efficacy of the Acucise device versus ureteroscopic electroincision are yet to be conducted. A prospective study is under way in our institution comparing outcomes achieved after retrograde endopyelotomy under direct visual control with rigid instruments and those attained with a cutting balloon device in female patients.

The majority of ureteral strictures affect the distal third of the ureter. Options for treatment of the strictured mid or lower ureteral segment include retrograde dilation with serial rigid dilators (Rusch), balloon dilatation, endoureterotomy (hot or cold knife incision through the scar tissue), Acucise balloon-wire incision, laparoscopic or open surgical excision, and reanastomosis. Strictures longer than 1.5 cm are best treated by excision and ureteroneocystostomy. Short strictures of the lower ureter can be incised with a hot or cold knife in a retrograde fashion. Benign strictures of the intramural ureter (which are not uncommon after previous balloon dilatation of the ureteral orifice) are intubated with safety and working guidewires. After insulation of each wire by a 5 Fr angiographic catheter (which also helps to tent the roof of the stricture), the incision can be made toward the bladder lumen in an oblique manner with the Collings knife using cutting electrocautery current to marsupialize the strictured ureteral segment into the bladder. A recent alternative is stricturotomy using a 3 Fr Holmium laser bare fiber (Versapulse, Coherent [Fig. 48–12]), which has a tissue penetration of 0.5 mm in contact mode and permits precision cutting of tissues by vaporization of scar tissue. This reusable flexible quartz fiber transmits laser energy from a crystalline source at a wavelength of 2140 nm, which is rapidly absorbed by water and can be introduced through the work channel of either rigid or flexible instruments (Fig. 48–13). Long-term outcomes with this laser are unknown at this time.

Reflux may occur in a small percentage of patients after any incisional treatment of an intramural ure-

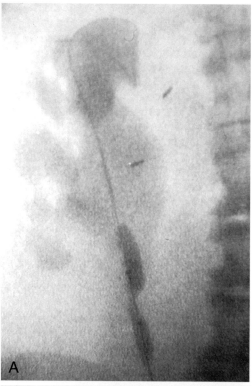

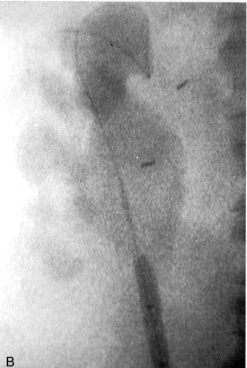

Figure 48-11 Composite showing "waisting" before balloon dilatation *(A)* and disappearance of "waisting" as the end point *(B)*.

teral stricture. Fibrous strictures tend to become hypovascular with time (usually after more than 3 months), and dilatation only serves to increase the density of the scar tissue in the long term.[55] Satisfactory results were therefore obtained in only half the

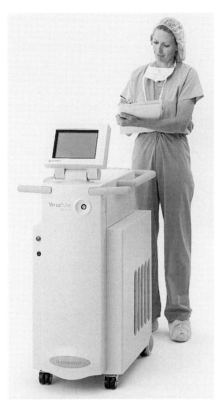

Figure 48-12 Versapulse laser system. (Courtesy of Coherent Medical Group, Palo Alto, California.)

cases in which treatment was delayed.[31] These studies reaffirm the fact that early intervention is desirable to obtain the best outcome in patients with lower ureteral strictures. After stricturotomy we customarily place two parallel 7 Fr indwelling ureteral stents to maintain separation at the incision site for 6 weeks so that mature healing occurs across the distracted cut edges around these. The ideal end result is a greater luminal diameter. Follow-up urography is essential at 3 months; thereafter, the patient may be followed by serial ultrasound examinations of the upper tract and annual isotope (MAG3) scans. One must be aware that residual dilatation of the upper tract may be present on follow-up sonography if chronic obstruction has preceded stricturotomy, but progressive dilatation of the renal pelvis and calyces is an ominous finding that requires prompt action. If a nephrostomy tube was placed and retained after definitive stricture treatment, an antegrade pyelogram made to evaluate outcome after stent removal should not overdistend the renal pelvis because this may paralyze residual proximal pacemaker activity in a redundant collecting system. In these cases, a small volume of contrast (20 to 30 ml) should be slowly instilled under gravitational drainage and one film made immediately; further films should be delayed until the nephrostomy tube has been clamped and the patient has ambulated for 20 to 30 minutes. Furthermore, the sterility of the urine should be confirmed before drainage of the upper tract is evaluated because it is known from in vitro studies that human

urinary pathogens can paralyze human calyceal pacemaker activity.[56]

Rigid dilation is useful only for gaining access to a narrow ureteral segment. Because considerable resistance may be encountered when attempting to dilate a stricture in this manner, a floppy-tipped Bentson guidewire may not provide sufficient fulcrum. In this situation it must be exchanged for a floppy-tipped but stiffer Lunderqvist guidewire over which serial dilators may be more readily passed across the stricture. Although Van Andel catheters[57] have been used for malignant strictures, these may be more likely to telescope the ureteral mucosa and increase the risk of epithelial stripping with serial passage compared to the tapered tipped (Rusch) dilators that we prefer. If an unsuspected stricture in the lower or mid ureter is encountered and requires such dilatation before diagnostic or therapeutic ureteroscopy can be performed using the two-wire technique we have previously described, postoperative CT scans are advisable to exclude extrinsic ureteral compression from occult coexisting disease. Long-term success is unlikely with this technique.

Balloon dilatation is also rarely successful for longstanding hypovascular fibrous strictures of the distal or mid ureter. In this situation this technique has an overall success rate of 20 to 40%. Only strictures shorter than 1.0 cm and of very short duration respond well to treatment with balloon dilatation (up to 70%). Furthermore, there has been little consensus on the best parameters to be used for size of balloon, duration of inflation, number of inflation episodes, and use, size, number, and duration of ureteral stents. Netto Junior and coworkers were able to improve the results of balloon dilatation with ureteral incision using special endoureterotomy scissors.[58] In our experience, balloons are best used for the treatment of fresh iatrogenic strictures secondary to pelvic surgery (e.g., partial ureteral obstruction by a periureteral suture).

All endoscopic ureterotomies and pyelotomies performed in our unit share a common final pathway, namely, the placement of two indwelling ureteral stents to minimize extravasation of urine into the retroperitoneum. These stents are retained for 6 weeks, as previously described. Other practitioners

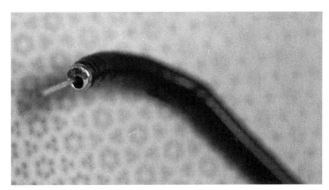

Figure 48-13 Bare Holmium laser fiber emanating from the work channel of a flexible ureteroscope.

use specialized ureteral stents for endopyelotomy (14 Fr proximally tapering to 7 Fr in the distal half). Research from the minipig animal model has shown that the longitudinally incised, partially resected ureter heals in a patent fashion around a stent, with regeneration of both the urothelial and muscular layers occurring in a matter of 6 weeks.[59] As to the effect of stent duration on ureteral healing after endourologic incision, no statistically significant difference was found when the mean values of the overall healing scores were compared at 1, 3, and 6 weeks. Interestingly, the overall healing scores at 1 week were better than those at 6 weeks for strictures longer than 2 cm that required more than one incision. This finding suggests that in this model, the inflammation associated with a chronic indwelling stent may act as a stimulus of late fibrosis after endoureterotomy. It is unknown whether the same dictum holds true for the human ureter.

Both endoscopic and open surgical stricture repair enjoy high success rates in excess of 80%, yet the individual healing response cannot be predicted with certainty. Failure is usually recognized within the first 3 to 6 months, and late failure is seen only in about 10 to 15% of patients. Therefore, extended follow-up for at least 1 year is of utmost importance in these patients. Management of ureteral strictures can to a large extent be achieved endoscopically in the majority of patients. Proper patient selection, meticulous endourologic technique with minimal extravasation of infected urine, and extended follow-up are invariably followed by success. Open surgery is reserved for complex stricture problems and occasional endoscopic treatment failures.

Laparoscopy in the Etiology and Management of Ureteral Injuries

Laparoscopic procedures have long been a mainstay in the gynecologic surgical armamentarium and have recently become popular in other surgical disciplines. The last few years have witnessed an explosion of new laparoscopic procedures, and with them, inherent complications have increased as surgeons experience the learning curve. Diathermic injury to the ureter during laparoscopic sterilization and ablation of endometriosis is a well known problem.[60–64] All reported injuries were recognized postoperatively. Patients presented either within the first 3 days of surgery with signs of peritonitis or later with a fistula. After diagnosis, the majority of ureters were repaired with open surgery. Partial or complete inadvertent transection of the ureter during laparoscopic pelvic surgery such as lymphadenectomy and hemicolectomy has also been reported. Early recognition and confirmation of the diagnosis favors an endourologic remedy provided that the ureter has not been completely transected. If ureteral transection is recognized intraoperatively, it may be repaired laparo-

scopically over an indwelling ureteral stent with interrupted intracorporeal 4–0 chromic catgut sutures.

Sporadic reports of laparoscopic excision and reanastomosis for ureteropelvic junction[65] and ureteral strictures[66] are currently appearing in the world literature. At the present time, however, these procedures must be considered experimental because even in proficient hands intracorporeal suturing is difficult and very time consuming. Refinements in instrumentation and new anastomotic techniques (e.g., magnetic anastomosis) may hold the promise of reducing these long operating times. Open surgical repair is mandatory if any difficulty is encountered with the laparoscopic technique.

It is only a matter of time before laparoscopic retroperitoneoscopy and direct ureteral occlusion in skilled hands are added to the ever-growing list of minimally invasive procedures available in the surgical armamentarium for the treatment of ureteral fistulas. One case of urinary diversion performed by laparoscopic ureterocutaneostomy has already been described.[67]

In patients with hydronephrosis and unsalvageable symptomatic end-stage renal disease after ureteral injury, laparoscopic simple nephrectomy has been firmly established as a safe and effective treatment in experienced hands. Such surgery should not be attempted by the unsupervised novice or those without experience in complex laparoscopic procedures involving dissection of major vessels.

Summary

Advances in endoscopic, percutaneous, and laparoscopic approaches to the urinary tract during the last decade now offer the skilled endourologist (assisted by an able interventional uroradiologist) a variety of minimally invasive options with which to manage ureteral pathology. Judicious application of these diagnostic and therapeutic methods based on individual patient circumstances should facilitate the management of ureteral obstruction, injuries, and their sequelae. In this manner, the ultimate goals of therapy—preservation of renal function and improved quality of life—can be optimized.

REFERENCES

1. Sampson JA: Complications arising from freeing the ureters in the more radical operations for carcimoma cervicis uteri with special reference to postoperative ureteral necrosis. Johns Hopkins Hosp Bull 15:123–134, 1904.
2. Newell QU: Injury to the ureters during pelvic operations. Ann Surg 109:981–986, 1939.
3. St. Martin EC, Trichel BE, Campbell JH, Locke CH: Ureteral injuries in gynecologic surgery. J Urol 70:51–57, 1953.
4. Conger K, Beecham CT, Horrax TM: Ureteral injury in pelvic surgery: Current thought on incidence pathogenesis, prophylaxis and treatment. Obstet Gynecol 3:343–357, 1954.
5. Higgins CC: Ureteral injury during surgery. JAMA 199:82–88, 1967.

6. Bunkin IA: Prevention of uretral injury in gynecologic surgery. Clin Obstet Gynecol 8:383–398, 1965.

7. Gangai MP, Agee RE, Spence CR: Surgical injury to the ureter. Urology 8:22–27, 1976.

8. Zinman LM, Libertino JA, Roth RA: Management of operative ureteral injury. Urology 12:290–303, 1978.

9. Hoch WH, Kursh ED, Persky L: Early, aggressive management of intraoperative ureteral injuries. J Urol 114:530–532, 1975.

10. Bright TC, Peters P: Ureteral injuries secondary to operative procedures. Urology 9:22–26, 1977.

11. Mendez R, McGinty D: The management of delayed recognized ureteral injuries. J Urol 119(2):192–193, 1978.

12. Guerriero WG: Ureteral injury. Urol Clin North Am 16(2)237–248, 1989.

13. Smith PJB, Williams RE, DeDombal AT: Genitourinary fistulae complicating Crohn's disease. Br J Urol 44:657–661, 1972.

14. Lang EK: Diagnosis and management of ureteral fistulas by percutaneous nephrostomy and antegrade stent catheter. Radiology 138:311–317, 1981.

15. Wrigley JV, Prem KA, Fraley EE: Pelvic exenteration: Complications of urinary diversion. J Urol 116:428–430, 1976.

16. Peterson DD, Lucey DT, Fried FA: Nonsurgical management of uretero-vaginal fistula. Urology 4(6):677–680, 1974.

17. Lang EK, Lanasa JA, Garrett J, et al: The management of urinary fistulas and strictures with percutaneous ureteral stent catheters. J Urol 122(5):736–740, 1979.

18. Mazer MJ, LeVeen RF, Call JE, et al: Permanent percutaneous anterograde ureteral stent placement without transurethral assistance. Urology 14(4):413–419, 1979.

19. Kearney GP, Mahoney EM, Brown HP: Useful technique for long-term urinary drainage by inlying ureteral stent. Six-year experience. Urology 14:126–134, 1979.

20. Gray RJ, Intriere L, Dolmatch BL, et al: Combined retrograde-antegrade ureteral stent passage: Salvage procedure for a ureteral leak. J Vasc Interv Radiol 3(3):557–558, 1992.

21. Gunther R, Klose K, Alken P: Transrenal ureteral occlusion with a detachable balloon. Radiology 142:521–523, 1982.

22. Reddy PK, Moore L, Hunter D, Amplatz K: Percutaneous ureteral fulgeration: A nonsurgical technique for ureteral occlusion. J Urol 138:724–726, 1987.

23. Papanicolaou N, Pfister RC, Yoder IC: Percutaneous occlusion of ureteral leaks and fistulae using nondetachable balloons. Urol Radiol 7:28–31, 1985.

24. Gunther R, Marberger M, Klose K: Transrenal ureteral embolization. Radiology 132:317–319, 1979.

25. Wanner K, Marx FJ: Erfahrungen mit der transrenalen ureterokklusion. Urologe Ausgabe [A] 20(5):265–268, 1981.

26. Kinn AC, Ohlsen H, Brehmer-Andersson E, Brundin J: Therapeutic ureteral occlusion in advanced pelvic malignant tumors. J Urol 135:29–32, 1986.

27. Gumpinger R, Miller K, Fuchs G, Eisenberger F: Antegrade ureteroscopy for stone removal. Eur Urol 11(3):199–202, 1985.

28. Clayman RV, Preminger GM, Franklin JF, et al: Percutaneous ureterolithotomy. J Urol 133:671–673, 1985.

29. Smith AD, Moldwin R, Karlin G: Percutaneous ureterostomy J Urol 138:286–288, 1987.

30. Darcy MD, Lund GB, Smith TP, et al: Percutaneously applied ureteral clips: Treatment of vesico-vaginal fistula. Radiology 163:819–821, 1987.

31. Cormio L, Ruutu M, Sevaggi FP: Prognostic factors in the management of ureteric injuries. Ann Chirurg Gynecol 83(1):41–44, 1994.

32. Meretyk S, Albala DM, Clayman RV, et al: Endoureterotomy for treatment of ureteral strictures. J Urol 147:1502–1506, 1992.

33. Kasulke RJ: Accurate intraoperative identification of the ureters with the use of ureteral illumination. Am Surg 49(9):501, 1983.

34. Harshman MW, Pollack HM, Banner MP, Wein AJ: Conservative management of ureteral obstruction secondary to suture entrapment. J Urol 127:121–123, 1982.

35. Clark DE: Surgical suture materials. Contemp Surg 17:33–48, 1980.

36. Lu DS, Papanicolaou N, Girard M, et al: Percutaneous internal ureteral stent placement: Review of technical issues and solutions in 50 consecutive cases. Clin Radiol 49(4):256–261, 1994.

37. Docimo SG, Dewolf WC: High failure rate of indwelling ureteral stents in patients with extrinsic obstruction: Experience at two institutions. J Urol 142(2):277–279, 1989.

38. Pauer W, Lugmayr H: Metallic Wallstents: A new therapy for extrinsic ureteral obstruction. J Urol 148:281–284, 1992.

39. Desgrandchamps F, Cussenot O, Meria P, et al: Anterior cutaneous nephrostomy: A new palliative urinary diversion. J Endourol 8(Suppl 1):P9–236, S111, 1994.

40. Desgrandchamps F, Cussenot O, Meria P, et al: Clinical experience of subcutaneous nephrovesical bypass. J Endourol 8(Suppl 1):P9–240, S112, 1994.

41. Harvey EB, Boice JD, Honeyman M, Flannery JT: Prenatal x-ray exposure and childhood cancer in twins. N Engl J Med 312:541–545, 1985.

42. Gluck CD, Benson CB, Bundy AL, et al: Renal sonography for placement and monitoring of ureteral stents during pregnancy. J Endourol 5:241–243, 1991.

43. Eisenkop SM, Richman R, Platt LD, Paul RH: Urinary tract injury during cesarean section. Obstet Gynecol 60(5):591–596, 1982.

44. Cormio L, Ruutu M, Traficante A, et al: Management of bilateral ureteric injuries after gynecological and obstetric procedures. Int Urol Nephrol 25(6):551–555, 1993.

45. Dykhuizen RF, Roberts JA: The ovarian vein syndrome. Surg Gynecol Obstet 130:443–452, 1970.

46. Sampaio FJB: Endopyelotomy, guided by meticulous anatomy. Contemp Urol 6(7):23–26, 1994.

47. Meretyk I, Meretyk S, Clayman RV: Endopyelotomy: Comparison of ureteroscopic retrograde and antegrade percutaneous techniques. J Urol 148:775–783, 1992.

48. Thomas R, Cherry R: Ureteroscopic endopyelotomy for management of ureteropelvic junction obstruction. J Endourol 4:S141, 1990.

49. Gallucci M, Alpi G, Ricciuti GP, et al: Retrograde cold-knife endopyelotomy in secondary stenosis of the ureteropelvic junction. J Endourol 5:49–50, 1991.

50. Chowdhury SD, Kenogbon J: Rigid ureteroscopic endopyelotomy without external drainage. J Endourol 6(5):357–360, 1992.

51. Kadir S, White RI Jr, Engel R: Balloon dilatation of a ureteropelvic junction obstruction. Radiology 143:263–264, 1982.

52. Beckmann CF, Roth RA, Bihrle W: Dilation of benign ureteral strictures. Radiology 172(2):437–441, 1989.

53. O'Flynn K, Hehir M, McKelvie G, et al: Endoballoon rupture and stenting for pelviureteric junction obstruction. Technique and early results. Br J Urol 64:572–574, 1989.

54. Nadler RB, Pearle MS, Nakada SY, et al: Acucise endopyelotomy: Two year follow-up report. J Endourol in press, 1995.

55. Hoe JW: Benign ureteric strictures—management by percutaneous interventional uro-radiological techniques. Ann Acad Med (Sing) 22(5):670–674, 1993.

56. Patel A: An experimental and clinical study of acute pyonephrosis in man with specific reference to human calyceal "pacemaker" contractility. MS Thesis, University of London, July, 1994.

57. Alexander RB, Thompson N, Pockaj BA, Chang R: Dilation of lower ureteral strictures with Van Andel catheters. J Urol 152(1):68–69, 1994.

58. Netto Junior NR, Ferreira U, Lemos GC, Claro JF: Endourological management of ureteral strictures. J Urol 144(3):631–634, 1990.

59. Kerbl K, Chandhoke PS, Figenshau RS, et al: Effect of stent duration on ureteral healing following endoureterectomy in an animal model. J Urol 150(4):1302–1305, 1993.

60. Irvin TT, Golingher JC, Scott JS: Injury to the ureter during laparoscopic tubal sterilization. Arch Surg 110:1501–1503, 1975.

61. Stengel JN, Felderman ES, Zamora D: Ureteral injury: Complication of laparoscopic sterilization. Urology 4:341–342, 1974.

62. Winslow PH, Kreger R, Ebbesson B, Oster E: Conservative management of electrical burn injury to ureter secondary to laparoscopy. Urology 27:60–62, 1986.
63. Baumann H, Jaeger P, Huch A: Ureteral injury after laparoscopic tubal sterilization by bipolar electrocoagulation. Obstet Gynecol 71(3):2, 483–485, 1988.
64. Grainger DA, Soderstrom RM, Schiff SF, et al: Ureteral injuries at laparoscopy: Insights into diagnosis, management and prevention. Obstet Gynecol 75:839–843, 1990.

65. Schuessler WW, Grune MT, Tecuanhuey LV, Preminger GM: Laparoscopic dismembered pyeloplasty. J Urol 150(6):1795–1799, 1993.
66. Adams JB, Moore RG, Clayman RV, Kavoussi LR: Laparoscopic ureteral reconstruction. J Endourol 8(Suppl 1):P2–82, S84, 1994.
67. Carmignani G, De Stefani S, Simonato A, Corbu C: Laparoscopic ureterocutaneostomy. J Endourol 8(Suppl 1):P2–84, S84, 1994.

CHAPTER 49

Hormonal Influences in the Lower Urinary Tract

Mauro Cervigni, M.D.

The physiology of the female urinary tract is influenced by sex hormones. Clinical and urodynamic changes are apparent in the female urinary tract system during pregnancy, in the menstrual cycle, and at menopause. This chapter reviews the physiology of the female genitourinary tract with particular emphasis on the origin and effect of gonadal steroids on the genital tract.

The Biochemistry of Sex Hormones

At least six different natural estrogens have been isolated from the plasma of women, but only three are present in significant quantities: (1) beta-estradiol, (2) estrone, and (3) estriol. Both beta-estradiol and estrone are present in large quantities in the venous blood from the ovaries, and estriol is an oxidative product derived from these first two, the conversion occurring mainly in the liver but also to some extent elsewhere in the body (Fig. 49–1). Beta-estradiol is considered the major estrogen, but the estrogenic effects of estrone are far from negligible.

Estrogens are synthesized in the ovaries from cholesterol or acetyl-coenzyme A, the acetate units of which can be conjugated to form the appropriate steroid nuclei. It is particularly interesting that progesterone and testosterone are synthesized first and then converted into the estrogens. The liver plays an important role in removing estrogens from the blood by conjugating them to form glucuronides and sulfates. About one-fifth of these conjugated products are excreted in the bile, and most of the remainder are excreted in the urine.

Progesterone has a molecular structure not far different from that of the estrogens. It is probably synthesized principally from acetyl-coenzyme A. However, it can also be formed from cholesterol. The potency of progesterone per unit of weight is much less than that of estrogens. Within a few minutes after secretion, almost all of the progesterone is degraded by the liver to other steroids that have no progesteronic effect. The major end product of progesterone degradation is pregnanediol.

Female Sex Hormones and the Lower Urinary Tract

Female sex hormones act on the lower urinary tract through two distinct mechanisms: (1) direct effect on target organs, and (2) interaction with neurotransmitter receptors.

DIRECT EFFECT ON TARGET ORGANS

The direct effect on target organs is mediated mostly by an interaction of estrogens with cellular DNA, the so-called genomic effect (Fig. 49–2). The hormone, which is soluble in the lipids of the cell membrane, enters the cell by diffusion. The hormone receptor is complexed with an inhibitor that is displaced after hormone receptor interaction. A dimer of the receptor protein bound to the hormone enters the nucleus and binds to DNA response elements, thus activating transcription of the dependent gene. This effect is exerted on various tissues of the female urinary tract.

Iosif and colleagues in 1981 demonstrated for the first time the existence of estrogen (estradiol) receptors in the female lower urinary tract in four patients.[1] High-affinity estradiol receptors could be detected in both cytosolic and nuclear fractions of the urethra and partially by specimens from the trigone,

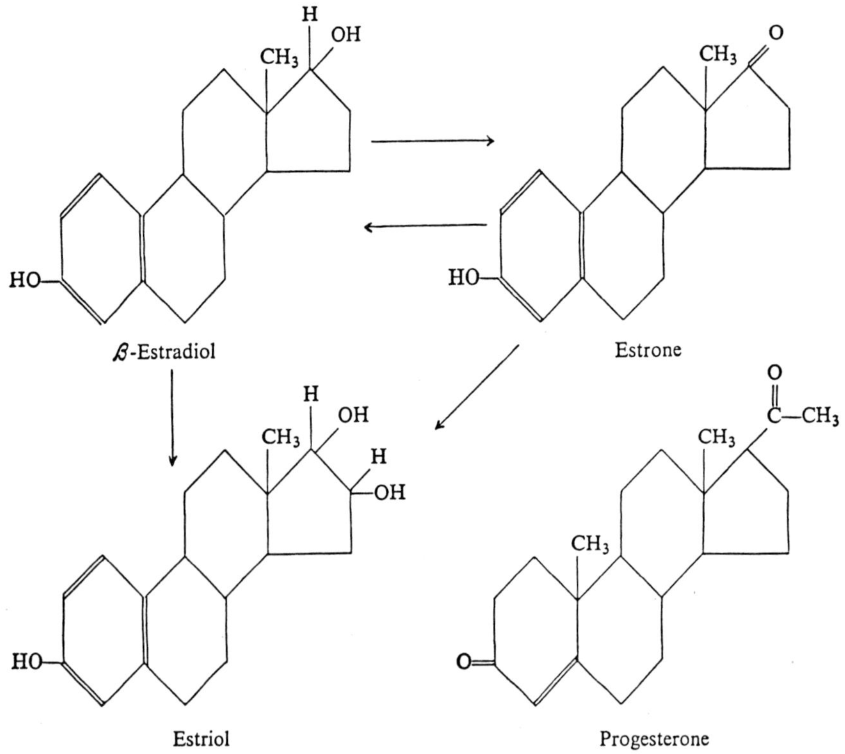

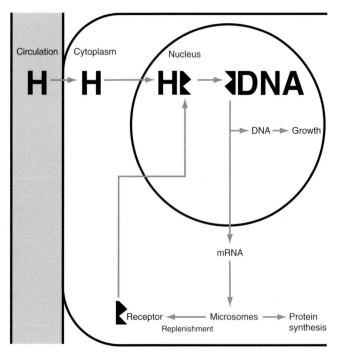

Figure 49-1 Structures of steroids.

Figure 49-2 Mechanism of action of steroid hormones. H, hormone; R, receptor. (From Speroff L, Glass RH, Kase NG: Hormone biosynthesis, metabolism, and mechanism of action. *In* Clinical Gynecologic Endocrinology and Infertility, 5th ed. Baltimore, Williams & Wilkins, 1994.)

whereas these receptors were evident in only the nuclear fractions of the bladder. The receptor concentrations in both trigone and bladder were lower than those in the urethra.[2] It has also been demonstrated in both animals and humans that estrogen receptors are present in the urethra in a concentration similar to that of the vagina.[3]

The various tissues of the urogenital tract, particularly those involved in maintaining urethral closure (urethral epithelium, vasculature and mucosa, paraurethral connective tissue, ligaments, and pelvic floor muscles), may result in incontinence once estrogen levels fall after menopause.

INTERACTION WITH NEUROTRANSMITTER RECEPTORS

MODIFICATION OF ADRENERGIC RECEPTORS The function of the lower urinary tract is mediated by neurotransmitters associated with the autonomic nervous system.[4] The activity of the lower urinary tract can be pharmacologically manipulated by agents that regulate the density of neurotransmitter receptors. Sex steroid hormones that act in various target tissues also modulate the neurotransmitter receptor density in the lower urinary tract.[5-9]

In very much the same manner as in the reproductive system, sex hormones may influence the urinary tract by modifying responses to adrenergic stimulation. Depending on the prevailing hormonal environment, the response to catecholamine shifts changes from contraction to relaxation. A contraction (alpha-adrenoreceptor–mediated) can be caused in the uterus of estrogen-pretreated rabbits[10] or rats[11] by a sympathetic stimulation that, in the uterus of progesterone-pretreated rats[12] and rabbits,[9] causes relaxation (beta-adrenergic–mediated). This change is due to a change in the relative prevalence of one or another of the adrenergic receptor types.

Beta-adrenoreceptors are predominant in the detrusor muscle. Stimulation of beta-adrenoreceptors produces relaxation in isolated strips of detrusor muscle in the human and cat, whereas alpha-adrenoreceptor stimulation produces detrusor contraction in human[13] and rabbit tissue.[4] On the other hand, the bladder neck, urethra, and bladder base contain a predominance of alpha-adrenoreceptors. The stimulation of adrenergic receptors increases urethral pressure in vivo[14, 15] and produces contraction in isolated human and cat preparations. Beta-adrenoreceptor stimulation produces relaxation of isolated preparations in both humans and cats and decreases urethral pressure in vivo in dogs.[16, 17] High doses of estrogens can also alter the normal characteristics of micturition, and in fact consecutive injections of pharmacologic doses of estradiol have induced urinary retention in male and female mice. This retention could well be attributed to the stratification of the epithelium, to fibrosis, or to both.[18] Insofar as estrogens have been shown to heighten alpha-adrenergic activity in the urinary tract,[5, 10, 19] at least part

of the urinary retention may be explained by the bolstering of alpha-adrenergic activity.

Sex hormones can interact with adrenergic receptors in different ways:

1. They can increase innervation and receptorial density. As reported by Levin and associates, estrogenic treatment induced a marked increase in the adrenergic innervation of the female rabbit bladder detrusor.[20] Estrogens also increase the amount of fluorescent adrenergic nerve terminals in the rabbit uterus and vagina, whereas pregnancy reduces catecholamine hystofluorescence in the adrenergic nerves.[21]
2. They can induce membrane potential changes. Some of the facilitation or increase in smooth muscle alpha-adrenergic responses due to estrogen administration and in beta-adrenergic responses due to progesterone depends on complementary action on the electrolyte shunt across smooth muscle membranes.[22] By creating an electrolyte change like beta-adrenoreceptor stimulation, progesterone hyperpolarizes the rat membrane myometrium,[23] whereas estrogen causes the hypopolarization of rabbit urethral smooth muscle[24] owing to electrolyte changes similar to alpha-adrenergic stimulation.
3. They can induce blockade of the extraneuronal reuptake of catecholamines. Estrogens can block the active transport system in the presynaptic nerve endings that is responsible for the extraneuronal reuptake of the released amine neurotransmitter norepinephrine. Adrenergic nerve terminals carry out their action in the synaptic area through a rapid reuptake of noradrenaline into neuronal (reuptake$_1$) and extraneuronal (reuptake$_2$) tissue.[25] Although reuptake$_2$ is not a major pathway for the disposition of innervated tissue, it does play an important role in those tissues with sparse adrenergic nerves.[26] Tricyclic antidepressants, particularly imipramine, are most useful in inhibiting reuptake$_1$ and have a profound effect in strengthening the response of sympathetically innervated organs. Likewise, the blockade of reuptake$_2$ has been shown to strengthen the sympathetic stimulation response.

INTERACTION WITH CHOLINERGIC RECEPTORS Estrogens heighten the rabbit detrusor muscle response to muscarinic cholinergic receptors (MChR). Levin and colleagues demonstrated that the administration of estrogen to immature female rabbits for 4 days resulted in both increased sensitivity of the bladder to muscarinic cholinergic agonists and increased MChR density.[27]

In a very refined study, Shapiro examined the effect of long-term estrogen treatment on the MChR in the adult female rabbit bladder and urethra.[28] Estrogen treatment was associated with a decrease in the MChR density in rabbit bladder bodies that led to a reduction in detrusor tone and an increase in bladder capacity. The conflicting results between the former study and the latter may be explained by the different intervals of estrogen administration used (Levin's short-term versus Shapiro's long-term therapy). The estrogen-induced down-regulation of the MChR density in the bladder could be another mechanism explaining the improvement in lower urinary tract symptoms in postmenopausal women.

INTERACTION WITH PROSTAGLANDINS Prostaglandins (PGs) are autacoids synthesized from the bladder tissue of several species, including humans, that are able to modify the contraction of smooth muscle. Prostaglandin types E and F are involved in the contraction of the urinary bladder.[29] The bladder neck and urethra are also affected by prostaglandins, with $PGF_{2\alpha}$ producing contraction and PGE_2 relaxation.[30] It was recently shown that the urinary bladder of estrous animals was more reactive to E series prostaglandins than were the muscles of ovariectomized rats.[31, 32] Quite suggestive, therefore, is the fact that some postmenopausal urinary problems (e.g., voiding difficulties) may be due in part to reduced prostaglandin sensitivity as a result of diminished estrogen levels.

PROGESTERONE AND THE URINARY TRACT

The effects of progesterone on the urinary tract are not thoroughly discussed in the literature except with respect to hydronephrosis of pregnancy. The hydroureter of pregnancy, the increased bladder capacity, and the increased incidence of genuine stress incontinence (GSI) are all thought to be due in some degree to the effect of progesterone. The changes are attributed to the relaxing effect of progesterone on the smooth muscle of the urinary system. Raz and associates, in a classic set of animal experiments, were able to demonstrate that progesterone facilitates beta-adrenergic activity in the ureter and in the urethra.[33] Progesterone may also have an anticholinergic effect in the bladder. Levin and colleagues showed that the bladder muscle of pregnant rabbits generated 50% less contractile response than virgin controls when exposed to bethanecol.[34] Furthermore, the bladder base showed a reduced contractile response to methoxamine (an alpha-adrenergic agonist).[35] Thus, progesterone, even if not well defined, seems to have a beta-adrenergic, an anti–alpha-adrenergic, and an anticholinergic effect on the lower urinary tract.

TESTOSTERONE AND THE LOWER URINARY TRACT

There is still no evidence of testosterone receptors or specific action on the female lower urinary tract. The effect of testosterone propionate (25 mg three times a week) on the urinary bladder was evaluated on urodynamic examination. The drug resulted in increased intravesical pressure throughout the cystometrogram curve. Males taking testosterone have an increased ability to void, have a better stream, and initiate micturition without difficulty.[36] In paraple-

gics, testosterone propionate has been used for its anabolic action. The drug did not interfere with micturition in any of 2000 patients. It has been suggested that testosterone may be used in women with GSI in order to increase the quality of periurethral tissues in response to testosterone therapy.[37]

Normal Hormonal Balance

In women of reproductive age the complex interplay of hormonal and neuroendocrine events results in a variety of cyclic physiologic changes known as the menstrual cycle.

MENSTRUAL CYCLE

The normal menstrual cycle length varies from 25 to 30 days with a slight decrease in mean length as a woman ages. It can be divided into two phases straddling ovulation. The first half of the cycle, the follicular phase, is dominated by the development of the mature oocyte in an ovarian follicle; there is an associated increase in estradiol. This phase of the cycle is also known as the proliferative phase because of the characteristic proliferation of the endometrium in response to estradiol. The second half of the cycle, the luteal phase, is dominated by the presence of an active corpus luteum derived from the ovulating follicle and the production of progesterone. This is also known as the secretory phase because of the characteristic endometrial response of progesterone to the gland secretion.

HORMONAL PATTERNS

The principal estrogen produced is estradiol-17-beta. Normal ovulatory cycles result in serum estradiol levels ranging from 40 pg/ml in the early follicular phase to 250 pg/ml at midcycle and 100 pg/ml during the midluteal phase. The dominant follicle and corpus luteum account for more than 95% of the circulatory estradiol in premenopausal women. Peripheral conversion of estrone to estradiol accounts for most of the remaining circulating estradiol. Estrone, the second major human estrogen, is derived principally from the metabolism of estradiol and from the aromatization of androstenedione in adipose tissue. A small quantity is secreted directly by the ovary and the adrenal gland. Serum levels during the menstrual cycle vary from 40 to 170 pg/ml, paralleling estradiol levels. The estradiol-to-estrone ratio is greater than 1.0 in premenopausal women.

The menstrual cycle induces important changes in several compartments of the female body including the hypothalamus, pituitary, ovaries, uterus and cervix, vagina, and vulva. The response of the lower urinary tract to cyclic events is also relevant. Gonadotropin-releasing hormone (GnRH) is the hypothalamic-releasing factor controlling the secretion of the pituitary gonadotropins, follicle-stimulating hormone (FSH) and luteinizing hormone (LH). GnRH is secreted in a pulsatile fashion under a variety of conditions and particularly throughout the menstrual cycle. The GnRH pulse frequency in the follicular phase has been shown to increase from about one pulse every 90 to 100 minutes during menses to one pulse every 50 to 60 minutes just before ovulation. The initially less frequent pulses favor the release of FSH from the pituitary, and the more rapid pulses later in the follicular phase favor LH release and ultimately an LH surge. Following ovulation, the GnRH pulse generator begins to slow down throughout the luteal phase, reaching a frequency of one pulse every 4 to 6 hours in the late luteal phase. This slowing down is largely influenced by estradiol and progesterone. At the end of the luteal phase the hypothalamus begins to speed up and initiate follicular development for the next cycle.

The ovary is both a target organ for gonadotropin stimulation and an endocrine organ producing a large amount of gonadal steroids. Oocytes are stored in the ovaries, induced to develop, and released in a process coordinated to facilitate pregnancy. A group of follicles is recruited before the onset of the menstrual cycle and begins gonadotropin-independent follicular development. Under the influence of the increasing FSH level, this cohort is induced to select a dominant follicle in the midfollicular phase. The dominant follicle is destined to ovulate, whereas the remainder of the cohort undergoes atresia. Estradiol production by the granulosa cells lining the dominant follicle reaches peak levels approximately 2 days before ovulation and contributes both negative feedback that suppresses FHS release and positive feedback that increases LH release. The LH surge initiates the final maturation events of the oocyte, changes the estradiol-producing granulosa cells to estradiol- and progesterone-producing luteal cells, and triggers ovulation. Luteinizing cells begin to produce increasing amounts of progesterone in addition to estradiol, reaching peak levels in the midluteal phase and steadily declining thereafter. The life span of the corpus luteum is about 14 days; an uncertain mechanism dictates its decline.

The uterus provides the most visible evidence of the reproductive cycle as the source of menstrual bleeding. The endometrium undergoes characteristic histologic and biochemical changes throughout the menstrual cycle in response to gonadal steroids and other factors. The first half of the menstrual cycle is characterized by the proliferation of endometrium from the relatively stable basal layer under the influence of increasing levels of estradiol.

Estrogen receptors are always present in the endometrium and increase under the influence of rising estradiol. Estradiol also induces the development of progesterone receptors. In the proliferative phase, the three main components of the endometrium—epithelial glands, stroma, and blood vessels—proliferate and increase the thickness of the endome-

trium five- to tenfold. This secretion is used to support the blastocyst before implantation, which occurs about 1 week after ovulation if conception has occurred. In the latter part of the secretory phase the endometrial stroma undergoes changes termed pseudodecidualization in which enlarged cells form an adequate matrix for a developing implantation. If pregnancy does not occur, estradiol and progesterone secretion from the corpus luteum decline. The most dramatic effect is the marked vasomotor response of the endometrial arteries, with rhythmic vasoconstriction eventually leading to ischemia of the upper two-thirds of the endometrium. Endometrial desquamation occurs within the first 24 hours of menses with visible bleeding lasting 3 to 5 days.

The cervix also demonstrates characteristic changes throughout the menstrual cycle in response to gonadal steroids. The two most prominent changes in the cervix involve the diameter of the internal os and the character of the cervical mucus secretion. The internal cervical os is constricted except under the influence of peak levels of estradiol in the immediate preovulatory period, when the diameter increases. Cervical mucus produced by endocervical glands is generally thick, sticky, and resistant to the passage of sperm or bacteria. Under the influence of estradiol the protein of the cervical mucus increases its water content, resulting in a copious, clear, slippery mucus that, together with the increased diameter of the internal cervical os, facilitates the migration of motile sperm through the cervix to allow conception. Cyclic vaginal changes are less obvious than those seen in the endometrium or cervix. The stratified squamous vaginal epithelium, however, demonstrates the characteristic growth pattern of such epithelium with continuous desquamation of surface cells and replenishment from basal cells. Studies of urethral smears have demonstrated the presence of cyclic changes throughout the menstrual cycle similar to those seen in vaginal epithelium. Cytologic studies of urethral cells of urinary sediment have confirmed these findings and have been used to detect ovulation.

Urinary symptoms, particularly stress incontinence, vary in premenopausal women according to the phase of the menstrual cycle, becoming worse during periods of progesterone dominance. Several papers have examined the relationship between the hormonal patterns of the menstrual cycle and the functional changes that occur in the bladder and urethra. Gitsch and Branstetter demonstrated an increase in bladder tone during the follicular phase and a decrease in tone during the secretory phase of the menstrual cycle,[38] whereas Schreiter and colleagues reported an increase in urethral pressure and length and the amplitude of periurethral pulsations during the follicular phase with a decrease occurring in all these parameters premenstrually.[39] Van Geelen and associates found a significant correlation between the increase in urethral length and periurethral pulsation and serum estradiol levels in healthy premenopausal women.[40]

Pregnancy and the Urinary Tract

Embryonic development begins under the influence of rising levels of progesterone. In the endometrial cavity the bulk of the embryo becomes a trophoblast, which begins to produce an increasing amount of beta-human chorionic gonadotropin (beta-HCG). Circulating levels of beta-HCG can be detected with sensitive assays within 8 to 9 days after ovulation and fertilization and before the first missed menses. Beta-HCG induces the corpus luteum to produce increasing amounts of progesterone, which in turn maintains the endometrium to allow support of the developing fetus. Trophoblast-placental development provides an increasing amount of progesterone to continue the support of pregnancy, and beta-HCG levels continue to rise throughout the first trimester, reaching a peak at about 12 weeks and declining steadily thereafter. In response to the change in the hormonal milieu, the female genital tract undergoes several changes including uterine hypertrophy, ovarian quiescence, an increased blood supply to the entire pelvis, and finally, relaxation of the supporting ligaments.

Pregnancy may precipitate urologic symptoms in apparently healthy women.[41, 42] Progesterone action predominates at the cellular and receptor levels, resulting in suppression of the estrogen receptors. Antagonism between estrogen and progesterone at the receptor and genomic levels in the lower urinary tract greatly depresses the estrogen receptor concentration in the urethra and myometrium during pregnancy. The low level of estrogen receptor, together with a complex set of nongenomic antiestrogenic actions of progesterone, such as a direct effect on the smooth muscle cell membrane,[43] should reduce the estrogenic influence during pregnancy that could be the basis of urologic symptoms experienced in late pregnancy.

The elevated levels of progesterone in pregnancy, by facilitating beta-adrenergic responses, contribute to the hypotonicity of the ureter in the gravid state. During times of a high estrogen-progesterone ratio, such as occurs at the end of pregnancy, endogenous uterine prostaglandin production increases, resulting in an increase in spontaneous uterine contractions.[44] On fluorescent microscopy in rabbits, pregnancy results in a loss of noradrenaline fluorescence in the adrenergic nerves of the uterus and vagina, whereas estrogen treatment enhances the intensity and quantity of fluorescent adrenergic nerve terminals.[21] In female rabbits pregnancy also enhances the sensitivity of the bladder.[5]

Progesterone has been shown recently to antagonize estrogen-induced increases in urethral blood flow that contribute positively to the maintenance of continence. Therefore, progesterone dominance during pregnancy would promote urinary incontinence.

Menopause and Hormonal Changes

The average age at the onset of menopause has increased since the turn of the century and is currently about 52 years. With menopause the ovaries no longer secrete progesterone and 17 beta-estradiol in appreciable quantities. Estrone is the predominant estrogen in postmenopausal women. Most of it is synthesized in the periphery, predominantly in adipose tissue, by the conversion of androstenedione to estrone (Fig. 49–3). As the negative feedback effect of the estrogens and progesterone is reduced, secretion of FSH and LH is increased, and plasma FSH and LH rise to a high level. Measurements of serum concentrations of estrogen in postmenopausal women have shown that the serum level is independent of the length of the postmenopausal period or the age of the subject.[45]

The tissues of organs directly affected by this relative estrogen deficiency are those with specific estrogen receptors; the vaginal epithelium and the urethral epithelium, which have the same embryologic origin (the urogenital sinus), are subject to estrogenic action,[46] as are the ovaries, endometrium, hypothalamus, and skin. Other tissues in which estrogen receptors have not been consistently identified, such as bone, are nevertheless affected by a lack of estrogen. Urogenital atrophy, "hot flashes," osteoporosis, and

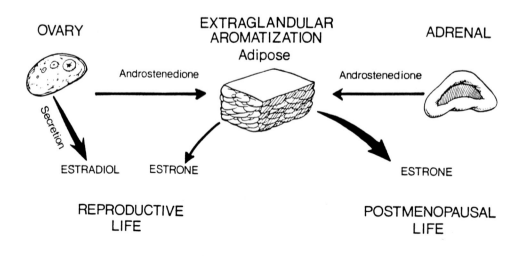

Figure 49–3 Sources of estrogen during reproductive and postmenopausal life. (From Carr BR, MacDonald PC: Estrogen treatment of postmenopausal women. Adv Intern Med 28:491–508, 1983.)

various psychological symptoms are common after ovarian function has ceased. Postmenopausal urinary symptoms mostly become manifest later than other climacteric symptoms, and the estrogen-related aging effect in the urethral mucosa does not occur promptly after menopause (Fig. 49–4).

The risk of cardiovascular disease is higher in men than in age-matched women before the age of 40 to 45 years. During the perimenopausal period the risk of cardiovascular disease in women begins to increase to a rate similar to that in men. The decrease in estrogen production is thought to be responsible for this acceleration of risk. In recent years, repeated studies have demonstrated an increase in high-density lipoprotein (HDL) levels and a concomitant decrease in low-density lipoprotein (LDL) levels associated with the postmenopausal administration of oral estrogens. This alteration in the lipoprotein fraction has had a beneficial effect on the occurrence of coronary artery disease and strokes. In women receiving postmenopausal low-dose estrogen supplements, the risk of myocardial infarction, stroke, and death resulting from these complications is reduced by at least 50%. After cardiovascular disease, the most significant problem related to estrogen deficiency is osteoporosis.

Urogenital disorders are common in postmenopausal women. In a group of 902 women in southern Sweden, Iosif and Bekassy reported the presence of urinary incontinence in 29.2%; the number with mixed incontinence was 9.5%, whereas 27.3% had urge incontinence, 13% had recurrent urinary tract infections, and 48.8% had such lower genital tract disorders as vaginal dryness, dyspareunia, pain, itch, or discharge.[47] Patients with GSI or urge symptoms reported vaginal dryness ($p < .001$). Urogenital disorders are also particularly frequent among elderly women treated in geriatric hospitals and often lead to urosepsis and bronchopneumonia.[48]

VAGINA

The vaginal epithelium of women deprived of estrogen loses its normal rugose appearance and becomes attenuated, pale, and transparent. The depth of the vaginal vault is shortened, and the upper third begins to constrict. The supporting ligaments of the uterus and the elastic tissue of the vagina also lose their tensile strength when deprived of estrogens. This may result in partial or complete uterine prolapse, cystocele, or rectocele.

Local symptoms resulting from vaginal atrophy include vaginal discharge, dryness, itching, burning, bleeding, vaginismus, dyspareunia, and sensations of pelvic heaviness. Usually, less estrogen is required to prevent atrophy of the genital tissues than is necessary to prevent hot flashes, heart attacks, and so on. Administered vaginally, estrogens are absorbed efficiently and increase the thickness of the vaginal epithelium and the tensile strength of the elastic tissue in the vagina. Intermittent therapy two or three times a week is usually sufficient to maintain a well-estrogenized vaginal epithelium.

URETHRA

The epithelium of the urethra becomes thin and the periurethral connective tissue becomes sclerotic. A significant consequence of urethral atrophy is the occurrence of dysuria, frequency, and urge incontinence. Three factors contribute to the maintenance of urinary continence in women: (1) resistance by the urethral epithelium, (2) the intra-abdominal location of the proximal urethra, and (3) contraction of the striated periurethral muscle fibers at times of stress. In postmenopausal women changes in all three factors diminish the capacity for urinary continence. The decrease in tensile strength of the elastic tissue surrounding the vagina leads to a prolapse of the urethrovesical junction, resulting in its removal from the intra-abdominal pressure sphere above the pelvic diaphragm. A poorly supported urethra also does not permit effective contraction of the striated periurethral muscle fibers at times of stress. Owing to a combination of attenuation of the urethral epithelium, loss of the intra-abdominal location of the proximal urethra, and loss of the striated periurethral muscle fiber tension, many postmenopausal women are unable to control urination. The muscles of the pelvis lose their vigor and the pelvic ligament its elasticity, which results in lower pressure in the urethra. Even if the pressure transmission ratio (PTR) is influenced by age very little or not at all,[49] the urethral closing pressure (UCP) decreases with age owing to urethral deterioration of elastic and vascular tissues, deterioration of smooth muscle fibers, and fibrosis. Once estrogen levels of various tissues decrease after menopause, this decline is variable, with some women exhibiting evidence of estrogen stimulation for many years afterward.[50]

Mucosal Changes

After birth, the proximal urethra is usually covered by transitional epithelium as an extension of the inner layer of the bladder. The distal urethra is

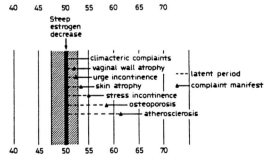

Figure 49–4 The climacteric complaints appearing during and after menopause. (From Van Keep P, and Lauritzen C: Ageing and Estrogens. Basel, Karger, 1973.)

coated by nonkeratinized squamous epithelium, which extends during the reproductive period[51] until it may eventually cover the entire urethra and trigone.[52] During the reproductive years the urethral mucosa undergoes cyclic variations during the menstrual cycle.[53] The atrophic changes that occur in the vagina during the postmenopausal years affect the epithelium of the trigone and the urethra. The squamous cell lining in the distal urethral epithelium is replaced by parabasal cells. Zinner and colleagues in 1980 emphasized the importance of the "mucosal seal" due to the enfolding and apposition of the mucosal layer,[54] which is hormonally dependent, decreases in thickness, and atrophies along with other estrogen-sensitive tissues after menopause.[55, 56] Everett first reported in 1941 the strict correlation between lower urinary tract symptoms and atrophic vaginitis that invariably resulted in atrophic urethritis with functional urethral stenosis.[57]

Another significant effect of estrogen deprivation in menopause is the decrease in the main layer of the mucopolysaccharide coating of the urothelium, which is estrogen-sensitive. Bacterial adhesion is enhanced by the reduction of this layer, partially explaining the increase in urinary tract infections seen in postmenopausal women.[58]

Urethral Vasculature

In the submucosal layer there are two vascular plexuses—the distal plexus, which is just proximal to the urethral meatus and does not change with age, and the proximal plexus, which is near the bladder neck, like the corpus spongiosum in males, and is modified by the menstrual cycle and menopause. These large vessels seem quite disproportionate to the needs of the normal blood supply of the urethral tissue and seem to constitute a vascular cushion to the mucosal lining.

The vascular component of the submucosal venous plexus accounts for approximately one-third of the resting intraurethral closure pressure in women.[55, 56] The urethral vascular pulsation varies with different phases of the menstrual cycle, being greatest during periods of follicular-phase estrogen dominance[39, 40] and declining in the postmenopausal years.[55] But estrogen replacement therapy can reverse this decline.[59]

Urethral Smooth Muscle

The smooth muscles are sensitive to estradiol, which acts on the tone of the urethral smooth muscles, strengthening them,[60] and to progesterone, which inhibits spontaneous muscular activity and contractions.[61] With aging, the urethra is subjected to estrogen and progesterone modulation. In addition to atrophy of the urethral epithelium and submucosal vasculature, hormonal depletion reduces the tone of the smooth muscles.[5, 62]

Estrogen deprivation may cause the reduced tone of the urethral smooth muscles, because it has been shown in animals that the contractile response of isolated urethral strips to α-adrenergic agonists is heightened by estrogen pretreatment.[24] In some clinical studies the urethral response to adrenergic agonists is enhanced by estrogen replacement therapy,[39, 63] although there is some debate about this.[64]

CONNECTIVE TISSUE AND SUPPORTS

Versi and colleagues showed that connective tissue collagen contributes to the generation of urethral pressure and that the beneficial effect of estrogens on urethral function may be mediated by collagen.[65] There is a statistically significant correlation between thigh skin collagen content and various variables of the urethral pressure profile; greater sphincteric function was associated with a higher collagen content of skin.

Structural collagen in the urethra is the same type as that in the skin, namely, types I and III. It has been shown that skin collagen content and skin thickness decline after menopause[66, 67] but can be restored following estrogen replacement therapy.[68] In fact, the increased urethral pressure seen with hormonal replacement therapy could be an effect of estrogen on urethral collagen.[63, 69–72] Gosling showed that connective tissue could also be involved in one of the functional elements of the urethra.[73]

Estrogen receptors have also been identified on skin fibroblasts,[74] and there is a positive correlation between skin collagen and parameters of the urethral pressure profile.[75]

Lack of estrogen affects the connective tissue, especially that of the transverse cervical and uterosacral ligaments, with loss of the usual support of the pelvic organs. The ligament and supports of the urethra may also be estrogen-dependent.[76] Improvement of uterovaginal prolapse following estrogen therapy has been reported.[77, 78]

STRIATED MUSCLES OF THE PELVIC FLOOR

It is widely accepted that the striated urethral sphincter and the pelvic floor muscles also possess estrogen receptors.[79–81] Because anal competence in women is reduced after the age of 50 years, it too may be dependent on the effect of estrogens. In fact, in a study by Haaden and colleagues, estrogen receptors were found to be present in the external anal sphincter at a median concentration of 5.0 fmol/mg in women compared with 1.1 fmol/mg in men.[82]

The striated muscle of the pelvic floor is important in maintaining urethral closure, accounting for one-third of the urethral closure pressure.[83, 84] In fact, the transmission of intra-abdominal pressure to the urethra, which is a measure of the effectiveness of pelvic floor function, improves in postmenopausal women with stress incontinence following estrogen therapy.[72, 85]

The neuromuscular functional decline due to aging tissues that occurs in postmenopausal women lowers the tone of the striated muscles, which shows an increase in interstitial connective tissue.

Hormonal Replacement Therapy

Hormonal replacement therapy (HRT) reverses the majority of postmenopausal genital tract atrophic changes. It also prevents postmenopausal osteoporosis and has beneficial cardiovascular effects through its influence on circulating lipids. All women who develop estrogen deficiency should be considered for HRT. After careful evaluation and counseling, the vast majority of patients are willing to accept the occasional side effects and minimal health risk of HRT in exchange for the symptomatic relief as well as the long-term benefits it provides. Estrogens are known to have a major effect on many aspects of the quality of life, and their administration in postmenopausal women produces subjective improvement,[72, 86, 87] yet no objective evidence has revealed the mechanism by which this subjective improvement occurs. Endometrium responds to HRT with proliferation. Therefore, it is imperative to counteract the unchecked proliferative effect of estrogen with progesterone to protect against endometrial hyperplasia and neoplasia.

THE EFFECT OF HORMONES ON HUMAN ENDOMETRIAL CELL PROLIFERATION

Estrogens have a "promoting effect" on existing endometrial tumor cells, but if used in routinely therapeutic doses, the natural estrogens, estradiol and estriol, have less promoting effects than synthetic and conjugated estrogens.[88] They are therefore preferred for HRT. Estriol in particular has a better effect on the genital soft tissue and has a less pronounced effect on the endometrium compared with other estrogen hormones.[89, 90] In patients with a uterus, oral medroxyprogesterone acetate, 5 to 10 mg daily for 10 to 14 days per month, should be added to prevent the development of endometrial hyperplasia and adenocarcinoma. Progesterone and synthetic related compounds have proved their ability to prevent the occurrence of endometrial hyperplasia, which is believed to precede the most frequent type of endometrial carcinoma.[91] Approximately 80 to 85% of endometrial carcinomas defined as type 1 appear to have estrogen-dependent precursors; these cancers are generally low grade, are slow growing, and have limited metastatic potential. They are often associated with a history of unopposed estrogen stimulation. However, approximately 15 to 20% of endometrial carcinomas are defined as type 2. This type of cancer in postmenopausal women occurs at a median age of 65. Estrogen stimulation is unlikely to be an etiologic factor in the development of this type of cancer, which is not associated with a specific hormonal risk factor or a history of endometrial hyperplasia. This cancer is generally highly malignant and deeply invasive and usually does not respond to hormonal manipulation. In women who decline therapy because of regular withdrawal bleeding, a continuous daily combination of conjugated equine estrogen, 0.625 mg, with medroxyprogesterone acetate, 2.5 mg, will lead to persistent amenorrhea within 3 to 6 months in more than 90% of patients. Most women experience unscheduled vaginal bleeding and spotting during the first month of use. Although such regimens appear to protect against osteoporosis and to prevent symptoms of estrogen deficiency, to date the possible negative long-term effects of low-dose continuous progestin therapy have been inadequately evaluated. Elderly women tend to welcome the return of regular vaginal bleeding. Therefore, if continuous estrogen therapy is used alone, careful clinical follow-up is recommended and any bleeding during treatment is an indication to stop therapy and conduct further investigations. Nevertheless, all women receiving HRT should have an annual history and complete physical examination. Pap smears should be performed annually on all women with a uterus. Endometrial sampling should be reserved for women with abnormal bleeding or those not receiving progestin therapy. Biannual mammography for women under age 50 and yearly mammography in those over 50 should be performed.

HRT AND BREAST CANCER

In the past 15 years more than 20 studies exploring the relationship between HRT and breast cancer have been done. None of these studies has demonstrated any dramatic increase in breast cancer associated with the use of estrogen replacement therapy (ERT), even after an extended duration of treatment. Investigators at the Centers for Disease Control and Prevention in Atlanta, Georgia, conducted a meta-analysis of the relationship between ERT and breast cancer.[92] They concluded that there was some evidence of a duration-related increase in breast cancer risk associated with ERT, but that this effect was of a relatively small magnitude, with about a 10% increase in risk for each 5 years of therapy; another meta-analysis concluded that, if any risk exists at all, it is even smaller.[93]

The use of oral contraceptive therapy may also slightly increase the risk of breast cancer in premenopausal women,[94] but there is little evidence to suggest an increased risk in postmenopausal women.

Bergkvist and colleagues and Persson and colleagues, in an analysis of the effect of conjugated estrogen plus progestin, provided some data showing that the effect of this combination on breast cancer risk was higher than any found for ERT users. Therefore, progestin increases risk further.[95, 96] The data on combination therapy are, however, very sparse at the current time.

CONTRAINDICATIONS AND SIDE EFFECTS

The presence of abnormal uterine or vaginal bleeding without tissue diagnosis, endometriosis, thromboembolic disease, severe liver renal or cardiac disease, severe hypertension, or estrogen-dependent tumors is a contraindication to initiation of estrogen therapy. In women with active migraine headaches or active seizure disorders, HRT may aggravate the problem. Existing breast cancer or endometrial cancer is a contraindication to estrogen therapy, although there is debate about whether previous successfully treated endometrial cancer constitutes a contraindication.

Commonly, about 5 to 10% of women given low-dose estrogen-progestin report side effects, which are more prevalent with synthetic estrogens. These include breast pain and swelling, exacerbation of cardiac failure, difficulty in controlling diabetes and hypertension, nausea, thrombophlebitis, withdrawal bleeding, and weight gain. Many of these side effects can be effectively controlled by reducing the dose of estrogen.

Most symptoms decrease after several months of therapy. If patients continue to have side effects, changing the prescribed dose or the specific estrogen or progestin used usually allows the patient to better tolerate the replacement regimen. With cyclic administration of estrogen and progesterone about 90% of patients have period-like withdrawal bleeding. If patients are well educated about the benefits of HRT they tolerate the mild side effects and the scheduled breakthrough bleeding they usually experience.

EFFECT OF THERAPY

The clinical effect of estrogens in the treatment of female urinary disorders is still controversial. In fact, it is difficult to draw definite conclusions because of the great disparity of results (the success rate varies from 34 to 80%, and the majority of these results are subjective[97]) and the urodynamic variations. There are several correlated problems: (1) the lack of inclusion criteria, (2) the limited number of available subjects and the absence of multicenter trials, (3) the variability of urodynamic techniques used to evaluate sphincteric function (fluid perfusion system, microtip transducers, and so on), (4) the variety and doses of estrogens used, (5) the outcome criteria, and (6) the existence of a limited number of controlled clinical trials.[69, 71, 72, 86, 98] The objectivity of trials is important because the feeling of subjective well-being obtained with HRT may confuse the results. One possible explanation may be related to the fact that the burning sensation caused by urinary loss on the atrophic vaginal mucosa after HRT may be perceived with less stimulus, as postulated by Rud.[56] Moreover, the variety of results reported in the literature is correlated with the dosage of the estrogens used and their administration. Walter,[70] Ek,[99] and Samsioe[100] and their colleagues reported limited or no results because they used a low dose of estrogen, whereas with a higher dose of estriol, for example, Schreiter and colleagues[39] and Rud[56] reported much more encouraging results.

ESTROGENS AND GENUINE STRESS INCONTINENCE

The physiologic role of estrogens in maintaining continence is still debated. Six women with proven premature ovarian failure were evaluated urodynamically before and after administration of oral and vaginal estrogen to study the effect of estradiol on lower urinary tract function.[101] The only change found was a significant increase in PTR to the proximal urethra. Therefore, these investigators concluded that estrogen alone, in the absence of aging and other known precipitating factors for GSI, is of minimal importance in maintaining normal urinary tract physiology.

Langer and colleagues studied the relationship between the onset of menopause and the appearance of lower urinary tract symptoms in 12 premenopausal women in whom hypoestrogenism was induced by treatment with GnRH.[102] No urodynamic changes were observed, so they concluded that estrogen deficiency in the absence of aging and other factors leading to urinary symptoms is probably of minimal importance as a cause of low urinary tract imbalance.

Longhurst and associates found that ovariectomy has no effect on micturition or bladder mass in the female rat[103]; however, it causes a significant decrease in contractile responsiveness of the bladder body, which also decreased in castrated rats, thereby indicating that the effects of castration are general phenomena and not necessarily linked to specific receptor changes. So, at least in the rat, decreases in sex hormones have a negligible effect on bladder function. Nevertheless, several studies have reported the use of HRT in the treatment of stress urinary incontinence. Regimens include oral or combined therapy, vaginal therapy, and, more recently, transdermal therapy and vaginal rings.

The rationale for estrogen treatment involves the hormone's ability to cause proliferation and increased thickness of the urethral mucosa, thereby increasing tension in the venous sinusoids secondary to increased vaginal vascular flow and increasing urethral resistance.[104, 105] Estrogen also has a positive effect on the "urethral softness factor." In addition, there may be other effects related to the fibroelastic tissue, periurethral musculature, and pelvic floor.[60, 106]

Oral Therapy

Raz and associates observed symptomatic improvement in GSI in 65% of cases using oral treatment of 2.5 mg/day of conjugated estrogens; there was a corresponding increase in maximum urethral closing pressure (MUCP).[107] On the other hand, administration of medroxyprogesterone acetate of 20 mg/day caused an increase in symptoms in 60% of cases. They attributed the positive effect of estrogens to mucosal proliferation, which led to an improved mucosal seal effect and enhancement of the alpha-adrenergic contractile response of the urethral smooth musculature to endogenous catecholamines. Rud in 1980 observed in 27 postmenopausal women a significant increase in maximum urethral pressure (MUP) and functional urethral length (FUL) at rest and an improvement in the PTR to the urethra following estrogenic oral therapy.[56] In terms of a clinical or urodynamic response, he saw no difference with the oral administration of either 4 mg/day of estradiol or 8 mg/day of estriol. Even though in 70% of cases subjective improvement was reported, he did not observe any significant correlation between subjective improvement in GSI and the increase in pressure profile and urethral length. Faber and Heidenreich in 1977 obtained subjective improvement in GSI in 34% of cases with the use of 2 mg/day of estriol, but no patient became continent even though in 95% of cases an increase in the urethral pressure profile was observed.[69] In a different investigation Ek and colleagues did not obtain a positive effect on parameters of importance for female stress incontinence in 13 postmenopausal women after treatment with 2 mg/day of oral estradiol.[108] Samsioe and colleagues conducted in 34 postmenopausal women a double-blind cross-over study using a dose of estriol of 3 mg/day; they noted that the treatment was effective in alleviating urgency and mixed incontinence but not in improving GSI.[100] Walter and co-workers, in a double-blind clinical trial using estradiol 2 mg/day combined with estriol 1 mg/day, noted subjective improvement in frequency, urgency, and urge incontinence, although GSI was unaffected and there were no significant changes in urethral pressure or urethral length.[109]

High doses of orally administered estrogens result in a significant increase in MUP and urethral length and an improved PTR over the urethra,[71] but no effects of low-dose oral contraceptives on the variables of the urethral pressure profile have been observed.[110]

Fantl and colleagues recently published a meta-analysis on ERT in the management of urinary incontinence in postmenopausal women.[111] From a review of 166 articles, only 23 were evaluated for strictly included criteria. Meta-analysis found an overall significant effect of estrogen therapy on subjective improvement for all subjects ($p < .01$) and for subjects with GSI alone ($p < .05$). Although the results showed no significant effect on quantity of fluid lost, they did reveal a significant effect ($p < .05$) on MUCP. Therefore, ERT has an effect only on subjective symptoms, and the mechanism of action of estrogen at the cellular level is still poorly understood.

Combined Therapy

Kinn and Lindskog in 1988 treated 36 postmenopausal women affected by GSI with oral estriol, 2 mg/day, and phenylpropanolamine (PPA), 50 mg/day, alone and in combination in a study with a crossover design.[112] MUCP increased after the use of PPA or PPA in combination with estriol, but not with estriol alone. Estriol alone has also caused an increase in MUCP in patients with low urethral pressure, confirming the theory of an insufficient tightening of the urethral walls, unlike patients with a PTR defect due to a weakness of the pelvic floor.

Beisland and colleagues, in a randomized crossover trial, treated 20 postmenopausal women suffering from urinary incontinence due to poor urethral closing pressure with a normal PTR.[113] PPA, 100 mg/day, and estriol cream, 1 mg/day, were administered separately and in combination. Both PPA and E_3 (estriol cream) increased the MUCP, but combined treatment was substantially more effective. With combined treatment eight patients became completely continent, nine improved, and only one remained unchanged. Even though there was a significant increase in urethral pressure, there was no meaningful correlation between clinical improvement and the urodynamic pattern.

Walter and associates, in a randomized double-blind placebo-controlled study, treated a group of 28 postmenopausal women affected by GSI by using oral estriol, 4 mg/day, or PPA, 50 mg/day, alone or in combination.[114] Two patients became continent on PPA, two on estriol, and 12 of 28 on combined treatment. Hilton and colleagues in a double-blind study compared oral and vaginal estrogens (conjugated estrogens in a dose of 1.25 mg/day) and placebo, alone and in combination with PPA, 100 mg/day.[98] Frequency and nocturia were both reduced with vaginal estrogen therapy and enhanced by the addition of PPA. GSI improved mainly with the combined treatment, but urodynamic parameters did not change in accordance with clinical improvement.

Schreiter and colleagues found that MUP increased after a single dose of 300 mg of phenylephrine.[39] Administration of 2 mg of estriol after 10 days in patients affected by GSI caused a marked increase in FUL and PTR; as a result, the patients became continent both subjectively and clinically.

Combined treatment is certainly more effective than treatment with the same drugs separately, but this enhanced effect is very moderate compared with the effect of PPA alone and therefore raises some doubt about combined treatment because of the risk of adverse side effects.

Vaginal Therapy

Whitehead and associates showed that the vaginal epithelium cleaves the sulfate radicals from estrone, increasing its conversion into estradiol to a greater degree than what occurs in the gastrointestinal tract.[115] Therefore, it is possible that the estrone-estradiol ratio after vaginal administration of estrogens has a greater estrogenizing effect on pelvic tissues than that occurring after oral administration.[72] Estrogens in the vaginal creams (estriol) are systematically absorbed, however, yielding physiologic premenopausal levels of estrogens that can suppress serum gonadotropins by as much as 30%.[116, 117] Estriol is a short-acting estrogen that does not bind firmly to plasma proteins,[118] and most of the unconjugated plasma estriol fraction is probably biologically active. Estriol binds to the same receptor as estradiol,[119, 120] but in contrast to estradiol it causes a brief monophasic increase in the nuclear estrogen-receptor complex[121] that is more effective than the oral route.

Vaginal administration of estriol is preferred[122] because oral administration has been found to have a minimal effect on urethral pressure. There are some advantages to vaginal administration of estriol to postmenopausal women, namely, the great difference in absorption and pharmacokinetics (0.5 to 1 mg estriol given vaginally does not differ significantly from 8 to 12 mg estriol given orally) and avoidance of the first liver passage in the enterohepatic recirculation.[123] Moreover, various authors believe that estriol is relatively danger-free in stimulating sex hormone-binding globulin,[124] coagulation factors,[125] HDL cholesterol and triglycerides,[97] and plasma renin activity.[126]

The effect of estriol on urethral and vaginal epithelium can be accurately evaluated by using the karyopyknotic index, which is a method of assessing quantitatively the biologic power of estrogenic activity.[127] In treatment with estrogens the difficulty is not how to achieve a therapeutic effect but how to avoid giving too large a dose and how to minimize the risk of undesirable side effects. This result is achieved by using the lowest possible therapeutic effective dosage. A dose of 0.5 to 1 mg one to two times daily is often needed, whereas for maintenance the same dose only two or three times a week is required.

Many studies have shown that vaginally administered estriol in low doses induces proliferation of the vaginal epithelium without affecting the endometrium.[128, 129] Kicovic and colleagues gave 0.5 mg estriol daily for 2 to 3 weeks, followed by a maintenance dosage of 0.5 mg twice a week.[128] After 16 weeks of treatment, no endometrial proliferation was found.[127] Mattsson and Cullberg reported that after 0.5 mg estriol daily for 14 days, no endometrial stimulation was seen.[129] Other studies have shown that some stimulation, albeit minimal, occurs with low-dose vaginal estriol even though side effects are absent. Englund and associates reported that 0.5 mg estriol administered once a day for 16 days induced an estrogenic effect in the surface of the endometrium.[130] Fink and colleagues reported that after 3 months of treatment with 0.5 mg estriol daily, some of the women showed ultrastructural changes in the endometrium similar to those seen in the midproliferation phase of the menstrual cycle.[131]

In vaginal treatment with estrogens, the dosages administered and the results obtained have varied considerably. In a prospective study Bhatia and colleagues treated a group of 11 postmenopausal women affected by GSI with 2 g of conjugated estrogen vaginal cream administered daily for a total of 6 weeks.[132] Cure resulted in 54.5% with increased MUCP and improved PTR to the proximal urethra. The use of estrogen vaginal cream resulted in a twofold increase in circulating estradiol levels and a threefold increase in estrone levels. The favorable clinical response correlated either with urodynamic findings of increased UCP and improved PTR to the proximal urethra or with urethral cytologic findings. The number of urethral transitional cells at the midurethra decreased significantly in women who responded favorably, and increased numbers of intermediate and squamous cells were noted. A favorable estrogen effect was achieved by a process of squamous metaplasia. A decreased number of estrogen receptors in the urethral mucosa could account for the poor response in women who were nonresponsive to vaginal therapy.

Hilton and Stanton observed that conjugated estrogen cream, 2 g/day, improved the symptoms of GSI, urgency, and voiding difficulties but caused no change in the resting urethral pressure, only an improvement in the PTR, which was observable as well, however, in patients who had no improvement in symptomatology.[72] These authors advanced the hypothesis that the improved PTR that occurs in the midurethra after estrogen therapy is probably due to extraurethral factors such as improved efficiency of the pelvic floor reflex. Indirect confirmation of this idea comes from a urodynamic investigation of continent women before and after treatment with danazol (an antiestrogen drug). It was found that despite considerably decreased plasma estrogens, the urethral pressure profile at rest was almost unaffected, whereas the PTR decreased in several patients.[133]

Iosif in 1992 studied the effectiveness of protracted vaginal administration of estriol (0.5 mg twice a week for a period ranging from 1 to 10 years) in a group of 80 postmenopausal women.[42] Clinically, 30 of 40 patients (75%) with GSI symptoms reported subjective improvement or cure of their incontinence. No significant change was observed in urethral pressure or functional length except for a significant increase in the PTR to the proximal urethra in patients who improved or were cured ($p < .01$).

Moreover, the amount of estrogen as well as the duration of treatment is important for the proliferation of the urethral epithelium. Heimer and Englund in 1992 studied 40 postmenopausal women to determine the effect of estriol on the vaginal and urethral epithelia.[34] They used two different intravaginal doses (0.5 mg/weekly and 0.5 mg/twice weekly) for a period of 6 weeks. Despite the initial epithelial maturation in the vagina and urethra (significant increase in karyopyknotic index, $p < .001$), this effect did not last long, and in 4 weeks the epithelia returned to pretreatment values. According to a study by Semmens and colleagues, the vaginal blood flow, pH, and transvaginal electropotential require 18 to 24 months of estrogen treatment to reach their maximum response. All these findings may indicate that estrogen treatment in elderly women with urogenital disorders should be of long duration, perhaps even lifelong.

Transdermal Therapy

In transdermal estrogen therapy (TET) a continuous and constant controlled release through the skin of 17 beta-estradiol at a substantially lower daily dose than that given orally (measured in micrograms instead of milligrams) is used. The release of estradiol directly into the circulatory system, avoiding first-pass liver metabolism, does not cause hepatic synthesis activation of angiotensinogen and therefore does not increase the risk of arterial hypertension.

The quantity of estradiol administered depends on the diameter of the contact surface of the system. The dose available varies from 25 to 100 µg/day applied two times a week for a period of no less than 3 weeks, followed by an interval of 1 week. This dose may or may not be associated with a sequential progestin during the last 10 to 12 days of each estrogen cycle. Some authors contend, however, that eliminating the first-pass effect on the liver that occurs with oral estrogens reduces the beneficial rise in HDL levels that is seen with oral estrogen replacement. Two recent studies have shown that patients have a high level of compliance with TET, which produced high success rates in relieving subjective symptoms. Mueck and colleagues treated a group of 118 postmenopausal women suffering from severe urogenital complaints and reported that 79% were symptom-free 6 months after treatment.[136] In another study of 21 postmenopausal women suffering from GSI, a TET dose of 50 µg proved to be highly successful in 16 of 21 patients (76%).[137]

Injection Therapy

Injectable estrogens, composed of a synthetic ester of estradiol, are available in depot preparations. The release rate is not constant (being very high initially and then abruptly decreasing), and more frequent injections may be needed to control symptoms. Thus, thermosensory and other areas of the brain and nervous system are up-regulated and fixed at a higher level. Therefore, routine use of this pharmacologic elevation of estrogen is a matter of concern because of hyperestrogenism (thrombosis and hormonal related cancers).[138]

New Treatment Modalities

Newer sustained-release subcutaneous estrogen pellets (25 or 50 mg) may be available. 17-beta-estradiol is delivered with these pellets, and the level remains fairly constant for 3 to 6 months, although it may be so highly elevated that it requires monitoring of blood levels. Vaginal rings that release 8 µg of estradiol per 24 hours for 90 days are a new device developed for the treatment of urogenital atrophy. In a Swedish multiple-center independent trial[139] carried out in 222 postmenopausal women with an estradiol vaginal ring, cure or improvement of symptoms and signs was obtained in 90% of patients. The great majority of patients (>90%) showed good acceptability of the device.

ESTROGENS AND SENSORY DISORDERS

Irritative symptoms due to sensory disorders (urgency-frequency syndrome, atrophic urethritis, and urethral syndrome) in postmenopausal women with or without incontinence seem to respond to ERT.[140, 141] Everett was the first to observe an association between senile atrophic vaginitis and lower urinary tract symptoms and suggested that the urinary symptoms were due to a change in the urethra linked to the estrogenic deficiency.[46] Natural variations in estrogenic activity affect the squamous epithelium that covers the distal urethra. In the absence of hormones an atrophic change in the urethral mucosa takes place similar to that occurring in the vagina. Although the atrophic urethritis may be asymptomatic, it is often associated with urethral syndrome characterized by recurrent episodes of frequency, urgency, nocturia, and dysuria.[48] Bent and colleagues, in an initial diagnosis in 100 postmenopausal women, showed that the urethral syndrome was first in order of frequency prior to 70 years of age (occurring in 40% of cases) and then declined to 14% after that age.[142] Also in postmenopausal women, Smith observed that both urinary symptoms and urethral cytologic results responded positively to HRT, but that treatment had to take place within 1 year after the beginning of the symptoms.[143] Otherwise, at a later stage, the dystrophic inflammation might first cause a fibrosis and later a stricture. Walter, in a double-blind trial on 29 postmenopausal women given estriol plus estradiol administered orally, observed subjective healing in 63% of the patients affected by sensory urge incontinence.[114] This result was also observed by Salmon and colleagues, Geist and Salmon, and Siegel and associates in noncontrolled treatment series.[145–147] Samsioe and associates, using an oral treatment of 3 mg/day of estriol, obtained subjective improvement in 65% of patients affected by sensory disorders.[100] A recent study by Fantl and colleagues highlighted the role played by estrogens in sensory disorders.[144] They hypothesized that hypoestrogenism affects the sensory threshold of the urinary tract, and therefore estrogens have a beneficial effect on the proprioceptive sensory threshold.

ESTROGENS AND DETRUSOR INSTABILITY

Although estrogens are useful in treating sensory urge incontinence, information on their potential use in the treatment of motor urge incontinence is scarce. The response of the bladder during pregnancy and the menstrual cycle and the potentiating effect of estrogen pretreatment on the contractile response of isolated animal detrusor muscle to alpha-agonists, prostaglandins, and cholinergic drugs suggest that estrogens might exacerbate bladder instability. Progesterone, on the other hand, based on animal studies[148] and urodynamic studies performed during the menstrual cycle,[38] may be of therapeutic use, although this has never been tested in clinical trials; it might, however, aggravate any associated stress incontinence.

Endometriosis

Endometriosis is a disorder in which abnormal growth tissue histologically resembling the endometrium is present in locations other than the uterine lining. Endometriosis is found almost exclusively in women of reproductive age. The lesions are usually found on the peritoneal surface of the reproductive organs and adjacent structures of the pelvis, but they can occur anywhere in the body.

EPIDEMIOLOGY

The incidence and prevalence in the population range from 1 to 50%.[149–151] The wide range results from the basic difficulty of collecting data. It is a common belief that the widespread knowledge and use of laparoscopic techniques may lead to better diagnosis, especially for patients with minimal and mild disease. Retrospective studies are not reliable, especially in mild cases. Endometriosis is the most common single gynecologic diagnosis responsible for hospitalization of women aged 15 to 44, being found in more than 6.2% of patients.[152]

PATHOGENESIS

The cause of endometriosis is unknown. More than a dozen theories have been offered in an attempt to explain it, but none have satisfactorily explained all of the features of the disease. Traditionally, the theories fall into the following groups:

1. Tubal regurgitation of menstrual epithelium. It has been proposed that fragments of müllerian mucosa arising from the uterus or oviduct are carried into the peritoneal cavity with menstrual fluid, where they become implanted on various structures and maintain the histologic characteristics of normal uterine tissue.
2. Lymphatic or vascular metastasis. This theory proposes that endometrium is transported via the lymphatic channels and the vascular system. The theory attempts to explain the finding of aberrant implants in lymph nodes, lungs, and pleura (i.e., documented sites of disease that cannot reasonably be explained by the theory of regurgitant menstrual flow).
3. Coelomic metaplasia. This theory is based on the observation that the peritoneal mesothelium, the müllerian epithelium, and the germinal epithelium of the ovary are all derived from a common embryonic tissue. It is suggested that these tissues retain the potential for further differentiation. The rare occurrence of endometriosis in men is often taken as proof of this theory. In certain conditions germinal epithelium or peritoneum may undergo metaplasia to form functioning endometrium.
4. Immune system alteration. The immune system plays a role in the pathophysiology of endometriosis,[153] and some patterns commonly seen in other autoimmune diseases are more frequent in women's family history and multiorgan involvement. According to Dmowsky and colleagues, endometriosis is a disorder of "immune surveillance recognition and destruction of endometrial cells."[153] During this process, in nonendometriotic women, endometrial self-antigens are eliminated by monocytes, T-helper cells activating T and B cells, and then macrophages. Macrophages inhibit endometrial cell proliferation. Natural killer cells and T cells are cytotoxic, and B cells may produce autoantibodies against normal endometrial antigens. Endometriotic patients have an abnormal response—the immune system does not stop the disease, producing prostaglandins, interleukin-1, growth cells, and autoantibodies that enhance endometrial ectopic cell proliferation. Danazol, a drug often used by gynecologists in the treatment of endometriosis as a hormonal or antihormonal agent, has some unforeseen effects on the monocyte-macrophage system (suppressing it) and on the B-cell level (it inhibits cellular activation and autoantibody production)[153] in endometriosis. Gonadotropin-releasing hormone agonists (GnRH-a) have less or no effect on the concentration of autoantibodies.[154, 155]

Natural killer cell activity, cytotoxicity, and peritoneal macrophages are decreased in patients with endometriosis.[156–159] Peritoneal macrophages are supposed to stimulate proliferation of endometrial cells.[160]

INVASION MECHANISM

ADHESION AND LOCAL PROTEOLYSIS Laminin, a glycoprotein found in the basilemma, together with fibronectins, acts as a bridge for the fixation of endometriotic cells to the peritoneum.[161, 162] The second stage is that of C local proteolysis, in which the role of collagenase type IV is thought to be important, just as it is in oncology.[163] It is also thought that some of the aggressive processes characteristic of tumor cells are active in this process, leading to a certain local aggression. This datum is supported by clinical experience.[164, 165]

C-MYC PROTO-ONCOGENES The proto-oncogenes are genes assigned to regulate cell division and differentiation and are thus very similar to some viral oncogenes present in some tumors.[165] The C-myc gene codifies a protein whose quantity is directly correlated with cellular proliferation and DNA production and is inversely correlated with cellular differentiation. Estrogens cause a rapid and transitory expression of the C-myc gene in some tissues. Using the polymerase chain reaction (PCR) and immunohistochemistry, an attempt was made to determine whether the C-myc polypeptide was in any way involved in the control mechanisms of healthy endometrial cells and endometriotic cells.[164] Preliminary histochemical studies showed that the C-myc gene is expressed in normal endometrial cells, and, to a lesser degree and in a less homogeneous way, in endometriotic cells. These data have been confirmed by PCR studies.[166–169] The next step will be to check the interaction between hormones, growth factors, and C-myc genes. It is expected that specific monoclonal antibodies able to selectively inhibit DNA and DNA-polymerase synthesis will be synthesized and that C-myc gene microinjections or transfers may induce dormant cells to begin the cellular cycle.

CLINICAL PRESENTATION

Endometriosis may present with a variety of manifestations, the frequency and severity of which appear to correlate better with the location than with the extent of the disease. Classic symptoms include cyclic pelvic pain, dysmenorrhea, dyspareunia, and infertility. Cyclic pelvic pain is believed to be related to the sequential swelling and extravasation of blood and menstrual debris into the surrounding tissues. However, pelvic pain may occur at any time during the cycle and frequently becomes chronic. Dyspareunia is a common symptom, especially in patients whose disease involves the posterior cul-de-sac, uterosacral ligaments, rectovaginal septum, or upper vagina; in addition, postcoital pain is frequently reported in this group of patients. Infertility may be present in the absence of other symptoms of endometriosis and affects 30 to 40% of women with diagnosed endometriosis (approximately two times the incidence in the general population). The urinary tract is affected in approximately 1% of cases. Of these, the bladder is affected in 19% and the ureter in 15% of patients; renal involvement is rare, but progression to uremia is serious.

SYMPTOMS AND SIGNS

Endometriosis of the bladder entails discomfort or suprapubic pain in 78% of patients and irritative symptoms (e.g., frequency, urgency, dysuria) in 71%.[170, 171] The timing of symptoms varies from a week before until the end of menstruation. Hematuria during menstruation is a characteristic symptom, but only 20 to 30% of patients have macrohematuria.[170] Bladder lesions ordinarily exist along with lesions in other pelvic locations. O'Conor and Greenhill report that only in 12% of cases does the bladder constitute the sole location of endometriosis.[172]

Involvement of the ureter is the most serious complication of endometriosis. In fact, in more than 25% of cases the ureteral location leads to permanent renal insufficiency. In less than 15% of cases is it bilateral,[173] and in the majority of cases the distal third of the ureter is involved, although some clinical work has reported involvement of the proximal ureter.[174]

Ureteral involvement is characterized by menstrual disturbances, specific abdominal or side pains, and macrohematuria.[175] Approximately 14% of cases are completely asymptomatic.

Ureteral endometriosis has classically been divided into intrinsic and extrinsic types, with a 1:4 ratio of intrinsic to extrinsic.[176] *Intrinsic endometriosis* consists of infiltrating implants involving the ureteral muscle or the lamina propria, or both, and may extend into the lumen, simulating a polypoid ureteral neoplasm. *Extrinsic endometriosis* consists of foci located around the adventitia and surrounding structures that can also compress "ab extrinsico."[177] Vesical locations in the uterosacral ligament or in adjacent pelvic structures may cause an obstruction extrinsic to the ureter.

It is interesting to note that, unlike vesical or intestinal endometriosis, ureteral endometriosis is not necessarily of the same cyclic nature as menstruation.[178]

Involvement of the upper urinary tract with obstructions becomes manifest by the appearance of headaches, backaches, and hypertension; the appearance of pyelonephritis, however, is rare, and a progressive renal insufficiency may arise in a stealthy way.[179]

Endometriosis located in the kidney has the most insidious course and most frequently involves side pains during menstruation as well as macro- or microhematuria. A urethral location of endometriosis is extremely rare, and the current literature reports only one case, characterized clinically by vaginal pain and occasional loss of urine without hematuria or puruloid urethral secretions.[180]

DIAGNOSIS

PHYSICAL EXAMINATION Essential for diagnosis is a physical examination that includes rectal and vaginal exploration. In fact, as reported by Abeshouse and Abeshouse, vaginal exploration reveals palpable masses in approximately 50% of patients with genitourinary and vesical endometriosis.[170] An accurate assessment of the uterosacral and cardinal ligaments is useful for the appraisal of possible extrinsic compression on the ureter or kidneys.

LABORATORY TESTS The first step in diagnosis is the urine test, which most frequently reveals a macrohematuria; pyuria is often present in patients with vesical endometriosis.

MARKERS A vast amount of research conducted for many years has focused energy on the search for an ideal marker that can determine the course of the disease in a sensitive and specified way. As often occurs in other fields of biology, this ideal marker has yet to be identified.

STUDY OF PERITONEAL FLUIDS The peritoneal fluid has been considered an ultrafiltrate of plasma and under normal conditions is present in a very limited quantity (up to 5 ml). During the periovular period this quantity increases to approximately 20 ml. In patients affected by endometriosis an alteration in the components of this fluid occurs that is yet to be studied in depth or understood in full. The most frequently studied components of peritoneal fluids are[181] C3-complement, alpha-2 macroglobulin, Ca 125, and dependent progesterone endometrial protein.

IMAGING TECHNIQUES For patients with urologic symptoms, appropriate radiologic and endoscopic investigations can be conducted. Radiologic investigations should be used for the identification of pelvic masses that compress or shift the adjacent organs. These are best performed during menstruation. In particular, intravenous pyelography can reveal an obstruction of the distal third of the ureter with or without the hydronephrosis or hydroureteronephrosis characteristic of ureteral endometriosis, and it can reveal a "minus" or a vesical compression.[182] Retrograde ureteropyelography helps to differentiate between extrinsic and intrinsic ureteral involvement, and endoscopy can also help in differential diagnosis. Entities important in differential diagnosis include radiotransparent ureteral calculi, neoplasms, ureteral stenosis, and cystic ureteritis. Computed tomography (CT) scans and magnetic resonance imaging (MRI) are not diagnostic but may be useful in monitoring disease progression or regression.

Ultrasonography is the most commonly used means of diagnosis. It can ascertain the presence and dimensions of a possible pelvic mass and establish whether it is solid or cystic without exposing the patient to ionizing radiation. This method, however, does not have very high sensitivity. Friedman and colleagues correlated the reliability of ultrasonography with that of laparoscopy and found that ultrasonography is capable of diagnosing only 11% of endometriosis in patients with nonpalpable masses.[183]

CT scans add little to ultrasound diagnosis and present the added risk of exposure to radiation. MRI, on the other hand, has the advantage of producing multilayer images and has a good sensitivity to "blood," and this often permits a preoperative diagnosis of endometriosis. In fact, it has a sensitivity of between 60 and 70% and a specificity of between 70 and 80%.[184, 185] It is nonetheless important to emphasize that it remains difficult to differentiate endometriosis from teratoma, hemorrhagic cystitis, and cystadenoma.

LAPAROSCOPY Definitive diagnosis can be performed through direct visualization and, in several cases, through biopsy during laparoscopy. In fact, laparoscopy is the gold standard for diagnosis. The most common sites for endometriosis in the pelvis are, in order of frequency, the ovaries (60%), posterior broad ligaments, posterior cul-de-sac, uterosacral ligaments, and anterior cul-de-sac. Hemosiderine-stained "powder burns" and ovarian chocolate cysts are the classic lesions described. Laparoscopic photography or video recording may be helpful if available. The extent of disease should be classified according to the revised American Fertility Society classification of endometriosis (R AFS 1985)[186] from stage 1 to stage 4: normal, mild, moderate, and severe. This is the most accepted and well-known classification of endometriotic lesions, although it does not include the recently studied peritoneal abnormalities related to the disease.[187–190]

CYSTOSCOPY The key examination in patients with vesical endometriosis is cystoscopy with biopsy. Cystoscopy is indicated in all patients with hematuria during menstruation and in those in whom vesical symptoms become worse during menstruation. Cystoscopy should be performed immediately before or at the beginning of menstruation; the endometriotic lesion appears as a swollen and bluish cystic lesion, ordinarily located at the vesical base, trigone, or dome. If the overlying mucosa is ulcerated, bleeding may appear. After menstruation the lesion will be less turgescent, less swollen, and less reddish. The lesion is ordinarily isolated and approximately 1 cm long, although some may be small and closely grouped cysts of a few millimeters.

The biopsy must reveal both the endometrial stroma and the glands. The most important entity in the differential diagnosis of vesical endometriosis is primitive cancer of the bladder. Because the lesion is ordinarily submucosal, a superficial biopsy may show only a cystitis or may even be normal. If the endoscopic evaluation is discordant with the biopsy that reveals only an inflamed area, it is imperative to repeat the examination and the biopsy during another phase of the menstrual cycle. When there is a strong suspicion of endometriosis, it is advisable to perform the cystoscopy in conjunction with laparoscopy.

THERAPY

Treatment of patients with endometriosis should be based on patient age, severity of symptoms, extent of disease, duration of infertility, presence of pelvic pain, and urinary referral symptoms.[177] A conservative approach is recommended for patients who are symptom-free or are only mildly symptomatic and have minimal pelvic findings. Regular examinations should be carried out at intervals of 6 months. Evidence of progression of the disease requires more specific treatment.

The range of therapies includes (1) danazol, (2) progestins, (3) GnRH analogs, (4) laparoscopic surgery, and (5) surgical reconstruction. Hormonal treatment with estrogens, androgens, and hormonal derivatives is often used in patients with recent endometriosis who are free of ovarian enlargement or who have moderate vesical involvement or low-grade ureteral involvement.

DANAZOL Danazol, an orally active synthetic derivative of 17-ethinyl testosterone, is the most effective approved drug for suppression of endometriosis.[191] Several theories about its mode of action have been proposed; there is evidence of effects on the hypothalamus, pituitary, ovary, and endometrium, as well as on endometriotic lesions. Both plasma LH and FSH levels, especially the midcycle surges, are suppressed, probably through inhibition of the release of gonadotropins from the pituitary. In addition danazol directly inhibits enzymes involved in steroidogenesis. Finally, the drug interacts with other cytosolic hormone receptors, explaining in part the androgenic, progestational, glucocorticoid, and estrogenic activities of danazol. Then again, even if the standard dose is 400 to 800 mg per day orally for 6 months, doses of less than 800 mg are not able to induce amenorrhea.[192] Side effects in 85% of cases include weight gain, acne, and hirsutism. Fortunately, these symptoms rapidly disappear on suspension of therapy, except for voice changes, which are not always reversible.

PROGESTIN REGIMEN Progestins such as medroxyprogesterone acetate, 10 to 30 mg orally per day, cause decidualization and eventual atrophy of endometriotic implants. Side effects include breakthrough bleeding (50%), weight gain, fluid retention, and depression.

GNRH ANALOGS The most recent advance in the medical management of endometriosis is the use of GnRH analogs that induce a transient rise in FSH and LH followed by a profound hypogonadotropic hypogonadism due to pituitary receptor down-regulation. The castrate levels of estrogens result in glandular involution and stromal atrophy of endometriotic implants. Side effects include hot flashes, sweats, vaginal dryness, and trabecular bone loss.

SURGICAL TREATMENT The surgical approach to endometriosis includes conservative surgery, mostly by laser with the preservation of the uterus and as much ovarian tissue as possible, and radical surgery in patients for whom fertility is no longer an issue. For lower urinary tract localization several reconstructive procedures have been devised.

In patients with vesical endometriosis Abeshouse and Abeshouse advocate localized excision of the endometriotic area or a partial cystectomy in patients in whom (1) the lesion is limited to the bladder with no involvement of other pelvic organs; (2) the vesical lesions are accompanied by other lesions affecting the pelvic organs; or (3) the vesical lesions are accompanied by a serious involvement of the upper urinary tract or a malignancy affecting the endometrial vesical lesions.[170]

Endometriosis that involves the bladder or the pelvis can lead to a gradual unilateral or bilateral ureteral obstruction causing serious damage to the upper urinary tract. The preferred treatment for ureteral endometriosis is revision of the concerned area, the restoration of the urinary tract's continuity, and bilateral adnexectomy with or without hysterectomy. In fact, mainly in patients with longstanding endometriosis, a large amount of collagen and scar tissue that is not responsive to hormonal treatment can be observed.[193] In patients who are hopeful for future pregnancy the conservation of the ovaries is imperative. However, many authors have reported that when the ovaries are conserved, 27% of patients require further surgery, whereas less than 3% of patients who undergo abdominal hysterectomy with bilateral oophorectomy require further surgery for the treatment of endometriosis.[194]

Many authors have stressed the importance of ureterolysis compared with ureteral resection in cases of moderate endometriosis. In fact, however, this procedure is indicated in patients with extrinsic endometriosis when, following decompression of the obstructed tract, there is a recovery of peristalsis testifying to morphologic and functional integrity.

Preoperative hormonal treatment can reduce the risk of endometrial implants, and postoperative hormonal treatment is recommended in patients undergoing ureterolysis. If any impairment in blood flow or fibrosis with persistent hydroureteronephrosis has occurred, resection of the tract of the involved ureter is preferred. Because the stenosis is ordinarily situated at the level of the distal ureter, the treatment preferred is a ureterocystoneostomy, eventually associated with a psoas hitch. A ureteroureteroanastomosis has also been proposed, but this entails a higher risk of vascular complications owing to the complex and delicate nature of the vascularization of the distal ureter. In some cases it is possible to use a Boari flap, a transureteroureteroanastomosis of the ileal ureter. The most severe complication of ureteral involvement during endometriosis is irreversible kidney damage.

In a 1987 review of the published literature, Gehr and Sica reported that at the time of diagnosis of ureteral obstruction due to endometriosis, 32% of the kidneys involved were lost.[195] A later review by Klein and Cattolica concluded that many of these kidneys could have been saved.[175] They attributed this loss to excessive diagnostic delay in 46% of cases and erroneous diagnosis in 30% of cases. If there is any possibility of functional rehabilitation it is advisable to insert a nephrostomy. If, however, normal function of the kidney is irreversibly compromised, the preferred procedure is nephrectomy.

REFERENCES

1. Iosif CS, Batra S, Anders E, et al: Estrogen receptors in the human female lower urinary tract. Am J Obstet Gynecol 141:817, 1981.

2. Batra S, Iosif CS: Female urethra: A target for estrogen action. J Urol 129:418, 1983.
3. Batra S, Iosif S: Functional estrogen receptors in the female urethra. *In* Proceedings of the 2nd Joint Meeting of the International Continence Society and Urodynamic Society, 1983, p 548.
4. Andersson KE, Sjögren C: Aspects of the physiology and pharmacology of the bladder and urethra. Prog Neurobiol 19:71, 1982.
5. Hodgson BJ, Dumas S, Bolling DR, et al: Effect of estrogen or sensitivity of rabbit bladder and urethra to phenylephrine. Invest Urol 16:67, 1978.
6. Downie JW, Dean DM, Carro-Ciampi G, et al: A difference in sensitivity in alpha-adrenergic agonists exhibited by detrusor and bladder neck of rabbit. Can J Physiol Pharmacol 53:525, 1975.
7. Roberts JM, Insel PA, Goldfien A: The regulation of myometrial adrenoceptors and adrenergic response by sex steroids. Mol Pharmacol 20:52, 1981.
8. Bleisch W, Luine VN, Nottebahm F: Modification of synapses in androgen-sensitive muscle. Hormonal regulation of acetylcholine receptor number in the songbird syrinx. J Neurosci 4:786, 1984.
9. Gejman PV, Cardinali DP: Hormone effects on muscarinic cholinergic binding in bovine and rat sympathetic superior cervical ganglia. Life Sci 32:965, 1983.
10. Roberts JM, Insel PA, Goldfien RD, Goldfien A: Alpha receptors but not beta receptors increase in rabbit uterus with oestrogen. Nature 270:624, 1977.
11. Diamond J, Brody TM: Hormonal alteration of the response of the rat uterus to catecholamines. Life Sci 5:2187, 1966.
12. Raz S, Zeigler M, Adoni A: Hormonal environment and uterine response to epinephrine. Am J Obstet Gynecol 111:345, 1971.
13. Coupar JM, Turner P: Relative potencies of sympathetic amines in human smooth muscle. Br J Pharmacol 36:213, 1969.
14. Awad SA, Downie JW, Kinuluta HG: Alpha-adrenergic agents in urinary disorders of the proximal urethra. Part 1: Sphincteric incontinence. Br J Urol 50:332, 1978.
15. Castleden CM, George CF, Renwick AG, et al: Imipramine a possible alternative to current therapy for urinary incontinence in the elderly. J Urol 125:318, 1981.
16. Awad SA, Bruce AW, Carro-Ciampi G, et al: Distribution of α and β adrenoceptors in human urinary bladder. Br J Pharmacol 50:525, 1974.
17. Nergardh A, Boreus LO: Autonomic receptor function in the lower urinary tract of man and cat. Scand J Urol 8:32, 1972.
18. Kuroda H, Kohrogy T, Uchida N, et al: Urinary retention induced by estrogen injections in mice: An analytical model. J Urol 134:1268, 1985.
19. Williams LT, Lefkowitz RJ: Regulation of rabbit myometrial alpha adrenergic receptors by estrogen and progesterone. J Clin Invest 60:815, 1977.
20. Levin RM, Jacobowitz DJ, Wein AJ: Autonomic innervation of the rabbit urinary bladder following estrogen administration. Urology 17:449, 1981.
21. Sjöberg NO: The adrenergic transmitter of the female reproductive tract: Distribution and functional change. Acta Physiol Scand (Suppl 305) 1, 1968.
22. Bulbring E, Tomita T: The effects of catecholamines on the membrane resistance and spike generation in the smooth muscle of guinea pig *Taenia coli*. J Physiol 194:74, 1968.
23. Kuriyama H, Csapo A: A study of the parturient uterus with a microelectrode technique. Endocrinology 68:1010, 1961.
24. Callahan SM, Creed KE: The effects of estrogens on spontaneous activity and responses to phenylephrine of the mammalian urethra. J Physiol 358:35, 1985.
25. Iversen LL: Role of the transmitter uptake mechanisms in synaptic transmission. Br J Pharmacol 41:571, 1971.
26. Gillespie JS: Uptake of noradrenaline by smooth muscle. Br Med Bull 29:136, 1973.
27. Levin RM, Shofer SF, Wein AJ: Estrogen induced alteration in the autonomic response of the rabbit urinary bladder. J Pharmacol Exp Ther 215:614, 1980.
28. Shapiro E: Effect of estrogens on the weight and muscarinic cholinergic receptor density of the rabbit bladder and urethra. J Urol 135:1084, 1986.
29. Hills NH: Prostaglandins and the tone in isolated strips of mammalian bladder. Br J Pharmacol 57:464, 1976.
30. Andersson KE, Henriksson L, Ulmsten U: Effects of prostaglandin E$_2$ applied locally on intravesical and intraurethral pressures in women. Eur Urol 4:366, 1978.
31. Bultitude MI, Hill NH, Shuttleworth KED: Clinical and experimental studies on the action of prostaglandins and their synthesis inhibitors on detrusor muscle in vivo and in vitro. Br J Urol 48:631, 1976.
32. Borda E, Chaud M, Gutnisky R, et al: Relationships between prostaglandins and estrogens on the motility of isolated rings from the rat urinary bladder. J Urol 129:1250, 1983.
33. Raz S, Zeigler M, Caine M: Hormonal influence on the adrenergic receptors of the ureter. Br J Urol 44:405, 1972.
34. Levin RM, Tong YC, Wein AJ: Effect of pregnancy on the autonomic response of the rabbit urinary bladder. Neurourol Urodyn 10:313, 1991.
35. Zderic SA, Plzak JE, Duckett JW, et al: Effect of pregnancy on rabbit urinary bladder physiology. Effects of extracellular calcium. Pharmacology 41:124, 1990.
36. Muellner SB, Hamilton JB: The effect of testosterone propionate on the tonus of the urinary bladder. J Urol 52:139, 1944.
37. Bors E, Comarr AE: Neurological Urology. Baltimore, University Park Press, 1971.
38. Gitsch E, Branstetter F: Phasen-sphinctero-cystometrie. Zentralbl Gynäkol 76:1746, 1954.
39. Schreiter E, Fuchs P, Stockamp K: Estrogenic sensitivity of α receptors in the urethral musculature. Urol Int 31:13, 1976.
40. Van Geelen JM, Doesburg WH, Thomas CMG, et al: Urodynamic studies in the normal menstrual cycle: The relationship between hormonal changes during the menstrual cycle and the urethral pressure profile. Am J Obstet Gynecol 15:384, 1981.
41. Stanton SL, Kerr-Wilson R, Harris VV: The incidence of urological symptoms in normal pregnancy. Br J Obstet Gynecol 87:897, 1980.
42. Iosif S: Stress incontinence during pregnancy and puerperium. Int J Gynecol Obstet 19:13, 1981.
43. Batra SC: Estrogen and smooth muscle function. Trends Pharmacol Sci 1:388, 1980.
44. Vane JR, Williams KJ: The contribution of prostaglandin production to contractions of the isolated uterus of the rat. Br J Pharmacol 48:629, 1973.
45. Faber P, Heidenreich J: Treatment of stress incontinence with estrogen in postmenopausal women. Urol Int 32:221, 1977.
46. Everett HS: Urology in the female. Am J Surg 52:521, 1941.
47. Iosif CS, Bekassy Z: Prevalence of genito-urinary symptoms in the late menopause. Acta Obstet Gynecol Scand 63:257, 1984.
48. Smith PJB: The effect of estrogens on bladder function in the female. *In* Campbell S (ed): The Management of the Menopause and Post-Menopausal Years. Edinburgh, Clark, 1976, p 296.
49. Le Contour X, Jouffroy C, Beuscart R, et al: Influence de la grossesse et de l'accouchement sur le function de clôture cervico-uréthrale. Etude rétrospective des conséquences tardives du traumatisme obstétrical. J Gynécol Obstét Biol Reprod (Paris) 13:775, 1984.
50. McLennan MT, McLennan CE: Oestrogenic status of menstruating and postmenopausal women assessed by cervicovaginal smears. Obstet Gynecol 37:325, 1971.
51. Huisman AB: Morfologie van de vrouwelijke urethra. Thesis, University of Groningen, The Netherlands, 1979.
52. Packham DA: The epithelial lining of the female trigone and urethra. Br J Urol 43:201, 1971.
53. Del Castillo EB, Argonz J, Galli Mainini CG: Cytological cycle of the urinary sediment and its parallelism with the vaginal cycle. J Clin Endocrinol Metab 8:76, 1948.
54. Zinner NR, Sterling AM, Ritter RC: Role of inner urethral softness in urinary incontinence. *In* Proceedings of the 9th Annual Meeting of the International Continence Society, 1979, pp 153–157.

55. Caine M, Raz S: The role of female hormones in stress incontinence. 16th Soc Int Urol Congress, Amsterdam, 1973.
56. Rud T: Urethral profile in continent women from childhood to old age. Acta Obstet Gynecol Scand 59:331, 1980.
57. Everett HS: Urology in the female. Am J Surg 52:521, 1941.
58. Bergström H: Estriol in recurrent urinary tract infection in elderly women? Acta Obstet Gynecol Scand Suppl 140:79, 1984.
59. Versi E, Cardozo LD: Urethral vascular pulsations. Proceedings of the International Continence Society, London, 1985, pp 503–594.
60. Bohler JL, Jacquetin B, Renaud RE: Physiologie du système de clôture cervico-uréthrale. Rev Fr Gynécol Obstet 74:239, 1979.
61. Batra S: Estrogen and smooth muscle function. Trends Pharmacol Sci 1:388, 1980.
62. Carlson AJ: Physiologic changes of normal aging. *In* Stieglitz EJ (ed): Geriatric Medicine, 2nd ed. Philadelphia, WB Saunders, 1949, p 47.
63. Beisland HO, Fossberg E, Moer A, et al: Urethral sphincteric insufficiency in postmenopausal females: Treatment with phenylpropanolamine and estriol separately and in combination. Urol Int 39:211, 1984.
64. Ek A, Andersson KE, Gullberg G, et al: Effects of oestradiol and combined norephredin and oestradiol treatment on female stress incontinence. Zentralbl Gynäkol 102:839, 1980.
65. Versi E, Cardozo L, Brincat M, et al: Correlation of urethral physiology and skin collagen in postmenopausal women. Br J Obstet Gynecol 95:147, 1988.
66. Brincat M, Moniz CF, Studd JWW, et al: The long term effects of the menopause and the administration of sex hormones on skin collagen and skin thickness. Br J Obstet Gynecol 92:256, 1985.
67. Brincat M, Moniz CF, Kabalan S, et al: Decline in skin collagen content and metacarpal index at the menopause and its prevention with sex hormone replacement. Br J Obstet Gynecol 94:126, 1987.
68. Brincat M, Moniz CF, Studd JWW, et al: Sex hormones and skin collagen content in post-menopausal women. Br Med J 287:1337, 1983.
69. Faber P, Heidenreich J: Treatment of stress incontinence with estrogen in menopausal women. Urol Int 32:221, 1977.
70. Walter S, Wolf H, Barlebo H, et al: Urinary incontinence in postmenopausal women treated with estrogens. Urol Int 33:125, 1978.
71. Rud T: The effect of estrogens and gestagens on urethral pressure profile in urinary continent and stress incontinent women. Acta Obstet Gynecol Scand 59:265, 1980.
72. Hilton P, Stanton SL: The use of intravaginal oestrogen cream in genuine stress incontinence. Br J Obstet Gynecol 90:940, 1983.
73. Gosling JA: The structure of the bladder and urethra in relation to function. Urol Clin North Am 6:31, 1979.
74. Stumpf WE, Madhabananda S, Joshi SG: Estrogen target cells in the skin. Experientia 30:196, 1974.
75. Versi E, Cardozo L, Brincat M, et al: Lower urinary tract symptoms, urodynamic findings and skin collagen in normal postmenopausal women. Maturitas 6:204, 1984.
76. Suntzeff V, Babcock RS, Loeb: Reversibility of hyalinization in mouse uterus produced by injections of oestrogen and changes in mammary gland and ovaries after cessation of injections. Am J Cancer 38:217, 1940.
77. Eckerling B, Goldman JA: Conservative treatment of uterovaginal prolapse and stress urinary incontinence. Int Surg 57:221, 1972.
78. Greenhill JP: The non surgical management of vaginal relaxation. Clin Obstet Gynecol 15:1083, 1972.
79. Dube JY, Lesage R, Tremblay RR: Androgen and estrogen binding in rat skeletal and perineal muscles. Can J Biochem 54:50, 1976.
80. Dionne FT, Lesage RL, Dube JY: Estrogen binding proteins in rat skeletal and perineal muscles: In vitro and in vivo studies. J Steroid Biochem 11:1073, 1979.
81. Ingelman Sundberg A: Cytosol oestrogen receptors in the urogenital tissues in stress incontinent women. Acta Obstet Gynecol Scand 60:585, 1981.
82. Haaden K, Ling L, Ferno M, et al: Estrogen receptors in the external anal sphincter. Am J Obstet Gynecol 164:609, 1991.
83. Raz S, Kaufman JJ: Carbon dioxide urethral pressure profile in female incontinence. J Urol 117:765, 1977.
84. Rud T, Andersson KE, Asmussen M, et al: Factors maintaining the intraurethral pressure in women. Invest Urol 17:343, 1980.
85. Rud T: The effects of estrogens and gestagens on the urethral pressure profile in the urinary continent and stress incontinent women. Acta Obstet Gynecol Scand 59:265, 1980.
86. Musaini U: A partially successful attempt at medical treatment of urinary stress incontinence in women. Urol Int 27:405, 1972.
87. Faber P, Heidenreich J: Treatment of stress incontinence with estrogen in postmenopausal women. Urol Int 33:135, 1978.
88. Salmi T: Risk factors in the endometrial carcinoma with special reference to use of oestrogens. Acta Obstet Gynecol Scand (Suppl 86):1, 1979.
89. Lauritzen CH: The female climacteric syndrome: Significance, problems and treatment. Acta Obstet Gynecol 53 (Suppl):47, 1976.
90. Tzingounis VA, Aksu MF, Greenblatt RB: Estriol in the management of the menopause. JAMA 239:1638, 1978.
91. Gambrell RD, Massey FM, Castaneda TA: Use of progestogen challenge to reduce the risk of endometrial cancer. Obstet Gynecol 55:732, 1980.
92. Steinberg K, Thacker SB, Smith SJ, et al: A meta-analysis of the effect of estrogen replacement therapy on the risk of breast cancer. JAMA 265:1985, 1991.
93. Dupont WD, Page DL: Menopausal estrogen replacement therapy and breast cancer. Arch Intern Med 151:67, 1991.
94. Lawson DH, Iick H, Hunter JR, et al: Exogenous oestrogens and breast cancer. Am J Epidemiol 114:710, 1981.
95. Bergkvist L, Adami H-O, Persson I, et al: The risk of breast cancer after estrogen and estrogen-progestin replacement. N Engl J Med 321:293, 1989.
96. Persson I, Yuen J, Bergkvist L, et al: Combined oestrogen-progestogen replacement and breast cancer risk. Lancet 340:1044, 1992.
97. Versi E, Cardozo LD: Oestrogens and lower urinary tract function. *In* Studd JWW, Whitehead MI (eds): The Menopause. Oxford, Blackwell Scientific, 1988, p 76.
98. Hilton P, Tweddell AL, Mayne C: Oral and intravaginal estrogens alone and in combination with alpha-adrenergic stimulation in genuine stress incontinence. Int Urogynecol J 1:80, 1990.
99. Ek A, Alm P, Andersson KE, et al: Adrenergic and cholinergic nerves of the human urethra and urinary bladder: A histochemical study. Acta Physiol Scand 99:345, 1977.
100. Samsioe G, Jansson I, Mellstrom D, et al: Occurrence, nature, and treatment of urinary incontinence in a 70 year old female population. Maturitas 7:335, 1985.
101. Karram MM, Yeko TR, Sauer MV, et al: Urodynamic changes following hormonal replacement therapy in women with premature ovarian failure. Obstet Gynecol 74:208, 1989.
102. Langer R, Golan A, Neuman M, et al: The absence and effect of induced menopause by gonadotropin-releasing hormone analogs on lower urinary tract symptoms and urodynamic parameters. Fertil Steril 55:751, 1991.
103. Longhurst PA, Kauer J, Leggett RE, et al: The influence of ovariectomy and estradiol replacement on urinary bladder function in rats. J Urol 148:915, 1992.
104. Zinner NN, Sterling AM, Ritter RC: Role of urethral softness in urinary incontinence. Urology 16:115, 1980.
105. Zinner NN, Sterling AM, Ritter RC: Evaluation of inner urethral softness. Urology 22:446, 1983.
106. Slunsky R: Beitrag zur Kombination mehrerer Behandlungsverfahren des insuffizienten Blasenverschlusses bei alten Frauen. Zentralbl Gynaekol 6:225, 1974.
107. Raz S, Zeigler M, Caine M: The role of female hormones in stress incontinence. Proceedings of the 16th Congress Societe Internationale d'Urologie, Vol. 1. Paris, Doin, 1973, p 397.
108. Ek A, Andersson KE, Gullberg B, et al: The effects of long-term treatment with estradiol and estradiol in combination

with norephedrine on stress incontinence and urethral pressure profile. Zentralbl Gynaekol 101:839, 1980.

109. Walter S, Wolf H, Barlebo H, et al: Urinary incontinence in post-menopausal women treated with estrogens. A double blind clinical trial. Urol Int 33:135, 1978.

110. Van Geelen JM, Doesburg WH, Martin Jr CB: Female urethral pressure profile: Reproducibility, axial variation and effects of low dose oral contraceptives. J Urol Gynecol 131:394, 1984.

111. Fantl JA, Cardozo L, McClish DK, et al: Estrogen therapy in the management of urinary incontinence in postmenopausal women: A meta-analysis. First report of the Hormones and Urogenital Therapy Committee. Obstet Gynecol 83:12, 1994.

112. Kinn AC, Lindskog M: Estrogens and phenylpropanolamine in combination for stress urinary incontinence in postmenopausal women. Urology 32:273, 1988.

113. Beisland HO, Fossberg E, Moer A, et al: Urethral sphincteric insufficiency in postmenopausal females: Treatment with phenylpropanolamine and estriol separately and in combination. Urol Int 39:296, 1980.

114. Walter S, Kjaergaard B, Lose G, et al: Stress urinary incontinence in postmenopausal women treated with oral estrogen (estriol) and alpha-adrenoceptor-stimulating agent (phenylpropanolamine): A randomized double-blind placebo-controlled study. Int Urogynecol J 1:74, 1990.

115. Whitehead ML, Minardi J, Kitchin Y, et al: Systemic absorption of estrogen from Premarin vaginal cream. In Cook ID (ed): The Role of Oestrogen/Progesterone in the Management of the Menopause. Lancaster, England, MTP Press, 1978.

116. Rigg LA, Hermann H, Yen SSC: Absorption of estrogens from vaginal creams. N Engl J Med 298:195, 1978.

117. Schiff I, Tulchinsky D, Ryan KJ: Vaginal absorption of estrone and 17-beta estradiol. Fertil Steril 28:1063, 1977.

118. Vermeulen AJ, Verdonck L: Studies on the binding of testosterone to human plasma. Steroid 11:609, 1968.

119. Anderson JN, Peck EJ Jr, Clark JH: Estrogen-induced uterine responses and growth: Relationship to receptor estrogen binding by uterine nuclei. Endocrinology 96:160, 1975.

120. Clark JH, Peck EJ Jr, Andersson JN: Estrogen-receptor binding: relationship to estrogen-induced responses. J Toxicol Environ Health 1:561, 1976.

121. Clark JH, Paszko Z, Peck EJ Jr: Nuclear binding and retention of the receptor estrogen complex: Relation to the agonist and antagonist properties of estriol. Endocrinology 100:91, 1977.

122. Hilton P, Stanton SL: Intravaginal estrogen cream in genuine stress incontinence. Clinical and urodynamic results. Proceedings of the 12th Annual Meeting of the International Continence Society, Leiden, 1982, p 120.

123. Saez S, Martin PM: Evidence of estrogen receptors in the trigone area of human urinary bladder. J Steroid Biochem 15:317, 1981.

124. Bergink EW, Crona N, Dahlgren, et al: Effect of oestriol, oestradiol valerate and ethyniloestradiol on serum proteins in oestrogen-deficient women. Maturitas 3:241, 1981.

125. Campagnoli C, Prelato, Tonsiju, et al: Effects of conjugated equine oestrogen and oestriol on blood clotting, plasma lipids and endometrial proliferation in postmenopausal women. Maturitas 3:135, 1981.

126. Errkola R, Lammintansta R, Punnonen R, et al: The effect of estriol succinate therapy on plasma renin activity and urinary aldosterone in postmenopausal women. Maturitas 1:9, 1978.

127. Hammond DO: Cytological assessments of climacteric patients. Clin Obstet Gynecol 4:49, 1977.

128. Kicovic PM, Cortes-Prieto J, Milojevic, et al: The treatment of postmenopausal vaginal atrophy with ovestin vaginal cream or suppositories: Clinical, endocrinological and safety aspects. Maturitas 2:275, 1980.

129. Mattsson LA, Cullberg G: A clinical evaluation of treatment with estriol vaginal cream versus suppository in postmenopausal women. Acta Obstet Gynecol Scand 62:397, 1983.

130. Englund DE, Johansson EDB: Endometrial effect of oral oestriol treatment in postmenopausal women. Acta Obstet Gynecol Scand 59:449, 1980.

131. Fink RS, Collins WP, Papadaki L, et al: Vaginal oestriol: Effective menopausal therapy not associated with endometrial hyperplasia. J Gynaecol Endocrinol 1–2:1, 1985.

132. Bhatia NN, Bergman A, Karram MM: Effects of estrogen on urethral function in women with urinary incontinence. Am J Obstet Gynecol 160:176, 1989.

133. Mellqvist P, Yossif S, Forman A, et al: The effect of danazol on the female urethral pressure profile. Acta Obstet Gynecol Scand 1979.

134. Heimer GM, Englund DE: Effects of vaginally administered oestriol on post-menopausal urogenital disorders: A cytohormonal study. Maturitas 14:171, 1992.

135. Semmens JP, Tsai C, Curtis Semmens E, et al: Effects of estrogen therapy on vaginal physiology during menopause. Obstet Gynecol 66:15, 1985.

136. Mueck AO, Rabe T, Grunwald K, et al: Urogenital symptoms in postmenopausal women treated with estradiol patch and a new oral two-monthly interval-gestagen regimen. Abstracts from the 7th Congress European Association of Gynecology and Obstetrics, Helsinki, July 1992, p 72.

137. Maekinen J, Pitkaenen Y, Salmi T, et al: Transdermal estrogen for stress urinary incontinence. Abstracts from the 7th Congress European Association of Gynecology and Obstetrics, Helsinki, July 1992, p 133.

138. Lobo AR: Treatment of the postmenopausal woman: Where are we today? In Lobo RA (ed): Treatment of the Postmenopausal Woman: Basic and Clinical Aspects. New York, Raven Press, 1994, pp 427–432.

139. Smith P: Clinical experience with an estradiol vaginal ring. In Urogenital aging, Part II: Physiology and low-dose estrogen treatment. Acts of the Kabi Pharmacia Symposium, Stockholm, 1993, p 10.

140. Rashbaum M, Mandlbaum CC: Nonoperative treatment of urinary incontinence in women. Am J Obstet Gynecol 56:777, 1948.

141. Youngblood VH, Tomlin EM, Davis JB: Senile urethritis in women. J Urol 78:150, 1957.

142. Bent AE, Richardson DA, Ostergard DR: Diagnosis of lower urinary tract disorders in postmenopausal patients. Am J Obstet Gynecol 145:218, 1983.

143. Smith P: Age changes in the female urethra. Br J Urol 44:667, 1972.

144. Fantl JA, Wyman JF, Anderson RL, et al: Postmenopausal urinary incontinence: Comparison between non-estrogen-supplemented and estrogen-supplemented women. Obstet Gynecol 71:823, 1988.

145. Salmon UJ, Walter RI, Geist SH: The use of etrogens in the treatment of dysuria and incontinence in postmenopausal women. Am J Obstet Gynecol 42:845, 1941.

146. Geist SH, Salmon UJ: The relationship of estrogens to dysuria and incontinence in post-menopausal women. J Mt Sinai Hosp 10:208, 1943.

147. Siegel I, Zelinger BB, Kanter AE: Estrogen therapy for urogenital condition in the aged. Am J Obstet Gynecol 84:505, 1962.

148. Langworthy OR, Brack CB: Effect of pregnancy and corpus luteum upon vesical muscle. Am J Obstet Gynecol 37:121, 1939.

149. Vercellini P, Crosignani PG: Epidemiology of endometriosis. The current status of endometriosis: research and management. Proceedings of the 3rd World Congress on Endometriosis, Brussels, June 1992.

150. Burns WN, Schenken RS: Pathophysiology. In Schenken RS (ed): Endometriosis: Contemporary Concepts in Clinical Management. Philadelphia, JB Lippincott, 1989, pp 83–126.

151. Vasquez G, Cornillie F, Brosens IA: Peritoneal endometriosis: Scanning electron microscopy and histology of minimal pelvic endometriotic lesions. Fertil Steril 42:696, 1984.

152. Boling RO, Abbasi R, Ackerman G, et al: Disability from endometriosis in the United States Army. J Reprod Med 33:49–52, 1988.

153. Dmowski WP, Braun DP, Gebel H: Manipulation of the immune system in endometriosis. In Brosens I, Donnez J (eds): Endometriosis Research and Management. Brussels, ICSS, 1992, pp 257–268.

154. Roeiy EL, Dmowski WP, Gleicher WP, et al: Danazol but not gonadotrophin-releasing hormone agonist suppresses auto-antibodies in endometriosis. Fertil Steril 50:864, 1988.
155. Haney AF: Alterations in cell-mediated immunity in women with endometriosis: Immunology or phenomenology? *In* Brosens I, Donnez J (eds): Endometriosis Research and Management. Brussels, ICSS, 1992, pp 249–256.
156. Steele RW, Dmowski WP, Marmer DJ: Immunologic aspects of human endometriosis. Am J Reprod Immunol 6:33, 1984.
157. Dmowski WP, Steele RW, Baker GF: Deficient cellular immunity in endometriosis. Am J Obstet Gynecol 141:377, 1981.
158. Oosterlynck DJ, Cornillie FJ, Waer M, et al: Women with endometriosis show a deficit in natural killer activity resulting in a decreased cytotoxicity to autologous endometrium. Fertil Steril 56:45, 1991.
159. Braun DP, Muriana A, Gebel H, et al: Stimulation of endometrial cell proliferation by peripheral blood monocytes from women with endometriosis. 47th Annual Meet of the American Fertility Society, 1991, S79.
160. Halme J, Becker S, Haskill S: Altered maturation and function of peritoneal macrophages: Possible role in pathogenesis of endometriosis. Am J Obstet Gynecol 156:783, 1987.
161. Engel J, Odermatt E, Engel A, et al: Shapes, domain, organization, and flexibility of laminin and fibronectin: Two multifunctional proteins of the extracellular matrix. Mol Biol 150:97, 1981.
162. Foidart IM, Beliard A, Donnez J: Endometriosis and invasion. *In* Brosens I, Donnez J (eds): Endometriosis Research and Management. Brussels, ICSS, 1992, pp 35–40.
163. Vernon MW: Biochemical activity: Differential responsiveness of endometriotic implants. *In* Brosens I, Donnez J (eds): Endometriosis Research and Management. Brussels, ICSS, 1992, pp 185–206.
164. Schenken RS, Johnson JV, Rao TR: C-myc proto-oncogene expression in endometriosis. *In* Brosens I, Donnez J (eds): Endometriosis Research and Management. Brussels, ICSS, 1992, pp 41–53.
165. Cole MD: The myc oncogene: Its role in transformation and differentiation. Annu Rev Genet 20:361, 1986.
166. Odom LD, Barrett IM, Pantazis CG, et al: Immunocytochemical study of ras and myc proto-oncogene polypeptide expression in the human menstrual cycle. Am J Obstet Gynecol 161:1663, 1989.
167. Kelly K, Cochran B, Stiles C, et al: The regulation of c-myc by growth signals. Curr Top Microbiol Immunol 113:117, 1984.
168. Kaczmarek L, Hyland J, Watt R, et al: Microinjected c-myc as a competence factor. Science 228:1313, 1985.
169. Armelin HA, Armelin MCS, Kelly K, et al: Functional role for c-myc in mitogenic response to platelet-derived growth factor. Nature (London) 310:655, 1984.
170. Abeshouse BS, Abeshouse G: Endometriosis of urinary tract. J Int Coll Surg 34(1):43–63, 1960.
171. Fein RL, Horton BF: Vesical endometriosis: A case report and review of the literature. J Urol 95:45–50, 1966.
172. O'Conor VJ, Greenhill JP: Endometriosis of the bladder and ureter. Surg Gynecol Obstet 80(2):113–119, 1945.
173. Denes FT, Pompeo ACL, Momtelatto NID, Lopes RN: Ureteral endometriosis. Int Urol Nefrol 12:205, 1980.
174. Rosenberg SK, Jacob H: Endometriosis of the upper ureter. J Urol 121:512, 1979.
175. Klein RS, Cattolica EV: Ureteral endometriosis. Urology 13:477, 1979.
176. Stiehm WD, Becker JA, Weiss RM: Ureteral endometriosis. Radiology 102:563–564, 1972.
177. Slutsky JN, Callahan D: Endometriosis of the ureter can present as renal failure: A case report and review of endometriosis affecting the ureters. J Urol 120:336–337, 1983.
178. Geraci E, Annoscia S, Lozzi C, et al: Endometriosi ureterale estrinseca: Descrizione di un caso. Arch Ital Urol 62:369–373, 1980.
179. Meyer EG: Unilateral ureteral obstruction due to endometriosis. Can J Surg 3:171, 1960.
180. Palagiri A: Urethral diverticulum with endometriosis. Urology 11:271, 1978.
181. Ronnberg L: Peritoneal fluid proteins. *In* Brosens I, Donnez J (eds): Endometriosis Research and Management. Brussels, 1992, pp 207–210.
182. Meyer EG: Unilateral ureteral obstruction due to endometriosis. Can J Surg 3:171, 1960.
183. Friedman H, Vogelzang RL, Mendelson EB, et al: Endometriosis detection by US with laparoscopic correlation. Radiology 157:217–220, 1985.
184. Arrive L, Hricak H, Martin MC: Pelvic endometriosis: MR imaging. Radiology 171:687–692, 1989.
185. Zawn M, McCarthy S, Scoutt L, et al: Endometriosis: Appearance and detection at MR imaging. Radiology 171:693–696, 1989.
186. American Fertility Society: Revised American Fertility Society classification of endometriosis. Fertil Steril 43:35, 1985.
187. Hendrickson MR, Kempson RL: Surgical Pathology of the Uterine Corpus. Philadelphia, WB Saunders, 1980, p 36.
188. Robbins SL: Pathologic Basis of Disease. Philadelphia, WB Saunders, 1974, pp 81, 1227.
189. Chatterjee SK: Scar endometriosis: A clinico-pathologic study of 17 cases. Obstet Gynecol 56:81, 1980.
190. Querleu D, Lecuru F, Subtil D: Endometriosis-associated infertility: An epidemiological approach. The current status of endometriosis: Research and management. Proceedings of the 3rd World Congress on Endometriosis, Brussels, June 1992.
191. Buttram VC, Reiter RC, Ward S: Treatment of endometriosis with danazol: Report of 6-year prospective study. Fertil Steril 43:356, 1985.
192. Cohen MR: Laparoscopic diagnosis and pseudomenopause treatment of endometriosis with danazol. Clin Obstet Gynecol 23:901, 1980.
193. Laube DW, Calderwood GW, Benda JA: Endometriosis causing ureteral obstruction. Obstet Gynecol 65:69–71, 1985.
194. Kane C, Drouin P: Obstructive uropathy associated with endometriosis. Am J Obstet Gynecol 151:207–211, 1985.
195. Gehr TWB, Sica DA: Case report and review of the literature: Ureteral endometriosis. Am J Med Sci 294(5):346, 1987.

CHAPTER 50

Caruncle and Prolapse of the Urethral Mucosa

Remigio Vela-Navarrete, M.D.

Urethral Caruncle

Urethral caruncle is a frequent finding during examination of the genital area of the menopausal woman.[1] It appears as a red nodular growth that contrasts with the pale edges of the urethral meatus, situated particularly on the posterior lip. Its vascular appearance has earned it the name "urethral hemorrhoid." In most cases the process is asymptomatic and requires no treatment (Fig. 50–1).

PATHOGENESIS

The origin of the urethral caruncle appears to be related to a slight prolapse or sliding of the urethral mucosa that everts from the meatus. Rubbing against underwear and other factors facilitate evolution toward a process that is similar to an inflammatory granuloma, although it has a notable vascular component. In its genesis there must be a factor related to the estrogen reduction in the menopausal woman.[2] Caruncles in a woman's fertile period and in girls and adolescents are exceptional,[3] and, when present, they must be carefully evaluated to avoid diagnostic errors.

Caruncles affect only the distal portion of the urethra and are not usually associated with inflammatory polyps of the vesical neck. Endoscopic examination reveals no other associated alterations. Congenital origin of caruncles by intestinal heterotopy of the urethral mucosa has been suggested.[4]

CLINICAL FINDINGS

Most caruncles are asymptomatic and are detected during a gynecologic exploration or for other reasons, although the woman may be aware of something abnormal in the urethral area. On occasion, underwear spotting occurs. Less often, the caruncle causes micturition syndrome with burning, a feeling of fullness, and an increase in frequency.

DIFFERENTIAL DIAGNOSIS

Diagnosis is normally easy because of the characteristic appearance of the caruncle. In the classic case it is basically found in the lower portion of the urethra, is the size of a pea, and is bright red. On occasion it may occupy the whole circumference of the meatus. Palpation of the urethra exaggerates the herniation of the mucosa and facilitates recognition of the caruncle.

The same procedure reveals induration or diverticula in the urethra, facilitating differential diagnosis with other processes such as senile urethritis, prolapse of the urethra, and urethral tumors[5] (Table 50–1 and Fig. 50–2). In case of doubt, diagnostic confirmation is achieved by biopsy. Cases of non-Hodgkin's lymphoma[6] and myeloid metaplasia[7] masquerading as a caruncle have been described and reported. The most common finding is vascular pyogenic granulation tissue covered by a transitional or squamous epithelial layer. Occasionally an angiomatous reaction is dominant, and in other cases a papillary reaction is present with very marked hyperplasia of the transitional or squamous epithelium. The folds of the hyperplastic epithelium may extend deeply into the stroma, resembling a carcinoma.

TREATMENT

Treatment is not required when the lesion is asymptomatic, although locally applied creams or oint-

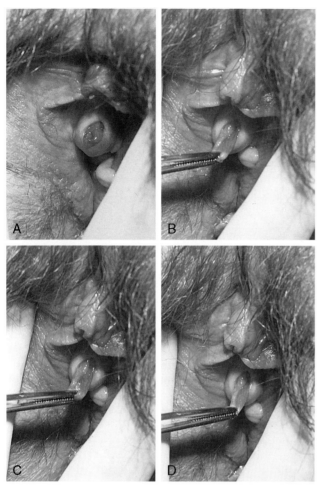

Figure 50-1 Caruncle. The distal part of the urethra appears occupied by a reddish mass covering mainly the posterior lip of the meatus. Traction exaggerates the sliding effect of the urethral mucosa.

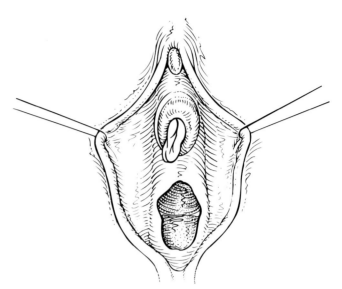

Figure 50-2 Carnosities at the external urethral meatus. Different pathologic conditions should be considered in the diagnosis of urethral caruncle (see Table 50–1).

thral venous plexus. It is advisable to leave a Foley catheter in place for 24 to 48 hours. Meatal stenosis rarely follows caruncle excision.

Prolapse of the Urethral Mucosa

Prolapse of the urethral mucosa is usually seen in two different circumstances—in young girls and in elderly women. In young girls, most frequently young black girls, it is thought to be caused by sliding of the urethral mucosa on the loose tissue of the lamina itself owing to lack of a specific attachment to the aponeurotic muscle structure. In elderly women the cause must be related to submucous edema caused by congestion in the area, occasionally associated with thrombosis of the urethral venous plexus (Fig. 50–3).

CLINICAL FINDINGS

Prolapse of the urethral mucosa in girls and adolescents has been widely discussed in the literature.[8–11] The physician is consulted when a mucus-like, pinkish excrescence appears in the urethral meatus. It is of varying size and may or may not be associated

ments containing estrogens or anti-inflammatory agents may be used. Indications for surgery are exceptional. The operation may be performed with a local anesthetic and must be preceded by an endoscopic examination or voiding cystourethrography to ensure normality in the rest of the urethra because the caruncle is exclusively distal. Electroresection or simple excision of the caruncle is sufficient.

Traction of the caruncle with Kocher or Allis clamps allows exteriorization, and two stay sutures, above and below, prevent retraction of the urethral mucosa once the caruncle has been excised. The cut should be deep and should include part of the ure-

TABLE 50–1
Carnosities at the External Urethral Meatus

	Caruncle	Senile Urethritis	Prolapse	Tumor
Presentation	Pain, spotting	Urethral syndrome	Sudden pain and appearance of a mass at the urethral meatus	Spotting, pain
Diagnosis	Typical aspect Biopsy	Estrogen status Replacement therapy	Sudden onset Typical aspect	Induration, biopsy

with slight bleeding. Differential diagnosis with ure-terocele prolapse should be done.

In elderly women the appearance of a urethral mucosal prolapse is usually sudden and apparently not related to effort. Discomfort is not noteworthy, and the patient consults the physician basically because of the sudden appearance of a mass in the vagina. On examination the urethral mucosa appears prolapsed all around the meatus, covering it. Usually the mucosa is pinkish; however, depending on the vascular component, it may be darker, more like a thrombosis. Differential diagnosis in these circumstances is usually simple because of the clinical presentation and the sudden appearance. Endoscopy shows that the problem is situated in the distal part of the urethra, the rest of the urethra, including the vesical neck, being normal.

TREATMENT

In childhood and adolescence, prolapse of the urethral mucosa tends to be recurrent, so methods of treatment that fix the mucous layer to the aponeurotic muscle have been proposed. In elderly women the condition must be corrected because it can progress to necrosis and gangrene.[12] Electroresection with local anesthetic may be sufficient. Nevertheless, in our experience, circumcision of the prolapsed mucosa, placing four interrupted equidistant sutures under a local anesthetic and leaving an indwelling catheter in place for 24 hours, has produced excellent results.

Thrombosis of the Urethral Veins

Thrombosis of the distal venous plexus of the female urethra has a spectacular clinical picture, in which severe urethral pain coincides with the sudden ap-

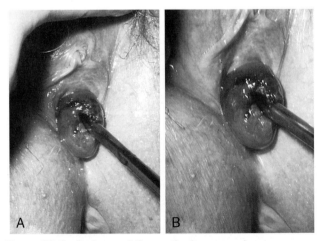

Figure 50-3 Prolapse of the urethral mucosa. A mass was noticed suddenly in the vagina. The mass was pale, soft, and easily depressed by a finger. Black spots appeared secondarily. A metal sound could be passed easily to the bladder.

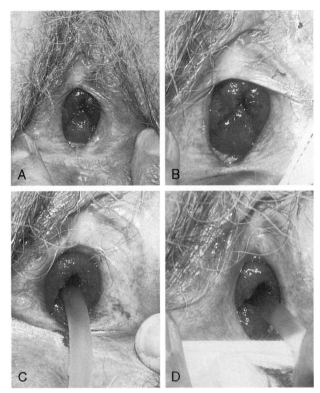

Figure 50-4 Thrombosis with prolapse of the urethral mucosa. The patient experienced acute pain in the urethra simultaneously with the appearance of a red mass in the vagina. Almost the entire introitus was occupied by this bluish-red, friable mass that oozed blood.

pearance of a mass that makes micturition difficult.[13] Examination reveals a prolapse of the urethral mucosa that finely covers a mass of thrombosed veins that give the mucosa a wine-red color much darker than that observed in a simple prolapse of the urethral mucosa. The congestive process usually causes a slight hemorrhage. Urethral palpation with a finger reveals no significant alteration other than this mass of soft tissue inside the urethra, and the spasm of the urethral meatus can also be recognized. Urethral catheterization is easy, and urethroscopy shows that the only area affected is the distal part (Fig. 50–4).

Although conservative measures with local anti-inflammatory agents and rest would probably be sufficient to correct this situation, surgery appears quicker and more efficient. Using a local anesthetic, circumcision of the prolapsed and thrombosed area is performed, and equidistant sutures are fixed in different points of the meatus.

REFERENCES

1. Marshall FC, Uson AC, Melicow MM: Neoplasms and caruncles of the female urethra. Surg Gynecol Obstet 110:723, 1960.
2. Smith P: Age changes in the female urethra. Br J Urol 44:667, 1972.
3. Türkeri L, Simsek F, Akdas A: Urethral caruncle in an unusual location occurring in prepubertal girl. Eur Urol 16:153, 1989.

4. Jarvi OH, Marin S, de Boer WG: Further studies of intestinal heterotopia in urethral caruncle. Acta Pathol Microbiol Immunol Scand A 92:469, 1984.
5. Neilson D, Grant JB, Smith CE: Squamous intraepithelial neoplasia presenting as a urethral caruncle. Br J Urol 64:200, 1989.
6. Vogeli T, Engstfeld EJ: Non-Hodgkin lymphoma of the female urethra. Scand J Urol Nephrol 26:111, 1992.
7. Balogh K, O'Hara CJ: Myeloid metaplasia masquerading as a urethral caruncle. J Urol 135:789, 1986.
8. Turner RW: Urethral prolapse in female children. Urology 2:530, 1973.
9. López C, Bochereau G, Eymeri JC: Le prolapsus muqueux uretral chez la fille. A propos de 24 cas. Chir Pédiatr 31:169, 1990.
10. Gerry F, Pascal-Mousselard H, Roudier M: Le prolapsus de la muqueuse uretrale chez la fille. Pédiatrie 45:259, 1990.
11. Johnson CF: Prolapse of the urethra: Confusion of clinical and anatomic characteristics with sexual abuse. Pediatrics 87:722, 1991.
12. Golomb J, Merimsky E, Braf Z: Strangulated prolapse of the urethra in the elderly female. Int J Gynaecol Obstet 23:61, 1985.
13. Harrow BR: The thrombosed urethral hemorroid: Three case reports. J Urol 98:482, 1967.

CHAPTER 51

Management of Vesicoureteral Reflux in Adults and Children

Samir S. Taneja, M.D.
Richard M. Ehrlich, M.D.

Along with the progression of knowledge about the etiology and clinical significance of vesicoureteral reflux (VUR) has come growing controversy about its management. Increasing insight into the long-term sequelae of reflux and the mechanism by which they occur has given rise to questions about the necessity for long-established methods of surgical correction. It is true that surgeons understood and perfected the craft of ureteral reimplantation long before the pathophysiology of VUR was well delineated. Currently, alternative means of managing reflux patients are well established, but the question of which patients are appropriate candidates for these alternative therapeutic modalities remains difficult to answer.

In this chapter the evolution of thought pertaining to vesicoureteral reflux, along with its impact on reflux management, is discussed. A basic approach to the reflux patient, and the subsequent decision-making process used in establishing conservative or interventional management, is described. Although the appreciation of the complexity of the disease process has changed since early descriptions, many of the fundamental concepts in evaluating the patient remain the same.

Described as early as 1883,[1] reflux took on significance in the 1950s when surgeons began to note the potential for renal damage and strongly advocated surgical repair.[2] At this time, reflux was thought to represent a phenomenon secondary to distal obstruction. Eventually it became understood that in the majority of children with the disease, reflux is indeed a primary concept secondary to incompetence of the ureterovesical junction. The comprehension of a shortened intramural ureteral segment as the primary cause gave way to better understanding of the pathophysiology of VUR and the concepts of ureteral reimplantation.

Evident even in early descriptions was the idea that hydronephrosis, upper tract infection, renal scarring, and compromise in renal function were potential serious sequelae of VUR. Hodson and Edwards described the cause of reflux nephropathy as intrarenal reflux.[3] In subsequent studies, Hodson and his colleagues demonstrated that surgically induced reflux in pigs produced intrarenal reflux with eventual interstitial fibrosis in the absence of infection.[4, 5] Ransley postulated that intrarenal reflux was dependent on papillary morphology with scarring occurring only in regions of flat or concave papillae and open papillary ducts.[6, 7] The sharp contrast of Ransley's work with that of Hodson is the assertion that infection, in combination with intrarenal reflux, is absolutely necessary to produce scarring. It is currently accepted that infection is a key factor in the development of reflux nephropathy[8]; however, the long-term effects of continued sterile reflux on the upper urinary tract remain to be elucidated.

VUR occurs far more frequently in women than in men. It is predominantly a disease of children in its primary form.[9] In adults the disease is frequently a sequela of functional or anatomic lower tract abnormalities, and it is now becoming more obvious that this may be true of children as well. Multiple studies have suggested a genetic predisposition to reflux, with a higher frequency of reflux in sibling patients with clinically detected VUR.[10–13] Recent follow-up studies in adults treated as children for reflux show a higher incidence of VUR among offspring than in the general population,[14] suggesting the possibility of a more direct penetrance than was previously suspected.

The most frequent presentation of VUR is urinary tract infection, with 29 to 50% of children with urinary tract infection having some degree of VUR.[15] Thirty percent of these children show evidence of renal scarring at presentation. This number increases to approximately 50% in children with reflux of moderate grade. This demonstrates a difficult issue in the management of VUR in that much of the damage is already done prior to the institution of therapy.

Conservative Management of Primary Reflux

From the idea that urinary tract infection, and not reflux itself, is the primary cause of reflux nephropathy in the VUR patient has come the logic of conservative management. It is well accepted that low-dose antibacterial prophylaxis or chemoprophylaxis prevents the recurrence of urinary tract infection in patients with low-grade reflux. The natural history of low-grade primary reflux in children is such that spontaneous cessation will occur in the majority. The time course to resolution of reflux is variable, and the road to that end point is fraught with significant danger in the form of recurrent infection and permanent renal damage. Herein lies the rationale of chemoprophylaxis with careful monitoring of reflux progression, infection, and renal damage.

Several studies have established the validity of conservative management of VUR in the pediatric population. King and associates presented data on 323 children followed by surveillance for VUR. Fifty-one percent of ureters in these children had spontaneous cessation of reflux.[16] Also advocated was the use of intramural ureteral length as the single best variable in predicting spontaneous resolution. It is estimated that 50 to 60% of ureters with a tunnel greater than 5 mm and 33% of ureters with a tunnel of 2 to 5 mm will show eventual resolution of reflux without correction.[17] Edwards and colleagues reported a 79% overall disappearance of reflux in patients followed for 7 to 15 years.[18] These patients were treated with chemoprophylaxis, and new scars developed only in 2 of 121 kidneys. Cessation of reflux occurred in 85% of nondilated ureters and 41% of dilated ureters. Smellie reported resolution in 75% of nondilated and 45% of dilated ureters.[19] This regimen included intensive efforts at bladder training in addition to standard chemoprophylaxis.

Lenaghan and associates delineated the importance of continuous chemoprophylaxis by showing a 21% rate of new scar development and a 66% rate of progression of established scars in patients treated with short-course intermittent antibiotic therapy.[20]

Early data on the natural history of nondilated low-grade VUR has brought conservative management into acceptance for this subset of patients. Using medical therapy, Arant reports 82% resolution in grade 1 reflux and 80% resolution in grade 2 with a further 8% showing downgrading.[21] In comparison, there was a 46% rate of resolution among patients with grade 3 reflux. Unlike with low-grade reflux,

controversy continues about the use of medical therapy in patients with moderate or severe reflux.

Definitive data about the conservative management of vesicoureteral reflux has come from the International Reflux Study in Children (IRSC). This multicenter prospective randomized study stratified children with regard to severity of reflux and clinical findings at the time of presentation and followed them, measuring for evidence of continued reflux, recurrent infections, progression or development of renal scars, and appearance of hypertension. Children in both European and American centers were randomized to either surgical or medical management and followed for 5 years.

Within the European group, 235 children were conservatively treated with chemoprophylaxis. Of these, 80 patients, consisting of patients in whom reflux spontaneously downgraded prior to entrance into the study, were followed as a sideline group. One hundred and fifty-one children (237 ureters) were managed surgically by reimplantation. All children had grade 3 to 4 reflux and a previous history of urinary tract infection. During follow-up 38% of medically treated patients and 39% of surgically treated children developed breakthrough infections.[22] Pyelonephritis episodes occurred significantly more often in the medically treated patients (21%) than in the surgical patients (10%). New renal scars developed in 12% of medical patients and 13% of surgical patients, with 6% and 10% of these patients, respectively, showing new renal parenchymal thinning.[23] A higher incidence of new scars was seen in children of younger age groups and in patients with parenchymal thinning at presentation. Five-year follow-up revealed no reflux in 97.5% of surgically treated patients compared to a 16% rate of cessation in the medical group.[24] Reflux was more likely to resolve in those with unilateral reflux (54%) and in patients in the sideline group with lower-grade reflux.

The United States group had similar results with no significant difference in recurrence of infection or occurrence of new renal scarring between surgical and medical groups.[25] Pyelonephritis episodes among the medical group were almost three times those in surgically treated patients. Seventy-five percent of medically treated patients still had reflux at follow-up compared to resolution of reflux in 86 of 87 surgically treated patients (average follow-up, 3.9 years).

The role of conservative management in the adult patient is somewhat different from that in the child. Unlike children, adults often have significant signs of progressive renal insufficiency, with or without recurrent infection, at the time of presentation. The preservation of renal function is a central issue in the management of these patients. Malek and colleagues reviewed 67 adult patients with primary reflux who underwent bilateral ureteroneocystostomy for VUR.[26] Although it was successful in terminating reflux in 97% of patients, surgical correction had no beneficial effect on renal size, scars, or significant proteinuria. A significant correlation was found between severity of reflux and degree of scarring at the time of surgery.

The preoperative level of proteinuria seemed to predict the likelihood of progression to renal insufficiency. The recurrence of pyelonephritis, however, was nicely abrogated. Fifty percent of patients with previous UTI had recurrent episodes of cystitis, and only 4 of these 54 patients showed clinical evidence of pyelonephritis. A follow-up study from Neves and colleagues compared 27 conservatively treated patients with the Malek group.[27] No significant differences in postoperative progression of scarring, hypertension, or renal insufficiency were noted. Again, the level of renal impairment at the time of initiation of therapy seemed to predict the likelihood of progression to end-stage renal disease. Of 12 patients treated with chemoprophylaxis, three had episodes of recurrent cystitis despite therapy. No patients showed evidence of recurrent pyelonephritis.

Conservative management necessitates strict follow-up with frequent visits to the physician's office and many diagnostic procedures. Many parents are concerned that repeated catheterizations and cystograms may be emotionally and psychologically traumatic to the female child. Parents often think that a voiding cystourethrogram performed by an adult x-ray technician, often male, is percieved by the child as an assault episode. For this reason, they are reluctant to return for multiple repeat studies and often opt for early surgery.

Other potential sequelae of chronic antibiotic therapy exist. The effect of long-term therapy, particularly in women of childbearing age, remains unknown. Many documented cases of drug reactions exist, including rash, anaphylaxis, marrow suppression, and even Stephens-Johnson syndrome. This emphasizes the fact that even conservative treatment is not without the potential for harm.

When evaluating a patient with VUR it is incumbent on the physician to identify any lower tract dysfunction. Failure to do so may result in poor results with the chosen therapy. Once the problem has been identified as primary reflux, a treatment strategy must be developed based on multiple factors. In children, the approach must be an aggressive one because renal development and lifelong renal function hang in the balance. The severity of reflux in the absence of infection should be carefully scored by cystogram. The history of infection and recurrence frequency should be considered in determining the need for intervention. The presence of renal scarring at the time of presentation can help to predict the potential for further renal damage in the presence of recurrent pyelonephritis. The desires and emotional resilience of the patient and parents must be assessed. In the adult population, conservative therapy seems to be satisfactory in ameliorating recurrent infection in the large majority of patients with primary reflux. The severity of reflux and the degree of renal damage at the time of presentation are important determinants in the response to therapy. Again, careful discussion with the patient, with emphasis on the potential impact of lifelong antibiotic therapy, is crucial in ensuring the feasibility of medical management in an individual patient.

A conservative approach should consist most importantly of meticulous monitoring for evidence of recurrent infection, renal scarring, hypertension, and deterioration in renal function. Chemoprophylaxis should consist of low-toxicity oral agents administered at relatively low doses. The potential for side effects and allergic reactions should be kept in mind, particularly in children. Initially, repeat studies for persistence or progression of reflux should be carried out at intervals of 3 months. In no worsening occurs or if reflux resolves, studies can be carried out at lengthened intervals. Nuclear cystography is ideal for follow-up because it carries far less radiation exposure than conventional cystography and has increased relative sensitivity. DMSA scanning can be used to follow renal scarring.[28] Scars seen on DMSA scans but not previously seen at the time of intravenous urography may simply represent the increased sensitivity of DMSA scanning rather than progressive renal damage. The length of follow-up remains controversial, but follow-up probably should continue through adolescent life in children with resolution of reflux, indefinitely in adults, and certainly throughout the period of ongoing reflux in any patient. Failure of resolution by puberty should cause the physician to reevaluate the patient and possibly proceed to surgical management.

Any evidence of recurrent upper urinary tract infection while on chemoprophylaxis mandates reevaluation and probable surgical intervention. Progressive renal deterioration in patients in whom reflux nephropathy was present initially should, at the very least, cause alarm and bring about further discussion with the patient and parents about reimplantation. New-onset hypertension, although rare, can be a sign of failure of therapy. Any evidence of scarring in kidneys in which scarring was not previously present or of infections in patients who were previously without infection should mandate reconsideration of strategy with a strong leaning toward surgical correction. Breakthrough infection remains the finding of most concern in this patient population.

Conservative Management of Secondary Reflux

Prior to selecting a therapeutic strategy for the patient with VUR, it is important to identify any evidence of lower urinary tract dysfunction producing secondary reflux. Included in this category are neurogenic bladder disease, dysfunctional voiding patterns and non-neurogenic neurogenic bladder (Hinman's syndrome), bladder neck obstruction, ureterocele, and bladder diverticulum. In the majority of these conditions, treatment of the primary process frequently results in spontaneous cessation of reflux, and failure to recognize the primary process may result in failure of therapy for VUR.

NEUROGENIC BLADDER DISEASE

Neurogenic bladder disease encompasses a wide variety of lower tract disorders including low-capacity, noncompliant bladders, high-capacity, atonic bladders, and gradations of such disease. Of particular concern is the low-capacity, poorly compliant bladder associated with myelodyplasia or spinal cord injury.[29] Hackler and colleagues found reflux in 46% of spinal cord injury patients with low bladder compliance compared to only 6% of such patients with normal bladder compliance.[30] These bladders tend to exhibit patterns of high-pressure voiding, instability of the detrusor, and occasional dyssynergy of the external striated sphincter. High intravesical pressure is also seen in the areflexic bladder. In a review of neurogenic bladder patients, Gerridzen and associates found that 17.5% of areflexic bladder patients had significant upper tract deterioration, whereas 16% of those with hyperreflexic bladders had upper tract damage.[31] Urodynamic evaluation in both types of bladder dysfunction revealed higher intravesical pressures among patients with damaged upper tracts than in patients with normal tracts. McGuire and coworkers found that 68% of myelodyplasia patients with areflexic bladders and a urethral leak pressure of greater than 40 cm H_2O had VUR, and 81% had upper tract dilatation.[32] In contrast, no patients with a low urethral leak pressure and atonic areflexic bladders had VUR. The primary cause of reflux in these patients is high intravesical pressure, not primary ureterovesical junction dysfunction. This point is further emphasized by the low incidence of reflux seen in newborns with myelodyplasia, suggesting an acquired mechanism.[33, 34] Many children treated with temporary vesicostomy show resolution of reflux, which then recurs on closure. High intravesical pressures can lead eventually to decompensation of the ureterovesical junction and reflux. This is especially true in patients with a previously marginally competent antireflux mechanism. The management of these patients is difficult owing to the high rate of therapeutic failure in both conservatively and surgically treated patients.

Management of these patients has evolved from indwelling catheters and urinary diversion to intermittent catheterization, anticholinergics, and bladder augmentation with or without antireflux procedures. Many authors have reported some resolution of reflux in patients treated conservatively with intermittent catheterization.[35–38] Sullivan and colleagues noted resolution of reflux in 35% of ureters in patients treated by intermittent catheterization, with an additional 13% showing improvement in grade of reflux.[39] Interestingly, 48% of patients treated with close observation alone showed improvement as well. Kass and colleagues noted resolution in 31% of ureters treated by intermittent bladder catheterization.[40] Of the 17% of patients with continued reflux in whom no surgical therapy was undertaken, no febrile urinary tract infections or signs of progressive renal deterioration were seen. Cass and coworkers found cessation of reflux in 35% and stabilization in 40% of children with neurogenic bladder disease who were followed with antimicrobials and intermittent catheterization.[41] Worsening reflux was seen in 25%. Upper tract dilatation improved in 12.5% of patients and remained unchanged in the remainder. Kaplan and colleagues reported that 62% of children with concomitant myelodysplasia and VUR experienced resolution or improvement in symptoms while on intermittent catheterization.[42]

Intermittent catheterization does carry some morbidity in that children may have soreness of the urethra, urethral bleeding, and urethral discharge. Also reported is genital swelling and even stone formation from inserted hair.[35] Patients must be chosen carefully because a regular schedule and parental or patient compliance are mandatory for good results. Intermittent catheterization may help by lowering intravesical pressure and decreasing the frequency of voiding during which intravesical pressures are high. Certainly many of these patients display increasing pressure during filling secondary to poor compliance. Despite carefully monitored catheterization, a large number of these patients will continue to experience worsening reflux and increasing upper tract deterioration that mandate surgical intervention.

The fundamental concept in the treatment of these patients is lowering the intravesical pressure by both reducing bladder instability and decompressing the bladder during filling. Initial evaluation includes urodynamic studies for evaluation of bladder capacity as well as generated pressures during filling and at capacity. Initial therapy should be focused on the use of timed intermittent catheterization in an effort to reduce or stabilize upper tract deterioration. Detrusor instability or hyperreflexia should be identified at presentation, and if necessary, anticholinergic agents should be instituted as part of the conservative regimen. The Crede maneuver is to be discouraged because voiding through increased intra-abdominal pressure only increases the transmitted intravesical pressure. Antibiotics should be used in patients with recurrent urinary tract infection. This may possibly reduce inflammation and restore competence to a marginally competent ureter. The severity of reflux, the length of the intramural tunnel, and the appearance of the orifice all help in deciding how aggressive therapy needs to be. Failure of these measures to control reflux or recurrent upper tract infection should lead to surgical efforts to decompress the bladder and, in cases of severe reflux, to repair the ureterovesical junction.

DYSFUNCTIONAL VOIDING

Hinman and Baumman introduced the idea that VUR is an acquired mechanism secondary to a lack of coordination between the involuntary detrusor and the striated sphincter.[43] This incoordination was postulated to cause bladder hypertrophy and decompensation leading to subsequent upper tract deterioration. These findings parallel the ultimate sequelae of obstructive uropathy. Recently it has been understood that the non-neurogenic neurogenic bladder described by Hinman is probably the extreme end of a wide spectrum of dysfunctional voiding patterns.[44]

Normal maturation of the bladder involves a shift from the spontaneous volume-induced contraction style of voiding seen in neonates and infants to the controlled voluntary detrusor contraction accompanied by simultaneous sphincter relaxation seen in adults. Dysfunctional voiding is caused by delay in maturation of the bladder past the age of toilet training. The social need to maintain continence forces these children to induce sphincter dyssynergy during uninhibited detrusor contraction, thereby potentially damaging their own urinary tract. Further urodynamic studies have shown that the difference between non-neurogenic neurogenic bladders and dysfunctional voiders may lie in the voiding pattern. Unlike the dysfunctional voider, who shows compensatory pelvic floor contraction during the filling phase but normal sphincter synergy during voiding, the child with a non-neurogenic neurogenic bladder shows poor detrusor-sphincter synergy during voiding, with bladder emptying occurring against a closed sphincter.[45] As a result, the bladders in these children often become decompensated, explaining the findings of a massively dilated bladder and upper urinary tract (Fig. 51–1). This voluntary sphincter contraction probably represents a learned behavior initiated during an earlier period of dysfunctional voiding.

Griffiths and Scholtmeijer went one step further and identified two patterns of dysfunctional voiding.[46] The first is characterized by bladder instability with high-pressure contractions accompanied by reflux, which is usually unilateral. The second is characterized by weak detrusor contractions in a usually stable bladder and increased activity of the sphincter closure mechanism. These patients frequently have bilateral reflux, and upper tract deterioration is not uncommon. This pattern seems to parallel the non-neurogenic neurogenic bladder and may simply represent a progression to bladder decompensation from the pattern seen in the first group.

Van Gool and colleagues described four patterns of dysfunctional voiding.[47] The urge syndrome involves frequent episodes of urgent necessity to void accompanied by hold maneuvers and some incontinence. Staccato voiding occurs in patients with an unstable bladder; additional episodes of increased pelvic floor activity during voiding produce an intermittent stream. Fractionated and incomplete voiding is seen in patients with a hypoactive detrusor and resulting high levels of residual urine. Finally, voiding postponement is seen in a group of children who urinate infrequently and hold urine to the point of unbearable urge, often resulting in incontinence. Again, these groups probably represent points on a spectrum of the natural history of this disorder.

It has recently been noted that a number of chil-

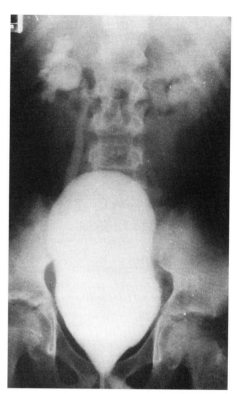

Figure 51–1 Cystogram of child with non-neurogenic neurogenic bladder disease showing the commonly seen presenting findings of dilated decompensated bladder and upper tracts. (From Allen TD: The non-neurogenic bladder. J Urol 117:235, 1976.)

dren believed to have primary reflux on the basis of radiologic findings and a normal neurologic examination are actually dysfunctional voiders. These children characteristically have detrusor instability with or without induced sphincter dyssynergy. Koff and colleagues evaluated urodynamically 363 children with urinary tract infection by simultaneous cystometrogram and periurethral striated muscle electromyography (EMG).[48] Fifty-three children with uninhibited bladder contractions and no neurologic abnormality were identified. EMG revealed voluntarily induced sphincter dyssynergy, which generated high intravesical pressures, when these children were instructed not to void. Urinary incontinence was identified in 68% of these 53 children, with 58% displaying daytime and nighttime wetting. A more striking finding was that 32% of these 53 children were completely continent. Methods of maintaining continence ranged from voluntary sphincter contraction to Vincent's curtsy (in which the child squats down during the uninhibited contraction, holding the heel of the foot against the perineum and urethra). Further analysis of these children revealed VUR in 47%. And of those without reflux, abnormal ureteral orifices by Lyon's criteria[49] were seen in 30%. Reflux was noted in 32 of 70 incontinent children and 9 of 17 children maintaining continence. These initial studies gave way to two fundamental questions: (1) will therapy directed at the uninhibited bladder cause any resolution in VUR as seen in neurogenic bladder disease, and (2) is there a role for screening urodynamic evaluation in children with urinary tract infection.

In an effort to address the first question, Koff and Murtagh evaluated 62 children (60 girls) with history of urinary tract infection and documented VUR on resolution of infection.[50] Uninhibited bladder contractions were noted in 34 children on urodynamic evaluation. Of these, 26 children were started on a regimen of antibiotic prophylaxis, bladder training, and anticholinergic bladder relaxants. The remaining eight children were unable to tolerate the anticholinergic agents because of side effects and were followed as a separate group. Children with normal cystometrograms were treated with chemoprophylaxis only. Urinary tract infection recurred in 16% of children with treated uninhibited bladder contractions compared to 63% of children not tolerating anticholinergic agents and 71% of those with normal cystometrograms. In these three groups, VUR resolved in 44%, 33%, and 17% of patients, respectively. Among children taking anticholinergic agents for uninhibited bladder contractions, 16% showed improvement of reflux to grade 1. Necessity for surgical reimplantation among these groups occurred in 33%, 67%, and 57% of patients, respectively.

Seruca prospectively followed 53 children with bladder instability and VUR.[51] Children were treated with antibiotic prophylaxis, anticholinergics for uninhibited detrusor contractions, and skeletal muscle relaxants for sphincter dyssynergy. The children were treated for a total of 12 to 30 months, during which time no progression of renal scarring or development of new renal scarring occurred. At the end of therapy, repeat cystograms revealed resolution of reflux in 92% of ureters and improvement in reflux in the remaining 8%. Normal urodynamic parameters were found in 87% of patients. Seruca also noted that children with residual disease often started with severe grades of reflux and had continued high intravesical pressures on completion of therapy.

Multiple studies have confirmed the suggestion that dysfunctional voiding contributes significantly to the development of childhood VUR.[52, 53] A large number of children presenting with urinary tract infection have bladder instability. Not only is vesicoperineal incoordination important in the development of reflux, but it may also have a negative impact on the success of various modalities of therapy for VUR. Noe, on reviewing 305 children undergoing ureteral reimplantation for primary reflux, noted that failures and complications could be directly attributed to bladder instability and dysfunctional voiding not recognized prior to surgery.[55] He concluded that bladder instability is the greatest risk factor for failure of reimplantation. In the second half of the aforementioned Seruca study, the results of a retrospective study of 48 children treated medically for primary VUR over a period of 5 years were reported.[51] Fifty-four percent of ureters showed resolution of reflux with chemoprophylaxis. Urodynamic evaluation of the children with continued reflux revealed bladder instability or vesicoperineal discoordination in all cases.

The significance of lower urinary tract dysfunction in the severity of VUR was further emphasized by Nielson and colleagues, who noted that enuretic children had a significantly lower incidence of reflux nephropathy than comparable nonenuretic children.[56] In children under the age of 10, 25% of kidneys with refluxing ureters in enuretic children were found to have reflux nephropathy on intravenous pyelography (IVP) compared to 31% of kidneys in nonenuretic children. In children over the age of 10 the findings were more impressive. Reflux nephropathy occurred in 28% of enuretic patients' kidneys and 76% of nonenuretic patients' kidneys. This idea of enuresis serving as a "pop-off valve" that protects the upper tracts is intriguing because it further serves to emphasize the importance of bladder training.

The second question about the role of urodynamic testing in the evaluation of reflux patients is more difficult to answer. Of particular concern is the finding by Koff that 32% of children with bladder instability are completely continent.[48] This emphasizes the importance of careful history taking. Van Gool and colleagues identified bladder instability in an additional 18% of children enrolled in the IRSC European branch by means of an extensive questionnaire on voiding habits.[47] This was a study in which dysfunctional voiding or bladder instability was an exclusion criterion for entry. Although many authors use urodynamic testing in a screening fashion for presumed reflux patients, the use of a history and physical examination for identification of a subset of patients at risk is preferable.

When evaluating the child with VUR initially, it is mandatory to look for the signs and symptoms of a dysfunctional voider. Daytime wetting, nocturnal enuresis, abdominal cramps, infrequent urination, frequent urination, urgency, and hold maneuvers such as Vincent's curtsy are all important indicators of bladder dysfunction. As such, these signs and symptoms must be elicited through careful history taking from both patient and parents. A history of bowel habits that include chronic constipation, encopresis, and fecal soiling, which are commonly seen in these children, can add to the physician's suspicion of bladder dysfunction. Additionally, many children with dysfunctional voiding patterns appear to come from social situations involving a dominant parent who is potentially demeaning to the child's self-esteem. Emotional and behavioral disturbances in the child's interactive skills and ability to function in school are not uncommon. Assessment of ongoing psychological stressors in the child's life is a necessary component of the complete evaluation.

Examination of the patient should stress identification of neurologic abnormalities as well as urinary pattern. Neurologic examination including a spinal and back examination, bulbocavernosus reflex, and evaluation of sphincter tone will help to identify the subset of patients who are at high risk for neurogenic bladder disease. Palpation for bladder distention as well as observation of the urinary stream may help. Urodynamic evaluation for detrusor instability, urine flow, voiding patterns, and emptying capacity should probably be reserved for patients in whom a suspicion of lower tract dysfunction exists. The actual process of testing can induce significant emotional stress in both patient and parent.

Conservative management of the dysfunctional voider revolves around bladder training. Frequent voiding (every 2 to 3 hours), fluid restriction, voiding with every urge, and relaxation during micturition to produce a continuous stream remain the major components of therapy. Antibiotics are given as a prophylactic measure to prevent recurrence of infection. The use of anticholinergic therapy directed at controlling bladder wall instability and skeletal relaxants for sphincter spasm can be useful adjuncts to bladder training. The use of these agents can increase the rate of spontaneous cessation of reflux and reduce the number of recurrent infections. These pharmacologic measures are strictly additions to bladder training, not replacements for it. Not only will stabilization of these bladders serve as means of treating reflux, it will also improve the outcome in patients who do require reimplantation.

ANATOMIC ABNORMALITIES OF THE LOWER TRACT

Many anatomic abnormalities of the lower urinary tract can cause or worsen reflux. Management of these patients should take into consideration the special situation. Failure to do so may result in failure of therapy.

VUR often occurs in patients with a duplicated ureteral system. The most frequently seen anomaly is reflux into a lower pole moiety or upper ureteral orifice. Reflux can also occur in ectopically placed orifices. The role of conservative management in these patients has been controversial because it results in a lower rate of cessation than in patients with primary reflux and a single ureter. Husmann and Ollen compared conservative management of reflux in patients with duplicated systems and single ureteral systems.[60] In 2 years of observation with chemoprophylaxis, 10% of patients with duplicated systems showed cessation of reflux compared with 35% of patients with single ureters. No difference was noted between groups in breakthrough infection or upper tract deterioration. Peppas and colleagues reported an 18% rate of resolution among duplicated refluxing systems during a 42-month observation period.[61] Infection was well controlled with antibiotics. Most often resolution of reflux occurred in patients with low- to moderate-grade reflux. It appears that a combination of chemoprophylaxis and observation is an acceptable first-line therapy in patients with duplicated ureteral systems and VUR, particularly patients with low-grade reflux. Persistence of reflux

through puberty and certainly breakthrough upper tract infection should lead to surgical intervention.

Bladder diverticula may be associated with VUR as described by Hutch.[2] These acquired diverticula most frequently occur as sequelae of elevated intravesical pressure. Paraureteral positioning of the diverticulum leads to either impingement on the ureteral orifice or stretching of the distal ureter causing destruction of the antireflux mechanism. Diverticula at sites distant from the orifice can provide a constant nidus for infection, thereby perpetuating reflux or causing decompensation of the marginally competent ureterovesical valve. Therapy of diverticula is mainly surgical, which explains some of the failure observed with conservative management.

Reflux is also seen following incision of ureterocele. This fact has led to the assertion that in children ureterocele should be managed by excision rather than incision.

Surgical Management of Vesicoureteral Reflux

Surgical management remains the cornerstone of VUR therapy. Patients who fail to respond to a conservative approach must be treated aggressively. Several options exist for the surgical correction of reflux.

ENDOSCOPIC SUBURETERAL INJECTION AS AN ALTERNATIVE THERAPY

In view of the growing controversy about the need for open surgical management of VUR, many surgeons have investigated alternative methods of surgical correction. In the mid-1980s, O'Donnell and Puri reported success in curing reflux using the technique of subureteral polytetrafluoroethylene (Teflon) injection.[63, 64] Initial studies of the so-called sting procedure were conducted in pigs in which VUR had been induced.[65] Successful abatement of reflux was achieved, and histologic studies revealed conformity of the shape and position of the Teflon. The authors then reported cure in 75% of ureters following a single injection and in 89% after multiple injections.[66] A further 8% of ureters showed significant improvement in the grade of reflux. At follow-up, 15% of ureters showed recurrent reflux. In a second study of patients with grade 4 and 5 disease, reflux abated in 67% of ureters following a single injection and in 92% after multiple injections, with 84% remaining reflux-free at follow-up ranging from 6 to 30 months.[67]

Since the initial reports, many centers have evaluated the technique of endoscopic Teflon injection with variable results.[68–71] With few exceptions, most groups report success rates of 85 to 95% following two to three injections in patients with primary reflux. Kaplan and colleagues reported a 95% correction or improvement in patients with primary reflux managed by a single injection.[72] Brown, on the other hand, reported only a 70% elimination of reflux with multiple Teflon injections compared to 98% elimination by standard surgical reimplantation in a comparable patient group.[73] A recent multicenter European survey reported an 82% rate of correction in 1290 ureters with either primary or secondary reflux after single injection.[74] Twenty-seven percent of ureters had grade 3 reflux, and 4% had grade 4, of which 24% and 36% failed, respectively. Results with duplicated ureters appear to be less satisfactory.

It is thought that subureteral injection of Teflon corrects reflux by providing a solid backing for the intramural ureter. This cannot be provided by the detrusor muscle in the presence of a shortened intramural tunnel. Failure of therapy has been attributed largely to either improper positioning of the Teflon globule or an insufficient amount of injection material. The latter may be occur with reabsorption of the glycerin component of the injected Teflon paste and may explain the need for frequent reinjections. Fortunately, reinjection is technically quite easy.

The technique of subureteral injection has been modified several times; however, it remains similar to the original description provided by O'Donnell and Puri.[64, 75] The instrumentation essentially involves either a "stinger" consisting of a rigid cannula and attached 22-gauge needle that inserts directly into an angled lens cystoscope, or a 5 Fr flexible cannula with a swaged-on needle inserted through a standard cystoscope (Fig. 51–2). Each is firmly attached to a metal or glass syringe for injection. A zero-degree lens is utilized for visualizing the ureteral orifices. The "stinger" is primed with either sterile oil or glycerin to facilitate ease of injection.

The operation is performed under general anesthesia. The patient is placed in the lithotomy position with the thighs generously abducted to flatten the bladder floor. The bladder is filled with a small amount of irrigation fluid to optimize visualization of the orifice. O'Donnell and Puri recommend insertion of a ureteral catheter into the orifice during injection. A Fogarty balloon catheter can be used in larger orifices to provide traction and added length to the intramural ureter. The needle is then inserted submucosally beneath the ureter in the 6 o'clock position (Fig. 51–3). Attention to detail is necessary to ensure that the needle is exactly at 6 o'clock because misplacement is a potential source of treatment failure. The needle is inserted 6 to 10 mm, taking great care not to enter the detrusor or perforate the ureter. Gentle upward traction on the needle allows the surgeon to visualize the position of the needle and inject the Teflon paste under direct visualization. The needle should penetrate at least 5 mm beneath the ureter. Injection of 0.2 to 0.8 ml of Teflon paste is then slowly performed. The end point of injection is determined by an inverted crescentic appearance of the orifice with good coaptation of the ureteral walls. An additional 0.1 ml of paste can be injected to compen-

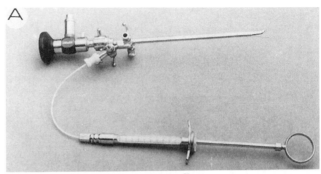

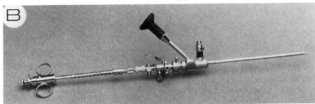

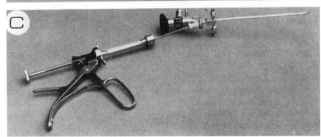

Figure 51–2 Instrumentation used for subureteral collagen injection. *A,* Flexible cannula with swaged-on needle inserted through standard cystoscope. *B,* Cystoscope with offset lens. *C,* Teflon injection gun inserted through modified cystoscope. (From O'Donnell B, Puri P: Technical refinements in endoscopic correction of vesicoureteral reflux. J Urol 140:1102, 1988.)

sate for the expected contraction of the paste due to glycerin absorption. The needle is held in place for a short time following injection to prevent immediate backflow of paste. Irrigation of the needle hole is carried out after the needle has been removed.

Bleeding, infection, and ureteral obstruction do not seem to be significant concerns with this procedure. Recurrent reflux is easily treated with repeated injections, taking care to correct any misalignment of the Teflon globule and to enlarge the globule as necessary to produce good coaptation of the orifice. Advocates of the procedure are quick to point out that the injected material does not in any way hamper subsequent reimplantation and simply "shells out" at the time of surgery.[65, 76] However, there have been many anecdotal reports of granulomatous reaction causing severe inflammation throughout the floor of the bladder.

Proponents of injection therapy believe that it is superior to open surgery for many reasons including the absence of abdominal incision and cystotomy; a lack of postoperative pain, bladder irritability, hematuria, and cumbersome drains and catheters; a decrease in time needed for anesthesia (roughly 15 minutes); and finally, no need for a hospital stay because this is an outpatient procedure.

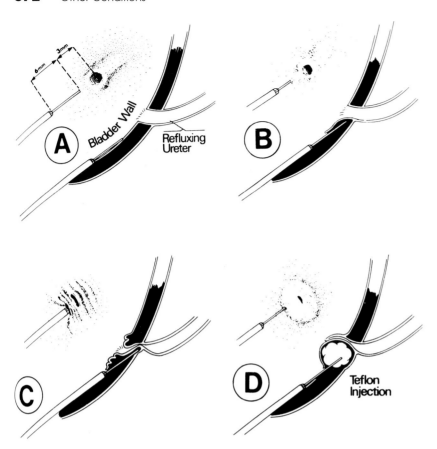

Figure 51–3 Technique of subureteral injection for vesicoureteral reflux. *A,* Needle is inserted under direct visualization. *B,* Needle is advanced, taking care not to perforate the ureter and to remain directly beneath the orifice. *C,* By lifting the needle gently, the depth and angle of insertion can be assessed. *D,* Once the needle is in place, slow injection is carried out. (From Farkas A, Moriel E, Lupa S: Endoscopic correction of vesicoureteral reflux: Our experience with 115 ureters. J Urol 144:535, 1990.)

Although much of this is true, many practitioners believe that the shortcomings of the procedure outweigh the advantages. The long-term cessation of reflux in injected patients remains to be seen, most series reporting follow-up ranging from only 6 to 36 months. There have been a large number of recurrences mandating either repeat injection or further surgery. On the whole, most series have reported that a large number of injected ureters have had only grade 1 to 2 reflux and have been treated in conjunction with a contralateral ureter of a higher grade reflux. The inclusion of this subset of patients with ureters that normally would not be reimplanted and may in fact experience resolution of reflux spontaneously falsely elevates both the short-term and long-term cure rates. In fact, despite the initial high success rate with ureters of grade 4 to 5 reflux reported by O'Donnell and Puri,[67] it appears that the majority of ureters in which failures and recurrences occur belong to this select group, composed of patients in whom some form of surgical correction will be necessary. These are the patients that will probably require multiple repeat injections (and possibly subsequent reimplantation) as opposed to a single reimplant.

Much criticism of the sting procedure has arisen because of the relative lack of knowledge about the long-term systemic effects of Teflon in patients. Teflon has been used for vocal cord and periurethral injections. There have been reports in the literature of migration of Teflon particles to distant sites including the lungs, brain, and lymph nodes.[77–79] A recent report suggested that Teflon migration to the lungs was responsible for fever and local pulmonary inflammation.[80] Other local complications such as perineal abscess and urethritis have been seen.[81] Proponents of the "sting" procedure believe that the subureteral injection site is an anatomically low-risk site that has much less chance of hematogenous or lymphatic spread. Histologic studies have revealed that the injected Teflon is surrounded by a dense reactive pseudocapsule that shows no local migration.[65, 82] The true long-term effects of this material remain to be elucidated.

Currently, many studies are being conducted in an effort to identify a more suitable injection material. A promising alternative appears to be glutaraldehyde cross-linked bovine collagen, a compound with low antigenicity that produces a minimal inflammatory reaction. Many series with provocative results have been reported.[83–87] Frey and colleagues reported recently a 59% cure after one injection and 77% after two injections.[88] Additionally, among patients with ureters undergoing one and two injections, respectively, 9 and 12% showed significant improvement in grade of reflux. Histologic studies have revealed that bovine collagen is eventually replaced with human collagen.[89–91] Difficulties have arisen with long-term recurrence that probably results from volume loss within the injected material. Similar problems with volume loss secondary to resorption occur with injected fat and fibroblasts.[92, 93] An intriguing report from Atala and associates directly addresses the issue of migration of injected material.[94] They reported the use of an inflatable silicon balloon that can be placed subureterally while deflated and then filled with a quick-drying polymer (Fig. 51–4). Initial results of this treatment in pigs with surgically induced reflux show successful resolution of reflux. Potential problems include balloon rupture during insertion and misplacement of the balloon, with subsequent treatment failure necessitating repeat injection. More recently, Atala and associates have reported the use of chondrocyte-seeded alginate suspensions for injection with the ultimate goal of creating cartilaginous support of the intramural ureter.[62] Initial studies in mice show the material to be safe and suitable for injection.

The role of injection therapy in secondary reflux has been addressed. Once again the results seem to be variable, with success rates of approximately 70%.[95, 96] Puri and Guiney reported successful treatment in 13 of 15 ureters in children with neuropathic bladders.[97] Although it may be tempting to approach chronically obstructed or neurogenic bladders endoscopically owing to the technical difficulty encountered with open reimplantation, one must be wary of the potential for failure with the high-pressure bladder. The fundamentals of managing secondary reflux in this situation by reducing intravesical pressure must be followed despite the ease of injection therapy.

The idea of a less-invasive procedure with a short-

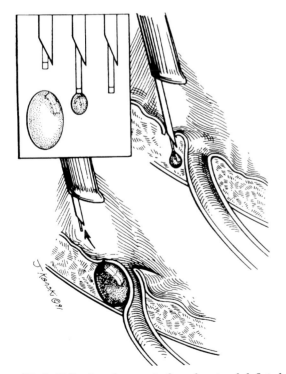

Figure 51–4 Following placement of a subureteral deflated silicon balloon, an injection of quick-drying polymer is used to distend the balloon to an appropriate size. (From Atala A, Peters CA, Retik AB, Mandell J: Endoscopic treatment of vesicoureteral reflux with a self-detachable balloon system. J Urol 148 [2pt 2]:592, 1992.)

ened hospital stay is inviting; however, repeated anesthesia and hospital visits may be potentially traumatic emotionally to the patient and parents. Brown showed that patients undergoing the sting procedure required significantly more follow-up cystograms compared with reimplant patients.[73] This may be unsettling to patients and parents who often have been through a long series of urinary tract infections and are eager to "get everything taken care of." Inability to effect a permanent cure may produce unnecessary anxiety on the part of the patient and may arouse distrust of the physician.

The role of endoscopic management of reflux is controversial. It does not serve as a substitute for reimplantation surgery. However, it is foolish to ascribe no value to a procedure of minimal invasiveness and morbidity. King points out that the procedure may be ideal for failed reimplantation by providing greater backing for the intramural ureter.[9] The experience with injection in adults has been limited but may be ideal for patients who are reluctant to undergo major open surgery. Many investigators believe that endoscopic examination of the orifice, noting its laterality and size as well as the length of the intramural ureter, may be a useful means of predicting which ureters will respond favorably to injection therapy. The greatest concern with Teflon injection remains the potential for systemic morbidity secondary to migration of the injected material. Unlike incontinent patients, most VUR patients are children with an anticipated postoperative course that is extremely long. The possibility of damaging the long-term health and even the longevity of the patient makes this procedure unattractive to the majority of pediatric surgeons.

When the data are stratified and patients with higher grade reflux are compared directly, injection therapy does not achieve the results seen with open reimplantation. A definite learning curve exists with regard to patient outcome after injection therapy, and in certain centers this may be an acceptable means of managing patients with persistent moderate grade reflux. In the hands of most surgeons, however, the procedure may be associated with frustration for both physician and patient. Most important, patients and parents should be aware of the potential for further reflux and the need for multiple procedures.

OPEN SURGICAL REIMPLANTATION

Surgical reimplantation of the ureter remains the gold standard for the therapy of VUR. Through the years, refinement of the technique has produced a procedure that allows high success rates with minimal morbidity. In many circumstances, failure of the procedure has been attributable to failure of preoperative assessment of the patient rather than unsatisfactory technique. Recent reports have suggested that in the hands of an experienced surgeon, excellent results can be achieved with a variety of techniques as long as the fundamental principles of reimplantation are observed.

The history of antireflux surgery dates back to the nineteenth century, but it was not until the midtwentieth century that the operation was truly refined. At this time reimplantation came into vogue as the potentially deleterious effects of reflux were noted. A progression in preferred technique has occurred, and the originally described extravesical vesicoureteroplasty has been virtually replaced by the intravesical ureteroneocystostomy in the United States. The extravesical procedure is still actively practiced in Europe and has nearly equivalent success rates in experienced hands.

TECHNIQUE

The decision of which technique of ureteral reimplantation to use is difficult to make and has generated much controversy. The commonly employed extravesical techniques include the Lich-Gregoire operation and extravesical detrusorraphy. The Paquin procedure employs a combined intravesical and extravesical approach. Intravesical procedures include the Leadbetter-Politano reimplantation, the Cohen crosstrigonal reimplantation, the Glenn-Anderson ureteral advancement, the Gil-Vernet trigonoplasty, and a variety of other modifications on a similar theme. The consensus appears to be that any of these techniques can be used successfully provided that the fundamental principles of reimplantation set forth by Paquin are adhered to.[98] These include creation of an adequate length of intramural ureter (preferably five times the length of the orifice diameter), an anastomosis free of tension, and adequate muscular support of the intramural ureter provided by the detrusor. In choosing a technique, the training and experience of the surgeon are probably the most important factors; however, subtle differences among these techniques do exist.

The Lich-Gregoire technique (Fig. 51–5), described in 1961,[99] is an extravesical extraperitoneal approach to the ureter. The ureter is freed to its vesical insertion. The detrusor is incised extramucosally in a cephalad direction, taking care not to enter the bladder. The ureter is then laid into this new bed and the detrusor is closed over it, providing lengthening of the intramural ureter with good detrusor support. Initial success rates with this procedure were very high, with a 96% resolution rate in refluxing ureters not accompanied by neurogenic bladder disease.[100] Marberger and colleagues reported a 98% rate of cessation of VUR with the Lich-Gregoire technique.[101] Limitations include an inability to gauge the tightness of the detrusor closure and therefore the pressure applied to the distal ureter. Additionally, the achievable tunnel length is limited by kinking of the distal ureter, making this procedure less attractive for significantly dilated ureters. Both these shortcomings make postoperative ureteral obstruction a significant concern, particularly in the hands

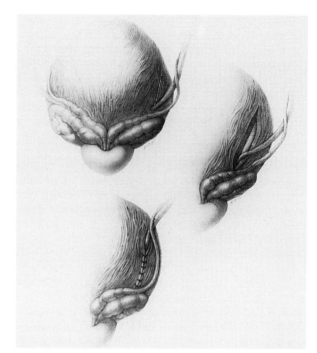

Figure 51-5 The Lich-Gregoire extravesical vesicoureteroplasty. An incision is made in the detrusor, preserving the mucosal layer, after which the ureter is laid into the created groove. (From Fowler JE [ed]: Urologic Surgery. Boston, Little, Brown & Company, 1992.)

of an inexperienced surgeon. Advantages of the extravesical approach include ease of ureteral mobilization, a reduction in postoperative bladder spasm, and a shorter and less complicated recovery period with less hematuria and no need for catheter drainage, stenting, or pelvic drains.

There has been renewed interest in the Lich-Gregoire extravesical approach with the idea of laparoscopic antireflux surgery. Reports of laparoscopic vesicoureteroplasty in animals have appeared,[58] and recently the first two human laparoscopic antireflux procedures were performed at UCLA.[59] The procedures were performed without complications and with minimal blood loss. Early follow-up revealed resolution of reflux in both patients. Perhaps attempts at laparoscopic correction of reflux will be accompanied by further refinements in extravesical vesicoureteroplasty.

In an effort to incorporate the idea of ureteral advancement with the extravesical approach and perhaps improve on the Lich-Gregoire technique, Daines and Hodges reported a new technique of extravesical repair.[102] The so-called detrusorraphy involves dissection of the ureter to its mucosal insertion followed by creation of a submucosal plane beneath the detrusor muscle (Fig. 51–6). Sutures are then placed from the mouth of the ureter to the most distant point of the mobilized detrusor. These sutures are then used to pull the ureter distally into the sleeve created by the detrusor and mucosa, thereby creating a ureteral advancement. The detrusor is then closed over the ureter to provide a strong back-

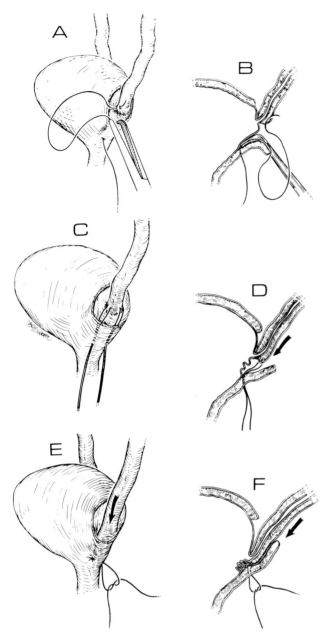

Figure 51-6 The detrusorrhaphy method of extravesical repair. *A* and *B,* Following elevation of the detrusor from the intact mucosa, sutures are placed from the distal ureteral musculature into the created pocket of detrusor. *C* and *D,* Using these sutures for traction, the ureter is advanced beneath the raised flap of detrusor to lengthen the intramural tunnel. *E* and *F,* The sutures are then tied down, and the overlying detrusor is closed. (From Zaontz MR, Maizels M, Sugar EC, et al: Detrusorrhaphy: Extravesical ureteral advancement to correct vesicoureteral reflux in children. J Urol 138:948, 1987.)

ing.[103] Zaontz and coworkers performed this procedure on 79 children with 120 refluxing ureters.[104] Resolution of reflux was noted in 93% of ureters with failures occurring predominantly in patients with higher grades of reflux, megaureter, and neuropathic bladders. These results again serve to emphasize the shortcomings of the extravesical approach. These limitations among others have led to a shift of prefer-

ence among surgeons away from the extravesical approach.

Paquin described a technique of combined intravesical and extravesical repair.[98] The extravesical portion involves dissection and mobilization of the ureter followed by transection at the ureterovesical junction (Fig. 51-7). The ureter is then tunneled submucosally intravesically, and a ureteral backing is created by closure of the detrusor extravesically. It is now realized that this extensive procedure is probably not necessary in most circumstances. In reoperation on failed ureteral reimplants, extravesical dissection of the ureter may allow the surgeon to assess adequately the feasibility of various intravesical reimplantation techniques as determined by the available length of the ureter.

In 1952 Politano and Leadbetter described a new technique of ureteroneocystostomy that employed dissection of the extravesical ureter from an intravesical approach.[105] This procedure, which is now one of the most commonly performed procedures, revolutionized ureteral reimplantation by bringing intravesical procedures to center stage. A circumferential mucosal incision is made around the ureteral orifice. Submucosal dissection is carried transmurally in an effort to mobilize the ureter as proximally as possible. A second and more cephalad muscular hiatus is then created. The ureter is then passed from its initial hiatus through the created hiatus into the bladder (Fig. 51-8). Following closure of the original muscular hiatus, the ureter is tunneled

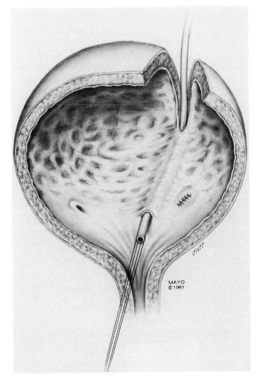

Figure 51-7 The Paquin combined extravesical/intravesical procedure. (From Kelalis PP, King LR, Belman AB [eds]: Clinical Pediatric Urology. Philadelphia, WB Saunders, 1985. By permission of Mayo Foundation.)

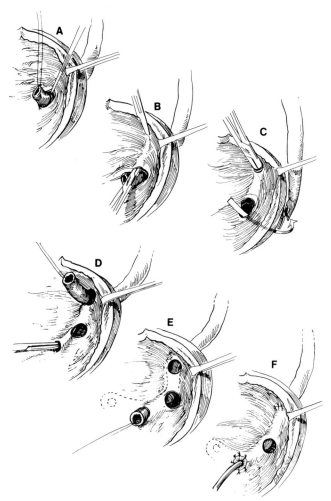

Figure 51-8 The Politano-Leadbetter technique of ureteral reimplantation. *A,* The refluxing ureter is mobilized until it is completely freed of all detrusor attachments. *B,* A submucosal tunnel is created to the point of a new muscular hiatus. *C,* The distal ureter is passed extravesically to the newly created superior muscular hiatus. *D* and *E,* The ureter is advanced through the new submucosal tunnel to the new mucosal hiatus. *F,* The mucosal anastomosis is completed with interrupted sutures. (From Walsh PC, Retik AB, Stamey TA, Vaughan ED Jr [eds]: Campbell's Urology, 6th ed. Philadelphia, WB Saunders, 1992.)

submucosally from the new hiatus to the old hiatus and beyond to a point of distal ureteral advancement. If greater length is required, the posterior bladder can be mobilized extravesically to achieve a more cephalad muscular hiatus. This will also reduce the potential risk of kinking at the site of entry into the muscular hiatus. Care must be taken to place the hiatus posteromedially rather than posterolaterally. In his initial review, Politano reported a 94% success rate in 100 patients undergoing the procedure.[106] Limitations of the procedure include the possibility of angulation of the ureter at the muscular hiatus. This makes the operation unsuitable for patients with a thick bladder wall or dilated ureters that require great tunnel length. Some practitioners have reported that this technique is of greater technical difficulty and requires greater experience with the procedure.[109]

The Gil-Vernet method,[107] or trigonoplasty, is an intravesical procedure in which the ureteral orifices are simply medialized to advance the intramural ureter (Fig. 51–9). A single transverse incision through the trigonal mucosa is employed. The internal lip of each ureter is then advanced across the trigone using tacking sutures to the exposed contralateral trigonal musculature. Since the original description, many groups have shown interest in this procedure with minor modifications. The initial results showed resolution of reflux in 90 to 97% of patients.[130–132] It is questionable how much intramural ureteral length

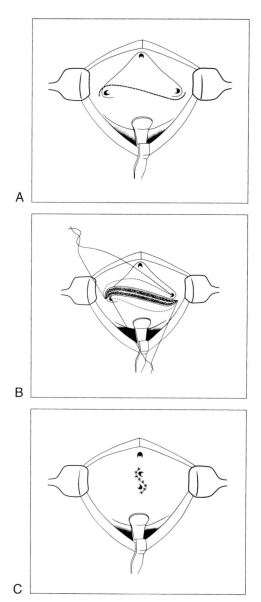

Figure 51-9 Bilateral medialization of the ureteral orifices by the method of Gil-Vernet. *A,* A transverse S-shaped incision is made across the trigonal mucosa. *B,* Sutures are placed laterally within a full-thickness incision of the trigonal muscle to the contralateral ureteral orifice. *C,* On completion of the procedure, the orifices are juxtaposed at midtrigone. (From Carini M, Selli C, Lenzi R, et al: Surgical treatment of vesicoureteral reflux with bilateral medialization of the ureteral orifices. Eur Urol 11:182, 1985. With permission from S. Karger AG, Basel.)

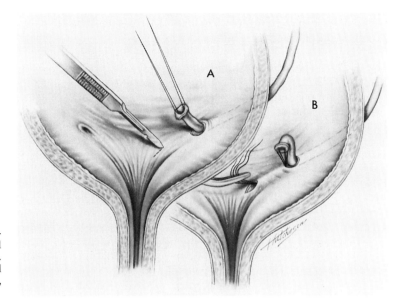

Figure 51-10 Distal ureteral advancement as described by Glenn and Anderson. The ureter is freed of all attachments and advanced within a submucosal tunnel. (From Kelalis PP, King LR, Belman AB [eds]: Clinical Pediatric Urology, 3rd ed. Philadelphia, WB Saunders, 1992. By permission of Mayo Foundation.)

can be achieved without remodeling the detrusor to provide additional support. Certain modifications have addressed this issue.[54] Recently one group reported the use of laparoscopic trocars placed suprapubically along with a standard cystoscope to perform an endoscopic trigonoplasty.[108]

Intravesical ureteral advancement procedures have been described by many authors. Perhaps the most well known of these is the Glenn-Anderson technique, initially described in 1967.[110] In this procedure the ureter is mobilized from the intravesical vantage (Fig. 51–10). Dissection is carried as far proximally as possible. A submucosal tunnel is then created, preserving the original muscular hiatus and advancing the ureter within. This procedure has the disadvantage of requiring a large trigonal area to provide sufficient tunnel length. Again, ureteral diameter plays a significant role in selection of patients for ureteral advancement.

The Cohen cross-trigonal reimplantation technique[111] has become the most commonly employed technique of ureteroneocystostomy and is used in a wide variety of patient groups. In this technique the ureter is advanced within a submucosal tunnel across the trigone to a position contralateral to its original insertion (Fig. 51–11). Adequate length can almost always be achieved, making the procedure suitable for dilated as well as nondilated ureters. The original muscular hiatus is preserved, thereby adding to the simplicity of the operation and reducing the chance of kinking at the entry site, as occurs in the Leadbetter-Politano operation. The orifice is cannulated initially with a 5 Fr feeding tube sutured to both lips of the ureter. This catheter provides traction during the procedure and allows easy visualization of the submucosal course of the ureter on dissection. During dissection of the intramural ureter, all bladder attachments are taken down from the ureteral wall. Once freed completely, the ureter is advanced through the created tunnel just superior to

the trigone. A single wide tunnel can be used in cases of bilateral repair. The muscular hiatus must be closed at the site of dissection to provide detrusor backing for the ureter. Caution must be exerted to avoid making too tight a closure of the hiatus because this can create obstruction postoperatively. Another common error is twisting the ureter as it crosses the

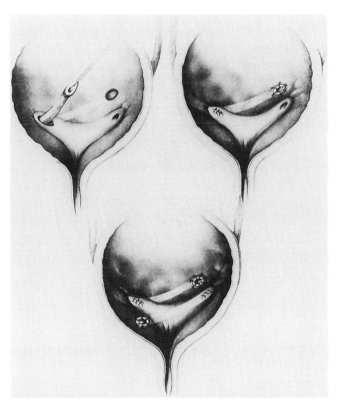

Figure 51-11 The Cohen technique of ureteroneocystostomy. Ureters are advanced across the trigone in a submucosal tunnel, resulting in a contralateral position for each ureter. (From Fowler JE [ed]: Urologic Surgery. Boston, Little, Brown & Company, 1992.)

trigone within its tunnel (Fig. 51–12); this can be easily avoided by paying attention to detail.

Many series have reported excellent results with the Cohen operation. Ahmed performed the procedure in 131 ureters in 92 children.[112] Persistent reflux was noted in only one ureter. One case of postoperative obstruction occurred, requiring percutaneous drainage. This obstruction resolved spontaneously 1 week later and was attributed to edema. Wacksman noted resolution of reflux in all but 1 of 157 ureters reimplanted by the Cohen technique.[113] One ureter displayed persistent but stable hydronephrosis at follow-up. Ehrlich reimplanted 229 ureters in children with primary reflux, reporting a 98.7% success rate with no postoperative obstruction.[114] Additionally, 109 ureters in patients with either anatomic abnormality or reoperation for failed ureteroneocystostomy were reimplanted by the Cohen technique. A 94.5% success rate was observed. Again, no ureteral obstruction occurred postoperatively.

Much of the criticism of the Cohen procedure arises from the difficulty encountered in postoperative ureteral instrumentation due to the contralateral displacement of the orifice. Many techniques have been devised to overcome this difficulty.[115–117] Suprapubic puncture for endoscopy allows easy visualization and cannulation. Specific catheters have been created for this purpose. The need for ureteral instrumentation in this subset of patients is rare. However, when necessary, current endourologic technology makes instrumentation possible, and ureteral instrumentation following the Cohen operation is apparently no longer a significant problem.

Questions have arisen about the ease of the Politano-Leadbetter procedure compared with cross-trigonal advancement. Many authors suggest that the Cohen procedure carries far less morbidity, higher success rates, and greater technical ease in the hands of most surgeons. Carpentier and colleagues reviewed 100 reimplantations performed by the Cohen technique and the Politano-Leadbetter operation in relatively comparable groups.[10] A 97% success rate in the Cohen group was noted, compared to 88% in the Politano-Leadbetter group. Contradictory data were published by Burbige showing a 97.8% success rate in 52 Cohen-treated patients and a 96.7% success rate in 70 Politano-Leadbetter–treated patients.[118] Burbige suggested that the lower success rates previously reported with the Politano-Leadbetter procedure may simply reflect the inexperience of the surgeon. Certainly with several potential sources for failure with this more difficult procedure, one must be experienced with the procedure. Prior to selecting patients for the Politano-Leadbetter method, the surgeon must be sure that adequate length can be achieved without angulation of the ureter at the new muscular hiatus. Although long-term cessation rates of reflux are similar for both procedures, hydronephrosis resolves more quickly in Cohen-treated patients. The likelihood of postoperative obstruction seems to be less as well.

When choosing an operation for reflux, the surgeon must take several factors into account. The dilatation of the ureter must be assessed because it predicts the length of the intramural tunnel that will be required (five times the ureteral diameter). Dilatation of greater than 8 to 10 mm probably requires tapering prior to reimplantation, in which case a low-risk, tension-free anastomosis is of paramount importance. Ureteral advancement procedures and extravesical procedures are limited in regard to the length of intramural ureter that can be created. These procedures are more appropriate for moderate grade reflux with relatively minimal ureteral dilatation. The experience of the surgeon with any given procedure is the most important factor because this influences the success of the surgery. The Cohen procedure is the most versatile of the operations and allows most surgeons satisfactory success rates.

Reoperative ureteroneocystostomy is a more complex procedure and should be performed only by those extremely familiar with the operation. Six months from the original reimplantation should elapse to allow time for inflammation to resolve and neovascularization of the distal ureter to occur. The use of a combined extravesical and intravesical approach is advisable if there is any question of available ureteral length. After careful extravesical dissection of the ureter, intravesical reimplantation can be performed if it is deemed technically possible. Boari flap creation, psoas hitch, transureteroureterostomy, ileal ureter construction, and even autotransplantation may be necessary on rare occasions. Hendren reviewed cases of failed reimplantation at the time of reexploration and found that causes included lateral placement of the orifice, too short an intramural tunnel, and fistula formation from the distal ureter to the bladder at the proximal tunnel.[119] Mesrobian and colleagues found that a short tunnel was the predominant cause of failure in 48 reviewed cases of failure.[120] Certainly unrecognized lower tract dysfunction, particularly neurogenic bladder, can be a cause of continued reflux. Careful reevaluation, with

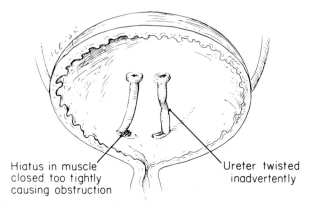

Hiatus in muscle closed too tightly causing obstruction

Ureter twisted inadvertently

Figure 51-12 Potential complications of the Cohen transtrigonal ureteral advancement: inadvertent twisting of the ureter within the submucosal tunnel or tight closure of the muscular hiatus. Both are easily avoided by paying attention to detail. (From Ehrlich RM: Success of the transvesical advancement technique for vesicoureteral reflux. J Urol 126:555, 1982.)

urodynamic studies if indicated, is prudent prior to reoperation.

Results of Reimplantation

A recent critical review of surgical reimplantation as a therapy for VUR was conducted through the IRSC. In the United States branch 87 children underwent ureteral reimplantation for grades 3 and 4 reflux.[121] In 80% of these children, reimplantation was performed bilaterally, making the total number of treated ureters 154. The Cohen reimplantation was the most commonly employed technique. Resolution of reflux occurred in all but five ureters. Spontaneous resolution had occurred in four of these five ureters by 13 months follow-up. No episodes of postoperative obstruction occurred. The European branch noted similar results.[122] One hundred and fifty-one children were treated surgically with a total of 237 ureters. Resolution of reflux was noted in 97.5% of ureters at 5 years follow-up. Ten episodes of postoperative obstruction occurred, requiring seven reoperations.

With the current standard of care, a rate of reflux cessation of less than 98% is unacceptable. Most series, regardless of the chosen technique, report high levels of success with minimal morbidity. Commonly seen complications of reimplantation include postoperative ureteral obstruction, hematuria, infection, bladder spasm, and residual reflux. An increased risk of urinary tract infection during pregnancy has been noted in women who have previously undergone ureteral reimplantation. Austenfeld and Snow reviewed the records of 30 women with previous ureteroneocystostomy who subsequently became pregnant.[123] Fifty-seven percent of women had a urinary tract infection during pregnancy and 17% had an episode of pyelonephritis. Eight of the women underwent spontaneous abortion, and one patient required percutaneous drainage for severe obstruction. These rates of infection are significantly higher than the accepted 4 to 7% rate of asymptomatic bacteriuria seen in the general population during pregnancy. This may be explained simply by the higher predilection of the reflux patient for development of urinary tract infection.

The most serious of the above-mentioned complications is postoperative obstruction. Most series report obstruction in less than 5% of patients. A significant number of episodes of postoperative obstruction may be secondary to anastomotic edema and may resolve prior to reoperation. Hendren observed several possible causes of postoperative obstruction in the patients he treated with reoperation.[119] Angulation of the ureter at the muscular hiatus was the most common cause. This can often be corrected simply by incising the hiatus itself. Also noted were a fibrotic distal ureteral segment secondary to ischemia. Care must be exercised during the operation to avoid picking up the ureter with forceps and to mobilize the ureter with adequate periureteral tissue. Reoperation in these cases is difficult owing to the shortened

length of available ureter, which often requires a psoas hitch or Boari flap. Finally, Hendren reported some cases in which the ureter had been brought across the cul-de-sac and through bowel serosa, forming an occlusive band. Most of these complications can be avoided by using the Cohen operation. These causes were confirmed in a review by Mesrobian and coworkers, who found that mechanical factors accounted for 61% of cases of obstruction and ureteral ischemia accounted for another 31%.[120] Certainly the potential for obstruction is greater in patients with megaureter that requires tapering. Stenting of such anastomoses is highly recommended.

Intraoperative and Postoperative Management

The use of ureteral stents postoperatively has become largely an issue of the surgeon's preference. Valid arguments in favor of and against stenting exist. In cases of ureteral advancement in which the ureterovesical junction is not disturbed, such as extravesical and trigonalization procedures, stenting is not necessary. The creation of a ureterovesical anastomosis provides greater potential for edema and concomitant obstruction. If used, stents should remain in place for only a short time while the patient is in the hospital and should exit percutaneously for ease of removal. Ureteral tapering or reoperation is an absolute indication for stenting. Suboptimal anastomoses with a potential for tension should be stented if tension cannot be released. In the majority of cases with uncomplicated ureteroneocystostomy, stenting is not necessary.

Suprapubic bladder drainage is recommended in most cases. In healthy bladder tissue most cystostomy closures heal quickly if they are closed meticulously; however, suprapubic drainage provides excellent drainage of the bladder and eliminates the need for uncomfortable urethral catheters in these children. Further episodes of postoperative retention can be treated quickly and with minimal discomfort. The tube need only remain for a short period once adequate healing of the ureteral anastomosis can be ensured. A retropubic drain need not be placed unless bladder closure is suboptimal or unhealthy tissue is present.

Postoperative management should include oral antibiotic prophylaxis until documentation of reflux cessation is obtained. Breakthrough infections should be treated aggressively with the strong suspicion of a partial obstruction. In the absence of flank pain, prolonged postoperative fever, elevation of creatinine level, or oliguria, follow-up studies can be obtained 3 months postoperatively.

Voiding cystourethrogram and renal ultrasound complete the follow-up. Repeat studies should be obtained at the end of the first postoperative year. The frequency of studies is determined by the presence and severity of continued reflux. Rarely does reflux recur following a normal vesicoureterogram at 3 months, particularly in the absence of worsening symptoms or infection. Reoperation should be performed with little hesitation when indicated, and the procedure should take place within the first year of continued significant reflux, particularly in the presence of recurrent urinary tract infection.

Special Surgical Considerations

In the presence of lower urinary tract abnormalities, specific plans must be made prior to reimplantation. Failure of the operation is a potential sequela of poor strategy in regard to anatomic abnormalities.

Duplicated ureteral systems can be managed by several options.[123, 124] Preoperative evaluation should include documentation of the segment or ureter that is refluxing and the degree of function present at the time of reimplantation. Most commonly, en bloc reimplantation of both ureteral orifices through an intravesical approach is ideal. With this method the lower pole–ureter is lengthened in its intramural course and the juxtaposition of the orifices is preserved. In cases of lateral or caudad displacement of the refluxing ureter, ureteroureterostomy may be ideal for preservation of the nonrefluxing orifice. Heminephrectomy is indicated in cases of nonfunction.

Bladder diverticula are often associated with and can cause VUR, mandating simultaneous excision at the time of ureteroneocystostomy. Paraureteral diverticula can cause failure of reimplantation if they are unrecognized. Reflux often resolves following bladder diverticulectomy without the need for a simultaneous reimplantation procedure, particularly when the diverticulum serves as a nidus of infection.[125] If the orifice is impinged on by the diverticulum or actually drains into it, ureteroneocystostomy is advisable and usually necessary because reflux may not abate or may actually become worse, particularly if a ureteral fistula tract is created during mobilization of the diverticulum. The clinical situation may dictate the overall management strategy, with the severity of infection or renal deterioration determining the aggressiveness used at the initial procedure.

Neurogenic bladder accompanied by VUR is a clinical scenario that presents many challenges in management. Operations for reflux in this setting are technically difficult and carry a high risk of failure. The thickened bladder wall in patients with spastic bladder can create technical difficulty by causing tension on the anastomosis, causing ureteral angulation at the muscular hiatus and making creation of a submucosal tunnel and ureterovesical anastomosis difficult. In patients who have had previous lower tract decompression procedures, the use of an extravesical procedure may be prudent to avoid intravesical inflammation and possible bacterial contamination. In many early series before the importance of lower tract dysfunction was understood, many reported failed reimplants were secondary to neuro-genic bladder dysfunction. With an understanding of intravesical pressure elevation as a causative factor in secondary VUR, the idea of decompressive surgery as a first-line management was conceived.

In patients with high intravesical pressures due to instability and low bladder compliance, the first tenet of therapy is conversion of the bladder to a low-pressure reservoir. Many authors propose that decompression alone should produce resolution of concomitant VUR. Nasrallah and Aliabadi performed bladder augmentation procedures in 14 patients with grade 2 to 4 reflux who had failed conservative attempts to lower intravesical pressure.[126] Of these patients, 12 had resolution of reflux, and postoperative urodynamic evaluation revealed low pressures and normal reservoir capacity. The authors concluded that persistent reflux following augmentation reflects inadequate reduction in intravesical pressure. Sidi and colleagues reviewed the treatment of 30 children with myelodysplasia and VUR.[36] Twelve of fourteen children required an antireflux procedure despite decompressive measures. The number requiring antireflux surgery among patients with low-grade reflux was much lower. Decompressive measures consisted of intermittent catheterization or vesicostomy. This group concluded that children with high-grade reflux and low-compliance reservoirs should undergo antireflux surgery early in management because they are at high risk for failure from decompressive procedures alone. The failures in this series may reflect the inability of vesicostomy to provide a low-pressure reservoir. The true predicting factor for response to decompressive therapy alone may be the condition of the ureterovesical junction at the time of surgery. In patients with normal-appearing orifices and an adequate length of intramural tunnel, augmentation alone may be enough to improve or resolve reflux. If there is evidence of deterioration of the competence of the ureterovesical valve or if the tunnel appears short, strong consideration should be given to simultaneous augmentation and reimplantation.

Several authors have reported good results with reimplantation in patients with a neurogenic bladder. Kaplan and Firlit reported a 96% rate of resolution with reimplantation.[127] Best results were achieved in the smooth-walled atonic bladder; however, trabeculation is not a contraindication. Kaplan and Firlit believe that the Cohen procedure is ideal because it avoids the trabeculated wall, and the trigone is often the only area suitable for a submucosal tunnel. Several authors have reported similar excellent results.[37, 128, 129]

CONCLUSIONS

The management of VUR is controversial and challenging. The physician must assess many variables in the nature of the reflux and the wishes of the patient prior to selecting a suitable therapeutic regimen. In children, therapy must be aggressive and should progress to surgical intervention as soon as upper tract deterioration or breakthrough upper tract infection occurs. Care must be exercised to identify any evidence of lower tract dysfunction. Surgical management must take into account the experience of the surgeon with a given procedure and the severity of reflux and upper tract dilatation. With careful selection of surgical technique and careful follow-up, excellent results with preservation of renal function can be achieved.

REFERENCES

1. Pozzi S: Ureterverletzang bei Laparotomie. Zentralb Gynaekol 17:97, 1893.
2. Hutch JA: Vesico-ureteral reflux in the paraplegic: Cause and correction. J Urol 68:457, 1952.
3. Hodson CJ, Edwards D: Chronic pyelonephritis and vesicoureteral reflux. Clin Radiol 11:219, 1960.
4. Hodson CJ, Maling TM, McManamon PJ, et al: The pathogenesis of reflux nephropathy. Br J Radiol Suppl 13:1, 1975.
5. Hodson CJ, Kincaid-Smith P: Lesions in the pig kidney with chronic pyelonephritis. In Hodson J, Kincaid-Smith P (eds): Reflux Nephropathy. New York, Masson, 1979, pp 197–212.
6. Ransley PG: Intrarenal reflux: Anatomical, dynamic and radiological studies—Part I. Urol Res 5:61, 1977.
7. Ransley PG, Risdon RA: Reflux and renal scarring. Br J Radiol 14(Suppl):1, 1978.
8. Duckett JW: Update on vesicoureteral reflux. AUA Update Series 12(5):34, 1993.
9. King LR: Vesicoureteral reflux, megaureter, and ureteral reimplantation. In Walsh PC, Retik AB, Stamey TA, Vaughan ED Jr (eds): Campbell's Urology, 6th ed. Philadelphia, WB Saunders, 1992, pp 1689–1742.
10. Bredin HC, Winchester P, McGovern HH, et al: Family study of vesicoureteral reflux. J Urol 113:623, 1975.
11. Jerkins GR, Noe HN: Family vesicoureteral reflux: A prospective study. J Urol 128:774, 1982.
12. Van den Abbele AD, Treves ST, Lebowitz RL, et al: Vesicoureteral reflux in asymptomatic siblings of patients with known reflux: Radionuclide study. Pediatrics 79:147, 1987.
13. De Vargas A, Evans K, Rausky P, et al: A family study of vesicoureteric reflux. J Med Genet 15:85, 1978.
14. Noe HN, Wyatt RJ, Peeden JN, et al: The transmission of vesicoureteral reflux from parent to child. J Urol 148:1869, 1992.
15. Weiss R, Tamminen-Mobius T, Koskimies H, et al: Characteristics at entry of children with severe vesicoureteral reflux recruited for a multicenter, international therapeutic trial comparing medical and surgical management. J Urol 148(pt 2):1644, 1992.
16. King LR, Kazmi SO, Belman AB: Natural history of vesicoureteral reflux. Urol Clin North Am 1:441, 1974.
17. King LR: Vesicoureteral reflux: History etiology, and conservative management. In Kelalis PP, King LR (eds.): Clinical Pediatric Urology. Philadelphia, WB Saunders, 1976, pp 342–365.
18. Edwards D, Normand ICS, Prescod N, et al: Disappearance of reflux during longterm prophylaxis of urinary tract infections in children. Br J Med 2:285, 1977.
19. Smellie JM: Commentary: Management of children with severe vesicoureteral reflux. J Urol 148:1676, 1992.
20. Lenaghan JD, Whitaker G, Johnson F, et al: The natural history of reflux and long term effects of reflux on the kidney. J Urol 115:728, 1976.
21. Arant BS: Medical management of mild and moderate reflux: Followup studies of infants and young children. A preliminary report of the Southwest Pediatric Nephrology Study Group. J Urol 148(pt. 2):1683, 1992.
22. Jodal U, Koskimies O, Hanson E, et al: Infection pattern in children with vesicoureteral reflux randomly allocated to operation or longterm antibacterial prophylaxis. J Urol 148(pt 2):1650, 1992.
23. Olbing H, Claesson I, Ebel KD, et al: Renal scars and parenchymal thinning in children with vesicoureteral reflux: 5 year report of International Reflux Study in Children (European branch). J Urol 148(pt. 2):1653, 1992.
24. Brunier E, Ebel KD, Lebowitz R, et al: Cessation of vesicoureteral reflux for 5 years in children allocated to medical treatment. J Urol 148(pt. 2):1662, 1992.
25. Weiss R, Duckett JW, Spitzer A: Results of randomized clinical trial of medical versus surgical management of infants and children with grades III and IV primary vesicoureteral reflux. J Urol 148(pt. 2):1667, 1992.
26. Malek RS, Svensson J, Neves RJ, et al: Vesicoureteral reflux in the adult. III. Surgical correction: Risks and benefits. J Urol 130:882, 1983.
27. Neves RJ, Torres VE, Malek RS, et al: Vesicoureeral reflux in the adult. IV. Medical versus surgical management. J Urol 132:882, 1984.
28. Smellie JS: The DMSA scan and intravenous urography in the detection of renal scarring. Pediatr Nephrol 3:6, 1989.
29. Ghoniem GM, Bloom DA, McGuire EJ, et al: Bladder compliance in meningomyelocele children. J Urol 141:1404, 1989.
30. Hackler RH, Hall MK, Zampieri TA: Bladder hypocompliance in the spinal cord injury population. J Urol 141:1391, 1989.
31. Gerridzen RG, Thijssen AM, Dehoux E: Risk factors for upper tract deterioration in chronic spinal cord injury patients. J Urol 147:416, 1992.
32. McGuire EJ, Woodside JR, Borden TA: Prognostic value of urodyanamic testing in myelodysplastic patients. J Urol 126:205, 1981.
33. Magnus RV: Vesicoureteral reflux in babies with myelomeningocele. J Urol 114:122, 1975.
34. Levitt SB, Sandler HJ: The absence of vesicoureteral reflux in the neonate with myelomeningocele. J Urol 114:118, 1975.
35. Cass AS, Luxenberg M, Johnson CF, et al: Management of the neurogenic bladder in 413 children. J Urol 132:521, 1984.
36. Sidi AA, Peng W, Gonzalez R: Vesicoureteral refluxing children with myelodysplasia: Natural history and results of treatment. J Urol 136:329, 1986.
37. Bauer SB, Colodny AH, Retik AB: The management of vesicoureteral reflux in children with myelodysplasia. J Urol 128:102, 1982.
38. Brock WA, So EP, Harbach LB, et al: Intermittent catheterization in the management of neurogenic vesical dysfunction in children. J Urol 125:391, 1981.
39. Sullivan T, Purcell MM, Gregory JG: The management of vesicoureteral reflux in the pediatric neurogenic bladder. J Urol 125:65, 1981.
40. Kass EJ, Koff SA, Diokno AC: Fate of vesicoureteral reflux in children with neuropathic bladders managed by intermittent catheterization. J Urol 125:63, 1981.
41. Cass AS, Luxenberg M, Gleich P, et al: Clean intermittent catheterization in the management of the neurogenic bladder in children. J Urol 132:526, 1984.
42. Kaplan WE, Sugar EC, Firlit CF: Effectiveness of intermittent catheterization in the myelomeningocele patient (abstract 276). Annual meeting of American Urological Association, Boston, Massachusetts, May 10–14, 1981.
43. Hinman F, Baumman FW: Vesical and ureteral damage from voiding dysfunction in boys without neurologic or obstructive disease. J Urol 109:727, 1973.
44. Allen TD: The non-neurogenic neurogenic bladder. J Urol 117:232, 1977.
45. Koff SA: Relationship between dysfunctional voiding and reflux. J Urol 148(pt. 2):1703, 1992.
46. Griffiths DJ, Scholtmeijer RJ: Vesicoureteral reflux and lower urinary tract dysfunction: Evidence for two different reflux/dysfunction complexes. J Urol 137:240, 1987.
47. Van Gool JD, Hjalmas K, Tamminen-Mobius T, et al: Historical clues to the complex of dysfunctional voiding, urinary tract infection and vesicoureteral reflux. J Urol 148(pt. 2):1699, 1992.
48. Koff SA, Lapides J, Piazza DH: Association of urinary tract infection and reflux with uninhibited bladder contractions and voluntary sphincteric obstruction. J Urol 122:374, 1979.
49. Lyon RP, Marshall S, Tanagho EA: The ureteral orifice: Its configuration and competency. J Urol 102:504, 1969.

50. Koff SA, Murtagh DS: The uninhibited bladder in children: Effect of treatment on recurrence of urinary tract infection and on resolution of vesicoureteral reflux. J Urol 130:1138, 1983.

51. Seruca H: Vesicoureteral reflux and voiding dysfunction: A prospective study. J Urol 142:494, 1989.

52. Nasrallah PH, Simon JW: Reflux and voiding abnormalities in children. Urology 24:243, 1984.

53. Homsy YL, Nsouli I, Hamburger B, et al: Effects of oxybutynin on vesicoureteral reflux in children. J Urol 134:1168, 1985.

54. Orikasa S: A new antireflux operation. Eur Urol 17:330, 1990.

55. Noe HN: The role of dysfunctional voiding in failure or complication of ureteral reimplantation for primary reflux. J Urol 134:1173, 1985.

56. Nielsen JB, Norgaard JP, Djurhuus JC: Enuresis as protective factor in vesicoureteral reflux. Urology 26:316, 1985.

57. Allen TD: Commentary: Voiding dysfunction and reflux. J Urol 148(pt. 2):1706, 1992.

58. Atala A, Kavoussi LR, Goldstein DS, et al: Laparoscopic correction of vesicoureteral reflux. J Urol 150:748, 1993.

59. Ehrlich RM, Gershman A, Fuchs G: Laparoscopic vesicoureteroplasty in children. Urology 43:255, 1994.

60. Husmann DA, Allen TD: Resolution of vesicoureteral reflux in completely duplicated systems: Fact or fiction. J Urol 145:1022, 1991.

61. Peppas DS, Skoog SJ, Canning DA, et al: Nonsurgical management of primary vesicoureteral reflux in complete ureteral duplication: Is it justified? J Urol 146:1594, 1991.

62. Atala A, Cima LG, Kim W, et al: Injectable alginate seeded with chondrocytes as a potential treatment for vesicoureteral reflux. J Urol 150:745, 1993.

63. O'Donnell B, Puri P: Treatment of vesicoureteric reflux by endoscopic injection of Teflon. Br Med J 289:7, 1984.

64. O'Donnell B, Puri P: Endoscopic correction of primary vesicoureteric reflux: Results in 94 ureters. Br Med J 293:1404, 1986.

65. Puri P, O'Donnell B: Correction of experimentally produced vesicoureteric reflux in the piglet by intravesical injection of Teflon. Br Med J 289:5, 1984.

66. O'Donnell B, Puri P: endoscopic correction of primary vesicouretric reflux. Br J Urol 58:601, 1986.

67. Puri P, O'Donnell B: Endoscopic correction of grades IV and V primary vesicoureteric reflux: Six to 30 month follow-up in 42 ureters. J Pediatr Surg 22:1087, 1987.

68. Schulman CC, Simon J, Pamart D, et al: Endoscopic treatment of vesicoureteral reflux in children. J Urol 138:950, 1987.

69. Farkas A, Moriel E, Lupa S: Endoscopic correction of vesicoureteral reflux: Our experience with 115 ureters. J Urol 144:534, 1990.

70. Dodat H, Takvorian P: Treatment of vesicoureteral reflux in children by endoscopic injection of Teflon. Eur Urol 17:304, 1990.

71. Sauvage P, Geiss S, Saussine C, et al: Analysis and perspectives of endoscopic treatment of vesicoureteral reflux in children with a 20 month follow-up. Eur Urol 17:310, 1990.

72. Kaplan WE, Dalton DP, Firlit CS: The endoscopic correction of reflux by polytetraflouroethylene injection. J Urol 138:953, 1987.

73. Brown S: Open versus endoscopic surgery in the treatment of vesicoureteral reflux. J Urol 142:499, 1989.

74. Geiss S, Alessandrini P, Allouch G, et al: Multicenter survey of endoscopic treatment of vesicoureteral reflux in children. Eur Urol 17:328, 1990.

75. O'Donnell B, Puri P: Technical refinements in endoscopic correction of vesicoureteric reflux. J Urol 140:1101, 1988.

76. Lacombe A: Ureterovesical reimplantation after failure of endoscopic treatment of reflux by submucosal injection of Polytef paste. Eur Urol 17:318, 1990.

77. Malizia AA Jr, Reiman HM, Myers RP, et al: Migration and granulomatous reaction after periurethral injection of Polytef (Teflon). JAMA 251:3277, 1984.

78. Kaufman M, Lockhart JL, Silverstein MJ, et al: Transurethral polytetrafluoroethylene injection for postprostatectomy urinary incontinence. J Urol 132:463, 1984.

79. Mittleman RE, Marracini JV: Pulmonary Teflon granulomas following periurethral Teflon injection for urinary incontinence. Arch Pathol Lab Med 107:611, 1983.

80. Claes H, Stroobants D, Van Meerbeek J, et al: Pulmonary migration following periurethral polytetrafluoroethylene injection for urinary incontinence. J Urol 142:821, 1989.

81. Politano VA, Small MP, Harper JM, et al: Periurethral Teflon injection for urinary incontinence. J Urol 111:180, 1974.

82. Marcellin L, Geiss S, Laustriat S, et al: Ureteral lesions due to endoscopic treatment of vesicoureteral reflux by injection of Teflon: Pathological study. Eur Urol 17:325, 1990.

83. Lipsky H: Endoscopic treatment of vesicoureteral reflux with bovine collagen. Eur Urol 18:52, 1990.

84. Frey P, Jenny P, Herzog B: Endoscopic subureteric collagen injection (SCIN): A new alternative treatment of vesicoureteric reflux in children. Experience in 82 refluxing ureters. Pediatr Surg Int 6:287, 1991.

85. Leonard MP, Canning DA, Peters CA, et al: Endoscopic injection of glutaraldehyde cross-linked bovine dermal collagen for correction of vesicoureteral reflux. J Urol 145:115, 1991.

86. Lipsky H: Endoscopic treatment of vesicoureteric reflux with collagen. Pediatr Surg Int 6:301, 1991.

87. Cendron M, Leonard MP, Gearhart JP, et al: Endoscopic treatment of vesicoureteral reflux using cross-linked bovine dermal collagen. Pediatr Surg Int 6:295, 1991.

88. Frey P, Berger D, Jenny P, et al: Subureteral collagen injection for the endoscopic treatment of vesicoureteral reflux in children. Followup study of 97 treated ureters and histological analysis of collagen implants. J Urol 148:718, 1992.

89. Frey P, Curschellas E, Kaeslin M: The longterm histological results following glutaraldehyde cross-linked collagen injection into the suburothelial space of the mini-pig bladder. Pediatr Surg Int 6:252, 1991.

90. Kempter F, Mohring K, Bersch W: Results of the endoscopic subureteric collagen injection for reflux correction in pigs and dogs. Pediatr Surg Int 6:261, 1991.

91. Reunanen MS, Toikkanen S, Viljanto J: Longterm followup of tissue reactions caused by Teflon paste and cross-linked collagen in rats. Pediatr Surg Int 6:241, 1991.

92. Canning DA, Gearhat JP, Jeffs RD: Persistence of suburothelial autologous fat transplants in the rabbit bladder. Presented at the American Society for Dermatologic Surgery, Ft. Lauderdale, Florida, March 1989.

93. Remmler D, Thomas JR, Mazoujian G, et al: Use of injectable cultured human fibroblasts for percutaneous tissue implantation. An experimental study. Arch Otolaryngol Head Neck Surg 115:837, 1989.

94. Atala A, Peters CA, Retik AB, et al: Endoscopic treatment of vesicoureteral reflux with a self-detachable balloon system. J Urol 148(pt. 2):724, 1992.

95. Kaminetsky JC, Hanna MK: Endoscopic treatment of vesicoureteral reflux in children with neurogenic bladder. Urology 37:244, 1991.

96. Aubert D, Zoupanos G, Destuynder O, et al: 'Sting' procedure in the treatment of secondary reflux in children. Eur Urol 17:307, 1990.

97. Puri P, Guiney EJ: Endoscopic correction of vesicoureteric reflux secondary to neuropathic bladder. Br J Urol 58:504, 1986.

98. Paquin AJ Jr.: Ureterovesical anastomosis: The description and evaluation of a technique. J Urol 82:573, 1959.

99. Lich R Jr, Howerton LW, Davis LA: Recurrent urosepsis in children. J Urol 86:554, 1961.

100. Gregoir W: Le traitement chirurgical des reflux vesicoureteral congenital. Acta Chir Belg 63:431, 1964.

101. Marberger M, Aitwein JC, Strach G: The Lich-Gregoir antireflux plasty: Experiences with 371 children. J Urol 120:216, 1978.

102. Daines SL, Hodges NB: Management of reflux in total duplication anomalies. J Urol 105:720, 1971.

103. Houle AM, McLorie GA, Heritz DM, et al: Extravesical non-dismembered ureteroplasty with detrusorrhaphy: Renewed

technique to correct vesicoureteral reflux in children. J Urol 148:704, 1992.

104. Zaontz MR, Maizels M, Sugar EC, et al: Detrusorrhaphy: Extravesical ureteral advancement to correct vesicoureteral reflux in children. J Urol 138(pt. 2):947, 1987.
105. Politano VA, Leadbetter WF: An operative technique for the correction of vesicoureteral reflux. J Urol 79:932, 1958.
106. Politano VA: One hundred reimplantations and five years. J Urol 90:696, 1963.
107. Gil-Vernet JM: A new technique for surgical correction of vesicoureteral reflux. J Urol 131:456, 1984.
108. Okamura K, Ono Y, Yamada Y, et al: Endoscopic trigonoplasty for primary vesicoureteral reflux: Initial case report. Presented at the annual meeting of the American Urological Association, San Antonio, Texas, May, 1993.
109. Carpentier PJ, Bettink PJ, Hop WCJ, et al: Reflux—a retrospective study of 100 ureteric reimplantations by the Politano-Leadbetter method and 100 by the Cohen technique. Br J Urol 54:230, 1982.
110. Glenn JF, Anderson EE: Distal tunnel reimplantation. J Urol 97:623, 1967.
111. Cohen SJ: Ureteroneocystostomy. Read at the annual meeting of the British Association of Paediatric Surgeons, Manchester, England, 1970.
112. Ahmed S: Ureteral reimplantation by the transverse advancement technique. J Urol 119:547, 1978.
113. Wacksman J: Initial results with the Cohen cross-trigonal ureteroneocystostomy. J Urol 129:1198, 1983.
114. Ehrlich RM: Success of the transvesical advancement technique for vesicoureteral reflux. J Urol 128:554, 1982.
115. Lamesch AJ: Retrograde catheterization of the ureter after antireflux plasty by the Cohen technique of transverse advancement. J Urol 125:73, 1981.
116. Ehrlich RM: Re:A special trocar for retrograde catheterization of the ureter following antireflux plasty by the Cohen technique of transverse advancement. J Urol 129:614, 1983.
117. Argueso LR, Kelalis PP, Patterson DE: Strategies for ureteral catheterization after the technique of transverse advancement. J Urol 146:1583, 1991.
118. Burbige KA: Ureteral reimplantation: A comparison of results with the cross-trigonal and Politano-Leadbetter techniques in 120 patients. J Urol 146:1352, 1991.
119. Hendren WH: Reoperation for failed ureteral reimplantation. J Urol 111:403, 1974.
120. Mesrobian HJ, Kramer SA, Kelalis PP: Reoperative ureteroneocystostomy: Review of 69 patients. J Urol 133:388, 1985.
121. Duckett JW, Walker RD, Weiss R: Surgical results: International Reflux Study in Children, United States branch. J Urol 148(pt. 2):1674, 1992.
122. Hjalmas K, Lohr G, Tamminen-Mobius T, et al: Surgical results in International Reflux Study in Children (Europe). J Urol 148(pt. 2):1657, 1992.
123. Austenfeld MS, Snow BW: Complications of pregnancy in women after reimplantation for vesicoureteral reflux. J Urol 140:1103, 1988.
124. Barrett DM, Malek RS, Kelalis PP: Problems and solutions in surgical treatment of 100 consecutive ureteral duplications in children. J Urol 114:126, 1975.
125. Ahmed S, Boucaut HA: Vesicoureteral reflux in complete ureteral duplication: Surgical options. J Urol 140:1092, 1988.
126. Nasrallah PF, Aliabadi HA: Bladder augmentation in patients with neurogenic bladder and vesicoureteral reflux. J Urol 146:563, 1991.
127. Kaplan WE, Firlit CF: Management of reflux in the myelodysplastic child. J Urol 129:1196, 1983.
128. Jeffs RD, Jonas P, Schillinger JF: Surgical correction of vesicoureteral reflux in children with neurogenic bladder. J Urol 115:449, 1976.
129. Woodard JR, Anderson AM III, Parrott TS: Ureteral reimplantation in myelodysplasia children. J Urol 126:387, 1981.
130. De Gennaro M, Appetito C, Lais A, et al: Effectiveness of trigonoplasty to treat primary vesicoureteral reflux. J Urol 146:636, 1991.
131. Kliment J, Fetisov I, Svitac J: Surgical management of vesicoureteral reflux by modified Gil-Vernet method. Int Urol Nephrol 22:531, 1990.
132. Carini M, Selli C, Barbagli G, et al: Surgical treatment of vesicoureteral reflux with bilateral medialization of the ureteral orifices. Eur Urol 11:181, 1985.

CHAPTER 52

Reconstruction of the Damaged Urethra

Jerry G. Blaivas, M.D., F.A.C.S.
Dianne M. Heritz, M.D., F.R.C.S.C.

Extensive damage to the female urethra is an uncommon occurrence that has two main causes—obstetrical injury and surgical trauma. In the industrialized countries, obstetrical injuries are exceedingly uncommon, but in the Third World, particularly Africa and Asia, childbirth injuries continue to exact a toll of enormous social and medical consequence. Damage to the trigone, vesical neck, and urethra during childbirth is usually the result of prolonged labor, most often associated with maternal-fetal disproportion. The bladder and urethra are thought to be compressed against the undersurface of the pubis by the fetal head, resulting in ischemic necrosis.

The compassion and surgical skills of Anna Ward and Lawson in Nigeria and the Hamlins in Ethiopia are renowned among urologists and gynecologists. Their routine success in treating the most extensive childbirth fistulas is well known. When the vesical neck and urethra are involved, incontinence all too often remains a devastating problem, which almost invariably results in social ostracism.

Surgical damage may occur during any of the Pereyra-type bladder neck suspension procedures, anterior colporrhaphy, urethral diverticulectomy, and, much less commonly, vaginal hysterectomy. In our experience, urethral diverticulectomy is the most common cause of extensive urethral damage. This most likely results from failure to obtain a tension-free closure of the urethral defect owing to excision of the diverticulum. During bladder neck suspension, inadvertent injury to the bladder or urethra may occur, or an errant suture may result in fistula formation or tissue necrosis. We have also seen several patients who sustained extensive loss of the urethra, vesical neck, and trigone after a seemingly simple Kelly plication. It is postulated that the plication sutures were tied too tightly around a urethral catheter and resulted in pressure necrosis.

Injudicious use of indwelling urethral catheters resulting in pressure necrosis of the urethra is most commonly seen in quadriplegic or paraplegic women but is occasionally encountered in neurologically normal women who have had a prolonged recovery after a devastating illness or injury. This form of injury is particularly disconcerting because it is preventable by routine hygiene and observation.

Occasionally, trauma to the pelvis may result in fracture or separation of the symphysis pubis that lacerates the urethra or vesical neck. Rarely there may be local invasion of these tissues from carcinoma of the cervix or damage from radiation treatment.

Regardless of the cause of urethral damage, the diagnostic and therapeutic challenges to the surgeon are considerable. The goals of surgical correction are to create a continent neourethra that permits the unobstructed passage of urine and is sufficiently long to ensure that the patient does not void into the vagina. It is our belief that these goals can almost always be accomplished by a single operative procedure. Rarely is a staged procedure necessary.

There are three generic approaches to urethral reconstruction: (1) anterior bladder flaps (Tanagho procedure), (2) posterior bladder flaps (Young-Dees-Leadbetter procedure), and (3) vaginal wall flaps. These techniques appear to be comparable with respect to creation of a neourethra or repair of a urethral fistula.

Whenever the vesical neck and proximal urethra are involved, which is usually the case, postoperative incontinence rates of about 50% should be expected unless a concomitant anti-incontinence procedure is performed.[1-30] We believe that vaginal reconstruction is considerably easier and faster, is much more amenable to concomitant anti-incontinence surgery, and is associated with much less morbidity than the bladder flap operations.

Preoperative Evaluation

Laboratory evaluation should include a blood urea nitrogen (BUN), serum creatinine, urinalysis, and culture. An elevated BUN and creatinine suggests the probability of ureteral obstruction. Urinalysis very often shows hematuria or pyuria. Urine cultures are often positive, but if the patient is asymptomatic, antibiotic treatment may be deferred until just prior to diagnostic cystoscopy or ureteral catheterization.

In all of these injuries, one must have a high index of suspicion for the presence of concomitant abnormalities such as ureterovaginal or vesicovaginal fistulas, ureteral obstruction, low bladder compliance, and urethral sphincteric deficiency. A careful evaluation to exclude each of these potential conditions should be undertaken prior to surgery. In addition, detrusor compromise in the form of impaired detrusor contractility or detrusor instability may be present, but these conditions generally do not require evaluation unless they persist postoperatively.

We believe that intravenous pyelography should be performed in all patients except those in whom it is contraindicated. Although renal ultrasound is adequate to evaluate the possibility of hydronephrosis, neither ureterovaginal fistulas nor partial ureteral obstruction may be apparent with this technique. If there is any suspicion of ureteral injury, retrograde pyelography should be performed even in women with normal-appearing intravenous pyelograms.

Cystoscopy and pelvic examination are essential to evaluate (1) the extent of the anatomic defect, (2) the possibility of unrecognized secondary fistulas, (3) the pliability of local tissue, (4) the need for securing bulk-ensuring tissue pedicle flaps, (5) the need for concomitant pelvic reconstructive surgery, and (6) the timing of surgery. At the time of cystoscopy, retrograde pyelography may be performed when indicated, and the integrity of the urethral sphincter should be tested while the bladder is full.

Secondary vesicovaginal fistulas are usually apparent at cystoscopic examination. If a vesicovaginal fistula is suspected but not seen at the time of cystoscopy, the bladder should be filled with fluid to which a dye such as indigo carmine or methylene blue has been added. The vagina should then be inspected for signs of urinary leakage with the urethra occluded by a Foley balloon catheter or the surgeon's examining finger to prevent urethral leakage.

Urinary incontinence is not always due to what appears to be the most overt lesion. For example, neither a urethrovaginal fistula nor a destroyed distal urethra should cause urinary incontinence unless the proximal urethra and vesical neck are also damaged. A careful stepwise evaluation should be carried out in all patients to delineate the pathophysiology underlying incontinence. Other causes of urinary incontinence commonly seen in these patients include (1) a previously undiagnosed vesicovaginal or ureterovaginal fistula, (2) detrusor instability, (3) low bladder compliance, and (4) sphincteric abnormalities.

Detrusor instability should be suspected from the history. These patients usually complain of urinary frequency, urgency, and urge incontinence. The diagnosis is confirmed by cystometry. Low bladder compliance is essentially a cystometric diagnosis that is confirmed by noting a steep rise in pressure during bladder filling. Although it is important to document the presence of detrusor instability or low bladder compliance preoperatively, it has been our experience that after surgery these conditions abate in the great majority of women. Accordingly, we do not recommend concomitant surgical interventions to treat these conditions at the time of urethral reconstruction.

There are two generic types of sphincteric incontinence—urethral hypermobility and intrinsic sphincter deficiency. Urinary incontinence due to urethral hypermobility is usually apparent on physical examination. With a full bladder the patient is asked to cough and bear down. Urethral hypermobility incontinence is apparent as a rotational descent of the bladder base, proximal urethra, and vesical neck associated with visible urinary loss during sudden increases in abdominal pressure. If, during the sudden increase in pressure, urinary loss is unaccompanied by significant descent or if there is obvious urinary leakage with a minimal increase in pressure, an intrinsic sphincteric deficiency should be suspected. The diagnosis may be confirmed by cystography or videourodynamic examination.

When sphincteric incontinence is present preoperatively, we believe that it should be surgically corrected at the time of urethral reconstruction. In general, we prefer to construct a fascial pubovaginal sling[32-53] with an interposed free graft of labial fat pad[2, 4-6, 8, 26, 37, 30, 54, 55] between the sling and the reconstructed vesical neck, but other authors have recommended the modified Pereyra technique in patients with less extensive anatomic damage and incontinence due to urethral hypermobility.

General Principles of Surgical Technique

Women with urethrovaginal fistula or anatomic urethral damage have usually undergone one or more prior vaginal operations and have urinary incontinence that is very difficult to manage. The vaginal tissues are often scarred, fibrotic, and ischemic. Prior to surgery careful examination of the vagina is necessary to determine the actual extent of urethral tissue loss and to assess the availability of local tissue for use in the reconstruction. In most instances there is sufficient tissue in the anterior vaginal wall to use as pedicled flaps for urethral reconstruction. If the vaginal tissue is extensively scarred, ischemic, or atrophied, other potential donor sites should be considered. These include labial, perineal, rectus, and gracilis pedicle flaps. Alternatively, an anterior bladder flap can be used.[2, 4-6, 17, 26, 30, 37, 54-57]

After reconstruction of the urethra or fistula repair it is usually advisable to interpose a well-vascularized pedicle flap. This can almost always be obtained from the labial fat pad (Martius flap), but occasionally other pedicled flaps may be more appropriate (see earlier discussion).

The most important surgical principles are (1) clear visualization and exposure of the operative site, (2) creation of a tension-free, multiple-layered closure, (3) assurance of an adequate blood supply, and (4) adequate bladder drainage. Operative exposure often requires two or more assistants and the use of self-retaining retractors. A tension-free closure can usually be accomplished by performing wide mobilization of the surrounding tissue, but sometimes it requires the use of local pedicle flaps or relaxing incisions in the anterior vaginal wall. Bladder drainage is best accomplished by using a large suprapubic catheter.

Timing of Surgery and Preoperative Management

In the past, much controversy surrounded the timing of surgical repair. For decades it had been taught that surgery should be delayed for 3 to 6 months or longer to allow adequate time for tissue inflammation and edema to subside. In our experience, surgery can be safely performed as soon as the vaginal wound is free of infection and inflammation and the tissues are reasonably pliable. It is usually possible to perform the surgery within 3 to 6 weeks after the original surgery.

Management of incontinence while waiting for healing of the vaginal tissue is sometimes a difficult problem. In most patients Foley catheter drainage is sufficient. If significant leakage occurs with a Foley catheter in place we generally recommend that the catheter be discontinued and the patient be managed with superabsorbent pads that are changed frequently throughout the day.

Surgical Technique of Vaginal Urethral Reconstruction

The patient is placed in the dorsal lithotomy position, and cystourethroscopy is performed to assess the relationship of the ureteral orifices to the damaged urethra. If the ureteral orifices are in close proximity to the fistula, single-J ureteral stents are left indwelling. A percutaneous suprapubic cystotomy tube is placed and sewn to the anterior abdominal wall. A 16 Fr Foley catheter is inserted into the bladder, and the balloon is inflated with enough fluid to hold it securely at the vesical neck.

The choice of incision depends on the local anatomy of the tissue loss. In most instances an inverted U

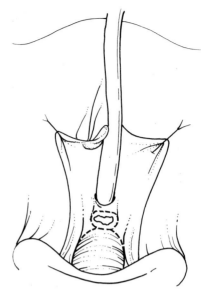

Figure 52–1 An inverted U incision is made in the anterior vaginal wall with the apex of the U at the vesical neck. In this case, a urethral fistula is present and it is circumscribed. (From Blaivas JG: Vaginal flap neourethra: An alternative to bladder flap urethral reconstruction. J Urol 141:542–545, 1989.)

vaginal flap incision is outlined on the anterior vaginal wall just proximal to the distal end of the damaged urethra (Fig. 52–1). The flap is mobilized with Metzenbaum scissors and reflected posteriorly (Fig. 52–2). At the end of the procedure this flap is advanced to cover the reconstructed urethra. If an anti-incontinence operation is to be done (we prefer the pubovaginal sling procedure), the dissection is completed and the sling is passed around the site of the vesical neck at this time. The sutures are not tied.

The technique of pubovaginal sling is as follows:

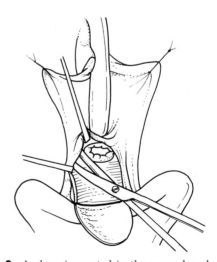

Figure 52–2 A plane is created in the avascular plane just underneath the vaginal epithelium, and the vaginal wall flap is reflected posteriorly. If a pubovaginal sling or other anti-incontinence procedure is to be performed, dissection into the retropubic space is completed at this time. (From Blaivas JG: Vaginal flap neourethra: An alternative to bladder flap urethral reconstruction. J Urol 141:542–545, 1989.)

the lateral edges of the vaginal wound are grasped with Allis clamps and retracted laterally. The dissection continues just beneath the vaginal epithelium with Metzenbaum scissors pointed in the direction of the patient's ipsilateral shoulder until the periosteum of the pubis or ischium is palpated with the tip of the scissors (Fig. 52–3). During this part of the dissection, it is important to stay as far laterally as possible. This is best accomplished by dissecting with the concavity of the scissor pointing laterally and by exerting constant lateral pressure with the tips of the scissor against the undersurface of the vaginal epithelium. Once the periosteum is reached, the endopelvic fascia is perforated and the retropubic space entered. In most instances this is easily accomplished by blunt dissection with the surgeon's index finger (Fig. 52–4). The tip of the finger, opposite the nail, palpates the periosteum. With the back edge of the fingertip the bladder and urethra are mobilized medially as the finger advances and perforates the fascia. This completely mobilizes the vesical neck and proximal urethra, releasing these structures from their vaginal attachments. In some instances this dissection must be performed sharply with Metzenbaum scissors.

A Pfannenstiel skin incision is made and carried down to the rectus fascia (Fig. 52–5). The surface of the rectus fascia is dissected free of subcutaneous tissue, and a suitable site is selected for excision of the fascial strip, which will be used as a free graft for creation of the sling. Two parallel horizontal incisions, 2 to 3 cm apart, are made near the midline in the rectus fascia. The incisions are extended superiorly and laterally for the entire width of the wound,

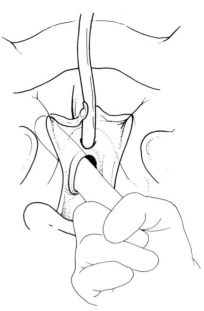

Figure 52–4 The endopelvic fascia is perforated with the index finger, and the retropubic space is entered. (Modified from Blaivas JG: Pubovaginal sling procedure. *In* Whitehead ED [ed]: Current Operative Urology. Philadelphia, JB Lippincott, 1990, pp 93–101.)

following the direction of the fascial fibers. The undersurface of the fascia is freed from muscle and scar tissue (Fig. 52–6). Prior to excising the strip, each end of the fascia is secured with a long 2–0 monofilament nonabsorbable suture using a running horizontal mattress suture placed at right angles to the direction of the fascial fibers. Each end of the fascial strip is transected approximately 1 cm lateral to the sutures and placed in saline (Fig. 52–7). No attempt is made to mobilize the bladder or vesical neck from above. The fascial defect is closed with 2–0 PDS suture.

The surgeon's right index finger is reinserted in the vaginal wound to retract the vesical neck and bladder medially. The tip of the finger indents the

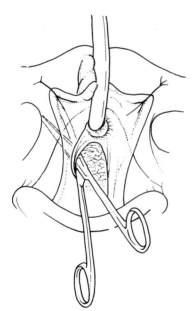

Figure 52–3 Dissection is begun with Metzenbaum scissors in the avascular plane just beneath the vaginal epithelium. The tips of the scissors are directed toward the patient's ipsilateral shoulder. (Modified from Blaivas JG: Pubovaginal sling procedure. *In* Whitehead ED [ed]: Current Operative Urology. Philadelphia, JB Lippincott, 1990, pp 93–101.)

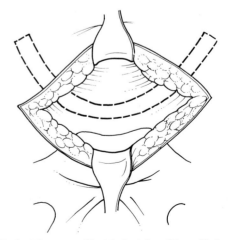

Figure 52–5 Pfannensteil's skin incision. (From Blaivas JG: Pubovaginal sling procedure. *In* Whitehead ED [ed]: Current Operative Urology. Philadelphia, JB Lippincott, 1990, pp 93–101.)

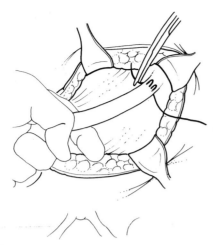

Figure 52–6 A 2- to 3-cm-wide graft is outlined, keeping the incision parallel to the direction of the fascial fibers. The incision is extended laterally to the point where the rectus fascia divides and passes to the internal and external oblique muscles. (From Blaivas JG: Pubovaginal sling procedure. *In* Whitehead ED [ed]: Current Operative Urology. Philadelphia, JB Lippincott, 1990, pp 93–101.)

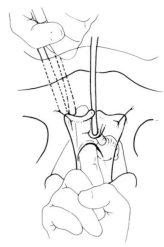

Figure 52–8 A long DeBakey clamp is passed from the abdominal to the vaginal wound lateral to the urethra. (Modified from Blaivas JG: Pubovaginal sling procedure. *In* Whitehead ED [ed]: Current Operative Urology. Philadelphia, JB Lippincott, 1990, pp 93–101.)

undersurface of the rectus and is palpated by the index finger of the left hand in the abdominal wound. A tiny incision is made in the rectus fascia at the site where the left index finger was palpated. This is just above the pubis and lateral to the midline on each side. A long sharp curved (DeBakey) clamp is inserted into the incision and directed to the undersurface of the pubis. The tip of the clamp is pressed against the periosteum and directed toward the index finger that is retracting the vesical neck and bladder medially through the vaginal incision (Fig. 52–8). In this fashion, the clamp is guided into the vaginal wound. When the tip of the clamp is visible, one end of the long suture, which is attached to the fascial graft, is grasped and pulled into the abdominal wound (Fig. 52–9). The procedure is repeated on the other side. The fascial sling is now positioned from the abdominal wall on one side around the undersurface of the vesical neck and back to the abdominal wall on the other side. The fascial sling is left loosely in position, and attention is turned to the urethral reconstruction. If a urethral fistula is present we prefer to retain the bridge of tissue and close the fistula to preserve the local blood supply. The fistula, which had been circumscribed during the initial incision, is closed by approximating its edges with interrupted sutures of 4–0 chromic catgut (Fig. 52–10).

If there is adequate vaginal tissue, two parallel incisions are made on each side of the urethral cathe-

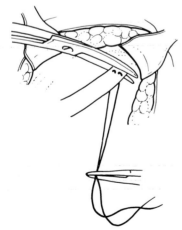

Figure 52–7 A 2–0 nonabsorbable running horizontal mattress suture is placed across the lateralmost portion of the graft, and the ends are left long. Each end of the fascial graft is transected approximately 1 cm lateral to the mattress suture. (From Blaivas JG: Pubovaginal sling procedure. *In* Whitehead ED [ed]: Current Operative Urology. Philadelphia, JB Lippincott, 1990, pp 93–101.)

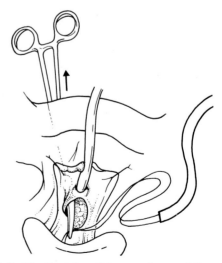

Figure 52–9 The fascial graft is passed around the urethra and brought out to the abdominal wound on either side. (From Blaivas JG: Pubovaginal sling procedure. *In* Whitehead ED [ed]: Current Operative Urology. Philadelphia, JB Lippincott, 1990, pp 93–101.)

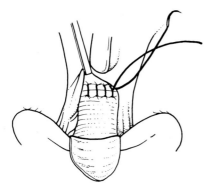

Figure 52-10 The urethrovaginal fistula is closed with interrupted sutures of 3–0 or 4–0 chromic catgut. (From Blaivas JG: Vaginal flap neurourethra: An alternative to bladder flap urethral reconstruction. J Urol 141:542–545, 1989.)

ter for construction of the neourethra (Fig. 52–11). The flaps are mobilized from lateral to medial, rolled into a tube over the urethral catheter, and sutured in the midline with 4–0 chromic catgut (Fig. 52–12). We prefer chromic catgut to longer-acting synthetic absorbable sutures because in our experience the latter often make voiding or urethral instrumentation painful.

A labial fat pad (Martius) flap is prepared to provide a second layer of tissue over the neourethra. A vertical incision is made over the labia majora, and the fat pad is mobilized. The fat pad is tunneled underneath the vaginal epithelium and sewn in place over the suture lines of the neourethra (Fig. 52–13). If a single labial fat pad flap does not provide adequate coverage, a second flap may be obtained from the other side, or a gracilis, perineal, or rectus pedicle flap may be harvested. The flap is placed between the sling and the reconstructed urethra.

The long sutures attached to each end of the sling are tied together in the midline over the rectus fascia with no tension at all (Fig. 52–14). Next, the inverted

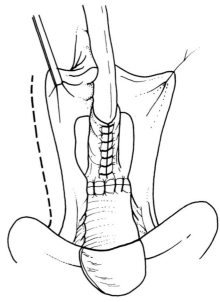

Figure 52-12 The edges of the flaps are approximated in the midline over the Foley catheter, creating the neourethra. (From Blaivas JG: Vaginal flap neurourethra: An alternative to bladder flap urethral reconstruction. J Urol 141:542–545, 1989.)

U flap is advanced over the entire reconstructed urethra. The vaginal and labial wounds are closed, and a $\frac{1}{4}$-inch Penrose drain is left in the labial wound (Fig. 52–15). The Foley catheter is taped to the anterior abdominal wall with a gentle loop to ensure that undue tension is not placed on the neourethra. Failure to maintain the correct position of the catheter may result in necrosis of the neourethra.

The Penrose drain is removed on the first postoper-

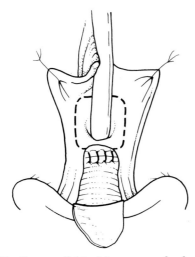

Figure 52-11 Two parallel incisions are made alongside the Foley catheter, and medially based flaps are created. (From Blaivas JG: Vaginal flap neurourethra: An alternative to bladder flap urethral reconstruction. J Urol 141:542–545, 1989.)

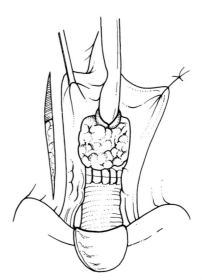

Figure 52-13 A vertical incision is made over the labia majora to gain access to the labial fat pad graft. The fat pad is mobilized and tunneled beneath the vaginal epithelium and is sutured in place over the site of the neourethra. If a pubovaginal sling was constructed, the fat pad is placed between the vesical neck and the sling. (From Blaivas JG: Vaginal flap neurourethra: An alternative to bladder flap urethral reconstruction. J Urol 141:542–545, 1989.)

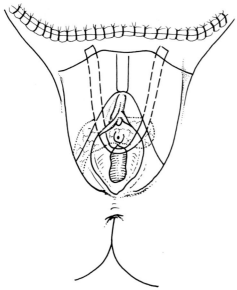

Figure 52-14 The long sutures attached to each end of the sling are tied together in the midline over the rectus fascia without tension. (Modified from Blaivas JG: Pubovaginal sling procedure. *In* Whitehead ED [ed]: Current Operative Urology. Philadelphia, JB Lippincott, 1990, pp 93–101.)

ative day. The urethral catheter is removed as soon as feasible, usually on the first or second postoperative day. A voiding cystourethrogram is performed through the suprapubic catheter at day 14. If the patient voids satisfactorily and there is no extravasation of urine, the suprapubic tube is removed. If not, the tube is left in place, and another voiding trial is undertaken 2 to 4 weeks postoperatively.

In our experience, the technique described here is appropriate for the great majority of cases. However, if there is insufficient tissue to create lateral vaginal wall flaps to roll into a tube for the urethral recon-

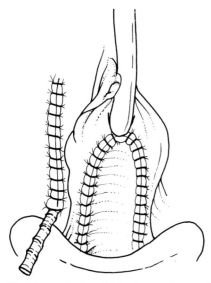

Figure 52-15 The vaginal and labial wounds are closed. (From Blaivas JG: Vaginal flap neurourethra: An alternative to bladder flap urethral reconstruction. J Urol 141:542–545, 1989.)

struction, there are several alternatives.[9, 12, 14, 24, 25, 55] A U-shaped incision can be made in whatever adjacent portion of the vagina is supple and of adequate dimension. A flap of vaginal wall is raised, rotated, and sutured to the anterior vaginal wall around the urethral catheter (Fig. 52–16). Sometimes the vaginal wall defect may be closed primarily, with or without lateral-based relaxing incisions (Fig. 52–17). If it is not possible to close the vaginal incision primarily, a labia minora (hair-free) pedicle graft may suffice; rarely, a gracilis myocutaneous graft may be necessary to cover the defect. However, it is not necessary to provide an epithelial covering for all of these reconstructions. If the defect is not too large and there is a good local blood supply, it is acceptable to let the remainder of the wound heal by secondary intention.

Results

A vaginal neourethral reconstruction was reported by Harris in 1935.[12] He used a U-shaped vaginal incision and created lateral flaps that were rolled into a tube to form the new urethra. Ellis and Hodges described further modifications of this technique and recommended a combined vaginal and retropubic approach but reported cure of incontinence in only one of six patients.[58] O'Conor further refined both the retropubic and vaginal approaches to neourethra reconstruction.[24]

To date there have been few series in the literature that assess urinary incontinence after urethral reconstruction; most authors have discussed only cure of the fistula or survival of the reconstruction.[1, 2, 9, 12–14, 15, 17, 24, 26, 59] Of the series that do describe postoperative incontinence, none do so in a systematic manner. Most imply that incontinence is sphincteric, and detrusor instability is not routinely reported. When incontinence is assessed in these series, the incidence ranges from 20 to 70%. Patil and colleagues reported a 20% incidence of incontinence after repair of urethrovaginal fistula in nine women.[26] Fistulas involving the middle and distal thirds of the urethra were closed by rolling the vaginal wall into a tube over a 22 Fr Foley catheter and covering the defect with a labial (Martius) fat pad flap. When the proximal urethra and trigone were involved, the fistula was closed in layers and covered with a gracilis muscle flap.

Sixteen percent of the patients in the series of Hamlin and Nicholson were incontinent after a single operation to repair the fistula, but incontinence was usually cured after a second procedure.[15] In Gray's series, 5 of 10 patients with urethrovaginal fistulas were still incontinent after a single operation that successfully cured the fistula.[14] Hendren reported the use of a full-thickness perineal flap in the construction of a neourethra in five girls up to the age of 18 who had undergone extensive prior surgery because of congenital abnormalities of the lower urinary tract.[17] The neourethra was purposely created

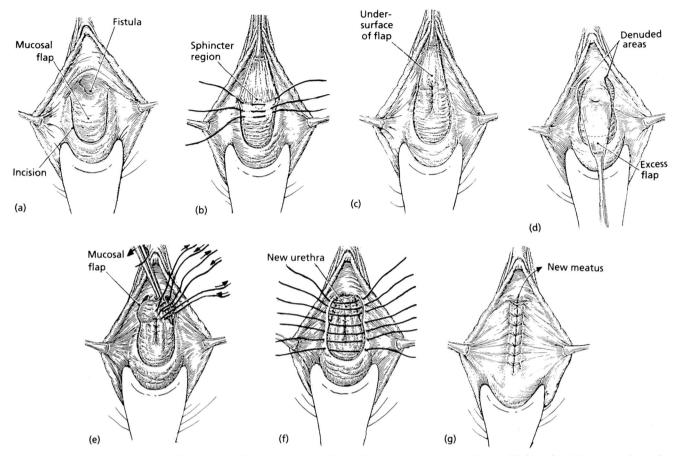

Figure 52-16 If there was insufficient vaginal tissue to create lateral flaps to form a neourethra, a U-shaped incision is made in the anterior vaginal wall. The vaginal wall flap is reflected anteriorly and sutured around the Foley catheter to form the neourethra. (Modified from Thompson JD, Rock JA: Vesicovaginal fistulas. *In* Mattingly RF, Thompson JD (eds): TeLinde's Operative Gynecology. Philadelphia, JB Lippincott, 1992, pp 810–811.)

to extend to the base of the clitoris. Three of the patients were completely continent, and two had mild degrees of stress incontinence.

Birkhoff and colleagues described their experience with closure of vesicovaginal and urethrovaginal fistulas in 10 women, four of whom had urethrovaginal fistulas.[2] They emphasized the use of the Martius flap and complete excision of the fistulous tract. Three of the four patients with urethrovaginal fistulas had urinary incontinence preoperatively, and all were cured after a single operation. All patients were cured of the fistula. The authors believe that the Martius flap itself contributed to continence in these patients.

Elkins and associates reviewed the results of 36 vesicovaginal or urethrovaginal fistula repairs performed by American visiting professors in West Africa.[60] All of the vesical neck and urethral fistulas resulted from obstructed labor. In this series, 2 of 13 proximal urethral fistulas were complicated by "severe stress urinary incontinence" postoperatively.

To date we have operated on 46 women with extensive anatomic vesical neck and urethral defects due to complications from urethral diverticulectomy, anterior colporrhaphy, and anti-incontinence surgery.[4, 5, 61] The patients ranged in age from 31 to 80 years, and follow-up ranged from 3 months to 8 years. We have previously published the results of surgery on our first 24 patients.[4, 5] A concomitant anti-incontinence procedure was performed in all but one patient. In the first 10 women, a pubovaginal sling procedure was done in six, a needle suspension in three, and a modified Kelly plication in one. Twenty-five of the subsequent twenty-six women underwent concomitant pubovaginal sling. In all patients who underwent pubovaginal sling, a pedicle flap was placed between the fascial sling and the neourethra. A unilateral Martius pedicle graft was used in 30, a bilateral Martius graft in 1, and a gracilis flap in 1.

Overall, an excellent (continent) result was obtained after a single operation in 30 patients (83%). Two patients developed necrosis of the vaginal flaps. One of these, an 80-year-old woman with extensive loss of the urethra, vesical neck, and trigone after a Kelly plication, was the only patient who did not undergo a concomitant anti-incontinence procedure because her vaginal tissues seemed so flimsy. She subsequently underwent a successful secondary neourethral reconstruction procedure using a gracilis muscle flap. The second patient had severe incontinence due to detrusor instability. Despite the breakdown of the neourethra, she did not develop sphincteric incontinence. She failed to respond to anticholinergic

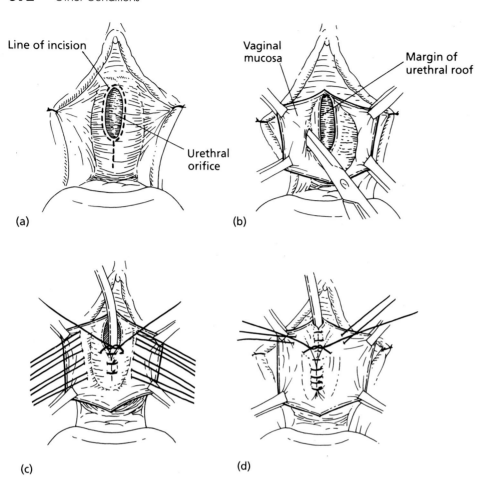

Line of incision

Urethral orifice

Vaginal mucosa

Margin of urethral roof

(a)

(b)

(c)

(d)

Figure 52–17 Primary closure of the neourethra and vaginal wall. (Modified from Thompson JD, Rock JA: Vesicovaginal fistulas. *In* Mattingly RF, Thompson JD [eds]: TeLinde's Operative Gynecology. Philadelphia, JB Lippincott, 1992, p 812.)

therapy, declined further surgery, and was treated with an indwelling catheter.

One woman had urinary incontinence due to detrusor instability postoperatively. At urodynamic evaluation she was found to have urethral obstruction. Despite the urethral obstruction, she is able to void with small postvoid residuals. Nevertheless, she is currently managed with anticholinergic therapy and intermittent self-catheterization.

One patient, who had undergone 19 prior anti-incontinence operations, had a previously undiagnosed vesicovaginal fistula that was not recognized until after the urethral reconstruction. She was cured after vesicovaginal fistula repair. Two of the three patients who underwent Raz urethropexy at the time of urethral reconstruction developed stress incontinence due to intrinsic sphincter deficiency and were successfully treated with a pubovaginal sling. In addition to the woman described earlier, intermittent catheterization was required temporarily in three other patients.

We believe that one of the most common reasons for operative failure is inadequate surgical exposure. In our experience, the dorsal lithotomy position, with steep Trendelenburg angulation, is sufficient in the vast majority of patients. Other authors have favored the Sims or Lawson position for more extensive fistula repair.[20] We believe that the use of vascularized pedicle grafts greatly enhances the likelihood of a

successful outcome with respect to both healing of the reconstruction and postoperative continence. In most instances, a modification of the Martius graft is sufficient, but occasionally a gracilis muscle graft or myocutaneous graft may prove necessary.[2, 4–6, 26, 30, 37, 54, 55]

In the original description, the Martius flap was prepared by dissection of the bulbocavernosus muscle through an incision over the labia minora[54] (Fig. 52–18). This dissection is sometimes associated with considerable bleeding, particularly if the erectile tissue of the vestibular bulb is entered. Hoskins and associates modified the approach and secured a full-thickness island graft from the labia minora.[37] This afforded a cutaneous covering of the vaginal wound (Fig. 52–19). Symmonds and Hill described a full-thickness graft of both the labia minora and the labia majora.[27] Currently, most authors, including ourselves, use a labial fat pad graft excluding the bulbocavernosus muscle from the dissection. This is prepared by a vertical incision in the lateral aspect of the labia majora. Elkins and colleagues reported their experience with a modified Martius (labial fat pad) graft in 37 women with vesicovaginal, urethrovaginal, and rectovaginal fistulas.[60, 61] In addition, they described the results of a cadaver dissection of the tissue used in their graft technique. They demonstrated a rich blood supply derived from the external pudendal artery anteriorly and the internal pudendal

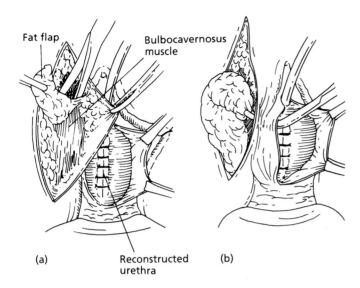

(a)

(b)

Reconstructed urethra

Fat flap

Bulbocavernosus muscle

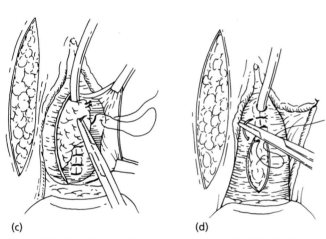

(c)

(d)

Figure 52-18 Martius fibrofatty pedical graft. (Modified from Thompson JD, Rock JA: Vesicovaginal fistulas. *In* Mattingly RF, Thompson JD [eds]: TeLinde's Operative Gynecology. Philadelphia, JB Lippincott, 1992, p 815.)

artery posteriorly. There is an extensive anastomosis between the two vessels. Clinically, because of the dual blood supply it was possible to detach the fat pad flap either superiorly or inferiorly with equal success. The graft itself is composed of fibrofatty tissue. The adipose tissue is interspersed with numerous fibrous septa that afford it a much stronger consistency than adipose tissue from other parts of the body. Moreover, because of the ability of the labial fat pad flap to form granulation tissue and to heal by secondary intention, it is not always necessary to cover it with an epithelial surface. When there is insufficient vaginal epithelium to close the wound, the fat pad flap may be left open to heal by secondary intention. However, in the Elkin series, there appeared to be an increased incidence of vaginal stricture and cellulitis when the wound was not closed primarily. This did not, however, affect the final result of the fistula repair.

Another advantage of the Martius flap technique is that the vertical labial incision can be extended

well into the abdominal wall to achieve almost any length of graft necessary to cover even the most extensive of vaginal wounds.

Bladder Flap Techniques

Successful urethral reconstruction using a bladder flap technique was first reported by Young in 1919. In 1922 Young reported a series of 13 children with epispadias, 12 of whom were said to be continent after a single reconstruction.[31] The essential feature of this operation was to plicate the urethra over a silver probe, thus narrowing its lumen. A modification of Young's technique was reported by Dees in 1949.[7] In this procedure a triangular wedge of tissue is excised from the roof and each lateral wall of the posterior urethra and adjacent bladder wall. Subsequent closure results in a snug internal and external sphincter and a tubular rather than a conical urethra. The urethra was closed with a continuous chromic catgut suture over an 8 or 10 Fr catheter. Dees reported that "good or perfect urinary control" was achieved in five boys and one girl with congenital epispadias.

Leadbetter modified the procedure further by routine reimplantation of the ureters:[22] "Even though the ureters may appear to be normally inserted far enough superiorly, experience has taught us not to succumb to the temptation and omit the reimplantation because the added length of bladder gained by reimplantation may be crucial for achieving continence . . . it is emphasized that no attempt is made to constrict the urethral or bladder lumen as has been previously described. . . ." Leadbetter noted that none of the patients achieved continence until 3 to 8 weeks after surgery and suggested that the cause was "probably bladder irritation and spasm . . . a parasympatholytic agent such as tincture of belladonna has been helpful." All five patients in this

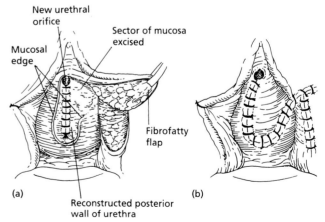

New urethral orifice

Sector of mucosa excised

Mucosal edge

Fibrofatty flap

(a)

Reconstructed posterior wall of urethra

(b)

Figure 52-19 Full-thickness labial-fibrofatty pedical graft. (Modified from Thompson JD, Rock JA: Vesicovaginal fistulas. *In* Mattingly RF, Thompson JD [eds]: TeLinde's Operative Gynecology. Philadelphia, JB Lippincott, 1992, p 813.)

series were girls. With a follow-up of 4 months to 2 years, two were completely dry, two had very mild stress incontinence that did not require pads, and one had what sounds like urge incontinence or low bladder compliance. She had a bladder capacity of only 45 to 60 ml, which was attributed to the fact that the "dog ears" were excised at the time of the original reconstruction. With the passage of time, the procedure that evolved from the ingenuity of these surgical pioneers became known as the Young-Dees-Leadbetter operation (Fig. 52–20).

In 1949 Barnes and Wilson reported the use of an anterior bladder flap to create a neourethra[1] (Fig. 52–21). Tanagho and colleagues in 1969 described a similar technique that did not require ureteroneocys-tostomy.[28] They used an anterior bladder flap that was rolled into a tube over a catheter and anasto-mosed to the distal urethra in patients with sphinc-teric incontinence: "After complete severance of the bladder from the urethra at the level of the internal meatus an anterior bladder flap 1 inch wide and 1 inch long is developed. The flap is turned into a

tube around a 14 to 16 Fr Foley catheter and is anastomosed to the cut end of the urethra. The blad-der outlet is reconstructed by suturing the apex of the trigone to the base of the flap, then suturing the remaining part of the bladder outlet in an inverted V fashion" (Fig. 52–22).

Until this time, it was generally agreed that the sphincteric function of the urethra was simply a func-tion of its length and width—that is, the longer and narrower the urethra, the more likely was a success-ful outcome. Of course, if it were too long or too narrow, outlet obstruction occurred, possibly account-ing for the genesis of refractory detrusor instability, which was a significant cause of failure. Tanagho challenged this length-width theory. He postulated that the muscular properties of the tube were suffi-cient to provide sphincteric function. He reported his 10-year experience with this procedure in 56 patients and compared the results with those from an addi-tional 25 patients who underwent a posterior bladder flap repair during the same time period at the same institution.[28] Overall, 65% of the patients had an

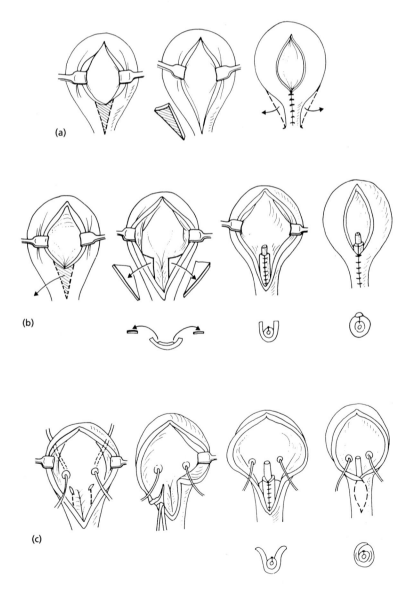

Figure 52-20 Young-Dees-Leadbetter urethral recon-struction. *A,* Young's urethral plication procedure. *B,* Dees' urethral lengthening. *C,* Leadbetter's urethral lengthening and reimplantation of ureters. (Modified from Gunst MA, Ackermann D, Zingg EG: Eur Urol 13:62–69, 1987, with permission from S. Karger AG, Basel.)

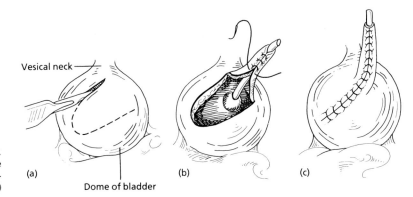

Figure 52-21 Barnes' bladder flap urethroplasty. (Modified from O'Conor VJ, Kropp KA: Surgery of the female urethra. *In* Glenn JF, Boyce WH [eds]: Urologic Surgery. New York, Harper Collins, 1969, p 568.)

"excellent or good result" after a single operation, of whom 30% were completely continent and voided without difficulty. Twenty-five of these patients were women, but the results were not further broken down according to gender. Koraitim reported his experience with variations of the anterior bladder flap.[19] In a series of 27 patients, 7 were women, and 1 of whom had extensive urethral disruption. Five of the seven women had good results, and 1 had satisfactory results. In a subsequent series, he reported a retropubic, retrourethral approach for the repair of large vesical neck and urethral fistulas with partially destroyed urethras. The procedure was a further modification of the Tanagho operation and incorporated the use of an omental flap to buttress the repair. Two patients were reported and both were continent 1 year after a single operation. Hanash and Sieck reported a single case of a large vesicourethrovaginal fistula that was successfully repaired using a modified anterior bladder flap and omental flap interposition. Postoperatively, the patient developed complete urinary retention owing to a stenotic vesical neck; this was successfully treated with a retropubic incision of the stenosis and interposition of another bladder flap. One year postoperatively, the patient was

continent and had a normal intravenous pyelogram and voiding cystourethrogram.

In 1985 Leadbetter reported a retrospective 10- to 22-year follow-up of 34 patients who underwent "ureteral reimplantation and tubularization of the trigone as described by Leadbetter."[22] Success was defined as a patient who wore no pads and claimed to be continent. A patient who wore one to three pads per day that were moist or damp was considered a partial success. Using these criteria, 57% of seven adults and 70% of 27 children were successes, and 29% and 3%, respectively, were partial successes.

Elkins and colleagues recently reported their experience with a Tanagho-like procedure in 20 West African women with extensive vesicourethrovaginal fistulas subsequent to obstructed labor.[61] These patients all had large vesicovaginal fistulas, and because of extensive scarring they were not suitable for vaginal flap techniques. The procedure was performed entirely through the vaginal approach. "The anterior and lateral fistula edges are dissected sharply away from the pubic bone beneath the arch of the pubic ramus, thus entering the retropubic space. . . . from the vagina . . . the anterior bladder wall is dissected free of surrounding tissues to the

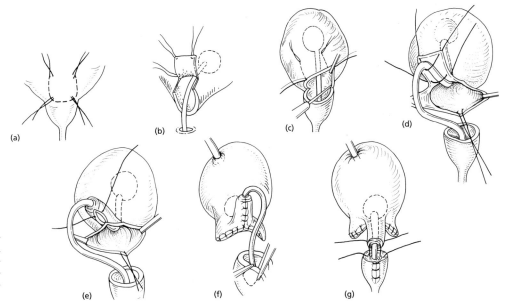

Figure 52-22 Anterior bladder flap urethroplasty. (From Tanagho EA: Bladder neck reconstruction for total urinary incontinence: 10 years of experience. J Urol 125:321, 1981.)

level of the peritoneal reflection." The anterior bladder was mobilized, and a 3- by 3-cm flap was raised and rolled into a tube over a 16 Fr catheter. The new urethra was sutured to either the remaining distal urethra or the site of the new meatus. The posterior edges of the vesicovaginal fistula were approximated, and "fixation sutures are placed through the top portion of the neo-urethra to reattach the urethra to the base of the pubic periosteum." In the last three patients a modified Pereyra procedure was performed instead. A Martius fat pad graft was then placed beneath the suture lines.

Eighteen of the twenty women had a satisfactory anatomic repair of the fistula, but 4 of the 18 had persistent stress incontinence that required further surgery. Two others had refractory detrusor instability or low bladder compliance.

We believe that these published results favor the vaginal flap techniques in patients who have sufficient vaginal tissue for a vaginal flap reconstruction. However, in patients with extensive vaginal scarring, such as those reported by Elkins and colleagues, bladder flap techniques appear to offer the best chance for a successful outcome.

REFERENCES

1. Barnes RW, Wilson WW: Reconstruction of the urethra with a tube from bladder flap. Urol Cutan Rev 53:604, 1949.
2. Birkhoff JD, Wechsler M, Romas NA: Urinary fistulas: Vaginal repair using labial fat pad. J Urol 117:595, 1977.
3. Bissada NK, McDonald D: Management of giant vesicovaginal and vesicourethrovaginal fistulas. J Urol 130:1073, 1983.
4. Blaivas JG: Vaginal flap neurourethra: An alternative to bladder flap urethral reconstruction. J Urol 141:542, 1989.
5. Blaivas JG: Treatment of female incontinence secondary to urethral damage or loss. Urol Clin North Am 18:355, 1991.
6. Davis RS, Linke CA, Kraemer GK: Use of labial tissue in repair of urethrovaginal fistula and injury. Arch Surg 115:628, 1980.
7. Dees JE: Congenital epispadias with incontinence. J Urol 62:513, 1949.
8. Diokno AC, Hollander HB, Alderson TP: Artificial urinary sphincter for recurrent female urinary incontinence: Indications and results. J Urol 138:778, 1987.
9. Elkins TE, Drescher C, Martey JO, Fort D: Vesicovaginal fistula revisited. Obstet Gynecol 72:307, 1988.
10. Falk HC, Tancer ML: Urethrovesicovaginal fistula. Obstet Gynecol 33:422, 1969.
11. Falk HC, Tancer ML: Loss of urethra: Report of three cases. Obstet Gynecol 9:458, 1957.
12. Harris SH: Reconstruction of the female urethra. Surg Gynecol Obstet 61:366, 1935.
13. Goodwin WE, Scardino PT: Vesicovaginal and urethrovaginal fistulas: A summary of 25 years of experience. J Urol 123:370, 1980.
14. Gray LA: Urethrovaginal fistulas. Am J Obstet Gynecol 101:28, 1968.
15. Hamlin RHJ, Nicholson EC: Reconstruction of urethra totally destroyed in labor. Br Med J 1:147, 1969.
16. Hanash KA, Sieck U: Successful repair of a large vesicovaginal fistula with associated urethral loss using the anterior bladder flap technique. J Urol 130:775, 1983.
17. Hendren WH: Construction of female urethra from vaginal wall and a perineal flap. J Urol 123:657, 1980.
18. Koraitim MA: A new retropubic retrourethral approach for large vesico-urethrovaginal fistulas. J Urol 134:1122, 1985.
19. Koraitim M: Anterior bladder tube: Four forms for incontinence of different etiology. J Urol 134:269, 1985.
20. Lawson JB: Tropical Obstetrics and Gynecology. London, Oxford Press, 1970.
21. Leadbetter GW Jr: Surgical correction of total urinary incontinence. J Urol 91:261, 1964.
22. Leadbetter GW Jr: Surgical reconstruction for complete urinary incontinence. J Urol 133:205, 1985.
23. Morgan JE, Farrow GA, Sims RH: The sloughed urethra syndrome. Am J Obstet Gynecol 130:521, 1978.
24. O'Conor VJ Jr: Repair of vesicovaginal fistula with associated urethral loss. Surg Gynecol Obstet 146:250, 1978.
25. O'Conor VJ Jr, Kropp KA: Surgery of the female urethra. In: Glenn JF, Boyce WH (eds): Urologic Surgery. New York, Harper & Row, 1969.
26. Patil U, Waterhouse K, Laungani G: Management of 18 difficult vesicovaginal and urethrovaginal fistulas with a modified Ingleman-Sundberg and Martius operations. J Urol 123:653, 1980.
27. Symmonds, RE, Hill LM: Loss of the urethra: A report on 50 patients. Am J Obstet Gynecol 130:130, 1978.
28. Tanagho EA, Smith DR, Meyers FH, Fisher R: Mechanism of urinary continence. II. Technique for surgical correction of incontinence. J Urol 101:305, 1969.
29. Tanagho EA: Bladder neck reconstruction for total urinary incontinence: 10 years of experience. J Urol 125:321, 1981.
30. Webster GD, Sihelnik SA, Stone AR: Urethrovaginal fistula: A review of the surgical management. J Urol 132:460, 1984.
31. Young HH: An operation for the cure of incontinence associated with epispadias. J Urol 7:1, 1922.
32. Aldridge AH: Transplantation of fascia for relief of urinary stress incontinence. Am J Obstet Gynecol 44:398, 1942.
33. Blaivas JG: Pubovaginal sling procedure. In Whitehead ED (ed): Current Operative Urology. Philadelphia, JB Lippincott, 1990, pp 93–101.
34. Frangenheim P: Zur operativen Behandlung der Incontinenz männlichen Harnröhre. Verh Dtsch Ges Chir 43:149, 1914.
35. Goebel R: Zur operativen Beseitigung der angelborenen Incontinenz vesicae. Z Gynakol 207:2:187, 1910.
36. Hohenfellner T, Petri E: Sling procedures. In Stanton SL, Tanagho EA (eds): Surgery of Female Incontinence. Berlin, Springer-Verlag, 1980.
37. Hoskins WJ, Park RC, Long R, et al. Repair of urinary tract fistulas with bulbocavernosus myocutaneous flaps. Obstet Gynecol 63:588, 1984.
38. Iosif CS: Porcine corium sling in the treatment of urinary stress incontiennce. Arch Gynecol 240:131, 1987.
39. Irving M, Lee R: Delayed transection of urethra by mersilene tape. Urology 8:580, 1976.
40. Jeffcoate TNA: The results of the Aldridge sling operation for stress incontinence. J Obstet Gynecol Br Empire 63:36, 1956.
41. McGuire EM, Lytton B: The pubovaginal sling in stress urinary incontinence. J Urol 119:82, 1978.
42. McGuire EM, Wang C, Usitalo H, Savastano J: Modified pubovaginal sling in girls with myelodysplasia. J Urol 135:94, 1986.
43. McGuire EM, Bennett CJ, Konnak JA, et al: Experience with pubovaginal slings for urinary incontinence at University of Michigan. J Urol 138:525, 1987.
44. Moir JC: The Guaze-Hammock operation. J Obstet Gynecol Br Commonw 75:1, 1968.
45. Morgan JE: A sling operation using Marlex polypropylene mesh for treatment of recurrent stress incontinence. Am J Obstet Gynecol 106:369, 1970.
46. Morgan JE, Farrow GA: Recurrent stress urinary incontinence in the female. Br J Urol 49:37, 1970.
47. Morgan JE, Farrow GA, Stewart FE: The Marlex sling operation for the treatment of recurrent stress urinary incontinence. Am J Obstet Gynecol 151:224, 1985.
48. Narik G, Palmrich AH: A simplified sling operation suitable for routine use. Am J Obstet Gynecol 84:400, 1962.
49. Sloan WR, Barwin BN: Stress incontinence of urine: A retrospective study of the complications and late results of simple suprapubic suburethral fascial slings. J Urol 110:533, 1973.
50. Stanton SL, Brindley GS, Holmes DM: Silastic sling for urethral sphincter incompetence in women. Br J Obstet Gynecol 92:747, 1985.

51. Stoeckel W: Über die Verwendung der Musculi pyrimidales bei der operativen Behandlung der Incontinentia urinae. Zentralbl Gynaekol 41:11, 1917.
52. Studdiford WE: Transplantation of abdominal fascia for the relief of urinary stress incontinence. Am J Obstet Gynecol 47:764, 1944.
53. Williams TJ, TeLinde RW: The sling operation for urinary incontinence using mersilene ribbon: Obstet Gynecol 19:241, 1962.
54. Martius H: Die operative Wiederherstelllung der vollkommen fehlenden Harnohare und des schliessmuskels Derselben. Zentralbl Gynaekol 52:480, 1928.
55. Mattingly RF, Thompson JD (eds): TeLinde's Operative Gynecology. Philadelphia, JB Lippincott, 1985.
56. Fleischmann J, Picha G: Abdominal approach for gracilis muscle interposition and repair of recurrent vesicovaginal fistula. J Urol 140:552, 1980.
57. Heckler F: Gracilis myocutaneous and muscle flaps. Clin Plast Surg 7:27, 1980.
58. Ellis LR, Hodges CV: Experience with female urethral reconstruction. J Urol 102:214, 1969.
59. Gunst MA, Ackermann D, Zingg EJ: Urethral reconstruction in females. Eur Urol 13:62, 1987.
60. Elkins TE, DeLancey JO, McGuire EJ: The use of modified Martius graft as an adjunctive technique in vesicovaginal and rectovaginal fistula repair. Obstet Gynecol 75:727, 1990.
61. Elkins TE, Ghosh TS, Tagoe GA, Stocker R: Transvaginal mobilization and utilization of the anterior bladder wall to repair vesicovaginal fistulas involving the urethra. Obstet Gynecol 79:455, 1992.

CHAPTER 53

Surgical Closure of the Bladder Neck

Lynn Stothers, M.D., M.H.Sc., F.R.C.S.C.
Ashok Chopra, M.D.
Shlomo Raz, M.D.

Destruction of the bladder neck with subsequent incontinence is infrequent but devastating to the patient. Although this complication has been described as early as 6 months after continuous urethral catheterization, the typical patient history is one of long-term drainage for over 5 years.[1–10] The medical conditions leading to continuous urethral catheterization in female patients include central and peripheral nervous system disorders, spinal cord injury, dementia, and multiple sclerosis.[1–3] In addition to long-term catheterization in patients with neurologic disease, the bladder neck may also be destroyed by pelvic trauma, complications of labor and delivery, or numerous repairs for stress urinary incontinence or vesicovaginal fistula.

The mechanism of destruction of the urethra is pressure necrosis of the bladder neck, which results from the use of ever-increasing sizes of catheters and balloons in attempts to decrease leakage around the catheter. A second contributing factor is bladder spasms, which can be strong enough to expel the Foley catheter through the bladder neck with the balloon intact. Initially the bladder neck widens, and the urethra becomes foreshortened. Bladder capacity may decrease with time. In its most severe form, the urethra is no longer visible, and the wide-open bladder neck allows visualization of the trigone and ureteral orifices.

On physical examination one may insert a sterile gloved finger through the bladder neck region without difficulty. The condition of the perineal skin should be noted because erosions or skin sloughing may have occurred owing to continuous wetness. Patients with neurologic disease require inspection for pressure sores, which may be infected. Such a dramatic appearance on physical examination makes the diagnosis of bladder neck destruction straightforward (Fig. 53–1).

When destruction of the outlet is evident on physical examination, further evaluation of the patient is required. Imaging of the kidneys and ureters as well as cystoscopy should be carried out. At the time of cystoscopy any coexisting pathology should be ruled out. This includes cytologic examination of the urine as well as a bladder biopsy to rule out bladder neoplasia, which is a recognized complication of long-term indwelling catheterization. Bladder capacity should be noted, and the ureteral orifices should be carefully inspected to note their location in relation to the opening of the bladder outlet.

Indications for and Contraindications to Surgical Closure of the Bladder Neck

A decision to close the bladder neck rather than reconstruct the urethra is made on an individual basis according to the patient's level of physical and mental ability. Even a short urethra can be reconstructed under the right circumstances. Preoperative conditions requiring consideration in each patient include life expectancy, ease of mobility getting into and out of bed, ability to transfer to the toilet, mental status, manual dexterity in performing intermittent catheterization, spasticity of the lower extremities (which would make intermittent catheterization difficult), and tissue quality. Coexisting medical conditions such as congestive heart failure may also limit a patient's life expectancy or mobility. Intractable incontinence around progressively larger Foley catheters with perineal skin sloughing or infected pressure sores are further indications.

Female paraplegic and quadriplegic patients with

vaginal wall to facilitate dissection. A circumscribing incision and an inverted U–type incision are made as shown in Figure 53–3.

STEP 2 A vaginal flap is created by sharply dissecting the anterior vaginal wall away from the perivesical fascia. The dissection is then continued to circumscribe the area of the destroyed bladder neck, as seen in Figure 53–4.

STEP 3 The bladder is freed from its attachments to the pubic and lateral pelvic walls with sharp dissection. The retroperitoneal space is opened sharply as in bladder neck suspension procedures to complete this dissection. The pubourethral ligaments are transected to free the bladder from its attachments to the symphysis pubis (Fig. 53–5).

STEP 4 The location of the ureteral orifices and their relationship to the remaining bladder neck are demonstrated with the use of intravenous indigo carmine. Remnants of any scarred remaining urethra are then excised to provide a well-vascularized margin for closure. The bladder neck area should be adequately mobilized by this point to allow closure in a tension-free manner (Fig. 53–6).

STEP 5 The bladder neck is closed in a vertical anteroposterior direction using continuous locking 2–0 polyglycolic acid sutures (Fig. 53–7). Adequate tissue around the bladder neck should be included to result in a watertight closure.

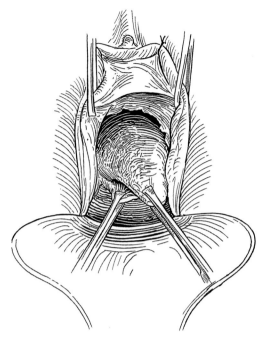

Figure 53–5 The pubourethral ligaments, which extend from the undersurface of the symphysis pubis to the area of the midurethra, are divided sharply. The transection allows complete mobilization of the bladder outlet from the symphysis pubis. (From Raz S: Atlas of Transvaginal Surgery. Philadelphia, WB Saunders, 1992.)

STEP 6 A second layer of continuous locking 2–0 polyglycolic acid sutures is placed in a transverse fashion approximating the bladder neck and anterior bladder wall to just behind the symphysis pubis. This suture line is at right angles to the first layer, which

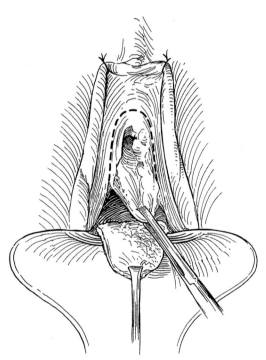

Figure 53–4 Creation of the anterior vaginal wall flap. An Allis clamp is used to provide gentle downward retraction, and sharp dissection is used to create the flap. A second Allis clamp is placed on the edge of the incision circumscribing the open bladder neck. Dissection is extended around the open bladder neck and advanced laterally toward the rami of the pubic bone. As in bladder neck suspension, the urethropelvic ligaments are exposed by detaching them from their fascial insertion into the tendinous arch of the obturator. Adequate mobilization is essential to provide a tension-free closure of the bladder neck. (From Raz S: Atlas of Transvaginal Surgery. Philadelphia, WB Saunders, 1992.)

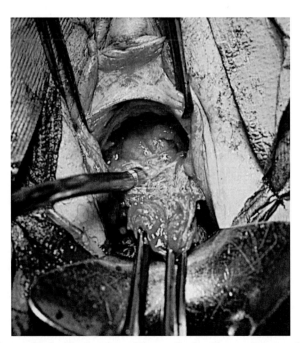

Figure 53–6 The location of the urethral orifices and their relationship to the remaining bladder neck is demonstrated using indigo carmine. Any remnants of the scarred remaining urethra are excised. (From Raz S: Atlas of Transvaginal Surgery. Philadelphia, WB Saunders, 1992.)

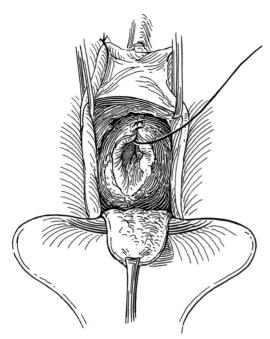

Figure 53-7 The bladder neck is closed in the vertical anterioposterior direction with a continuous polyglycolic acid suture. (From Raz S: Atlas of Transvaginal Surgery. Philadelphia, WB Saunders, 1992.)

was closed in an anteroposterior direction. This allows minimal overlap of suture lines. Following the second layer of closure, the closed bladder neck should be located in the retropubic space high behind the symphysis pubis (Fig. 53–8).

STEP 7 The vaginal defect is closed by advancing the inverted U–shaped vaginal flap (Fig. 53–9). The vagina is packed for 24 hours with ribbon packing covered in antibiotic cream. Irrigation of the suprapubic catheter confirms that it has proper drainage. Adequate drainage of urine through the suprapubic catheter is vital to prevent overdistention of the bladder and to allow healing of the suture lines without tension or subsequent fistula formation. A Martius flap may be used when necessary to add a further layer of closure. (Details of the fibrofatty labial [Martius] flap technique are given in Chapter 52.) A drain is left in the retroperitoneal space.

Complications

The frequency of complications following bladder neck closure varies widely in the literature and is reported to range from 0 to 100%. Most series report an overall complication rate of approximately 20%. The most common complication with both the abdominal and vaginal techniques is vesicovaginal fistula. Bleeding and infection may also occur. Feneley reported one patient with persistent perineal pain following the vaginal approach to closure.[1]

The potential complications related to access of the bladder differ depending on whether a suprapubic

catheter, a continent stoma, or an incontinent stoma has been used. The use of suprapubic catheters may be associated with blockage, urinary tract infection, and bladder stones. Suprapubic catheters should be changed every 3 weeks, and cystoscopy should be carried out on a yearly basis to rule out bladder stones or other pathology. Hulecki and Hackler described persistent leakage around the suprapubic catheter when the bladder capacity is small or when a hypercontractile neurogenic bladder is present.[3] Bladder antispasmodics can be tried; if these fail, an augmentation cystoplasty should be created. Herschorn and colleagues reported a 22% stomal revision rate for the hemi-Kock ileocystoplasty with a continent stoma.[7] This rate is similar to those cited in other reports in the literature. Stomal leakage, stricture, inability to catheterize, and parastomal hernias are the most frequently encountered problems that can be successfully managed with minor revision procedures. Rupture of an augmented bladder with a closed bladder neck has been reported in one patient who failed to catheterize after an alcoholic binge.

Outcome

When destruction of the bladder neck has occurred, a suprapubic catheter alone fails to achieve continence in the majority of patients. Feneley reported on 32 women with destruction of the bladder neck

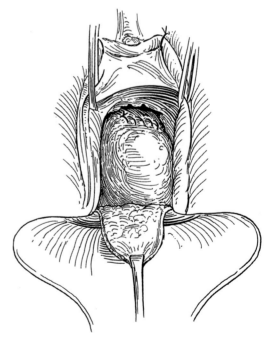

Figure 53-8 A second layer of continuous closing sutures is placed in a transverse fashion approximating the bladder neck and anterior bladder wall to just behind the symphysis pubis. This transfers the underlying closed bladder neck to the retropubic space. Following placement of this second layer of sutures, the closed bladder neck should be located high behind the symphysis pubis. (From Raz S: Atlas of Transvaginal Surgery. Philadelphia, WB Saunders, 1992.)

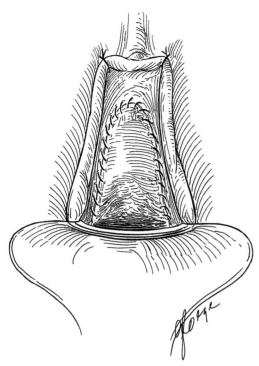

Figure 53-9 The vaginal defect is closed by advancing the inverted U–shaped vaginal flap. The vagina is packed for 24 hours with ribbon packing that has been covered in antibiotic cream. Irrigation of the suprapubis confirms that it has proper drainage. A drain is left in the retroperitoneal space. (From Raz S: Atlas of Transvaginal Surgery. Philadelphia, WB Saunders, 1992.)

who were treated initially with a suprapubic catheter.[1] Twenty-four subsequently required closure of the bladder neck to achieve continence. Feneley emphasized the need to close the bladder outlet to achieve a dry perineum.

Augmentation cystoplasty with a continent stoma and closure of the bladder neck is preferable to cystectomy and continent diversion. Cystectomy carries with it a higher morbidity than augmentation cystoplasty. The ureters are left in situ with an augmentation cystoplasty and do not require reimplantation

with its related potential complications of reflux, stenosis, and dehiscence. The natural bladder may aid in sensation to indicate when the reservoir is full. Renal function is reported to be preserved in patients with augmentation cystoplasty, whereas continent neobladders may have associated renal dysfunction.[3]

The transvaginal approach to closure of the bladder neck provides a simple method of bladder neck closure that is less invasive than the abdominal approach. Long-term follow-up over 5 years has revealed no recurrence of perineal leakage.[8]

REFERENCES

1. Feneley RCL: The management of female incontinence by suprapubic catheterization, with or without urethral closure. Br J Urol 55:203–207, 1983.
2. Reid R, Schneider K, Fruchtman B: Closure of the bladder neck in patients undergoing continent vesicostomy for urinary incontinence. J Urol 120:40–42, 1978.
3. Hulecki SJ, Hackler RH: Closure of the bladder neck in spinal cord injury patients with urethral sphincteric incompetence and irreparable urethral pathological conditions. J Urol 131:1119–1121, 1984.
4. Desmond AD, Shuttleworth KED: The results of urinary diversion in multiple sclerosis. Br J Urol 49:495, 1977.
5. Dunn M, Roberts JBM, Smith PJB, Slade N: The long-term results of ileal conduit urinary diversion in children. Br J Urol 51:458, 1979.
6. Goldwasser B, Ben-Chaim J, Golomb J, et al: Bladder neck closure with an Indiana stoma outlet as a technique for continent vesicostomy. Surg Gynecol Obstet 177:448–450, 1993.
7. Herschorn S, Thijssen AJ, Radomski SB: Experience with hemi-Kock ileocystoplasty with a continent abdominal stoma. J Urol 149:998–1001, 1993.
8. Zimmern PE, Hadley HR, Leack GE, Raz S: Transvaginal closure of the bladder neck and placement of a suprapubic catheter for destroyed urethra after long-term indwelling catheterization. J Urol 134:554–557, 1985.
9. Chancellor M, Erhard MJ, Kiilholma PJ, et al: Functional urethral closure with pubovaginal sling for destroyed female urethra after long-term urethral catheterization. Urology 43:499–505, 1994.
10. Kreder K, Das AK, Webster GD: The hemi-Kock ileocystoplasty: A versatile procedure in reconstructive urology. J Urol 147:1248–1251, 1992.

CHAPTER 54

Vaginal Reconstruction

Malcolm A. Lesavoy, M.D.
Eugene J. Carter, M.D.

Reconstruction of the vagina has become a standard procedure performed by plastic surgeons, gynecologists, and urologists. The most common indication for vaginal reconstruction is congenital absence of the vagina. However, there are other situations for performing this procedure including various intersex and transsexual conditions, previous ablative surgery for various perineal malignancies, and, on occasion, for relief of pain following radiation therapy.

In general, the results of vaginal reconstruction are satisfactory; however, potential problems can include inadequate genital wound coverage owing to foreshortened graft or flap harvest, fecal contamination if preoperative bowel preparation has not been adequate, adjacent urethral injuries during dissection of the new vaginal pocket, and difficult immobilization of the patient in the postoperative period.

Counseller reported that congenital absence of the vagina occurs in approximately 1 in every 4000 births and that these abnormalities usually coexist with uterus and urinary tract abnormalities.[1] Usually, however, the ovaries are not affected, and the secondary sex characteristics develop normally. Embryologically, because the cervix and vagina initially form a solid unit, the lack of cavitation and cell death needed to form a vagina is the reason for vaginal agenesis.[1] However, the hormonal factors that stimulate cavitation are not known.

History

In 1573, a student of Vesalius, Realdus Colombus, first reported vaginal agenesis, and it was not until 1872 that Heppner described vaginal reconstruction using the labia.[2] However, the true landmark report for vaginal reconstruction is credited to Abbé in 1898.[3] In one patient, Abbé described dissecting a canal and lining it with split-thickness skin grafts.

These skin grafts were placed over a rubber stent packed with gauze. After 10 days, the stent was removed, and the skin grafts were found to be completely vascularized. The patient was asked to wear a vaginal conformer postoperatively, and evidently intercourse was possible. However, Abbé's report was lost for almost 40 years until McIndoe popularized the Abbé technique by lining the new vaginal canal with partial-thickness skin grafts.[4] McIndoe reported an impressive array of 63 cases,[5] and subsequently Counseller in 1948 reported 70 cases.[1] Other methods of vaginal reconstruction have been attempted, but most have had undesirable effects, specifically when segments of the gastrointestinal tract have been used for lining the new vaginal canal. Conway and Stark in 1953 described use of the rectum[6] (earlier Sneguireff,[7] Popow,[8] and Schubert[9] had described the same thing). Baldwin in 1904 even described using a loop of ileum.[10] However, obvious difficulties with bowel transposition such as necrosis, infection, and abscess formation occurred. If the procedure was successful, the type of secretions arising from the bowel lining were mostly inappropriate and unwanted. The added morbidity of an intra-abdominal procedure, various bowel anastomoses, the possibility of vascular compromise, and undesired mucosal secretions account for the lack of popularity of these procedures.

The Frank procedure, a nonoperative technique, has been successful in some cases of incomplete vaginal atresia. In 1927 Frank and Geist demonstrated the use of intermittent pressure at the perineal dimple between the anus and the urethra where the vagina should be.[11] This pressure is applied until the patient feels mild discomfort by a series of graduated obturators in the form of increasing sizes of test tubes. The pressure is relieved and then reapplied. The patient gradually stretches this skin inwardly in the same way that a skin expander works with an

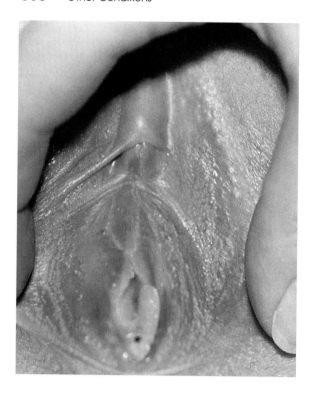

Figure 54–1 Congenital vaginal aplasia with an enlarged urethral meatus below the clitoris.

outward force. This process continues for weeks until the largest dilator can be introduced within the neovagina and worn comfortably. This procedure requires a very compliant and persistent patient and an anatomy that is consistent with incomplete vaginal agenesis. Obviously, the skin lining the new vagina is cutaneous squamous epithelium and must be lubricated externally to allow intercourse.

Procedure

ABBÉ-McINDOE PROCEDURE

Over the years, the Abbé-McIndoe procedure evolved to become the easiest and most successful method of vaginal reconstruction, avoiding the risks and disadvantages of laparotomy (Figs. 54–1, 54–2). The procedure must be performed under general or spinal anesthesia. A Y incision is made along the median raphe between the urethra and the anus. A catheter is placed in the urethra, and dissection is carried cephaloposteriorly. This dissection can be done relatively bluntly, and safety is ensured by keeping a gloved finger in the rectum for tactile ease of dissection. The Y incision allows three cutaneous flaps to be enfolded into the vaginal canal so that circumferential scar contraction can be avoided. The depth of dissection should be somewhat exaggerated and is in the range of 10 to 14 cm in the adult. The surgeon must overcorrect somewhat because of the expected subsequent contraction (Fig. 54–3).

After the vaginal canal has been bluntly dissected, a partial-thickness skin graft is harvested from the buttock-hip area. Obviously, one must keep in mind the subsequent scar that will definitely ensue from this partial-thickness skin graft, and one should avoid harvesting the graft from an area low on the thigh just for the surgeon's convenience. The skin

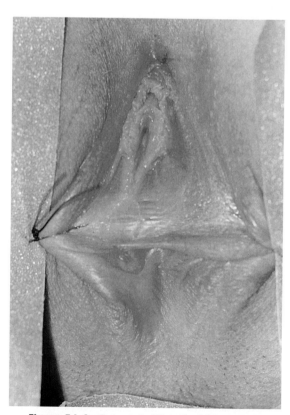

Figure 54–2 Sutures holding the labia majora.

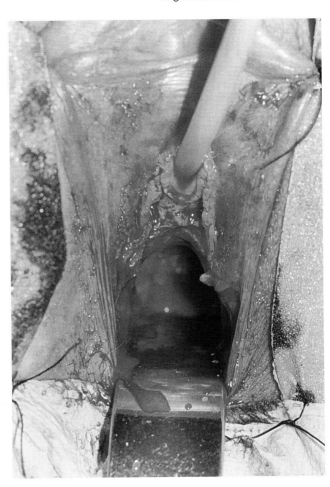

Figure 54-3 Catheter in the urethra and dissection of the neovaginal canal.

graft can be taken with any type of dermatome, and frequently two or three sheets of skin are needed to achieve a total dimension of approximately 14 by 7 cm.

A number of techniques have been developed to apply the skin graft to the vaginal canal. Historically, candle wax, carved balsa wood, gauze packing, syringe casing, dental wax, and hard plastic conformers have been used. Recently, the Heyer-Schulte Company has produced a soft, pliable, and expandable vaginal conformer that works very well in our opinion. This stent has a central semirigid foam core and a surrounding silicone envelope that can be expanded with air or saline (Fig. 54–4). There is also a central drain site through the core of the stent. Once the graft has been harvested, the vaginal stent should be inflated with air and lubricated with mineral oil.

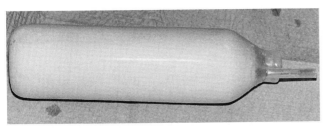

Figure 54-4 Heyer-Schulte inflatable vaginal stent.

The skin graft sheets are then sutured to each other and placed over this stent with the raw dermal sides *out* (Fig. 54–5). This means that the epidermal side of the skin is adjacent to the stent. Subsequently, hemostasis is checked in the neovaginal canal, and the now-deflated stent and overlying skin grafts are eased into the canal (Fig. 54–6). It may be necessary to deflate the vaginal stent while slowly rotating and pushing the stent and skin graft into the vaginal canal, but once the stent is seated to the depth of the dissection, it should again be inflated to spread out the skin graft, ensure direct apposition to the raw walls, and provide an excellent bolster for the ensuing neovascularization of the skin graft.

Following this, the flaps from the Y incision are sutured to the superficial ends of the skin graft in a tacking fashion with absorbable sutures. Fluff gauze is then packed around the perineum under compression, and the labia majora are sutured to each other to ensure that the stent does not slide out of the canal.

Postoperatively, the patient remains in bed for a minimum of 5 days and is medically constipated (a lower bowel preparation is required preoperatively). On the fifth or sixth postoperative day, the patient is sedated in bed, and the labial sutures are removed. The skin graft can then be checked by aspirating the outer lumen of the Heyer-Schulte vaginal

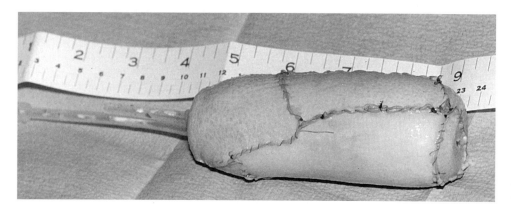

Figure 54-5 Split-thickness skin graft sutured around the vaginal stent with the epithelial side inward next to the stent and the raw side out.

stent and actually deflating it, gently removing the stent and leaving the skin graft intact within the vaginal vault. If there is any difficulty with this maneuver, mineral oil can be injected between the

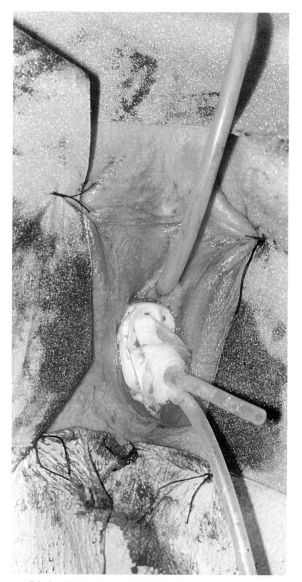

Figure 54-6 Vaginal stent with the skin graft invaginated into the neovaginal canal.

stent and the skin graft using a soft rubber catheter. This allows lubrication of the interface between the stent and the skin graft so that disruption and shearing of the skin graft are avoided when the stent is removed. The perineum can then be cleansed, and the stent can be washed and replaced immediately. Subsequently, a perineal binder can be applied, and the patient can be allowed to ambulate; the constipating medicine is then discontinued.

The vaginal stent is checked every other day, and the patient is usually discharged on the seventh or eighth day postoperatively. The patient should be fully aware of the mechanics of the stent so that she can remove, wash, and reintroduce the stent daily while at home.

It is extremely important in vaginal reconstruction that the patient be fully aware that a conformer must be worn for a minimum of 6 months postoperatively. If this is not done, contraction of the vaginal vault will definitely ensue. After 3 or 4 months, as the skin graft matures, vaginal intercourse should be encouraged. As a matter of fact, this procedure should not be done unless intercourse is anticipated. Intercourse, obviously, is an excellent obturator and conformer. After 6 months, the conformer can be eliminated during the day but should be worn at night. If the patient is active sexually and has intercourse two to three times per week, the conformer can be eliminated. However, if there is a time when intercourse is not anticipated for weeks or months, the conformer should be worn at night (Figs. 54-7 to 54-10). Because the skin grafts do not have the same properties as normal vaginal mucosa and do not have secretory abilities, most patients require the application of lubricants prior to intercourse.[30, 31]

FULL-THICKNESS SKIN GRAFTS

Full-thickness skin grafts are important for certain types of vaginal reconstruction (i.e., vaginal aplasia, vaginal stenosis, intersex conditions, and iatrogenic disease). One advantage of these grafts is that they allow reconstruction at an earlier age (anytime after puberty), providing psychological reassurance as the

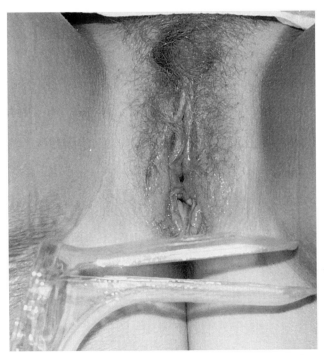

Figure 54-7 Photograph taken 3 months postoperatively showing the normal-looking vulva and the size of the speculum that can be inserted into the vagina.

child develops that she is normal. They also reduce postoperative stenting time and minimize vaginal stenosis by decreasing postoperative vaginal contraction. They improve the cosmesis of the donor site, and a full-thickness skin graft grows with the body proportionately.[12, 13] Inguinal donor sites are used for full-thickness skin grafts, and the donor site closure occurs primarily.

FLAPS

Vulvobulbocavernosus Myocutaneous Flap

The vulvobulbocavernosus myocutaneous flap was described by Knapstein and colleagues in 1990.[14] This flap is based on the skin fat and underlying vulvobulbocavernosus erectile muscle and tissue and is useful because of the low axis of the flap. It is not easily used for transfer into the upper pelvis, but it is best for reconstruction of the vagina after a pelvic exenteration that removes the perineal body and the anus (i.e., a lower pelvic defect). This is a relatively new procedure and should be considered especially for patients with anterior or total exenteration with low rectal anastomosis.

Generally, the vulvobulbocavernosus myocutaneous flap is not large enough to form a complete vaginal canal. The anterior edges of the flap are sewn together to form the anterior margins of the newly formed vaginal cylinder. Its disadvantage is the retention of vulvar hair, which results in vaginal discharge and strong odor. The blood and nerve supply comes from the pudendals.[15]

Gracilis Myocutaneous Flaps

The gracilis muscle is the most common flap used after pelvic exenteration for vaginal reconstruction.[16, 17] Following pelvic exenteration, an abdominoperineal resection, or the sequela of vaginal radiation (Fig. 54-11), the patient is usually left with a large vaginal defect. Use of a gracilis island myocutaneous flap can enhance vaginal reconstruction. It also provides adequate vaginal length and is an expendable muscle for the most part.

The gracilis myocutaneous flap provides sufficient bulk to fill the empty pelvic space and simultaneously brings its own new blood supply, leading to a softness and pliability not achievable with skin graft techniques. The disadvantage of the gracilis may include a loss of approximately 10 to 20% of the flap due to vascular compromise of the flap resulting from potential tension of its small-caliber vascular pedicle when transposed into the pelvic defect. Residual scarring on the legs may also be a common source of minor complaints.[18–20]

The principle of employing muscle with its overly-

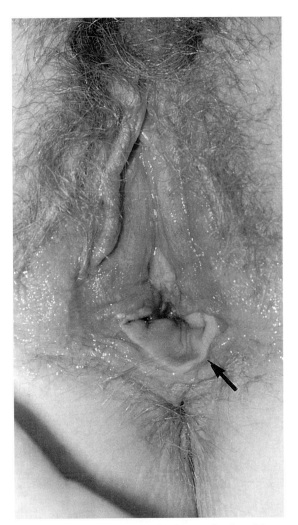

Figure 54-8 The discrepancy in the skin graft color of the neovagina.

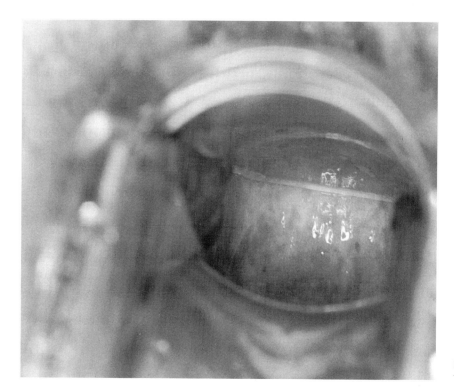

Figure 54-9 Depth of the neovagina as seen through the plastic speculum.

ing skin, vascularized by the muscular perforators, has been well documented in the plastic and reconstructive surgical literature by Owens (1955),[21] Bakamjian (1963),[22] Hueston and McConchie (1968),[23] and McCraw and his associates (1976).[24] McCraw and associates were the first to describe the principle of the "skin island" over the muscle unit, and this principle is applicable to vaginal reconstruction. Interestingly, McCraw's paper on vaginal reconstruction was one of the landmark works in the plastic surgery literature that opened the floodgate to the revived use of myocutaneous flaps.

The operation begins with the patient in the lithotomy position (Fig. 54-12). Either unilateral or bilateral island gracilis myocutaneous flaps are harvested

(Fig. 54-13) based on their superior neurovascular pedicles (Fig. 54-14). The flap can then be tunneled (Fig. 54-15) under intact perineal skin (Fig. 54-16) and "invaginated" into the neovaginal canal. A conformer is not needed, and the donor sites are closed

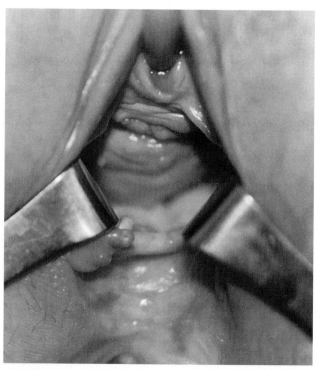

Figure 54-11 Case of radiation vaginitis with severe pain, drainage, fibrosis, and contraction.

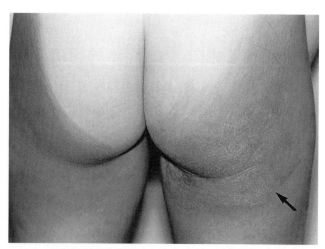

Figure 54-10 Donor site on the right buttock.

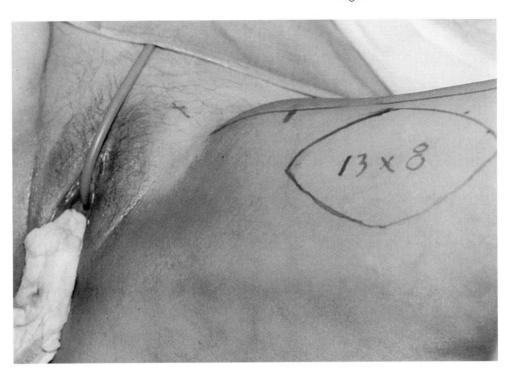

Figure 54-12 After excision of radiation-damaged tissue and a pack in the vaginal vault, a 13-by 8-cm gracilis myocutaneous island flap is outlined on the left medial thigh.

in a linear fashion with primary approximation along the medial thigh area (see Fig. 54–15).

The illustrative case presented (see Figs. 54–11 to 54–16) shows the use of a unilateral gracilis myocutaneous flap for radiation contracture and pain of the vaginal vault. Sensibility of the skin of the gracilis myocutaneous island is maintained by way of the sensory branches of the obturator nerve as described by Lesavoy and colleagues.[25] However, sensitivity of the transposed skin is not the same as that of a normal vagina. Sensitivity to pressure is excellent, but tactile sensitivity is diminished.[26] (Sexual sensitivity is mostly cerebral.)

Rectus Abdominis Myocutaneous Flap

Recently popularized because of its success in breast reconstruction, the rectus abdominis myocutaneous flap can also be used for vaginal reconstruction. Its major and primary arterial blood supply is the inferior epigastric vessels. Two island flaps can be harvested: (1) the horizontally oriented lower abdominal myocutaneous flap[27] or (2) the vertically oriented upper abdominal myocutaneous flap.[28] The transverse and vertical rectus abdominis myocutaneous flaps, because of the extended length of their vascular pedicles, allow a high arc of rotation. The axis is deter-

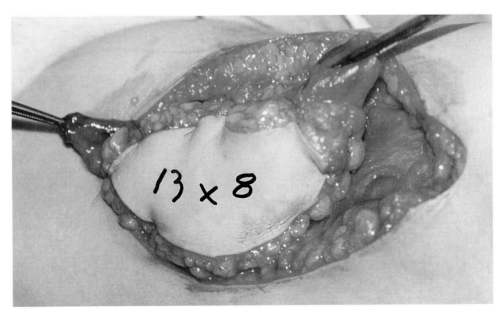

Figure 54-13 The gracilis muscle and island skin flap are isolated.

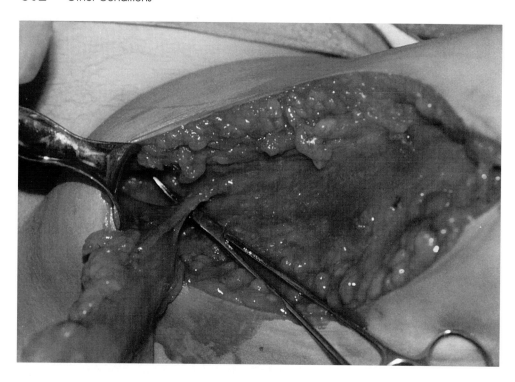

Figure 54-14 The undersurface of the gracilis myocutaneous island flap and its neurovascular bundle.

mined by the vascular supply and is transferred intra-abdominally through the posterior rectus sheath. This need for laparotomy is one of the obvious negative aspects of this procedure. A vertically oriented flap may be preferred when it is necessary to maintain an intact lower abdominal rectus muscle for exit sites of stomas on the contralateral side.

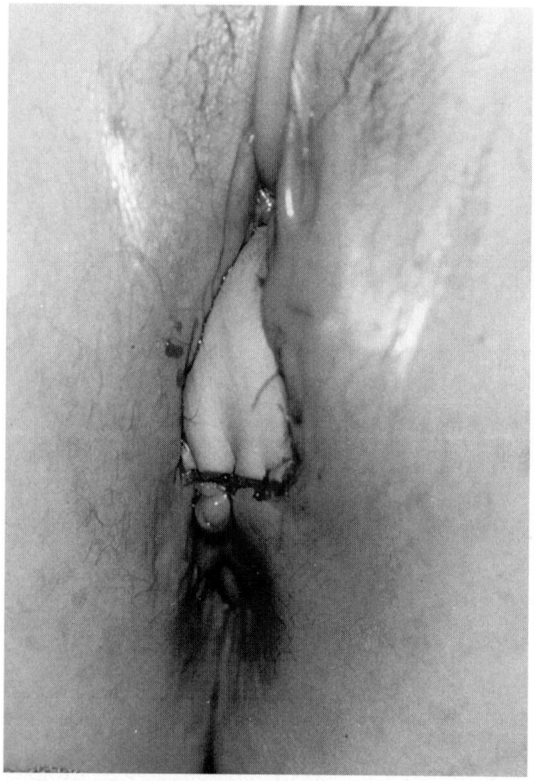

Among the many advantages of this flap are a very reliable blood supply[19] and the ability to resurface a defect with a *single* flap. This flap also provides ease of mobilization without tension and a low incidence of vascular compromise.[18, 29] In a series of 22 patients there was little tissue loss and an acceptable donor site, and return to sexual activity was possible in 80% of patients.[28]

PROCEDURE After completion of the exenteration procedure, attention is directed toward harvesting the myocutaneous flap from the abdomen. Centered just to the left or right of the umbilicus, a transverse rectus abdominal myocutaneous (TRAM) flap is harvested measuring approximately 9 cm long by 12 cm wide. The flap should include skin, subcutaneous tissue, a strip of anterior rectus sheath, and the rectus muscle itself (Fig. 54–17). The initial incision should commence at the lateral apex of the TRAM (which corresponds to the anterior axillary line) and should extend medially to include all of the above-mentioned flap components. The rectus muscle is identified and carefully dissected laterally to the region of the deep inferior epigastric perforating vessels, with identification of the inferior epigastric vascular pedicle at its origin on the external iliac vessels. This ensures adequate flap mobilization when the flap is isolated. At this point, the superior and inferior margins of the rectus muscle are divided (Fig. 54–18). A vaginal tube is then created from the flap by means of continuous and interrupted sutures to approximate the superior and inferior margins of skin and muscle with the raw side out (Fig. 54–19).

The manually formed vaginal cone is then mobilized and transferred through the posterior rectus

Figure 54-15 Inset of the flap into the vaginal defect. The donor site is closed primarily.

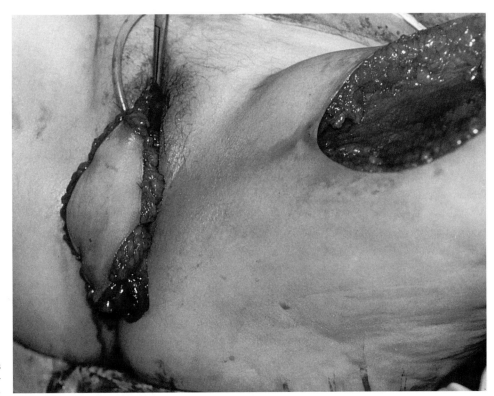

Figure 54-16 The myocutaneous island flap is transferred subcutaneously and is prepared to be inset.

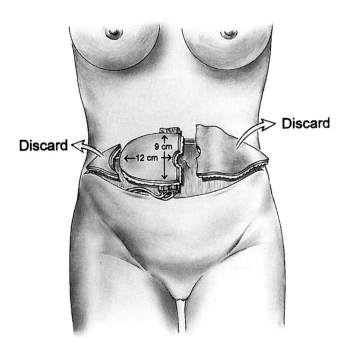

Figure 54-17 Harvesting of right rectus abdominis myocutaneous flap for vaginal reconstruction.

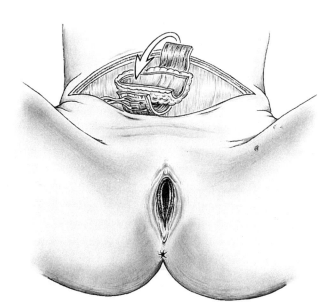

Figure 54-18 The flap is mobilized and formed into a tube.

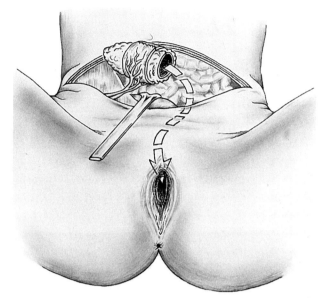

Figure 54-19   The mobilized myocutaneous flap is sutured together to form a blind tube of sufficient length and diameter to serve as a functional vagina. It is then transferred through the posterior rectus sheath to reach the vaginal defect.

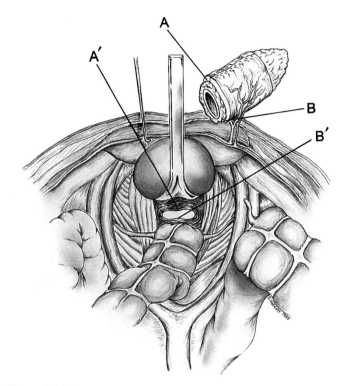

Figure 54-20   View after a laparotomy incision is made through the peritoneum at the origin of the deep inferior epigastric vessels into the pelvis to reach the vaginal defect.

sheath after a laparotomy incision is made through the peritoneum at the origin of the deep inferior epigastric vessels into the pelvis to reach the vaginal defect (Figs. 54–19 and 54–20). The lateralmost portion of the flap becomes the apex of the vagina. Care must be taken when placing the flap to ensure that no tension is placed on the vascular pedicle. The neovagina is then attached to the introitus with interrupted sutures (Fig. 54–21).[15, 18] An estrogen cream is spread on the mold, which is placed in the vagina and sutured in place.[18] On day 5, the mold is removed, and a vaginal dilator is worn three times per week for 3 months in conjunction with estrogen cream.[18]

The initial procedure is concluded with primary closure of the fascial defect with interrupted or continuous permanent sutures. The closure of subcutaneous tissue after a horizontal (TRAM) harvest is best achieved with the patient in a 30-degree semi-Fowler position to assist with approximation. A subcutaneous drain is placed beneath the mobilized skin flaps and is externalized through a separate incision.

It is advisable postoperatively to maintain strict bed rest for 48 hours with the hips flexed 30 degrees to decrease abdominal wall fascial tension at the repair site. The vertical rectus abdominis myocutaneous (VRAM) flap has all the advantages of the TRAM flap, but it leaves a single para-midline scar at closure rather than the additional horizontal lateral scar.

Intestinal Flaps

For the sake of completeness, other methods of vaginal reconstruction, such as flaps of small intestine,

ascending colon, sigmoid colon, and sigmoid and lower rectum may be briefly described here, since they have been used with varying degrees of success for vaginal reconstruction. The patient requires hospitalization 2 days before the operation to allow time to prepare and sterilize the bowel adequately. With the patient in the lithotomy position, a vaginal tract is first dissected from the perineum into the perito-

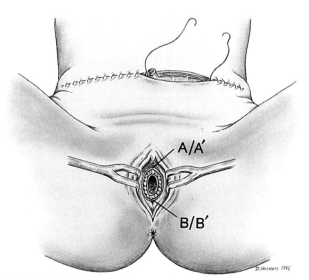

Figure 54-21   The myocutaneous flap is transposed into the pelvis and sutured to the perineal (introital) incision.

neum, and the tract is widened laterally. When hemostasis is satisfactory, the vaginal tract is packed and the abdomen opened. The sigmoid is generally mobile enough to allow a satisfactory vascular pedicle to be developed. With proper planning, an adequate length of intestine (12 to 15 cm) can be isolated, an oblique end-to-end anastomosis performed, and the bowel segment drawn through the vaginal tract. The patient is returned to a lithotomy position. The end of the bowel is incised on an angle to gain additional room and is then attached to the introitus.

Advantages of the intestinal neovagina include the absence of a need for frequent dilatation or stent wearing. However, the disadvantages include excessive mucus formation, especially when the small intestine is used, and a mortality rate of between 1 and 2%.[12]

Summary

Vaginal reconstruction can be an uncomplicated and straightforward procedure when attention to detail is maintained. The Abbé-McIndoe procedure of lining the neovaginal canal with split-thickness skin grafts has become the standard. Use of the inflatable Heyer-Schulte vaginal stent provides comfort for the patient and ease for the surgeon in maintaining skin graft approximation.

For large vaginal and perineal defects, myocutaneous flaps such as the gracilis island flap have been extremely useful for correction of radiation-damaged tissue to the perineum and for the reconstruction of large ablative defects. Minimal morbidity and scarring ensue because the donor site can be closed primarily.

The gracilis has sufficient bulk to fill the pelvis, thus decreasing the incidence of herniation or possible obstruction. It also provides vaginal length, is an expendable muscle, and generally is out of the irradiated field. Limitations may be its 10 to 20% incidence of vascular compromise due to the vessel's small caliber, which results in tension as the flap is moved into the pelvic defect.

The use of the transverse rectus abdominis myocutaneous flap is a newer technique to create a functional vagina. Its advantage over the gracilis is its variable vascular pedicle caliber and length. Of paramount importance are its extremely reliable blood supply and its potentially long vascular pedicle, which provides flap versatility with a resulting low incidence of vascular compromise. This flap augments the surgical options available for pelvic and vaginal reconstruction.

An absolute contraindication to rectus harvest is a history of potential vascular disruption of the inferior epigastric vessels. Obesity may be a relative contraindication because the thick subcutaneous tissue prohibits flap flexibility and mobilization into the pelvic space.

There remains a wide range of procedures from which to choose for the correction of congenital absence of the vagina, and unfortunately no consensus has been reached about which of these is best. Each case must be evaluated on an individual basis.

With all vaginal reconstructions, a compliant patient is a necessity. The patient must wear a vaginal obturator for a minimum of 3 to 6 months postoperatively and is encouraged to use intercourse as an excellent obturator. In general, vaginal reconstruction can be an extremely gratifying procedure that enhances the functional and emotional well-being of these patients. In short, vaginal reconstruction can be successful in patients with either congenital or ablative vaginal absence, and it can be a functional and emotional plus for all concerned. Attention to detail and support are necessary in all cases.

REFERENCES

1. Counseller VS: Congenital absence of the vagina. JAMA 136:861, 1948.
2. Heppner (1872): Cited by Paunz A: Formation of an artificial vagina to remedy a congenital defect. Zentralbl Gynakol 47:833, 1923.
3. Abbé R: New method of creating a vagina in a case of congenital absence. Med Rec Dec. 10, 1898.
4. McIndoe A: The application of cavity grafting. Surgery 1:535, 1937.
5. McIndoe A: The treatment of congenital absence and obliterative conditions of the vagina. Br J Plast Surg 2:254, 1950.
6. Conway H, Stark RB: Construction and reconstruction of the vagina. Surg Gynecol Obstet 97:573, 1953.
7. Sneguireff WF: Zewei neu Fälle von Restitutio Vaginiae per Transplantationen Ani et Recti. Zentralbl Gynakol 28:772, 1904.
8. Popow DD (1910): Cited by Meyer HW: Kolpo-plastik. Zentralbl Gynakol 37:639, 1918.
9. Schubert G: Concerning the formation of a new vagina in the case of congenital malformation. Surg Gynecol Obstet 193:376, 1914.
10. Balwin JF: The formation of an artificial vagina by intestinal transplantation. Ann Surg 40:398, 1904.
11. Frank RT, Geist SH: Formation of an artificial vagina by a new plastic technique. Am J Obstet Gynecol 14:712, 1927.
12. Horton CE, Sadove RC, McCraw JB: Reconstruction of female genital defects. Plast Surg 6:4203–4212, 1990.
13. Sadove RC, Horton CE: Utilizing full thickness skin grafts for vaginal reconstruction. Clin Plast Surg 15(3):443–448, 1988.
14. Knapstein PG, Friedberg V, Sevin BU: Reconstructive Surgery in Gynecology. New York, Georg Thieme, 1990, pp 30–32.
15. Hatch KD: Construction of a neovagina after exenteration using the vulvobulbocavernosus myocutaneous graft. Obstet Gynecol 63:110–114, 1984.
16. Wee JT, Joseph VT: A new technique for vaginal reconstruction using neurovascular pudendal thigh flaps: A preliminary report. Plast Reconstr Surg 83:701–709, 1989.
17. Soper JT, Berchuck A, Creasman WT, Clarke-Pearson DL: Pelvic exenteration: Factors associated with major surgical morbidity. Gynecol Oncol 35:93–98, 1989.
18. Carlson JW, Soisson AP, Fowler JM, et al: Rectus abdominis myocutaneous flap for primary vaginal reconstruction. Gynecol Oncol 51(3):323–329, 1993.
19. Benson C, Soisson AP, Carlson J, et al: Neovaginal reconstruction with a rectus abdominis myocutaneous flap. Obstet Gynecol 81(5 pt 2):871–875, 1993.
20. Lacey MD, Jeffery L, Stern MD, et al: Vaginal reconstruction after exenteration with use of gracilis myocutaneous flaps. The University of California, San Francisco experience. Am J Obstet Gynecol 158(6 pt 1):1278–1284, 1988.

21. Owens N: A compound neck pedicle designed for the repair of massive facial defects. Plast Reconstr Surg 15:369, 1955.
22. Bakamjian V: A technique for primary reconstruction of the palate after radical maxillectomy for cancer. Plast Reconstr Surg 31:103, 1963.
23. Hueston JJ, McConchie IH: A compound pectoral flap. Aust NZJ Surg 38:61, 1968.
24. McCraw J, Massey F, Shankin K, Horton C: Vaginal reconstruction using gracilis myocutaneous flaps. Plast Reconstr Surg 58:176, 1976.
25. Lesavoy MA, Korn HN, Castro DJ, Cedars MG: Sensible flap coverage for pressure sores in patients with meningomyelocele. Plast Reconst Surg 85(3):390–394, 1990.
26. Hatch KD: Neovaginal reconstruction. Cancer 15, 71(4 Suppl): 1660–1663, 1993.
27. McCraw J, Kemp G, Givens F, Horton CE: Correction of high pelvic defects with the inferiorly based rectus abdominis myocutaneous flap. Clin Plast Surg 15:449–454, 1988.
28. Pursell SH, Day TG Jr, Tobin GR: Distally based rectus abdominis flap for reconstruction in radical gynecologic procedures. Gynecol Oncol 37:234–238, 1990.
29. Tobin GR, Day TG: Vaginal and pelvic reconstruction with distally based rectus abdominis myocutaneous flaps. Plast Reconstr Surg 81(1):62–73, 1988.
30. Lesavoy MA: Vaginal reconstruction. Clin Obstet Gynecol 12(2):515–525, 1985.
31. Lesavoy MA: Vaginal reconstruction. Urol Clin North Am 12(2):369–379, 1985.

Acknowledgments

The authors wish to express their gratitude to Mr. Don Hockett, to Mr. Tin Syiau for helping in drafting the illustrations, and to Ms. Juanita Navarette for the manuscript preparations.

CHAPTER 55

Complications of Vaginal Surgery

Gregory R. Wahle, M.D.
George P. H. Young, M.D.
Shlomo Raz, M.D.

The most effective method of management of surgical complications is to avoid them. Prevention of complications requires exact knowledge of the patient's medical and surgical history, familiarity with the relevant anatomy, and thorough awareness of the most common difficulties that may arise during the planned procedure. Appropriate use of preoperative diagnostic methods, such as voiding cystography, intravenous urography, and ultrasonography, allows visualization of the urinary tract prior to performing transvaginal surgery; interpretation of the findings helps to avoid potential intraoperative problems. In addition, adequate preoperative preparation facilitates accurate identification of a complication intraoperatively. Timely recognition and prompt treatment of a complication will prevent untoward late sequelae. Satisfactory results are much more likely if an injury is recognized and repaired at the time of occurrence and not addressed at a later date after the discomfort and inconvenience of a protracted and costly postoperative course.

Despite adequate preoperative preparation, even the most conscientious surgeon armed with precise knowledge of anatomic details and great surgical skill occasionally experiences surgical complications. Specifically, the reported incidence of injury of the urinary or intestinal tract during gynecologic surgery ranges from 5 to 8%.[1, 2]

This chapter first considers the management of intraoperative complications such as surgical injuries to the ureter, bladder, and bowel that may occur during vaginal surgery, including those recognized intraoperatively as well as those presenting during the period of recovery as a source of unanticipated postoperative morbidity. Additional postoperative complications that may be encountered after surgical procedures, including those specific to transvaginal surgery, are discussed last.

Intraoperative Complications

URETERAL INJURIES

Injuries Recognized Intraoperatively

In general, the risk of intraoperative ureteral injury during vaginal surgery is very low if the total number of vaginal procedures performed is taken into account. It is generally reported that the incidence of injury to the ureter during transvaginal procedures is between 0.5 and 1.5%,[3, 4] although precise numbers are not known. Risk factors for ureteral injury include a history of prior abdominal or pelvic surgery, the presence of vaginal prolapse such as an enterocele or a large cystocele defect, and a history of multiple prior vaginal surgeries.

Dissection of the anterior vagina should always be undertaken with caution because of the intimate association between the anterior vaginal wall and the base of the bladder. Use of a Foley catheter with careful palpation of the balloon during dissection will assist the surgeon in keeping the location of the bladder neck and trigone in mind. In addition to direct trauma occurring during dissection, ureteral injury may also be caused by clamping, coagulation, and incorporation into ligatures or suture lines. The importance of careful intraoperative cystoscopic examination of the ureteral orifices following intravascular injection of indigo carmine or methylene blue during any vaginal procedure involving dissection in proximity to the ureters cannot be overemphasized. If the efflux of dye-stained urine is not visualized, intraoperative ureteral injury should be suspected and ureteral catheterization, retrograde ureteropyelography, or uteroscopy should then be performed.

INCISIONAL INJURIES A small ureterotomy may be easily corrected if the cut edges are clean and can be seen clearly. To preserve the blood supply, care must be taken not to dissect the adjacent periureteral tissue extensively. Interrupted fine sutures of 4–0 or 5–0 absorbable suture material should be used. The ureter should be repaired over an indwelling stent, and the area should be properly drained. This drain should exit via the suprapubic area and not through the vagina to decrease the risk of vaginal fistula formation. The drain may be inserted by passing a long clamp under finger control from a small suprapubic puncture to the vaginal area. The end of the clamp is then used to grasp the drain, which is then transferred to the suprapubic area. After proper positioning and securing of the drain, the vaginal wall may be closed.[5]

Reanastomosis of the severed ends of a completely transected ureter may be performed using an oblique or spatulated technique.[6] A normal thin, nondilated ureter can be easily reanastomosed with five or six interrupted, absorbable 4–0 or 5–0 sutures. The use of too many sutures or tying them too tightly may lead to ischemia of the anastomotic site, with subsequent leakage or stricture formation. The anastomosis should be properly drained and performed over an indwelling stent inserted for proper modeling. With proper exposure, end-to-end anastomosis or ureteral reimplantation may be done transvaginally, but as a rule it is simpler and safer to perform the repair transabdominally. Proper dissection of the proximal ureter will provide a tension-free ureteroureterostomy. If ureteral length is sufficient, a direct antireflux ureteroneocystostomy may be performed.[7] If the proximal ureteral stump is too short to allow a tension-free reimplantation, a psoas hitch or Boari-type bladder flap can be used for the antireflux reimplantation.[8, 9]

SUTURE AND CLAMP INJURIES If the ureter has been captured incompletely by a suture that is removed immediately, surgical repair is generally not required. Nevertheless, a double-J stent should be inserted because the extent of the ischemic damage is never known for certain. On removal of the injuring suture, the ureter should be observed to estimate its color and shape. If the affected area is discolored, narrow, or adynamic, resection of the ischemic area is recommended. Either spatulated reanastomosis over an indwelling stent or reimplantation, depending on the location and extent of the injury, should then be performed.[10]

Short-term clamping of the ureter during vaginal surgery may not always lead to ischemic damage.[11] In general, the clamping is incomplete, and some periureteral tissue is also captured. If atraumatic clamps have been used and the ureter is clamped for a short period of time (less than 30 minutes), a double-J stent may be inserted and should remain in place for a period of at least 1 week after surgery. If the ureter has been clamped for a longer period of time (more than 30 minutes), it must be assumed that more extensive ischemic damage has occurred. A lesion of this nature requires exposure of the clamped

portion of the ureter, resection of the damaged area, and either ureteroureterostomy or reimplantation.

CAUTERY-RELATED INJURIES As in suture or clamp injuries, damage to the ureter from excessive fulguration during surgery must be carefully assessed. Although low-grade defects may be managed with stent placement, coagulative damage is frequently severe, and consideration must be given to resection of the involved segment of ureter with indicated reanastomosis or reimplantation.[11]

Injuries Presenting Postoperatively

Seventy to eighty percent of ureteral injuries occurring during surgical procedures present postoperatively.[10] In the postoperative period, the most common manifestations of previously unrecognized ureteral injury are those of obstruction or extravasation. Postoperative flank pain and tenderness of the costovertebral angle are signs of ureteral obstruction. Postoperative parenteral analgesia may mask these symptoms, and a rise in creatinine,[12] diffuse abdominal pain, or paralytic ileus, all of which are uncommon after vaginal surgery, should lead to consideration of possible ureteral injury.[5] Urinary extravasation may also result in a lack of pain despite significant ureteral injury.

A high index of suspicion is therefore required to consider the possibility of ureteral injury in the early postoperative period and to enact appropriate measures of evaluation. Ultrasonography may discover hydronephrosis or a perirenal or intrapelvic urinary collection. Intravenous pyelography is usually diagnostic[13] and may reveal hydronephrosis or poor kidney visualization, indicating obstructive impairment of renal function. In cases of complete or partial ureteral disruption or transection, the pyelogram may be normal but contrast material is subsequently seen outside the urinary tract in delayed films, representing urinary extravasation. Retrograde ureteropyelography may assist in defining the nature and extent of the ureteral trauma.

When a diagnosis of ureteral injury is made postoperatively, and particularly if it is the result of an incomplete lesion, passage of a stent should be the first therapeutic maneuver. If a guidewire cannot be inserted past the site of injury under fluoroscopic control, it may be possible to negotiate a guidewire and stent under direct vision with the use of ureteroscopy.[10] Small ureteral leaks may resolve spontaneously with stent drainage but may require subsequent operative repair. If a diagnosis of complete ureteral obstruction is made, percutaneous nephrostomy drainage is arranged. In addition to relieving the obstruction, percutaneous nephrostomy access may allow successful stent placement by antegrade techniques despite failure of attempts using retrograde approaches.[14] In rare cases, the obstructive process may resolve spontaneously after absorption of the periureteral suture material, but areas of persistent ureteral strictures are the rule. Although these may be managed conservatively through endoscopic balloon dilatation[15] or endoureterotomy,[16] open surgical repair may be required.

BLADDER INJURY

Injuries Recognized Intraoperatively

As with ureteral injuries, intraoperative damage to the bladder during vaginal surgery may result from direct dissection, suturing, clamping, or excessive use of electrocautery. Risk factors for inadvertent bladder injury during transvaginal procedures include a past history of multiple pelvic or vaginal surgeries, tissue atrophy from ischemia or hormonal trophic changes, and a history of previous pelvic radiation therapy. Most intraoperative lesions occur at the bladder base adjacent to the anterior vaginal dissection, but with the increased popularity of needle bladder neck suspension procedures, lesions of the bladder neck are becoming more common.[5] Measures that aid in the prevention of intraoperative bladder injury during vaginal surgery include the use of delicate, precise dissection, familiarity with and strict adherence to known anatomic landmarks, and avoidance of undue retraction or fulguration.

The intraoperative use of a transurethral balloon catheter (and suprapubic tube) is strongly recommended. As discussed previously, the urethral catheter aids in location of the urethra, bladder neck, and trigone. Optimal catheter drainage limits urine collection and distention of the bladder during surgery. The appearance of bloody drainage through a catheter that previously drained clear urine at the beginning of the procedure should lead to a suspicion of bladder injury. In addition, urine generally appears in the surgical field if the bladder lumen has been opened inadvertently. Normal saline, methylene blue, or indigo carmine solutions may be instilled through either catheter to further assist in determining the presence and location of a suspected bladder injury. Cystoscopy may help in further identifying the nature and extent of the injury and in assessing the possibility of ureteral involvement.

INCISIONAL INJURIES If a cystotomy injury is diagnosed at the time of surgery, the defect and adjacent bladder wall must be exposed sufficiently. A tension-free, two-layer closure is required for successful repair, using a running inner layer of 3–0 or 4–0 absorbable suture and an interrupted second layer, also of absorbable suture material, which includes the perivesical fascia.[11] If required, a fibrofatty labial flap as described by Martius[17] can be used to reinforce the repair. On completion of the closure, cystoscopy must be performed after intravenous injection of indigo carmine or methylene blue to ensure that the ureters remain patent. Bladder irrigation should also be performed to demonstrate that the suture lines are watertight and that the closure is adequate. The repair should be drained through the suprapubic area (as described in the section on ureteral injuries)

and not through the vagina to avoid potential vesicovaginal fistula formation. Uninterrupted suprapubic and urethral catheter drainage of urine for at least 10 days is essential to further limit the risk of fistula formation. A cystogram should confirm good bladder emptying and the absence of extravasation prior to removal of the catheters.

SUTURE-, CLAMP-, AND CAUTERY-RELATED INJURIES In the unlikely event of a significant crush or fulguration injury of the bladder during vaginal surgery, the area should be exposed sufficiently to allow adequate debridement and a tension-free, two-layer repair as described previously. Use of a fibrofatty flap should be considered in cases in which tissue quality appears to be suboptimal. Suprapubic drainage of the repair, maximal bladder drainage through suprapubic and urethral catheters, and cystography prior to catheter removal are similarly required.

PERFORATION INJURIES With the recent increase in popularity of transvaginal needle suspension procedures for stress urinary incontinence, intraoperative penetration of the bladder by ligature carrier needles and nonabsorbable suture material has become common. It is therefore extremely important to perform a careful, systematic cystoscopic examination of the bladder prior to completion of vaginal surgery. The sutures can easily be removed and repositioned without increasing the risk of postoperative complications,[18, 19] although several days of catheter drainage may be considered. On rare occasions, delayed perforation of the bladder through erosion of the nonabsorbable suspension suture may occur, even months after the surgery. The new onset of such symptoms as severe urgency, frequency, and repeated or relapsing urinary tract infections in the late postoperative period should be thoroughly investigated. Cystoscopy will confirm the presence of a foreign body or adherent stone along the wall of the bladder. In general, the sutures can be removed under local anesthesia in the office using cystoscopic scissors.[5]

Injuries Presenting Postoperatively

Bladder injury that is unrecognized at the time of surgery is one of the most important complications of transvaginal procedures. Prolonged postoperative hematuria, vaginal or urethral leakage of urine despite adequate bladder drainage, severe frequency and urgency on removal of the urinary catheters, and severe pain in the vaginal and suprapubic areas all indicate the possibility of undiagnosed bladder injury.[11] A cystogram may demonstrate extravasation of urine, and cystoscopy generally confirms the presence of a bladder injury and further delineates its location and extent. Adequate bladder drainage must be obtained, and on rare occasions in which a large amount of leakage into the prevesical space occurs, percutaneous insertion of a drain through the suprapubic area may be required. Depending on the nature and extent of the bladder injury, prolonged catheter drainage may be sufficient to result in complete healing of the defect. Some patients develop a chronic vesicovaginal fistula despite an adequate period of optimal drainage. After exhausting routine methods of conservative therapy, the fistula may be approached surgically. These topics are discussed in Chapter 46.

Unrecognized placement of nonabsorbable suture material into the lumen of the urinary tract during vaginal surgery generally results in development of irritative voiding symptoms, recurrent urinary tract infections, or pain in the postoperative period. Evaluation and treatment should proceed as described earlier in the section on perforation injuries of the bladder.

BOWEL INJURY

Bowel injury occurring at the time of vaginal surgery is another major complication of vaginal surgery and may result in significant morbidity, particularly if the patient has not received bowel preparation prior to surgery. Risk factors for bowel damage include a history of multiple prior surgical procedures, radiation therapy, and intrinsic bowel disease. Familiarity with vaginal anatomy (especially if distorted by prolapse), proper placement of vaginal retractors, and the use of precise, delicate dissection in the isolation of enterocele defects and in the area of the posterior vaginal wall over the rectum all minimize the risk of intraoperative bowel injury. Whenever the need for rectocele or enterocele repair is anticipated, the patient should receive standard lower bowel preparation, including 48 hours of a clear liquid diet preoperatively, laxatives administered the day before surgery, and enemas if necessary.[5] We also advocate routine insertion of a Betadine-soaked sponge in the rectum prior to draping, which permits palpation of the rectal wall at the time of posterior vaginal repair, thereby facilitating the dissection. In general, if the patient has had adequate preoperative bowel preparation and the injury can be easily identified, repair of iatrogenic injury of the rectum or small bowel can be performed at the time of the injury according to established tenets of general and urologic surgery without increasing perioperative morbidity.[20]

Injuries Recognized Intraoperatively

If a bowel laceration is recognized immediately and can be adequately exposed, direct multiple-layer closure should be performed. Clamp or cautery injury should be clearly identified and debrided prior to closure, if necessary. Placement of a finger in the rectum may assist in the exposure and repair of a rectal injury.[11] Following repair of a clean rectal laceration, dilatation of the anal sphincter is recommended as well.[21] In the presence of an extensive injury of the rectum with significant spillage of stool into the surgical field or in a patient with a history

of significant previous radiation therapy, creation of a temporary diverting colostomy should be considered.

Injuries Presenting Postoperatively

Unrecognized bowel injury may be the source of distressing postoperative morbidity, including prolonged ileus, intestinal obstruction, or fistulas between the injured segment of bowel and the vagina or urinary tract. As in the case of unrecognized intraoperative urologic trauma, a high index of suspicion may be required to diagnose promptly and treat a surgical bowel injury that presents during the postoperative period. Plain films, computed tomography, and antegrade and retrograde contrast studies of the intestinal and urinary tracts may be used to define the problem and plan appropriate treatment.

BLEEDING

Efforts toward preventing perioperative bleeding begin during the preoperative evaluation. A prior history of unusual bleeding in response to trauma or associated with prior surgery must be evaluated. Medications with adverse effects on platelet function, such as aspirin or nonsteroidal anti-inflammatory drugs, should be discontinued at least 2 weeks prior to elective surgery. The use of appropriate screening laboratory studies, including platelet count, prothrombin time, partial thromboplastin time, and bleeding time, lessens the chance of encountering abnormal bleeding in a patient with an undiagnosed clotting abnormality. Careful attention should be paid to anatomic landmarks intraoperatively, and areas of potential vascular injury should be avoided or treated with extreme caution.

Injuries Recognized Intraoperatively

Ignoring significant intraoperative bleeding during vaginal surgery in the hope that "venous" bleeding can be stopped by extrinsic pressure is a dangerous practice. The retropubic and pararectal spaces are not confined and will not tamponade bleeding, even if it is from a venous source. At the end of surgery and prior to the closure of the vaginal wall, the surgical field must be free of bleeding. To avoid damage to adjacent structures, coagulation should be used with extreme caution and only for well-defined, small bleeding vessels. Precise placement of fine suture ligatures is generally preferable to indiscriminate use of cautery. Minor vaginal oozing can be controlled by the use of a vaginal pack. If diffuse bleeding is heavier, a Foley catheter with 50 to 60 ml of fluid instilled into a 30-ml balloon can be positioned against the vaginal packing[5] (Fig. 55–1).

Injuries Presenting Postoperatively

Although significant postoperative bleeding following vaginal surgery is unusual, it is essential to monitor

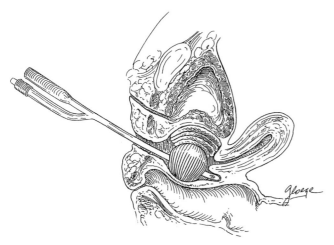

Figure 55-1 Diagram showing the hemostasis maneuver used after vaginal surgery when venous bleeding or oozing is a problem. A large Foley catheter balloon is inserted posterior to the vaginal packing. (From Raz S. Complications of vaginal surgery. *In* Raz S [ed]: Atlas of Transvaginal Surgery. Philadelphia, WB Saunders, 1992.)

the patient's vital signs closely in the immediate postoperative period. A drop in the patient's blood pressure accompanied by tachycardia and a drop in hematocrit in the absence of significant external vaginal bleeding strongly suggests active retropubic or retroperitoneal bleeding. Appropriate resuscitation maneuvers should be instituted. If the patient is stable, ultrasonography or computed tomography may help in locating the bleeding source. In selected cases, pelvic angiography and embolization of an arterial bleeder may correct the problem. In patients with substantial persistent postoperative bleeding, reexploration is generally required, in some cases through formal laparotomy. If massive pelvic hemorrhage without an obvious source is encountered, bilateral ligation of the internal iliac artery may be necessary.[11]

Late onset of postoperative vaginal bleeding, occurring more than 5 days after vaginal surgery, is rare and usually resolves with the application of vaginal packing or an intravaginal Foley catheter as described earlier. Delayed bleeding may be the result of a local infection, and appropriate antibiotic therapy should be prescribed.[22]

NEUROLOGIC INJURY

Significant direct injury to major neurologic structures during vaginal surgery is unusual and typically presents postoperatively. Owing to its proximity to the sacrospinalis ligament, injury of the pudendal nerve can occur during sacrospinalis fixation procedures used to address vaginal vault prolapse.[23] Proper exposure of the pararectal space, unambiguous palpation of the ischial spine, and placement of the fixation sutures at least 2 cm medial to the ischial spine minimize the risk of this complication. Obturator nerve damage can result from aggressive

lateral retropubic dissection. Entrapment or injury of the sciatic nerve may occur during placement of hemostatic sutures in an attempt to control brisk bleeding from the internal iliac vessels.[11]

Common peroneal nerve palsy, femoral neurapraxia, and development of lower extremity compartment syndromes resulting from retraction or positioning are rare complications of the lithotomy position used for routine vaginal surgery.[24] Nevertheless, the patient should be carefully positioned and padded to avoid compressive or tractive lower extremity neurologic trauma. Despite careful attention to proper positioning, the lithotomy position itself may create nerve injury despite proper padding and support, particularly in long procedures. Recovery from these injuries is usually spontaneous and complete but may be prolonged over several months.

Denervation of the bladder can occur after extensive vaginal surgery[25] and may contribute to prolonged or permanent postoperative urinary retention. The cause of bladder instability after vaginal surgery is not clear but does not appear to be related to bladder wall denervation.

Postoperative Complications

THROMBOEMBOLISM

Although the perioperative risk of lower extremity deep venous thrombosis and pulmonary thromboembolism after vaginal surgery is low compared with that seen with thoracic or abdominal intervention,[22] the complications are well known and dreaded and must be prevented.

Positioning of the patient on the operating table must be done carefully. Compression of the lower extremities can generate stasis, thereby predisposing to venous thrombosis. The use of ankle stirrups (which suspend the patient's legs) rather than potentially compressive supporting stirrups is therefore strongly recommended to avoid this problem. Although we do not use them routinely, perioperative prophylactic low-dose heparin administered subcutaneously or intermittent pneumatic compression stockings should be considered in patients thought to be at significantly increased risk for the development of venous thrombosis.[26]

The patient should be instructed to move her legs freely while in bed, and early mobilization with ambulation the morning after surgery is strongly encouraged. Excessive analgesia and sedation may impair mobility and increase the tendency toward venous stasis, and should therefore be avoided.

If venous thrombosis and pulmonary embolism become clinically evident, diagnostic studies should be performed, and intravenous heparinization should begin immediately.[27] After an intravenous loading dose of 5000 units of heparin, intravenous heparin is given continuously, starting at an infusion rate of 1000 units an hour with careful monitoring to keep the patient's partial thromboplastin time between 1.5 and 2 times its normal value. The patient is eventually switched to oral Coumadin, which is typically continued for 3 months.[28]

INFECTION

The vagina is a potential source of contamination by various types of microorganisms. The vaginal bacterial flora vary with the patient's age, the time of the menstrual cycle, sexual activity, and social environment.[24] Preoperative cleansing of the vagina by douching with antibacterial soaps is therefore recommended to reduce the number of bacteria. Vaginitis, cervicitis, urethritis, and urinary tract infection should be aggressively treated, and, optimally, a sterile urine culture should be obtained before performing elective vaginal surgery.

The use of antibacterial prophylaxis in patients undergoing elective urologic surgery with documented sterile urine is controversial.[29, 30, 31] In our practice, the majority of patients undergoing vaginal surgery for incontinence or prolapse are elderly and frequently debilitated, the procedures usually involve urologic manipulation and placement of permanent suture material through a vaginal incision and the retropubic space, and the patients have indwelling urinary catheters postoperatively. Because infection may result in significant adverse effects on the patient's health and the potential for success of the procedure, we routinely use antibacterial prophylaxis in vaginal surgery for incontinence and pelvic floor relaxation.[5] A combination of an extended-spectrum penicillin or cephalosporin (vancomycin is used in patients with an allergy to penicillin) in conjunction with an aminoglycoside is generally given preoperatively and continued for 24 hours postoperatively to provide broad-spectrum, synergistic antibacterial coverage that includes both gram-positive and gram-negative organisms.[32] Metronidazole is added to the regimen to include anaerobic bacteria in patients scheduled for hysterectomy, repair of rectocele or enterocele defects, or planned reconstructive procedures involving the use of bowel.

Fever in the first 48 hours following vaginal surgery is a frequent source of concern. The urine should be examined and cultured for possible urinary tract infection, which should be aggressively treated if present. Lung atelectasis and infection of intravenous catheter sites should be considered and ruled out. Flank or lumbar pain may indicate pyelonephritis or unrecognized intraoperative ureteral injury, and intravenous pyelography should be considered to evaluate the possibility of ureteral obstruction or fistula. Prolonged fever after vaginal hysterectomy, sacrospinalis fixation, or rectocele repair can be due to a pelvic abscess. Pelvic ultrasonography or computed tomography should be performed to rule out urinary tract obstruction, pelvic fluid collection, or other local pathology. If there is limited clinical response to antibiotic therapy in a patient with a post-

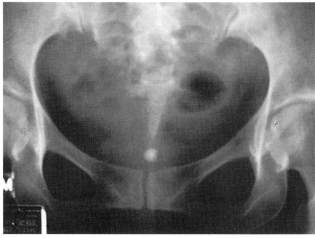

Figure 55-2 X-ray of the pelvis showing a bladder stone in a patient with recurrent urinary tract infections after a Marshall-Marchetti procedure. A nonabsorbable intravesical suture was found to be the nidus for the stone. (From Raz S: Complications of vaginal surgery. *In* Raz S [ed]: Atlas of Transvaginal Surgery. Philadelphia, WB Saunders, 1992.)

operative fluid collection, percutaneous, transvaginal, or surgical drainage should be performed.[5]

Pain and swelling in the suprapubic area several weeks after a vaginal suspension procedure should alert the surgeon to the possibility of cellulitis or a subcutaneous abscess at the site of the suspension suture knots, which may require incision and drainage if antibiotic therapy is unsuccessful.

Lower urinary tract infection after vaginal surgery is common and generally responds well to a short course of antibiotics. Recurrent or persistent infection after vaginal surgery requires a detailed evaluation including cystogram and cystoscopy, as previously discussed in the section on bladder injury (Figs. 55–2 and 55–3).

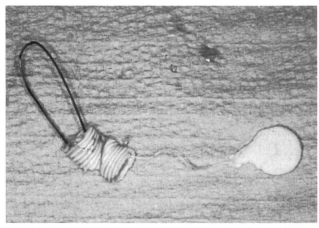

Figure 55-3 The Dacron graft and nylon suture have penetrated the bladder (forming a stone) 6 months after a Stamey suspension in a patient with recurrent urinary tract infections. (From Raz S: Complications of vaginal surgery. *In* Raz S [ed]: Atlas of Transvaginal Surgery. Philadelphia, WB Saunders, 1992.)

POSTOPERATIVE PAIN

Relatively significant discomfort in the immediate postoperative period after vaginal surgery is normal and should be treated with appropriate analgesic measures. Unusual or persistent pain following common transvaginal procedures may be experienced in the suprapubic, vaginal, or rectal area and should be thoroughly evaluated.

Suprapubic Pain

Suprapubic pain may be related to the insertion of a suprapubic catheter. A cystogram may be required to confirm proper catheter placement and rule out any complication due to the catheter or its placement. Bladder spasms and urgency are often felt as intermittent suprapubic pain and can be successfully treated with cholinolytic agents.

Another source of most distressing pain in the suprapubic area is related to the suspension sutures used in stress incontinence and transvaginal cystocele repair procedures. The pain is often related to activity and may be severe but is generally transitory, requiring several weeks before it subsides completely. Pain related to suspension sutures may be due to cellulitis or subcutaneous abscess, osteitis pubis (if the sutures are anchored to the bone), nerve or muscle entrapment, overly vigorous tying of the sutures, or placement of the sutures in a mobile portion of the anterior abdominal wall, which creates tension over the rectus muscle and fascia during activity. If suspension sutures used in vaginal procedures are transferred in the midline and kept as close to the pubic bone as possible, suprapubic pain after needle suspension will be very rare.[5]

In some cases of severe persistent suprapubic pain, the symptoms may be relieved by cutting the suspension sutures through a small suprapubic incision under a local anesthetic. The patient must be informed of the small risk of recurrent incontinence that this procedure carries.

Vaginal Pain

Vaginal pain after transvaginal surgery is rare but may be due to local hematoma or infection, which should resolve with appropriate treatment. A more unusual cause of persistent vaginal pain is the inclusion of the levator muscles in the transvaginal repair.[5] Such a patient typically complains of pain that increases with intercourse or certain movements, and her symptoms can be reproduced by palpation of the levator plate during a vaginal examination. Vaginal pain during intercourse may also be related to stenosis, shortening, or inflammation of the vaginal wall. A suture granuloma may lead to a chronic local infection or sinus tract that may result in vaginal pain. Minor vaginal procedures should be sufficient to treat these conditions successfully.

Rectal Pain

Extensive rectal or perineal repair during vaginal surgery may lead to temporary perirectal pain. The most common sources of persistent rectal pain following vaginal surgery are hematoma and infection in the rectovaginal space. The diagnosis is typically made on physical examination, and the process generally resolves with time. In rare cases, infection or hematoma may be associated with abscess or fluid collection that can be demonstrated on imaging studies, and percutaneous, transvaginal, or surgical drainage may be necessary.

VOIDING DYSFUNCTION

A certain degree of voiding abnormality can be expected during the normal recovery period after vaginal surgery. Prior to surgery, the patient should be informed about common postoperative voiding disorders, including transient urinary retention and mild symptoms of bladder irritability, and should be reassured that in the great majority of cases, normal voiding can be completely resumed within a short period of time. Persistent voiding dysfunction should be taken seriously and carefully evaluated.

Urinary Retention

Urinary retention after vaginal surgery is in general a temporary event. Surgical pain, pain medication, postoperative edema, and response to surgical manipulation of the bladder all contribute to impaired voiding in the immediate postoperative period. Urinary or vaginal infection, hematoma, or the presence of suspension sutures in close proximity to the bladder neck can induce prolonged urinary retention.[11] Because of the relatively high incidence of voiding impairment in the immediate postoperative period following vaginal surgery, we prefer to place a suprapubic catheter during surgery, which is then left plugged for the first 1 to 2 postoperative weeks so that the patient can attempt to void naturally and comfortably check the residual of urine. Intermittent self-catheterization may also be performed by the patient but can be painful and difficult in the immediate postoperative period. The suprapubic tube should be removed and intermittent self-catheterization initiated if urinary retention is still present 2 to 3 weeks after surgery.

Permanent urinary retention after routine vaginal surgery is very rare.[33–35] Although, as discussed previously, retention may result from bladder denervation, the most common cause is postoperative urethral obstruction (Fig. 55–4). Obstruction after an anterior repair is generally due to extensive and tight plication of the periurethral tissues. After vaginal or abdominal bladder neck suspension, sutures in the proximity of the urethra can impede the normal funneling, relaxation, or shortening of the bladder neck

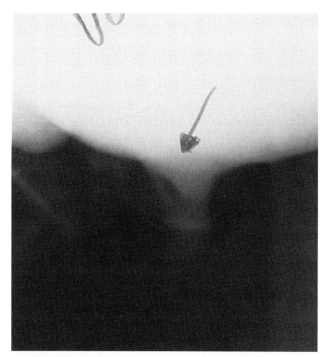

Figure 55–4 Voiding cystogram in a patient with severe urinary obstruction after a bladder neck suspension. A suture crossed the area of the proximal urethra. Endoscopic removal of the suture corrected the problem. (From Raz S: Complications of vaginal surgery. *In* Raz S [ed]: Atlas of Transvaginal Surgery. Philadelphia, WB Saunders, 1992.)

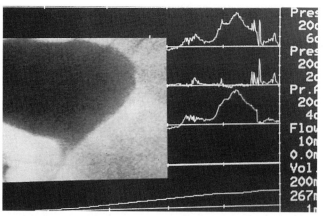

Figure 55–5 Videourodynamic evaluation of a patient with severe incontinence after stress incontinence surgery. The upper graph records the bladder pressure; just below it the abdominal and true detrusor pressures obtained by electronic subtraction are shown. Flow was not recorded. The patient had severe early-filling bladder instability that required medication. (From Raz S: Complications of vaginal surgery. *In* Raz S [ed]: Atlas of Transvaginal Surgery. Philadelphia, WB Saunders, 1992.)

during voiding.[36] Another common source of obstruction after bladder neck suspension is misplacement of the sutures in the midurethral area rather than at the bladder neck.

Complete urodynamic evaluation is necessary in cases of urinary retention that persists past the first 3 postoperative months.[5] A combined pressure-flow study may reveal a pattern of high pressure and low flow during attempts to void, which is typical of obstruction. In other instances, the urodynamic examination is negative for obstruction and may reveal an absence of voluntary bladder contractions.

If clinically indicated, urethrolysis should be performed after several months. In our experience, patients with persistent postoperative urinary retention who demonstrate an absence of detrusor function on urodynamic evaluation but voided normally prior to vaginal surgery have a high likelihood of regaining the ability to void if urethrolysis is performed within the first 6 postoperative months.

Bladder Instability

Although de novo detrusor instability is a recognized complication of transvaginal surgery, the most common explanation for symptoms of detrusor instability after vaginal surgery is their persistence from the preoperative period. Most elderly women undergoing surgical repair of stress incontinence have symptoms of detrusor instability as well, and although most

experience improvement or resolution of frequency, urgency, and urge incontinence, some do not.[37, 38] Symptoms of postoperative frequency, urgency, and urge incontinence are in general only temporary after vaginal surgery and resolve with time. Outlet obstruction may lead to de novo symptoms of bladder instability, but in most cases no clear cause of persistent frequency, urgency, and urge incontinence beyond the first 3 months after surgery can be found (Figs. 55–5 and 55–6). Sling procedures and bladder neck suspension procedures in the elderly, although well indicated and properly performed, appear to be particularly likely to be associated with the development of persistent symptoms of instability postoperatively.[5] Extensive vaginal surgeries, in particular repair of large cystocele defects, may induce inflam-

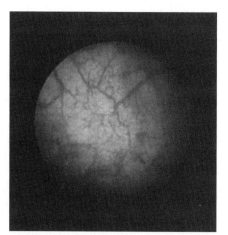

Figure 55–6 Cystoscopy findings in a patient with persistent frequency and urgency after a successful bladder neck suspension. Biopsy of the lesions revealed carcinoma in situ. (From Raz S: Complications of vaginal surgery. *In* Raz S [ed]: Atlas of Transvaginal Surgery. Philadelphia, WB Saunders, 1992.)

mation of the bladder base or irritative neuropathy, but this is unusual.

Treatment measures include fluid restriction, pelvic floor exercises, cholinolytic medications, and electrical stimulation.[25] In some cases of persistent severe detrusor instability, augmentation cystoplasty may be considered.

Stress Incontinence

The development of de novo stress urinary incontinence may be a complication of vaginal surgery in patients undergoing cystocele repair in whom concomitant bladder neck suspension is not performed.[39] We therefore recommend that a procedure to elevate and support the bladder neck and urethra be performed in every patient with cystocele repair in whom bladder neck and urethral hypermobility is demonstrated on preoperative physical examination or urodynamic evaluation, whether or not the patient complains of stress incontinence. If this is not done, the urethra will remain hypermobile, facilitating the development (or unmasking) of stress incontinence.

Persistent or recurrent stress incontinence following transvaginal bladder neck suspension requires a complete urodynamic evaluation. The most common cause is recurrent (or persistent) malposition and hypermobility of an otherwise functional bladder neck and urethra[5] (Fig. 55–7). In these cases, successful repositioning of the intrinsically normal sphincteric unit to a well-supported retropubic location will cure the stress incontinence. In other instances, evaluation of persistent or recurrent stress incontinence (which is often worse than the situation that existed prior to the failed procedure) reveals a well-supported urethra and bladder neck or other evidence of intrinsic sphincteric dysfunction. Measures designed to restore compression and coaptation of the outlet, including periurethral injection of bulk-ing agents, sling procedures, or artificial urinary sphincter devices, should then be considered. These are discussed elsewhere in this book.

ENTEROCELE AND GENITAL PROLAPSE

Postoperative genital prolapse may occur (or recur) after properly selected and well-performed vaginal reconstructive surgery. Poor quality of tissue, a history of multiple failed vaginal procedures, the presence of vaginal infection or hematoma, radiation exposure, and poor general and nutritional condition of the patient all increase the risk for postoperative prolapse.

The development of a secondary enterocele, not present prior to surgery, is a complication of any procedure that alters the vaginal depth and orientation, including bladder neck suspension procedures. Suspension of the anterior vaginal wall or uterus may transfer the axis of the vagina, placing the cul-de-sac into a more dependent part of the pelvis. Subsequent increases in intra-abdominal pressures may place stress on the vaginal vault and facilitate the formation of a pulsion enterocele defect,[40] which has been reported as a postoperative complication in as many as 15 to 25% of patients after a Burch colposuspension.[23, 41] Measures designed to prevent the formation of a secondary enterocele defect, including cul-de-sac obliteration and reapproximation of the cardinal-sacrouterine ligament complex, are discussed elsewhere in this book.

VAGINAL STENOSIS OR SHORTENING

Excessive excision of the vaginal wall may lead to narrowing or shortening of the vagina on closure. During repair of cystocele, enterocele, and rectocele defects, excision of vaginal tissue should be mini-

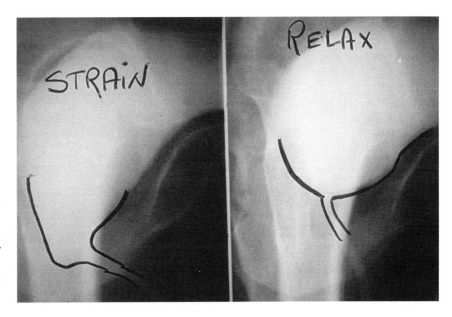

Figure 55-7 Lateral straining and relaxed cystogram in a patient with recurrent anatomic stress incontinence after a failed bladder neck suspension. The bladder base and urethra are hypermobile owing to the loss of support and fixation. (From Raz S: Complications of vaginal surgery. *In* Raz S [ed]: Atlas of Transvaginal Surgery. Philadelphia, WB Saunders, 1992.)

mized. The excised vaginal wall should be kept in sterile normal saline until the end of the procedure and may be used as a free graft when difficulties in closing the vagina without narrowing or tension are encountered. Excessive plication of the vaginal epithelium during closure and undue tension of the vaginal suture line should be avoided to limit the risk of ischemic contraction. At the end of a vaginal procedure, in particular one involving rectocele repair, the vaginal wall should be smooth, without bumps or constricting rings, and should easily allow the insertion of at least two fingers. Hematoma involving the vaginal wall may also lead to late scarring and subsequent deformity of the vaginal canal, so complete hemostasis must be ensured prior to vaginal closure.

A history of dyspareunia, pelvic or vaginal pain, and the findings from a careful physical examination are usually sufficient to make the diagnosis of vaginal stenosis or shortening. Longitudinal relaxing incisions in the lateral vaginal wall with transverse closure are generally adequate to correct mild vaginal stenosis.[11] In cases of severe stenosis or shortening of the vaginal canal, free skin grafts or vascular flaps may be required. An expandable, intravaginal conformer should be used until the graft has healed completely.[42]

REFERENCES

1. Everett HS, Williams TI: Urology in the female. *In* Campbell MF, Harrison JH (eds): Urology, vol 3. Philadelphia, WB Saunders, 1970, pp 1957–2014.
2. Nichols DH: Preface. *In* Nichols DH (ed): Clinical Problems, Injuries, and Complications of Gynecologic Surgery. Baltimore, Williams & Wilkins, 1983, p ix.
3. Mann WJ, Arato M, Patsner B, Stone ML: Ureteral injuries in an obstetrics and gynecology training program: etiology and management. Obstet Gynecol 72:82, 1988.
4. Daly J, Higgins KA: Injury to the ureter during gynecologic surgical procedures. Surg Gynecol Obstet 167:19, 1988.
5. Raz S: Complications of vaginal surgery. *In* Raz S (ed): Atlas of Transvaginal Surgery. Philadelphia, WB Saunders, 1992.
6. Marshall FF: Ureteral injuries. *In* Marshall FF (ed): Urologic Complications. St. Louis, Mosby-Year Book, 1990, pp 261–273.
7. Politano VA, Leadbetter WF: An operative technique for the correction of vesicoureteral reflux. J Urol 79:932, 1958.
8. Turner-Warwick R, Worth PHL: The psoas bladder hitch procedure for replacement of the lower third of the ureter. Br J Urol 41:701, 1969.
9. Williams JL, Porter RW: The Boari flap in lower ureteric injuries. Br J Urol 38:528, 1966.
10. St. Lezin MA, Stoller ML: Surgical ureteral injuries. Urology 38(6):497, 1991.
11. Schmidtbauer CP, et al: Complications of vaginal surgery. Semin Urol 4(1):51, 1986.
12. Stanhope CR, Wilson TO, Utz WJ, et al: Suture entrapment and secondary ureteral obstruction. Am J Obstet Gynecol 164 (6 pt 1):1513, 1991.
13. Dowling RA, Corriere JN Jr, Sandler CM: Iatrogenic ureteral injury. J Urol 135:912, 1986.
14. Chang R, Marshall FF, Mitchell S: Percutaneous management of benign ureteral strictures and fistulas. J Urol 137:1126, 1987.
15. Kramolowsky EV, Tucker RD, Nelson CMK: Management of benign ureteral strictures: open surgical repair or endoscopic dilatation? J Urol 141:285, 1989.
16. Clayman RV, Kavoussi LR: Endosurgical techniques for the diagnosis and treatment of noncalculous disease of the ureter and kidney. *In* Walsh PC, Retik AB, Stamey TA, Vaughan ED (eds): Campbell's Urology, 6th ed. Philadelphia, WB Saunders, 1992, pp 2231–2312.
17. Martius H: Supplementary surgery with bulbocavernosus fat flap. *In* McCall ML, Bolton KA (eds): Martius' Gynecological Operations. Boston, Little, Brown, 1956, pp 322–334.
18. Stamey TA: Urinary incontinence in the female: The Stamey endoscopic suspension of the vesical neck for stress urinary incontinence. *In* Walsh PC, Retik AB, Stamey TA, Vaughan ED (eds): Campbell's Urology, 6th ed. Philadelphia, WB Saunders, 1992, pp 2829–2850.
19. Staskin DR: Complications of female anti-incontinence surgery. *In* Smith RB, Ehrlich RM (eds): Complications of Urologic Surgery, 2nd ed. Philadelphia, WB Saunders, 1990, pp 499–517.
20. Goodwin WE, Turner RD, Winter CC: Rectourinary fistula: Principles of management and a technique of surgical closure. J Urol 80:246, 1958.
21. Walsh PC: Radical retropubic prostatectomy. *In* Walsh PC, Retik AB, Stamey TA, Vaughan ED (eds): Campbell's Urology, 6th ed. Philadelphia, WB Saunders, 1992, pp 2865–2886.
22. Ledger WJ: Infection in the Female. Philadelphia, Lea & Febiger, 1977.
23. Nichols DH: Complications and sequelae of vaginal surgery. *In* Nichols DH, Randall CL (eds): Vaginal Surgery. Baltimore, Williams & Wilkins, 1983.
24. Angermeir KW, Jordan GH: Complications of the exaggerated lithotomy position: A review of 177 cases. J Urol 151:866, 1994.
25. Wein AJ: Neuromuscular dysfunction of the lower urinary tract. *In* Walsh PC, Retik AB, Stamey TA, Vaughan ED (eds): Campbell's Urology, 6th ed. Philadelphia, WB Saunders, 1992, pp 573–642.
26. Coe NP, Collins REC, Klein LA: Prevention of deep vein thrombosis in urological patients: A controlled randomized trial of low dose heparin and external pneumatic compression boots. Surgery 83:230, 1978.
27. Hull RD, Raskob GE, Hirsh J: The diagnosis of clinically suspected pulmonary embolism: Practical approaches. Chest 89 (Suppl):417, 1986.
28. Hyers TM, Hull RD, Wez JG: Antithrombotic therapy for venous thromboembolic disease. Chest 89 (Suppl):26, 1986.
29. Antimicrobial prophylaxis in surgery. Medical Lett 29:91, 1987.
30. Madsen PO, Larsen EH, Dorflinger T: The role of antibacterial prophylaxis in urologic surgery. Urology 26 (Suppl):38, 1985.
31. Larsen EH, Gasser TC, Madsen PO: Antimicrobial prophylaxis in urologic surgery. Urol Clin North Am 13:591, 1986.
32. Marrien R, Valenti AJ, Madri JA: Gram-negative endocarditis following cystoscopy. J Urol 119:134, 1978.
33. Raz S, Sussman EM, Erickson DB, et al: The Raz bladder neck suspension: Results in 206 patients. J Urol 148:845, 1992.
34. Raz S, Siegel AL, Short JL, Snyder JA: Vaginal wall sling. J Urol 141:43, 1989.
35. McGuire EJ, Bennett CJ, Konnak JA, et al: Experience with pubovaginal slings for urinary incontinence at the University of Michigan. J Urol 138:525, 1987.
36. Maggio AJ, Raz S: Why vesicourethral suspension works or fails. *In* Raz S (ed): Female Urology, 1st ed. Philadelphia, WB Saunders, 1983, pp 299–307.
37. McGuire EJ: Bladder instability and stress incontinence. Neurourol Urodyn 7:563, 1989.
38. Nitti VW, Bregg KJ, Sussman EM, Raz S: The Raz bladder neck suspension in patients 65 years old and older. J Urol 149:802, 1993.
39. Nichols DH: Vaginal prolapse affecting bladder function. Urol Clin North Am 12 (2):329–338, 1985.
40. Zaccharin RF: Pelvic Floor Anatomy and the Surgery of Pulsion Enterocele. New York, Springer-Verlag, 1985.
41. Wiskind AK, Creighton SM, Stanton SL: The incidence of genital prolapse following the Burch colposuspension operation (abstract). Neurourol Urodyn 10:453, 1991.
42. Lesavoy MA: Vaginal reconstruction. Clin Obstet Gynecol 12:515, 1985.

CHAPTER 56

Benign Cystic Lesions of the Vagina and Vulva

Ashok Chopra, M.D.
Shlomo Raz, M.D.
Lynn Stothers, M.D., M.H.Sc., F.R.C.S.C.

Cystic lesions of the vagina and vulvar areas generally reflect benign pathologies. An inclusive classification as outlined by Kaufman is shown in Table 56–1.[1]

TABLE 56–1
Classification of Cysts of Vagina and Vulva

Epidermal origin
Epidermal inclusion cysts
Pilonidal cysts

Epidermal appendage origin
Sebaceous cysts
Hidradenoma
Fox-Fordyce disease
Syringoma

Embryonic remnant origin
Mesonephric (Gartner's) cysts
Paramesonephric (müllerian) cysts
Urogenital sinus cysts
Cysts of canal of Nuck
Adenosis
Cysts of supernumerary mammary glands
Dermoid cysts

Bartholin's gland origin
Duct cysts
Abscesses

Urethral and paraurethral cysts
Paraurethral (Skene's duct) cysts
Urethral diverticula

Miscellaneous origin
Endometriosis
Cystic lymphangioma
Liquefied hematoma
Vaginitis emphysematosa

Cystic Lesions of Epidermal Origin

Cysts of epidermal origin have the common histologic finding of viable keratinizing stratified squamous epithelium.[2] If these tissues are enveloped beneath normal skin or mucosa they may proliferate to form inclusion cysts. Depisch and colleagues, in a review of 64 vaginal cysts, found that this histologic type accounted for 34.[3]

The most common form of vaginal inclusion cyst reflects traumatic displacement of tissue following laceration or incision. In contrast, cysts of the vulva with a similar histology are rarely associated with trauma, and various theories have been put forward to account for their presence.

Epidermal cysts are described as round and whitish, yellow, or orange. They are often visible through the vaginal mucosa. Their contents appear as thick mucopurulent material. Generally, epidermal cysts become symptomatic only if they become superinfected or if they achieve an unusually large size. Treatment is reserved for symptomatic cases and involves excision.

Pilonidal cysts are a second form of epidermal cyst. These may be found, albeit rarely, in the vulva. Symptoms and treatment are similar to symptoms and management of pilonidal cysts in the sacral area.

Epidermal Appendage Cysts

Epidermal appendage cysts do not involve the vagina but are lesions of the vulva. Generally speaking, these lesions include syringoma, hidradenoma, and Fox-Fordyce disease. These entities reflect benign pathology of the apocrine or eccrine structures. The reader is referred to other sources for further data.[4]

Cysts of Embryonic Origin

These cysts are classified by source of embryonic origin as mesonephric, paramesonephric, or urogenital sinus cysts. Studdiford and associates found a prevalence of .006% in 20,000 patients admitted to Bellevue Hospital.[5] As one would expect, mesonephric and paramesonephric cysts are most commonly found in the vagina; urogenital sinus cysts are more commonly found in the vestibule.

Mesonephric (Gartner's) cysts form when portions of the mesonephric ducts persist and remain functional (Fig. 56–1). They are lined by cuboidal or low columnar, non–mucin-producing cells. In Deppisch's paper they accounted for 3 of 64 cysts.[3] Paramesonephric cysts, in contrast, reflect persistence of müllerian epithelium after the vaginal epithelium has been replaced by stratified squamous cells.[3] These cysts are lined by columnar or cuboidal, mucin-producing cells. In Deppisch's paper they accounted for 22 of 64 vaginal cysts.[3] Cysts of urogenital origin are rare and are lined by transitional or stratified columnar cells.[2] Differentiation of mesonephric and paramesonephric cysts is best made on the basis of histochemical staining for mucin.[1]

Clinical features of the three cyst types are similar except for location. Generally they are less than 2 cm

in size, single, and asymptomatic. Gartner's duct cysts are located from the cervix to the introitus and in the anterolateral portion of the vagina. They may be multiple on occasion and may have the appearance of linked sausages as they extend toward the introitus. Cysts of müllerian origin are also located in the anterior vagina, most commonly in the distal third. Cysts of urogenital origin most commonly occur in the vestibule, as one would expect based on fetal development.

Cysts of embryologic origin are rarely symptomatic unless they achieve a very large size or become infected. Both mesonephric and paramesonephric cysts may extend anteriorly between the vagina and the lower urinary tract; in such cases they may cause dysuria. Even more rarely, Gartner's duct cysts may grow and contact the ureter or bladder. Treatment of these lesions is dependent on symptoms and hence is rarely needed. Excision is the primary treatment in such cases, although there are reports of sclerotherapy and aspiration.[6]

Adenosis

Adenosis is defined as the presence of mucin-containing columnar epithelium or its products in the vagina.[1] There is general agreement that these cells represent remnants of embryonic müllerian epithelium.[1] Some authors do not distinguish between paramesonephric cysts and adenosis.[1] This entity has been the source of much investigation since Herbst's work in 1971 suggesting that a link existed between maternal DES and adenocarcinoma and adenosis of the vagina in female offspring.[7]

Vaginal adenosis is usually asymptomatic and hence is usually an incidental finding. Symptoms, when present, include postcoital bleeding, dyspareunia, and excessive mucoid discharge. Grossly, the lesions appear as red patches, usually confluent, on the cervix; on colposcopy they have a grapelike appearance. Diagnosis is suggested by the presence of columnar epithelial cells in vaginal scrapings, although biopsy is more definitive.

Treatment consists of close follow-up with surveillance directed toward metaplastic progression. Replacement of the normal cell lining with squamous epithelium implies metaplastic progression.[1] Nodular changes in the gross appearance of the lesions may herald progression and require biopsy. Profound mucorrhea may require treatment with laser, cryotherapy, or other ablative therapy.

Bartholin's Gland (Duct) Cysts

Lesions of Bartholin's gland or duct are the most frequently diagnosed cysts of the vulvar area. These are seen in approximately 2% of new gynecologic

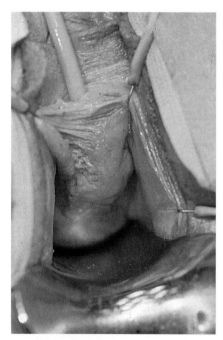

Figure 56–1 Gartner's duct cyst.

patients.[1] The disease process generally reflects obstruction of the duct followed by bacterial infection and abscess formation. Organisms involved include a broad variety of bacteria; however, cultures may be sterile.[8] The histologic appearance varies with site of origin. Acinar lesions consist of cuboidal or mucinous columnar epithelium; ductal lesions are lined by transitional or squamous cells. Symptoms may vary greatly. Most patients have small lesions and are completely asymptomatic; others may present with severe vulvar pain and dyspareunia. On physical examination the classic finding is a crescent-shaped introitus. Noninfected cysts are generally palpable in the midline of the labia minora. Superimposed infections may cause the lesion to become exquisitely tender and may distort the architecture of the introitus to a greater degree. On rare occasions these infected cysts may spread beyond the area of the introitus proper.

Treatment usually reflects the severity of symptoms. Small cysts generally require no therapy, but larger lesions and those complicated by infection are managed with surgery and antibiotics. Treatment options include excision, marsupialization, aspiration, maintenance of the ostia by dilatation, or creation of a new ostia.[9, 10] Marsupialization is generally the treatment of choice because it is technically straightforward, preserves function, has low morbidity, and is associated with a low incidence of clinical recurrence. Excision is often technically difficult and may be complicated by severe hemorrhage from the vestibular bulb or injury to adjacent organs.[11] Exceptional situations that might push the surgeon toward excision include multilocular cysts and a suggestion of tumefaction (i.e., postmenopausal onset). One technique of marsupialization or excision as outlined by Raz is described below.[11]

Marsupialization of a Bartholin's cyst is performed with a longitudinal incision in the vaginal wall overlying the cyst along its entire length. Using 2–0 Vicryl, the cut edges are approximated to the surrounding vaginal wall. If significant inflammation and edema of the surrounding tissues are noted, larger and more encompassing sutures may be required. The cyst cavity is next irrigated and packed with an antibiotic-soaked pack. Excision of a Bartholin's cyst requires similar steps in the initial set-up. The cyst is elevated by gentle pressure from the genitofemoral sulcus by the assistant. The incision is placed at the lateral vaginal wall at the medial aspect of the labium minus in a longitudinal fashion. The lower pole is generally mobilized first. This maneuver allows one to use traction on the lower pole when tackling the more vascularized upper pole. The cyst is mobilized by staying as close to the wall as possible to avoid bleeding. Dissection of a lower pole cyst may require placement of a finger in the rectum to avoid injury. Glandular epithelium may extend beneath the bulbocavernosus muscle and may be difficult to remove if hemostasis is suboptimal. Vicryl 3–0 is used to make a multilayered closure of the defect. Penrose drains should be used if hemostasis is in doubt.

Skene's Duct Cysts

Skene's ducts empty adjacent to the external urethral meatus (Fig. 56–2). The ducts are lined with stratified squamous epithelium or transitional epithelium. Clinically significant lesions, although unusual, develop while the cyst is small because of the ducts' proximity to the urethra. Indeed, cysts larger than 2 cm are unusual because the patient is usually profoundly symptomatic by this point. Symptoms include obstruction, dyspareunia, and dysuria. Superimposed infection may cause significant discomfort as well. Physical examination generally reveals a clear discharge of purulent material from Skene's glands. Often no distinct collection or cyst is seen. Cystoscopy is usually normal as well. Treatment usually consists of antibiotic management. In cases refractory to long-term antibiotic use, excision is the treatment of choice. Incision and drainage may be used as a temporizing measure if the gland is thought to be significantly infected and inflamed. In all instances care must be given to the urethra.[11] One technique of excision as outlined by Raz is described below.[11]

A Foley catheter is placed, and then an oblique incision is made over the cyst. Dissection is carried out around the cyst, and the occluded communication to the distal meatus is exposed and excised. The vaginal wall is closed without drainage. If the gland is actively infected and inflamed the approach is modified. Initially, a small semicircular incision is made in the vaginal wall just proximal to the meatus. A flap of vaginal wall is thus created and dissected free. A wedge resection of the distal urethra is performed next. This generally includes the entire urethral wall and the Skene's gland openings. The flap of vaginal wall is advanced forward and approximated to the urethral incision using absorbable su-

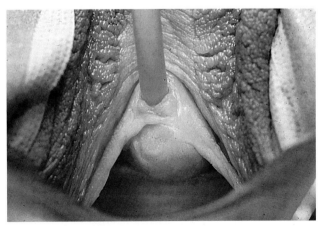

Figure 56–2 Skene's duct cyst.

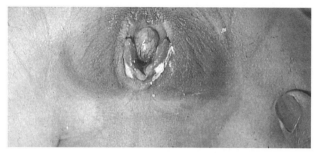

Figure 56-3 Ectopic ureterocele in a female infant.

ture. This maneuver has the effect of creating a slightly hypospadic, larger meatus. A Foley catheter and vaginal pack are left in place for 2 to 3 hours.

Miscellaneous Lesions of the Vagina and Vulva

Brief mention should be made of other lesions that may present as cystic masses of the vagina and vulva. These include urethral diverticulum, ectopic ureterocele (Fig. 56–3), urethral prolapse, ectopic mammary tissue, hydroceles, endometriosis, cystic lymphangioma, vaginitis emphysematosa, and prolapsed fallopian tube. For various reasons these have not been addressed in this chapter.

REFERENCES

1. Kaufman, Friedrich, Gardner: Benign Diseases of the Vagina and Vulva, 3rd ed., Chicago, Year-Book, 1989.
2. Gompel, Silverberg: Pathology in Gynecology and Obstetrics, 4th ed. Philadelphia, JB Lippincott, 1994, p 15.
3. Deppisch LM: Cysts of the vagina. Obstet Gynecol 45:632–637, 1975.
4. Woodworth H, et al: Papillary hidradenoma of the vulva. A clinical pathologic study of 69 cases. Am J Obstet Gynecol 110:501–508, 1971.
5. Studdiford WE: Vaginal lesions of adenomatous origin. Am J Obstet Gynecol 73:641, 1947.
6. Abd-Rabbo MS et al. Aspiration and tetracycline sclerotherapy: A novel method for management of vaginal and vulvar Gartner cysts. Int J Gynaecol Obstet 35(3):235–237, 1991.
7. Herbst AL: Vaginal and cervical abnormalities after exposure to stilbestrol in utero. Obstet Gynecol 40:287–298, 1972.
8. Lee YH, Rankin JS, Alpert S, et al: Microbiological investigation of Bartholin's gland abscesses and cysts. Am J Obstet Gynecol 129:150, 1977.
9. Cheetham DR: Bartholin's cyst: Marsupialization or aspiration. Am J Obstet Gynecol 152:567–570, 1985.
10. Davis GD: Management of Bartholin duct cysts with the carbon dioxide laser. Obstet Gynecol 65:279, 1985.
11. Raz S: Atlas of Transvaginal Surgery. Philadelphia, WB Saunders, 1992.

CHAPTER 57

Continent Urinary Diversion

Stephen D. Mark, M.B., F.R.A.C.S.
George D. Webster, M.B., F.R.C.S.

Orthotopic bladder replacement is the optimal urinary "diversion" for men; however, for a variety of reasons it has not yet gained widespread acceptance for use in women. The most important reason cited is the current philosophy that in women with bladder cancer undergoing cystectomy, urethrectomy and removal of a portion of the anterior vaginal wall are required to optimize the outcome. Obviously, this removes the continence mechanism, and, although the diversion reservoir can be anastomosed to the native urethral meatal site and an artificial sphincter can be placed around the bowel for continence, such techniques are extremely complex and are prone to complications. Hence, optimal urinary diversion in women is currently thought to be construction of a continent catheterizable urinary reservoir with a "dry" abdominal wall stoma.

The ideal urinary diversion should mimic bladder function as closely as possible. It should provide a low-pressure, capacious reservoir, achieve continence, and allow complete emptying by either voluntary expulsion or easy catheterization. In addition, it should protect the upper tracts from reflux or obstruction and avoid metabolic disturbance and subsequent malignant change. It is doubtful whether any current continent diversion can consistently achieve these goals; however, compared with the standard ileal conduit diversion, a continent diversion promotes an improved quality of life and body image, fostering psychological well-being by more closely mirroring normal bladder function. It is also probable that these goals of continent urinary diversion can be achieved with low morbidity in properly selected patients.

Patient Selection

Urinary diversion of any type is becoming less commonly performed as the indications shrink primarily to those patients undergoing extirpative procedures for pelvic malignancy. In the past, intractable voiding symptoms, incontinence, and upper tract deterioration due to structurally or functionally altered bladders of congenital or neurologic etiology were managed by diversion. However, advances in urodynamics have led to a better understanding of bladder and outlet dysfunction, and the development of successful reconstructive techniques, the acceptance of clean intermittent catheterization, and the development of the artificial urinary sphincter have led to a decline in urinary diversion.[1] Many patients who had previously undergone diversion to an appliance-dependent urostomy and who cannot be returned to use of their native bladder, because of either prior cystectomy or other structural difficulties, often elect to undergo conversion to a catheterizable stoma because of its superior personal and social acceptance. Patient selection criteria may be divided into patient factors, renal factors, bowel factors, and bladder (disease-specific) factors (Table 57–1).

PATIENT FACTORS

In this modern surgical era it is our belief that any patient who is a candidate for "surgery" that requires urinary diversion is a candidate for a continent diversion, provided that certain prerequisites are observed. Age alone does not constitute a contraindication to such procedures; however, cognitive ability is required to understand the complexities of caring for the bladder replacement and its attendant risks and lifestyle changes. Patients should be sufficiently dexterous to be able to perform clean intermittent catheterization of the abdominal stoma or should have family support to assist with this. The presence of a progressive neurologic disorder involving the upper extremities is a contraindication to the creation of a continent urinary diversion because the patient who

TABLE 57–1
**Relative Indications and
Contraindications for Continent
Urinary Diversion**

Patient Factors
Life expectancy ≥1 year
Adequate social support
Intelligence
Manual dexterity
Absence of progressive neurologic disease
Renal Factors
Creatinine clearance ≥25 ml/second
Bowel Factors
Previously normal bowel function
Adequate bowel availability
Mobile mesentry
Absence of bowel pathology
Bladder (Disease-Specific) Factors
Organ-confined malignancy

is unable to catheterize herself is placed in a more dependent position than would be the case if a non-continent urinary diversion were performed. A life expectancy of at least 1 year should be presumed before undertaking a continent urinary diversion.

RENAL FACTORS

Continent urinary reservoirs have the potential for significant resorption and secretion of fluid and electrolytes because the reservoir allows increased contact time with urine compared with the standard ileal conduit. The metabolic changes most often seen are hyperchloremic metabolic acidosis due primarily to resorption of urinary acid compounds and some secretion of bicarbonates.[2] It is therefore important that patients have a satisfactory reserve of renal function to compensate for these changes; as a general rule, a creatinine clearance of more than 25 ml/minute is required for patients being considered for a continent urinary diversion.

BOWEL FACTORS

All continent urinary diversion procedures necessitate resection of a considerable length of bowel. Technical factors such as nonavailability of the desired segment due to prior bowel resection, extensive intestinal adhesions, or bowel pathology such as ulcerative colitis or Crohn's colitis may make fashioning of a continent reservoir impossible. A short, fat, or diseased mesentery may limit bowel mobilization and remodeling, precluding formation of a continent urinary diversion. Preoperative radiologic studies of the bowel are recommended when symptoms suggest bowel dysfunction.

It is important to recognize that resection of a significant length of intestine may also alter bowel habit. In our experience, short-term bowel dysfunc-

tion may occur in a majority of patients; however, this has been troublesome only in neurologically impaired patients in whom anal sphincter dysfunction may lead to fecal incontinence if stool consistency becomes too soft.[3] We have also found that resection of the ileocecal valve may lead to significant bowel dysfunction involving short transit times in this patient population, and therefore we prefer to perform a continent diversion using ileum alone.

Intestinal malabsorption and prior abdominal or pelvic radiation therapy may contraindicate continent urinary diversion, particularly if the radiation dose was high or if prior surgery caused bowel fixation in the radiation field.

BLADDER (DISEASE-SPECIFIC) FACTORS

Metastatic carcinoma is a relative contraindication to the formation of a continent urinary diversion. Life expectancy, however, is an important consideration, and learning new techniques such as intermittent catheterization can become time consuming and laborious to someone who quickly develops terminal disease. It adds one more form of dependency to an already dependent and difficult limited life style. We prefer, therefore, to perform continent diversions only in patients who have organ-confined malignant disease rather than those with metastasis.

Bowel Segment Selection and Reconfiguration

The propulsion of intestinal contents in the small and large intestines occurs by peristalsis and mass contraction, respectively, the main stimulus for that activity being distention. Detubularization of the bowel and remodeling of the intestine used for reservoir construction should aim to create a spheroidal shape that will reduce the amplitude of contractions. The creation of a spheroidal reservoir has a number of advantages including achievement of the maximum capacity for any given intestinal surface. An antimesenteric intestinal incision and spherical reconfiguration of the segment also result in uncoordinated and asynchronous bowel contractions, effectively nullifying and dissipating the effects of peristalsis. According to Laplace's law, the larger the radius of a sphere the lower the pressures within, and therefore an effort should be made to achieve this. A spheroidal reservoir with a capacity of 500 ml can be created from 40 cm of ileum.[4] Previous studies have shown that colonic reservoirs develop higher pressures than those made solely from ileum.[5] The evidence suggests that a spherically reconfigured detubularized ileal segment provides the most docile and capacious system.

Continence Mechanisms

Construction of the continence mechanism presents the most variable and challenging area in the construction of a continent urinary reservoir (Table 57–2). The system must be durable, easy to catheterize, and continent. A number of alternative systems have been used including an intussuscepted ileal nipple, a tapered and reinforced ileocecal valve, a hydraulic valve, the flap value (Mitrofanoff principle), and use of an artificial urinary sphincter. Each system has its proponents and critics, and currently the ideal technique has yet to be identified.

NIPPLE VALVES

The stapled intussuscepted ileal nipple valve, as described by Kock and modified by Skinner, has proved to be quite successful for continence and is based on the principle of sphincteric compression.[6, 7] Mean resting intussuscepted ileocecal valve pressures in empty and filled pouch states were 39 cm H_2O (range, 32 to 50) and 57 cm H_2O (range, 28 to 120), respectively, exceeding reservoir pressures at all times and providing excellent continence.[8] Over the years Skinner has devised numerous modifications to improve reliability, including stapling of the nipple valve to the sidewall of the pouch, replacing the Marlex collar with a polyglycolic acid (PGA)-mesh around the base of the nipple, and stripping the mesentery from the portion of ileum (about 8 cm) to be intussuscepted. Exposed metal staples have, however, shown a predisposition to stone formation in the reservoir, although modifications to the Ta 55 staple cartridge by removal of the distal six staples have reduced this problem.

Other problems associated with this technique include nipple prolapse and desusception, nipple fistula, a tendency to parastomal hernia formation, nipple splitting at the staple line, and catheterization difficulties due to irregularities or distortions of the efferent limb just outside the nipple.

In experienced hands this technique offers extremely good results; however, it is not the popular choice of most urologists performing continent diversions.

TABLE 57–2
Classification of Continent Urinary Diversion by Site of Continence Mechanism

Anal sphincter
Native urethral sphincter
Catheterizable abdominal stoma
Artificial bladder and sphincter

PLICATED AND TAPERED TERMINAL ILEUM WITH REINFORCED ILEOCECAL VALVE

Rowland and coworkers have popularized the technique of suture plication of the terminal ileum, and, when associated with a competent ileocecal valve, this method has provided an effective continence mechanism for an ileocecal reservoir.[10] This technique has been further developed by a number of workers. Lockhart suture reinforced the ileocecal valve, and the Bejani staple reduced the terminal ileum together with suture reinforcement of the valve.[11, 12] This latter technique provides reliable continence with rare catheterization difficulties and remains the most widely used technique.

FLAP VALVES

The flap valve (Mitrofanoff principle) utilizes a tube with a narrow lumen, such as an appendix or ureter, implanted in a submucosal tunnel in the reservoir wall.[13] Continence is good with this technique, and it may be adapted to a variety of reservoir types. Studies have shown that resting pressures generated in a Mitrofanoff conduit are two to three times higher than the highest pressure generated within the reservoir.[14] Stomal stenosis has, however, been frequent, although this should be overcome by regular catheterization. The major drawback to this technique is the fact that the small catheter of the efferent limb requires the use of a small catheter that provides slow drainage and may be prone to mucus plugging.

Patient Preparation and Counseling

As intimated earlier, careful patient selection is paramount in the success of these operations, and thorough preoperative counseling ensures that the patient has realistic expectations of the outcome and is not surprised by any untoward event. A simple diagram explaining the difference between an ileal conduit and a continent diversion is useful in preoperative counseling. The patient should be informed about the more common early and late complications of the operation and the ways in which her lifestyle will change, especially the need for regular intermittent catheterization, which uncommonly can be as often as every 3 to 4 hours. In this endeavor we are assisted by a nurse clinician who functions as an enterostomal therapist and is often able to present an important alternative perspective to the patient that differs from that of the surgeon. Most patients find it extremely helpful to speak with a patient who has undergone a similar procedure. It has been our experience that a number of patients will decline a continent diversion in lieu of a simple urinary ileostomy based on honest reporting to them of the duration of surgery and hospitalization and the incidence of early and late complications. Having a high drop-out rate is certainly better than dealing with an unhappy and poorly informed patient who has encountered problems!

Preoperative studies will to some degree be determined by the cause of the disease leading to the continent urinary diversion. Assessment of renal function should include a serum creatinine level and imaging of the upper urinary tracts, preferably by urography. If abnormalities are found, creatinine clearance should be measured by a diethylenetriomene penta-acetic acid (DPTA) renogram. A bowel contrast study should be performed in patients in whom bowel pathology is suspected or in whom prior intestinal surgery may influence one's choice of bowel segment to be used.

Preoperatively, the enterostomal therapist should mark the patient for an appropriate stoma site for an appliance-dependent ostomy if intraoperative findings dictate this course. The continent stoma, on the other hand, has few rigid siting criteria, although bringing it through the rectus muscle may reduce the incidence of parastomal hernia. Most patients prefer an unobtrusive site low on the abdominal wall, even in a skin crease, to improve concealability.

Prior to surgery the intestines are prepared by lavage or mechanical preparation and antibiotics according to the surgeon's preference. We prefer to begin a diet consisting solely of clear fluids by mouth 2 days prior to surgery; GoLYTELY, a polyethylene glycol electrolyte gastrointestinal lavage solution, is used the day before surgery. For adults, a volume of up to 4000 ml may be required to lavage the bowel until the rectal efflux is clear. Dehydration should be avoided by starting intravenous fluids the day before surgery. Patients with poor nutrition may benefit from a period of preoperative hyperalimentation.

Surgical Techniques

CONTINENT RIGHT COLON RESERVOIR (WITH STAPLE-TAPERED TERMINAL ILEUM AND SUTURE-REINFORCED ILEOCECAL VALVE CONTINENCE MECHANISM)

All currently used right colon reservoirs are based on the original work by Gilchrist and colleagues.[15] However, as noted earlier, many workers have modified the procedure, particularly during this decade, and it has evolved into a reliable diversion that is simple to perform and is well within the capability of most urologists. The most important changes have been detubularization of the bowel segment to improve its pressure characteristics and functional capacity, reinforcement of the ileocecal valve to improve continence, and stapled tapering of the terminal ileum to facilitate trouble-free intermittent catheterization.

If cystectomy is to be performed simultaneously, it should be completed prior to commencing the continent diversion. The abdomen is entered through a midline incision extending from above the umbilicus to the symphysis pubis. The left ureter is mobilized and transferred beneath the sigmoid mesocolon to approximate the right. The ends of the ureters may be obstructed with a hemoclip to allow them to dilate while pouch construction proceeds, thus facilitating the anastomosis to the reservoir. Distal ureteral margins should be free of any tumor, and therefore frozen section biopsies should be routinely performed prior to anastomosis in patients with bladder cancer.

In patients undergoing conversion from a previous conduit diversion, the stoma should be circumscribed and the conduit freed from the abdominal wall and surrounding adhesions. If appropriate, the base of the conduit with its implanted ureters and mesentery intact may be saved for later anastomosis as an afferent limb of the reservoir.[16]

The segment of colon and ileum to be used is supplied by the ileocolic and right colon vessels and includes the terminal 10 cm of ileum and the colon to between the right colic and middle colic vessels (Fig. 57–1). This includes the hepatic flexure, which must be mobilized by incision of the hepatocolic and duodenocolic attachments. The right colon is mobilized from its retroperitoneal attachment by incision of the peritoneum alongside the right colon along the

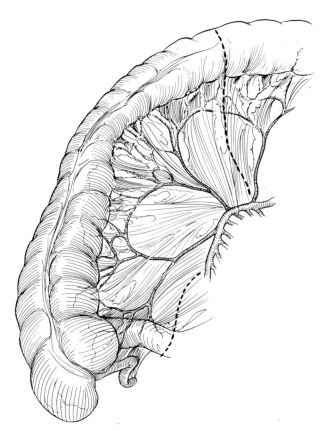

Figure 57–1 A length of right colon based on the ileocolic and right colic vessels is raised. The ileal tail should be approximately 10 cm in length.

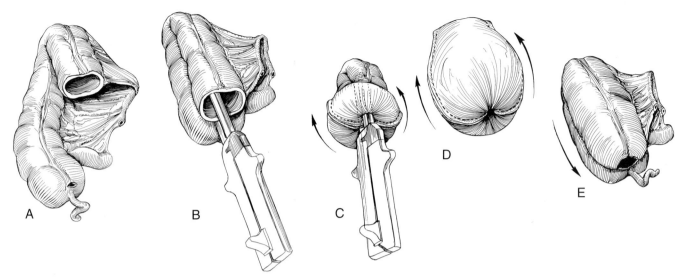

Figure 57-2 *A,* The isolated segment is folded on itself. *B–D,* Using an absorbable stapler, a side-to-side anastomosis is accomplished. *E,* Completed reservoir.

line of Toldt. The small bowel mesentery is incised down the avascular watershed between the ileocolic and superior mesenteric (ileal) blood supplies. Ileocolic reanastomosis after isolation of the bowel segment may be performed by sutures or staples.

The isolated ileocecal segment is irrigated with antibiotic solution, and the large bowel is detubularized by an incision made along a tenia. Construction of the reservoir is performed by folding the opened colon on itself (transverse colon to cecum), usually along the anterior tenia, and completing two anastomotic closures in two layers of running interlocking 3–0 PGA suture (Fig. 57–2). An alternative method is to perform the reservoir construction using absorbable gastrointestinal anastomosis (GIA) staples,

which both opens and anastomoses the bowel and certainly saves considerable time (Fig. 57–3).[17]

Attention is then turned to tapering the terminal ileum and plicating the ileocecal valve. A 12 Fr red rubber catheter is placed along the ileum through the ileocecal valve into the opened pouch and snugged against the mesenteric border of the terminal ileum, aided by Babcock clamps (Fig. 57–4 to Fig. 57–7). Using a GIA stapling device, tapering is accomplished using the 12 Fr catheter as a stent, so that the lumen of the terminal ileum is reduced to approximately its size. Although the stent used is 12 Fr, the system will subsequently be catheterized by an 18 Fr straight catheter. Stapling is stopped immediately short of the ileocecal junction, and, depending on the

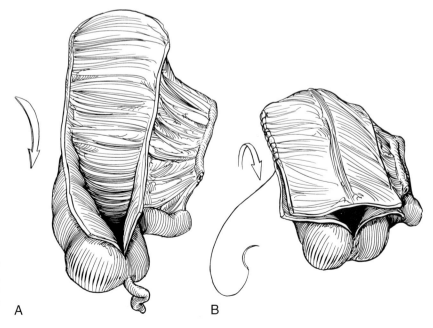

Figure 57-3 The alternative to a stapled anastomosis is a sutured reservoir construction. *A,* The colon is opened along its anterior tinea. *B,* The reservoir is constructed with a two-layer, continuous absorbable suture closure.

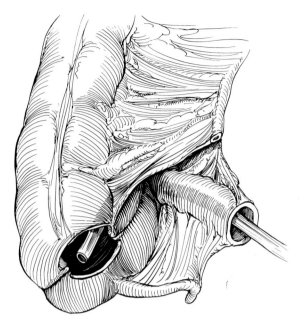

Figure 57-4 A 12 Fr stenting catheter is passed along the afferent ileal limb and through the ileocecal valve.

length of the ileum, one or two staple cartridges are used. The separated ileum is removed with a further run of GIA staples placed obliquely along the ileocecal valve but not including the cecal wall. Lembert plicating sutures of 3–0 silk are then used to invert this last staple line, effectively augmenting and reinforcing the natural ileocecal valve. A further two or three circumferential pursestring serosal sutures of 2–0 silk may be placed around the terminal ileum in the manner described by Begani and Politano.[11] The

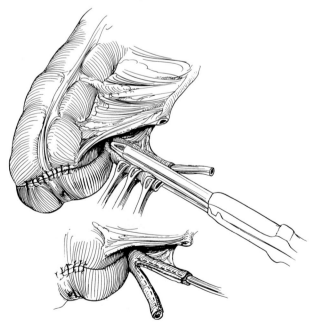

Figure 57-5 With the stent snugged against the mesenteric border of the afferent ileal limb and using a GIA staple-device with metal staples, the ileum is staple-reduced to a smaller size.

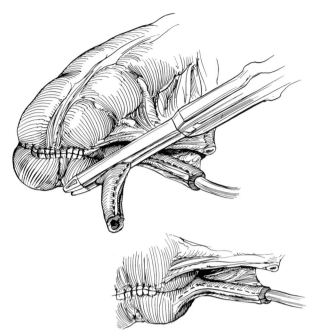

Figure 57-6 The redundant ileum is excised with a GIA stapler close to the ileocecal valve.

first suture is close to the tapered ileocecal junction, and subsequent sutures are 5 mm apart. The 12 Fr stenting catheter is replaced with an 18 Fr catheter prior to placing these sutures, which are snugged down loosely on the shaft of the catheter. These nonabsorbable sutures must pick up only serosa because intraluminal silk would predispose to stone formation. It must be noted that this step is not performed by many who construct right colon reservoirs; however, it does have the potential to improve continence. Once the efferent limb has been completed, trial catheterization with an 18 Fr catheter should be easy. If the catheter does not pass smoothly, loosening of the circumferential purse-string sutures in the most terminal ileum is usually required.

Prior to completing closure of the remaining open end of the reservoir, the ureteral anastomosis to the reservoir is completed. We prefer to use nonrefluxing tunneled reimplants after the fashion of the Leadbetter-Nesbit technique, performed from outside the reservoir (Fig. 57–8); however, many authors perform a simple, potentially refluxing end-to-side anastomosis. Anastomoses are performed with 4–0 PGA suture and are stented with 8 Fr stents fixed to the ureter with a 5–0 CCG suture that transfixes the ureter and stent. Stents either are brought through the reservoir and anterior abdominal wall to external drainage or are fixed to the tip of the reservoir drainage catheter, internalizing urine drainage postoperatively. The remaining opening in the reservoir is sutured closed, and the pouch is tested for watertightness and continence.

Attention is now directed to construction of the stoma. The site is selected so that the tapered efferent ileal limb has a perpendicular course from the intra-abdominal reservoir through the abdominal

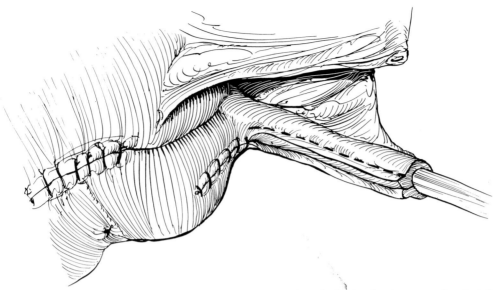

Figure 57-7 Using interrupted 3–0 silk sutures, the staple line is imbricated, and additional sutures are placed at the ileocecal valve to reinforce the valve.

wall to the stoma site. A small button of skin is excised, a narrowed tract is incised in the abdominal wall, and the efferent nipple is brought through to the skin. The pouch is snugged against the anterior abdominal wall, and any excess tapered ileum is excised above the skin (Fig. 57–9); the open end is sutured flush to the skin with interrupted 4–0 PGA suture. The pouch is fixed to the peritoneal surface of the anterior abdominal wall at the stoma site, and a 20 Fr suprapubic tube is inserted through a separate abdominal entry. Two Jackson-Pratt drains are placed in the vicinity of the pouch and ureteral anastomosis, and a 12 Fr red rubber catheter is left in the stoma for postoperative stenting. This catheter is

tied off near the stoma. The abdomen is then closed in the customary fashion.

A 24-hour period of postoperative intensive care nursing is advised. Broad-spectrum antibiotics are continued for 3 postoperative days, and nasogastric or gastrostomy tube drainage is continued for 4 to 7 postoperative days until intestinal motility returns and graduated oral feeding is commenced. Catheter and stent irrigation is performed at least every 4 hours depending on the catheter drainage technique used. The suction drains are removed sequentially, the first on postoperative day 7 or 8, the second on postoperative day 9 or 10. The patient is usually discharged between days 9 and 11 with the reservoir

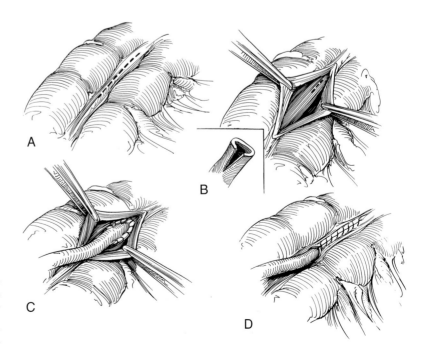

Figure 57-8 If nonrefluxing ureteral anastomoses are used they are preferably attached to a tinea, but not necessarily. *A,* Incision in tinea. *B,* Small hiatus made in underlying reservoir mucosa. *C,* Spatulated ureteral anastomosis to mucosal hiatus. *D,* Tineal muscle closed over ureter to create tunnel.

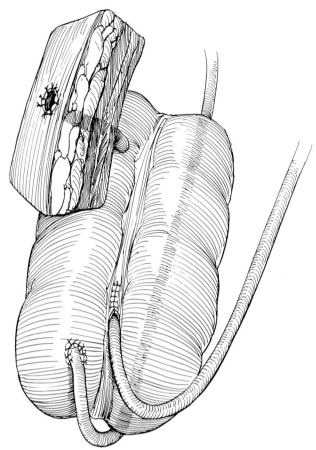

Figure 57–9 The staple-reduced ileal limb is brought through the abdominal wall and matured to the skin. The reservoir is snugged against the anterior abdominal wall at this location with no redundancy.

those procedure-specific complications peculiar to urinary diversion (Table 57–3). General complications such as pneumonia, deep venous thrombosis, and wound infection may be minimized by preoperative prophylactic management. Procedure-specific complications include prolonged gastrointestinal motility disturbances in up to 20% of patients, ileal anastomotic leaks requiring reoperation in 0.5%, intra-abdominal abscess in 1.5%, and temporary obstruction of the upper tracts requiring percutaneous stents in 7%.[18]

LATE COMPLICATIONS

Ureteral Anastomotic Obstruction and Reflux

Anastomotic stricture occurs with an incidence of approximately 7% in patients with a right colon reservoir construction[12]; patients with tunneled, nonrefluxing anastomoses are more likely to suffer this complication than those with simple end-to-side anastomoses. Early strictures may be successfully managed by endoscopic techniques; however, late strictures usually require open repair.

At present, it is still debated whether an antireflux technique is required in these diversion techniques; however, we believe that restoration of functional anatomy as close to the native system is warranted, and therefore we pursue an antireflux system in all patients other than those with a poor prognosis or with large dilated ureters.

drained by its percutaneous catheter and with the stomal stent in place.

Three weeks after surgery the patient returns for reservoir activation. Under parenteral antibiotic cover a pouchogram and ureteral stentograms are performed to ensure anastomotic healing. If this is confirmed, the stomal stent is removed; the reservoir Malecot catheter is plugged, and the patient is taught self-catheterization of the stoma using a 16 or 18 Fr catheter. If successful, the Malecot catheter is removed, and the patient commences self-catheterization, initially at 2-hour intervals, which are increased by 1 hour a week until a satisfactory reservoir volume is attained. An intravenous pyelogram as well as serum chemistries are performed at 3 months, and an annual ultrasound examination is subsequently performed if these are normal.

Potential Complications

EARLY COMPLICATIONS

Early complications encompass the general complications expected after major abdominal surgery and

TABLE 57–3
Potential Complications of Continent Urinary Diversion

Early
   General
   Procedure-specific
     Prolonged ileus
     Bowel anastomotic leak
     Reservoir leak
     Temporary upper tract obstruction
Late
   Procedure-specific
     Ureteral
       Stenosis
       Reflux
     Reservoir
       High pressure
       Calculi
       Mucus obstruction
       Perforation
     Outlet
       Incontinence
       Catheterization difficulties
       Fistulas
       Parastomal hernias
   Infection
   Gastrointestinal disturbances
   Metabolic disturbances
   Secondary malignancy

Reservoir Complications

Renal function may deteriorate as a result of ureteral obstruction or reflux of infected urine and recurrent pyelonephritis. Identification of the cause is achieved with pouchogram and upper tract studies.

HIGH PRESSURE High pressure may result from reservoir hypercontractility perhaps due to inadequate bowel detubularization and reconfiguration from a small capacity reservoir, or from reduced reservoir compliance. This uncommonly leads to incontinence provided that the efferent continence mechanism is competent and catheterization fully empties the reservoir. If urodynamic studies suggest reservoir hyperactivity, anticholinergic medications or diphenoxylate hydrochloride (Lomotil) may be given either orally or into the neobladder with moderate success.[19] Reservoir augmentation using an ileal patch may be tried in exceptional cases.

RESERVOIR CALCULI Asymptomatic calculi may form around exposed staples or may result from urine stasis and mucus inspissated in the reservoir. These are usually removed endoscopically under local anesthesia, but if they are large or inaccessible they may require open removal. Pouch access for endoscopic management may be difficult in the Mitrofanoff system owing to the small size of the efferent limb.

RESERVOIR PERFORATION Rupture of a continent urinary diversion has not yet been reported; however, rupture of the augmented bladder is an uncommon but well-recognized and dangerous complication. Signs may be nonspecific, especially in the neurologically impaired patient, and require a high index of suspicion. Diagnosis may be aided by abdominal ultrasound and computed tomography, cystography and pouchography, and paracentesis with creatinine estimation of free peritoneal fluid. Management is achieved by immediate laparotomy for drainage and repair.

MUCUS FORMATION Mucus accumulation within the reservoir occurs in all patients but is rarely troublesome; however, rarely it may predispose to infection, stone formation, and poor emptying. It is thought to decrease with time. Pouch tamponade by mucus plug has been described as an early complication in patients with ileoneobladders,[20] and one case of rupture of an ileoneobladder due to mucus plug obstruction has been reported.[21] Not all patients with significant mucus production require treatment, periodic irrigation sufficing in most; however, the use of N-acetylcysteine or ranitidine has been reported to be effective in reducing the problem.

Reservoir Outlet Malfunction

Outlet malfunction is the most common long-term complication of continent urinary diversion leading to incontinence, catheterization difficulties, or peristomal hernia.

In patients with a Kock pouch the incidence of efferent nipple complications in the first 250 patients reported by Skinner was approximately 40%; however, this figure was reduced to approximately 7 to 10% by a variety of technical modifications. A similar low rate is reported for continent diversions using the modified ileocecal valve for continence.[22] In these procedures, hand-sewn plications have been reported to lead to luminal irregularities and small diverticula in the catheterizable limb, resulting in catheterization difficulties. This problem occurs less frequently with the staple tapered system described earlier. It is important that the efferent catheterizable limb from the reservoir be made as short as possible to avoid redundancy, which will also lead to catheterization problems. Stomal and continence mechanism problems frequently require reoperation. These procedures may be long and tedious and sometimes require total reconstruction of the continence mechanism using a new bowel segment.

Infection

All catheterized continent urinary reservoirs are colonized with bacteria, leading to pyuria, bacteriuria, and positive urine cultures. However, if the reservoir is emptied completely at regular intervals, and if reflux (or ureteral obstruction) is absent, symptomatic pouchitis or pyelonephritis rarely occurs.

Gastrointestinal Disturbance

There is a significant early incidence of bowel dysfunction with frequent loose bowel movements and a short transit time; however, this usually resolves within 3 months of continent urinary diversion construction. In a few patients, especially those with neurogenic bowel dysfunction in whom the ileocecal valve was removed, loose bowel movements may be persistent and troublesome. Malabsorption is uncommon, but vitamin B_{12} deficiency has been reported in a small number of patients.[23] It is recommended that vitamin B_{12} levels be determined on an annual basis in these patients; replacement may be required in approximately one-third. Cholestyramine, a substance that binds bile acids, may be useful in patients with frequent loose bowel movements, as may bulking agents and Lomotil. A higher incidence of cholelithiasis has been reported in these patients, probably due to impaired intrahepatic circulation and decreased ileal absorption of bile salts.[24]

Metabolic Disturbance

Hyperchloremic metabolic acidosis is the common metabolic abnormality seen; however, it is rarely clinically significant and rarely requires therapy. Patients with renal impairment have a much higher risk of development of electrolyte and metabolic disturbances, and the pathophysiology and complications associated with these conditions are described in more detail elsewhere.[2]

Secondary Malignancy

Filmer and Spencer recently reviewed several series with long-term follow-up and found carcinoma at or near the ureterocolic anastomosis in 5 to 13% of patients undergoing ureterosigmoidostomy who were followed for 10 or more years.[25] It is postulated that this carcinoma is due to the formation of carcinogenic nitrozo compounds resulting from enteric bacteria acting on normally occurring nitrates in the urine. Tumors have also been reported infrequently in bladders augmented with intestinal segments. Follow-up of continent urinary reservoirs is short; however, currently there have been no reports of tumor formation, but long-term vigilance is required.

Conclusion

Although the appliance-dependent urinary ileostomy is still considered the gold standard in urinary diversion, it must be recognized that continent urinary reservoirs have evolved to a point of reliability and simplicity, demanding that they be offered as an alternative in the majority of patients. They offer a significantly better quality of life, self-image, and sexual attractiveness and have complication rates comparable to those of the appliance-dependent urostomy. Undoubtedly, the field will continue to evolve; however, at the present time the right colon reservoir using a reinforced ileocecal valve continence mechanism offers the best results when performed by the average urologist.

REFERENCES

1. Webster GD: Achieving the goals of bladder reconstruction by enterocystoplasty. Prob Urol 1(2):337–362, 1987.
2. Koch MD, McDougal WS, Reddy PK, Lange PH: Metabolic alterations following continent urinary diversion through colonic segments. J Urol 145:270, 1991.
3. Mark SD, MacDiarmid SA, Webster GD: Factors associated with bowel dysfunction following cystoplasty: Analysis of 253 patients. J Urol 149:370A, 1993.
4. Studer UE, Gerber E, Springer J, Zing EJ: Bladder reconstruction with bowel after radical cystectomy. World J Urol 10:11–19, 1992.
5. Goldwasser B, Barrett DM, Webster GD, Kramer SA: Cystometric properties of ileum and right colon after bladder aug-

mentation, substitution, or replacement. J Urol 138:1007, 1987.
6. Kock NG, Norland L, Philipson BM, et al: The continent ileal reservoir (Kock pouch) for urinary diversion. World J Urol 3:146, 1985.
7. Skinner DG, Lieskovsky G, Boyd SD: Continuing experience with the continent ileal reservoir (Kock pouch) as an alternative to cutaneous urinary diversion: An update after 250 cases. J Urol 137:1140, 1987.
8. Lowe BA, Woodside JR: Urodynamic evaluation of patients with continent urinary diversion using cecal reservoir and intussuscepted ileocecal valve. Urology 35:544, 1990.
9. Boyd SD, Skinner DG, Lieskovsky G: Kock pouch: Update of USC technique and result. In King, LR, Stone AR, Webster GD (Eds): Bladder Reconstruction and Continent Urinary Diversion. Chicago, Mosby-Year Book, 1992, pp 272–282.
10. Rowland RG, Mitchell ME, Bihrie R, et al: Indiana continent urinary reservoir. J Urol 137:1136–1139, 1987.
11. Bejani DE, Politano VA: Stapled and nonstapled distal ileum for construction of continent colonic urinary reservoir. J Urol 140:491, 1988.
12. Lockhart JL, Pow-Sang J, Persky L, et al: A continent colonic urinary reservoir: The Florida Pouch. J Urol 144:864–867, 1990.
13. Mitrofanoff P: Cystostomi continente trans-appendiculaire dans le traitement des vessies neurologiques. Chir Pediatr 21:297–305, 1980.
14. Woodhouse CRJ: The Mitrofanoff technique for a continent stoma. In King LR, Stone AR, Webster GD (eds): Bladder Reconstruction and Continent Urinary Diversion. Chicago, Mosby-Year-Book, 1992, pp 299–307.
15. Gilchrist RK, Merricks JW, Hamlin HH, Reger IT: Construction of substitute bladder and urethra. Surg Gynecol Obstet 97:52–76, 1950.
16. Pow-Sang JM, Helal M, Figueroa TE, et al: Conversion from external appliance wearing or internal urinary diversion to a continent urinary reservoir (Florida pouch I and II): Surgical technique, indications and complications. J Urol 147:356–360, 1992.
17. Kirsch AJ, Hensle TW, Olsson CA: Rapid construction of right colon pouch: Initial clinical experience. Urology 43:228–231, 1994.
18. Donohue JP, Bihrle R, Hautmann RE, Skinner DG: After continent diversion, ensuring function and satisfaction. Sympos Contemp Urol 41:49, 1993.
19. Anderson KE, Headlund H, Mansson W: Pharmacologic treatment of bladder hyperactivity after augmentation and substitution enterocystoplasty. Scand J Urol Nephrol (Suppl) 142:42–46, 1992.
20. Hautmann RE, Windroth UK: Ileoneobladder. In Rowland RG, (ed): Problems in Urology. Philadelphia, JB Lippincott, 1991, pp 336–346.
21. Haupt G, Pannek J, Knopf HJ, et al: Rupture of an ileal neobladder due to urethral obstruction by mucous plug. J Urol 144:740–741, 1990.
22. Skinner DG: Intussuscepted ileal nipple valve—development and present status. Scand J Urol Nephrol (Suppl) 142:63–65, 1992.
23. Steiner MS, Morton RA, Marshall FF: Vitamin B12 deficiency in patients with ileocolic neobladders. J Urol 149:255–257, 1993.
24. Hensley TW, Ring KS: Total bladder replacement in children. In King LR, Stone AR, Webster GD (eds): Bladder Reconstruction and Continent Urinary Diversion. Chicago, Mosby-Year Book, 1992, pp 347–356.
25. Filmer RB, Spencer JR: Malignancies in bladder augmentation and intestinal conduits. J Urol 143:671–678, 1990.

Neurosurgical Intervention for Female Lower Urinary Tract Dysfunction

CHAPTER 58

Clinical Value of Neurostimulation: A Urologic Viewpoint

Richard A. Schmidt, M.D.

Physiologic Principles

The neural regulation of the pelvic organs is unique in the nervous system. The pelvis is the only part of our anatomy wherein diverse functions are intimately linked by the origins of the nerves controlling them. There is no visceral or somatic parallel elsewhere in the body. It is the complexity of the reflex coordination involving somatic, parasympathetic, and sympathetic branches of the peripheral nervous system that places the lower urinary tract at high risk for dysfunction.

It should therefore not be surprising that patients with symptomatic voiding dysfunction are often found to have simultaneous dysfunction of the reproductive organs, lower bowel, or both. Although it is easy to appreciate the pathologic causes of micturition dysregulation, it is also quite possible that functionally driven instabilities in pelvic muscles can permanently disturb the central coordination of micturition.[1] Correction of pelvic muscle dysfunction is therefore of primary importance and is a major goal of treatment of symptomatic bladder dysfunction.

The rationale and motivation for the clinical use of electrical stimulation are based on the following observations:

1. Most dysfunctional voiding syndromes are associated with an exaggerated activity within the sacral reflex arcs controlling the bladder. Neural stimulation is intrinsically inhibitory (through gating) to this type of activity. It is therefore associated with a therapeutic benefit.
2. Most voiding syndromes are associated with the loss of efficient pelvic muscle behavior. There is thus a functional disconnection in proper regulation of pelvic muscle behavior by the conscious mind. Neural stimulation helps to restore higher center awareness of the pelvic muscles. Improvements in central coordination of bladder function then follow.
3. Direct stimulation of the motor nerves to the bladder has the ability to restore bladder emptying in the patient with spinal injury.
4. Neural stimulation can promote growth of tissue. It therefore has the potential to allow nerve regeneration.

THE MODULATION PRINCIPLE

There are many reports in the literature documenting the clinical benefits of nerve stimulation. All approaches have a common mechanism of therapeutic benefit, which lies in the intrinsic inhibitory action of electrical stimulation.

This principle of action is true of acupuncture, transcutaneous electrical nerve stimulation (TENS), vaginal or rectal devices, and implantable sacral foramen electrodes. Techniques that contract the pelvic muscles have an additional benefit of educating patients about correct methods of pelvic muscle contraction. Virtually all patients with bladder symptoms have inefficient pelvic floor muscle behavior. Patients cannot be relied on to suddenly reverse long-standing habits. They must be given an understanding of what constitutes proper muscle behavior. Stimulation works best in younger patients with healthy muscles and nerves. It can decrease exaggerated reflex activity by directly reeducating conscious control, by increasing the degree of inhibitory reflex activity within the sacral segments, or both.

Neurostimulation has been shown to have a useful role in managing many voiding disorders regardless of cause. At times, symptoms responding to neurostimulation may seem to be incongruous—for example, incontinence and retention. The answer to this paradox lies in the capacity of neurostimulation to modulate the excitability of reflex activity using electrical stimulation of selected nerve pathways.

The aim of this chapter is to discuss the current role of neuroprosthetics in urology.

Understanding the Pelvic Floor

The pelvic floor is a well-described anatomic entity. Functionally, it is best understood through an appreciation of its neurologic control. The pelvic floor muscles can be subdivided into two functional layers—the levator ani, innervated by S_3–S_4, and the true sphincters, innervated by the pudendal nerve (S_2–S_3). Motion within these two functional layers is quite different. The levator is attached to the pelvic brim and forms a sling around the rectum. Contraction and relaxation of the levator therefore deepens and flattens the buttock crease. This creates a bellows-like motion of the perineum. The sphincters, on the other hand, squeeze the perineum from front to back in a clamplike action. This movement occurs in a different plane than that produced by the levators. Both muscle groups are consciously controlled and are used in the voluntary regulation of the bowel and bladder. They are the key to proper reflex regulation of bowel, bladder, and sexual function. Behavioral dysfunction of either or both of these systems is found in virtually all patients with bladder symptoms. Correction of the behavioral dysfunction provides the best chance for therapeutic success.

INNERVATION OF THE PELVIC MUSCLES

Six sacral nerves are concerned with the innervation of the pelvic tissues—S_2, S_3, and S_4 bilaterally.[2] S_2 is much larger than S_3 and provides a much larger contribution to the sciatic as well as the pudendal nerve. The S_3 nerves predictably supply the more anterior levator muscle groupings by way of pelvic branches that leave the nerve trunk before contributions to the sciatic and pudendal nerves cross the ischial spine. S_3 is unique in that it provides motor control to both skeletal and smooth muscle. There is no significant skin sensation associated with this nerve. Assessment is therefore best made by observing for the bellows-like contraction or by palpating the levator ani on rectal examination during a voluntarily initiated hold. In men, stimulation produces referred sensations to the scrotum, testes, and groin, especially when there is a postfixation of the sacral spinal nuclei.

The S_4 nerves do not contribute to the pudendal innervation of the pelvis or to the sciatic nerves. Pain symptoms related to this nerve refer to the coccygeal region or the posterior anal area.

SACRAL NERVE TEST STIMULATION

Test stimulation of the various sacral nerves is very helpful in understanding the degree of dysfunction in the pelvic musculature (Table 58–1). One can com-

pare stimulation-induced pelvic muscle activity with the patient's voluntary effort to quantify distinct inefficiency in the use of the pelvic muscles. The specific dysfunctional components of pelvic floor activity (e.g., bellows-like S_3 or a viselike clamp effect of S_2) can be identified. A very high percentage of patients with urge-frequency syndromes, prostatism, pelvic pain, incontinence, interstitial cystitis, and even bowel dysfunction lack proper control and use of the pelvic musculature. Conversely, improvement in symptoms is paralleled by improvement in perineal muscle behavior. This observation raises the possibility that long-standing inefficiency in perineal muscle activity could predispose patients to these various conditions. It remains to be proved, however, whether the inefficient behavior so common to these conditions is causative or is simply part of the overall problem.

Percutaneous testing of the sacral nerve roots appears to be benign. Although there are a number of potential risks associated with the technique, no significant difficulties have been encountered. Testing also helps to establish whether neurostimulation has a therapeutic role.

Candidates for Functional Electrical Stimulation

Functional electrical stimulation (FES) has been used extensively in Europe,[3] but experience in the United States has been much more limited. This approach has been used to manage patients with urge frequency disorders, pelvic pain, and urinary incontinence. It is a simple approach that has few if any side effects, and the literature is strongly supportive of its effectiveness.

Many of the patients presenting to a urologic service (or an obstetrics-gynecology or gastrointestinal service) have symptoms linked to inefficient behavior of the pelvic floor muscles. Therapy therefore needs to include structured reeducation of pelvic muscle control. Without this approach, treatment successes are likely to be of limited merit or of short duration. Tension in the pelvic muscles is a strong determinant of physiologic function of the bowel or bladder. Improper postures (e.g., excessive holding), improper voiding techniques (e.g., hovering to void), or improper bowel evacuation methods (e.g., excessive straining at stool) cannot be corrected without conscious, voluntary, efficient identification of the action of these muscles. Most patients, when asked to perform a Kegel movement, either cannot correlate the movement with the levator muscle or do so in a flimsy, erratic, or inconsistent fashion. Stimulation of the pelvic musculature can be a very effective teaching tool. Similarly, biofeedback treatment sessions in themselves can be severely limited or doomed to failure in their therapeutic potential without the use of pelvic stimulation techniques. Many patients simply cannot regain this control without the direct assistance of stimulation. The principle of performing Kegel exercises is sound. However, the benefit results

TABLE 58–1

Key Sensations and Contractile Responses Associated with the S$_2$ to S$_4$ Nerves

S$_2$ Sensation Deficiency	S$_2$ Stimulation Referral	S$_2$ Motor Responses	S$_2$–S$_3$ Associated Referred Pains	S$_3$ Stimulation Referred Sensations	S$_3$ Motor Responses	S$_4$ Stimulation Referred Sensations	S$_4$ Motor Responses
All perineal skin Glans penis and clitoris Lateral toes Arches	Distal foot Glans penis and clitoris Scrotum and labia Soles of feet, all toes, lateral side of foot, calf	Toe flexion—all Anal clamp Urethral squeeze	Scrotum, testes Anal, rectal, vaginal Groin, lower abdomen Flank, upper abdomen Soles of feet	Scrotum, testes Rectum, vagina Distal foot, large toes	Large toe flexion Anal bellows Urethral lift	Rectum	Anal bellows Urethral lift

645

not so much from strengthening the muscle as from improving the coordination of movements based on neurologic integrity.

EVOKED POTENTIAL MONITORING

A useful aid in assessing the effectiveness and efficiency of sacral nerve stimulation is to monitor the motor-evoked activity of the pelvic floor muscles. An electromyographic (EMG) signal from the deep and superficial anal sphincters is obtained using surface or needle electrodes. This provides a sensitive monitor of any contractile activity occurring in the levator (S_3) or superficial anal sphincter (S_2 or pudendal nerve). There is a clear separation in the recording of these responses (Fig. 58–1). Levator responses are restricted to stimulation of the S_3 and S_4 nerves. Superficial anal sphincter responses are restricted to stimulation of the S_2 and pudendal nerves. There are diagnostic and therapeutic advantages to this information. The motor-evoked response (MEP) quantitates the amount of muscle recruited and hence provides information about the integrity of the perineal muscle. This information is helpful in patients who have a suspected nerve injury resulting from spinal surgery or patchy neural deficits associated with neural disease.

On a technical level, it can be very difficult to appreciate the efficiency of pelvic floor stimulation in patients who are obese or are apprehensive and tense. At the time of a permanent implant, the MEP can be used as a guide to duplicate the type of stimulation response known to have produced a beneficial effect on symptoms. After the implantation of a permanent neuroprosthesis, the MEP is helpful in selecting the ideal parameters of stimulation. The threshold response and the point of maximum recruitment can be defined. The peak MEP response (below the pain threshold yet close to the maximum response possible) can be accurately selected. Overstimulation, leading to pain or wasted energy, is therefore avoided, and the life of the battery used in the permanent implant is optimized.

The MEP provides a clear documentation of a response that can be correlated with clinical benefit. It can be used as a marker of nerve integrity and can facilitate a decision about whether the electrode should be revised owing to malfunction or positioning problems.

TRIAL STIMULATION

A test or trial period of stimulation has proved to be an effective way to assess the therapeutic potential

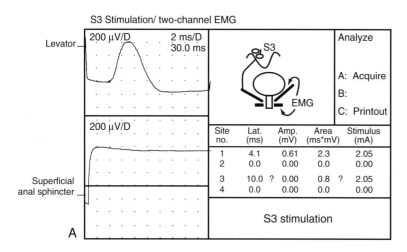

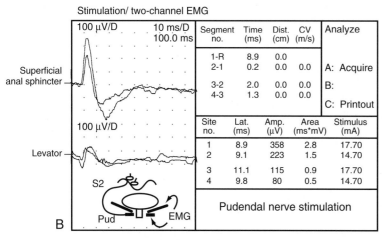

Figure 58-1 Motor-evoked recordings (simultaneous evoked response recording). *A,* Direct S_3 nerve root stimulation. *B,* Stimulation of the pudendal nerve, which arises from the S_2 nerve. Note the differences in the motor-evoked responses between the levator (excellent in *A,* and poor in *B*) and the superficial anal sphincter (absent in *A,* excellent in *B*). The evoked response is useful in quantifying the integrity of the individual S_3 and pudendal neuromuscular units. In *B,* note the effect of amplitude. Frequency = 3 cps. Lat., latency; CV, conduction velocity.

of chronic sacral nerve stimulation.[4] The S_3 nerve is used most frequently, the S_4 infrequently, and the S_2 rarely. The aim is to achieve as comfortable and as full a contraction of the perineal musculature as possible while causing minimal or no foot or toe recruitment. Without good and consistent muscular recruitment, the value of therapeutic stimulation is generally limited (Figs. 58–2 and 58–3).

After screening for a suitable response, a thin wire

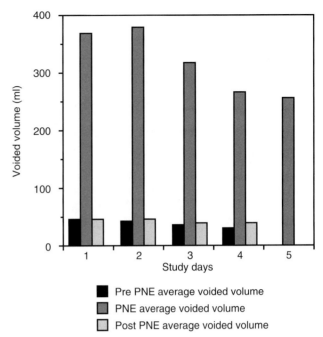

Figure 58-3 Voiding diary from a female patient with hesitant, frequent voiding that was unchanged by a bladder augmentation procedure. Note dramatic change in void volumes during stimulation trial period.

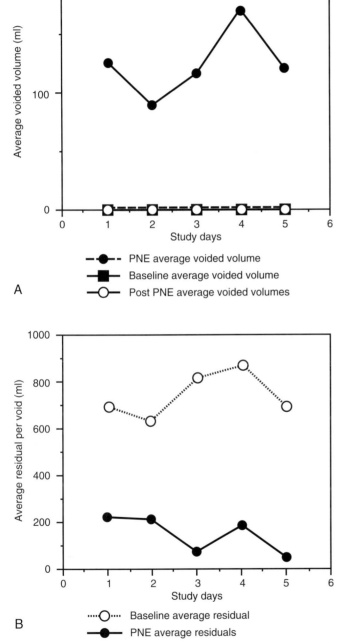

Figure 58-2 Voiding diary of average voided volume *(A)* and residual *(B)* in a female patient with idiopathic urinary retention. Compare voiding behavior before, during, and after a trial of S_3 stimulation. Note dramatic improvement in voided volumes and postvoid residuals during stimulation trial. PNE, percutaneous nerve examination.

electrode (3–0 Flexon pacer wire) is inserted into the foramen through the angiocatheter guide, coiled in place, and secured with Tegaderm. It is then coupled to a pulse generator for 3 to 7 days. Positional adjustments may be necessary after the wire has been placed. If inserted too deeply, it can be pulled back carefully; if too superficial, it should be withdrawn and reinserted. Conclusions about the therapeutic benefit of stimulation cannot be made without a 4- to 7-day period of consistent perineal muscle stimulation. Thus, daily monitoring of both technical and physiologic results are necessary for proper conclusions about the test to be made.

The location and number of temporary wires inserted varies from patient to patient. Variables that determine the number and location of wires include (1) the neurologic and mental status of the patient, (2) the laterality and location of pelvic pain, (3) the severity of voiding dysfunction, (4) patient anatomy and habitus, (5) the time available for the evaluation, (6) available technical support, and, most importantly, (7) the skill of the treating urologist.

If the initial trial fails despite achieving the appropriate muscle response (e.g., if partial control of symptoms was achieved), consideration should be given to testing another nerve or a combination of nerves.

If the trial is successful, there are three options: (1) no further testing, (2) a second trial at another date, or (3) a permanently implanted device. The choice varies with the effectiveness of stimulation to modify symptoms, both during the trial and afterward.

ADVANTAGES OF PELVIC FLOOR MONITORING IN FORAMEN IMPLANT CANDIDATES

1. Quantitates the amount of muscle contraction.
2. Identifies the muscles and region being stimulated.
3. Allows comparisons of response over time.
4. Provides objective documentation of the stimulation result. This helps in the following circumstances: (a) when it is difficult to appreciate pelvic floor movement in response to stimulation visually (in obese or tense individuals), and (b) when it is necessary to compare a percutaneous retest result after implantation with the implanted electrode response in patients in whom a revision seems needed.

Surgical Implantation

Once a decision has been made to implant a neural prosthesis permanently, there is then the choice of placing an electrode either at the foramen level, usually at one of the S_3s nerves, or in the ischial fossa on the pudendal nerve. The actual site chosen varies and depends somewhat on the response obtained in the temporary trial. The S_3 foramen site is attractive in that it is technically much easier than exposure of the pudendal nerve. Patients can be screened for both approaches, starting with the S_3 foramen.

As a rule, one electrode implant is sufficient to produce the desired effect. The modulation principle works quite well in patients with milder degrees of symptomatic voiding dysfunction (pelvic pain, recurrent urinary tract infection, urgency and frequency, dribbling, incontinence, or intermittent retention). However, there are occasional patients (e.g., those with incontinence associated with detrusor instability or those with bilateral pelvic pain) who may benefit from two or more electrode implants. However, from a standpoint of cost effectiveness only, it is less practical. Also, it may not become apparent for several weeks or months after use of the first implant whether a dual implant will be useful. Eventually, as pulse generators become programmed to control more than one electrode site, and as electrode designs are simplified, dual implants will become a more realistic possibility.

The procedure is done as a short-term stay unless there are extenuating circumstances. Patients are requested to take antiseptic (Betadine or pHisoHex) showers twice a day for 3 days prior to the procedure. A preoperative bowel movement with the assistance of a suppository if necessary is recommended. Antibiotic prophylaxis is also recommended.

At the time of the electrode implant, it is important to recheck the position of the temporary wire placement on the radiograph and to cross-check this with the muscle responses obtained in the temporary trial. How much foot and toe activity was there? Was the S_3 response atypical in being more like that of S_2 or

S_4? These observations are extremely useful in sorting out which foramen level should be the site of the implant. The aim of the surgery is to recruit the identical response with the permanent electrode that produced the clinical effect seen during the temporary trial.

General anesthesia is preferred. The operation generally lasts about 3 hours. It is difficult for an awake patient to remain comfortable on the table for this length of time.

The anesthesiologist should be counseled not to use long-acting muscle relaxants to avoid impairing the surgeon's ability to stimulate the muscles to determine the level and site of placement of the electrode.

OPERATIVE TECHNIQUE

The patient is positioned prone on the operating room table over a Wilson frame. This allows flattening of the lumbosacral arch and comfortable flexion of the hips and knees. This position greatly facilitates assessment of perineal muscle responses to stimulation of individual sacral roots.

The skin overlying the sacrum is given a 10-minute Betadine scrub, followed by application of an iodine or Betadine paint. Drapes are applied to allow visual access to the pelvic floor and the feet and to allow adequate room for tunneling the electrode lead toward the posterior superior iliac spine of one side. The buttock crease is prepared and left partially exposed to view. An EMG monitor is set up to record evoked activity from the levator muscles.

The surgeon should work on the patient's right side if he or she is right-handed, and on the patient's left side if he or she is left-handed. This provides a technical advantage for inserting the electrode into a foramen. The side associated with symptoms, or a foramen providing a healthy perineal muscle response similar to that noted in the trial implant is chosen for the permanent implant.

Once the implant location has been selected, an incision is made from the high point of the sacrum cephalad for 4 inches. The fascia on one side is cleared using a peanut sponge or a gauze sponge for blunt dissection. The upper edge of the gluteus muscle, which comes into view at this point, usually marks the level of the S_3 foraman. The paraspinal muscles should then be split 1 cm from the midline with sharp and blunt dissection. The muscle is opened for the length of the wound until the surface of the sacrum is visualized. Scott retractor hooks are used to maintain the exposure.

It is important to preserve the periosteum overlying the sacrum because it is used in fixation of the implanted lead. The implant location is then confirmed using a small current (2 mA) applied to an insulated needle as it is inserted into the various foramens. One should minimize the number and depth of needle insertions to avoid the risk of inducing a neurapraxia before the electrode is properly positioned.

When the level has been identified, an Itrel quadlead is prepared. The fascial cover of the foramen is carefully punctured with the tips of a Gerald forceps. The puncture should be no more than 3 mm deep. A quadlead (i.e., electrode) is pushed bluntly into the foramen. It should then pass smoothly without any springback.

Generally, one likes to see a perineal muscle response in the range of 0.5 to 2 v or mA. This ensures an adequate space between the nerve and the electrode, which minimizes pressure on the nerve and ensures a comfortable perception of stimulation. Once positioned, the electrode is fixed in place using the friction collars. At this point the quadlead is tunneled subcutaneously toward the left posterior superior iliac spine. The quadlead is exited through a small incision in the vicinity of the posterior superior iliac spine, and the tip is left in a subcutaneous pocket. Wounds are closed and covered with Tegaderm.

The first stage of electrode implantation has now been completed, and the drapes are removed. The patient is rotated to the lateral decubitus position within the Wilson frame but angled 75 degrees from the table to keep weight off the shoulder. The flank and abdomen are reprepared and draped. The Itrel generator is implanted in a subcutaneous pocket approximately three fingers below the ribs and overlying the lateral edge of the rectus muscle. An extension lead is then tunneled between the front and back incisions to establish a connection between the generator and the quadlead.

Postoperatively, antibiotic coverage should be continued for a minimum of three doses. A lateral and an anteroposterior sacral radiograph are taken to document the electrode location. The implant can be programmed and the patient normally discharged within 36 to 48 hours of the procedure.

SAFETY

Animal experiments[5] have shown that a 50-Hz rectangular pulse, applied to a peripheral nerve continuously for a period as short as 16 hours, will result in a significant loss of large-diameter axons. This change is not seen at frequencies of 20 Hz or less. Presumably, there is a progressively higher risk of nerve injury as the frequency increases above 20 Hz, but by how much and over what length of time have not yet been determined. Nerve damage may result from overdrive of the peripheral nerve rather than from the amplitude of the current delivered. Lower frequencies more closely mimic the normal neuromuscular physiologic functions and therefore would logically be safer. This view of the cause of neural injury is new. Nevertheless, the maximum current density should not exceed 45 $\mu C/cm^2$.

Patient tolerance for stimulation declines precipitously above 15 Hz. Fortunately, a healthy fused recruitment of muscle contraction occurs at 15 Hz and a therapeutically acceptable one at 10 Hz. These ranges are also those safest for long-term stimulation. Frequency adjustments between 2 and 15 Hz can be made for any one patient. The initial setting should be 10 Hz because it is sufficiently therapeutic, is the most comfortable frequency range, and prolongs battery life of the implanted generator.

More than 400 implants have now been made worldwide, and there have been no reported instances of permanent adverse change in perineal sensation or micturition behavior as a result of long-term stimulation. Some patients have accumulated more than 40,000 total hours of stimulation without experiencing a decline in stimulation. There have been instances of decline in perineal muscle recruitment, but these have not been associated with any change in sensation or micturition physiology. Such changes are explained by tissue impedance shifts at the electrode site.

The ability to maintain a muscular response to stimulation may reflect the integrity of the underlying neural metabolism more than the physical effects of the current delivered to the tissues. Healthy neuromuscular units have shown no predisposition to response deterioration. These points suggest that patients who do not demonstrate a strong contraction of the perineum with initial stimulation are poor candidates for long-term stimulation.

There is a much higher tolerance level for stimulation when the muscle contracts than when it does not. A pure sensory effect, without visually apparent muscle contraction, does not effectively modulate voiding dysfunction and is associated with a very narrow patient tolerance level. This observation suggests that direct stimulation of afferent nerves results only in pain and is not therapeutic. It does not, however, negate the possible indirect influence of the muscle afferents as a result of muscle stimulation. Thus a patient should be able to tolerate the effect of stimulation for long periods without annoying distraction or discomfort.

The exact pattern of stimulation and time of use vary from patient to patient. Patients are free to determine the amount of "on" time they believe is necessary to keep their symptoms under control. Because experimental data suggest that damage from neurostimulation is greater with continuous stimulation than from intermittent patterns of use, a cycle pattern is used at first. A cycle of 10 seconds on and 5 seconds off is selected at the initiation of stimulation (Table 58–2). The cycle pattern can be varied to accommodate patient comfort. There is no magic formula. The goal is to provide sufficient on time to achieve a modulation effect. This on time should be therapeutic, within the parameters that have been shown to be safe, and comfortable, to avoid discouraging the patient from using the implant. Patients should be encouraged to use the implant only as much as necessary to control symptoms. Generally, less on time is needed 6 months after the implant than in the initial months.

TABLE 58–2
Advantages of 10-Hz Stimulation Parameters

1. Effective fused contraction of perineal muscles
2. Inhibition of labile sphincter behavior contributing to voiding dysfunction
3. Safety with long-term stimulation
4. Maximum patient comfort
   Minimal fatigue of stimulated muscle
   Preserved sense of muscle activity and awareness of stimulation
5. Effective conversion of fast-twitch muscle to slow-twitch muscle

SURGERY AND NERVE INJURY

The greatest risk of nerve injury occurs at the time of implantation of an electrode. This risk is much greater for an electrode placed around a nerve (as with a bladder pacemaker implant) than alongside it (as with the foramen implant). Excessive pressure on the nerve, either from a cuff wrapped around a nerve or from cable tension after placement of an electrode, is obviously detrimental. Great care must be taken to fix the electrodes and leads to minimize this risk. Sufficient lead length should be left whenever possible to allow for strain relief.

Other Methods of Treatment

BIOFEEDBACK

The essential goal of biofeedback is to help the patient to relax and to ease tension in the pelvic musculature.[6] It is important for patients to be made aware of the adverse effects of uncontrolled anxiety on symptoms. They should be counseled about methods of dealing with stress and about lifestyle patterns that contribute to unnecessary anxiety.

Resting tension in the pelvic muscles and their sphincter components is regulated involuntarily. Voluntary regulation of this tension is exercised usually only at times of voiding or defecation Even these are somewhat unconscious actions. Patients do not consciously consider the efficiency of pelvic muscle relaxation. Inefficiency in the use of these muscles can lead to or contribute to soreness. The goal of biofeedback is to restore appropriate concepts of pelvic muscle relaxation. This can be as simple as a suggestion to take one's time with voiding and never to push, strain, or rush the event. Many times, however, patients simply have no concept of how to relax these muscles. They may not be able to identify these muscles or to exert any voluntary control over their behavior. In these situations, patients need more specific instruction.

The rectal examination can be very useful in helping patients to learn to control their pelvic muscles. Patients can be asked to tighten and relax on the gloved finger in such a way that the physician can assess the efficiency and specificity of this control. Patients should practice easing pelvic tension at regular intervals on a daily basis. If relaxation is successful, there should be a precipitous decline in the tenderness of the levator muscles on rectal examination, and the patient should report a decrease in such symptoms as hesitancy, intermittency, and slowness of the urinary stream. Unfortunately, only the more mildly symptomatic patients respond well enough to this treatment for this to be the only therapy necessary. Progress should be monitored because patients often discontinue this behavior.

MODULATION OF PAIN

Within the dorsal horns of the spinal cord, pain transmission results from a complex summation of nociceptive and non-nociceptive activity on the interneurons.[7] Large-diameter axons can exert a considerable inhibitory influence over nociceptive transmission within the dorsal horns of the spinal cord. These large-diameter axons have a normal role in modulation of afferent transmission. As a therapy, selective stimulation of only large-diameter axons can be very effective in reducing symptoms—for example, using TENS to reduce postoperative pain. The greater the input from the larger afferents and the closer the input to the spinal segments involved in the symptoms, the more effective the gating of the abnormal afferent input causing the symptoms.

ACUPUNCTURE

Acupuncture needles placed above the medial malleolus on the inside of the leg and direct S_3 nerve root stimulation have been found to suppress pelvic pain.[34, 35] The mechanism is probably direct activation of the larger muscle efferents, which effectively modulate pain transmission on the spinal cord. The technique is simple to administer and complements biofeedback and drug therapy. For reasons that are unclear, the technique is most effective if the needles are placed through the skin at the point of lowest skin impedance, 4 cm above the medial malleolus and just behind the tibia (post-tibial nerve).

TRANSCUTANEOUS NERVE STIMULATION THERAPY

TENS has been established as a valuable tool in the treatment of incontinence and pain disorders during the last 15 years.[8, 9] The technique is simple and virtually risk-free. Electrical stimulation is applied to critical areas within the sacral dermatomes. Sites reported to be associated with beneficial results include the sacrum and the suprapubic, common peroneal, and posterior tibial nerves. Large skin afferents are stimulated, and these in turn suppress spastic reflexes within the same dermatome.[10, 11] Vaginal[12] and intravesical[13–16] devices have also been reported to be effective. The techniques are simple and should definitely be considered before or as part of more aggressive surgical procedures.

Although it is encouraging to know that relatively simple approaches can be effective, these approaches do have drawbacks. As a general rule, the effects of neurostimulation do not last. When it is effective, patients are dependent on frequent treatments. In addition, the results of superficial stimulation are rather unpredictable in individual patients, and the devices often prove to be too uncomfortable for prolonged use.

IMPLANTED DEVICES

Implanted devices[17] are cosmetically acceptable and circumvent many of the inconvenient drawbacks of TENS therapy. The device are easy to activate and can be used regardless of the time or place.

A period of testing is required to determine whether stimulation of a sacral nerve fiber can be used on a continuing basis to control symptoms.[17] An insulated needle is positioned in one or more of the sacral foramina. Stimulation is applied by gradually increasing (ramping) the current to a comfortable intensity. When a suitable response is identified, a temporary electrode is inserted into the foramen through the test needle and is left in place for 3 to 7 days. If the patient does well during this period of trial stimulation, the options are to place the electrode permanently or to wait and repeat the trial. The reason for considering a permanent electrode implant is that few patients who benefit from the stimulation will remain in remission from the symptoms once the stimulation therapy is withdrawn. Trial therapies lasting several days have been performed in more than 1000 patients for a variety of reasons. Permanent implants have been performed in more than 300 of these patients. None of the patients have demonstrated evidence of nerve injury attributable to the stimulation. Thus, the techniques of evaluation and subsequent chronic stimulation do not appear to present undue risks to the patient.

Dorsal Column and Epidural Stimulation

The overall results of treatment for pain are reported to be in the 30 to 50% range.[18] However, the technique does not work at all for pelvic pain. Technically and functionally, it is just not possible to project the stimulus into the perineum or pelvic viscera with this approach.

Neural stimulation has both advantages and disadvantages (Table 58–3).

Modulation Through Pelvic Muscle Stimulation: Approach and Advantages

1. Active pelvic muscle contraction allows patients to better identify the pelvic floor and urethral sphincter muscles. Most patients have a very poor idea of pelvic floor regulation and have identifiable problems in using these muscles. Reeducation, therefore, must correct this deficiency as much as possible.
2. Training by demonstration isolates the pelvic muscles for retraining and defines their contractile capability. This training provides the patient with some comparative guidelines to follow and goals to achieve.
3. The patient gains freedom from dependency on visits to a medical center.
4. Convenience is an advantage; devices can be used in the privacy of one's home at a convenient time of day.
5. Patients can lose the ability to hold urine with very full bladders (i.e., pelvic afference suppresses pudendal efference). Very full bladders can gate out the ability of higher centers to control the pelvic muscles. Stimulation can always recruit these muscles and therefore can prevent urinary incontinence or inappropriate urge.

Screening for Those Who May Benefit

The effectiveness of modulation is determined by two variables. The first is the degree of detrusor instability. Very unstable bladders or poorly compliant bladders will not respond to stimulation. Low-pressure instability of the bladder or urethral sphincter can be modulated very well. The second variable is strong recruitment of the pelvic floor muscles. Recruitment of these muscles is essential to successful modulation of dysfunctional micturition reflexes. The pathways of inhibition are reinforced by stimulation of the pelvic floor.

Electrical stimulation can be used effectively to modulate unstable reflexes that cause inappropriate relaxation of the urethra (with problematic incontinence) or high, unstable urethral sphincter pressures (with symptoms of frequency, urgency, and pain). Efficiency of voluntary control over the pelvic floor and urethral sphincter are essential to long-term success.

TABLE 58–3
Results of Neurostimulation

Advantages

Stimulation is targeted therapy, unlike medications
It does not harm nerves
It is trophic to virtually all tissue—bone, wounds, nerves
It can be used to condition tissue prior to surgery to obtain better results
It does not exclude any other therapy
It has a strong scientific and biologic basis for application

Disadvantages

Biologic—When used within proper parameters, no risk has been demonstrated
Technical—Related to the nature of the device. External devices present problems (inconvenience to the patient)

Discussion

Neuromodulation is a nonspecific stimulus that causes both afferent and efferent impulses to be carried in the pelvic somatic nerves. These impulses are routed via interneurons to the detrusor motor nuclei and the pudendal nuclei.[19] There is an increase in CNS synaptic activity that blocks or gates out the excitatory pathways. This results in an inhibitory influence on the motor output from the spinal nuclei controlling the bladder and sphincter, thereby decreasing symptoms.[20]

The neurophysiologic principles are fundamentally sound and have been demonstrated independently and repeatedly by numerous investigators.[21–23] The therapeutic effectiveness of the treatment is due to (1) increased pudendal nerve afferent feedback, (2) an increase in striated urethral sphincter activity, or (3) an improved pelvic floor behavior dynamic. An increase in afferent inhibitory feedback occurs with any form of peripheral nerve stimulation. Stimulation may be mechanical (e.g., acupuncture) or electrical depolarization of 1a and 1d nerve afferents. Active contraction of muscle and the targeting of specific muscles (e.g., the urethral striated muscle versus the levator) will result in more efficient suppression of instability.

The whole subject of electrical nerve stimulation continues to intrigue yet baffle the treating physician.[24] There are numerous reports in the literature that describe the wonders of stimulation as a therapeutic tool. However, the devices and approaches used for stimulation continue to be enmeshed in controversy. This is partly due to limited access to the devices. Hence, there has been limited opportunity for physicians to gain enough hands-on experience to draw their own conclusions. A larger issue is the education of physicians in the principles that guide usage of neurostimulation methodologies.

The Bladder Pacemaker

Implanted neuroprosthetics were developed primarily to benefit the patient with a spinal cord injury.[25–30] The dorsal roots of S_2–S_4 are divided, and electrodes are placed around the ventral S_3 nerve roots. Dorsal rhizotomy greatly reduces spasticity, thereby increasing bladder storage capacity, restoring continence, and reducing risk to the upper tracts.[31] Because dyssynergic sphincter behavior is reduced, there is a more efficient detrusor contraction with stimulation and more efficient emptying. Erection and bowel evacuation patterns are affected but surprisingly often are preserved. Only the lability with which sacral reflexes govern these varied functions is affected. On occasion they may even improve, as if excess reflex inhibition existed within that dermatome prior to the dorsal rhizotomy.

CANDIDATES FOR A BLADDER PACEMAKER

The primary candidates for this procedure are patients with spinal cord injuries. Patients with neurologic disabilities, such as multiple sclerosis or transverse myelitis, may be considered. There are two main limitations for bladder stimulation: (1) pain elicited by the current required to stimulate the bladder, and (2) the contractility of the bladder. There are many other factors to consider as well before a patient can be considered a good candidate:

Completeness of injury. Complete spinal cord injury patients do better than those with incomplete injuries. Stimulus amplitude is not limited by pain, and as a rule the bladder contractions are easier to produce.

Level of injury. Patients with a spinal cord injury between the levels of T_{10} and L_2 often are ideal candidates for a bladder pacemaker. Detrusor responsivity to stimulation may be insufficient to empty the bladder in the patient with high quadriplegia or in cauda equina lesions.

Psychological status. Patients must be emotionally prepared to interact with their device and the treating physician.

General medical health. Serious medical problems (e.g., decubitus ulcers, kidney stones, or pulmonary difficulties) need to be addressed prior to consideration of an implant.

Age. Age limits are those of the available technology.

Time from injury. Although there is no time exclusion, the experience to date suggests that patients are better served over the long term by having an implant early, even within the first year of injury.

Mobility. Patients must be able to achieve suitable and convenient collection of the voided urine. Female patients thus must be able to transfer to a toilet facility. Male patients can opt to void into a condom catheter and leg bag.

UROLOGIC CONSIDERATIONS

DETRUSOR REFLEX CONTRACTILITY For successful electromicturition, a detrusor contraction of 75 to 100 cm H_2O must be achieved. Hence, the integrity of detrusor contractility must be assessed prior to implantation. This can be done by a simple cystometrogram, obstructing the urethra of the bladder temporarily to measure peak detrusor pressure as a guide to the maximal contractile force. If intravesicular pressures remain low (<50 cm H_2O), direct stimulation of the sacral roots can be performed to assess the potential for voiding.

COMPETENCE OF URETHRAL SPHINCTER Implant patients must have the potential for continence. Female patients who are incontinent secondary to an intrinsically weak sphincter are not good candidates, but males with partial incontinence due to a failed sphincterotomy are.

DETRUSOR MORPHOLOGY Bladders that are mildly hy-

TABLE 58–4

Comparison of Intradural Versus Extradural Approaches to Bladder Pacemaking

	Surgical Risk	Exact Anatomic Identification of Roots	Functional Identification of Roots	Anatomic Identification of Dorsal Roots	Functional Identification of Dorsal Roots	Ease of Electrode Application	Repair of Damaged Lead	Risk of Surgical Nerve Damage	Bladder Contractions	Sphincter and Lower Leg Contractions
Sacral	Very small (sacrum is fused, dura not opened, roots protected)	Very easy	Very easy—bladder monitor not essential	Very certain	Includes all dorsal branches with and without a detrusor response	Easy	Electrodes all replaceable	Low—nerves protected by epineurium	Strong	Strong
Lumbar	Moderate—lumbar laminectomy risks sacral curvature; must open dura, roots are unprotected	Not possible	Easy with bladder monitoring	Uncertain	Includes only those nerves not giving a detrusor response	Easy	Intradural repair not possible	High—nerves unprotected by epineurium	Strong	Modest to strong

pertrophic secondary to unstable behavior respond much better to stimulation than thin-walled bladders. Contracted and poorly compliant bladders do not have the potential for sufficient storage.

STATUS OF UPPER TRACTS Upper tract pathology, principally stones, should be ruled out or treated before considering the patient for an implant. Urinary reflux may improve or disappear after a dorsal rhizotomy. Renal parenchymal loss, unless the patient is left with marginal kidney function, does not disqualify a patient from an implant.

FUNCTIONAL STATUS OF ERECTIONS Approximately 50% of patients retain the ability to have a reflex erection after a dorsal rhizotomy. Brindley and colleagues report a 60% success in producing an erection via stimulation.[30]

BOWEL EVACUATION PROGRAM Sacral rhizotomies have a variable dampening effect on the use of trigger techniques for achieving bowel movement. Spontaneous movements can be induced or coaxed via suppositories and are aided by electrostimulation.

DISCUSSION

Both the intradural and the extradural approach have been successful in restoring bladder evacuation (Table 58–4). The intradural approach presently enjoys greater worldwide familiarity, primarily because of the availability of the Brindley device rather than as a result of a true comparative assessment of the two approaches. There are important differences between the approaches that have yet to be sorted out—(1) the vertebral column may be subject to curvature as a result of lumbar laminectomy, and (2) intradurally the roots are unprotected by epineurium. The somatic fibers are therefore more susceptible to surgical and mechanical injury. This may prove to be an advantage of the intradural approach given the associated compromise of sphincter contractility. However, it is difficult to control this, and it may prove to be a disadvantage over the long-term as the nervous system ages. The results have nonetheless been dramatically successful over a 10-year span.

It is important to keep a scientifically balanced perspective. More information is needed to avoid the dangerous precedent of allowing bias to set a standard. The extradural approach, from a purely academic perspective, is safer and hence preferable to the intradural approach. The extradural roots have epineural protection, there is no risk of spinal scoliosis with aging, electrode repairs are possible, and excellent recruitment of the bladder and rectum can be achieved.

The exciting aspect of the bladder pacemaker approach to management of the bladder in a patient with spinal injury is that the technique works very well. Dorsal rhizotomy is a valuable surgical procedure in itself for treating bladder instability. Technology continues to offer better hardware options. Better devices will become available, and exciting research is being done on direct stimulation of the spinal cord

micturition center. There is therefore a need for more medical centers to encourage the expertise needed to use these devices and a need for more surgeons with the appropriate background to perform these procedures.

REFERENCES

1. Simons DG, Travell JG: Myofascial pain syndromes. *In* Wall PD, Melzack R (eds): Textbook of Pain. Edinburgh, Churchill Livingstone, 1984, p 368.
2. Juenemann KP, Schmidt RA, et al: Clinical significance of sacral and pudendal nerve anatomy. J Urol 139:74, 1988.
3. Fall M: Does electrostimulation cure urinary incontinence? J Urol 131:664–667, 1984.
4. Mortimer JT: Electrical excitability: The basis for applied neural control. Eng Med Biol 2:12–13, 1983.
5. McCreery D, Agnew WF: Mechanisms of stimulation induced neural damage and their relation to guidelines for safe stimulation. *In* Agnew DD, McCreery DD (eds): Neural Prostheses: Fundamental Studies. Englewood Cliffs, NJ, Prentice Hall, 1990.
6. Jessup BA: Biofeedback. *In* Wall PD, Melzack R (eds): Textbook of Pain. Edinburgh, Churchill Livingstone, 1984, G 2.
7. Fields HL, Levine JD: Pain—mechanisms and management. West J Med 141:347–357, 1984.
8. Mendelson G: Acupuncture analgesia. I. Review of clinical studies. Aust NZJ Med 7:642–648, 1977.
9. Stoller ML, Copeland S, Millard RJ, Murnaghan GF: The efficacy of acupuncture in reversing the unstable bladder in pig-tailed monkeys. J Urol 137:104A, 1987.
10. Wolf CJ: Transcutaneous and implanted nerve stimulation. *In* Wall PD, Melzack R (eds): Textbook of Pain. Edinburgh, Churchill Livingstone, 1984, D1.
11. McGuire EJ, Shi-Chun Z, Horwinski ER, Lytton B: Urological neurology and urodynamics. J Urol 129:78, 1983.
12. Fall M, Lindstrom S: Electrical stimulation: A physiologic approach to the treatment of urinary incontinence. Urol Clin North Am 18:393–407, 1991.
13. Ebner A, Lindstrom S, Jiang CH: Intravesical electrostimulation: How does it work? An experimental study. J Neurol Urodyn 10:281–282, 1991.
14. Katona F: Stages of vegetative afferentation in reorganization of bladder control during electrotherapy. Urol Int 30:192–203, 1975.
15. Kaplan WE, Richards I: Intravesical transurethral electrotherapy for the neurogenic bladder. J Urol 136(1 pt 2):243–246, 1986.
16. Madesbacher H, Pauer W, Reiner E: Rehabilitation of micturition by transurethral electrostimulation of the bladder in patients with incomplete spinal cord lesions. Paraplegia 20:191, 1982.
17. Schmidt RA: Advances in genitourinary neurostimulation. Neurosurgery 18(6):1041–1044, 1986.
18. Krainick JU, Thoden U: Dorsal column stimulation. *In* Wall PD, Melzack R (eds): Textbook of Pain. Edinburgh, Churchill Livingstone, 1984, D3.
19. Hillman P, Wall PD: Inhibitory and excitatory factors influencing the receptive field of lamina 5 spinal cord cells. Exp Brain Res 9:284–306, 1969.
20. Wall PD: The gate control theory of pain mechanisms. A restatement and re-examination. Brain 191:1–18, 1978.
21. Vodusek DB, et al: Detrusor inhibition induced by stimulation of pudendal nerve afferents. Neurourol Urodyn 5:381–389, 1986.
22. Lindstrom S, et al: J Urol 148:920–924, 1992.
23. De Groat WC, Ryall RW: Reflexes to sacral parasympathetic neurones concerned with micturition in the cat. J Physiol (Lond) 200:87–108, 1969.
24. Bradley WE, Timm GW, Chou SN: A decade of experience with electronic stimulation of the micturition reflex. Urol Int 26:283, 1971.

25. Hald T, Meier W, Khalili A., et al: Clinical experience with a radio-linked bladder stimulator. J Urol 97:73, 1967.
26. Jonas U, et al: Studies on the feasibility of urinary bladder evacuation by direct stimulation of the spinal cord. II. Post stimulus voiding: A way to overcome outflow resistance. Invest Urol 13:151, 1975.
27. Jonas U, Honefellner R: Late results of bladder stimulation in 11 patients: Follow up to 4 years. J Urol 120:565, 1978.
28. Schmidt RA, et al: Extradural approach to bladder pacemaker. World J Urol 9:109–166, 1991.
29. Thuroff JW, Schmidt RA, et al: Chronic stimulation of the sacral roots in dogs. Eur Urol 9:102–108, 1983.
30. Brindley GS, Polky CE, Rushton DN, Cardozo L: Sacral anterior root stimulators for bladder control in paraplegia. The first 50 cases. J Neurol Neurosurg Psychol 49:1104, 1986.
31. Gasparini ME, Schmidt RA, Tanagho EA: Selective sacral rhizotomy in the management of the reflex neuropathic bladder: A report on 17 patients with long-term follow-up. J Urol, 1990.

CHAPTER 59

The Use of Nerve Deafferentation and Stimulation in the Paraplegic Female Patient

Dieter H. Sauerwein, M.D.

In patients with lesions accompanied by the loss of functionality of the spinal nerves of the conus medullaris, it is usually possible to regain urinary continence. Bladder emptying in these cases is achieved by clean intermittent catheterization (CIC), which does not constitute a higher demand on the patient, because men as well as women quickly learn this technique, even without sensory perception at the urethra.

Patients with lesions causing paraplegia above the level of the conus medullaris suffer from spasticity of the bladder. The loss of corticospinal control and the influence of external stimuli trigger noncoordinated and uncontrolled contractions in the muscles of the lower urinary tract. With time, a hyperreflexia of the detrusor with detrusor-sphincter dyssynergia (DSD) develops—the so-called spastic bladder.

The continuous contractions of the detrusor with wavelike pressure modulations result in ineffective micturition and lead to further worsening of the hyperreflexia (Fig. 59–1). This vicious circle causes the spasticity to set in at ever lower bladder fill volumes, and the constant involuntary contractions of the detrusor leads to its hypertrophy. The final outcome of this development is complete decompensation along with deterioration of the lower and upper urinary tracts.

Uncontrollable incontinence, recurrent urinary tract infections (UTIs), progressing kidney insufficiency, and autonomic dysreflexia leading to blood pressure crises are common clinical findings in paraplegic and quadriplegic patients with DSD. In this way spasticity causes a large number of secondary conditions, which eventually all lead to terminal kidney failure.

One of the first demands of the patient is to become continent. Female paraplegic patients depend on wearing pads, which, consciously or unconsciously, sets them back to the state of an infant. The psychological strain on these women often dictates day-to-day life, a problem almost always grossly underestimated by the physician. Men, on the other hand, are able to hide their incontinence by the aid of urinary condoms and the urinal. Control of the spastic bladder is therefore the top priority in neurourologic treatment.

Numerous attempts have been made to convert the spastic reaction of the detrusor into an areflexia such as occurs with sacral nerve blockades or selective neurotomy. For example, as reported by Torring and colleagues in 1988,[1] reflex incontinence may be temporarily improved in 50% of patients, with hyperreflexic detrusor action recurring within 2 years.

Recently, the advent of effective anticholinergic drugs has supplied us with a means of successfully

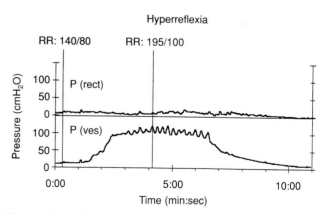

Figure 59-1 Hyperreflexic detrusor action with autonomic dysreflexia. The bladder fill volume is 240 ml. The high blood pressure is accompanied by a sensation of pressure in the ears. RR, blood pressure; P (rect), pressure rectum; P (ves), bladder pressure.

suppressing the spasticity of the bladder.[2] With this treatment, the effects of the general suppression of the parasympathetic system and intermittent catheterization must be accepted. However, frequently no reliable continence is achievable with bladder fill volumes of over 400 ml.

In the past, an ileocystoplasty with concurrent subtotal resection of the detrusor was an alternative. By forming a new low-pressure reservoir, the damage caused by high pressure within the urinary tract could be avoided. In the mostly young patients with a long life expectancy, however, the added risk of recurring UTIs and possible malignant degeneration of the bowel tissue used for the cystoplasty is still not sufficiently known. As with anticholinergic therapy, intermittent catheterization must be accepted. Furthermore, this treatment includes the replacement of healthy bladder tissue or bladder muscle tissue only because detrusor *control* is malfunctioning.

In 1972, Brindley described a transmitter-controlled stimulator that activates the spinal nerves controlling the bladder.[3] In 1979 and 1983, the Tanagho group reported attempts to activate the spinal micturition center by stimulation in laboratory animals.[4, 5] Even with prolonged stimulation, the authors did not observe nervous or muscular damage in the dog model.

Brindley and colleagues reported on the first 50 patients in whom a stimulator was placed on the sacral anterior root in 1986.[6] The patients were described as continent with frequent transmitter-controlled micturition. Neurotomy at the posterior roots was done on either one or two spinal nerves only or not performed at all. In 1984 Cardozo and associates reported urodynamic findings in 13 patients previously treated by Brindley.[7] Five of these showed no relief from hyperreflexia and thus were incontinent.

A new neurourologic method for treatment of the spastic bladder must consider the following clinically important questions:

1. Bladder dysfunction in the paraplegic patient converts the organ into a high-pressure reservoir. Is an intervention on the spinal micturition center (sacral deafferentation [SDAF]) capable of permanently restoring a normal low-pressure reservoir?
2. Among the symptoms of autonomic dysreflexia are the annoying ones of sweating and goose pimples. However, a sudden blood pressure crisis can be the expression of autonomic dysreflexia and represents a serious and, in advanced age, life-threatening complication. Can the treatment eliminate autonomic dysreflexia?
3. Stimulation of the anterior motor root provided Brindley with a way to trigger micturition. Can electrical stimulation establish a way to achieve bladder emptying permanently in paraplegic patients?
4. Is an operation combining SDAF to eliminate urinary bladder spasticity and electrical sacral anterior root stimulation (SARS) to empty the bladder possible? Is it physiologically lasting?

5. Does the combination of SDAF and SARS have a positive influence on recurring UTIs, the progressive morphologic damage, and kidney failure?

It is the aim of the following chapter to point out the operative therapeutic methods to control bladder spasticity in paraplegic patients available today.

Therapeutic Concepts

Experience with sacral nerve blockades gathered at this hospital showed only temporary success. However, an operative method designed to relieve bladder spasticity permanently seemed to be viable. It promised to restore urinary continence and preserve the natural reservoir function of the bladder while making possible a lower urinary tract not prone to pressure damage.

The encouraging findings reported by Cardozo and colleagues[7] suggest that it should be possible to gain transmitter control of micturition.

SACRAL DEAFFERENTATION

The parasympathetic system of the body is mainly supplied by the vagus nerve. The lower sacral spinal cord from S_2 to S_5 houses a second parasympathetic center controlling the bladder, the rectum, and erection. Above S2 no parasympathetic nerve fibers are found.

Consequently, parasympathetic deafferentation of all spinal nerves from S_2 to S_5 completely prevents the arrival of stimuli from the bowel or bladder. The result is suppression of all autonomic spasticity in these organs. However, the procedure does not alter the sympathetic system with its positive influence on the reservoir function of bladder and bowel. The sparing of the motor fibers conserves the unit of nerve cell, nervous motor fiber, and muscle. The effect is a normal adaptation of the bladder to the varying fill states up to the natural limit.

This procedure was designed and initiated by the author[8] and has, up to 1993, been performed successfully about 500 times worldwide.

SACRAL ANTERIOR ROOT STIMULATION

As reported by Brindley and Tanagho and colleagues,[4-6] transmitter-controlled activation of the parasympathetic motor sacral nerves yields detrusor contraction. It seemed that with a modified stimulation strategy it should be possible to overcome DSD. Because the bowel is controlled by the same spinal center, defecation should be achievable by stimulation as well. (Furthermore, Brindley obtained an erection in 60% of the male patients by anterior root stimulation.)

Prerequisites for SDAF–SARS

Female paraplegic patients must meet two requirements to profit from this new procedure:

1. Most paraplegic patients show signs of anatomic damage to the lower urinary tract after years of the presence of the lesion. However, a detrusor capable of reflexic contraction is a requirement.
2. The presence of the bulbus cavernosus reflex along with a hyperreflexic detrusor (as seen in the urodynamic measurement) are indications of a functional reflex loop. Even when the reflex loop is intact it may be possible to overlook detrusor action—for example, if the applied stimuli are too weak.

If the detrusor itself is not capable of contracting, or if there are anatomic alterations like fibrosis of the muscle tissue, SDAF and SARS cannot restore bladder function. In such cases methods like ileocystoplasty must be used to create a low-pressure reservoir.

DIAGNOSTIC TOOLS

A strongly reduced compliance of the bladder not always is an indication for a fibrotic detrusor. On the other hand, routine urodynamic examination may frequently give the impression of an areflexia.

Urodynamics Under Lumbar Anesthesia

Spastic malcontrol may mimic fibrosis of the bladder. Urodynamic measurement performed during spinal anesthesia is the tool of choice to clarify the situation. If under these conditions compliance improves by at least a factor of 2 compared with the value obtained immediately before anesthesia, SDAF also can be expected to improve reservoir function. A simple way of checking whether anesthesia is sufficient and whether it has been performed at the correct level is to check the anal reflex; it should be completely suppressed during the examination.

If autonomic dysreflexia developed as a consequence of bladder spasticity, it will not be detectable under spinal anesthesia. This diagnostic aid indicates whether the relief of bladder spasticity by SDAF can also improve other symptoms such as blood pressure crises.

Cystometric examination under spinal anesthesia is a better indicator of the extent of bladder spasticity than a histologic examination of the detrusor tissue for direct detection of fibrotic alterations.

Provocational Tests

Cystometry performed with ice water or filling with high flow rates enhances stimulation of the detrusor, making hyperreflexic detrusor contractions detectable. Alternatively, the use of special electrodes applied transrectally can be used to stimulate the parasympathetic spinal nerves directly. Direct percutaneous stimulation[9] is the tool of choice to test for intact motor nerve fibers. A positive finding indicates that transmitter-controlled bladder emptying is possible.

Patients with incomplete paraplegia who retain partial sensory function in the sacral dermatomes may find that stimulation is accompanied by pain. This fact initially represented a contraindication to the implantation of an anterior root stimulator. The various stimulation tests performed transrectally and transcutaneously give a good idea of whether future stimulation with the implant will be painful. If very high pain levels are to be expected, the patient must be informed prior to the operation that, to empty the bladder, CIC will have to be performed. However, the more important part of the procedure, SDAF with its restoration of the normal reservoir function, is unaltered by pain level.

The Anterior Root Stimulator

The investment of 10 years of development work by Brindley[3, 6, 7] led to an anterior root stimulator that became available commercially in 1986. The implanted receiver block consists of three receiver coils with cable connections to the electrodes. Transmission of power and pulse is accomplished by the use of radio frequencies of 7 to 9 MHz. The electrodes themselves are book-shaped to permit the enclosure of the spinal nerves for the bladder and rectum. Depending on the anatomic necessities, a one-, two-, or three-channel implant can be used (Fig. 59–2).

The external part of the system consists of three transmitter coils with a cable connection to the pulse generator. Two types of pulse generators are available. An older model by Brindley is based on analog technology and allows three combinations of stimulation. We developed a newer digital pulse generator that gives access to 10 different stimulation settings. These are typically used for micturition, defecation, erection, lubrication, and muscle training of the gluteus medius to avoid decubital ulcers.

In the battery-powered pulse generator, electrical pulses are generated. The transmitter block converts these into high-frequency signals, which in turn are sent to the implanted receivers. Here, the original electrical signals are recovered and then arrive at the electrodes via three cables. In this way, selective activation of spinal nerves S_2 to S_5 is possible. The receiver block is encased in silicone rubber. The chosen production technique avoids corrosion of the metallic parts of the implant.

Following computer-aided entry of the stimulation parameters during urodynamic monitoring, the digital control box allows the patient to choose between 10 different stimulation settings. For each of these,

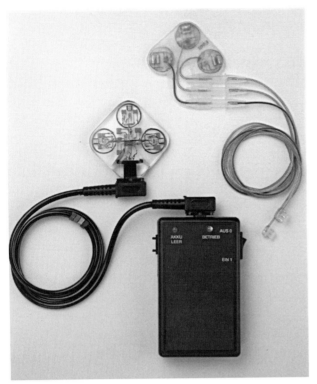

Figure 59–2 Anterior root stimulator with a three-channel implant consisting of electrodes, receiver and transmitter blocks, and digital bladder control box.

every channel can be configured depending on the desired function and the individual susceptibility of the nerves. The pulse generator inside the control box limits the current output to 1.5 mA and allows the setting of mode (either pulsed or continuous), pulse frequency (8 to 200 Hz), amplitude (0 to 40 volts), shape (sawtooth or square wave), and pulse width of the individual pulses in the pulse train (from 50 to 800 μs).

The Operation

In paraplegic patients an operation involving implants presents a high risk of infection. Special preoperative precautions must be taken in acknowledgement of that fact (see later in this chapter under Complications). The type of procedure makes special training in handling the nervous structures necessary.

INTRADURAL APPROACH

Access to the lower spinal canal is gained by performing a laminectomy from L_4 to S_3. Opening of the dura and arachnoidea is performed with the patient positioned with the head low to minimize the loss of cerebrospinal fluid and damage to the brain stem in the region of the foramen magnum.

It is then simple to classify the spinal nerves. Differentiation of the anterior and posterior roots is accomplished with the help of a magnifying glass or a microscope. The bundles are stimulated, noting the resulting motor responses. Somatomotorically, toe and plantar flexion as well as pelvic floor contraction and activity in the gluteus muscles are seen. Detrusor and rectum actions are recorded by the accompanying pressure increase. When stimulating the posterior roots, the blood pressure increase is monitored as well. After the fibers of the posterior roots have been correctly identified, coagulation and resection are performed.

It is vital to achieve complete deafferentation of the spinal nerves from S_2 to S_5 to relieve the spasticity of the bladder. If stimulation of the root at S_5 yields a visceromotor response, deafferentation at S_5 must also be attempted. If monitoring of S_5 is not possible, the entire approximately hair-sized root of S_5 is squeezed or resected to suppress all afferent fibers and achieve a normal filling phase for the bladder.

The sacral anterior roots are embedded in the electrodes and fixed at the vertebral level at approximately L_4. A chimney-shaped flange serves as the duct from the intradural space to the outside. With the aid of silicone rubber glue the cables are attached within the flange, which also helps to prevent cerebrospinal fluid fistulas. The dura is then closed using a continuous watertight suture.

After the dura and the musculature are closed, the cables are subcutaneously led to the position of the receiver block chosen by the patient (above the costal arch or the lower abdomen) using a tubular trocar. If the patient chose a position in the lower abdominal region, the cables are stored in a temporary location (Fig. 59–3) and the patient is repositioned in the supine position before the receiver block is implanted.

EXTRADURAL APPROACH

If the intradural approach is contraindicated, laminectomy is performed from L_5 to S_4. It is easy to find the spinal nerves S_2 to S_5. After opening the perineurium, an injection of physiologic sodium chloride solution simplifies the separation of posterior and anterior roots. The separation must be done between the dura and the spinal ganglion because at the distal side and within the ganglia the afferent and efferent fibers are intermingled.

Although identifying these fibers is straightforward at the levels of S_2 to S_3, it becomes very difficult at S_4 and impossible at S_5.[10] However, only *complete* deafferentation of all afferent parasympathetic paths can guarantee the suppression of the hyperreflexia of the detrusor. Because the extradural approach is not capable of securely reaching this goal, the further use of it is not recommended. The extradural attachment of the spiral- or stripe-shaped electrodes is a simple task. The following steps then parallel those used in the intradural method.

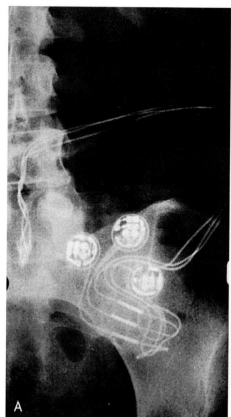
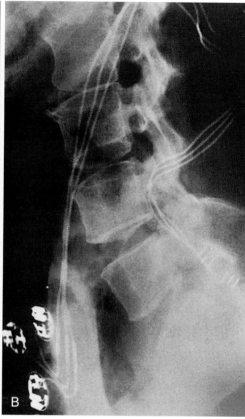

Figure 59-3   Anteroposterior (*A*) and lateral (*B*) radiographs showing a three-channel implant. Note the electrodes in the lower spinal canal with their cable connections to the receiver block in the left lower abdomen.

Results

SDAF in combination with SARS was inaugurated by the author in 1986. Since then, it has been performed worldwide on 700 patients in 22 centers.[11]

The major aim of the treatment is the permanent suppression of bladder spasticity in order to restore a normal, physiologic reservoir function. Secondary complications such as recurrent UTIs, damage to the lower urinary tract, and loss of kidney function become a dominant part of the disability if this goal is not reached. If, in contrast, the lower urinary tract can once again fulfill its normal reservoir function, which is its job during 99% of our lifetime, the first prerequisite for a healthy urinary tract is returned to the patient.

PATIENT GROUP

Since the start of SDAF plus SARS in September 1986, 180 patients have been treated in this department of Neuro-Urology in the Werner-Wicker-Klinik, Bad Wildungen, Germany. For 162 patients, follow-up data of 3 months or longer postoperatively are available.

As expected from the fact that an accident is the most frequent cause of the lesion, the patients are young at the time of the lesion. Whenever possible, during the first 2 years after the lesion patients are treated with anticholinergic drugs and advised to perform CIC. They are also informed about the option of deafferentation with implantation of an anterior root stimulator.

SDAF and SARS may be indicated earlier if management by anticholinergic therapy and CIC is not possible, or if autonomic dysreflexia in the form of high blood pressure crises is uncontrollable.

Besides the urodynamic methods described here, magnetic resonance imaging (MRI) and computed tomography (CT) have been used to gain knowledge about the lower spinal canal. The results of these investigations are discussed in a preoperative consultation with orthopedic surgeons and neurosurgeons, whose advice helps to determine the optimum course of the operation. An unstable spinal column is operatively stabilized by these colleagues in the same procedure.

ROOT RESPONSE IN SARS

Systematic testing of the spinal roots during the operation reveals which roots are the most important for detrusor action. The results of these electrostimulation tests are shown graphically in Figure 59–4.

Earlier beliefs in the field of neurology were that stimulation of the root of S_2 results in activity in the region of the gluteus muscles, the musculus biceps femoris, and the perineal muscles. In contrast to textbook knowledge, however, with stimulation of the roots at the levels of S_3 and S_4 not only the bladder

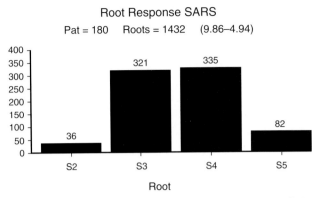

Root Response SARS

Pat = 180   Roots = 1432   (9.86–4.94)

Figure 59–4 Response to intraoperative electrical stimulation. The ordinate shows the absolute numbers of roots that, when stimulated, give an intravesical pressure increase.

and rectum respond, but, with the exception of the flexor hallucis longus, plantar and digital flexion is routinely found as well.

RESULTS OF SDAF

Hyperreflexia

Postoperatively, in 152 of the 162 patients, complete areflexia of the detrusor was observed. Bladder capacities exceeded the 500-ml mark. Neither spontaneously nor as a result of various provocational stimuli (e.g., ice water, mechanical triggering) could detrusor actions be effected. Normal reservoir function in 95% of the patients was restored.

In eight cases no complete deafferentation was achieved. Five patients received a second deafferentation at the level of the conus medullaris, which resulted in the desired areflexia. The remaining three patients showed hyperreflexia above a filling volume of 400 ml with a moderate pressure increase within the bladder, which at the present time is tolerable for these patients.

Urinary Continence

One hundred and thirty-seven patients are completely continent. Their voiding volumes are above 500 ml. Generally, the damaged detrusor muscle limits the bladder capacity, above which incontinence may persist. Three women are continent only up to a 400-ml filling volume for that reason. An open bladder neck was diagnosed in 11 women. In all of these cases a second procedure encompassing the implantation of an artificial sphincter was able to control the stress incontinence. The mean time interval between SDAF and this second operation was 8 months.

All patients remain rectally continent.

Dysreflexia

The often underestimated autonomic dysreflexia disappeared immediately following the SDAF procedure

as far as the high blood pressure crises are concerned. Other typical symptoms such as sweating, goose pimples, and increased somatomotor spasticity persisted initially but were not reported by the patients in the 6-month follow-up examination.

Reflux

Preoperatively, 39 reflux units in 32 patients were diagnosed. Postoperative urinary tract infections can cause uteric reflux and bladder spasticity to reappear. One low-pressure reflux to the kidney remained postoperatively, caused by a dystopic uteric orifice. It was successfully treated with an antireflux operation. Six uteric units had persistent low-grade reflux and did not require therapy. Postoperatively, a UTI can cause the spastic action of the bladder to reappear. Long wavelike detrusor contractions as well as reflux are once more detectable. A combined antibiotic and anticholinergic treatment for the duration of the UTI completely restores the areflexic no-reflux condition.

Urinary Tract Infections

All patients have fewer or no UTIs. It is interesting to observe that even with complete areflexia a UTI lowers the bladder capacity. During the time of infection, incontinence occurs at otherwise safe filling volumes. In one patient increased reflex activity was observed during the infection (see earlier section). Successful antibiotic therapy completely restored the preinfection condition. If reflux was observed preoperatively, an anticholinergic drug should accompany the antibiotic in the therapy for UTI. Bladder emptying should be done by CIC during this time. Because SDAF reduces the infection rate from 7 to 1.2 per year, a prophylactic antireflux procedure is not recommended.

Renal Function

Generally, the progressive deterioration of kidney function is arrested after the procedure. Only one male patient with poor kidney function (creatinin clearance of 18 ml/minute) showed further worsening. Some patients show stagnation, but in most of them kidney function improves. The short mean follow-up time of 2.5 years (range, 3 months to 8.5 years) does not allow a conclusive evaluation. However, together with the morphologic evaluation of the infusion pyelogram the urinary tract may be safely assumed to be stabilized.

RESULTS OF SARS

Even very careful intraoperative handling of the sacral nerves does not exclude occasional damage to the fibers. Loss of nervous function, if it occurs, generally

Micturition by SARS

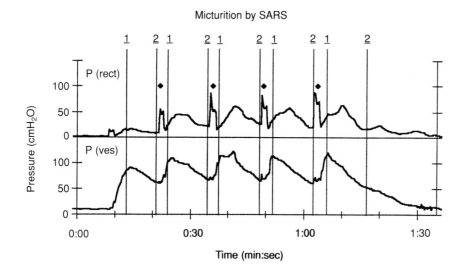

Figure 59-5 Micturition via sacral anterior root stimulation (SARS). Section of a urodynamic measurement 11 months postoperatively. 1, Start micturition; 2, stop micturition; ♦, anal sphincter contraction. The left edge starts at a filling volume of 500 ml after filling with a fill rate of 20 ml/minute. Note that compliance is 50 at that point.

persists up to 6 months. The quality of the operating surgeon manifests itself in the rate of damage.

Stimulation of the Bladder

Follow-up examination confirms the results obtained intraoperatively in that it shows that S_3 and S_4 roots are the most important for detrusor action. For micturition the intravesical pressures are easily adjusted to values between 50 and 90 cm H_2O. If more than one root produces a response in the bladder, a combination of all of these is chosen.

In no case was continuous stimulation of the pelvic floor necessary to achieve urinary continence.

Earlier fears that simultaneous stimulation of the somatomotor musculature and the external sphincter should again lead to DSD proved groundless. The immediate contraction and relaxation of the striated musculature responsible for closing the urethra combines with the slower responding (smooth muscle) detrusor contraction, which, after the stimulation burst, results in low-resistance voiding. Figure 59–5 shows the urodynamic measurement during micturition by SARS. The beginning and end of the stimulation bursts are accompanied by direct action of the anal sphincter. The delayed detrusor response to stimulation is evident in the intravesical pressure increase and the resulting micturition. The area under the curve between markers *1* and *2* corresponds to the *effective* detrusor energy, i.e., the energy that is converted into micturition. These results show that micturition by means of SARS, called post-stimulus voiding by some authors, is very similar to the normal bladder emptying of nonparalyzed patients.

The morphology of micturition by SARS avoiding DSD is easily depicted in a micturition cystourethrogram under stimulation in a male patient (Fig. 59–6).

The majority of the patients (97%) use the anterior root stimulator exclusively for micturition. The average voiding volume is 500 ml and the mean frequency of voiding is 3.6 voids per day. Eighty-six percent of

all patients use SARS exclusively and are completely continent. Only seven patients occasionally use CIC to check residual volumes, which are in the range of 50 to 95 ml.

Long-term follow-up data allow the conclusion that no change in voiding frequency or volume occurs as the result of this mode of micturition.

Rectum Stimulation Response (Table 59–1)

In the past, the possibility of defecation by way of SARS was viewed merely as a bonus in addition to bladder emptying. Patient polls indicated, however, that this is generally viewed as a major factor enhancing their quality of life. The results from video-urodynamic evaluation show that the same nerves

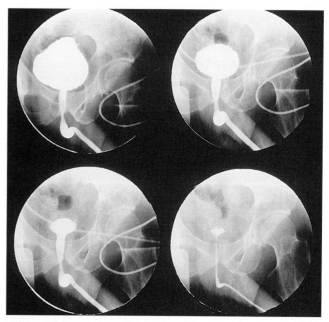

Figure 59-6 Radiographic micturition cystourethrogram with SARS.

TABLE 59–1
**Voiding and Defecation with the
Use of SARS**

	Voiding	Defecation
Stimulator in use	139 patients	130 patients
Frequency	3.6 times/day	4.3 times/week
Volume	500 ml	
Residuals <40 ml	132 patients	
Residuals >40 ml (50–95 ml)	7 patients	

162 patients total.

that supply the detrusor are also responsible for activation of the bowel. The differentiation is achieved by minor adjustments of the stimulation parameters.

Bowel emptying with the anterior root stimulator is used by 130 patients with a mean frequency of 4.3 per week. Preoperatively, defecation took a mean of 75 minutes and cholinergic drugs were necessary in more than half the patients. SARS accelerates the process to 25 minutes postoperatively. Simple aids like manual control and volume-increasing laxatives are sufficient; drugs are not necessary. Although several patients have asked for the operation for these reasons, we do not perform the operation for this indication.

Complications

In general, operations on the paraplegic patient mean a high risk. Special care must be taken pre- and postoperatively as described earlier. Especially postoperatively, regular repositioning of the patient to avoid delayed wound healing and pressure sores is an absolute necessity. If these precautions are taken, the complication rate is expected to be comparable to that seen in nonparalyzed patients.

EARLY COMPLICATIONS

The number of postoperative complications with the SDAF–SARS method has been very low. The Bad Wildungen center has treated the largest patient group and has over 200 individuals under regular and prospective control. In two cases a cerebrospinal fluid fistula had to be closed operatively. Among these patients, no implant infection has occurred so far, setting the infection rate to below 0.5%. Twice postoperative bleeding in the receiver location made a revision necessary. In no case has the anterior root stimulator or parts of it needed to be removed in consequence of an early complication.

Avoiding Infections

An implant infection poses a great risk for the patient and would make the removal of the stimulator

necessary. Although after such a revision the benefit of deafferentation would remain, the aid of micturition by stimulation would have to be given up for at least some time. Bladder emptying once more would have to be achieved by CIC. Whole body disinfection is performed daily starting 3 days prior to the operation using an aqueous 0.05% chlorhexidine solution. Patient compliance with this procedure is very high because they know it guarantees their safety. A silicone coat of an antibiotic against gram-positive germs is applied to the implant 3 days prior to sterilization.[12] A bacteriologic check using *Bacillus subtilis* after the removal of a defective receiver block 7 years after implantation showed that the antibiotic was still active.

Avoiding Cerebrospinal Fluid Fistulas

To avoid cerebrospinal fluid fistulas the patient is positioned head down at 15 degrees during the operation and for 3 days postoperatively. As in microsurgery the use of swabs is replaced by cleansing with physiologic saline solution. A Y-shaped drainage system at the lowest point above the proximal opening of the dura provides continuous removal of the cleansing solution. This makes liberal use of solution possible and avoids the entry of blood into the spinal canal. Cerebrospinal fluid loss is minimized thanks to these precautions.

Closure of the dura incorporating the chimney-shaped cable flange is performed with the help of magnifying glasses using continuous monofilic thread with a long resorption time. Real-time control of tightness is achieved by beginning the suture distally allowing the fluid level to rise continuously.

LATE COMPLICATIONS

Even years of using the anterior root stimulator have no negative effects on the urinary tract. All late complications have been caused by technical failures. Among the first 500 implants used worldwide, defects of some kind occurred in 98 patients.[13] The total implanted time was 1922 years, and the mean time after which the failure occurred was 19.9 years.

In the Bad Wildungen center 14 of 162 patients have required a revision because of defective implants. The most frequent cause has been breakage of a cable lead, which occurred after an implant time of more than 4 years. When the breakage point can be removed from the entry into the spinal canal the cable can be repaired. In other cases a simple repair was not possible and required an extra set of electrodes to be attached extradurally. In all cases it was possible to restore the desired stimulation function.

Reducing Health Care Costs

Restoration of a normal reservoir function of the urinary bladder is responsible for a sizable reduction in health care costs. The rate of urinary infections is lowered from 7 to 1 per year, which translates into a decreased use of antibiotics. Independence from CIC means lowered costs for the aids necessary for that technique. Last but certainly not least, the secure continence of the patient makes the use and purchase of pads (diapers) superfluous. Deafferentation stops the progressive loss of kidney function, which in turn saves the costs involved in the management of these patients.

New Developments—Research Outlook

The therapy described constitutes a major advance in the treatment of the spastic bladder and helps to minimize the patient's morbidity rate. Future research must strive to further enhance this patient group's independence from medical aids and personnel. New paths promise to achieve this goal.

Judging from the worldwide results, it unfortunately is not rare for the sacral anterior roots to be damaged during the operation. However, even with one or two roots damaged, typically it is still possible to achieve satisfactory micturition using the remaining fibers. Damage to *all* roots rarely happens. Furthermore, a root damaged intraoperatively frequently regenerates within a time span of several months. Still, it should be noted that 45 of the first 500 patients who underwent SDAF with SARS[13] were not able to use their stimulators, and nerve fiber damage was the cause in 23 of them.

Surgeons who have considerable experience in performing implants less frequently damage the anterior roots. If the operation is not to be performed exclusively by these experts, a method involving a lower risk must be found. One possible procedure would be to cut the posterior roots of S_2 to S_5 at the level of the conus medullaris. For this procedure, laminectomy at T_{11}–T_{12} to L_1–L_2 is necessary. Extradural implantation of the stimulator can then be easily performed without damaging the motor fibers. This procedure has been used by several centers in 23 patients. In eight of these patients a careful investigation of the muscular regions of the foot, leg, and pelvic floor shows no evidence of anterior root damage. Further studies are necessary to elucidate the viability of this method.

The potentially lower risk of damage of the anterior roots with this method goes with the risk of instability of the thoracolumbal region of the spinal column. Many orthopedic paraplegiologists fear that instability with formation of a gibbus may be the possible result of this operation. The orthopedic stabilizing procedure involves fixation of these vertebrae, causing a severe limitation in the mobility of

these patients. Laminectomy from L_4–L_5 to S_3, as is necessary for the intrathecal approach, has never led to any deformations of the spinal column. Because it is still too early to make any final decisions or decisive recommendations, the risk of gibbus formation must be weighed against the damage of roots by inexperienced surgeons.

Benefit for the Paraplegic Woman

1. In women with a spastic bladder, deafferentation of the spinal nerves S_2 to S_5 restores the low-pressure reservoir function of the bladder.
2. For the patient this means the acquisition of permanent reliable continence. There is no usable urinal available for women. After a successful SDAF they are independent of urinary pads.
3. Unlike men, who may lose a reflex erection due to deafferentation, women suffer no losses.
4. SARS once again allows bladder emptying under the patient's control.
5. Independence from the handicap of the spastic bladder, the ability to regain control over micturition, and lower morbidity mean a better quality of life for these patients.

REFERENCES

1. Torring J, Petersen T, Klemar B, Sogard J: Selective sacral anterior rootlet neurectomy in treatment of hyperreflexia. J Neurosurg 68:241, 1988.
2. Moisey C, Stephenson T, Brendler C: The urodynamic and subjective results of treatment of detrosor instabitity with oxybutinin chloride. Br J Urol 52:452, 1988.
3. Brindley GS: Electrode arrays for making long-lasting electrical connections to spinal roots. J Physiol 222:135, 1972.
4. Schmidt RA, Tanagho AE: Feasibility of controlled micturation through electric stimulation. Urol Int 34:199, 1979.
5. Thüroff JW, Schmidt RA, Bazeed MA, Tanagho EA: Chronic stimulation of the sacral roots in dogs. Eur Urol 9:102, 1983.
6. Brindley GS, Polkey CE, Rushton DN, Cardozo L: Sacral anterior root stimulators for bladder control in paraplegia: The first 50 cases. J Neurol Neurosurg Psychiatry 49:1104, 1986.
7. Cardozo L, Krishnan KR, Polkey CE, et al: Urodynamic observations on patients with sacral anterior root stimulators. Paraplegia 22:201, 1984.
8. Sauerwein D: Die operative Behandlung der spastischen Blasenlähmung bei Querschnittlähmung Sakrale Deafferentation (SDAF) mit der Implantation eines sakralen Vorderwurzelstimulators (SARS) Urologe [A] 29:196–203, 1990.
9. Schmidt RA: Advances in genitourinary neurostimulation. Neurosurgery 18:1041–1044, 1988.
10. Sauerwein D, Ingunza W, Fischer J, et al: Extradural implantation of sacral anterior root stimulators. J Neurol Neurosurg Psychiatry 53:681–684, 1990.
11. Van Kerrebroeck PEV, Koldewijn EL, Debruyne FMJ: Worldwide experience with the Finetech-Brindley sacral anterior root stimulator. Neurourol Urodyn 12:497–503, 1993.
12. Rushton DN, Brindley GS, Polkey CE, Browning GV: Implant infections and antibiotic-impregnated silicone rubber coating. J Neurol Neurosurg Psychiatry 52:223–229, 1989.
13. Brindley GS: Private communication, January, 1995.

Index

Note: Page numbers in *italics* refer to illustrations; page numbers followed by t refer to tables.

665

ISBN 0-7216-6723-6

90038